Handbook of LGBT Elders

Debra A. Harley · Pamela B. Teaster
Editors

Handbook of LGBT Elders

An Interdisciplinary Approach
to Principles, Practices, and Policies

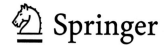 Springer

Editors
Debra A. Harley
University of Kentucky
Lexington, KY
USA

Pamela B. Teaster
Virginia Tech
Blacksburg, VA
USA

ISBN 978-3-319-03622-9   ISBN 978-3-319-03623-6   (eBook)
DOI 10.1007/978-3-319-03623-6

Library of Congress Control Number: 2015943054

Springer Cham Heidelberg New York Dordrecht London

Printed on acid-free paper

Springer International Publishing AG Switzerland is part of Springer Science+Business Media (www.springer.com)

Foreword

Every so often, a book comes along that substantially contributes to much-needed broader and deeper understanding of a minority group and to clarifying and addressing multiple pressing questions of social justice regarding that group. This is one of those books.

Contributing editors, Debra A. Harley and Pamela B. Teaster, have created a collection of all new essays on LGBT persons and aging that easily moves among elucidating the sometimes fluid boundaries of LGBT communities and individuals within those communities, to explanations and applications of basic principles ranging from queer theory to moral theory in addressing the issues facing LGBT persons and aging. And this is all done with an unblinking transnational eye. The collection's reach is, in fact, a model for transnational studies including, as it does, discussions of LGBT persons and politics the worldwide, with special attention to aging.

The collection is rightly titled as a handbook, put together expressly for those who work with LGBT persons and policy in a variety of human services, including social work, physical and mental health care, the military and criminal justice systems, and education. But its reach is even farther than that. Anyone at all interested in the social positionality of LGBT persons will be well served by reading the essays gathered here.

Beginning with a clarification of who LGBT elders are and how being sexual/gender minorities influence social relationships from the most public to the most private, the collection moves through the complicated world of multiple identities, including race, age, health status, and how the intersections of these identities often subject LGBT persons to multiple forms of oppression and exclusion. For example, in the contemporary USA, class, race, age, sexual orientation, and gender identity and presentation bestow privileges on some (namely, the middle and upper economic classes, Caucasians, the young, heterosexuals, and those whose gender identity and presentation matches their "given" sex), and oppression and exclusion on others (namely, the poor, nonwhites, the elderly, gay men, and lesbian women, and trans persons). Every individual has multiple identities, and with those identities in a given society come benefits and burdens, many unique to certain identity combinations. So, for example, the life experiences of a white, middle class, lesbian elder will be importantly different from those of an African American, poor, transgender elder. This book takes such differences very seriously.

The collection also takes very seriously the reality that in so many areas, discrimination according to these categories is even firmly protected by law—laws that not just allow, but actually promote, discrimination in housing, employment, and public accommodation. And even if not formally protected by law, customary exclusions on the basis of biases such as racism, classism, ageism, homophobia, and transphobia continue to thrive as this book goes to press in 2015, which is likely to be the year when, according to the US Supreme Court, marriage equality (the legal recognition of same-sex marriages) becomes the law of the land. The contributing authors of this collection know well that if/when that happens, homophobia will not go away. Indeed, as this decision by the US Supreme Court comes to seem inevitable, there is a "frontlash" taking place as more and more US municipalities introduce laws that will allow frank exclusion of sexual and gender minorities specifically on the basis of religious belief. So, even if marriage equality comes into the legal light as this book goes to press, the need for this unique collection will remain compelling.

By getting to the heart and effects of bias against sexual and gender minorities and their multiple identities as aged persons, this book makes an enormous and exquisitely timely contribution, not just to the empirical, theoretical, and practical literatures for service professionals, but to the literatures on social justice, as well. We are all well served by it.

Joan Callahan
Professor Emerita
Department of Philosophy
Department of Gender and Women's Studies
University of Kentucky

Preface

As editors of this text, Pamela and I have over 40 years of combined experience in service delivery; education; and research in aging, human rights, disability, and social services. Beginning in 2013, we collaborated on a chapter, *Aging and Mistreatment: Victimization of Older Adults in the United States,* and as part of that chapter, we wrote about LGBT elders. Afterward, we discussed the lack of focus and collaboration across disciplines in addressing LGBT elders. Although discipline-specific books have been published about LGBT populations, aging, health care, and human and social service, we decided that the time had come for a comprehensive text that addressed the challenges faced by LGBT elders. Our goal for this book is to discuss both LGBT elders who are from groups for which research was conducted often and groups rarely included in mainstream research (e.g., racial and ethnic groups, persons living in rural and remote areas, veterans, [ex]-offender populations, immigrants, and persons with disabilities). In addition, we decided to cover issues that impact LGBT persons individually and collectively. Our 36 chapters cover the following topics pertaining to LGBT elders: theories and constructs, the nexus of sexual minority status and aging, family relationships, deconstruction of "isms," African American and Blacks, American Indians, Asian and Pacific Islanders, Europeans, Hispanics, veterans, [ex]-offenders, immigrants, transgendered persons, bisexual persons, mistreatment and victimization, bullying, healthcare reform and healthcare practices, residents of long-term care facilities, end-of-life issues, mental health, substance abuse, the impending US Supreme Court ruling on same-sex marriage, ethics and ethical standards, law enforcement and public safety, religious and faith communities, workplace issues, counseling, socialization and recreation, advocacy, disability, and trends and future directions. Our comprehensive handbook recognizes the intersection of identities because individuals do not exist or live their lives in separate compartments.

At the writing of this text (March 2015), we are awaiting the outcome of the Supreme Court ruling on same-sex marriage. The ruling has significant implications for LGBT elders in many areas of their lives, including housing, health insurance and benefits, medical decisions, and the definition of family and spouse. The timing of the ruling may shed a different perspective on the information presented in some of the chapters.

Our text provides an interdisciplinary perspective on LGBT elders. A unique feature is that the authors of the individual chapters represent an array of diverse backgrounds and expertise. Among the disciplinary perspectives represented are social work, public health, medicine, rehabilitation counseling, law, public policy, counseling, diversity consultation, gerontology, psychiatry, and education. The broad assemblage of disciplines is important in adequately addressing challenges, resiliency, and strengths of LGBT elders *vis a vis* an interdisciplinary perspective. Many of the chapters also include international perspectives about LGBT elders, populations, and cultures.

We do not present this text as inclusive of all aspects that impact LGBT elders, but rather, we hope that it will be an important contribution to the existing literature as well as a response to identified gaps in policy, practice, and research. Although texts on services and programs assisting older adults are readily available, they focus primarily on the general population and rarely if ever take into account the unique circumstances facing current and future LGBT elders. Our desire is for the text to serve as a useful and reliable resource for those studying and teaching for those involved in health care, human and social services programs, as well as in courses on diversity and gender and women's studies. Similarly, practitioners, policy and decision makers, advocates, community leaders, families, and LGBT elders themselves may benefit from this text.

Debra A. Harley
Pamela B. Teaster

Contents

Part VII   Conclusion

About the Editors

Debra A. Harley, Ph.D., CRC, LPC is a professor in the Department of Early Childhood, Special Education, and Rehabilitation Counseling at the University of Kentucky (UK). Professor Harley holds the distinction of Provost's Distinguished Service Professor. She is past editor of the Journal of Rehabilitation Counseling and the Journal of Rehabilitation Administration and guest editor of numerous special issues of rehabilitation journals. She is co-editor of a book, Contemporary Mental Health Issues Among African Americans. Professor Harley has published over 80 refereed articles and 26 book chapters. She has served on the certification board for rehabilitation counselors, the Certified Rehabilitation Counselor Commission, and the accreditation board rehabilitation counselor education programs, Council on Rehabilitation Education. Professor Harley is affiliate faculty with the Department of Gender and Women's Studies, the Center Research on Research on Violence Against Women, and the Human Development Institute at UK. She has received the Educator of the Year Award by the National Council on Rehabilitation Education and the Provost's Award for Outstanding Teaching by the University of Kentucky. Professor Harley's primary teaching assignment at UK is in rehabilitation counseling, in which she teaches courses and does research in the areas of cultural diversity, gender issues, and substance abuse.

Pamela B. Teaster is the associate director for Research at the Center for Gerontology and a professor in the Department of Human Development at Virginia Tech. She established the Kentucky Justice Center for Elders and Vulnerable Adults and the Kentucky Guardianship Association and was its first president. She is the secretary general of the International Network for the Prevention of Elder Abuse. She served as director and chairperson of the Graduate Center for Gerontology/Department of Gerontology as well as the director of Doctoral Studies and associate dean for Research for College of Public Health at the University of Kentucky. She serves on the editorial board of the *Journal of Elder Abuse and Neglect* and *Frontiers*. Dr. Teaster is a fellow of the Gerontological Society of America and the Association for Gerontology in Higher Education, a recipient of the Rosalie Wolf Award for Research on Elder Abuse, the Outstanding Affiliate Member Award (Kentucky Guardianship Association), and the Distinguished Educator Award (Kentucky Association for Gerontology). She has served as both board member and president of the National Committee for the Prevention of Elder Abuse. She has received funding from The Retirement Research Foundation, Administration on Aging, National Institute on Aging, Kentucky Cabinet for Families and Children, National Institute of Justice, Centers for Disease Control, National Institute of Occupational Safety and Health, Health Resources and Services Administration, and the Office of Victims of Crime. Her areas of scholarship include the mistreatment of elders and vulnerable adults, public and private guardianship, end-of-life issues and decision making, ethical treatment of vulnerable adults, human rights issues for vulnerable adults, public policy and public affairs, public health ethics, and quality of life. She is the co-author of two books and of over 100 peer-reviewed articles, reports, and book chapters.

Contributors

Katherine R. Allen is professor of Human Development at Virginia Tech, and a faculty affiliate of the Center for Gerontology, Faculty of Health Sciences, and the Women's and Gender Studies Program. She is a fellow of the Gerontological Society of America and the National Council on Family Relations. Her research involves the study of family diversity over the life course, family experiences of LGBT adults, feminist family studies, and sexuality in adulthood.

Reginald J. Alston, Ph.D., CRC, NCC is a professor and associate chancellor at the University of Illinois, Urbana-Champaign.

Robin P. Bonifas, Ph.D. is an associate professor at the Arizona State University School of Social Work. She has over 15 years of experience working with elders and their families in both long-term care and inpatient psychiatric settings. Her research focuses on enhancing psychosocial care for persons with chronic illness and disability, especially those with comorbid mental health conditions and those requiring long-term care. Her current projects examine elder social justice issues such as resident-to-resident aggression in nursing homes, late-life bullying, and other challenges to social relationships in senior care organizations.

William E. Burleson is the author of Bi America: Myths, Truths, and Struggles of an Invisible Community (Rutledge 2005), a book about the bisexual community and the bisexual experience. Burleson's work has appeared in the Lambda Book Report, the Journal of Bisexuality, and various print and online LGBT publications, and he has been a speaker at college campuses across the country (www.williamburleson.com).

Loree Cook-Daniels has been working on LGBT aging issues for more than four decades, focusing particularly on public policy and social change. She is the founder of the Transgender Aging Network and currently serves as policy and program director for FORGE, Inc.

Tracy Davis is an assistant professor at Rutgers University, School of Health Related Professions in the Department of Interdisciplinary Studies. She holds a Ph.D. from the University of Kentucky in gerontology. Her research interests include LGBT aging, HIV/AIDS and aging, health promotion, and disease prevention.

Lisa Dunkley, M.A., CRC is a doctoral student in Rehabilitation Counseling Program at the University of Kentucky.

Robert Espinoza is vice president of policy at Paraprofessional Healthcare Institute, a national organization focused on transforming eldercare and disability services by improving the lives of direct care workers—nearly 4 million home health aides, certified nurse aides, and personal care attendants. Espinoza currently serves on advisory boards for Story Corps, the Johns Hopkins School of Medicine, and Aging Today, the national newspaper for the American Society on Aging.

Anthony Fluty Jr., MSW, LCSW is a substance abuse counselor at Eastern State Hospital in Lexington, Kentucky. He has also had clinical experience working with senior adults in an intensive outpatient program conducting group psychotherapy.

Linda Gassaway, Ed.D is a lecturer in the Department of Early Childhood, Special Education, and Rehabilitation Counseling at the University of Kentucky.

Tracey L. Gendron is an assistant professor with the Department of Gerontology in the School of Allied Health Professions at Virginia Commonwealth University. Tracey has a Master of Science in gerontology, a Master of Science in psychology and a Ph.D. in developmental psychology. She teaches several graduate and undergraduate service-based courses including grant writing, research methods, and old is the new young. She is also a Service-Learning faculty fellow at Virginia Commonwealth University. Tracey takes an all-inclusive approach to teaching about aging, particularly highlighting those understudied and underrepresented groups that are at increased risk of negative health outcomes and discrimination. Her community-engaged research interests include the professional identity development and career commitment of gerontologists, education through community engagement and service-learning, aging anxiety, ageism and gerontophobia, LGBT aging and staff knowledge and quality of care.

David Godfrey, J.D. is a senior attorney to the ABA Commission on Law and Aging in Washington DC. He is responsible for the ABA's role in the Administration on Aging funded National Legal Resource Center and for producing the National Aging and Law Conference. He is a board member of the National Academy of Elder Law Attorneys. Prior to joining the Commission, he was responsible for elder law programming at Access to Justice Foundation in Kentucky.

Michael T. Hancock, M.A. is a doctoral student in the Rehabilitation Counseling Program at the University of Kentucky.

Steven D. Johnson, Ph.D., LCSW is vice-chair of Education for the Department of Psychiatry at the University of Kentucky. He works extensively with LGBTQ clients as well as teaching and supervising psychiatry residents in their psychotherapy training.

Sujee Kim is a doctoral student in the Adult Development and Aging Program at Virginia Tech. Her research interests include long-term caregiving and productive aging.

Eileen Klein, Ph.D. is an assistant professor at the Ramapo College Department of Social Work. Her research interests LGBT persons with serious mental health issues and culturally responsive and LGBT affirming treatment.

Ron Levine is a professional photographer and documentary maker. He is known for his Prisoners of Age photo exhibit.

Tina Maschi, Ph.D., LCSW, ACSW is an associate professor at the Fordham University Graduate School of Social Service with research interests at the intersection of trauma, mental health, and aging, especially related to vulnerable elders in the criminal justice system. She is the founder and president of Be the Evidence International: www.betheevidence.org.

Brian McNaught was named "the godfather of gay diversity training" by The New York Times. He has been brought to offices throughout the world to help managers create welcoming environments for LGBT employees. He is the author of several books and is featured in numerous DVDs on LGBT issues. He and his spouse, Ray Struble, have been together since 1976.

Thomas W. Miller, Ph.D., ABPP is professor emeritus, senior research scientist, master teacher, great teacher and university teaching fellow during forty-year tenure at the University of Kentucky College of Medicine, University of Connecticut, School of Allied Health, and Murray State University. Tenured in the Department of Psychiatry, he held joint appointments in the Department of Psychology, College of Arts and Sciences and the Department of Educational, School and Counseling Psychology, College of Education, University of Kentucky. He served as a career VA chief psychology service and developed the first APA-approved Psychology Internship in the Commonwealth of Kentucky. He received his doctorate from the State University of New York, is a diplomate of the American Board of Professional Psychology in Clinical Psychology, fellow of the American Psychological

Association, the Association of Psychological Science and the Royal Society of Medicine. He is editor and author of the Praeger Handbook on Veterans Health.

Melanie D. Otis, Ph.D. is the Richard K. Brautigam Professor of Criminal, Juvenile, and Social Justice in the College of Social Work at the University of Kentucky. Dr. Otis has served as editor-in-chief of the Journal of Gay and Lesbian Social Services since 2010.

Terrie Pendleton is a Licensed Clinical Social Worker (LCSW) in Richmond, Virginia. She received her master's degree in social work from Virginia Commonwealth University. Ms. Pendleton has held positions as an adjunct instructor and faculty field liaison with Virginia Commonwealth University, School of Social Work. She has served as a Steering Committee Member for the organization, Services and Advocacy for Gay, Lesbian, and Bisexual & Transgender Elders (SAGE) in Richmond VA and has provided clinical counseling and support to the LGBT community. Terrie lives happily with her partner of 22 years and their two dogs.

Jo Rees, Ph.D. is an assistant professor on Long Island University Department of Social Work. Her research interests lie at the intersection of LGBT issues, mental health, and the criminal justice system.

Karen A. Roberto is professor and director of the Center for Gerontology and the Institute for Society, Culture and Environment at Virginia Tech, and a faculty member in Human Development, the Faculty of Health Sciences, and in the Departments of Internal Medicine and Psychiatry and Behavioral Medicine at the Virginia Tech Carilion School of Medicine. She is a fellow of the American Psychological Association, the Gerontological Society of America, and the National Council on Family Relations. Her research focuses on health and social support in late life and includes studies of the health of rural older women, family relationships and caregiving, and elder abuse.

Tracy Robinson-Wood is a professor in the Department of Applied Psychology at Northeastern University. She is author of *The Convergence of Race, Ethnicity, and Gender: Multiple Identities in Counseling*. The fifth edition, to be published by SAGE, is anticipated in 2016. Her research interests focus on the intersections of race, gender, sexuality, and class in psychosocial identity development. She has developed the Resistance Modality Inventory (RMI), which is a psychometrically valid measure of resistance, a theory she co-developed for black girls and women to optimally push back against racism, sexism, classism, and other forms of oppression. Her research is also focused on parents' racial socialization messages within interracial families, and the relational, psychological, and physiological impact of microaggressions on highly educated racial, gender, and sexual minorities.

Amanda E. Sokan is an assistant professor (part-time) at University of Kentucky, Department of Health Management and Policy, in the College of

Public Health. She holds a Ph.D. in gerontology and masters in health administration from the University of Kentucky. Her research interests include elder rights and justice, elder abuse and mistreatment, LGBT aging, long-term care, aging and healthcare navigation, and health promotion.

Randy Thomas is a retired police officer having served for over 25 years in the law enforcement profession (Tampa Police Department, Richland County (SC) Sheriff's Office and South Carolina Department of Public Safety). He was a member of the South Carolina Adult Protection Coordinating Council and was instrumental in the passage of South Carolina's Omnibus Adult Protection Act. He received his bachelor's degree from Chaminade University (1971) and his master's degree in political science from the University of South Florida (Tampa 1974).

Amanda Weber is a doctoral student at Boston College in the department of Counseling Psychology. Her research interests include intersections of race, sexuality, gender and class as well as how trauma plays a role in people's lives.

John T. White is the director of Professional and Community Development for Virginia Commonwealth University's Department of Gerontology. He received a BA in American history from Washington and Lee University, a Master of Science (gerontology) from Virginia Commonwealth University and is completing a doctorate in educational leadership. Previous chapters, articles, and presentations include LGBT and aging, operationalizing person-centered care and culture change, team building in long-term care and organizational diversity.

Part I

Foundations of Aging and Sexual Identities

Theories, Constructs, and Applications in Working with LGBT Elders in Human Services

1

Debra A. Harley and Pamela B. Teaster

Abstract

This chapter presents an overview of select theories of sexual orientation and gender identity. Traditional theories of life span development offer a general framework within which to understand issues and experiences common to persons in later stages of life. The intent of this chapter is to discuss theoretical constructs and models of sexual identity, counseling, public health, gerontology, and social work that can be applied with aging LGBT populations. These theories underscore the necessity of helping present and future professionals who understand differences among LGBT elders and the complex nature of identity, their psychosocial adjustment, and ways in which stigma of sexual identity and gender identity affects their well-being. Although the various theories and models in this chapter are presented according to discipline, theories are not mutually exclusive to disciplines.

Keywords

LGBT theories · Sexual orientation identity development · Gender identity development · Life span development theories

Overview

This introductory chapter on theories, constructs, and applications in working with LGBT elders presents an overview of select theories of sexual orientation and gender identity. The reader is reminded that just as identities are culturally defined, theories of sexual identity are framed within cultural contexts as well. Thus, the terminology of the "LGBT" acronym may not accurately reflect how sexual minorities are discussed within certain cultures. However, Burleson (2005) nevertheless points out that "the sexual identity of bisexual, heterosexual, or homosexual is cultural; feelings of attraction are organic. People are hammered into molds, albeit their own culture's mold, the world over" (p. 37). Most of the models of sexual orientation and

D.A. Harley (✉)
University of Kentucky, Lexington, Kentucky, USA
e-mail: dharl00@email.uky.edu

P.B. Teaster
Virginia Tech, Blacksburg, VA, USA
e-mail: pteaster@vt.edu

gender identity are based on Eurocentric cultural models of sexuality. Traditional theories of life span development (e.g., Erikson 1950; Levinson 1978, 1996) offer general frameworks within which to understand issues and experiences common to persons in later stages of life (Hash and Rogers 2013).

Although it is beyond the scope of this chapter to include all theories, constructs, and applications in human services, our intent is to present an overview of select theoretical constructs and models of sexual identity, counseling, public health, gerontology, and social work that can be applied with aging LGBT populations. These theories underscore the necessity of helping present and future professionals who understand differences among LGBT elders and the complex nature of identity, their psychosocial adjustment, and ways in which the stigma of sexual identity and gender identity affects their well-being. Specific theories of late adulthood development and functional capacity are presented in Chap. 3. Also, it is not the intent of this chapter to present techniques for counseling LGBT elder in specific circumstances (e.g., couples or relationship, family, mental), nor to critique various theories. Although the various theories and models in this chapter are presented according to discipline, theories are not mutually exclusive to disciplines. A theory may easily be applied by various disciplines to investigate and explain behavior and phenomenon.

Learning Objectives

By the end of the chapter, the reader should be able to:

1. Understand the various theories of LGBT identity development.
2. Identify the counseling theories that can be applied effectively for work with LGBT elders.
3. Identify the theories of public health and practice.

4. Identify the social work theories that work effectively with LGBT elders.
5. Explain how various practice models can be integrated in working with LGBT elders.

Introduction

Theory is a general statement, proposition, or hypothesis about a real situation that can be supported by evidence obtained through a scientific method. A theory explains in a proven way why something happens and offers guidance in explaining and responding to forgoing problems (Gratwick et al. 2014). A construct is an idea, often referred to as a theory, which contains conceptual elements or parts that are put together in a logical order to explain something. Constructs are typically subjective and not based on empirical evidence. A model is a blueprint for implementation. It describes what happens in practice in a general way. Theory and models are influenced by perspective, a value position (Payne 1997). Every discipline has theories to explain particular phenomena upon which it operate to guide development of hypotheses, research, and recommendations for best practices and policy. In fact, Payne suggests that theory succeeds best when it contains all three elements —perspective, theory, and model/construct. Theory serves the function of providing practitioners a guide for behavior in very specific circumstances and making decisions.

Although various disciplines study aging, the study of older persons occurs primarily within the discipline of gerontology. Hooyman and Kiyak (2008) suggest that because of the multidisciplinary nature of gerontology, examination of aging on the societal, psychosocial, and biological levels. However, on all these levels, older sexual minorities (lesbian, gay, bisexual, transgender [LBGT]) have been relatively ignored in gerontological research (Grossman 2008; Orel 2004; Quam 2004). Similarly, very little content on specific care needs of LGBT persons exists in the nursing literature, especially for older adults. This lack of focus is particularly troubling because nurses and other such caregivers are the front line of care and are in a position to create health care environments that will meet the needs of LGBT elders (Jablonski et al. 2013). In addition, many other disciplines omit LGBT populations from curricula and research to the extent that it appears that sexual minorities do not even exist (Hall and Fine 2005; Harley et al. 2014). The lack of focus on LGBT elders in research and training programs frequently results in service providers who are inadequately to meet the needs of this population. According to Gratwick et al. (2014), "even when providers of aging services express willingness to become more responsive to the needs of LGBT older adults there is evidence that they do not take sufficient action" (p. 5). Hughes et al. (2011) report that of service providers affiliated with the National Association of Area Agencies on Aging, only 15 % provide services tailored to the need of older LGBT adults. Moreover, at the organizational level, LGBT older adults are literally not being seen, organizations are not directing resources to these populations, and it appears that there is agency resistance to acknowledging the distinctiveness of LGBT aging issues.

Considering the increase in the number of older persons in general and the projection for continued growth in numbers and anticipated growth in the one to three million individuals in the USA over age 65 who are already identified as LGBT, the lack of focus of multidisciplinary research relegates older LGBT persons to a status of invisibility. Mabey (2011) contends that the omission of LGBT elders in gerontological research "leaves professional counselors without a substantive bridge with which to connect resources with treatment planning when working with sexual minorities" (p. 57). Moreover, ageism as experienced in LGBT communities has

the additional impact of making a marginalized and stigmatized group feel even more of a minority.

Elderly LGBT Diversity, Identity, and Resilience

As an LGBT person and an older person, an LGBT elder does not belong to one homogenous group within the acronym. LGBT elders come from every race and ethnicity, nationality, gender, ability level, socioeconomic status, place, and space. Some LGBT elders have been married and have children, while other have either or neither. Thus, LGBT elders cannot be grouped or treated as one cohesive category (Mabey 2011). Older LGBT persons grew up during a time when homosexuality and gender nonconformity were viewed as a mental illness, a sin, or a sexual perversion. Open discussion about homosexuality, sexual identity, and gender identity was not done. Rather, secrecy about one's sexual desires and behaviors was the norm; to reveal that one's sexual orientation was other than heterosexual or one's gender identity was other than conforming to social expectations was not only vocationally and socially devastating, but patently unsafe. Negative attitudes and perceptions about LGBT persons are not only historical. Today, heterosexism, homophobia, transphobia, and biphobia continue to be intertwined in social customs, cultural beliefs, institutional structures, and policy development. It is both the long-term and ongoing socially sanctioned discrimination, prejudice, and stereotypes that present unique challenges and, ironically, opportunities for LGBT persons globally (e.g., Austria, Canada, England, Ireland, USA). Because of the diversity among LGBT elders, some of the stereotypes encompass the entire LGBT population such as its attempts to covert heterosexuals that the population is composed of pedophiles or that it is a threat to marriage and structure of the family. Other stereotypes are specific to subgroups of LGBT persons such as the belief that a lesbian cannot "get a man," gay men are responsible for HIV/AIDS, or that older LGBT persons are not attractive.

In a society that places an inordinate emphasis on youth, older adults face stigma and discrimination beyond that of their younger counterparts, especially ageism (Butler 1994) in addition to lifelong negative attitudes and poor treatment related to their sexual orientation and gender identity. Hash and Rogers (2013) acknowledge "while these difficult experiences can create a host of problems for LGBT individuals, they can also help them develop unique skill sets or strengths that their non-LGBT counterparts do not necessarily benefit from as they age" (p. 249). Further, Hash and Rogers suggest that despite difficulties associated with aging as LGBT persons, elders have successfully developed social networks, successfully developed a strong sense of identity through the coming-out process, and have successfully responded to discrimination and stigma to develop a positive sense of self and identity leading to stronger ego integrity. Despite the challenging and threatening context often associated with LGBT elders' earlier lives, most are now comfortable with their sexual orientation and gender identity and display a marked resilience to the minority stress they experienced in their lives (Irish Association of Social Workers 2011; Szymanski and Gupta 2009) (see especially Chaps. 6, 7, 8 and 10 in this book on resilience among LGBT elders of color).

The process of aging for LGBT persons presents the typical challenges and concerns related to health status, financial stability, loss of a spouse or partner, and so forth. We present the case of Maria, a Latina 73-year-old lesbian, to illustrate some of the challenges she faces.

As a member of the Latino culture Maria believes that the Latino community is less accepting of homosexuality. Maria recognizes that living in Los Angeles she faces the challenges of being invisible because of ageism, an LGBT community that values youth, and rejection of old persons. In addition, cultural barriers and being very self-reliant further isolate Latinos LGBT elders. In a needs assessment of older Hispanic LGBT adults, participants expressed varied experiences of aging as: (a) not different from that of the general population, with more self-acceptance, particularly if one is financially secure, (b) there is a great deal of rejection of older persons because they are persons in which people are not interested and, even why they do not have a support group even among themselves, (c) social isolation within their own families because of their identities as LGBT people, and (d) dual discrimination as Latinos and as members of the LGBT community (www.gallup/poll/158066/special-report-adults-identity-lgbt.aspx).

Case of Maria

Maria is a Latina 73-year-old lesbian. She and her partner of 40 years live in a small third floor apartment in Los Angles. The building is old and does not have an elevator. Maria has arthritis in her knees and hands, hypertension, and glaucoma. Here partner, Sophia, is in better health but has asthma. Neither Maria nor Sophia has children and both have been estranged from their families for most of their adult life. They consider themselves "closeted" and have identified themselves publically as sisters.

Maria worked for 55 years as a housekeeper for a wealthy family. She does not have retirement income and receives Social Security of $540 per month, Medicare, and food stamps. Sophia worked as a city bus driver for 30 years and receives retirement benefits, Social Security, and Medicare.

The two of them are concerned about the feasibility of continuing to live in their apartment, but know that it will be difficult to find other affordable housing. In addition, their share of cost for health care continues to increase. Although neither women have been diagnosed with depression, both express having feelings of depression.

Questions

What identity issues are confronting these two women?
Do they have a social network? How can they form a social network?
Can you identify resilience factors for Maria and Sophia?
What type of service would benefit Maria and Sophia?

As previously mentioned, the theories of Erikson (1950) and Levinson (1978, 1996) have foundational significance in explaining the psychological development of LGBT elders. In Erikson's final stage of psychosocial development, *Ego Integrity v. Despair*, older adults (age 60 and over) reflect upon and evaluate their lives. When confronted with loss, the older person must arrive at acceptance of his or her life or will fall into despair. The ability to accept one's life and self in the ego integrity stage may be more complicated for LGBT elders (Hash and Rogers 2013; Humphreys and Quam 1998). According to Humphreys and Quam, the social stigma experienced by LGBT elders can adversely affect how they view their identity and life. Despair can be influenced by the culmination of losses over a lifetime. Transgender persons may be at a greater risk for despair because of the indignity they face from society and lack of support from loved ones. Moreover, older LGBT adults may have struggled with development as reflected in earlier stages of Erikson's theory, which could impact developmental tasks during the final stage. Levinson's theories of life span development examine primary pattern of people's lives at particular points in time and the transitions necessary between eras in life for them to successfully develop into adulthood. Similar to Erikson, Levinson identifies the final era as older adulthood (age 60 and over). This era often involves significant adjustment to a significant change and acceptance of immortality. For LGBT elders, this late stage life transition may involve acceptance

and openness about sexual orientation and gender identity (Humphreys and Quam).

The remainder of this chapter concerns select theories and models used in the disciplines of counseling, public health, and selected social sciences. Sexual identity theories are also presented. As mentioned earlier, theories are not discipline specific; however, some disciplines may gravitate more toward certain theories and models.

Theories and Constructs on Sexual Identity

An introduction to theories of sexual identity must at least mention the work of Sigmund Freud (1949). According to Freud, homosexuality and bisexuality resulted from unresolved conflicts (fixation) occurring within one of the stages of psychosexual development. In addition, Freud hypothesized that all human beings are innately bisexual and it is the influence of family and environment that determines if one becomes homosexual or heterosexual. However, Freud never identified homosexuality or bisexuality as a mental disorder. Freud's theory is not empirically tested and is not used today in discussion of sexual identity formation.

Later, the work of Erving Goffman (1963), *Stigma: Notes on the Management of Spoiled Identity*, was one of the most important early works addressing minority self-identity (Eliason and Schope 2007). According to Goffman, social stigma is learned and internalized through childhood socialization and shapes the minority person's identity. The minority person shares the belief of the majority if it deems that he or she is a failure and abnormal. This belief leads to self-hate and self-derogation. Goffman proposed that formation of the minority sexual identity involves dealing with social expectations of what is considered normal. Conversely, Altman (1971) and Plummer (1973) offered explanations for the development of a stable "homosexual identity" (Eliason and Schope 2007). Altman suggested

Table 1.1 Plummer's stages of homosexual identity

Stage 1: Sensitization—thinks about one's sexual identity

Stage 2: Significance and disorientation—accepts the deviant label with all the potential social consequences. Social oppression creates disequilibrium where the homosexual person becomes stalled, perhaps for life, in this stage

Step 3: Coming-out—goes public with one's rebuilt sexual identity. Disclosure is linked to the person's willingness and ability to join the homosexual community

Stage 4: Stabilization—no longer questions one's homosexual identity

Adapted from Plummer (1973)

that self-disclosure of one's homosexuality was beneficial because coming-out meant dealing with the socially learned "internalization of oppression," which is liberating. Plummer's approach was one of individuals adopting a "homosexual way of life" or a "career type" of sexuality. Recognizing homosexuality as a social construct developed by the majority to restrict and pathologize a sexual minority, Plummer argued that all forms of deviancy need to be viewed within a historical and cultural context. He regarded current social hostility to homosexuality as responsible for many of what he labeled "pathologies." Plummer was one of the first theorists to present identifiable stages of "homosexual identity" (see Table 1.1) (Eliason and Schope).

Subsequent to Altman (1971) and Plummer's (1973) theories, an abundance of stage models on sexual identity formation evolved, the majority of which moved away from the deviance model to a focus on healthy consequences of accepting one's sexuality (see Table 1.2). Eliason and Schope (2007) identify two assumptions about stage model theorists. First, most assumed that one is or is not gay or lesbian and embraced the argument from an Essentialists' perspective. Second, most models are based on a review of the literature and are not empirically tested or are based on single case or small sample size.

Probably, one of the most influential and frequently cited theories of gay and lesbian identity development is that of Cass (1979). Cass describes a process of six stages of gay and lesbian development. Although these stages are sequential, some persons revisit stages at different points in their life. Each stage is accompanied by a task. Cass believes that coming-out is a lifelong process of exploring one's sexual orientation and lesbian or gay identity and sharing it with others. Table 1.3 contains Cass's model of identity formation.

Bisexual Identity Formation. Though limited research as been conducted on development of bisexual identity formation, probably the most important research on bisexuality was that of Alfred Kinsey with the publication of *Sexual Behavior in the Human Male* (Kinsey et al. 1948) and *Sexual Behavior in the Human Female* (Kinsey et al. 1953) (as cited by Burleson 2005). Kinsey developed the Kinsey scale, in which individuals can fall anywhere along a continuum of 0 (exclusively heterosexual) and 6 (exclusively homosexual). Burleson contends that Kinsey had created the present model of bisexuality without ever once using the word bisexual. In addition, Kinsey scale clarified two issues: (a) There is great variability of sexual orientation, and (b) an implication that perhaps all human beings on this continuum are ranked the same way (i.e., heterosexuality is not primary or held above other sexual orientations). Kinsey's work, while groundbreaking, was rudimentary and did not address the complexities of behavior and attraction and past behavior and future predictions. In response to questions of complexity, Fritz (1993) expanded on Kinsey's continuum model to measure a person's past and future sexual attraction, behavior, fantasies, emotional preference, social preference, lifestyle, and self-identification.

Stroms (1978) offers yet different model of sexual attraction, a multiple-variable model, in which sexual attraction to different genders is examined independently of each other. In this model, Stroms' scale has one end representing no attraction to one gender and the other end presenting high attraction to that gender. The continuum offers great variation within this model. Although this model did not include transgender persons, a scale could be created for them. In

Table 1.2 Stage theories of sexual identity formation

Theorists	Population	Stages of identity formation
Ponse (1978)	Lesbian	*"Gay trajectory"* Subjective feelings of difference from sexual/emotional desire for women Understanding feelings as lesbian Assuming a lesbian identity Seeking company of lesbians Engaging in lesbian relationship (sexual and/or emotional)
[a]Coleman (1982)		Precoming-out Coming-out Tolerance Acceptance Pride Integration
Minton and McDonald (1984)	Gay men	Egocentric Sociocentric Universalistic
[a]Faderman (1984)	Lesbian	Critical evaluation of societal norms and acceptance of lesbian identity Encounters with stigma Lesbian sexual experience (optional)
Sophie (1985/1986)	Lesbian	First awareness Testing/exploration Acceptance Integration
Chapman and Brannock (1987)	Lesbian	Same-sex orientation Incongruence Self-questioning Choice of lifestyle
Troiden (1988)	Men	*Spirals rather than linear* Sensitization Confusion Assumption Commitment
[a]Morales (1989)	Racial/ethnic minority LGB	Denial of conflicts Bisexual versus gay/lesbian identity Conflicts in allegiances Establish priorities in allegiances Integrate various communities
[a]Reynolds and Pope (1991)	Multiple identity formation	Passive acceptance of society's expectations for one aspect of self Conscious identification with one aspect of self Segmented identification with multiple aspects of self Intersection identities with multiple aspects of self
[a]Isaacs and McKendrick (1992)	Gay men	Identity diffusion Identity challenge Identity exploration Identity achievement Identity commitment Identity consolidation

(continued)

Table 1.2 (continued)

Theorists	Population	Stages of identity formation
[a]Siegel and Lowe (1994)	Gay men	Turning point Aware of difference Identify source of difference Coming-out Assumption Acceptance Celebration Maturing phase Reevaluation Renewal Mentoring
[a]Fox (1995)	Bisexual	First opposite-sex attractions, behaviors, relationships First same-sex attractions, behaviors, relationships First self-identification as bisexual Self-disclosure as bisexual
McCarn and Fassinger (1997); Fassinger and Miller (1996)	Lesbian and gay	Awareness Exploration Deepening/commitment Internalization/synthesis
[a]Eliason (1996)	Lesbian	Cycles/not linear Pre-identity Emerging identity Recognition/experiences with oppression Reevaluation/evolution of identities
[a]Nutterbrock et al. (2002)	Transgender	Awareness Performance Congruence Support
[a]Devor (2004)	Transgender	Abiding anxiety Confusion Comparison (birth sex/gender) Discover trans identity Confusion (trans) Comparison (trans) Tolerance (trans) Delay before acceptance Acceptance Delay before transition Transition Acceptance of post-transition gender/sex Integration Pride

Adapted from Eliason and Schope (2007)
[a]No empirical validation

addition, Strom's model includes people who tend toward asexuality. The model describes attraction to women and men as two separate variables (Burleson 2005).

Theoretical State Stage Models. In the USA, the 1970s ushered in a new era of research about sexual orientation identity development with the emergence of theoretical state stage models. The primary focus of these models was on the resolution of internal conflict related to identification as lesbian or gay and informed the "coming-out" process. Bilodeau and Renn (2005) describe these

Table 1.3 Cass model of gay and lesbian identity formation

Stage 1	**Identity Confusion**—Personalization of information regarding sexuality. "Could I be gay?" This stage begins with the person's first awareness of gay or lesbian thoughts, feelings, and attractions. The person typically feels confused and experience turmoil
Task	Who am I?—Accept, deny, reject
Stage 2	**Identity Comparison**—Accepts possibility one might be homosexual. "Maybe this does apply to me." In this stage, the person accepts the possibility of being gay or lesbian and examines the wider implications of that tentative commitment. Self-alienation becomes isolation
Task	Deal with social alienation
Stage 3	**Identity Tolerance**—Accepts probability of being homosexual and recognizes sexual/social/emotional needs of being homosexual. "I am not the only one." The person acknowledges that she or he is likely lesbian or gay and seeks out the other lesbian and gay people to combat feelings of isolation. There is increased commitment to being lesbian or gay
Task	Decrease social alienation by seeking out lesbian and gay persons
Stage 4	**Identity Acceptance**—Accepts (versus tolerates) homosexual self-image and has increased contact with lesbian/gay subculture and less with heterosexual. "I will be okay." The person attaches positive connotation to her or his lesbian or gay identity and accepts rather than tolerates it. There is continuing and increased contact with the lesbian and gay culture.
Task	Deal with inner tension of no longer subscribing to society's norm, attempt to bring congruence between private and public view of self
Stage 5	**Identity Pride**—Immersed in lesbian/gay subculture, less interaction with heterosexuals. Views world divided as "gay" or "not gay." "I've got to let people know who I am!" There is confrontation with heterosexual establishment and disclosure to family, friends, coworkers, etc
Task	Deal with incongruent views of heterosexuals
Stage 6	**Identity Synthesis**—Lesbian or gay identity is integrated with other aspects of self, and sexual orientation becomes only one aspect of self rather than the entire identity
Task	Integrate lesbian and gay identity so that instead of being the identity, it is an aspect of self

Adapted from Cass (1979)

models as having the following characteristics: (a) begin with a stage, (b) describe individuals using multiple defense strategies to deny recognition of personal homosexual feelings, (c) include a gradual recognition and tentative acceptance, (d) have a period of emotional and behavioral experimentation with homosexuality, (e) involve a time of identity crisis, and (f) marked by the coming-out process. Although difference exists among the stage models, which illustrate the difficulty of using one model to understand the complex psychosocial process of the development of sexual orientation identity, their predominance and persistence in the research literature and in current educational practice suggest that they represent with some accuracy the developmental process (Bilodeau and Renn 2005).

The minority stress model (Brooks 1981; Meyer 1995) is useful in understanding aspects of sexual minority identity development for older LGBT adults and the impact of sociocultural issues on their lives. Based on this model, individuals in minority groups experience additional minority-related stressors that individuals who are part of the majority do not have to contend. The minority stress model is a consolidation of several theories and models that propose that minority persons experience chronic stressors and these stressors can lead to negative psychosocial adjustment outcomes. According to Meyer (2010), the minority stress model does not attempt to imply that sexual minorities have higher rates of psychosocial issues because of their sexual orientation and gender identity; rather, the model identifies the pathogenic conditions that stigmatize LGBT persons and treat them as inferior to heterosexual individuals. Minority stressors for LGBT persons include experiences of discrimination, concealment or disclosure of sexual orientation/gender identity, expectations of prejudice and discrimination, and internalized homonegativity (Cox et al. 2011; Meyer 2003). Unlike ethnic and racial minority groups who experience minority stress, LGBT persons who experience sexual minority stress often do not receive support and understanding from their families of origin (Dziengel 2008). Minority stress in LGBT persons has been linked to higher levels of depression and negative health outcomes (Cox et al. 2009; Huebner and Davis 2007).

McCarn-Fassinger (1996) developed the lesbian identity development model, and Fassinger and Miller (1996) later validated the applicability of the theory with gay men (subsequently referenced in the literature as Fassinger's gay and lesbian identity development model), which examines identity development from a personal and a group perspective. The lesbian identity development model includes four phases: awareness, exploration, deepening/commitment, and internalization/synthesis. The use of "phases" is intentional to explicitly indicate flexibility that individuals revisit earlier phases in new or different contexts. The model explores attitudes of lesbians and gay men toward self, other sexual minorities and gender identity, and heterosexuals. A distinguishing aspect of Fassinger's model is that lesbians, gays, or bisexuals are not required to "come out" or to be actively involved in the lesbian, gay, or bisexual community.

A life span approach to sexual orientation development has been introduced an alternative to stage models. D'Augelli (1994) offers a "life span" model of sexual orientation development. This model takes social contexts into account in different ways than stage models. In addition, D'Augelli's model has the potential to represent a wider range of experiences than do the theories relating to specific racial, ethnic, or gender groups and addresses issues often ignored in other models. D'Augelli presents human development as unfolding in concurring and multiple paths, including the development of a person's self-concept, relationships with family, and connections to peer groups and community. This

Table 1.4 D'Augelli life span model of sexual orientation development

Exiting homosexuality
Developing a personal LGB identity
Developing an LGB social identity
Becoming an LGB offspring
Developing an LGB intimacy status
Entering an LGB community

D'Augelli (1994)

model suggests that sexual orientation may be fluid at certain times and more fixed at others and that human growth is intimately connected to and influenced by both biological and environmental factors. D'Augelli's model has six "identity processes" that function more or less independently and are not sequenced in stages (see Table 1.4). An individual may experience development in one process to a greater extent than another, and, depending on context and timing, he or she may be at different points of development in a given process (Bilodeau and Reen 2005).

Renn and Bilodeau (2005) extended D'Augelli's (1994) model and applied it to understanding corresponding processes in the formation of transgender identity development. Bilodeau (2005) found that transgender persons describe their gender identities in ways that reflect the six processes of D'Augelli's model.

Since the inclusion of gender identity disorder (GID) for the first time in the diagnostic and statistical manual of mental disorders (DSM) in 1980 as a mental illness, other theories on transgender identity formation have been proposed by Nutterbrock et al. (2002) and Devor (2004), bisexual identity formation by Fox (1995), and multiple identity formation by Reynolds and Pope (1991) (Table 1.2); however, none of these models have been empirically validated. In the fifth edition of the DSM, GID was deleted and replaced with gender dysphoria (GD), indicating that it is not a mental illness, rather a lifestyle with which individuals may need assistance in making adjustments. Feminist, postmodern, and queer theoretical theorists (e.g., Butler 1990, 1993; Creed 1995; Feinberg 1996,

Table 1.5 Lev's transgender emergence model

Stage 1	**Awareness**—Gender-variant people are often in great distress. The therapeutic task is the normalization of the experiences involved in emerging as transgender
Stage 2	**Seeking Information/Reaching Out**—Gender-variant people seek to gain education and support about transgenderism. The therapeutic task is to facilitate linkages and encourage outreach
Stage 3	**Disclosure to Significant Other**—Involves the disclosure of transgenderism to significant other. The therapeutic task involves supporting the transgendered person's integration in the family system
Stage 4	**Exploration (Identity and Self-Labeling)**—Involves the exploration of various (transgender) identities. The therapeutic task is to support the articulation and comfort with one's gendered identity
Stage 5	**Exploration (Transition Issues and Possible Body Modification)**—Involves exploring options for transition regarding identity, presentation, and body modification. The therapeutic task is the resolution of the decision and advocacy toward their manifestation
Stage 6	**Integration (Acceptance and Post-Transition Issues)**—The gender-variant person is able to integrate and synthesis (transgender) identity. The therapeutic task is to support adaptation to transition-related issues

Adapted from Lev (2004)

1998; Halberstam 1998; Wilchins 2002) have introduced alternatives to medical and psychiatric perspectives on gender identity. These theorists suggest that gender is not necessarily linked to biological sex assignment at birth, but is created through complex social inequities, and gender identity is more fluid. These theorists propose transgender identities and gender fluidity as normative as oppose to the binary, two-gender system and the influence of themes reflecting fluidity of gender that have emerged in the discipline of human development (Bilodeau and Renn 2005).

As an extension of sexual minority identity, in 2004 Lev introduced the transgender emergence model, a stage model that examines at how transgender people come to understand their identity. Lev's model comes from the perspective of a counseling or therapeutic point of view and focuses on what the individual is experiencing and the responsibility of the counselor or interventionist. As with other stage theories, Lev's model begins with the first stage as awareness. (see Table 1.5 for Lev's stages). Lev's clinical and philosophical ideology is based on the belief that transgenderism is a normal and potentially healthy variation of human expression. As postulated by Goldner (1988), gender dichotomies are not only restrictive, but also constitutive, with the gendering of social spheres constraining personal freedom and gender categories

determining what is possible to know. Lev's approach is to consider the ecosystem (i.e., influence of environment on perception and behavior) in working with transgender persons. According to Lev, "gender variance does not simply live within individuals but exists 'within' a larger matrix of relationships, families, and communities" (p. xx).

Lev offers three goals for therapists working with transgendered persons and their families. The first goal is "to accept that transgenderism is a normal expression of human potentiality." The second goal is "to place transgenderism within a larger social context that includes an overview of the existence of gender variance throughout history." The third goal is "to outline various etiological theories that impact assessment and diagnosis, as well as innovative, possibly iconoclastic treatment strategies to work with gender-dysphoric, gender-variant, transgendered, third-sexed, transsexual, and intersexed people as members of extended family systems" (pp. xx–xxi).

Counseling Theories and Practice for Older Adults

A commonly held view of older persons is that they are mentally incompetent. Although there is some cognitive decline associated with normal aging, the majority of older adults do not demonstrate significant mental decline. For LGBT elders, psychosocial issues arise from ongoing discrimination on the basis of their sexual orientation and gender identity, lack of acceptance from the heterosexual community and family members, and isolation and exclusion from LGBT communities because of ageism. The general lack of support in many political, educational, and religious institutions and the distinctively oppressive social climate for sexual minorities in which older LGBT generations live creates personal conflict that can manifest itself through internalized disorders (e.g., depression, homophobia) or externalized disorders (e.g., suicidal behavior) (Mabey 2007). Counseling or therapeutic intervention can help LGBT elders who experience multiple discrimination to come to terms with factors associated with ageism (Sue and Sue 2013) and how the historically negative climate of discrimination and oppression shapes their experiences with, and impressions of, their own sexual identity (Heaphy 2007; Porter et al. 2004). However, it is important for counselors not to view identity as necessarily problematic (Berger 1982; Mabey 2011). In fact, researchers have introduced the concept of "crisis competence" or "stigma competence" (Almvig 1982; Balsam and D'Augelli 2006; Vaughan and Waehler 2010), in which coming-out by LGBT persons allows them to develop a competency for dealing with other crises or stigma in the life span, including difficulties associated with aging (Heaphy 2007; Kimmel et al. 2006; Schope 2005). Stigma competence was first developed with regard to persons from racial and ethnic minority groups who have multiple minority statuses, including sexual minority identity. In a study testing the theory of stigma competence with lesbian, gay, and bisexual adults over age 60, Lawson-Ross (2013) found that older sexual minority adults who were more accepting of their sexual minority identities had lower levels of internalized ageism and had higher levels of life satisfaction and happiness than their peers who were less accepting of their sexual minority identities.

Counseling Approaches. In working with LGBT elders, the selection of the counseling approach should be based on the individual and his or her needs. Counselors tend to adapt their approaches to working with a client based on the person's developmental changes in life, the particular cohort to which the person belongs, and the social context in which the person lives (Blando 2011). Older persons fit into a contextual, cohort-based, maturity-specific change model (Knight 1996) that suggests they face particular challenges that are unique in later life. Older LGBT persons belong to a particular cohort with a collection of experiences and norms that differ from those of the present and from heterosexual elders (Blando). In the remainder of this section, we will present select counseling approaches that may be effective with older LGBT populations. These counseling approaches are not intended to be either inclusive or suggestive; rather, they are a starting point or serve as guidelines.

One of the most common forms of therapy with the general population and with older adults is cognitive-behavioral therapy (CBT). CBT may be particularly efficacious with older adults because of its focus on the present, strict structure, emphasis on self-monitoring, psychoeducational orientation, and goal oriented. Adjustment may need to be made for older adults who have developmental changes such as speed of processing in intellectual configuration (e.g., later life of crystalized over fluid intelligence), emotional changes (i.e., emotions are more nuanced and complex and may include co-experience of discrepant emotions such as being both happy and sad), and the person's worldview (Blando 2011). CBT examines the role thoughts play in maintaining a problem, stress, or concern. Emphasis is on changing dysfunctional thoughts that influence behavior. The application of CBT with LGBT elders may be effective in addressing behaviors stemming from past experiences of discrimination with institutions and service providers, fear of homophobia-based victimization, and also from fear or anticipation of discrimination. In addition, Satterfield and Crabb (2010) demonstrated the effectiveness of CBT for depression in an older gay man.

Guided autobiography is another approach that is effective with older adults. Guided autobiography is used to help people understand and make meaning from their past through reading and sharing brief, written essays about their lives, and sharing their thoughts about these stories. It promotes integration, fulfillment, and competence (Blando 2011). LGBT elders often have not had a safe venue in which to explore or express their feelings, self-concept, or self-identity. Guided autobiography offers them a private mechanism to do so.

Another approach applicable to working with LGBT elders is persons-centered therapy (PCT) by Rogers (1951). Rogers described people who are becoming increasingly actualized as having four characteristics: (a) an openness to experience, (b) a trust in themselves, (c) an internal source of evaluation, and (d) a willingness to continue growing. PCT has emphasized on how individuals can move forward in constructive directions and how they can successfully deal with obstacles both within themselves and outside of themselves that are blocking their growth. Through self-awareness, an individual learns to exercise choice. The therapeutic goal is for an individual to achieve a greater degree of independence and integration (Corey 2103).

Theories of Public Health and Practice

A number of important theories and approaches germane to public health are salient for LGBT elders. It is important that at least two distinguishing approaches are borne in mind regarding public health constructs. First, public health primarily concerns population health versus the health of individuals, and so, allowing for within-group differences, public health efforts concern the *population* of LGBT elders rather than the actions of individuals. Second, public health stresses the importance of prevention efforts above and beyond any other efforts. Though this is not to say that public health does not involve intervention, public health experts seek to improve the health of LGBT elders far earlier than most other discipline's current intervention efforts contemplate, for example, preventing poor health outcomes as a result of historic stressors and inequities, such as, until recently, the lack of health insurance coverage for same-sex partners. In this section, we explain four well-recognized approaches/theories to public health that have applicability to LGBT elders, in particular the socio-ecological model, the theory of reasoned action, the health belief model, and the transtheoretical model of change (DiClemente et al. 2013).

The first of these approaches is the socio-ecological model, most closely associated with Bronfenbrenner (1986). Applied to LGBT elders, the model places the elder at the center of four nested systems (depicted graphically as concentric circles), consistent with an "elder-centered" (Quandt et al. 1999) approach to prevention and intervention. The *microsystem*, which includes the older adult, includes biological and personal factors that converge to influence how individuals behave as well as risk factors for adverse health outcomes. Consideration of LGBT elders at the level of the *mesosystem* focuses on close relationships (e.g., family, friends, neighbors) in order to explore how such relationships either protect against or promote LGBT health and quality of life. The *exosystem* identifies community contexts in which social relationships occur (e.g., neighborhoods, service organizations). This system promotes how characteristics settings may affect LGBT elders' health and well-being. Finally, the *macrosystem* includes broad ideological values, norms, and institutional patterns that may foster a climate in which LGBT elders are either encouraged or prohibited, including changes in power and control dynamics (e.g., dominance of spouse/partner; reversal of child/parent roles) as well as age-related changes in social positions and financial resources.

One of the most well-known value-expectancy theories in public health is the theory of reasoned action, which grew out of research Ajzen (2002) and Ajzen and Fishbein (1980) on behavior and attitude. Central to this theory is that people have control over their lives and can consequently make a decision made about a behavior to adopt or discontinue. The authors contend that an elder's beliefs and attitudes shape his or her intent to take an action and that social influences or norms on LGBT elders also affect behavioral intent. For example, if an LGBT elder believes that stopping smoking is a goal but that society would offer little help for him or her to do so because of a pervasive attitude that the elder's sexual orientation is causing the problem, then he or she is unlikely to attempt the change because the cost of doing so is too high or difficult.

Another type of theory or perspective is those concerning a perceived threat. Perhaps the most well known is the health belief model, which has been used by public health practitioners and researchers for over 50 years. The health belief model has similarities to the value-expectancy model above, but it is also a departure, due to the insertion of a threat or fear that drives changes in health behavior as well as a person's perception of health severity and his or her perception of health susceptibility (Salazar et al. 2013), and, added to the model in the late 1980s, the concept of self-efficacy (Bandura 1977) or an older adult's conception of his or her own power or self-determination (Rosenstock et al. 1988). The cost-benefit valuation determines the course of action, as it also does with the theory of reasoned action described above. A fear appeal might be used to promote a health behavior change, such as the threat of susceptibility to HIV in older adult populations.

A fourth and well-known stage is the transtheoretical model of change, a model explaining how persons may change their health behavior and derived from more than 300 theories of psychotherapy (Prochaska 1979; Prochaska and Di-Clemente 1986). Five stages, in which persons can facilitate, comprise the model: precontemplation, contemplation, preparation, action, and maintenance. Precontemplation is the stage when a person is not ready to attempt a change at all. In the contemplation stage, an elder is thinking of embarking on a change, and the impetus to act or not is the fulcrum of decisional balance. The scale must tip in favor of attempting the change rather than impediments to doing so. Preparation

concerns undertaking some steps toward a change, such as talking to a doctor about a health condition or visiting another health professional to seek advice. The stage of action concerns undertaking an identifiable activity (e.g., walking, eating healthy foods, wearing a condom). Finally, the maintenance stage is when the change is adopted and the effort to continue the change diminishes from the action phase. Recidivism is possible, but continued progress decreases the chances of returning to the former and undesired behavior (Schneider 2013). High self-efficacy is critical to reach the maintenance stage (Bandura 1986).

Social Work Theories and Approaches

One of the unique concepts of social work practice is an understanding of the constant state of change of the contextual arena in which social workers operate. With the continuous change in environments and populations, social workers need to rethink how they deliver services in response to distinct alterations in family structures and functions, medical advances and aging, economic shifts, and shifting evolving professional and political ideologies (Allen 2005). Gratwick et al. (2014) contend that theoretically driven service models are crucial to effective service provision. Similar to the other disciplines mentioned previously, various theories and model are used in social work practice. Social work practice employs the developmental theories of moral reasoning (Kohlberg 1973; Gilligan 1982), cognition (Piaget 1932), stage theories (Erikson 1950), and transpersonal theories of human development (going beyond identity rooted in the individual body or ego to include higher levels of consciousness). Developmental theories focus on the changes and stability of behavior across the life span. The remainder of this section concerns a presentation of these theories, the primary perspectives, and current social work practice models. Infused throughout is discussion on social work practice with LGBT elders.

The major theories used in social work practice are systems theory, psychodynamic, social learning, and conflict theory. Systems theory

(Bertalanffy 1968) is the interdisciplinary study of systems to identify and understand principles that can be applied reciprocal relationships between parts or elements that constitute a whole, and the relationships among individuals, groups, organizations, or communities and mutually influencing factors in the environment. A system is a set of elements that interact with one another. The system is only as strong as its weakest part, and the system is greater than the sum of its parts. The focus of this theory is on the interconnectedness of elements with all living organisms (systems) in nature and social relationships (Gladding 2011). Bertalanffy's model assumes a single-dimension cause-and-effect relationship between social elements within the environment. A demarcation of systems in social work involves the designation of particular social systems as being microlevel (small-size social system such as individual or couples), mezzo-level (intermediate-size social system such as support networks), and macrolevel (large-size social system such as communities and organizations) (Friedman and Allen 2011). It appears that the systems model, as it is applied to social systems, provides the social work practitioner the means to view human behavior through a comprehensive lens that allows for the assessment of the person across a broad spectrum of human conditions (Lesser and Pope 2011).

Carsetensen et al. (1999) introduced socio-emotional selectivity theory (SST), which builds upon the idea that social networks have value and maintains that the perception of time systematically influences motivation. A basic tenet is that the perception of time affects how people regulate their social environment and that those people who perceive time as finite spend their time optimizing relationships that are emotionally fulfilling. Adults are expected to contact their social networks and avoid unbeneficial relationships. LGBT elders have significantly diminished traditional supports when compared to the general older population (Lancet 2011), which translates into a lack of traditional support networks that may not be replaced by the strength of other close friends or informal support networks with the LGBT community (Irish

Association of Social Workers 2011). Older LGBT adults suggest that they may not use or disclose when qualifying for or receiving services because they do not trust the social environment in which services are delivered or do not perceive potential relationships in these contexts to be emotionally supportive or fulfilling (Gratwick et al. 2014). Discussion Box 1.1 provides further information on the theoretical framework of SST. Older LGBT persons must perceive value in social networks in order to believe that they will benefit from them. Sullivan (2011) found that LGBT elders' decisions to enter LGBT senior housing were due to an LGBT-accepting social environment that increased their sense of safety to increase their social networks. The extent to which older LGBT individuals have social networks varies by gender. Schope (2005) found that the appearance of older gay men tended to be judged more negatively in the gay community, resulting in less social support. Conversely, lesbians tend to have more social networks comprised of lesbians across the age spectrum and are revered by younger lesbians for their insight and perceived political power. Older bisexual and transgender adult face greater challenges than their gay and lesbian peers with regard to stigma, discrimination and self-identity, and social networks because of their perceived lack of identity to either gay men or lesbians.

> **Discussion Box 1.1: Socioemotional Selectivity Theory (SST)** SST presumes that goals are always set in temporal contexts and that the relative importance of specific goals within this goal constellation changes as a function of perceived time.
>
> When the future is perceived as open-ended, future-oriented goals weigh most heavily and individuals pursue goals that optimize long-range outcomes.
>
> When endings are perceived, goal constellations are recognized such that emotionally meaningful goals (related to feelings) are prioritized because such goals have more immediate payoffs.

Although achieved more gradually, approaching old age is also associated with increasing recognition that time is, in some sense, running out.

SST was originally formulated to explain and predict age differences in motivation. Because chronological age is associated with perceived time left in life, the theory predicts systematic age differences in motivation.

Questions:

1. Why are individuals more motivated toward goal constellation as they age?
2. Does SST consider a continuum in which individuals optimize goal-oriented outcomes?
3. How does SST explain the role of social networks for LGBT elders?

Adapted from Fung and Carstensen (2006).

Another approach, psychodynamic theory, also known as insight-oriented theory, has its origin in psychoanalytic theory, similar to the transdisciplinary change model in public health. The psychodynamic approach includes all the theories in psychology that regard human functioning as based on how interaction, drive and emotions, particularly unconscious processes as manifested in a person's present behavior. The goal of psychodynamic intervention is to increase a person's self-awareness and understanding of the influence of the past on present behavior. A psychodynamic approach enables a person to examine unresolved conflicts and symptoms that arise from past dysfunctional relationships and manifest themselves in the need to engage in abusive and dysfunctional behavior (Haggerty 2006). The theory purports that emotions have a central place in human behavior and both conscious and unconscious mental activity serves as the motivating force in human behavior (McLeod 2007). Individuals may become overwhelmed by internal and/or external demands and frequently use ego defense mechanisms to avoid becoming overwhelmed. Social workers use this theory when addressing early attachment relationships and the developmental history of the individual, which includes past trauma. The therapeutic techniques used include transference, dream and daydream analysis, confrontation, focusing on strengths, life history, and complementarity. Typically linear, psychodynamic-oriented therapy focuses on cause-and-effect interactions (Gladding 2011).

Social learning theory (SLT) (Bandura 1971), also used by public health, operates from the hypothesis that human behavior is learned as individuals interact with their environment. People learn through observing others' behavior, attitudes, and outcomes. Individuals observe others and learn through modeling. From observing others, an elder forms an idea of how new behaviors are performed and later this coded information serves as a guide for action. SLT explains human behavior as continuous reciprocal interaction among cognitive, behavioral, and environmental influences (reciprocal determinism). SLT is regarded as a bridge between behaviorist and cognitive learning theories because it encompasses attention, retention, reproduction, and motivation. Problematic behavior is maintained by positive or negative reinforcement. Cognitive-behavioral therapy examines the role that thoughts play in maintaining a problem, and its emphasis is on changing dysfunctional thoughts, which influence behavior. Social learning theory has been used extensively with younger LGBT persons, especially in the area of career choice. SLT applied to LGBT elders can be effective in working with substance abusers. For example, Bowman and Bryant (2011) applied SLT to understand smoking behavior among LGBT persons because compared to the general population, LGBT adults have significantly higher smoking rates. One plausible explanation for the higher rates is that the tobacco industry targets the LGBT community. Bowman and Bryant found that LGBT persons often start smoking after "coming-out" in direct response to social stresses and gay culture, which seems to be support smoking behavior.

Conflict theory, introduced by Karl Marx (cited in Dobb 1979) as the name implies, involves conflict, dominance, and oppression in social life. Basically, groups and individuals attempt to advance their own interests over those of others. However, because power is unequally divided, social order is based on manipulation and control of non-dominant groups by dominant groups. In the case of LGBT elders, heterosexuals and younger groups exert domination through heterosexism and homophobia. Depending on other group affiliations of LGBT persons (e.g., race/ethnicity, socioeconomic status), they may be further dominated. Conflict theory is further characterized by a lack of open conflict as a sign of exploitation. Social change is driven by conflict, with periods of change interrupting long periods of stability. Social workers use conflict theory to understand those experiencing oppression in some form or another in society. Research indicates that LGBT elders experience oppression (e.g., political, religious, economic, cultural) and marginalization (e.g., sexual orientation, gender identity, age) from numerous sources. For example, in a study of the prevalence of mental disorders in LGBT persons, Meyer (2003) found a higher prevalence of mental disorders than in heterosexual persons. He attributed this to minority stress, explaining that stigma, prejudice, and discrimination create a hostile and stressful social environment that causes mental health problems. Application of conflict theory helps LGBT elders to deal with a history of homophobia and discrimination, experiences of antigay gay violence and hate crimes, addressing public opposition to gay marriage, expectations of rejection, internalized homophobia, hiding and concealing identity, and ameliorative coping processes.

Perspective in social work practice represents the specific aspects of a session that are emphasized. The primary perspectives used in social work practice include strengths (Saleeby 1996) or resilience, feminist, and ecosystem. The social worker believes that a person has multiple strengths that are assessed and incorporated into the helping relationship. Although resilience has various definitions, at times it is "defined as a psychological process developed in response to intense life stressors that facilitate healthy functioning" (Ballenger-Browing and Johnson 2010). Resilience has four prerequisites: (a) risk or predisposition to biopsychosocial or environmental conditions, (b) exposure to a high-magnitude stressor, (c) stress response, and (d) return to baseline functioning and symptom levels (Ballenger-Browning and Johnson 2010, p. 1). The feminist perspective takes into account the role of gender and the historical lack of power experienced by women in society. Social workers using this perspective emphasize equality and empowerment of women in society. Application of the feminist approach with LGBT elders would place emphasis on equality with regard to sexual orientation, gender identity, age, and other characteristics of the populations. Finally, the ecosystem (Germain 1973) is the person-to-environment concept presented earlier in this chapter. According to Mattaini and Meyer (2002), the ecological system has been almost universally accepted in social work practice because of its framework for understanding network complexities.

Social work practice model provides step-by-step guides for client sessions. The current social work practice models include problem-solving, task-centered, solution-focused, narrative, cognitive-behavioral, and crisis. In the problem-solving approach, one must first understand the presenting problem or issue and then brainstorm possible solutions. It is incumbent upon the person or client to select a solution, implement it, and evaluate its effectiveness. The task-centered model focuses on breaking down the problem into small manageable tasks, thus facilitating accomplishment. The solution-focused model takes the approach of identifying the solution first and having the person establish the process that will lead to the solution. Finally, the narrative model uses a variety of method for the person to express his or her thoughts.

Integration of Practice Models in Working with LGBT Elders

Understanding how models work can work effectively in support of LGBT elders is necessary to improving service outcomes. When drawing from theories from the disciplines represented in this chapter, it is efficacious to consider bringing them together from an interdisciplinary perspective (some cross one or more disciplines anyway). Tan (2009) suggests that many in the field of social work remain too focused on individual therapy and clinical practice when there is a need to shift more globally and holistically. Furthermore, progressive social work place more emphasizes on the need for the individual to be part of his or her own change (Mullaly 2002). Tan suggests that community development theory (CDT) is a practical framework. Community development theory is defined as "the employment of community structures to address social needs and empower groups of people" (Mendes 2008, p. 3). CDT is rooted in sociology. Its primary functions are to provide norms for the practitioner's actions and a model of practical help to communities. CDT depends heavily on general systems and on the conceptual frameworks of social systems, thus treating communities as systems (Cook 1994). Tan purports that the principles of CDT have implications for the ways clinicians view and engage with clients and ways social workers seek to make large-scale changes within the community.

A key to application of CDT to LGBT elders is the notion that people involved in a system have a sense and recognition of the relationships and areas of common concerns with other members. For LGBT elders, the community may be their immediate surroundings as well as regional, national, or international organizations with which they have affiliation or that provide services and advocacy on their behalf. Because many theories are used in community development, the holistic approach of CDT consciously attempts to emphasize on the functional relationship among the parts and the whole. Given the variety and degree of services that LGBT elders need, CDT offers a way of looking at the interconnectedness of services and activities from an operational level intended to improve outcomes. Moreover, CDT values and principles potentially empower LGBT elder to be involved in their community to have input on decisions that may influence them.

Several practice models have been developed to assist in older LGBT adults, ranging from guidelines for practice to specialized support groups and approaches to individual therapy (Hash and Rogers 2013). The American Psychological Association (APA) developed the Guidelines for Psychological Practice with Lesbian, Gay, and Bisexual Clients (www.apa.org/pi/lgbt/resources/guidelines.aspx) (APA 2012), the Association for Lesbian, Gay, Bisexual, and Transgender Issues in Counseling (ALGBTIC 2009) developed competencies for counseling LGBT clients, and ALGBTIC in conjunction with the American Counseling Association (ACA 2010) approved competencies for counseling transgender clients. The code of ethics of the National Association of Social Work (NASW 2008) (http://www.socialworkers.org/pubs/code.asp) emphasizes the importance of cultural competency and social diversity, including sexual orientation and gender identity, as does the Code for Professional Ethics for Rehabilitation Counselors (www.crccertification.com/filrbin/pdf/crcCodeOfEthics.prf) (CRCC 2010). The Centers for Disease Control (http://www.cdc.gov/lgbthealth/) emphasize the importance of addressing disease in the LGBT community across the life course, particularly as it concerns HIV and other sexually transmitted diseases as well as violence prevention and intervention (CDC 2014). The Council on Social Work Education (CSWE) has incorporated issues relevant to sexual orientation (www.cswc.org/File.aspx?id=25501) (CSWE 2008). Through an examination of the unique strengths and challenges faced by older LGBT adults, Crisp et al. (2008) constructed a profile and suggested an age-competent and gay affirmative model for practice, including culturally competent knowledge, attitudes, and skills for work with older LGBT adults in the USA.

Building social networks to address challenges faced by LGBT elders who share similar experiences and backgrounds is offered as a way to build an effective modality (Hash and Rogers 2013). In a technological era, the use of cyber counseling has the potential to deliver services to LGBT elders within their residential setting without requiring them to travel for services. However, it is important to recognize that some LGBT elders do not have access to technology or do not have technology literacy.

Summary

In conclusion, theories from the disciplines presented here (i.e., counseling, public health, and social work) are replete with theories that are discipline specific but also that draw upon other disciplines, in particular those from psychotherapy and sociology. Consistent among those presented is an understanding of LGBT elders from the perspectives of stages of development or progress, of interlocking systems and networks, of the influence of the environment, of costs and benefits, of holism, and of interdisciplinarity. Not intended to be exhaustive, this chapter has presented major theories, frameworks, and concepts necessary to provide human services for the LGBT population. These frameworks, either explicitly or implicitly, undergird the rest of the chapters of the book as well as provide a touchstone for understanding the unique perspective presented.

Learning Exercises

Self-Check Questions

1. What is the function of theory for practitioners?
2. Even when providers of aging services express willingness to become more responsive to the needs of LGBT older adults, what usually are the outcomes?
3. In which of Erikson's stages of psychosocial development is it more complicated for an LGBT elder to accept one's life and self? Explain why?
4. What are the similarities between Sigmund Freud and Erving Goffman's concepts about childhood development?
5. What is the difference between a theory, a construct, and a model?

Experiential Exercises

1. Select a theory and apply the concepts in a role-play situation to LGBT elders in a group counseling session or self-advocacy activity.
2. Given current theories, constructs, and models, identify what is a gap and propose a model for application to LGBT elders for counseling and/or service delivery.
3. Select a theory in a specific discipline and deconstruct it through a critical analysis in its shortcoming for application to LGBT elders.

Multiple-Choice Questions

1. Who was one of the first theorists to present identifiable stages of homosexual identity?
   (a) Rogers
   (b) Skinner
   (c) Plummer
   (d) Gladding
2. The Kinsey scale clarified which of the following issues about sexuality?
   (a) Individuals are strictly heterosexual or homosexual
   (b) There is greater variability of sexual orientation
   (c) Heterosexuality is not primary or held above other sexual orientations
   (d) Both B and C
   (e) All of the above
3. How does the minority stress model apply to LGBT persons?
   (a) Identifies pathogenic conditions that stigmatize LGBT persons and treat them as inferior to heterosexual individuals

    (b) Attempts to imply that sexual minorities have higher rates of psychosocial issues because of their sexual orientation and gender identity

    (c) Confirms LGBT sexual identity as a mental illness

    (d) Supports the notion that gender is socially defined

4. Which of the following developed the transgender emergence model?

    (a) McCarn-Fassinger

    (b) Lev

    (c) D'Augelli

    (d) Devor

5. Which therapy may be particularly effective with older adults because of its focus on the present, emphasis on self-monitoring, psychoeducational orientation, and goal orientation?

    (a) Person-centered therapy

    (b) Psychoanalytic therapy

    (c) Cognitive-behavioral therapy

    (d) Existential therapy

6. Which of the following is of primary concern for public health?

    (a) Health of individuals

    (b) Population health

    (c) Immigrant populations

    (d) Underserved groups

7. Which theory emphasizes that people have control over their lives and can consequently make a decision about a behavior to adopt or discontinue?

    (a) Theory of reasoned action

    (b) Centrality theory

    (c) Snowball theory

    (d) Gestalt theory

8. Which theory has as it basic tenet that the perception of time affects how people regulate their social environment and that those who perceive time as finite spend their time optimizing relationships that are emotionally fulfilling?

    (a) Reality theory

    (b) Feminist theory

    (c) Behavior theory

    (d) Socioemotional selective theory

9. Which theory hypothesizes that human behavior is learned through observing other's behaviors and through modeling?

    (a) Ecological theory

    (b) Systems theory

    (c) Social learning theory

    (d) Solution-focused theory

10. Which theory is defined as the use of community structures to address social needs and empower groups of people?

    (a) Community action theory

    (b) Community development theory

    (c) Family systems theory

    (d) Action development theory

Key

1-c
2-d
3-a
4-b
5-c
6-b
7-a
8-d
9-c
10-b

Resources

American Counseling Association: www.counseling.org.

Association for Adult Development and Aging: www.aadaweb.org.

Association for Lesbian, Gay, Bisexual, & Transgender Issues in Counseling: www.algbtic.org.

Association of Lesbian, Gay, Bisexual, & Transgender Issues in Counseling. (2009). *Competencies for counseling with transgender clients*. Alexandria, VA: Author.

Bockting, W., Knudson, G., & Goldberg, J. M. (2006). *Counseling and mental health care of transgender adults and loved ones*. Available at www.vch.ca/transhealth.

Dworkin, S. H., & Pope, M. (Eds.). (2012). *Casebook for counseling lesbian, gay, bisexual, and transgender persons and their families.* Alexandria, VA: American Counseling Association.

Institute of medicine. (2011). The health of lesbian, gay, bisexual, and transgender people: Building a foundation for better understanding. Available at http://www.jom.edu/Reports/2011/The-Health-of-Lesbian-Gay-Bisexual-and-Transgender-People.aspx.

National Association for Social Workers: www.socialworkers.org.

National Gerontological Society of America: www.geron.org.

References

Ajzen, I. (2002). Residual effects of past on later behavior: Habituation and reasoned action perspectives. *Personality and Social Psychology Review, 6*(2), 107–122.

Ajzen, I., & Fishbein, M. (1980). *Understanding attitudes and predicting social behavior.* Englewood Cliff, NJ: Prentice-Hall.

Allen, E. V. (2005). Teaching generalist practice in a rural context. In L. H. Ginsberg (Ed.), *Social work in rural communities* (pp. 445–463). Alexandria, VA: Council on Social Work Education.

Almvig, M. (1982). *The invisible minority: Aging and lesbianism.* Utica, NY: Institute of Gerontology.

Altman, D. (1971). *Homosexual: Oppression and liberation.* New York: E. P. Dutton.

American Counseling Association. (2010). Competencies for counseling with transgender clients. *Journal of LGBT Issues in Counseling, 4,* 135–159.

American Psychological Association. (2012). *Guidelines for practice with LGBT clients.* Available from http://www.apa.org/pi/lgbt/resources/guidelines.aspx.

Association for Lesbian, Gay, Bisexual, and Transgender Issues in Counseling. (2009). *Competencies for counseling with transgender clients.* Alexandria, VA: Author.

Ballenger-Browning, K., & Johnson, D. C. (2010). *Key facts of resilience.* San Diego, CA: Navel Center for Combat & Operational Stress Control.

Balsam, K., & D'Augelli, A. (2006). The victimization of older LGBT adults: Patterns, impact, and implications for intervention. In D. Kimmel, T. Rose, & S. Davis (Eds.), *Lesbian, gay, bisexual, and transgender aging: Research and clinical perspectives* (pp. 110–130). New York, NY: Columbia University Press.

Bandura, A. (1971). *Social learning theory.* New York: General Learning Press.

Bandura, A. (1977). Self-efficacy: Toward a unifying theory of behavioral change. *Psychological Review, 84*(2), 191.

Bandura, A. (1986). *Social foundations of though and action: A social cognitive theory.* Upper Sadle River, NJ: Prentice-Hall.

Berger, R. M. (1982). The unseen minority: Older gays and lesbians. *Social Work, 27*(3), 236–242.

von Bertalanffy, L. (1968). *General systems theory: Foundation, development, and application.* New York: Braziller.

Bilodeau, B. L. (2005). Beyond the gender binary: A case study of transgender college student development at a Midwestern university. *Journal of Gay and Lesbian Issues in Education, 3*(1), 29–44.

Bilodeau, B. L., & Renn, K. A. (2005). Analysis of LGBT identity development models and implications for practice. *New directions for Student Services, 111,* 25–39.

Blando, J. (2011). *Counseling older adults.* New York: Routledge.

Bowman, L., & Bryant, L. (2011). *The application of social learning theory to understanding smoking behavior among LGBTQ individuals.* Retrieved July 1, 2014 from www.adulter.org/Proceedings/2011/papers/bowman_bryant.pdf.

Bronfenbrenner, U. (1986). The ecology of the family as a context for human development: Research perspectives. *Developmental Psychology, 22,* 723–742.

Brooks, V. R. (1981). *Minority stress and lesbian women.* Lexington, MA: D. C. Health.

Burleson, W. E. (2005). *Bi America: Myths, truths, and struggles of an invisible community.* New York: Harrington Park Press.

Butler, J. (1990). *Gender trouble: Feminism and the subversion of identity.* New York: Routledge.

Butler, J. (1993). *Bodies that matter: On the discursive limits of sex.* New York: Routledge.

Butler, R. N. (1994). *Dispelling ageism: The cross-cutting intervention. Changing perceptions of aging and the aged.* New York, NY: Springer.

Carstensen, L. L., Isaacowitz, D. M., & Charles, S. T. (1999). Taking time seriously: A theory of socioemotional selectivity. *American Psychologist, 54*(3), 165–181.

Cass, V. C. (1979). Homosexual identity formation: A theoretical model. *Journal of Homosexuality, 4,* 219–235.

Cass, V. C. (1984). Homosexual identity: A concept in need of definition. *Journal of Homosexuality, 9*(2–3), 105–126.

Centers for Desiease Control. (2014). The sociological-ecological model: A framework for prevention. Available from http://www.cdc.gov/violencePrevention/overview/social-ecologicalmodel.html.

Chapman, B., & Brannock, J. (1987). Proposed model of lesbian identity development: An empirical examination. *Journal of Homosexuality, 14*(3/4), 69–80.

Coleman, E. (1982). Developmental stages of the coming-out process. W. Paul, J. D. Weinrich, J. C. Gonsiorek & M. E. Hotvedt (eds.), *Homosexuality: Social, psychological and biological issues*. Beverly Hills, CA: Sage.

Commission on Rehabilitation Counselor Certification. (2010). *Code of professional ethics for rehabilitation counselors*. Available from http://www.crccertification.com/filrbin/pdf/crcCodeOfEthics.pdf.

Cook, J. B. (1994). *Community development theory*. Retrieved June 30, 2014 from http://extension.missouri.edu/p/MP568.

Corey, G. (2103) *Theory and practice of counseling and psychotherapy*. Belmont, CA: Brooks Cole.

Cox, N., Dewaele, A., van Houtte, M., & Vincke, J. (2011). Stress-related growth, coming out, and internalized homonegativity in lesbian, gay, and bisexual youth. An experiment of stress-related growth within the minority stress model. *Journal of Homosexuality, 58*, 117–137.

Cox, N., Vanden Berghe, W., Dewaele, A., & Vincke, J. (2009). General and minority stress in an LGB population in Flanders. *Journal of LGBT Health Research, 4*(4), 181–194.

Creed, B. (1995). Lesbian bodies: Tribades, tomboys, and tarts. In E. Grosz & E. Probyn (Eds.), *Sexy bodies: The strange carnalities of feminism*. New York: Routledge.

Crisp, C., Wayland, S., & Gordon, T. (2008). Older gay, Lesbian, and bisexual adults: Tools for age-competent and gay affirmative practice. *Journal of Gay and Lesbian Social Services, 20*(1/2), 5–29.

D'Augelli, A. R. (1994). Identity development and sexual orientation: Toward a model of lesbian, gay, and bisexual development. In E. J. Trickett, R. J. Watts & D. Birman (Eds.), *Human diversity: Perspectives on people in context* (pp. 321–333). San Francisco: Jossey-Bass.

Devor, A. H. (2004). Witnessing and mirroring: A fourteen-stage model of transsexual identity formation. *Journal of Gay and Lesbian Psychiatry, 8*(1/2), 41–67.

DiClemente, R. J., Salazar, L. F., & Crosby, R. A. (2013). *Health behavior theory for public health: Principles, foundations, and applications*. Burlington, MA: Jones and Barlett Learning.

Dobb, M. (Ed.). (1979). *A contribution to the critique of political economy*. London, Lawrence & Whishart.

Dziengel, L. E. (2008). *Older same sex couples and ambiguous loss theory: The mutual existence of ambiguity and resiliency*. Doctoral dissertation. University of Minnesota, Minneapolis, MN.

Eliason, M. J. (1996). An inclusive model of lesbian identity. *Journal of Gay, Lesbian and Bisexual Identity, 1*(1), 3–19.

Eliason, M. J., & Schope, R. (2007). Shifting sands or solid foundation? Lesbian, gay, bisexual and transgender identity formation. In I. H. Meyer & M. E. Northridge (Eds.), *The health of sexual minorities* (pp. 3–26). New York: Springer.

Erikson, E. (1950). *Childhood and society*. New York: Norton.

Faderman, L. (1984). The "new gay" lesbians. *Journal of Homosexuality, 10*(3/4), 65–75.

Fassinger, R. E., & Miller, B. A. (1996). Validation of an inclusive model of sexual minority formation on a sample of gay men. *Journal of Homosexuality, 32*(2), 53–78.

Feinberg, L. (1996). *Transgender warriors: Making history from Joan of Arc to Dennis Rodman*. Boston: Beacon Press.

Feinberg, L. (1998). *Trans liberation: Beyond pink and blue*. Boston: Beacon Press.

Fox, R. C. (1995). Bisexual identities. In A. R. D'Augelli & C. J. Patterson (Eds.), *Lesbian, gay, and bisexual identities over the lifespan: Psychological perspectives* (pp. 48–86). New York: Oxford University Press.

Freud, S. (1949). *An outline of psychoanalysis*. New York, NY: Norton.

Friedman, B. D., & Allen, K. N. (2011). Systems theory. In J. Brandell (Ed.), *Theory and practice of clinical social work* (pp. 3–18). New York, NY: The Free Press.

Fritz, K. (1993). *The bisexual option* (2nd ed.). Binghamton, NY: The Haworth Press.

Fung, H. H., & Carstensen, L. L. (2006). Goals change when life's fragility is primed: Lessons learned from older adults, the September 11 attacks and SARS. *Social Cognition, 24*(3), 248–278.

Germain, C. B. (1973). An ecological perspective in case work. *Social Casework, 54*, 323–330.

Gilligan, C. (1982). *In a different voice*. Cambridge: Harvard University Press.

Gladding, S. T. (2011). *Family therapy: History, theory, and practice* (5th ed.). Upper Saddle River, NJ: Pearson.

Goffman, E. (1963). *Stigma: Notes on the management of spoiled identity*. New York: Simon & Schuster.

Goldner, V. (1988). Generation and gender: Normative and covert hierarchies. *Family Process, 27*, 17–31.

Gratwick, S., Jihanian, L. J., Holloway, I. W., Sanchez, M., & Sullivan, K. (2014). Social work practice with LBGT seniors. *Journal of Gerontological Social Work, 57*, 889. doi:10.1080/01634372.2014.885475.

Grossman, A. H. (2008). Conducting research among older lesbian, gay, and bisexual adults. *Journal of Gay and Lesbian Social Services, 20*(1/2), 51–67.

Haggerty, J. (2006). Psychodynamic therapy. *Psych central*. Retrieved July 1, 2014 From http://psycentral.com/lib/psychodynamic-therapy/0001 19.

Halberstam, J. (1998). *Female masculinity*. Durham: Duke University Press.

Hall, R. L., & Fine, M. (2005). The stories we tell: The lives and friendship of two older black lesbians. *Psychology of Women Quarterly, 29*, 177–187.

Harley, D. A., Stansbury, K., Nelson, M., & Espinosa, C. T. (2014). A profile of rural elderly African American lesbians: Meeting their needs. In H. F. O. Vakalahi, G. M. Simpson, & N. Giunta (Eds.), *The collective spirit of aging across cultures* (pp. 133–155). New York: Springer.

Hash, K. M., & Rogers, A. (2013). Clinical practice with older LGBT clients: Overcoming lifelong stigma through strength and resilience. *Clinical Social Work Journal, 41*(3), 249–257.

Heaphy, B. (2007). Sexualities, gender and ageing. *Current Sociology, 55*(2), 193–210.

Hooyman, N. R., & Kiyak, H. A. (2008). *Social gerontology: A multidisciplinary perspective* (8th ed.). Boston, MA: Pearson.

Huebner, D., & Davis, M. (2007). Perceived antigay discrimination and physical health outcomes. *Health Psychology, 26*, 627–634.

Hughes, A. K., Harold, R. D., & Boyer, J. (2011). Awareness of LGBT aging issues among aging services network providers. *Journal of Gerontological Social Work, 54*, 659–677.

Humphreys, N. A., & Quam, J. K. (1998). Middle-aged and old gay, lesbian, and bisexual adults. In G. A. Appleby & J. W. Anastas (Eds.), *Not just a passing phase: Social work with gay, lesbian, and bisexual people* (pp. 245–267). New York: Columbia University Press.

Irish Association of Social Workers. (2011). *Lesbian, gay and bisexual people: A guide to good practice for social workers*. Dublin: Health Service Executive.

Isaacs, G., & McKendricj, B. (1992). *Male homosexuality in South Africa: Identity formation, culture, and crisis*. Oxford University Press, USA.

Jablonski, R. A., Vance, D. E., & Beattie, E. (2013). The invisible elderly: Lesbian, gay, bisexual, and transgender older adults. *Journal of Gerontological Nursing, 39*(11), DOI: 10.3928/00989134-20130916-02.

Kimmel, D., Rose, T., & David, S. (Eds.). (2006). *Lesbian, gay, bisexual, and transgender aging: Research and clinical perspectives*. New York, NY: Columbia University Press.

Kinsey, A. C., Pomeroy, W. B., & Martin, C. E. (1948). *Sexual behavior in the human male*. Philadelphia: W. B. Saunders.

Kinsey, A. C., Pomeroy, W. B., Martin, C. E., & Gebhard, P. H. (1953). *Sexual behavior in the human female*. Philadelphia: W. B. Saunders.

Knight, B. (1996). *Psychotherapy with older adults* (2nd ed.). Thousand Oaks, CA: Sage.

Kohlberg, L. (1973). The claim to moral adequacy of a highest stage of moral judgment. *Journal of Philosophy, 70*(18), 630–646.

Lancet. (2011). Health of lesbian, gay, bisexual and transgender populations. *The Lancet, 377*, 1211.

Lawson-Ross, A. D. (2013, August). *Testing the theory of stigma competence with gay, lesbian and bisexual adults over age 60*. Dissertation, University of Akron, Akron, Ohio.

Lesser, J. G., & Pope, D. S. (2011). *Human behavior and the social environment: Theory and practice*. Upper Saddle River, NJ: Pearson.

Lev, A. I. (2004). *Transgender emergence: Therapeutic guidelines for working with gender-variant people and their families*. New York: Haworth Clinical Practice Press.

Levinson, D. J. (1978). *The seasons of a man's life*. New York: Knopf.

Levinson, D. J. (1996). *The seasons of a woman's life*. New York: Knopf.

Mabey, J. E. (2011). Counseling older adults in LGBT communities. *The professional Counselor: Research and Practice, 1*(1), 57–62.

Mattaini, M. A., & Meyer, C. H. (2002). The ecosystems perspective: Implications for practice. Retrieved July 1, 2014 from http://home.earthlink.net/~mattaini?Ecosystems.html.

Maybe, J. E. (2007). Spirituality and religion in the lives of gay men and lesbian women. In L. Badgett & J. Frank (Eds.), *Sexual orientation discrimination: An international perspective* (pp. 225–235). London: Routledge.

McCarn, S. R., & Fassinger, R. E. (1997). Revisioning sexual minority identity formation: A new model of lesbian identity and its implications for counseling and research. *The Counseling Psychologist, 24*(3), 508–534.

McLeod, S. (2007). Psychodynamic approach. *Simply Psychology*. Retrieved July 1, 2014 from http://www.simplypsychology.org/psychodynamic.html.

Mendes, P. P. (2008). Teaching community development to social work students: A critical reflection. *Community Development Journal, 44*(2), 248–262.

Meyer, I. H. (1995). Identity, stress, and resilience in lesbian, gay men, and bisexuals of color. *The Counseling Psychologist, 38*, 442–454.

Meyer, I. H. (2003). Prejudice, social stress, and mental health in lesbian, gay, and bisexual populations: Conceptual issues and research evidence. *Psychological Bulletin, 129*, 674–697.

Meyer, I. H. (2010). Identity, stress, and resilience in lesbians, gay men, and bisexuals of color. *The Counseling Psychologist, 38*, 442–454.

Minton, H. L., & McDonald, G. J. (1984). Homosexual identity formation as a developmental process. *Journal of Homosexuality, 8*(1), 47–60.

Morales, E. S. (1989). Ethnic minority families and minority gays and lesbians. *Journal of Homosexuality, 17*, 217–239.

Nutterbrock, L., Rosenblum, A., & Blumenstein, R. (2002). Transgender identity affirmation and mental health. *International Journal of Transgenderism, 6*(4), 237–256.

Mullaly, B. (2002). *Challenging oppression: A critical social work approach*. Canada: Oxford University Press.

Orel, N. A. (2004). Gay, lesbian, and bisexual elders. *Journal of Gerontological Social Work, 43*(2), 57–77.

Payne, M. (1997). *Modern social work theory*. Chicago, IL: Lyceum Books.

Piaget, J. (1932). *The moral judgment of the child*. London: Kegan, Paul, Trench. Trubner and Company.

Plummer, K. (1973). *Sexual stigma: An interactionist account*. Boston: Routledge & Kegan Paul.

Porter, M., Russell, C., & Sullivan, G. (2004). Gay, old, and poor: Service delivery to aging gay men in inner city Sydney, Australia. *Journal of Gay and Lesbian Social Services, 16*(2), 43–57.

Prochaska, J. O. (1979). *Sysyems of psychotherapy: A transtheoretical analysis.* Homewood, IL: Dorsey Press.

Prochaska, J. O., & DiClemente, C. C. (1986). *Toward a comprehensive model of change* (pp. 3–27). New York, NY: Springer.

Quam, J. K. (2004). Issues in gay, lesbian, bisexual, and transgender aging. In W. Swan (Ed.), *Handbook of gay, lesbian and transgender administration and policy* (pp. 137–156). New York: Marcel Dekker Inc.

Quandt, S. A., Mc Donald, J., Bell, R. A., & Arcury, T. A. (1999). Aging research in multiethnic rural communities: Gaining entree through communty involvement. *Journal of Cross-cultural Gerontology, 14*(2), 113–130.

Renn, K. A., & Bilodeau, B. (2005). Queer student leaders: A case study of identity development and lesbian, gay, bisexual, and transgender student involvement at a Midwestern research university. *Journal of Gay and Lesbian Issues in Education, 2*(4), 49–71.

Reynolds, A. I., & Pope, R. L. (1991). The complexities of diversity: Exploring multiple oppressions. *Journal of Counseling and Development, 70,* 174–180.

Rogers, C. (1951). *Client-centered therapy.* Boston: Houghton Mifflin.

Salazar, L. F., Stephenson, R. B., Sullivan, P. S., & Tarver, R. (2013). Development and validation of HIV-related dyadic measures for men who have sex with men. *Journal of Sex Research, 50*(2), 164–177.

Saleeby, D. (1996). *The strength perspective in social work practice.* Needham, MA: Allyn & Bacon.

Satterfield, J. M., & Crabb, R. (2010). Cognitive-behavioral therapy for depression in an older gay man: A clinical case study. *Cognitive and Behavioral Practice, 17*(1), 45–55.

Schneider, M. J. (2013). *Introduction to public health* (4th ed.). Burlington, VA: Jones & Barlett Learning.

Schope, R. D. (2005). Who's afraid of growing old? Gay and lesbian perception of aging. *Journal of Gerontological Social Work, 45*(4), 23–39.

Siegel, S., & Lowe, R., Jr. (1994). *Uncharted lives: Understanding the life passages of gay men.* New York: Dutton.

Storms, M. D. (1978). Sexual orientation and self-perception. In P. Pliner, K. R. Blanstein, I. M. Spigel, T. Alloway, & L. Krames (Eds.), *Perception of emotion in self and others: advances in the study of communication and affect* (Vol. 5, pp. 165–180). New York: Plenum.

Sue, D. W., & Sue, D. (2013). *Counseling the culturally diverse: Theory and practice* (6th ed.). Hoboken, NJ: John Wiley & Sons.

Sullivan, K. (2011). *The experience of senior housing for lesbian, gay, bisexual and transgender seniors: An exploratory study.* Portland, Oregon: Portland State University Press.

Szymanski, D. M., & Gupta, A. (2009). Examining the relationship between multiple internalized oppressions and African American lesbian, gay, bisexual, and questioning persons' self-esteem and psychological distress. *Journal of Counseling Psychology, 56*(1), 110–118.

Tan, A. (2009). *Community development theory and practice: Bridging the divide between 'micro' and 'macro' levels of social work.* Paper presented at the North American Association of Christian in Social Work. Indianapolis Indiana. Retrieved June 10, 2014 from www.nacsw.org/Publications/Proceedings2009/TanACommunity.pdf.

Troiden, R. (1988). *Gay and lesbian identity: A sociological analysis.* Dix Hills, NY: General Hall.

Vaughan, M., & Waehler, C. (2010). Coming out growth: Conceptualizing and measuring stress-related growth associated with coming out to others as a sexual minority. *Journal of Adult Development, 17,* 94–109.

Wilchins, R. A. (2002). Queerer bodies. In J. Nestle, C. Howell, & R. A. Wilchins (Eds.), *Genderqueer: Voices from beyond the sexual binary.* Alyson: Los Angeles.

Pamela B. Teaster, John T. White and Sujee Kim

Abstract

There are estimated to be between 1.4 and 3.8 million LGBT Americans over the age of 65. This population is expected to increase between 3.6 and 7.2 million due to the Baby Boom generation. The older adult population is the most rapidly growing age group in the United States and experiences normal age-related changes in cognition as well as in internal and external physical health. Although differences exist within and among groups, more minority elders live in more poverty and with lower incomes than their white counterparts. Emerging scholarship reveals that social isolation and discrimination experienced by many LGBT elders hinder them from aging well. Increasing diversity of the LGBT elder population has important implications for bolstering individual autonomy in the care environments.

Keywords

LGBT · Demographic characteristics · Theories of aging · Population

Overview

Older adults as a population are living longer than ever before in history. Because of this phenomenon, one relatively recent in history, our understanding of the population of older adults is becoming more nuanced as the once and parochially assumed homogeneity of older adults is disentangled to reveal a landscape that is increasingly heterogeneous. Scholars are increasingly examining the heterogeneity of the older adult population that identifies as LGBT. To that end,

P.B. Teaster (✉) · S. Kim
Virginia Tech, Blacksburg, VA, USA
e-mail: pteaster@vt.edu

S. Kim
e-mail: sujee@vt.edu

P.B. Teaster · J.T. White
Virginia Commonwealth University, Richmond, USA
e-mail: whitejt2@vcu.edu

© Springer International Publishing Switzerland 2016
D.A. Harley and P.B. Teaster (eds.), *Handbook of LGBT Elders*,
DOI 10.1007/978-3-319-03623-6_2

this chapter delineates an understanding of LGBT elders by providing information on a general aging population as well as on those elders who identify as being in a minority status, particularly those with a sexual minority status. We consider basic age-related changes as well as what they may mean for elders who are LGBT, and we consider current trends and future issues (e.g., health disparities and person-centered care).

Learning Objectives

By the end of the chapter, the reader should be able to:

1. Identify basic terms, including sexual orientation and gender identity, LGBT, unisex, queer, questioning, ally, sex, gender role, and gender expressing.
2. Understand relevant characteristics of African-American, Hispanic, and Asian elders.
3. Identify age-related changes.
4. Explain the nexus between aging and LGBT older adults.
5. Describe basic theories of aging salient for LGBT older adults.

Introduction

That older adults are living to longer ages are now culturally and historically accepted, but thinking beyond the fact that older adults comprise approximately a fifth of the US population still seem enigmatic to many. Though many policies and services dating back from the 1960s have evolved to reflect a more nuanced view of the population of adults who are age 65 and over, others have lagged behind, still regarding older adults as a homogenous group. In fact, nothing could be further from the truth. Our understanding of the current population of older adults tends to reveal great differences in race and ethnicity, which is further revealed in sexual orientation and gender identify, education, income, and physical and mental health measures. The population of elders who identify as lesbian, gay, bisexual, and transgender has come to the forefront as our understanding of the aging population becomes more nuanced than in previous generations and as individuals who are aging are coming out more than in previous generations. Legislative landmarks, such as the Defense of Marriage Act (DOMO 1996) and the ensuing state by state legislative and legal battles, heighten the overall awareness and need to understand both how individuals in the general population age as well as how those who are of sexual minority status age.

The purpose of this chapter is to help the reader understand the nexus of sexual minority status and aging. First, we provide definitions germane to those who identify as being members in the population with sexual minority status. Second, we characterize the population of elders, elders with a minority status, and the population of LGBT elders. Third, we explain age-related changes for the general population. Next, we discuss issues of aging for those in a sexual minority status. We explain theories of aging that are salient for the aging population and conclude with a discussion of future considerations for those who are aging and identify as LGBT.

Definitions

The nomenclature surrounding sexual orientation and gender identity, across the life span, is ever-expanding and increasingly complex. The decade between the Stonewall Riots in New York in 1969 and the Castro Riots in San Francisco in 1979 saw an emergence of the term "gay" to replace the largely derogatory term, "homosexual." Both terms served as an umbrella for "gay" men and women. At the same time, as gay women forged more public identities in conjunction with the second feminist movement for equal rights in the 1970s, the terms "gay and lesbian" emerged (Faderman 1991). The terms "bisexual" and "transgender" subsequently emerged also, as new and unique communities struggled for voice and identity from the macrostructural and overly inclusive "homosexual" umbrella.

Toward the latter part of the 1980s, the initials LGBT and GLBT evolved as inclusive of the lesbian, gay, bisexual, and transgender community in place of "gay" or "gay and lesbian." It is, however, important to note that significant strains of resistance to the inclusivity were present and remain, particularly among bisexual and transgender communities (Alexander and Yescavage 2004). These strains of resistance continue as the LGBT initials expand to include queer, questioning, unisex, intersex, asexual, and ally.

To enjoy a comprehensive understanding of the totality of the sexual orientation and gender identity umbrella of terms requires a nuanced understanding when engaging in a true person-centered approach to care for elders. For the purposes of this and the following chapters, it is important to understand that sexual orientation (LGB) and gender identity (T) are unique. Sexual orientation refers to one's sexual or romantic attraction and, in the case of LGB, refers to a sexual or romantic attraction to members of the same gender. Gender identity refers to someone's innate, psychological (not necessarily physical) identification as male, female, or other gender (see definitions for LGBTQUIA in Fig. 2.1).

Describing the Population

According to the National Gay and Lesbian Task Force (2011), there are currently between 1.4 and 3.8 million LGBT Americans over the age of 65. By 2030, this number is expected to increase to between 3.6 and 7.2 million LGBT Americans, as the Baby Boom population, those born between 1946 and 1964, ages. Although there is no definitive measure to determine the percentage of LGBT individuals in the USA, national organizations such as the Human Rights Campaign and the National Gay and Lesbian Task Force use 3.5 % as a measure.

Certainly, numerous limitations impact the LGBT census, not the least of which are individuals who do not recognize and report their sexual orientation or gender identity. Further, there are those whom the LGBT umbrella does not cover, such as persons who identify as unisex, intersex, and asexual. In addition, the Human Rights Campaign believes that the data based on the 2010 US Census do not represent a comprehensive picture, as the Census only counts individuals from gay- and lesbian-identified households (Gendron et al. 2013). Much of the data on LGBT individuals are aggregated from national, urban studies, many of which do not include older adults; individuals from rural communities; and those who do not, or have not as yet, identified as LGBT. This representation is only one component, however, of those individuals who are considered to be older adults.

Understanding the Older Adult Population

The very description of an older adult calls into question at what age one becomes an older adult. Historians have long recognized that persons as young as age 40 could be characterized as old as late as the early 1900s; the Age Discrimination in Employment Act (1967) covered discrimination of employees aged 40 and over. What does seem to be clear is that most people think of themselves as being "younger than" another person rather than "older than." This statement illustrates that being older is somewhat subjective as well as dependent on the population under examination. For example, the age at which a farmer is considered old is 50 (Amshoff and Reed 2005), which is also the age that HIV/AIDS researchers place research participants in the older adult category (Goodroad 2003). Despite numerous subgroups within the population, many of whom age differently, the age at which recipients qualified for full Social Security benefits was set at age 65 in 1935. In the 1960s, the US government again de facto established old age as being 65 years old or the age when most persons qualify for Older Americans Act, Medicare, and Medicaid dollars and services. These rough age delineations do little to encapsulate what it means to be an older adult who is

Lesbian- A woman who is attracted physically, romantically, emotionally and/or spiritually to other women.

Gay- Commonly used to describe a man who is attracted physically, romantically, emotionally and/or spiritually to other men. Some women prefer the term "gay" over "lesbian." Gay can also be an umbrella term for many people who identify within the LGBTQUIA realm.

Bisexual- A person who is attracted sexually and emotionally to members of both sexes. (Assumes a binary understanding of gender)

Transgender- A person whose gender identity and/or gender expression differs from the sex they were assigned at birth. A person who feels that the binary gender system (male/female) is an incomplete description of who they are. An umbrella term for people whose anatomies and/or appearance do not conform to predominant gender roles.

Unisex: a term referring to individuals who ascribe to both a male and female gender or have an outward expression of both the male and female gender.

Queer- A blanket term that some LGBTQUIA individuals use to describe themselves. It is preferred by some because it is inclusive of the entire LGBTQUIA community. Most often used as a self-identification by an LGBTQIA individual.

Questioning- A person who is in the process of determining sexual orientation or gender identity.
Intersex- A term to describe a person whose biological sex is ambiguous. There are many genetic, hormonal, and/or anatomical variations which cause someone to be intersex. The term intersex is preferred to "hermaphrodite," which is now considered a derogatory term.
Asexual- A person who does not experience sexual attraction towards anyone. Asexual individuals view their asexuality in different ways and are extremely diverse.

Ally- A member of the majority/dominant group who works to support and advocate for the LGBTQUIA population.

SEX, GENDER ROLE, GENDER IDENTITY, GENDER EXPRESSION:

Sex- Classification of a person as male or female, assigned at birth based on external genitalia. Most often sex is based on chromosomes that an individual is born with. Please notice that sex and gender are not interchangeable terms.

Gender Role- Set of roles and behaviors assigned to females and males by society.
Gender Identity- An individual's internal, personal sense of their gender.

Gender Expression- Refers to the ways in which people externally communicate their gender identity to others through behavior, clothing, haircut, voice, and emphasizing, de-emphasizing, or changing their bodies' characteristics.

Fig. 2.1 LGBTQUIA alphabet soup (adapted from St. Mary's College Intercultural Lounge)

not a member of the majority group of older adults (at this point, Caucasian), the face of which is rapidly changing (see, especially, Chaps. 6–10). The focus of this chapter is to consider older persons with a minority status, and in many cases, more than one.

In order to understand what it means to be a person in a minority status as well as a person in a sexual minority status, we characterize the older adult population and older adult LGBT population and then present a brief discussion of normal age-related changes that many, but not all persons experience. The population of older adults represents the most rapidly growing age group in the US. For example, in 1990, older adults composed 13 % of the total population. By 2020, that number is estimated to increase to 18 % and to 25 % in 2050 (McKinney and Young 1985). In 2012, persons aged 65+ numbered 43.1 million, for an increase of 21 % since 2002, a number is projected to grow to 79.7 million by 2040. Moreover, the 85+ population, the most rapidly growing age cohort, is projected to increase from 5.9 million in 2012 to 14.1 million in 2040.

Consequently, approximately one in every seven persons in the USA is an older adult: people aged 65+ represented 12.4 % of the population in the year 2000, a percentage projected to increase to 19 % by 2030 (West et al. 2014).

Persons who reach age 65 are projected to have an average life expectancy of an additional 19.2 years (20.4 years for females and 17.8 years for males). Because of their ability to live to longer, older women outnumber older men (24.3 to 18.8 million). Another reflection of that phenomenon is that in 2013, 36 % of older women were widows (Administration on Aging 2010). Also, older men are married far more frequently than are older women (i.e., 71 % of men vs. 45 % of women). About 28 % (12.1 million) of older persons live alone (8.4 million women and 3.7 million men); 45 % of women age 75+ live alone. In 2012, approximately 518,000 grandparents aged 65 or older assumed primary responsibility for their grandchildren who were living with them. In 2012, the median income of older persons was $27,612 for males and $16,040 for females, approximately 9.1 % of those persons were living below the poverty level (Administration on Aging 2010).

Within the older adult population are older adults who are LGBT. Mentioned in Chap. 1 and throughout this book, no accurate percentages of LGBT people in the US exist; however, most researchers estimate that approximately 3–7 % of the aging population are LGBT, most of whom identify as lesbians and gay men. Thus, between one and 3.5 million older lesbians and gay men, this number is expected to double by 2030 (Jackson et al. 2009). Individuals who are aging, those who are heterosexual and those who are LGBT, can expect to experience some age-related changes, typically starting around the fourth decade.

Age-Related Changes that May Affect Older Adults

Cognitive Changes. Changes in our understanding of the aging brain are among the most exciting in all of aging science. Though many

adults worry about becoming more forgetful and worry that it is the first sign of Alzheimer's Disease (AD), according to NIH Medline Plus (2007), scientists now know that people can remain both alert and able as they age, although it may take them longer to process their memories. The cognitive functions that aging affects most are attention and memory, which are not simultaneously affected—some aspects are relatively unaffected, while others may decline precipitously. Though the results of studies of psychometric testing of persons of older ages seem to paint a picture of overall cognitive decline, enormous variability exists across aging individuals. Many older people out-perform young people, at least on some cognitive tasks, and others of the same age do at least as well as their younger counterparts (Glisky 2007).

Internal Age-Related Changes. Internal changes occur as adults age. Although many changes occur gradually across an individual's lifetime, the rate is dependent on heredity as well as environment (Rowe and Kahn 1998). Many changes are inter-related; however, the body has a remarkable variety of compensatory abilities that adjust to insults experienced over time. Stressed in previous sections, high variability exists as to when these age-related changes present.

Heart. Age-related changes in heart muscle cells help explain alterations in the heart as a whole. As the heart ages, it thickens, becomes less elastic, and may become enlarged. An older heart is less able to relax completely between beats, and its pumping chambers stiffen. Because the heart is unable to pump as vigorously as it once did, it is less able to supply adequate blood and oxygen to muscles during exercise (Young 2002).

Lungs. Age-related changes to the pulmonary system are associated with structural changes leading to a decline in function. The reduction in the diameter of small airways and their tendency for closing early contributes to air trapping and ventilation problems. With age, the lungs stiffen, making it harder for them expand and contract. The chest wall becomes more rigid, and the diaphragm and other muscles of respiration become weaker. A decreased cough reflex and a reduction in the number of cilia that sweep mucous up and out of the lungs results in increased likelihood of infection (Medline Plus 2010).

External Physical Changes

Generally accepted physical changes that occur as persons age include a reduction in physical height, usually more pronounced in women than in men (Currey et al. 1996), a decline in total body weight due to a loss of lean body mass, a decrease in bone strength, wrinkling and dryer skin (often exacerbated by exposure to UV rays), and changes in hair color. As with the above, physical changes that older adults experience are subject to great variability. One of the most significant factors thought to slow such changes is physical activity, which is now recommended for in all ages, and in sharp contrast to the prevailing wisdom of the early 1900s, when elder adults were encouraged to rest frequently and preserve their (remaining) strength (Buchner 1997; Roig et al. 2010). Below, we discuss a few examples of common age-related sensory changes.

Sensory Changes. Starting roughly around the fourth decade, eyesight weakens; around the sixth decade, cataracts and macular degeneration may develop for some individuals. Hearing may also decline with age. Mentioned earlier, variability exists within the population of older adults.

Eyesight. Around age 40, most individuals encounter weakened eyesight, and some experience cataracts and glaucoma. Certain adults may be less able to see objects at close distances or read fine print than in earlier years. For most, reading glasses or contact lens address the problem. Other adults are less able to see objects at far distances, and eyeglasses or contact lenses are helpful. Some individuals develop cataracts, which affects nearly 22 million Americans age 40 and older; by age 80, more than half of all Americans have cataracts (National Eye Institute 2008). Corrective surgery is now one of the most common surgeries done in the US. Annual eye examinations can help older adults protect themselves from developing severe eye problems that may occur for some, but not all older adults. Preventive measures (e.g., proper nutrition, wearing sunglasses, and physical activity) can help mollify eye problems that some older adults experience.

Hearing. About one-third of Americans between the ages of 65 and 74 have age-related hearing problems, and about half of adults aged 85 and older have hearing loss (National Institute on Deafness and Other Communication Disorders 2010). Another common problem that some older adults encounter is ringing, roaring, or other noises inside the ears. This problem, known as tinnitus, may be diminished when certain medicines or other health problems (e.g., allergies or atherosclerosis) are addressed.

The central message about age-related changes is that variability exists among older adults. Some adults experience age-related changes so small as to be barely noticeable. Others, however, experience such difficulties that their health and quality of life are greatly diminished. Although some age-related changes do occur over time, there are many opportunities and strategies to mitigate their affects.

Aging and Minority Status

Along with the general trends for America's aging population and the age-related changes described earlier, many minority populations are living to older ages. In this section, we characterize the population of older adults living in a minority status. Below, we focus on older African-Americans, Hispanics, and Asians.

African-American Elders

In 2008, the African-American older population was 3.2 million in 2008 and is projected to grow to over 9.9 million by 2050, when African American elders will compose 11 % of the older population. In 2008, 50 % of black elderly people lived in eight states: New York (9.1 %), Florida (7.1 %), California (6.5 %), Texas

(6.4 %), Georgia (6.1 %), North Carolina (5.5 %), Illinois (5.4 %), and Virginia (4.4 %). In 2008, over 60 % of the black population aged 65 and older had completed high school, as compared with 1970, when only 9 % did so. Also in 2008, over 12 % of black older persons had a bachelor's degree or higher. In 2008, 54 % of older Black men lived with their spouses, 11 % lived with other relatives, 4 % lived with non-relatives, and 30 % lived alone (Fig. 2.2).

For older black women, 25 % lived with their spouses, 32 % lived with other relatives, 2 % lived with non-relatives, and 42 % lived alone. Households containing families headed by black persons aged 65+ reported a median income in 2008 of $35,025. The comparable figure for all older households was $44,188. The median personal income for black men was $19,161 and $12,499 for black women. Comparable figures for all elderly were $25,503 for men and $14,559 for women. The poverty rate in 2008 for black elders (65 and older) was 20 %, or more than twice the rate for all older adults (9.7 %). In 2007, black males had an average life expectancy at age 65 of an additional 15.3 years (to 80.3 years) and black women had a life expectancy of 18.7 additional years (to 83.7 years). These figures are 1.3 years less than the figures for all elderly men and 1.1 years less than the figure for all elderly women. (Administration for Community Living 2010) (see Chap. 7 for a discussion of African-American and LGBT elders).

Hispanic Elders

Making up 6.6 % of older adult, the Hispanic older population numbered 2.5 million in 2007 and is projected to grow to over 17 million by 2050, when they will compose 19.8 % of the older population. By 2019, Hispanic adults aged 65 and older will be the largest racial/ethnic minority in this age group. In 2007, 70 % of Hispanic persons aged 65 and over resided in four states: California (27 %), Texas (19 %), Florida (16 %), and New York (9 %). In 2007, about 42 percent of the Hispanic population aged 65 and older had finished high school, compared with 76 % of the total older population (Administration for Community Living 2010) (Fig. 2.3).

In 2007, 65 % of Hispanic older men lived with their spouses, 17 % lived with other relatives, 3 % lived with non-relatives, and 15 % lived alone. For older Hispanic older women, 39 % lived with their spouses, 33 % lived with other relatives, 2 % lived with non-relatives, and 26 % lived alone. The percent of Hispanic elderly men and women living alone is lower than that of the general population. Also, the percent of Hispanic older persons living with other relatives is nearly twice that of the total older population (Administration for Community Living 2010).

Households containing families headed by Hispanic persons 65+ reported a median income in 2007 of $31,544 (as compared to $43,654 for non-Hispanic Whites). Among such Hispanic

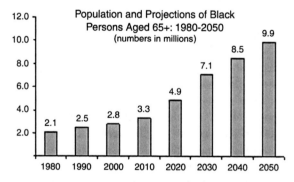

Fig. 2.2 Population and projections for black elders. *Source* Administration for Community Living (2010). A statistical profile of black older Americans aged 65+. Retrieved from http://www.aoa.acl.gov/Aging_Statistics/minority_aging/Facts-on-Black-Elderly-plain_format.aspx

Population and Projections of Hispanic
Persons Aged 65+ -- 1980-2050
(numbers in millions)

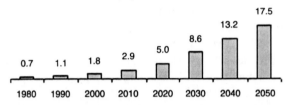

Fig. 2.3 Population and projections for Hispanic elders. *Source* Administration for Community Living (2010). A statistical profile of Hispanic older Americans aged 65+.

Retrieved from http://www.aoa.acl.gov/Aging_Statistics/minority_aging/Facts-on-Hispanic-Elderly.aspx

households, 16 % had an income of less than $15,000 (compared to 5.4 % for non-Hispanic Whites family households) and 45 % had incomes of $35,000 or more (compared to 62 % for non-Hispanic Whites). The poverty rate in 2007 for Hispanic older persons (65 and older) was 17.1 %. This was more than twice the percent for non-Hispanic Whites (7.4 %) (Administration for Community Living 2010) (see Chap. 10 for a discussion of Hispanic and LGBT elders).

Asian Elders

Older members of the older adult population who identified as Asian, Hawaiian, and Pacific Islander numbered over 1.3 million in 2008 (3.4 % of the older population) and is projected to grow to over 7.6 million by 2050, at that time accounting for 8.6 % of the older population. In 2008, almost 60 % of Asian, Hawaiian, and Pacific Island elders lived in just three states: California (40.5 %), Hawaii (9.6 %), and New York (9.2 %). In 2008, 74 % of the older Asian population aged 65 and older had finished high school. Also in 2008, almost 32 % of Asian older persons had a bachelor's degree or higher. The percent of high school graduates among older Asians is almost as high as the percent among all older persons (77 %). However, the percent of older Asians in 2008 who had a bachelor's degree or higher (32 %) was over 50 % higher than for the overall older population. Furthermore, the percent of male Asians who had a

bachelor's degree or higher (40 %) is almost 50 % higher than for the overall older population (27 %) (Administration for Community Living 2010) (Fig. 2.4).

In 2008, 84 % of older Asian men lived with their spouses, 6 % lived with other relatives, 2 % lived with non-relatives, and 8 % lived alone. For older Asian women, 47 % lived with their spouses, 30 % lived with other relatives, 3 % lived with non-relatives, and 20 % lived alone. Households containing families headed by Asian persons aged 65+ reported a median income in 2008 of $48,859. The comparable figure for all older households was $44,188. The median personal income for Asian men was $18,518 and $11,501 for Asian women. The comparable figures for all elderly were $25,503 for men and $14,559 for women. In 2008, the poverty rate in for Asian elders was 12.1 %; the rate for all elders was 9.7 %. The rate for Asian men was 11.1 %, and the rate for Asian women was 12.8 % (Administration for Community Living 2010) (see Chap. 8 for a discussion of Hispanic and LGBT elders).

The data above posted by the Administration for Community Living and distilled from the information reflected by the US Census indicate that there are both differences and similarities between and among older adults with a minority status and those who are Caucasian. In the main, minority status for elders means that they live in greater poverty and with lower incomes that do those with majority status. For older Asian-Americans, the educational level attained

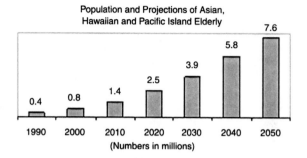

Fig. 2.4 Population and projections for Asian, Hawaiian, and Pacific Island elders. *Source* Administration for Community Living (2010). A statistical profile of Asian older Americans aged 65+. Retrieved from http://www.aoa.acl.gov/Aging_Statistics/minority_aging/Facts-on-API-Elderly2008-plain_format.aspx

is actually higher than that of the general population. All older adults of minority status live with their spouses more so than those of the general population. Also, the older adult population as a whole, whether or not they are members of minority groups, are living longer than were previous generations, a trend continuing until at least 2050. Statistics are but one way to understand what it is like to be a member of a minority population. Another are stressors, affecting both physical and mental health—much has been written on early and persistent stressors over the life course and will not be discussed here. However, one important stressor that will be discussed below are implications for being a member of a minority status and a member of a sexual minority.

Aging and Sexual Minority Status

In recent years, new scholarship has emerged on the barriers to positive aging faced by members of the LGBT population (e.g., Fredriksen-Goldsen et al. 2011). It has taken decades for this information to "come out" simply because it has been difficult to acquire data from this largely unseen and fragmented population. In a 2010 study, the National Resource Center on LGBT Aging reported that there are approximately 1.5 million lesbian, gay, bisexual, and transgender elders currently residing in the USA. Given the increase in the number of Baby Boomers, those born between 1946 and 1964, this number is expected

to increase to approximately 3.5 million by 2030. Among these elders, social isolation has been identified as affecting a disproportionate numbers as they continue to deal with stigma, discrimination ageism, homophobia, and transphobia (see Table 2.1).

LGBT Optimal Aging: Barriers and Opportunities

Older reports and other supporting data indicate rates of smoking, alcohol use, and obesity higher for the LGBT population than their heterosexual peers (Hughes and Evans 2003). Also, older data tend to support other antiquated stereotypes of the LGBT population: immersed in a culture of alcoholism, depression, and poor health habits. Examples of real evidence-based qualitative and quantitative studies on LGBT elders began to emerge in the 1990s and 2000s when membership from national organizations including the Human Rights Campaign, National Gay and Lesbian Task Force, and Services and Advocacy for GLBT Elders (SAGE) were queried. Although an improvement, the data were collected from members of the LGBT population who are active, enfranchised, engaged, and more likely to participate in "out and proud" organizations. Many of the previous studies lack statistical power due to small sample size and a high potential for participant bias. Therefore, it is unwise to unilaterally rely on research that is still emerging and calibrating. Although excellent,

Table 2.1 Support systems of LGBT elders and the general elderly population

Support system	LGBT elders (%)	General elder population (%)
Live alone	75	33
No children	90	20
Single	80	40

(Adapted from the Web site of services & advocacy for GLBT elders on social isolation. Retrieved from http://www.sageusa.org/issues/isolation.cfm)

rich, and statistically significant studies have recently been completed (Fredriksen-Goldsen et al. 2011), further research that supports a person-centered model of care and inquiry is needed.

Emerging scholarship tells us that elders who are isolated are at increased risk for abuse and premature death (Acierno et al. 2010; Pantell et al. 2013). Compounding this, according to SAGE, LGBT elders are at increased risk for isolation: LGBT elders are over twice as likely to live alone with thinner support networks, three to four times less likely to have children, and twice as likely to be single as compared to the heterosexual population. LGBT elders have higher disability rates, struggle with economic insecurity, and have increased mental health concerns manifest from a lifetime of discrimination (SAGE 2010).

The Caring and Aging with Pride Study (2011) gives additional information on why the barriers to inclusion and "othering" of LGBT elders are so real and profound. The study found that 82 % reported having been victimized at least once, with 64 % reporting experiencing victimization at least three times in their lives. The report notes: "The most common type of victimization is verbal insults (68 %), followed by threats of physical violence (43 %), and being hassled by the police (27 %). Nearly one in four (23 %) have had an object thrown at them, and one-fifth (20 %) have had their property damaged or destroyed. Nearly one in five (19 %) have been physically assaulted (i.e., punched, kicked, or beaten), 14 % threatened with a weapon, and 11 % have been sexually assaulted."

This discrimination continues into later life. According to a 2005 study of LGBT long-term care residents, LGBT elders fear discrimination from administration, direct care professionals, and other residents (Johnson et al. 2005). These responses varied widely with regard to the variables of age, income, gender, community size, and education level of the respondents but are concurrent with the notion, even among healthcare professionals and, arguably, younger members of the LGBT community, that LGBT elders are "homogeneous, isolated, lonely and without hope." (Johnson et al. p. 86).

According to the National Gay and Lesbian Task Force, the fear of isolation is real among LGBT elders. For many elders who have experienced marginalization and disenfranchisement over the life span, with advancing age comes an increasing reliance on public programs and social services. LGBT elders have less independence or ability to retreat from discrimination, consequently reinforcing isolative behaviors and leading to the negative health outcomes outlined above.

Further, as of this writing, housing discrimination based on sexual orientation and gender identity is prohibited in only 15 states and the District of Columbia: California, Colorado, Connecticut, the District of Columbia, Illinois, Iowa, Hawaii, Maine, Minnesota, New Jersey, Nevada, New Mexico, Oregon, Rhode Island, Vermont, and Washington. There are also six states that prohibit housing discrimination based on sexual orientation (but not gender identity): Delaware, Maryland, Massachusetts, New Hampshire, New York, and Wisconsin. In addition, many cities prohibit discrimination on the basis of sexual orientation, including Atlanta, Chicago, Detroit, Miami, New York, Pittsburgh, and Seattle. While the status of the LGBT population is changing, anti-discrimination is by no means universal.

When reviewed in its sum, there are few "usual and normal" phenomenon facing LGBT elders. Social isolation is a common occurance. Fear of healthcare professionals is a theme that is worthy of note. The lack of family caregivers is also a barrier for positive aging. But when evaluating sexual orientation, gender identity, and aging, there is much more to the story. While discrimination and fear are pervasive in these communities, there are examples of positive aging. In particular, studies by Frederiksen-Golden et al. (2011) and others are revealing the emergence of stronger scaffolding, with stories of resilience in the face of adversity (see Table 2.2).

Theories of Aging as Applied to LGBT Elders

Data discussed above demonstrate that diversity among elders is on the rise from racial, ethnic, sexual orientation, and gender identity perspectives. This is not only true from basic demographic data, but it is also true from gerontological theories that have applicability for the older adult LGBT population.

The Continuity Theory of Aging (Atchley 1989) suggests that, in making adaptive choices, middle-aged and older adults attempt to preserve and maintain existing internal and external structures. They prefer to accomplish this objective by using strategies tied to past experiences of themselves and their social world. Change is linked to the perceived past, producing continuity in inner psychological characteristics as well as in social behavior and in social circumstances. Continuity is thus a grand adaptive strategy that is promoted by both individual preference and social approval. In other words, what makes elders unique earlier in life will only be enhanced in later life, particularly true for LGBT elders?

Another salient theory for aging persons who are LGBT and that draws upon Continuity Theory is Carstensen et al. (2003) Socioemotional Selectivity Theory, which suggests that, with age and the realization of mortality, individuals focus on more personally relevant and meaningful pursuits and passions. As persons age, items that comprise individuality and uniqueness become more pronounced with age. As individuals age, regardless of race, ethnicity, and sexual orientation of gender identity, they tend to focus their attention on a more refined series of activities, experiences, emotions, and memories. Increasing the focus on "things" that make us unique that supports the inherent diversity of the aging population.

Though most research on LGBT elders examines those in community settings, the increasing diversity of the aging population also has profound implications for the long-term care continuum (Fig. 2.5).

One challenge is that the long-term care continuum, from independent living through skilled nursing facilities, has been developed in a medical model. The medical model suggests a top-down approach to direct care that supports uniformity and lack of participation in medical treatment, a model better suited to the generalizations alluded to in the previous section. The medical model ascribes to the philosophy that the dispensation of medication, the creation of

Table 2.2 Risks for elders lacking adequate social interaction

- Older people without adequate social interaction are twice as likely to die prematurely
- This increased risk of mortality is comparable to smoking **15** cigarettes per day, **6** alcoholic beverages per day, and it is twice as dangerous as obesity
- 43 % of elders experience social isolation
- 11.3 million elders live alone (8.1 million are women)
- Based on current demographic trends, 16 million elders will live alone by 2020
- Older adults without adequate social interaction are twice as likely to die prematurely

activities, the development of menus, and, really, the physical structure of the long-term care environment can be created on an assembly line.

Person-centered care is a holistic approach to care that recognizes and empowers the uniqueness of each individual. It supports individual autonomy throughout the long-term care continuum while creating environments conducive to independence, engagement, social confidence, respect, and diversity. (Barsness and White 2011). Scholars, educators, and employees who work in the long-term care continuum are seeing a culture-change movement that supports the redirection of care to a person-centered model. This approach is extremely important for members of the LGBT community because it creates an environment where apathy and even discrimination is unacceptable and where uniqueness is actually embraced.

The person-centered care movement to inform culture change in long-term care is by no means fully accepted by owners of long-term care communities, administrators, direct care professionals and regulators or inspectors. Efforts by organizations such as the Pioneer Network and initiatives such as the Eden Alternative (Thomas 1996) are far from universally acknowledged and integrated into regulations, organizational mission statements, care plans, and direct care practices. The push and pull of profitability versus person-centered care and culture change, to say the least of more historically conservative values and norms, should be considered when evaluating the following chapters.

Summary

The letters LGBT represent an initialism that indicates lesbian, gay, bisexual, and transgender community. National Gay and Lesbian Task Force (2011) reported that there are currently between 1.4 and 3.8 million LGBT Americans over the age of 65, and this population is expected to increase to between 3.6 and 7.2 million due to the Baby Boom generation.

We have discussed the characteristics of the older adult population in order to aid readers' understanding of elders with a sexual minority status. The older adult population is the most rapidly growing age group in the USA with

Graphic: Barriers to Health Care Access

According to the US Department of Health and Human Services, LGBT Adults are:

+ Less likely to have health insurance coverage

+ More likely to delay or not seek medical care

+ Facing barriers to access as older adults due to isolation and a **lack of culturally competent providers. One study found 13% of older LGBT adults were denied or provided inferior health care.**

+ More likely to **delay** or not get needed **prescription medications**

+ More likely to receive health care services in **emergency rooms**

+ Fail to receive screenings, diagnoses and treatment for important medical problems. 22% of LGBT older adults do not reveal sexual orientation to physicians. In some states health care providers can decline to treat or provide certain necessary treatments to individuals based on their sexual orientation or gender identity.

+ Particularly distressed in nursing homes. One study indicates elderly LGBT adults face distress from potentially **hostile staff and fellow residents**, denial of visits from partners and family of choice, and refusal to allow same-sex partners to room together

Fig. 2.5 Barriers to health care for LGBT elders. *Source* LGBT—health disparities impacting long-term care. Retrieved from http://longtermcare.gov/the-basics/lgbt/lgbt-health-disparities-impacting-ltc/

extended average life span. Older adults experience normal age-related changes in their cognition and internal and external physical health. Differences and similarities exist in the trends between elders in a minor racial/ethnic group, and those who are Caucasian, but, mainly, minority elders live in more poverty and with lower incomes.

Although scholarly attention to aging of LGBT elders is increasing, much research needs to be done to discover this largely isolated and fragmented population. Nevertheless, emerging scholarship has investigated how social isolation and discrimination experienced by LGBT elders hinder them from achieving positive aging (e.g., Caring and Aging with Pride Study 2011). Also, several gerontological theories have applicability for the LGBT elders including, the Continuity Theory of Aging (Atchley 1989) and the Socioemotional Selectivity Theory (Carstensen et al. 2003). Increasing diversity of the aging population, especially the LGBT elder population, has important implications for the continuum of long-term care, suggesting the necessity of bolstering individual autonomy in care environments.

Discussion Box 2.1: Barriers to Optimal Aging Encountered by LGBT Elders
Read the article below, "*LGBT Advocate Sees Hurdles Ahead,*" written by Michael Adams, Retrieved from the Web site of AARP: http://www.aarp.org/relationships/family/info-04-2011/biggest-issues-facing-older-lgbt-americans.html.

"*America's older population is growing, and so is the number of lesbian, gay, bisexual and transgender (LGBT) adults who are moving into their later years. In the next several decades, LGBT adults age 65 and above is expected to double, reaching more than 3 million by 2030. In my job as executive director of SAGE (that's for Services & Advocacy for Gay, Lesbian, Bisexual and Transgender Elders). I'm constantly hearing about the unique challenges facing our community.*

These are the five main things we need to change if we want our society to be prepared for the full diversity of its aging population:

1. *Basic Health Care*
   In the United States, about 80 percent of long-term care for older people is provided by family members, such as and spouses, children and other relatives. But LGBT elders are only half as likely as their heterosexual counterparts to have close family to lean on for help. This means that they rely heavily on the services of professional health care providers—doctors, pharmacists, or hospital and nursing home staff— who might be uncomfortable with or even hostile toward LGBT elders and who are not trained to work with them. In SAGE's experience, even when these providers are supportive, fear of discrimination prevents many LGBT older people from seeking out the care they need.

2. *Caregiving Issues*
   Can you imagine not being able to care for a longtime partner or spouse, or have any say in your loved one's medical care? It's unthinkable for most of us. Because the support systems of LGBT elders—their partners and their families of choice—often are not recognized under the law, LGBT people frequently are not granted family or medical leave to take care of a sick or terminally ill partner. Furthermore, LGBT people can be excluded from decision-making on a partner's medical care and funeral plans, unless they have put specific legal arrangements in place. Unfortunately, many people don't make such arrangements, either because they can't afford the legal costs or because they, like so many Americans, think they can put them off for another day. (Here's a link to resources

that can help you get those documents prepared.)

3. *Financial Insecurity*

   LGBT older people are less financially secure than American elders as a whole. For example, poverty rates among elder lesbian and gay couples are 9.1 and 4.9 %, respectively, compared with 4.6 % among elder heterosexual couples. Several factors contribute to higher poverty rates, including employment discrimination and barriers in Social Security, Medicaid, and pension and retirement plans that deny same-sex couples key retirement benefits afforded to the broader population. In addition, state laws can shut LGBT partners out of an inheritance, or can require them to pay steep taxes on an estate that a surviving heterosexual spouse would inherit tax-free.

4. *Social Isolation*

   Despite creating families of choice and other support networks, many LGBT older people still experience high rates of social isolation. They are twice as likely to be single and to live alone, and three to four times as likely to be childless. They are also less likely to feel welcome in the places where many older people socialize, such as senior centers, volunteer centers and places of worship. Research and SAGE's experience show that the harmful effects of this include depression, delayed care-seeking, poor nutrition and premature mortality.

5. *Access to Aging Services*

   LGBT older people often do not access aging services out of fear of harassment or hostility. Few aging services providers plan for, or reach out to, the LGBT community—and few are prepared to address insensitivity or discrimination aimed at LGBT elders by staff or other older people.

Fortunately, such attitudes are changing. A recent survey of aging services providers shows that a growing number of respondents would welcome LGBT elders, but lack the proper training. Resources such as the federally funded National Resource Center on LGBT Aging have been created to provide training and tools to aging providers, LGBT organizations and LGBT older people themselves, ensuring that our community increasingly will be able to age with the dignity and respect we all deserve."

Discussion Questions:

1. What are the five unique challenges faced by LGBT community?
2. Do you agree that those five challenges are prevalent in our society? Give specific examples.
3. What challenge do you think most problematic as a barrier to optimal aging for LGBT elders?
4. Think about how LGBT elders and heterosexual elders differently experience and deal with aging.

Discussion Box 2.2: Age-related Physical Changes

Visit the link, Columbia University's *Brave Old World* Web site (http://news21.com/columbia/2011/2010/growing-old/index.html) and watch the four videos on age-related changes in vision, hearing, mobility, and thinking. After watching each video, answer the following questions.

1. Describe the changes you see taking place with aging.
2. When, approximately at what age, do you expect to undergo each of these changes? Why you chose that age?
3. What strategies and/ or information do you know to slow the rate of these changes? Give examples for each condition.

4. Think about how you manage your life once these age-related changes occur in your 60s or 70s?

Learning Exercises

Questions to Consider

1. What makes me a unique individual?
2. How will these qualities and interests be important to me as I age?
3. What scaffolding will I need to ensure for myself and my loved ones to support aging in a person-centered environment?

Experiential Learning

Visit www.gensilent.com and view the film trailer and review the following statistics in Fig. 2.4. What do you find most startling from this brief introduction to these cases? Why would any elder wait until near the end of life to reach out for assistance?

Resources

National Resource Center on LGBT Aging: See more at http://lgbtagingcenter.org/.

Services & Advocacy for Gay, Lesbian, Bisexual & Transgender Elders (SAGE): See more at http://www.sageusa.org/issues/general.cfm.

Caring and Aging with Pride: Learn more about aging and health needs of LGBT elders at www.caringandaging.org#sthash.qYHm9484. dpuf, http://www.centerforpositiveaging.org/lgbt.html#sthash.qYHm9484.dpuf.

LGBT Aging Resources Clearinghouse of the American Society on Aging (ASA): See more at http://www.centerforpositiveaging.org/lgbt. html#sthash.qYHm9484.dpuf.

Age-related physical changes at Meldline Plus' Web site http://www.nlm.nih.gov/medline plus/seniorshealth.html.

Frequently asked questions answered by the American Psychological Association at http://www.apa.org/pubinfo/answers.html.

LGBT Aging Project at http://www.lgbtagingproject.org/.

References

Acierno, R., Hernandez, M. A., Amstadter, A. B., Resnick, H. S., Steve, K. & Muzzy, W., et al. (2010). Prevalence and correlates of emotional, physical, sexual, and financial abuse and potential neglect in the United States: The national elder mistreatment study. *American Journal of Public Health, 100*(2), 292–297. doi:10.2105/ajph.2009.163089.

Administration for Community Living. (2010). Minority aging facts. Retrieved on February 20, 2015 at http://www.aoa.acl.gov/Aging_Statistics/minority_aging/Facts-on-API-Elderly2008-plain_format.aspx.

Alexander, J. & Yescavage, J. (2004). Introduction. In J. Alexander & J. Yescavage (Eds.), *InterSEXions of the others: Bisexuality and transgenderism.* Binghamton: Haworth Press.

Amshoff, S. K. & Reed, D. B. (2005). Health, work, and safety of farmers ages 50 and older. *Geriatric Nursing, 26*(5), 304–308.

Atchley, R. C. (1989). A continuity theory of normal aging. *The Gerontologist, 29*(2), 183–190.

Barsness, S. & White, J. (2011). *Aging in place: A hallmark of person-centered care.* Retrieved from www.alzpossible.com.

Buchner, D. M. (1997). Preserving mobility in older adults. *Western Journal of Medicine, 167*(4), 258–264.

Carstensen, L. L., Fung, H. H., & Charles, S. T. (2003). Socioemotional selectivity theory and the regulation of emotion in the second half of life. *Motivation and Emotion, 27*(2), 103–123.

Currey, J. D., Brear, K., & Zioupos, P. (1996). The effects of ageing and changes in mineral content in degrading the toughness of human femora. *Journal of Biomechanics, 29*, 257–260.

Faderman, L. (1991). *Odd girls and twilight lovers.* New York: Columbia University Press.

Fredriksen-Goldsen, K. I., Kim, H. J., Emlet, C. A., Muraco, A., Erosheva, E. A., Hoy-Ellis, C.P. et al. (2011). *The aging and health report: Disparities and resilience among lesbian, gay, bisexual, and transgender older adults.* Seattle: Institute for Multigenerational Health.

Gendron, T., Maddux, S., Krinsky, L., White, J., Lockeman, K., Metcalfe, Y., & Aggarwal, S. (2013). Cultural competence trainings for healthcare professionals working with LGBT older adults. *Educational Gerontology, 39*(6), 454–463.

Glisky, E. L. (2007). Changes in cognitive function in human aging. *Brain aging: Models, methods, and mechanisms*, 3–20.

Goodroad, B. K. (2003). HIV and AIDS in people older than 50: A continuing concern. *Journal of Gerontological Nursing, 29*(4), 18–24.

Grant, J., Mottet, L., Tanis, J., Harrison, J., Herman, J., & Keisling, M. (2011). Injustice at every turn: A report of the national transgender discrimination survey. Washington: National Center for Transgender Equality and National Gay and Lesbian Task Force.

Hughes, C. & Evans, A. (2003). Health needs of women who have sex with women. British Medical Journal, *327*(7421), 939–940.

Johnson, M., Jackson, N., Arnette, J., & Koffman, S. (2005). Gay and lesbian perceptions of discrimination in retirement care facilities. *Journal of Homosexuality, 49*(2), 83–102.

National Eye Institute. (2008). Vision problems in the U. S.: Prevalence of adult vision impairment and age-related eye disease in America. Retrieved February 20, 2015 at http://www.preventblindness.org/vpus/2008_update/VPUS_2008_update.pdf].

National Institute on Deafness and Other Communication Disorders. (2010, June 7). Hearing loss and older adults. Retrieved July 8, 2010, from http://www.nidcd.nih.gov/health/hearing/older.asp.

NIH Medline Plus (2007). Eight areas of age-related change. http://www.nlm.nih.gov/medlineplus/magazine/issues/winter07/articles/winter07pg10-13.html.

Medline Plus. (2010). Aging changes in the lungs. Retrieved May 10, 2012 from http://www.nlm.nih.gov/medlineplus/ency/article/004011.htm.

Pantell, M., Rehkopf, D., Jutte, D., Syme, S., Balmes, J., & Adler, N. (2013). Social Isolation: A predictor of mortality comparable to traditional clinical risk factors. *American Journal of Public Health, 103*(11), 2056–2062.

Roig, M., MacIntyre, D. L., Eng, J. J., Narici, M. V., Maganaris, C. N., & Reid, W. D. (2010). Preservation of eccentric strength in older adults: Evidence, mechanisms and implications for training and rehabilitation. *Experimental Gerontology, 45*(6), 400–409. doi:10.1016/j.exger.2010.03.008.

Rowe, J. W., & Kahn, R. L. (1998). *Successful aging.* New York: Pantheon Books.

Thomas, W. H. (1996). *Life worth living: How someone you love can still enjoy life in a nursing home: The Eden alternative in action.* Acton: VanderWyk & Burnham.

United States Administration on Aging. (2010). A toolkit for serving diverse communities. Washington, DC: Author. http://digitalcommons.ilr.cornell.edu/key_workplace/734.

West, L.A., Cole, S., Goodkind, D., & He, W. (2014). 65 + in the United States: Current population reports. Washington: U.S. Department of the Census.

Young, L. (2002). Heart disease in the elderly (Chap. 21). Retrieved 28 February from http://www.atrainceu.com/course-module/2438910-141_elders-and-their-care-module-03.

Family Relationships of Older LGBT Adults

3

Katherine R. Allen and Karen A. Roberto

Abstract

The study of older lesbian, gay, bisexual, and transgender (LGBT) adults and their families is a growing area of research and practice. This field addresses intersections of social structure and personal experience, beginning with the interaction of family and sexual minority status, and complicated by gender, race, social class, ability status, and other social locations. Older LGBT adults experience families in normative and non-normative ways. They have families of origin (i.e., the family one is born into), families of procreation (i.e., the family one creates, typically, through a committed union and the children they rear), and families of choice (i.e., the family one creates through converting friends into kin). Yet, there are unique aspects of what it means to be an aging LGBT individual that affect the emotional dynamics of family relationships, including the historical treatment of LGBT individuals, the increasing social climate of self-affirmation and public acceptance, and the policies that impact their lives.

Keywords

LGBT families · Family of origin · Family of procreation · Family of choice · Chosen kin

Overview

The purpose of this chapter is to examine the relationships that older lesbian, gay, bisexual, and transgender (LGBT) adults have with their families, including biological, legal, and chosen kin (e.g., families of choice). We address classic and current research on family relationships for

K.R. Allen (✉) · K.A. Roberto
Virginia Tech, Blacksburg, USA
e-mail: kallen@vt.edu

K.A. Roberto
e-mail: kroberto@vt.edu

© Springer International Publishing Switzerland 2016
D.A. Harley and P.B. Teaster (eds.), *Handbook of LGBT Elders*,
DOI 10.1007/978-3-319-03623-6_3

individuals who identify as lesbian, gay, bisexual, or transgender, as shifting social norms have challenged conventional definitions of families and have helped produce greater diversity across and within families (Bianchi 2014). We examine LGBT family dynamics, including reliance on families of choice and the use of formal services and networks to meet older adults' care needs. We incorporate research and practice from primarily modern Western societies in North America and Northern Europe (e.g., the USA, Canada, and United Kingdom), and where it exists, include what is currently known regarding other LGBT families in countries on other continents. We acknowledge that cultural differences influence the perceptions, behaviors, and interactions of family members; however, it is not feasible to include representation of all cultures in this chapter. Finally, we provide an assessment of directions for expanding the research on older LGBT family relationships and address the future of service delivery and public policies affecting this ever-increasing population.

Learning Objectives

After reading this chapter, the reader should be able to:

1. Identify the similarities and differences between the family relationships of older LGBT individuals and the family relationships of older heterosexual individuals.
2. Explain the distinctions among families of origin and families of choice in the LGBT community.
3. Understand the history of research and activism regarding LGBT aging individuals and their families.
4. Identify the major issues and future directions for research on older LGBT individuals and their families.
5. Explain the service models and intervention strategies that are effective in addressing the practical and policy issues for LGBT elders and their families.

6. Locate national and international resources for working with older LGBT individuals and their families.

Introduction

The study of older LGBT adults and their families is a growing area of research and practice. This field addresses numerous intersections of social structure and personal experience, beginning with the ways in which aging, sexual orientation, and family experience interact, and is further complicated by gender, race, ethnicity, social class, ability status, among many other social locations. Given the lack of comprehensive data collected on the experiences of LGBT individuals and families, it is difficult to estimate the precise number of LGBT aging individuals and even more difficult to estimate their distribution by family structure (e.g., LGBT-parent families; older couples; aging parent–adult child relationships). Estimates, however, do suggest that approximately one to four million Americans aged 65 and older identify as LGBT (see Cahill et al. 2000; NGLTF 2015; Orel 2014). With the aging of the population and the increasing visibility of LGBT individuals, these numbers will nearly double by 2030.

Turning to the family relationships of older LGBT adults, it is clear that older LGBT adults experience families in both normative and non-normative ways. Structurally, older LGBT adults are not unlike non-LGBT adults: they have families of origin (i.e., the family one is born into), families of procreation (i.e., the family one creates, typically, through a committed union and the children they rear), and families of choice (i.e., the family one also creates through converting friends into kin). At the same time, there are some unique aspects of what it means to be an aging LGBT individual; thus, the emotional dynamics of family relationships may also vary from normative expectations, and for a variety of reasons. These reasons are associated with all aspects of life, including the historical treatment of LGBT individuals, the increasing social climate of self-affirmation and public acceptance, and the policies that impact their lives.

Historical Perspectives on the Family Relationships of Older LGBT Adults

Research on sexual orientation and aging began to appear in the late 1970s and 1980s. As with many new areas of research in the study of LGBT individuals and families (Allen and Demo 1995), the original papers that appeared in scholarly journals and books were primarily personal narratives and included a call to acknowledge and accept the study of aging of LGBT families as a legitimate area of investigation (Cohler and Hostetler 2002; Cooper 1997; Kimmel 1978, 1992).

In part, the attempt by scholars to address sexual orientation and aging was spurred by the political activism that was initiated with the Stonewall Riot on Friday, June 27, 1969. The moment that sparked a new era of activism for civil and legal rights was the death of Judy Garland, a beloved icon for the gay community. In the wake of mourning, gay men who dressed in drag and other patrons rebelled against Manhattan police raids of the popular bar (The Stonewall Inn) in Greenwich Village (Allen 2005; D'Emilio and Freedman 1997; Editors of the Harvard Law Review 1990). The uprising was the lighting rod that led to the emergence of the Gay Liberation Front, an activist movement that challenged heteronormativity and sought self-affirmation for lesbian and gay men in private and public realms (Engel 2002). The gay liberation movement mirrored other social movements in privileging men, but lesbians, too, fought back against the oppression that both condemned them and outlawed their sexual behavior and social relationships (Faderman 1991).

This gay-affirmative social activism led to increasing visibility of lesbian and gay individuals, with reverberations throughout society.

For example, in 1973, the American Psychiatric Association reversed its stance on homosexuality as a mental illness, setting the stage for more openly identifiable research and theorizing about the experience of LGBT aging individuals, couples, and their families. Also in the activist realm, Senior Action in a Gay Environment (SAGE; now Services and Advocacy for Gay, Lesbian, Bisexual, and Transgender Elders) was founded in 1978 in New York City in order to create a support network for older gay individuals. This pioneering group, co-founded by gerontologist Douglas Kimmel, has evolved into one of the largest member-led organizations in both the LBGT community and the aging community (SAGE 2015).

Case Study: Douglas Kimmel

Douglas C. Kimmel is one of the pioneers in LGBT aging. His research on adulthood and aging, in general, and aging gay and lesbian couples and families, in particular, has broken new ground and inspired young and old scholars alike. In addition to his research and scholarship, Dr. Kimmel is one of the founders of SAGE: Services and Advocacy for GLBT Elders. He is a champion of all of the values described in this chapter: aging well, valuing family, and working for social justice.

Dr. Kimmel was born in Denver in 1943. He received his PhD in Clinical Psychology from the University of Chicago in 1970. For many years, he was a professor in the Department of Psychology, at City College of the City University of New York. He has also served as a visiting scholar in universities around the world, particularly in Japan. He has received many prestigious awards for his research and service, including several from the American Psychological Association: the Distinguished Elder Award, the Distinguished Service Award, and the Distinguished Educational Contribution Award.

Currently, Dr. Kimmel lives in Maine with his husband, Ronald W. Schwizer. They were legally married on August 19, 2013, in Hancock, Maine, on the 44th anniversary of their earlier wedding in 1969 in Boulder Colorado. Dr. Kimmel's Web site includes photographs and slide shows of their weddings and their life together over the years.

Website: www.tamarackplace.com/kimmel

Discussion Questions:

1. In what ways does Dr. Kimmel integrate his professional work, his family life, and his activist work on behalf of social justice for LGBT rights?
2. As you view Dr. Kimmel's web site, how does he reveal his passions for social activism on behalf of LGBT issues?

The emerging scholarship on older LGBT individuals and their families reflected this bridge from lived experience to research. In 1980, Monica Kehoe, a self-identified lifelong lesbian, conducted one of the first studies of older lesbians (Kehoe 1986). She surveyed 50 lesbians aged 65 and older in order to examine their personal and social concerns and well-being. Beginning with the premise that older lesbians have a "triple threat" to their well-being, due to their gender, age, and sexual orientation, she grounded her study in the observation that aging lesbians are an unknown, invisible, and mysterious minority, ignored by gerontologists, feminists, and sexologists who studied homosexuality. Part of the difficulty in studying older lesbians, she demonstrated, was that older lesbians at that time were deeply closeted. Nevertheless, Kehoe was able to find women willing to be interviewed. Most of her participants were never married, childless, retired professional women living in California, and were not partnered. Most of the women had a positive self-image and considered themselves survivors of a culture that denigrated them. Yet, they also reported concerns about loneliness and

the need for more companionship within the lesbian community. Ultimately, Kehoe concluded that they were probably well equipped to deal with the challenges and adjustments needed in old age, having dealt with and survived, discrimination and prejudice related to their gender, age, and sexual orientation.

At about the same time, Berger (1984), a professor of social work, published one of the first studies on gay aging as a minority within a minority. Berger conducted a qualitative study of 18 older gays and lesbians (age range 40–72, with a median age of 54), identifying the themes of (a) stereotypes, (b) coming out, (c) love and family, (d) intergenerational attitudes, (e) discrimination, and (f) growing older. His findings on love and family for this small sample presage the complexity that is now acknowledged among LGBT families as well as scholars. Although there was very little social acceptance and no legal recognition of gay partnerships when his study was conducted, Berger reported that in the gay community, individuals shared a home and a social and sexual life with a partner (typically identified by the term, lover) in order to meet their needs for intimacy and lifelong companionship. Yet, not all of his participants were coupled in a gay or lesbian relationship. Some individuals did not live with their partners, and in one case, a man stayed in a heterosexual marriage despite identifying as gay. Berger's research, as well as Kehoe's (1986) study, attempted to uncover the normative aspects of family life for older gays and lesbians, and to debunk stereotypes of deviance, loneliness, and lack of intimate ties.

Turning to the gerontology literature, Lipman (1984) wrote the first article on "homosexuals" in one of the premier aging handbooks. Over time, as public and scholarly recognition of this topic emerged, so did the titles and focus of the chapters dealing with LGBT issues in the major gerontology handbooks. Although the lives of older LGBT individuals and their families still are not likely to be the subject of entire chapters in these authoritative handbooks (for an exception, see Allen 2005), their experiences are increasingly integrated into chapters dealing with relationships and families (for example, see Blieszner and Bedford 2012; Brock and Jennings 2007).

Despite these publications in scholarly venues, the lack of integration of the research on aging families and sexual orientation is an ongoing concern. For example, in a review of research in the last decade (2000–2010) on aging families, sexual orientation was only mentioned as an area that lacks attention (Silverstein and Giarrusso 2010). Similarly, in a review of research about LGBT families, older LGBT adults and their family relationships were not mentioned (Biblarz and Savci 2010). Sullivan (2014) and Witten and Eyler (2012), as well, identifies the dearth of research on aging in the LGBT community. Yet, we also see a great deal of promise in the emerging literature that addressing aging, sexuality, and family (see Kimmel et al. 2006). Perhaps now, gerontologists, family scholars, and LGBT scholars are discovering the importance of investigating lived experience at these intersections.

Theory, Research, and Policy Related to LGBT Aging and Families

Family relationships are typically defined by a legal or biological tie, as in legal marriage, in-law relationships, biological parenthood, or adoptive and step parenthood. Family relationships can also be matters of choice. In situations where LGBT individuals have been rejected by biological family members, they have turned to LGBT community members and converted them to kin-like relationships. Indeed, as Maupin (2015), author of the iconic novels, *Tales of the City*, is credited as saying, friends are the "logical" (compared to the biological) family for LGBT people. Families incorporate both structural (i.e., household) units and emotional ties. Older LGBT individuals, particularly those who came out before a new wave of significant social change began in the 1990s, have had to be creative in their family ties, given legal and social

constraints. Now that same-sex marriage is legal in most of the USA as well as many other countries (e.g., Argentina, Canada, France, New Zealand, Norway, South Africa, and Spain) (HRC 2015), the research will uncover more trends and issues facing older LGBT couples and families. Next, we address theory, research, and policy linked to variations in aging LGBT family relationships, in terms of coming out and developing intergenerational, intragenerational, and chosen kin relationships.

Theoretical Perspectives

Most of the research on older LGBT families was spurred by the articulation of the life course perspective, which provides a model for understanding individual, family, and social historical processes and change over time (Allen et al. 2000; Bengtson and Allen 1993; Bengtson et al. 2005). There are several key concepts from the life course perspective that are particularly relevant to the study of LGBT aging individuals and their families. The concept of linked lives refers to the ways that individual lives are connected "across the generations by bonds of kinship" (Bengtson et al. 2005, p. 494). A second key concept refers to the major life transitions that individuals and families experience, as well as their timing in each person's life (Bengtson and Allen 1993). For example, the first time one comes out to family members is an event that signals a major life transition. From that point forward, an individual is no longer seen as heterosexual, or as fitting into a normative model of development. A third key concept refers to the historical time, place, and context in which individuals experience major social changes. For example, as we describe later in this chapter, the issue of "same-sex marriage" is likely experienced very differently for persons who are currently age 65, compared to adults who are currently age 25. Older LGBT individuals partnered and established their families at a time when same-sex marriage was legally and socially prohibited. This social historical reality is a likely contribution to so many older LGBT individuals first marrying heterosexually, particularly in order to become a parent. In contrast, young LGBT adults are much more free to come out as a sexual minority and to have the opportunity to legally marry their same-sex partner, as well as to establish their own LGBT-parent family (Tasker 2013).

In an application of the life course perspective, Fredriksen-Goldsen and Muraco (2010) reviewed 58 empirical articles published between 1984 and 2008 that focused on the lives of LGB adults aged 50 and older. They found that much of the research addressed two themes central to the life course perspective: (a) the interplay of lives and historical times and (b) linked and interdependent lives. Early studies on LGB aging focused on stereotypes about the mental health status of these populations. Contrary to popular belief that older gay men and lesbians were depressed, felt sexually undesirable, and struggled with the normative aging process, the majority of the early articles describe positive psychosocial functioning among older gay men and lesbians (Berger 1984; Berger and Kelly 1986; Gray and Dressel 1985), with favorable feelings about aging (Whitford 1997), appearance (Gray and Dressel 1985), and sexuality (Pope and Schulz 1990). In fact, studies showed that older gay and lesbian adults typically rated their mental health as good or excellent (D'Augelli et al. 2001) and reported no more depressive symptoms than their heterosexual counterparts (Dorfman et al. 1995). With respect to social relationships, the research suggested that older gay male and lesbian women were not isolated but were actively engaged in supportive relationships with partners, friends, members of their families of origin, and the larger LGB communities (Brown et al. 2001; Grossman et al. 2000; Nystrom and Jones 2003; Whitford 1997).

Another major theoretical framework relevant to the study of LGBT aging and families is Minority Stress Theory. Developed by Meyer (2003), minority stress theory is a conceptual framework that explains how "stigma, prejudice, and discrimination create a hostile and stressful social environment that causes mental health problems" (p. 674). Minority stress for LGBT individuals is linked to alienation and problems with self-acceptance (that is, internalized homophobia). Aging-related stress is linked to concerns about the ability to maintain health and independence into old age, as well as fiscal concerns, such as outliving their income and having a place to live (MetLife Mature Market Institute 2010). Minority stress theory has been used to examine whether same-sex marriage is a protective factor against the combined effects of sexual minority stress and aging-related stress. For example, an analysis by Wight et al. (2012) of a subsample of gay men (age range of 44–75 years, with a mean age of 57 years) from the Multicenter AIDS Cohort Study, examined the impact of minority stress and aging-related stress on their lives. They found that legal marriage among HIV-negative and HIV-positive older gay men is indeed a protective factor that may offset the mental health issues associated with being gay and growing old.

Research Perspectives

LGBT families are varied. There is no "typical" LGBT family form any more than there is a typical heterosexual family form. In addition, cultural norms dictate additional family interactions for racial and ethnic minority LGBT persons (see Chaps. 6, 7, 8, and 10).

Families of origin. Family of origin relationships refers to biological or genetic ties within the context of marriage and parenthood. Family of origin relationships include, then, the relationships that LGBT adults have with their aging parents and adult siblings, as well as the relationships they have with their same-sex partners, same- or different-sex partners, children, and grandchildren. As we note throughout this chapter, it is very common for LGBT individuals to substitute chosen family relationships for biological ones, given the lack of acceptance and legal protection that has been the legacy of being gay, at least until very recently (Cohen and

Murray 2006). We discuss chosen family relationships in a subsequent section below and focus on the traditional understanding of "family of origin" in this section.

Considering a wide age span (65+) for older adulthood, elders who are 65 years old in 2015 were born in 1950; elders who are 85 years old in 2015 were born in 1930. Representatives of these two eras were thus born into the baby boom generation (1950s) and the children of the Great Depression generation (1930s). All of these individuals came of age when sexual minority status was illegal, prosecuted, and considered morally and mentally depraved. Being a sexual minority was a truly isolating and underground experience. Individuals hid their sexual orientation from their family members and employers in order to survive persecution and rejection. Thus, coming of age as an LGBT individual before the end of the twentieth century was a time when openness was dangerous to one's social standing and familial relationships.

As a result of the severely restricted social climate for LGBT individuals until the very late twentieth century, one of the most significant family of origin issues was "coming out" as lesbian or gay to parents and siblings (Cohen and Murray 2006; Jacobson and Grossman 1996; Orel 2014).

Until recently, LGBT individuals did not tend to come out until well into adulthood, after they had already experienced heterosexual marriage, and possibly parenthood. Although mothers and siblings were reported to be more accepting than fathers (a trend that continues to this day), many LGBT individuals lost their family of origin ties (Friend 1990). As they grew older, this lack of sustained biological family ties contributed to a need for chosen kin relationships, particularly the development of friendship ties as a substitute for family ties (Muraco and Fredriksen-Goldsen 2011). However, Connidis (2010) explains that coming out and experiencing rejection is not a lifelong legacy for LGBT adults; as time passes, "many gay and lesbian persons with families work out good relations with both their parents and siblings" (p. 239).

Although aging baby boomers are among the first to experience a more positive social and legal climate in which to grow old, the literature on LGBT elders has documented more challenges to their well being, compared to heterosexually identified elders (e.g., Fredriksen-Goldsen et al. 2013; Gabrielson and Holston 2014; Quam and Whitford 1992; Shenk and Fullmer 1996). A history of strained relationships with family of origin members can add additional stresses to aging-related concerns. Naples' (2001) autoethnography of coping with her father's funeral in the face of disapproving adult siblings is a powerful illustration of strained family ties. The good news is that because private life is inextricably linked to broader social and political trends, LGBT aging family relationships are likely to be less stressful as public acceptance increases.

Reczek (2014) examined the intergenerational relationships of 22 lesbian women and 28 gay men aged 40 and older who were in an intimate relationship for at least seven years. The participants' relationships with both their parents and parents-in-law included dimensions of support, conflict, and ambivalence. Supportive parents integrated the couple into their everyday lives and special family events (i.e., holidays, funerals), used inclusive language seen as evidence of acceptance of the relationships regardless of legal status, relied on the couple for instrumental and emotional support, and affirmed their gay or lesbian identity. Evidence of conflict in their relationship with at least one of their parents manifested as rejection in everyday life (e.g., unpleasant or absent interactions), rejection around traumatic events (e.g., changing will with the occurrence of a severe illness), and the threat of being usurped (e.g., not respecting wishes at illness or death). Some respondents acknowledged that their parents and parents-in-law experienced both support and strain simultaneously (e.g., acts of acceptance but words of disapproval). Identification of these dimensions in the families of aging LGBT individuals provides the groundwork for future research on parent–child relationships and the consequences for the well-being of aging LGBT adult children and their older adult parents.

Another life course issue that is complicated by sexual orientation diversity is the likelihood that older LGBT individuals, especially lesbians, are more likely called upon to care for aging parents. Although 43.5 million individuals in the USA provide care for a family member 50 years of age or older (Family Caregiver Alliance 2012), to date, there has been little empirical research on family of origin caregiving by LGBT adults. Based on available qualitative data and anecdotal accounts, LGBT caregivers' reasons for providing care (e.g., need; filial responsibility), types of caregiving tasks in which they engage (e.g., emotional and instrumental support), and concerns they have about caregiving (e.g., where to turn for help, how to access services, and what services are available) are very similar to heterosexual family caregivers. For example, Cantor et al. (2004) study of gay and lesbian adults caring for a relative from their family of origin identified three primary reasons their family member needed care: physical illness, frailty, and Alzheimer's disease. The types of care included providing emotional support and hands-on care, helping with decision making and financial management, serving as liaison with other family members, and arranging for medical care and support services. About half of the caregivers were women and about two-thirds of lesbian caregivers said that they were either the sole provider or provided most of the care. As with the general population of family caregivers, gay and lesbian caregivers reported significant burden and stress as a result of their caregiver role (e.g., juggling the demand of being employed and caregiving, limited time for self and other relationships, and conflicts or disagreements with other family members about the care of the older person).

While family caregivers often experience both positive and negative aspects of caregiving, LGBT caregivers may face additional challenges when their family has a negative view of their sexual orientation. Cohen and Murray (2006) cited findings from an unpublished study by

Murray in which lesbian caregivers described strained interpersonal family relationships because of a lack of acceptance of their sexual orientation or choice of partner. The following quote by two study participants illustrates the tension LGBT caregivers may face.

> Robin, single, age 46: As long as my Dad is alive, I cannot openly live as a lesbian. He has threatened to leave his estate to one of my male cousins if I act 'queer.' I thought that getting married would get him off my case about women, but it didn't. At this point in my life, it's just easier to have female friends rather than lovers (p. 293)
> Anne, partnered for 16 years, age 42: Although I'm the only one who has taken responsibility for Mom and Dad, they have cut me out of their will. Dad said that he wouldn't leave any money to his queer daughter. (Cohen and Murray, p. 293)

From a life course perspective, with its emphasis on linked lives, transitions, and trajectories over time, when a person comes out, there is also an impact on their siblings' lives. Thus, one person's coming out is likely to be a family event for heterosexual and LGBT individuals alike (Connidis 2010). One of the most exciting areas of new research is how sibling relationships are impacted by LGBT identity among family members throughout the life course. For example, Rothblum et al. (2004), in a study of 1254 LGB adults and their siblings, found that, in general, LGB adults were more highly educated, geographically mobile, less religious, and less likely to have or live with children than heterosexual siblings. Thus, understanding the nature of sibling ties among older adults, particularly in terms of companionship and caregiving, is an important issue for future study (Goldberg 2007; Gottlieb 2004; Grossman et al. 2000).

Intergenerational relationships with children and grandchildren. Although about one-half of lesbian and gay older adults have biological or adoptive children from previous heterosexual relationships (Heaphy 2009), little is known about older LGBT persons' relationships with their adult children. Coming out to children after years of hiding their sexual identity often happens indirectly and can be emotionally challenging for older adults (Hunter 2007). Yet,

Goldberg (2007) found that most of the 42 adult children with LGB parents in her study reported positive relationships with their parents.

The small, but growing literature on the experiences of gay and lesbian grandparents suggests that adult children are the key in determining the nature of the relationship between grandparents and their grandchildren (Orel 2014). Because adult children typically act as family gatekeepers, their acceptance and attitudes toward non-heterosexual identities and relationships often determine the amount of access grandparents have to their grandchildren (Orel and Fruhauf 2013). When adult children hold negative beliefs about homosexuality, many grandparents are reluctant to disclose their sexual identity to their children because they fear they may lose contact with their grandchildren. Conversely, supportive adult children often facilitate the process of coming out to grandchildren, which many gay and lesbian grandparents believe is important because it promotes tolerance and honesty.

In a qualitative study of 11 gay grandfathers, aged 40–79, Fruhauf et al. (2009) found that adult children played an active role in the men's coming-out process to grandchildren, with most adult children involved in explaining their fathers' relationship to their children. For example, Bruce relayed the following story.

> The family was over for dinner and my granddaughter turned to Eric, my life partner, who is Japanese-American. (So, hardly, you know, a match in terms of an obvious brother or something.) She said, "Why do you live here?" and I went like that, and my daughter said, "No, no, no, no, I'll deal with this." So, they left the table, came back about 15 min later, and everybody, you know, is terribly silent waiting to see what will happen. My granddaughter sits there, and she said after a few minutes, "Mommy says that Eric is daddy's special friend. When I'm older, Jessica will be my special friend." (p. 111)

The roles grandfathers played in the lives of their grandchildren also depended on their relationship with the grandchildren's parents (Fruhauf et al. 2009). Some grandfathers have no or limited contact with their adult children because they are unaccepting of their father's sexuality.

For example, Kerry explained that he recently reunited with his estranged son and had since become "more of a grandfather" to his five-year-old grandson. Conversely, Kerry's son-in-law does not accept Kerry's sexuality, which has influenced his relationship with his older grandsons with whom he does not have a close relationship.

With the increase in the number of LGBT adults who are parents and the aging of the population, "doing family" will require an openness to complex family structures and relationships (Perlesz et al. 2006). In their study of multi-generational family interviews with 20 lesbian-parented families living in Victoria, Australia, Perlesz et al. (2006) revealed that being a grandparent in a lesbian-parented family was not always comfortable and challenged the dominant discourse around the definition family. In one family, the non-biological grandfather initially made heterosexist jokes about his daughter "playing daddy" in her prospective lesbian co-parenting role. Yet, upon the birth of his grandchild, he adopted the title of "Pop" and embraced a grandparent role in relation to his non-biological granddaughter. The biological grandmother in this family initially also was negative about her daughter's decision to parent in a lesbian relationship, but after the child was born she embraced her role as a grandmother. The lesbian couple, while recognizing the existence of their parents' homophobia, was pleased that their parents engaged in positive relationships with their child (Perlesz et al. 2006, p. 193):

> Fiona: … you do think about your own parents, how you were parented when you have a child and like Jacqui's family, as much as they are a pain in the butt sometimes, they're actually, it's nice having them around you know. Like your mum, Imogen has a great time with your mum. Your mum is bloody atrocious sometimes with some of the stuff that she says but her relationship with Imogen is really good.
> Jacqui: Yeah it is good.
> Fiona: And it is great, it's fabulous seeing that….

LGBT intimate relationships in later life. About 60 % of older lesbian and bisexual women and about 40 % of older gay and bisexual men are in a coupled relationship (Heaphy et al. 2004). Historically, these couples were more likely than their heterosexual counterparts to maintain separate households (Barker et al. 2006), which allowed them to remain closeted to family and others. Issues of concern for LGBT couples include ageist attitudes, financial stability, long-term care, lack of access to legal marriage, and sexuality (Baumle 2014). The study highlighted in the research box provides an illustration of the fluidity of sexuality for older lesbians, particularly in terms of their perceptions of their romantic and sexual relationships over time (Averett et al. 2012).

Research Box: Older Lesbians and Sexual Intimacy

Averett et al. (2012). Older lesbian sexuality: Identity, sexual behavior, and the impact of aging. *Journal of Sex Research, 49*, 495–507. doi:10.1080/00224499.2011. 582543

Objective: To fill a void in the existing literature and to promote the experiences, needs, and concerns of a nearly invisible population, this study examined the sexual identity, romantic relationships, and experiences of discrimination of older lesbians.

Method: An online national survey was completed by a convenience sample of 456 lesbian women, ranging in age from 51 to 86. To be eligible for the study, participants had to have been involved in an emotional, physical, or sexual relationship with a woman at some point in their lives.

Results: At the time of the survey, 60.5 % of the women were involved in an emotional, physical, or sexual relationship with another woman. The average length of the relationship was of 15.4 years; 58 % of the women defined their relationship as a lifetime partner. Approximately 38 % of the women were satisfied with their sex life over the last year, 25 % were neither satisfied nor unsatisfied, and 37 % were unsatisfied. When asked to describe how

their relationships with women had differed since age 55, common themes were continuity (i.e., no change/difference), relationships were more stable and mature, and a decrease in the focus on the physical or sexual aspects of a relationship.

Conclusion: Researchers must continue to examine the needs of older lesbians in order to increase both understanding and competencies in working with this vulnerable population and to enhance and further conceptual ideas about sexuality identities, experiences, and needs in late life.

Discussion Questions:

1. How important is sexual intimacy in the lives of older lesbian women?
2. What is the relationship between older lesbian women's satisfaction with their sexual lives and attitudes toward aging?
3. What are the limitations of this research study?

de Vries (2007) addressed the diversity of coupled relationships for LGBT elders, including cohabiting and legal unions, as well as partnerships formed post-heterosexual divorce or post coming out as gay or lesbian. Herdt et al. (1997) estimated that for older adults age 55 and over, approximately one-third of gay men and one-half of lesbians had been married at one time to a different-sex spouse. Among the current cohort of older LGBT individuals, it was likely that at least one of the partners was previously married to a cross-sex spouse, because marriage was typically the only way to have children (Connidis 2010). While the growing recognition of same-sex marriages provides LGBT elders access to the personal benefits and social recognition of a formal marriage, some gay and lesbian adults view legalized marriage as a "sell out" to a heterosexist society, often fearing the loss of connection to their LGBT roots and social networks (Lannutti 2005). Bisexual individuals, of whom very little is known (Biblarz and Savci 2010; Rodriguez Rust 2012), particularly those in long-term committed heterosexual marriages, often experience stigma in both the heterosexual and the LGBT communities (de Vries 2007). Relationships in which an older adult is transitioning from male-to-female or female-to-male have added complexity as the gender-based socialization of the individuals and the couple is changed (Cook-Daniels 2006; Persson 2009).

Caregiving norms consistent with heterosexual marital relationships appear to govern same-sex partnerships and marriages as well. When the need for care arises, older LGB adults report that they would first turn to their partners, then to friends and other family members (Cahill et al. 2000). Muraco and Fredriksen-Goldsen (2014) interviewed 36 LGB dyads comprised of committed partners and friends aged 50 and older to understand care norms in varied relationship contexts. Most of the best caregiving experiences between committed partners were identified as expressions of love and commitment to the relationship. Care recipients described their partners' willingness to do anything that was necessary to meet their needs, both day-to-day and in times of crises. However, they also worried about being a burden to their partner. Caregiving partners identified their best caregiving experiences as engaging in meaningful activities with the care recipient (e.g., going to a social event) or providing financial and emotional support. Caregivers were also aware that their relationship with their partner was different and sometimes strained because of the illness, but felt they would survive the challenges. They also expressed concerns about care burdens, fearing that they may someday be unable to take care of their partner because of their own limitations or the worsening health of their partner.

Very little research has focused on the loss of a LGBT partner in late life. For couples who are not completely open about their relationship, the grief and loss experienced after the death of a partner has been described as disenfranchised grief (Doka 2002) because the loss is not openly acknowledged or validated by family, friends, or society. Discounting of the validity of the relationship and of the loss negatively impacts the remaining partner's ability to adequately grieve the loss.

Jenkins et al. (2014) examined bereavement issues of 55 older lesbians. Older lesbians faced emotional, social, legal, and financial obstacles following the death of their partner. Only two of the women reported positive experiences in responding to the death of their partner, which in one case was attributed to the support of the partner's family and in the second case, the support of friends, neighbors, children, and coworkers. The other women all discussed negative experiences after the death of their partner including disenfranchised grief, discriminatory actions, loneliness of isolation, and the frustration of relentless battles. The following quotes from several participants in Jenkins et al. study capture the essence of the lesbian women's experiences with the loss of their partners. *Disenfranchised grief* concerns the personal attitudes and responses that are a result of not giving equal value to a loss in this kind of relationship, as one woman stated, "Nobody was willing to honor my 30-year relationship with her in that I was not considered to be a 'widow' by them" (p. 258). *Discriminatory actions* concerns the refusal of rights—both legal and social—that would typically be granted to spousal partners in a heterosexual relationship, described by another woman as: "It was especially difficult dealing with her biological family in spite of all of the legal papers and arrangements we made in advance" (p. 279). Another woman explained:

> Even the newspaper refused to refer to me as her partner and instead listed me as one of many "friends," even though I had been the breadwinner for several years and was the primary caregiver and hospice caregiver the last 3 years of her life. (p. 281)

Regarding *the loneliness of isolation*, which is learning to live alone and isolation from their partner's family and other support systems, a woman stated that "the worst emotional toll was that her family pulled away and I don't get to see the grandkids I helped raise" (p. 281). Another woman said, "Because most of us become invisible as we become older, it becomes harder to find other lesbians to interact with" (p. 281). Finally, considering the theme of *frustration of relentless battles,* which are a constant stream of battles—with one's own emotions, with family and the partner's family, and with other individuals in the broader social system, a woman stated, "None of my family attended the funeral .... I have loads of anger about how I was treated by others over her passing" (p. 282). The authors concluded that until the legal status of same-sex marriage is widespread, it is important for service providers to develop appropriate means of helping lesbian women (as well as GBT individuals) deal with the issues surrounding the death of a partner.

Families of choice. The concept of "families of choice", which we have described throughout this chapter, was first articulated by Weston (1991). It is linked to fictive kin concepts, which have strong roots in the field of family gerontology (See Allen et al. 2011; Johnson 1999). Families of choice of older LGBT adults are characterized as ones comprised of a deep sense of belonging and feelings of safety, common values, and mutual trust (Gabrielson and Holston 2014). They provide many of the same supportive and care functions as family of origin. In fact, research suggests that older gay and lesbian individuals prefer to receive care from their chosen family instead of their biological family members (Fredriksen-Goldsen et al. 2011; Heaphy 2009). When receiving care from other LGBT people, older adults do not have to "de-sexualize" or eliminate evidence of their sexual orientation from their homes or the stories to appease or hide their identity from a heterosexual caregiver (Cronin et al. 2011).

Older LGBT care recipients rely upon their friends as a safety net that stands between them and an unmet need for care (Muraco and Fredriksen-Goldsen 2014). For example, an older gay man in this study explained that when he was hospitalized, none of his family members came to visit and, "all the things that they should have done, could have done, ought to have done—[my friend] did that" (p. 262). Caregiving friends acknowledged the benefits they received from providing care including feeling good about

themselves, perceiving improvement in their self-esteem, and engaging in typical friend activities (Muraco and Fredriksen-Goldsen 2014). Conversely, caregiving can create conflict between friends due to misunderstandings and short tempers. Depending on the nature of the conflict, it may negate the beneficial feelings that caregiving friends gain from providing care and ultimately threaten the duration of the caregiving relationship, leaving the care recipient vulnerable.

The federal Family Caregivers Support Program, created with the 2000 reauthorization of the Older Americans Act, and amended in 2006, expanded its definition of family caregivers so that extended LGBT family members qualify (Administration on Aging 2012). Eligibility for the program is no longer limited to a married partner or blood relative. As a consequence, LGBT people caring for partners or other members of their chosen families can benefit from services provided under the program, including individual counseling, support groups, caregiver training, respite care, and other supplemental assistance. Research has shown that these services can reduce caregiver depression, anxiety, and stress and enable them to provide care longer, thereby avoiding or delaying the need for institutional care (Wacker and Roberto 2014).

Service Delivery and Interdisciplinary Approaches

One of the major issues affecting older LGBT families is the invisibility and marginalization they face with respect to health care and supportive social services. Reports of discrimination, homophobia, hostility, bias, and general lack of understanding of lifestyle choices are common. Older LGBT adults often report anxiety around the prospect of requiring health or supportive care (Cohen and Murray 2006; Davies et al. 2006; Heaphy and Yip 2006; Price 2005) and fear having to come out to service providers or having to forcibly return to the closet (Brotman et al. 2007). They may be reluctant to seek mental health services, for fear of being invisible as LGBT, or if out, stigmatized (Blando 2001; Greene 2002).

Brotman et al. (2003) conducted four qualitative focus groups in three Canadian provinces (Quebec, Nova Scotia, and British Columbia) to assess their perceptions of health and social service providers. Participants included 21 gay and lesbian elders, and 11 familial and informal caregivers or service providers. All participants identified a profound marginalization and invisibility of gay and lesbian elders. Those who were gay and lesbian themselves described their lack of trust for health care services and professionals saying that issues of sexuality and the nature of gay and lesbian chosen family relationships were unacknowledged or denied. Similarly, responses to a survey completed by 569 LGBT adults attending the 2007 Palm Springs Pride weekend events revealed that older gay men and lesbians maintain some fear of openly disclosing their sexual orientation and some discomfort in their use of older adult social services (Gardner et al. 2014). The majority of respondents reported that they would feel more comfortable accessing LGBT friendly identified services and programs. Women reported being somewhat more likely to use those services publicly identified as LGBT friendly than respondents who were men.

For older LGBT families dealing with dementia, the entry of service providers into their lives is a pivotal point at which they need to decide whether or not to come out to professionals. Price (2010) conducted qualitative interviews in England with 21 gay and lesbian adults aged 20–69 who cared for a parent, partner, or friend with dementia. Participants used a mix of strategies for disclosure of their sexuality to care providers including: (a) active disclosure, where service providers were directly informed that the family caregiver was not heterosexual; (b) passive disclosure, where caregivers' sexual identity was suggested by way of clues given that relate to their sexuality; and (c) passive nondisclosure, where caregivers purposefully concealed aspects of their sexuality or actively avoided questions related to sexuality. The caregivers'

decision to disclose was mediated by three interlinked factors: experiences of negative reactions to and misunderstanding of their sexuality, their perceived feelings of discrimination, and their anticipation of negative responses. For example, a passive discloser who was a gay caregiver of a female friend that he and his partner took into their home so they could provide her care relayed the following experience. This excerpt reveals how the service provider's misconceptions and lack of understanding undermined the caregiver's efforts to ensure his friend's dignity:

> We were talking about getting her dressed and everything…and I was saying Yeah, 'cos we bought all her clothes, so we kind of erm, and, in a way, we made sure she was fantastic, you know what I mean, she wasn't just like, you know a lot of people who are like cared for, they just wear easy to wear clothes with elasticated things and t-shirts and stuff, but we liked, because she always did look fantastic, so we tried to keep that up as much as we could. …And somebody said to us, 'So, when you're getting her dressed then, do you love it? So, do you sometimes think, hey, I could wear that and I could put that on?' And I'm just like, 'No, no we don't think like that actually!' (p. 163–164)

The above example and others like it found in the literature reinforce the need for education and training for health and human service providers to eliminate discriminatory and oppressive practices and implement appropriate responses and care. Service providers must consider the extensive invisibility of older LGBT families and practice in a manner that is culturally sensitive and competent (Healy 2002). Culturally sensitive practices are affirming to LGBT families and include the use of language and behavior that validates, acknowledges, and accepts LGBT families. Culturally competent practice requires that service providers acquire knowledge about the diversity within the LGBT population, learn the resources available to LBGT families, gain an understanding of the unique challenges faced by LGBT families due to the laws and policies that discriminate against them, and be sensitive to the general impact of heterosexual assumptions in the health and social service system (Healy 2002).

Unfortunately, as highlighted by cases presented in the Discussion Box, such shifts in practices are slow to come about. Knochel et al. (2010) found that more than one-half of the 316 directors of Area Agencies on Aging (AAA) and State Units on Aging (SUAs) who responded to a nationwide survey had not offered or funded any LGBT aging training to staff and very few were providing any LGBT aging outreach. Agencies whose staff had received some form of LGBT training were twice as likely to receive a request to help an LGB individual and three times as likely to be requested to help a transgender older adult. Such findings provided evidence that cultural competency training could substantially improve the lives of many LGBT older adults.

Discussion Box: Older LGBT Families Providing Care and Seeking Services

Partners, families, and friends are the most preferred sources of support and daily care among older LGBT adults. When the need for help and assistance escalates, due to chronic health problems or cognitive decline, families may seek formal services to assist in meeting the older adult's care needs.

All too often LGBT families face discrimination and insensitive treatment when they seek help from formal health and community service providers, which makes many LGBT older adults reluctant to access mainstream aging services, and ultimately may put them at greater risk for worsening chronic health problems, depression and anxiety, social isolation, and premature mortality. For example, consider the experiences of Amirah who felt discriminated against by her doctor (http://www.lgbtmap.org/file/lgbt-older-adults-and-inhospitable-health-care-environments.pdf; p. 2), Lawrence and Alexandre who experienced hostility from paid home care providers (http://www.lgbtagingcenter.org/resources/resource.cfm?r=15), and Clay and Harold's poor treatment when Harold needed nursing

home care (http://www.lgbtmap.org/file/lgbt-older-adults-and-inhospitable-health-care-environments.pdf; p. 3).

Training care staff on how to identify and address the needs of LGBT older adults is one important key to making health care and supportive services more welcoming to older LGBT families and to ensure that they have access to appropriate care options.

Discussion Questions:

1. What recommendation do you have for training to help make positive changes in the health and formal care provision for LGBT elders and their families?
2. What specific knowledge and information should community services providers and long-term care providers, such as case managers, social workers, nurses, and nursing assistants, have in order to best assist older LGBT families meet their care needs?
3. In what ways can the LGBT families advocate for culturally sensitive and appropriate services and treatment by formal health and human service professionals?

In 2010, for the first time, the Administration on Aging (AoA), a federal agency that provides funds to state units on aging who in turn support local AAAs, publically recognized that older LGBT individuals have unique concerns and needs. To address these concerns and needs, the AoA provided a three-year grant to SAGE to create the National Resource Center for LGBT Aging. The initial objectives of the National Resource Center focused on both service organizations and LGBT individuals and families:

1. Educate aging network services organizations about the existence and special needs of LGBT older adults.
2. Sensitize LGBT organizations to the existence and special needs of older adults.

3. Educate LGBT individuals about the importance of planning ahead for future long-term care needs. (Meyer 2011, p. 25)

Establishing the National Resource Center for LGBT Aging was an integral first step in addressing the needs of LGBT elders and their families. While the education and training processes have shown initial signs of success, federal, state, and local agencies must continue to invest in this work in order to implement the necessary systemic changes to the aging service delivery system (Meyer 2011).

Issues to Be Resolved Through Research and Practice

Although promising strides have been made, much more research is needed about the various biological and chosen family relationships of aging LGBT individuals. As we have noted throughout this chapter, these relationships include those with same-sex and different-sex partners, with children and grandchildren, with aging parents and adult siblings, and with friends and informal relationships that are converted into family relationships. With the changing social and political context, as well as the aging of the LGBT population, conducting the research on LGBT families is increasingly possible. Social changes in marriage equality, legalized second parent adoption, and recognition of friends as informal caregivers are likely to contribute to new research and thinking about aging, sexual minority status, and families. With all of these changes, there will be an expansion of resources for LGBT older adults and their families, beyond the pioneering efforts that currently exist (e.g., Lambda Legal Defense 2015; SAGE 2015).

The challenges facing older LGBT individuals as members of families of origin, families of procreation, and families of choice are well documented. What is needed now are more studies about LGBT resilience over the life course (e.g., Oswald 2002) and successful aging (van Wagenen et al. 2013). Research on how LGBT adults bring their accumulated wisdom and adaptability into their later years in order to maintain emotional, physical, and relationship health is a promising pathway to deepen understanding about aging differently, and aging well.

Summary

Families are the most important institution for the care and nurturance of human beings; attention to family ties is crucial for professionals in all areas working with elders. Historically, the family experiences of LGBT aging individuals have been largely ignored and stigmatized given the social and legal prohibitions against sexual orientation minority status. Currently, however, this situation of exclusion is being rectified and now older LGBT family life is beginning to receive the theoretical, empirical, and practical attention it deserves.

Aging LGBT individuals have faced many stresses associated with the overlap between aging and being members of a sexual minority. As a result, these elders have developed very resilient strategies for constructing long-term kinship bonds, even when societal customs and laws have disallowed them. One of the strengths of this population is the activist spirit in the LGBT community. The desire to live an authentic life, despite prejudice and hardship has led older LGBT individuals to create a rich array of legal, biological, and fictive kin ties. Indeed, some "family" ties of older LGBT individuals are actually with their friends. Blurring the boundaries across biological and chosen kin ties is a legacy and a contribution of the LGBT aging community.

As the aging LGBT population increases, it is even more imperative that health care and social services professionals have up-to-date knowledge about similarities and differences in families where members are LGBT. They also need to be informed about the changing legal climate that impacts the family relationships of these elders so that they can ensure their access to the services that will improve their quality of life.

LGBT Older Adult Resources

United States

AARP (American Association of Retired Persons): AARP is a nonprofit, nonpartisan organization that advocates for consumers in the marketplace, including those who identify as LGBT. The AARP-Pride Web content provides consumers and families with information specific to LGBT older adults. Here, readers can find information on LGBT news, estate planning tips, social security, same-sex divorce, dating, history of LGBT rights, health and well-being, leisure activities, and read AARP's stance on LGBT issues. (http://www.aarp.org/relationships/friends-family/aarp-pride/).

ASA Clearinghouse (American Society on Aging LGBT Aging Resources Clearinghouse): The American Society on Aging has created a searchable database where LGBT older adults can find annotated listings of aging resources. The clearinghouse was created to provide access to information for elders, young persons, caregivers, students, researchers, and other professionals. Listings include reports and articles, links for ordering DVDs and books, service providers, community organizations, information sites, and other useful products. (http://asaging.org/lgbt_aging_resources_clearinghouse).

DEC (Diverse Elders Coalition): Founded in 2010, the Diverse Elders Coalition advocates for policies and programs that improve the lives of racially and ethnically diverse people (including American Indians and Alaska Natives) and LGBT people. This coalition was created to give voice to those often absent from policy-making conversations. Here, readers can find resources on research, information booklets, webinars, and policies affecting LGBT older adults. (http://www.diverseelders.org/learn/).

FORGE TAN (FORGE Transgender Aging Network): The FORGE organization advocates for the rights of transgender individuals and their significant others, friends, family, and allies (SOFFAs). The FORGE Trans Aging Network is a membership-based community that offers listservs, publications, training, and consultations on issues related to aging. (http://forge-forward.org/aging/).

LGBT FCA (Lesbian, Gay, Bisexual, and Transgender Family Caregiver Alliance): The Family Caregiver Alliance is a nonprofit organization dedicated to caregiver awareness and advocacy. The FCA has a section dedicated specifically to caregiving issues and strategies for LGBTQ populations. Here readers can find LGBT facts and tip sheets and access an online caregiver support group. (https://www.caregiver.org/special-issues/lgbtq).

NRC LGBT (National Resource Center on LGBT Aging): Founded in 2010, the National Resource Center on LGBT Aging is a self-described "technical assistance resource center" created to address the needs of older LGBT adults as they age. Here readers can access training documents, technical assistance, and educational resources. Topics include caregiving, intergenerational issues, and long-term care. (http://www.lgbtagingcenter.org/resources/index.cfm?s=3; http://www.lgbtagingcenter.org/resources/resources.cfm?s=16; http://www.lgbtagingcenter.org/resources/resources.cfm?s=15).

SAGE (Services and Advocacy for Gay, Lesbian, Bisexual, and Transgender Elders): Founded in 1978, SAGE is the US oldest and largest organization dedicated to serving the needs of LGBT older adults. SAGE offers services and programs to LGBT older adults nationwide, advocates at all levels of government (federal, state, and local) for inclusive public policy, provides training to service providers, and develops consumer resources to help older LGBT adults make informed decisions. Here readers can find information on their programs, advocacy, issues, and latest news. (http://www.sageusa.org/).

International

AUK (Age United Kingdom): Age UK is the largest charity organization consisting of over 170 local Age UKs across England. This organization aims to help all adults live out their later years to the best of their ability. Age UK provides older LGBT adults with access to services, tools for planning, and support group information. In addition, this organization has several international branches in more than 40 countries. (http://www.ageuk.org.uk/health-wellbeing/relationships-and-family/older-lesbian-gay-and-bisexual/).

Equal Aging (Seta—LGBTI Rights in Finland). Founded in 1974, Seta is a national human rights non-governmental organization (NGO) with local and national branches in Finland. Equal Aging is a three-year project run by Seta in cooperation with Fin-Bears and Mummolaasko. Here Finnish caregivers and students can find information on LGBTI care needs. In addition, this web site also includes a care for the elderly knowledge library. (http://seta.fi/yhdenvertainen-vanhuus/in-english/; http://seta.fi/yhdenvertainen-vanhuus/vanhustyon-tietokirjasto/).

National LGBTI Health Alliance. (National Lesbian, Gay, Bisexual, Transgender, and Intersex Health Alliance—Australia): The National LGBTI Health Alliance advocates for the improved health and well-being of LGBTI individuals across Australia. This coalition group is made up of individuals and organizations and was created in response to the expected increase in the demand for services for LGBTI older adults in Australia. The Alliance Web site provides information on the organization, their training initiatives, strategic documents, and a review of progress made in the previous calendar year. (http://lgbtihealth.org.au/ageing).

ODL (Opening Doors London): Opening Door London is one of the largest sources of support and information for older LGBT adults in the United Kingdom. Opening Doors London was created as a response to the high rates of isolation experienced by older LGBT adults. The program is aimed at LGBT men and women over the age of 50 and includes regular social activities, referral services, and information and guidance to service providers. (http://opening doorslondon.org.uk/).

RFSL Stockholm (Swedish Federation for Lesbian, Gay, Bisexual, Transgender, and Queer Rights): Founded in 1950, the RFSL is one of the oldest LGBT rights organizations in the world. It works to serve the needs of LGBT individuals and their relatives and friends. The organization carries out advocacy work, educational courses, and support groups. Here readers can find information on projects, health, and older adult and family support groups. (http://rfslstockholm.com/).

SPN (Senior Pride Network): The Senior Pride Network is a two-pronged service provider to LGBTQ Canadians aged 50+. This network-based organization is comprised of individuals, organizations, and community groups that serve or are committed to serving the needs of LGBT older adults. In addition, this Senior Pride Network also includes a six-person advisory committee that sets the network's priorities, strategic direction, and future initiatives. Here readers can access information on programs and services, training, and research. (http://www.seniorpridenetwork.com/home.htm).

Acknowledgment We thank Erin Lavender-Stott and Emma Potter for their research assistance.

Learning Exercises

Self-Check Questions

1. In what ways did the scholarship on LGBT elders and their families emerge out of the social activism on behalf of LGBT civil rights?
2. What are families of choice? How are they significant in the LGBT aging community?
3. What impact will the legalization of same-sex marriage have for current generations of LGBT individuals as they age?
4. What are the unique circumstances that older LGBT individuals and their family members must prepare for, due to their sexual minority status?
5. What knowledge do health care professionals and social service providers need to be able to ensure quality of care to aging LGBT individuals and their families?

6. What do aging LGBT individuals have to teach others about family relationships?

Experiential Exercises

1. Visit a GLBT senior center or a GLBT community center and interview staff members and participants about their experiences of "chosen family" in their community.
2. View the documentary, *Gen Silent*, and reflect on the issues facing the LGBT individuals and their partners as they consider long-term care. http://www.lgbtagingcenter.org/resources/resource.cfm?r=14
3. View the short video featuring Hilary Meyer, Director of the National Resource Center on LGBT Aging, discuss issues facing LGBT older adults (13.04 min). Identify 3-5 key caregiving issues in late life. http://www.lgbtagingcenter.org/resources/resource.cfm?r=13.

Multiple-Choice Questions

1. Families in which friends are converted into kin are called:
   (a) Families of procreation
   (b) Families of origin
   (c) Families of choice
   (d) Families of extension
2. Douglas Kimmel is one of the founders of:
   (a) SAGE
   (b) NLGTF
   (c) Gray Panthers
   (d) AARP
3. Which of the following US states has not allowed legal same-sex marriage?
   (a) Alabama
   (b) California
   (c) Montana
   (d) Virginia
4. "Personal attitudes and responses that are a result of not giving equal value to a loss in this kind of relationship" is the definition of:
   (a) Discriminatory action
   (b) Disenfranchised grief

   (c) Loneliness of isolation
   (d) Frustration of relentless battles
5. Family gatekeeper is a term that refers to what generation:
   (a) Grandparents
   (b) Adult children
   (c) Grandchildren
   (d) Great-grandchildren
6. Older LGBT adults' relationships with their parents and siblings are characterized by:
   (a) Ambivalence
   (b) Support
   (c) Conflict
   (d) All of the above
7. Which theory explains how stigma, prejudice, and discrimination create a hostile and stressful social environment that can cause mental health problems?
   (a) Life course theory
   (b) Social exchange theory
   (c) Minority stress theory
   (d) Activity theory
8. LGBT care providers who purposefully conceal aspects of their sexuality are called:
   (a) Active disclosure
   (b) Passive disclosure
   (c) Active nondisclosure
   (d) Passive nondisclosure
9. Which of the following does **not** appear to be a major concern for older LGBT adults:
   (a) Going on vacations
   (b) Moving into a nursing home
   (c) Relationships with biological family members
   (d) Chronic illness
10. This chapter addressed the intersections across the following social locations:
    (a) Age, nationality, and residence
    (b) Age, family, and sexual orientation
    (c) Age, disability, and gender
    (d) Age, ethnicity, and religion

Multiple-Choice Key

1. c
2. a
3. a

4. b
5. b
6. d
7. c
8. d
9. a
10. b

References

Administration on Aging. (2012). National Family Caregiver Support Program (OAA Title IIIE). Retrieved from http://www.aoa.gov/AoA_programs/HCLTC/Caregiver/index.aspx

Allen, K. R. (2005). Gay and lesbian elders. In M. Johnson, V. L. Bengtson, P. Coleman, & T. Kirkwood (Eds.), *The Cambridge handbook of age and aging* (pp. 483–489). Cambridge, UK: Cambridge University Press.

Allen, K. R., Blieszner, R., & Roberto, K. A. (2000). Families in the middle and later years: A review and critique of research in the 1990s. *Journal of Marriage and the Family, 62,* 911–926. doi:10.1111/j.1741-3737.2000.00911.x.

Allen, K. R., Blieszner, R., & Roberto, K. A. (2011). Perspectives on extended family and fictive kin in the later years: Strategies and meanings of kin reinterpretation. *Journal of Family Issues, 32,* 1156–1177. doi:10.1177/0192513X11404335.

Allen, K. R., & Demo, D. H. (1995). The families of lesbians and gay men: A new frontier in family research. *Journal of Marriage and the Family, 57,* 111–127. doi:10.2307/353821.

Averett, P., Yoon, I., & Jenkins, C. L. (2012). Older lesbian sexuality: Identity, sexual behavior, and the impact of aging. *Journal of Sex Research, 49,* 495–507. doi:10.1080/00224499.2011.582543.

Barker, J. C., Herdt, G., & de Vries, B. (2006). Social support in the lives of lesbians and gay men at midlife and later. *Sexuality Research & Social Policy, 3,* 1–23. doi:10.1525/srsp.2006.3.2.1.

Baumle, A. K. (2014). Same-sex cohabiting elders versus different-sex cohabiting and married elders: Effects of relationship status and sex of partner on economic and health outcomes. *Social Science Research, 43,* 60–73. doi:10.1016/j.ssresearch.2013.09.003.

Bengtson, V. L., & Allen, K. R. (1993). The life course perspective applied to families over time. *Sourcebook of family theories and methods* (pp. 469–499). New York, NY: Plenum.

Bengtson, V. L., Elder, G. H., & Putney, N. M. (2005). The lifecourse perspective on ageing: Linked lives, timing, and history. In M. Johnson, V. L. Bengtson,

P. Coleman, & T. Kirkwood (Eds.), *The Cambridge handbook of age and aging* (pp. 493–501). Cambridge, UK: Cambridge University Press.

Berger, R. M. (1984). Realities of gay and lesbian aging. *Social Work, 29,* 57–62.

Berger, R. M., & Kelly, J. J. (1986). Working with homosexuals of the older population. *Social Casework, 67,* 203–210.

Bianchi, S. M. (2014). A demographic perspective on family change. *Journal of Family Theory & Review, 6,* 35–44. doi:10.1111/jftr.12029.

Biblarz, T. J., & Savci, E. (2010). Lesbian, gay, bisexual, and transgender families. *Journal of Marriage and Family, 72,* 480–497. doi:10.1111/j.1741-3737.2010.00714.x.

Blando, J. A. (2001, Summer). Twice hidden: Older gay and lesbian couples, friends, and intimacy. *Generations, 25,* 87–89.

Blieszner, R., & Bedford, V. (Eds.). (2012). *Handbook of families and aging* (2nd ed.). Denver, CO: Praeger.

Brock, L. J., & Jennings, G. (2007). Sexuality & intimacy. In J. A. Blackburn & C. N. Dunn (Eds.), *Handbook of gerontology: Evidence-based approaches to theory, practice, and research* (pp. 244–268). Hoboken, NJ: Wiley.

Brotman, S., Ryan, B., Collins, S., Chamberland, L., Cormier, R., Julien, D. et al. (2007). Coming out to care: Caregivers of gay and lesbian seniors in Canada. *The Gerontologist, 47,* 490–503.

Brotman, S., Ryan, B., & Cormier, R. (2003). The health and social service needs of gay and lesbian elders and their families in Canada. *The Gerontologist, 43,* 192–202.

Brown, L. B., Alley, G. R., Sarosy, S., Quarto, G., & Cook, T. (2001). Gay men: Aging well! *Journal of Gay and Lesbian Social Services, 13*(4), 41–54.

Cahill, S., South, K., & Spade, J. (2000). *Outing age: Public policy issues affecting gay, lesbian, bisexual and transgender elders.* Washington, DC: National Gay and Lesbian Task Force Policy Institute.

Cantor, M. H., Brennan, M., & Shippy, R. A. (2004). *Caregiving among older lesbian, gay, bisexual, and transgender New Yorkers.* New York: National Gay and Lesbian Task Force Policy Institute. Retrieved from http://www.thetaskforce.org/static_html/downloads/reports/reports/CaregivingAmongOlderLGBT.pdf.

Cohen, H. L., & Murray, Y. (2006). Older lesbian and gay caregivers: Caring for families of choice and caring for families of origin. *Journal of Human Behavior in the Social Environment, 14*(1/2), 275–298. doi:10.1300/J137v14n01_14.

Cohler, B. J., & Hostetler, A. J. (2002). Aging, intimate relationships, and life story among gay men. In R. W. Weiss & S. A. Bass (Eds.), *Challenges of the third age: Meaning and purpose in later life* (pp. 137–160). New York, NY: Oxford University Press.

Connidis, I. A. (2010). *Family ties and aging* (2nd ed.). Los Angeles, CA: Pine Forge Press.

Cook-Daniels, L. (2006). Trans aging. In D. Kimmel, T. Rose, & S. David (Eds.), *Lesbian, gay, bisexual, and transgender aging: Research and clinical perspectives* (pp. 20–35). New York, NY: Columbia University Press.

Cooper, B. (1997). The view from over the hill. In M. Pearsall (Ed.), *The other within us: Feminist explorations of women and aging* (pp. 121–134). Boulder, CO: Westview Press.

Cronin, A., Ward, R., Pugh, S., King, A., & Price, E. (2011). Categories and their consequences: Understanding and supporting the caring relationships of older lesbian, gay and bisexual people. *International Social Work, 54*, 421–435. doi:10.1177/0020872810396261.

D'Augelli, A. R., Grossman, A. H., Hershberger, S. L., & O'Connell, T. S. (2001). Aspects of mental health among older lesbian, gay, and bisexual adults. *Aging and Mental Health, 5*, 149–158. doi:10.1080/713650002.

Davies, M., Addis, S., MacBride-Stewart, S., & Shepherd, M. (2006). *The health, social care and housing needs of lesbian, gay, bisexual and transgender older people: Literature review*. Cardiff, UK: Cardiff Institute of Society, Health and Ethics.

de Vries, B. (2007). LGBT couples in later life: A study in diversity. *Generations, 31*, 18–23.

D'Emilio, J., & Freedman, E. B. (1997). *Intimate matters: A history of sexuality in America* (2nd ed.). Chicago, IL: University of Chicago Press.

Doka, K. J. (Ed.). (2002). *Disenfranchised grief: New directions, challenges, and strategies for practice*. Champaign, IL: Research Press.

Dorfman, R., Walters, K., Burke, P., Hardin, L., Karanik, T., Raphael, J., & Silverstein, E. (1995). Old, sad and alone: The myth of the aging homosexual. *Journal of Gerontological Social Work, 24*(1/2), 29–44.

Editors of the *Harvard Law Review*. (1990). *Sexual orientation and the law*. Cambridge, MA: Harvard University Press.

Engel, S. (2002). Making a minority: Understanding the formation of the gay and lesbian movement in the United States. In D. Richardson & S. Seidman (Eds.), *Handbook of lesbian and gay studies* (pp. 377–402). Thousand Oaks, CA: Sage.

Faderman, L. (1991). *Odd girls and twilight lovers: A history of lesbian life in twentieth century America*. New York, NY: Penquin.

Family Caregiver Alliance. (2012). *Selected caregiver statistics*. Retrieved from https://www.caregiver.org/selected-caregiver-statistics.

Fredriksen-Goldsen, K. I., Cook-Daniels, L., Kim, H., Erosheva, E. A., Emlet, C. A., Hoy-Ellis, C. P., et al. (2013). Physical and mental health of transgender older adults: An at-risk and underserved population. *The Gerontologist, 54*, 488–500. doi:10.1093/geront/gnt021.

Fredriksen-Goldsen, K. I., Kim, H.-J., Emlet, C. A., Muraco, A., Erosheva, E. A., Hoy-Ellis, C., et al. (2011). *The aging and health report: Disparities and resilience among lesbian, gay, bisexual, and transgender older adults*. Seattle, WA: Institute for Multigenerational Health.

Fredriksen-Goldsen, K. I., & Muraco, A. (2010). Aging and sexual orientation: A 25-year review of the literature. *Research on Aging, 32*, 372–413. doi:10.1177/0164027509360355.

Friend, R. A. (1990). Older lesbian and gay people: Responding to homophobia. In F. W. Bozett & M. B. Sussman (Eds.), *Homosexuality and family relations* (pp. 241–263). New York, NY: Harrington Park Press.

Fruhauf, C., Orel, N., & Jenkins, D. (2009). The coming out process of gay grandfathers: Perceptions of their adult children's influence. *Journal of GLBT Family Studies, 5*, 99–118. doi:10.1080/15504280802595402.

Gabrielson, M. L., & Holston, E. C. (2014). Broadening definitions of family for older lesbians: Modifying the Lubben social network scale. *Journal of Gerontological Social Work, 57*, 198–217. doi:10.1080/01634372.2013.879683.

Gardner, A. T., de Vries, B., & Mockus, D. S. (2014). Aging out in the desert: Disclosure, acceptance, and service use among midlife and older lesbians and gay men. *Journal of Homosexuality, 61*, 129–144. doi:10.1080/00918369.2013.835240.

Goldberg, A. E. (2007). Talking about family: Disclosure practices of adults raised by lesbian, gay, and bisexual parents. *Journal of Family Issues, 28*, 100–131. doi:10.1177/0192513X06293606.

Gottlieb, A. R. (2004). *Side by side: On having a gay or lesbian sibling*. New York, NY: Haworth Press.

Gray, H., & Dressel, P. (1985). Alternative interpretations of aging among gay males. *The Gerontologist, 25*, 83–87.

Greene, B. (2002). Older lesbians' concerns and psychotherapy: Beyond a footnote to the footnote. In F. K. Trotman & C. M. Brody (Eds.), *Psychotherapy and counseling with older women: Cross-cultural, family, and end-of-life issues* (pp. 161–174). New York, NY: Springer.

Grossman, A. H., D'Augelli, A. R., & Hershberger, S. L. (2000). Social support networks of lesbian, gay, and bisexual adults 60 years of age and older. *Journal of Gerontology: Psychological Sciences, 55B*, 171–179. doi:10.1093/geronb/55.3.P171.

Healy, T. C. (2002). Culturally competent practice with elderly lesbians. *Geriatric Case Management Journal, 12*(3), 9–13.

Heaphy, B. (2009). Choice and its limits in older lesbian and gay narratives of relational life. *Journal of GLBT Family Studies, 5*(1–2), 119–138. doi:10.1080/15504280802595451.

Heaphy, B., & Yip, A. K. T. (2006). Policy implications of ageing sexualities. *Social Policy and Society, 5*, 443–451. doi:10.1017/S1474746406003150.

Heaphy, B., Yip, A. K., & Thompson, D. (2004). Ageing in a non-heterosexual context. *Ageing and Society, 24*, 881–902. doi:10.1017/S0144686X03001600.

Herdt, G., Beeler, J., & Rawls, T. (1997). Life course diversity among older lesbians and gay men: A study in Chicago. *Journal of Gay, Lesbian, and Bisexual Identity, 2*, 231–246. doi:10.1023/A:1026338004449.

Human Rights Campaign (HRC). (2015, January). *Marriage equality and other relationship recognition laws.* Retrieved from www.hrc.org

Hunter, S. (2007). *Coming out and disclosures: LGBT persons across the life span.* Binghamton, NY: Haworth Press.

Jacobson, S., & Grossman, A. H. (1996). Older lesbians and gay men: Old myths, new images, and future directions. In R. C. Savin-Williams & K. M. Cohen (Eds.), *The lives of lesbians, gays, and bisexuals: Children to adults* (pp. 345–373). Fort Worth, TX: Harcourt Brace.

Jenkins, C. L., Edmundson, A., Averett, P., & Yoon, I. (2014). Older lesbians and bereavement: Experiencing the loss of a partner. *Journal of Gerontological Social Work, 57*, 273–287. doi:10.1080/01634372.2013.850583.

Johnson, C. L. (1999). Fictive kin among oldest old African Americans in the San Francisco Bay area. *Journal of Gerontology: Social Sciences, 54B*, S368–S375. doi:10.1093/geronb/54B.6.S368.

Kehoe, M. (1986). Lesbians over 65: A triply invisible minority. *Journal of Homosexuality, 12*(3/4), 139–152. doi:10.1300/J082v12n03_12.

Kimmel, D. C. (1978). Adult development and aging: A gay perspective. *Journal of Social Issues, 34*(3), 113–130.

Kimmel, D. C. (1992). The families of older gay men and lesbians. *Generations, 17*(3), 37–38.

Kimmel, D., Rose, T., & David, S. (Eds.). (2006). *Lesbian, gay, bisexual, and transgender aging research and clinical perspectives.* New York, NY: Columbia University Press.

Knochel, A., Croghan, C., Moone, R., & Quam, J. (2010). *Ready to serve? The aging network of LGB and T older adults.* St. Paul, MN: Author. Retrieved from http://www.lgbtagingcenter.org/resources/pdfs/ReadyToServe.pdf.

Lambda Legal. (2015). *Seniors.* Retrieved from http://www.lambdalegal.org/issues/seniors.

Lannutti, P. J. (2005). For better or worse: Exploring the meanings of same-sex marriage within the lesbian, gay, bisexual, and transgendered community. *Journal of Social and Personal Relationships, 22*, 5–18. doi:10.1177/0265407505049319.

Lipman, A. (1984). Homosexuals. In E. Palmore (Ed.), *Handbook on the aged in the United States* (pp. 323–337). Westport, CT: Greenwood Press.

Maupin, A. (2015, January). *Books.* Retrieved from www.armisteadmaupin.com.

MetLife Mature Market Institute. (2010). *Still out, still aging: The Metlife study of lesbian, gay, bisexual, and transgender baby boomers.* Retrieved from www.metlife.com/mmi/research/still-out-still-aging.html.

Meyer, H. (2011). Safe spaces? The need for LGBT cultural competency in aging services. *Public Policy & Aging Report, 21*(3), 24–27.

Meyer, I. H. (2003). Prejudice, social stress, and mental health in lesbian, gay, and bisexual populations: Conceptual issues and research evidence. *Psychological Bulletin, 129*, 674–697. doi:10.1037/0033-2909.129.5.674.

Muraco, A., & Fredriksen-Goldsen, K. I. (2011). "That's what friends do": Informal caregiving for chronically ill LGBT elders. *Journal of Social and Personal Relationships, 28*, 1073–1092. doi:10.1177/0265407511402419.

Muraco, A., & Fredriksen-Goldsen, K. I. (2014). The highs and lows of caregiving for chronically ill lesbian, gay, and bisexual elders. *Journal of Gerontological Social Work, 57*, 251–272. doi:10.1080/01634372.2013.860652.

Naples, N. A. (2001). A member of the funeral: An introspective ethnography. In M. Bernstein & R. Reimann (Eds.), *Queer families, queer politics: Challenging culture and the state* (pp. 21–43). New York, NY: Columbia University Press.

National Gay and Lesbian Task Force (NGLTF). (2015). *FAQ sheet on LGBT elders & outing Age 2010.* Retrieved from www.thetaskforce.org.

Nystrom, N. M., & Jones, T. C. (2003). Community building with aging and old lesbians. *American Journal of Community Psychology, 32*, 293–300.

Orel, N. A. (2014). Investigating the needs and concerns of lesbian, gay, bisexual, and transgender older adults: The use of qualitative and quantitative methodology. *Journal of Homosexuality, 61*, 53–78. doi:10.1080/00918369.2013.835236.

Orel, N. A., & Fruhauf, C. A. (2013). Lesbian, gay, bisexual, and transgender grandparents. In A. E. Goldberg & K. R. Allen (Eds.), *LGBT-parent families: Innovations in research and implications for practice* (pp. 177–192). New York, NY: Springer.

Oswald, R. F. (2002). Resilience within the family networks of lesbians and gay men: Intentionality and redefinition. *Journal of Marriage and Family, 64*, 374–383. doi:10.1111/j.1741-3737.2002.00374.x.

Perlesz, A., Brown, R., Lindsay, J., McNair, R., De Vaus, D., & Pitts, M. (2006). Family in transition: parents, children and grandparents in lesbian families give meaning to 'doing family'. *Journal of Family Therapy, 28*, 175–199. doi:10.1111/j.1467-6427.2006.00345.x.

Persson, D. I. (2009). Unique challenges of transgender aging: Implications from the literature. *Journal of Gerontological Social Work, 52*, 633–646. doi:10.1080/01634370802609056.

Pope, M., & Schulz, R. (1990). Sexual attitudes and behavior in midlife and aging homosexual males. *Journal of Homosexuality, 20*, 169–177.

Price, E. (2005). All but invisible: older gay men and lesbians. *Nursing Older People, 17*(4), 16–18. doi:10.7748/nop2005.06.17.4.16.c2377.

Price, E. (2010). Coming out to care: Gay and lesbian carers' experiences of dementia services. *Health and Social Care in the Community, 18*, 160–168. doi:10.1111/j.1365-2524.2009.00884.x.

Quam, J. K., & Whitford, G. S. (1992). Adaptation and age-related expectations of older gay and lesbian adults. *The Gerontologist, 32*, 367–374.

Reczek, C. (2014). The intergenerational relationships of gay men and lesbian women. *Journals of Gerontology. Series B, Psychological Sciences and Social Sciences, 69*, 909–919. doi:10.1093/geronb/gbu042.

Rodriguez Rust, P. C. (2012). Aging in the bisexual community. In T. M. Witten & A. E. Eyler (Eds.), *Gay, lesbian, bisexual & transgender aging: Challenges in research, practice & policy* (pp. 162–186). Baltimore, MD: The Johns Hopkins University Press.

Rothblum, E. D., Balsam, K. F., & Mickey, R. M. (2004). Brothers and sisters of lesbians, gay men, and bisexuals as a demographic comparison group: An innovative research methodology to examine social change. *The Journal of Applied Behavioral Science, 40*, 283–301. doi:10.1177/0021886304266877.

SAGE: Services and Advocacy for Gay, Lesbian, Bisexual & Transgender Elders. (2015). Retrieved from www.sageusa.org/about/history.

Shenk, D., & Fullmer, E. (1996). Significant relationships among older women: Cultural and personal constructions of lesbianism. In K. A. Roberto (Ed.), *Relationships between women in later life* (pp. 75–89). New York, NY: Harrington Park Press.

Silverstein, M., & Giarrusso, R. (2010). Aging and family life: A decade review. *Journal of Marriage and Family, 72*, 1039–1058. doi:10.1111/j.1741-3737.2010.00749.x.

Sullivan, K. M. (2014). Acceptance in the domestic environment: The experience of senior housing for lesbian, gay, bisexual, and transgender seniors. *Journal of Gerontological Social Work, 57*, 235–250. doi:10.1080/01634372.2013.867002.

Tasker, F. (2013). Lesbian and gay parenting post-heterosexual divorce and separation. In A. E. Goldberg & K. R. Allen (Eds.), *LGBT-parent families: Innovations in research and implications for practice* (pp. 3–20). New York, NY: Springer.

van Wagenen, A., Driskell, J., & Bradford, J. (2013). "I'm still raring to go": Successful aging among lesbian, gay, bisexual, and transgender older adults. *Journal of Aging Studies, 27*, 1–14. doi:10.1016/j.jaging.2012.09.001.

Wacker, R. R., & Roberto, K. A. (2014). *Community resources for older adults: Programs and services in an era of change* (4th ed.). Thousand Oaks, CA: Sage.

Weston, K. (1991). *Families we choose: Lesbians, gays, kinship*. New York, NY: Cambridge University Press.

Whitford, G. S. (1997). Realities and hopes for older gay males. *Journal of Gay and Lesbian Social Services, 6*, 79–95.

Wight, R. G., LeBlanc, A. J., de Vries, B., & Detels, R. (2012). Stress and mental health among midlife and older gay-identified men. *American Journal of Public Health, 102*, 503–510. doi:10.2105/AJPH.2011.300384.

Witten, T. M., & Eyler, A. E. (2012). Transgender and aging: Beginnings and becomings. In T. M. Witten & A. E. Eyler (Eds.), *Gay, lesbian, bisexual & transgender aging: Challenges in research, practice & policy* (pp. 187–269). Baltimore, MD: The Johns Hopkins University Press.

Deconstructing Multiple Oppressions Among LGBT Older Adults

4

Tracy Robinson-Wood and Amanda Weber

Abstract

The purpose of this chapter is to interrogate oppression through an analysis of discourses related to lesbian, gay, bisexual, and transgender (LGBT) older adults. As part of our reflexive posture, we attend to the social constructions of meaning about age, ability, gender, race, and sex and their colossal impacts on LGBT older adults. We are mindful of the weight of oppression for LGBT older adults in general but in particular overlooked subgroups of this diverse population (e.g., people who are with low income, people of color, and people who are transgender and do not fit into the binary of woman or man, gay or straight). We confront multiple layers of discrimination by deconstructing cultural assumptions of normalcy (e.g., heteronormativity within the LGBT community) presented in visual form, verbal text, and within discourses.

Keywords

LGBT elders · Ageism · Racism · Homophobia · Transphobia · Multiple oppressions

Overview

In this chapter, we examine gender and sexuality, race, privileged queer identities, and policy issues affecting lesbian, gay, bisexual, and transgender (LGBT) older adults. A case study with discussion questions concludes our work. The following tenets guide our formulations and constructions of meaning: (1) Sexuality is fluid; (2) there is a difference between LGBT identity and same-sex behavior; (3) differences as well as inequities exist within the LGBT population and mirror the differences and inequities that exist among non-LGBT and the under-65 population; (4) there is inadequate attention devoted to ethnic and racial diversity among LGBT older adults; (5) there is inadequate attention devoted to transgender issues in the research on LGBT older adults; and (6) patriarchy and racism produce and

T. Robinson-Wood (✉)
Northeastern University, Boston, USA
e-mail: tr.robinson@neu.edu

A. Weber
Boston College, Chestnut Hill, Boston, MA 02467, USA
e-mail: weberai@bc.edu

perpetuate silence about race and transgender among LGBT older adults.

As authors, we bring our lens, biases, and positions to the writing of this chapter. We acknowledge our subjectivity informed by our location within multiple identities. We are heterosexual and lesbian, faculty member and graduate student in counseling psychology, black and white, married and single, and baby boomer and millennial. Despite our differences, our similarities are greater and galvanize us to speak truth to power. We monitor our proximity to a multitude of live discourses in our interactions with LGBT people and clients. We have queried ourselves and one another about the unconscious and/or unspoken discourses that lie beneath socially constructed categories of difference relative to LGBT older adults.

Learning Objectives

Upon completion of this chapter, the reader should be able to:

1. Understand the role of discourses in the lives of LGBT individuals in general and for LGBT elders, in particular.
2. Understand the multiple impacts of racism, sexism, homophobia, transphobia, and biphobia on the LGBT older adult population.
3. Understand the roles of policies and laws on older LGBT individuals.

Introduction

Within the last few years, the United States of America (USA) has witnessed dramatic changes regarding who can legally marry. As of the writing of this book, nineteen states now sanction marriage between two women or two men. The heterosexist discourse is being challenged that dictates that marriage between a normal XY male and a normal XX female is the only acceptable union that warrants legal protection. Another major cultural shift pertains to people with 65 years of age and older. Older adults are living and working longer than ever before. Although the actual numbers are inaccurate, millions of older adults are LGBT. In not being young and not being heterosexual, LGBT older adults are distinguished by multiple identities that run counter to the dominant culture's fascination with and insistence on youth, beauty, and traditional gender roles (Robinson-Wood 2013).

Ageism or age discrimination is fueled by a cultural belief that people who are middle-aged and older are past their prime, disabled and unproductive that denies the vast diversity among old LGBT adults. Although successful aging refers to the physical and emotional ability to thrive, cope, socialize, and learn (Van Wagenen et al. 2013), the USA culture places considerable emphasis on anti-aging, youth, and the body beautiful (Robinson-Wood 2013). Ageism and ableism intersect and are codependent on one another for their existence.

Gender prescriptions normalized by heterosexuals extend to LGBT populations. Moreover, the social construction of race is evident within the LGBT community. LGBT individuals of color experience more psychological distress, financial instability, limited access to culturally competent care, and housing inequality than their white counterparts.

Discrimination occurs among most LGBT older adults; however, vast intragroup differences exist and are related to disability, age, gender status, race, income, the quality of aging, and identity development. An LGBT older adult, who is transgender, single, working class, a person of color, and resides with friends in an apartment, lives in a society where his or her gender, sexuality, and marital status are inconsistent with cultural values such as patriarchy, heterosexual marriage, home ownership, economic success, and reproduction. Conversely, the middle-class gay male, who is married to and living with his husband, has children, and owns a home, occupies identity statuses that are culturally privileged and valued.

The purpose of this chapter is to interrogate oppression through an analysis of discourses related to LGBT older adults. As part of our reflexive posture, we attend to the social constructions of meaning about age, ability, gender, race, and sex and their colossal impacts on LGBT older adults. We are mindful of the weight of oppression for LGBT older adults in general but in particular overlooked subgroups of this diverse population (e.g., people who are with low income, people of color, and people who are transgender and do not fit into the binary of woman or man, gay or straight). We confront multiple layers of discrimination by deconstructing cultural assumptions of normalcy (e.g., heteronormativity within the LGBT community) presented in visual form, verbal text, and within discourses.

Self-Check Exercise: What kind of messages did you receive from your family about LGBT people and the elderly? What is your proximity to current discourses about LGBT elders? Do you know any persons who are LGBT elders?

Weedon (1987) defined *discourses* "as ways of constituting knowledge, together with the social practices, forms of subjectivity, and power relations which inhere in such knowledge and relations between them. Discourses are more than ways of thinking and producing meaning, they constitute the 'nature' of the body, unconscious and conscious mind, and emotional life of the subjects they seek to govern" (p. 105). Discourses can be subtle, yet they are pervasive throughout society and hold enormous power. Discourses can be unconscious. They can be insidious in that people are unaware of where they are located within and positioned by certain other discourses (Robinson-Wood 2013).

Discourses portray older people as homogenous, feeble, disabled, unproductive, asexual, unattractive, and forgetful (Robinson-Wood 2013). The tenets of patriarchy privilege LGBT older adults whose lives are most closely aligned with dominant cultural values and norms. In America, marriage, youth, gender conformity, wealth, ability, heterosexuality, and white skin operate as valued identities and commodities.

Falling outside of this cultural swath has significant implications for financial stability, employment, dating, marriage, access to and quality of health care, and social capital.

Discussion Box: Can you think of any movies (non-musicals) where LGBT elders have been depicted? What were their lives like? What race were they? How similar were their lives to cultural values? How do movies reinforce dominant cultural values and often perpetuate race, gender, and sexuality stereotypes?

LGBT Older Adults

Within the next 15 years, the number of older adults in the USA will nearly double, from 38 to 72 million. In 2030, one in five Americans will be 65 or older (Grant et al. 2010a). Between 2012 and 2030, the non-Hispanic white population is expected to increase by 54 % compared to 125 % for older racial and ethnic minority populations, including Hispanics (155 %), African Americans (104 %), American Indian and Native Alaskans (116 %), and Asians (119 %) (US Department of Health and Human Services 2012). Widely represented among LGBT older adults are people of color: black (non-Hispanic), Hispanic, American Indian or Native Alaskan, Asian or Pacific Islander. See Chaps. 6–8, and 10 respectfully, for further discussion on these groups.

Self-Check Exercise: What does deconstruction mean to you? How does deconstruction take place within society? Social construction suggests that society creates race, gender, and sexuality as meaningful categories of privilege and oppression among people. Society makes sense of these meanings, and difference is created rather than intrinsic to a phenomenon. Deconstruction is taking part; unlearning;

analyzing the way that meaning was constructed; and engaging in a different process of social construction with different meanings and outcomes.

Health and policy researchers have examined the implications of this dramatic increase in the numbers of older adults with respect to Medicare, the sustainability and availability of social security, healthcare affordability, retirement pensions, and tax revenues. LGBT older adults have recent scant attention from researchers. Approximately 3.5 % of the adult population or 8 million adults in the USA are lesbian, gay, or bisexual. Over 700,000 people are transgender (The Williams Institute, 2011). Due largely to advances in health care, aging baby boomers are living longer than those in previous decades. There are also significant numbers of LGBT people among aging baby boomers. Nonetheless, LGBT aging has been grossly understudied in health research.

Examining 2010 Census data, demographer Gary Gates (August 25, 2011) from the Williams Institute Study reports that in the USA there are 901,997 same-sex couples who are represented in 99 % of the counties. The 2010 Census included LGBT persons; however, marital status was queried but not sexual orientation. For instance, a woman living with another woman to whom she is not married could check the "unmarried partner" box. According to Gates (2011), as many as 15 % of same-sex couples were not identified as same-sex couples in the 2010 Census. Approximately 10 % of same-sex couples described their relationship as "roommates" or "non-relatives" and not as "spouses" or "unmarried couples." When queried further, researchers learned that confidentiality was a concern among one-quarter of respondents. One-third took issue with the Census for not asking about sexual orientation or gender identity. Some people were offended by the options presented to them.

The actual percentage of the LGBT population is a complex issue. People can and do, for a variety of reasons, conceal and/or camouflage their sexuality. The invisibility of LGBT sexuality and, in some cases, lack of disclosure about one's sexual status presents methodological obstacles to research investigations on aging. The fluidity of sexuality over time and the nebulous nature of defining LGBT identity confound the methodological difficulties involved with researching this population. Estimates of persons who report any lifetime same-sex sexual behavior and any same-sex sexual attraction are substantially higher than estimates of those who identify as lesbian, gay, or bisexual. The distinction between behavior and identity may be illuminating. An estimated 19 million Americans (8.2 %) report that they have engaged in same-sex sexual behavior. Nearly 25.6 million Americans (11 %) acknowledge at least some same-sex sexual attraction.

According to Rust (2006), a person's "sexual landscape might change, thus creating new opportunities for self-description while transforming or eliminating existing possibilities" (p. 174). LGBT individuals may be recently out, whereas others have been out for a lifetime since adolescence or early adulthood. Others lived primarily heterosexual lives and came out during middle adulthood. Some people have lived a portion of their lives according to a particular sexual orientation and have, with time, come to question their sexuality.

Methodological challenges withstanding in researching this largely invisible population (Shankle et al. 2003), recent research has begun to explore the unique issues LGBT older adults face. Pressing issues include these: (1) social isolation from communities of support; (2) identifying suitable and affordable LGBT-friendly housing; (3) elder abuse; (4) financial instability; and (5) health concerns related to aging (Grant et al. 2010a; Hash and Rogers 2013; Sargeant 2009; Fredriksen-Goldsen and Muraco 2010; Graham 2011; Hudson 2011; SAGE 2010). Research on the intersection of race and LGBT older adults has begun and is spearheaded by Services and Advocacy for GLBT Elders (SAGE) and the National Resource Center on LGBT Aging.

Gender and Sexuality

Gender refers to the complex interrelationship between those traits and one's internal sense of self as male, female, both, or neither as well as one's outward presentations and behaviors related to that perception (American Psychological Association 2006). Whereas sex refers to the XX and XY chromosome pairs for genetically healthy female or male (Atkinson and Hackett 1998), gender is a crucial part of identity presentation and representation across the life span. Although the meaning of gender varies among different cultures and changes throughout time (McCarthy and Holliday 2004), the most common definition refers to culturally determined attitudes, cognitions, and belief systems about females and males. Sex, gender, and gender expression are formed from interactions with parents, peers, and teachers and transmitted through the educational system, religious institutions, politics, and the media.

Gender marginalization can be found within the LGBT older adult community. Due to sexism or the institutionalized system of inequality based on the biological and social stratification of gender, LGBT individuals who are born male enjoy privileges that women and transgender persons do not. More specifically, power and privilege are conferred upon men who are viewed as masculine, powerful, and wealthy and conferred upon women who are regarded as attractive and emotionally available and pliable. As forms of expressions of one's gender, masculinity and femininity are shaped by traditional gender roles. Masculinity discourses embody men as aggressive, strong, and in control (much like America herself), whereas feminine discourses include female submission to men and masculinity validation. Lesbians, across age groups, suffer from gender discrimination by virtue of their sex and also due to a failure to compliment men as sexual and emotional partners (Sargeant 2009).

> **Discussion Box:** Lesbians, across age groups, suffer from gender discrimination by virtue of their sex and also due to a failure to compliment men as sexual and emotional partners (Sargeant 2009). Do you think this applies to lesbian elders?

Cisgender individuals are those who have gender-confirming identities where biological sex and gender match. This sex-gender congruity affords privilege and a cover of normalcy within society. Conversely, gender non-conformity refers to an individual's gender identity that does not align with biological sex; however, one's view of their sex is consistent with their sex at birth. Individuals who are gender non-conforming and transgender/transsexual (e.g., trans*) contest the dominant model of gender identity. People who are trans* may be biologically one sex but identify emotionally, physiologically, and psychologically with another sex or gender expression. They may identify as gay, lesbian, bisexual, or heterosexual. A male-to-female transsexual who has completed gender-confirming surgery might say: *I see myself being with a man, but I did not see myself as a man with a man. I saw myself as a woman with a man.*

According to the Diagnostic Statistic Manual of Mental Disorders (DSM)-5, people who are transgender have gender dysphoria. The DSM-5 is the diagnostic authority relied upon by all mental health clinicians to classify diagnostic codes for their patients, but this diagnosis can be controversial with people who are trans* and trans* rights advocates. Required for third-party billing, the DSM-5 has more than a 60-year history in the USA. Transgender is an umbrella term for people whose gender identity differs from that which is typically associated with their sexual assignment at birth. Often a source of confusion, transgender is not synonymous with homosexuality. Various transgender terms exist, including transsexual, genderqueer, transman, and transwomen.

Across race, class, culture, disability, and sexuality, gender influences what we believe about ourselves and others. Gender labels are applied to people, and, once assigned, people behave toward individuals based on a set of expectations for persons with the same label. Deviation from prescribed gender roles attracts notice and comment from a scrutinizing public. At the center of cultural and gender normativity is patriarchy through which gender oppression is maintained. Among older people, gender is eclipsed by age unless it is nestled within youthfulness or age defiance. Among people of color, gender tends to be obscured by race, in that race vies for more attention as the salient identity construct (Robinson-Wood 2013).

Social constructions of gender and sexual identity impact one's lived experience. The visible signs of aging that mark a person as undesirable or unappealing are a phenomenon in the LGBT community (Sargeant 2009). Ageism in the gay community is rampant with gay men being particularly vulnerable to becoming "too old" for relationships if over the age of 35 (Sargeant 2009). Gay and bisexual men are twice as likely to live alone as heterosexual men. Gay and bisexual men tend to have a harder time successfully aging, and they seemed to be overwhelmed and even depressed, in comparison with lesbian and bisexual women (Macdonald and Rich 1983; Schope 2005). Feminism has exerted a tremendous impact on the formation of lesbian and bisexual women's communities, thus inspiring resistance to and confrontation of ageism (Grant et al. 2010a).

Gay and bisexual men appear to have had little connection to dialogues in which queer women have participated (Grant et al. 2010a). The youth orientation of gay culture has helped to cultivate internalized ageism among some gay and bisexual men who feel rejected and isolated from the mainstream gay community. Schope (2005) took a different position and argues that gay men are actually better able to cope with aging than are heterosexual men.

Although lesbian and bisexual women are more likely to live alone than heterosexual women (Grant et al. 2010a), lesbians seem to fare better than their gay counterparts and have broader social support networks and community involvement. Many lesbians enjoy intimate and sexual relationships well into older adulthood (Kimmel et al. 2013) and are less likely to be viewed as unattractive as they age. The heteronormative standard of beauty has been critiqued by many older lesbians who refuse to be bound by body image ideals that harass heterosexual women (Kimmel et al. 2013). Although older lesbians are likely to be welcomed, respected, and even "treasured" by younger lesbians (Schope 2005), the challenge with this endearment is the perception of being patronized (Macdonald and Rich 1983).

Unlike the majority of lesbian, gay, and bisexual (LGB) individuals, many trans* individuals decide to transition later in life after retirement and after adult children have moved out of the house (Kimmel et al. 2013). The economic means to live one's gendered and sexual identity exists for many older trans* individuals; nonetheless, problems remain with dating, finding culturally competent healthcare providers, and coexisting within a marginalizing society. Little research is available on trans* individuals and how they live in older adulthood.

Privileged Queerness

Queer theorists have excluded LGBT older adults from their research in much the same way that LGBT older adults have been excluded from health care, policy, and mental health research. Brown (2009) argued that the producers of queer and gerontological theory communicate from a position of power that both silences and ignores the realities of LGBT older adults. She argues that homophobia, heterosexism in gerontology, and ageism in queer theory drive this production.

Halberstam (2005) identified two new terms in queer theory that have direct implications for LGBT older adults. Queer time and queer space is a model for minimizing the heteronormative gaze of aging. A new queer version centers on the present and is not focused on biological reproduction and the traditional family. Queer time and queer space questions the mainstream definition of healthy development and identity politics. Brown (2009) proposed that this perspective of living for today may have emanated from the AIDS epidemic during the 1980s, which had a profound and lasting impact on the LGBT community. Brown (2009) also postulates that queer theory has historically focused on the young, creating a power differential and a dismissal of LGBT older adults' voices, bodies, desires, and perspectives.

Research and media on LGBT individuals ignores stratification and diversity within the LGBT community. Television shows such as *The L Word* and *Will and Grace* made a valiant attempt to empower and give voice to LGBT individuals. LGBT portrayals were overwhelmingly problematic because they presented people in stereotypical and sensationalized fashion (Akita et al. 2013). Far too often, a preferred type of LGBT person blankets the media. Despite the number of prime time television shows that give voice to the LGBT experience, such as *Orange is the New Black* and *Gray's Anatomy,* more often than not, media reflect dominant discourses concerning which LGBT individuals are worthy of watching. People who are young, attractive, white, wealthy, promiscuous, dramatic, gender-conforming, and physically fit are iconic. Most LGBT individuals and heterosexuals do not resemble these unrealistic television images.

A bifurcated and binary system of gender and gender expression is still imposed at this point in the twenty-first century. Within this system some, albeit not all, LGBT individuals are positioned at the periphery of mainstream society, which can increase one's susceptibility to oppression, prejudice, and stereotyping. Adherence to a binary gender and sexuality system contributes to discrimination against bisexuals within the LGBT community. Men and women who identify as bisexual experience biphobia and may not be considered as serious romantic partners or are perceived to be in transition or experimenting sexually, similar to adolescence. Bisexuals and trans* individuals have historically been silenced and excluded with many regarding them as part of the "out group" within LGBT organizations and movements (Graham 2011). Little research is available on internalized transphobia and ageism within the trans* older adult population.

Internalized homophobia can cause serious mental health effects and is fairly prevalent in the LGBT older adult population. Although many LGBT older adults are typically well adjusted and mentally healthy (Graham 2011), the Aging Health Report (Fredriksen-Goldsen et al. 2011) stated that 26 % of the 2500 LGBT older adults in the project tried at one time or another to *not* be lesbian, gay, bisexual, or transgender. On a scale of 1–4 with 4 representing higher levels of stigma, the average level of stigma on a nine-item measure adapted from the Homosexuality-Related Stigma Scale was 1.5 for LGBT older adult participants; 1.3 for lesbians; 1.5 for bisexual women; 1.5 for bisexual men; and 1.8 for transgender older adults.

Multiple Oppressions Among and Between LGBT Older Adults

Defining systems of oppression is critical to a thoughtful analysis of the history of LGBT people during the twentieth and twenty-first centuries. Pre- and post-WWII era policies banned LGBT individuals from serving in the military. In 1952, the Diagnostic and Statistical Manual of Mental Disorders (DSM-I) published by the American Psychiatry Association referred to homosexuality, pedophilia, and sexual sadism (e.g., rape and mutilation) as sexual deviation. WWII and the DSM were watershed events that perpetuated a cultural belief about homosexuality—that it was pathological, immoral, deviant, and unpatriotic. LGBT individuals were banned from mainstream society; however, wartime accelerated social changes, providing recruits who joined the military with an opportunity to escape to large cities. Such an exodus served to jump-start the formation of large LGBT communities.

Senator McCarthy was intent on excising identifiable LGBT individuals from government positions through arrests, blackmail, and coercion. Many private businesses followed suit. LGBT individuals living through pre- and post-WWII were largely closeted. Exorbitant amounts of energy were spent cloaking the vestiges of their sexual orientation. Being out as a gay person was a serious threat to the state, personal safety, occupational, and residential security (Shankle et al. 2003).

A turning point for the social liberation of the LGBT community was Stonewall, a 1969 protest against police discrimination and brutality faced by countless openly LGBT individuals. The post-Stonewall generation is characterized by individuals who came of age during a period in history where homosexuality was less stigmatized (Shankle et al. 2003). In 1973, the American Psychiatry Association declassified homosexuality as a mental disorder.

During the 1980s' AIDS epidemic, the perception of gay men as deviant and unnatural was reified. Hudson (2011) states:

> Due to the perception of being lesbian, gay, bisexual, or transgender, 82 % of these older adults have been victimized at least once in their lives and nearly two-thirds at least three times. More than 66 % have experienced verbal insults; 42 % have been threatened with physical violence; 27 % have been hassled by police; 23 % faced the threat of being outed as LGBT; 22 % were not hired for a job; and 20 % had property damaged. Transgender older adults experience higher levels of victimization and discrimination than non-transgender older adults.

More so than in the past, the twenty-first century ushered in inclusive policies for the LGBT community, including the repeal of "Don't Ask; Don't Tell." Same-sex marriage is now legal across 19 states and the District of Columbia. Eight Native American tribes as well as nine states declare the ban on same-sex marriage as unconstitutional (Freedom to Marry 2013). On June 2, 2014, President Obama declared that gender confirmation surgery could be reviewed for possible Medicare coverage.

Policy Box: On June 2, 2014, President Obama declared that gender confirmation surgery could be reviewed by Medicare for coverage http://www.hhs.gov/dab/decisions/dabdecisions/dab2576.pdf.

Despite these important legal advancements, LGBT older adults face social isolation, high rates of suicidality, and depression. Among LGBT older adults, 59 % feel lonely and lack companionship, and 53 % feel isolated from others (Fredriksen-Goldsen et al. 2011). Recent research shows that lesbians, gay men, and bisexuals who have experienced prejudice-related life events were about three times more likely to have suffered a serious physical health problem over a one-year follow-up period compared to those who had not experienced such stressful events (Frost et al. 2011). The effects of prejudice-related events remain statistically significant after controlling for the experience of other stressful events and other factors known to affect physical health, such as age, gender, employment, and lifetime health history. Older LGBT adults have a lifetime of prejudice-related events as a function of living in a society that has struggled with extending equality to all people.

The Grand Master Status of Skin Color

Research is scarce on older adults of color who are LGBT. As a social construction, race is based on phenotype (i.e., hair, skin color, facial features). These variables do not accurately reflect one's race but rather represent a basis for assigning people to a particular racial group (Robinson-Wood 2013). Racism renders an explanation for why LGBT people of color are vulnerable to experiencing the worst outcomes and receiving the least institutional attention.

The aging concerns of LGBT older adults of color are virtually absent in national policy discussions on aging, health, and economic security (Auldridge and Espinoza 2013). LGBT older adults who are also people of color contend with racism and homophobia, which increases levels of psychological distress. Fredriksen-Goldsen et al. (2011) reported that Hispanic and Native American LGBT older adults are more likely to experience victimization than white LGBT older adults. She also reported that both Hispanic and Native American LGBT older adult participants report lower levels of general mental health, higher rates of depression, and more stress than do whites. The likelihood of neglect for Hispanic and black LGBT older adults is also greater. Compared to whites, Native Americans are more likely to experience anxiety, suicidal ideation, and loneliness. Asian/Pacific Islanders do not differ on mental health indicators from whites with one exception; Asian/Pacific Islanders have lower rates of suicidal ideation. The Center for Black Equity has hosted black LGBT Prides for years in an effort to grant LGBT people of color a separate voice outside of the mainstream LGBT community. Please visit the Center for Black Equity (http://centerforblackequity.org/) for more information on how this organization promotes social justice for black LGBT communities.

Some people of color understand the LGBT movement as complicit with an imperialistic culture in support of white superiority. A history of excluding some sexual, gender, and racial minorities influenced some people of color not to identify as LGBT but rather endorse other identifiers (e.g., third gender, down low, MSM, WSW, same gender-loving). Previous studies found that black men having sex with men (MSM) are generally less likely to self-identify as being "gay" when compared to white men, even when they are open about their sexuality (Han et al. 2014). Han et al. (2014) also found that black MSM do not identify as gay because of their marginalization in the larger gay community. Some black MSM men have come to reject what they perceive to be a narrow and non-inclusive definition of sexual relations with other men. Very little research has been conducted on marginalization among LGBT people of color in general and the trans* community of color in particular.

Racism is undeniable in the marginalization of far too many LGBT older adults of color. Research suggests that black and Latino elders experience poverty at twice the rate of the general US elder population. For LGBT elders, including many of color, a lifetime of employment discrimination translates into earning disparities, reduced lifelong earnings, smaller social security payments, and fewer opportunities to accumulate large pensions and retirement packages (Auldridge and Espinoza 2013).

Patriarchy and racism have contributed to the institutionalization of privilege for some and to disadvantage for others. Although context and situation are relevant, race occupies grand master status in that race has enormous power to eclipse other identities, such as socioeconomic class, professional dress, and title/position (Robinson-Wood 2013). LGBT older adults of color occupy multiple marginalized identities within a system where the grand master status of race is active with respect to one's position in society, experiences with discrimination, and overall treatment. Irrespective of gender and sexuality, elderly African Americans are more than three times as likely as elderly Caucasians to live in poverty, while elderly Hispanics are more likely than the older population to be poor and in need of long-term care. Elderly women also are highly vulnerable. Nearly three out of four older Americans who fall below the poverty line are women, and retirement incomes for older women average about 55 % of those for comparable men (SAGE 2010).

Internalized homophobia and transphobia exist among some LGBT people of color. Black men experience higher levels of internalized homophobia and are less likely to disclose their homosexual orientation. They are also more likely to perceive their friends and neighbors as disapproving of homosexuality (Graham 2011). In both the Latino and Asian American communities, cultural expectations surrounding family role obligations encourage the maintenance of strong ties to families of origin.

> ***Discussion Box***: Concerns about individual behavior that is outside of cultural dictates and subsequent implications for a family's honor or social standing can weigh heavily on groups characterized by a

collectivistic orientation. How has individualism or collectivism shaped your prescribed identities?

Cultural collectivism may discourage individuation that is commonly seen and necessary to the "coming out" process (Cochran et al. 2007). These cultural expectations may also cultivate internalized homophobia and transphobia experienced by some LGBT older adults.

LGBT Elder Policies in a Young, White, Rich, Straight, Valuing Culture

Half of Americans living with HIV will be over the age of 50 by 2015, and over 80 % of people with HIV are people of color (Hudson 2011). The National Hispanic Council on Aging (2013) recently released a report stating that HIV/AIDS disproportionately affects older gay men. Despite these disturbing data, HIV prevention programs targeted at older adults are virtually nonexistent. Doctors and other healthcare providers avoid talking with their older patients about HIV/AIDS risks (SAGE 2010; Davis 2013). Many healthcare providers endorse the belief that LGBT older adults are not sexually active or are not included in their patient database (National Resource Center on LGBT Aging 2013). Failure to provide adequate care to LGBT individuals is the unfortunate result.

Access to health insurance and to culturally competent healthcare providers is vital to LGBT older adults. That said, LGBT older adults use health care less often than their heterosexual counterparts (Graham 2011). LGBT individuals face stigma from the larger society and also at the physician's office. LGBT individuals face discrimination in the healthcare system that can lead to difficulty obtaining care, denial of care, or to the delivery of inadequate care (Graham 2011). The National Resource Center on LGBT Aging (2013) outlined a few misconceptions often heard from healthcare providers: (1) We do not have any LGBT older adult clients; (2) I can identify the LGBT individuals within my service population; (3) I treat everyone as equal; (4) there is not a distinction between gender and sexual identity; and (5) it is illegal to ask about a person's sexual orientation or gender identity. Healthcare providers' inability to recognize differences between the LGBT older population and the heterosexual population can be costly to LGBT older adults whose histories include an active substance abuse or chronic illness such as HIV/AIDS and/or depression. For trans* individuals, hormones must be monitored and adjusted as people age (Fredriksen-Goldsen et al. 2014).

Research Box: As individuals age, it is important for doctors to monitor trans* individuals' hormones and adjust testosterone and estrogen levels as they fluctuate with age. Estrogen and testosterone can have effects on menopause, osteoporosis, hair loss, weight distribution, and ovarian and breast cancer as adult age. See http://transhealth.ucsf.edu/trans?page=protocol-aging for more information. How do hormones play a role in trans* individuals' life? Are medical intake forms asking broad enough questions to understand possible medical issues that trans* individuals may face? How do black market hormones play a role in medical care?

In long-term care facilities where LGBT older adults are at their most vulnerable stage, discrimination endures. A recent national report with LGBT older adults found that more than half of the survey's respondents believed that staff or other residents would abuse or neglect an LGBT elder. The same study revealed that respondents reported a disproportionate amount of mistreatment in long-term care facilities out of fear of and hatred toward LGBT people, even among those who are elderly (Auldridge and Espinoza 2013). Many LGBT older adults continue to be forced into the closet and are forbidden to make essential choices about and for their partners. Because, in most cases, LGBT couples are not legally recognized, hospital visitation policies may exclude same-sex partners or other family members, which can impede or complicate critical health decision-making processes (Grant et al. 2010a). Although President Obama issued a memorandum (House 2010) allowing for LGBT couples to make decisions for each other, many hospitals and long-term care agencies refuse to follow suit.

Another challenge for LGBT older adults is financial insecurity as they enter retirement. Overall, 42 % of all LGBT elders indicated that "financial problems" are a big concern in their lives (SAGE 2010). Many LGBT individuals have faced historical employment discrimination that has resulted in lower levels of financial security throughout life and that directly affects retirement income and social security payouts. A recent article by *New York Times* economists Tara Siegel Bernard and Ron Lieber estimated the added costs incurred by a hypothetical same-sex couple between $41,196 and $467,562 (Grant et al. 2010a). The poverty rate for senior gay couples is 5 and 9 % for lesbian couples (SAGE 2010). Trans* individuals are more likely to live in extreme poverty and are nearly four times more likely to have a household income of less than $10,000/year as compared to the general population (Grant et al. 2010b). Employment discrimination against trans* individuals is rampant; 90 % of those surveyed reported harassment, mistreatment, or discrimination (Grant et al. 2010b) with no legal protection because the Employment Non-Discrimination Act (ENDA) has not passed through Congress yet. With the repeal of the Defense of Marriage Act (DOMA), LGBT older adults are able to receive retirement benefits, social security, benefits for military action, and Medicaid after their spouse is deceased. This important legislation does not alleviate the lost financial opportunities for LGBT older adults whose partners died prior to DOMA.

Recently, the US Department of Housing and Development (HUD) (Friedman et al. 2013) released a study about housing discrimination toward individuals who identify as LGBT. HUD (Friedman et al. 2013) concluded that gross estimates of discrimination, which reflect the extent to which heterosexual couples were consistently favored over gay male or lesbian couples, are 15.9 and 15.6 %, respectively. Sexual orientation and gender identity are not federally protected classes. In efforts to end housing discrimination against LGBT individuals, on February 3, 2012, HUD published its Final Rule, "Equal Access to Housing in HUD Programs regardless of Sexual Orientation or Gender Identity." This ruling prohibits HUD-assisted organizations from discriminating on the basis of sexuality or gender identity. There is very little recourse for LGBT individuals when other organizations continue to discriminate, particularly with laws written as they are.

Contending with financial insecurities, housing, and other types of chronic discrimination is a breeding ground for social isolation and depression. LGBT older adults may be denied housing, including residency in mainstream retirement communities, based on their sexual orientation, gender identity, and expression. This discrimination may separate LGBT older adults from beloved friends or partners or push them into homelessness (SAGE 2010). In response to systemic housing discrimination, some LGBT older adults have created non-mainstream retirement communities that honor diversity. LGBT older adults have even been able to erect small retirement communities and assisted living communities. For resources and advocacy groups, please visit theses Web sites for more information (Legal Resources: http://www.lambdalegal.org/ and http://www.hrc.org/resources/entry/maps-of-state-laws-policies.

Research Box: Research shows that the rate of homelessness among elders has increased in the last decade with about 2,960,000 elder adults who are homeless. Rates for LGBT older adults homelessness are currently not recorded, but 30 % of LGB older adult couples faced housing discrimination and 19 % of trans* older adults being denied a home or an apartment.

Policy Impact and Mental Health for LGBT Older Adults

As individuals transition into older adulthood, multiple challenges arise, such as disability and loss of loved ones. Compared to their heterosexual counterparts, lesbian, gay, and bisexual older adults are at an elevated risk of disability and psychological distress (Hudson 2011). A 2006 study reported evidence of higher levels of depression and psychological distress among midlife and older lesbians and gay men, which the researchers attribute to the accumulated effect of a lifetime of stigma (SAGE 2010).

Defined as chronic stress related to stigmatization and actual experiences of discrimination and violence, minority stress has been found to increase loneliness in LGBT older adults (SAGE 2010). An alarming 41 % (out of 6450 individuals) of trans* older respondents reported attempting suicide compared to 1.6 % in the general population (Grant et al. 2010a). In an effort to address disparities, former Secretary Kathleen Sebelius of the US Department of Health and Humans Services (HHS) announced on June 29, 2011, that HHS would begin collecting data through population health surveys to facilitate identification of health issues (National Resource Center on LGBT Aging 2013).

In light of the mental health disparities between heterosexual and LGBT older adults, there is a distinction between health policies that perpetuate marginalization and policies that protect human rights. Policy differences between state and federal governments are a hindrance to having full protection under federal mandates. Medicaid now offers benefits to legally married same-sex couples. Prior to 2014, this was not the case. Thousands of people have access to healthcare providers. The Institute of Medicine (IOM) defines access to health care as the "timely use of personal health services to achieve the best possible outcomes." With the passage of the Affordable Care Act (ACA), LGBT older adults will have health insurance previously unavailable. Moreover, the ACA has created an insurance-based system that allows LGBT individuals access to healthcare plans targeted for same-sex families and trans* individuals. Unfortunately, homophobia and multicultural incompetence from healthcare professionals have contributed to primary care underutilization for many LGBT individuals (Grant et al. 2010a).

The Federal Family Caregivers Support Program, which was created with the 2000 reauthorization of the Older Americans Act and amended in 2006, expanded its definition of family caregivers to include extended LGBT family members (Grant et al. 2010a). This program provides LGBT individuals who are caregivers to partners or family members by choice with the ability to utilize respite care, counseling, support groups, and training groups. This bill is significant for many reasons. First, it reflects social justice and basic human rights. Second, when the data are examined, it is evident that LGBT individuals are more likely than are heterosexuals to report a disability: 41 % aged 50 and older report a disability (Hudson 2011).

The Family Caregivers Support Program broadened the definition of families in 2006. In 2013, with the repeal of the Defense of Marriage Act (DOMA), individuals were protected by the Family Medical Leave Act (FMLA). FMLA allows people to take extended periods of paid leave to care for their partners (United States Department of Labor 2013). Family of choice is critical for caregiving given the substantial numbers of LGBT older adults receiving support from families of choice or partners; 27 % provide assistance to someone close to them with a health issue. A national survey of LGBT baby boomers by the MetLife Mature Market Institute found that 42 % of LGBT caregivers reported assisting partners, friends, neighbors, or others outside of their families of origin. Another recent study found 32 % of gay men and lesbians providing some sort of informal caregiving; 61 % of their care recipients were friends, and 13 % were partners (Grant et al. 2010a). There is a limited research on trans* individuals with respect to family of choice and caregiving. The National Center for Transgender Equality (Grant et al. 2010b) stated that 55 % of respondents experienced family rejection; 45 % of respondents reported that their family is as strong today as it was before coming out.

Case Study

In the case study of Ginger, we see a common story that is told among transwomen veterans. Pay close attention to the intersections of gender, race, age, religion, employment, and substance use in Ginger's life.

Ginger was born male. For as long as Ginger could remember, being male felt like a mistake. Ginger had a military career for over three decades. Once Ginger left the military, she went to culinary school and worked as a chef for ten years. Ginger is now retired. For the last two years, Ginger's outward appearance has been feminine with respect to appearance, hairstyle, makeup, dress, and mannerism. Ginger identified as a male for 60 years but did not identify as gay in her attraction to men. For her 65 birthday, Ginger's gift to herself is gender-confirming/reassignment surgery. Ginger's youngest sister is present to support Ginger before and after the surgery. Raised in a very devout Catholic, Puerto Rican family that vehemently denounced Ginger's interest in girls' toys and clothes, Ginger could not reconcile being openly transgender with her family. Out of respect for her parents' feelings and reputation, her plan was to come out after both her parents died. At the age of 60, Ginger decided the wait was over. Both her parents are in their late 80s and enjoy good health. Ginger is determined to live the remaining years of her life as authentically and honestly as possible. Married to a woman for 16 years, Ginger fathered three children who are now adults in their 40s. Her children have limited contact largely due to Ginger's emotional unavailability to them and her history of addiction. Ginger credits her sanity to a good therapist whom she has seen for three years. In therapy, Ginger learned that she was dying as she waited for her parents to die. She also came to realize that respect was not driving her decision to come out after her parents' deaths but fear,

deception, and shame. Therapy also helped Ginger think about what it means to be an older transsexual woman of color. Throughout her life, Ginger battled not only heterosexism but also racism, sexism, internalized self-hatred, and ageism. She also struggled with alcoholism but has been sober for eight years with the help of Alcoholics Anonymous. Therapy provided a space for Ginger to declare that she was a transfemale who has always been and is currently attracted to men. Her decision to undergo surgery was not attached to the presence of a life partner, although finding a loving relationship with a man is something that Ginger desires. She has found dating to be challenging, especially as she ages. Once Ginger came out as a transgender, Ginger's parents ceased communication, claiming that Manuel (Ginger's birth name) is dead to them.

Self-Check Exercise: Pair and share with another student in the classroom. Discuss your feelings about Ginger. How do you feel about her decision to marry when she knew she was queer? What are your feelings about Ginger's surgery at age 60? How do socially constructed notions of beauty, age, and sexuality collide for Ginger and/or impact your feelings about her life choices?

Discussion of Case Study

Trans* individuals may be less likely to disclose their sexuality than their heterosexual counterparts. Ginger resisted the asexualization of her sexuality by disclosing her sexuality and stepping into her life as the female that she knew she was. Disclosure of sexual and gender identity can lead to an array of social and community support in the LGBT community (Fredriksen-Goldsen et al. 2011). Mental healthcare providers are encouraged to be familiar with community resources. Knowledge of sexual identity development models (e.g., Cass 1979 and Troiden

1989) can assist the clinician in understanding phases and junctures of development, from fragmentation to affirmation (Robinson-Wood 2013). Ginger's therapist needs knowledge of the historical implications of homophobia and transphobia on transgender individuals, medical care concerns, particularly given Ginger's recent surgery and continued hormone use, and aspects of LGBT culture for older transwomen.

Hardacker et al. (2013) and the Howard Brown Health Center (HBHC) developed the nurses' Health Education About LGBT Elders (HEALE) curriculum, a 6-h cultural competency curriculum that focuses on providing training for nurses and other direct caregivers (for more information, visit http://www.nursesheale.org/curriculum/). Individuals who have been trained using the HEALE modules have shown increase in health care providers' confidence in administering culturally sensitive care to older LGBT individuals. There are six modules that would be helpful for Ginger's medical team to review: (1) introduction to the LGBT elder community; (2) barriers to health care and health disparity; (3) sex and sexuality of LGBT elders; (4) legal concerns for LGBT elders; (5) an introduction to transgender community; and (6) human immunodeficiency virus (HIV) and aging (Hardacker et al. 2013).

Interprofessional collaborations are needed to provide the best care for Ginger. A multipronged approach would encompass nursing, geriatric medicine, and psychosocial education. Ginger's multiculturally competent therapist needs the ability to create a holding environment for Ginger's excitement, fear, anger, and shame while facilitating the acquisition of skills needed to be healthy and whole as a transwoman of color in a society that struggles with extending justice and decency for Ginger and others like her.

Summary

LGBT older adults have faced a lifetime of discrimination yet continue to fight for equality and resist homophobia and ageism. A 63-year-old gay man quoted in The Aging Health Report (Fredriksen-Goldsen et al. 2011) said, "The LGBT community has stepped up in the past to address coming out, AIDS, and civil rights. The next wave has to be aging." LGBT older adults have a distinct experience of aging stemming from shared experiences in relation to the LGBT community, the lifelong process of coming out, the experience of sexual and gender minority stress, marginalization inside and outside LGBT communities, and LGBT pride and resilience (Van Wagenen et al. 2013).

LGBT older adults have created families of choice when biological family is physically removed or emotionally detached. Family of choice is one way that older LGBT adults thrive and alleviate isolation and depression. In many ways, the LGBT older adult community shows resilience (Fredriksen-Goldsen et al. 2011) and the ability to handle adversity and challenges successfully, which are important keys to maintaining good physical, social, and mental health. Meyer et al. (2011) found that participants spoke of the positive aspects of exposure to stigmatizing experiences. Some who identify as a LGBT individual, and for some, persons of color and women, felt like they were *better people* for surviving and thriving in the midst of oppression. It is possible that some LGBT older adults may be in a better position to age successfully compared to their heterosexual counterparts because some older LGBT adults have acquired strengths, including adaptability, self-reliance, advocacy skills, crisis competencies, and gender role flexibility (Hash and Rogers 2013).

Discussion Box

1. What are issues experienced by trans* individuals that may differ from those experienced by gay men or lesbians?
2. Is there a relationship between cumulative and multiple oppressions (racism, heterosexism, transphobia, ageism) and Ginger's addiction to alcohol?

3. What are the health implications of surgery and hormones at Ginger's age and as she continues to age?
4. Although sexual orientation is unlikely to change (APA 2009), some persons modify their identity (e.g., change their reference group or self-label behavior). What was the impact on Ginger in her early years when trying to deny her sexual and gender identities?

Experiential Exercises (3)

1. Draw four stick figures on the board and label them each as follows: sex, gender, sexual attraction, and sexual behaviors. As a group, have people draw what each of these four categories mean on the stick figures. After you are finished, discuss identities and how they intersect.
2. Create a character that embodies several of the identities in the chapter (older adult, LGB, trans*, and person of color). Have each individual partner up and role-play a scene that would be common in their profession (counselor, nurse, social worker). Ask each pair of individuals to discuss challenges in the conversation.
3. Watch "Gen Silent" and discuss how loss, health, sexuality, gender, and family play important roles in people's lives as they age.

Multiple-Choice Questions (5)

1. Based on the social stratification of gender, which of the following groups benefit from privilege among LGBT populations?
   a. Those born as female
   b. Those born as male

c. Those with gender reassignment
d. None of the above
2. Individuals who have gender-conforming identities where biological sex and gender match are referred to as:
   a. Bisexual
   b. Transgender
   c. Cisgender
   d. Questioning
3. Which of these is an instance of homophobia and elder abuse?
   a. An individual says that a woman with short hair looks like a man.
   b. An older gentleman is visiting his partner in a nursing home, a nurses aid enters the room and says please leave visitation rights are only for family members only.
   c. A grocery store bagger helps carry out an older woman's bags to her car.
   d. A doctor forgetting to ask about an older individual's sexual behaviors.
4. What are older LGBT individuals more at risk of developing than the older heterosexual population?
   a. More friendships
   b. Arthritis
   c. Dementia
   d. Depression
5. What are discourses?
   a. Ways of constituting knowledge, together with the social practices, forms of subjectivity.
   b. Power relations that inhere in such knowledge and relations between them.
   c. Practices based on knowledge
   d. a and b

Key

1-b
2-c
3-b
4-d
5-d

Resources

A Report of the National Transgender Discrimination Survey: http://endtransdiscrimination.org/.

Lambda Legal: www.lambdalegal.org/.

National Center for Lesbian Rights: http://www.nclrights.org/.

National Center for Transgender Equality: http://transequality.org/.

National Gay and Lesbian Task Force: http://www.thetaskforce.org/.

National Resource Center on LGBT Aging: http://lgbtagingcenter.org/.

Nurses HEALE Curriculum: http://www.nursesheale.org/curriculum/.

References

Akita, K., Besel, R. D., Comeforo, K., Drushel, B., Guthrie, J., Hidahl, B., & Zingsheim, J. (2013). *Queer media images: LGBT perspectives*. T. Carilli, & J. Campbell (Eds.). Lexington Books.

Auldridge, A., Espinoza, R. (2013). *Health equity and LGBT elders of color: Recommendations for policy and practice*. Retrieved from SAGE website: http://issuu.com/LGBTagingcenter/docs/sage_LGBT_healthequities/1?e=2766558/2092028.

American Psychological Association. (2006). *Answers to your questions about transgender individuals and gender identity*. Retrieved May, 17, 2014 from: http://www.whitehouse.gov/omb/fedreg_race-ethnicity.

Atkinson, D. R., & Hackett, G. (1998). *Counseling diverse populations*. McGraw-Hill.

Brown, M. T. (2009). LGBT aging and rhetorical silence. *Sexuality Research and Social Policy Journal of NSRC, 6*(2), 65–78.

Cass, V. C. (1979). Homosexual identity formation: a theoretical model. *Journal of Homosexuality, 9*, 219–235.

Cochran, S. D., Mays, V. M., Alegria, M., Ortega, A. N., & Takeuchi, D. (2007). Mental health and substance use disorders among Latino and Asian American lesbian, gay, and bisexual adults. *Journal of Consulting and Clinical Psychology, 75*(5), 785–794.

Davis, T., (2013). *An exploratory study of primary care providers' HIV prevention practices among older adults* (Unpublished doctoral dissertation). University of Kentucky, Lexington, KY.

Fredriksen-Goldsen, K. I., & Muraco, A. (2010). Aging and sexual orientation: A 25-year review of the literature. *Research on Aging, 32*(3), 372–413.

Fredriksen-Goldsen, K. I., Hoy-Ellis, C. P., Goldsen, J., Emlet, C. A., & Hooyman, N. R. (2014).Creating a vision for the future: Key competencies and strategies for culturally competent practice with lesbian, gay, bisexual, and transgender (LGBT) older adults in the health and human services. *Journal of Gerontological Social Work*, (ahead-of-print), 1–28.

Fredriksen-Goldsen, K. L., Kim, H., Emlet, A. C., Muraco, A., Erosheva, A. E., & Hoy-Ellis. (2011). *The aging and health report: Disparities and resilience among lesbian, gay, bisexual, and transgender older adults*. Retrieved from Caring and Aging with Pride website: http://caringandaging.org/wordpress/wp-content/uploads/2012/10/Full-report10-25-12.pdf.

Freedom to Marry. (2013). *Why marriage matters to native Americans*. Retrieved from http://www.freedomtomarry.org/communities/entry/c/native-americans.

Friedman, S., Reynolds, A., Scovill, S., Brassier, F. R., Campbell, R., & Ballou, M. (2013). *An estimate of housing discrimination against same-sex couples*. Available at SSRN.

Frost, D. M., Lehavot, K., & Meyer, I. H. (2011). Minority stress and physical health among sexual minorities. Poster Presented at the american Psychological Association, Washington, DC. Retrieved from https://escholarship.org/uc/item/6h25x5sh.

Gates, G. J. (2011). How many people are lesbian, gay, bisexual and transgender? Retrieved April 6, 2014 from http://williamsinstitute.law.ucla.edu/wpcontent/uploads/Gates-How-Many-People-LGBT-Apr-2011.pdf.

Graham, R. (2011). *The health of lesbian, gay, bisexual, and transgender people: Building a foundation for better understanding*. Washington, D.C: Institute of Medicine, The National Academic Press.

Grant, J. M., Koskovich, G., Frazer, S., & Bjerk, S. (2010a). *Outing age 2010: Public policy issues affecting gay, lesbian, bisexual, and transgender older adults*. National Gay and Lesbian Task Force.

Grant, J. M., Mottet, L. A., Tanis, J., Herman, J. L., Harrison, J., & Keisling, M. (2010b). National transgender discrimination survey report on health and health care. *National Center for Transgender Equality and National Gay and Lesbian Task Force*. Washington, DC, 1–23.

Halberstam, J. (2005). *In a queer time and place: Transgender bodies, subcultural lives*. NYU Press.

Hardacker, C. T., Rubinstein, B., Hotton, A., & Houlberg, M. (2013). Adding silver to the rainbow: The development of the nurses' health education about LGBT elders (HEALE) cultural competency curriculum. *Journal of Nursing Management, 22*, 257–266.

Hash, K. M., & Rogers, A. (2013). Clinical practice with older LGBT clients: Overcoming lifelong stigma through strength and resilience. *Clinical Social Work Journal, 41*(3), 249–257.

House, W. (2010). Presidential memorandum: Hospital visitation. Retrieved from https://www.whitehouse.

gov/the-press-office/presidential-memorandum-hospital-visitation.

Han, C. S., Rutledge, S. E., Bond, L., Lauby, J., & LaPollo, A. B. (2014). You're better respected when you carry yourself as a man": Black men's personal accounts of the down low "lifestyle. *Sexuality and Culture, 18*(1), 89–102.

Hudson, R. B. (2011). Integrating lesbian, gay, bisexual, and transgender older adults into aging policy and practice. *Public Policy and Aging Report, 21*(3), 1–35.

Kimmel, D. C., Rose, T., & David, S. (Eds.). (2013). *Lesbian, gay, bisexual, and transgender aging: Research and clinical perspectives.* Columbia University Press.

Macdonald, B., & Rich, C. (1983). *Look me in the eye: Old women, aging, and ageism.* Tallahassee: Spinsters Ink.

Meyer, I. H., Ouellette, S. C., Haile, R., & McFarlane, T. A. (2011). "We'd be free": Narratives of life without, or sexism. *Sexuality Research and Social Policy, 8*(3), 204–214.

McCarthy, J., & Holliday, E. L. (2004). Help-seeking and counseling within a traditional male gender role: An examination from multicultural perspective. *Journal of Counseling and Development, 82*, 25–30.

National Resource Center on LGBT Aging. (2013). *Inclusive questions for older adults: A practical guide to collecting data on sexual orientation and gender identity.* Retrieved from National Resource Center on LGBT Aging website: http://www.LGBTagingcenter.org/resources/resource.cfm?r=601.

Robinson-Wood, T. L. (2013). *The convergence of race, ethnicity, and gender: Multiple identities in counseling* (4th ed.). New Jersey: Pearson Education Inc.

Rust, P. C. (2006). Sexual identity adn bisexual identities: The struggle for self-description in a changing sexual landscape. In T. E. Orr (Ed.), *The social construction of difference and inequality: Race, class, gender and sexuality* (pp. 169–186). Boston: McGraw-Hill.

SAGE & MAP. (2010, March). *Improving the lives of GBT older adults.* New York and Denver, CO: Author.

Sargeant, M. (2009). Age discrimination, sexual orientation and gender identity: UK/US perspectives. *Equal Opportunities International, 28*(8), 634–645.

Schope, R. D. (2005). Who's afraid of growing old? Gay and lesbian perceptions of aging. *Journal of Gerontological Social Work, 45*(4), 23–39.

Shankle, M. D., Maxwell, C. A., Katzman, E. S., & Landers, S. (2003). An invisible population: Older lesbian, gay, bisexual, and transgender individuals. *Clinical Research and Regulatory Affairs, 20*(2), 159–182.

The National Hispanic Council on Aging. (2013). In their own words: A needs assessment of Hispanic LGBT older adults. Retrieved from The National Hispanic Council on Aging website: http://www.nhcoa.org/wp-content/uploads/2014/02/NHCOA-Hispanic-LGBT-Older-Adult-Needs-Assessment-In-Their-Own-Words.pdf.

Troiden, R. R. (1989). The formation of homosexual identities. *Journal of Homosexuality, 17*, 43–73.

United States Department of Labor. (2013). *Fact sheet #28F: Qualifying reasons for leave under the Family and Medical Leave Act.* Retrieved from http://www.dol.gov/whd/regs/compliance/whdfs28f.htm.

U.S. Department of Health and Human Services, Administration on Aging. (2012). A profile of older Americans: 2012. Retrieved May 15, 2014, from http://www.aoa.gov/Aging_Statistics/Profile/2012/docs/2012profile.pdf.

Van Wagenen, A., Driskell, J., & Bradford, J. (2013). "I'm still raring to go": Successful aging among lesbian, gay, bisexual, and transgender older adults. *Journal of Aging Studies, 27*(1), 1–14.

Weedon, C. (1987). *Feminist practice and poststructuralist theory.* New York: Blackwell Publishing.

The Intersection of Identities of LGBT Elders: Race, Age, Sexuality, and Care Network

Melanie D. Otis and Debra A. Harley

Abstract

This chapter focuses on the complexity of human identity by considering the multifaceted and intertwined relationships between sexuality, gender, race, ethnicity, socioeconomic status, and age, as well as other aspects of one's social and personal identity. To assist in illuminating our understanding of these relationships, the structural, political, and social factors that contribute to social inequality experienced by LGBT elders situated at the multidimensional intersections of different races, ethnicities, socioeconomic status (SES), sexes, and sexualities are explored. By simultaneously considering the multiplicity and fluidity of identity and exposing the diversity of experiences of LGBT elders, we are able to underscore some of the many reasons for extant research involving sexual minorities which must be carefully and critically evaluated.

Keywords

Intersection of identities · Multiple identities · Race · Age · Sexuality · Care network

Overview

To help us make sense of this multifaceted set of intertwined relationships, this chapter will begin by defining the foundational organizing constructs of *multiple identities* and *intersectionality* and providing some background on how these constructs have evolved into useful heuristic tools that can guide the conceptualization and execution of meaningful inquiry in the social and behavioral sciences (Bowleg 2008; Crenshaw 1993; Fish 2008). Once the core constructs of multiple identities and intersectionality have been defined, we explore the structural, political, and social factors that contribute to social inequality experienced by elderly LGBT persons situated at the multidimensional intersections of different races, ethnicities, socioeconomic status (SES), sexes, sexualities, and among others (Fukuyama and Ferguson 2000; Hancock 2007). Exposing the diversity of experience of elderly LGBT persons underscores some of the many reasons extant research involving sexual minorities must be carefully and critically evaluated, particularly

M.D. Otis (✉) · D.A. Harley
University of Kentucky, Lexington, USA
e-mail: Melanie.Otis@uky.edu

© Springer International Publishing Switzerland 2016
D.A. Harley and P.B. Teaster (eds.), *Handbook of LGBT Elders*,
DOI 10.1007/978-3-319-03623-6_5

when the predominant subjects of that research seem to mirror the longstanding stereotypical profile of young, white, gay, well-educated, middle-class, and urban dwelling (Albelda et al. 2009). To be fair, while this profile describes a segment of the population, it is most notable for the many LGBT persons it excludes—and for the fact that its persistence as a presumably adequate proxy for the population of sexual minorities as a whole is based on a tacit acceptance of the study participants as representative (Institute of medicine [IOM] 2011). Building on this platform, we explore the ways that racism, sexism, ageism, and heterosexism impact the processes through which individuals develop, experience, and manage their multifaceted social identities (Kertzner et al. 2009; Purdie-Vaughns and Eibach 2008; Settles 2006). With a clearer understanding of the diversity represented among elder LGBT persons, the chapter will consider the relevance of these factors for the development of informal support and caregiver networks, as well as their implications for the creation and maintenance of formal care networks that are responsive to the needs of the multidimensional population of elder LGBT persons with whom we will engage (Van Der Bergh and Crisp 2004). Finally, having established a foundation upon which we might build, suggestions for the development of models of culturally competent practice (Leyva et al. 2014), training of human service professionals (Hardacker et al. 2014; Hillman and Hinrichsen 2014), creation of effective and responsive communities of care and service organizations (Meyer and Johnston 2014), and the development of inclusive policies will be delineated (Auldridge and Espinoza 2013).

Learning Objectives

By the end of the chapter, the reader should be able to:

1. Understand the multiple dimensions of identities and their intersections.
2. Identify the stigmatization of "isms" with regard to race, age, and sexuality in informal and formal care networks.
3. Understand the diversity of relationships in the LGBT community.
4. Understand the complexities of families of choice as impacting intersectionality.
5. Summarize the convergence of race, age, sexuality, and service provision.

Introduction

A common theme and driving force behind this book is an acknowledgment that the elder LGBT community/population is made up of a complex and diverse collection of human beings about whom we know relatively little. Yet, if we are to effectively address the needs of such a diverse aging population, we must develop care networks, services, and programs that acknowledge and affirm the multiplicity of social identities that converge to create the unique human beings with whom we will work (Abes et al. 2007; Jones and McEwen 2000). In a very real sense, one can look to this book as a call to action for human service professionals—seeking to simultaneously educate and inspire them to become the very best practitioner possible while moving forward on their career paths. Throughout our careers, we are called upon to act as culturally competent professionals in a variety of practice settings. In an effort to rise to that challenge, we will turn to the scholarly professional literature to seek guidance on best practices and insights into the lived experiences of aging sexual minorities from diverse backgrounds. In the process, we are constantly confronted by the reality that our knowledge of this heterogeneous population of individuals who identify as lesbian, gay, bisexual, or transgender is based largely on a fairly monochromatic and unidimensional body of research (Huang et al. 2010; IOM 2011). In short, we know very little about the full spectrum of LGBT lives.

Until recently, the relative dearth of research focusing on diversity within the LGBT population drew little attention. Whether this was the result of a failure to acknowledge the actual diversity of the LGBT population, a level of satisfaction with the fact that there was finally an evolving body of LGBT-focused scholarship in general, a combination of the two, or something else entirely, LGBT-focused research tended to ignore the roles of potentially relevant issues such as race, ethnicity, social class, age, and among others, in the lives of sexual minorities (IOM 2011; Van Sluytman and Torres 2014; Young and Meyer 2005). Over the last twenty years, a growing number of studies have included more diverse samples, yet recent systematic reviews of the literature reveal that extant scholarship still offers only a limited look a more diverse LGBT population (Eliason et al. 2010; Fredriksen-Goldsen and Muraco 2010; Huang et al. 2010). When researchers do give consideration to differences related to race, ethnicity, age, sexual minority identity, gender identity, geographic location, and/or SES, this acknowledgment comes primarily in the form of a sample description that rarely translates into a more in-depth analysis (IOM 2011). Generally, when acknowledged, the absence of such analysis is a limitation that is attributed to having insufficient numbers of individuals representing specific demographic characteristics (IOM 2011). Among the very limited number of studies that seek to specifically address some aspect of the diversity *within* the LGBT population, we find research that is typically characterized by small sample sizes and a reliance on qualitative research methods (e.g., case studies, focus groups, interviews). While these studies provide us with valuable and useful information, the reality is that our knowledge of significant portions of the LGBT community is based on the experiences of a very small number of people whose experiences may or may not share commonalities with others who have a similar, much less different, demographic profile. Thus, we remain fairly uninformed about the lives of LGBT persons of color or elderly LGBT persons of any race/ethnicity and/or socioeconomic background, with scholars recently noting that amidst this limited scope of available research, transgender persons remain all but invisible in the vast majority of all sexual minority-focused scholarship (Averett

et al. 2012; Fredriksen-Goldsen and Muraco 2010; Siverskog 2014).

Against this less than satisfying backdrop, this chapter focuses on one of the more challenging aspects of understanding the lives of human beings—confronting the reality that each of us is much more than the sum of our parts, and amidst this complexity, we each experience our identities as simultaneously fluid, contextual, and in some ways, concrete (Diamond 2005; Fish 2008; Hancock 2007). If that description seems to suggest inherent contradictions, in reality, it only offers the tip of the iceberg of what makes the process of developing a meaningful understanding of human beings and the human condition so challenging. Of particular relevance to the current focus of inquiry, this task is made all the more difficult by the fact that sexual minorities confront stigma, prejudice, and discrimination on a daily basis and thus have often been justifiably reticent about participating in research (Bowleg 2008; DeBlaere et al. 2010; Moradi et al. 2009). Despite this reality, social scientists must continue to acknowledge the complex combination of factors that contribute to individual experiences, seek ways to measure these factors, and subsequently configure this newly acquired knowledge into a narrative that can guide human service professionals in areas of practice, program development, and policy to positively impact the lives of aging LGBT persons (Eliason et al. 2010; Van Der Bergh and Crisp 2004).

The Limitations of LGBT Scholarship Related to Diversity

As efforts are underway to increase the diversity of questions explored in research involving elder LGBT persons, certain identity-related assumptions that have influenced past scholarship have been exposed. First, the centrality of problem-focused inquiry in the literature involving LGBT persons has been well established (IOM 2011). Although this work has provided the basis for seeking funding for much-needed LGBT-focused services and programming, it has also been used to support politically and culturally charged arguments, suggesting that sexual minorities as a group are physically and mentally less healthy than heterosexual men and women (Bowleg et al. 2003; Purdie-Vaughns and Eibach 2008), and as such must be precluded from certain environments and/or activities (i.e., teaching young children, adoption/having children, serving in the military). Amidst this body of work sits a significant number of studies that focus on the centrality of the role of coming out as being either highly problematic, essential to well-being, and/or the indisputable foundation of a sexual minority person's identity (Hunter 2007). Conceptually, this work suggests that for persons who identify as lesbian, gay, bisexual, or transgender, one's sexuality is/should be the primary dimension defining one's identity. Given that some research suggests that elder LGBT persons who came out prior to the beginning of the gay rights movement (generally considered to be the day of the Stonewall riots—June 28, 1969) may not view publically acknowledging their sexuality (in any way) as necessary or appropriate, this assumption about the primacy of one's identification as a sexual minority may be highly problematic.

There can be little argument that each of these paths of inquiry has produced some important information that has enhanced our understanding of the lives of LGBT persons and that could (and does) assist in creating some form of positive change, for direct practice, programming, policy development, or community change (IOM 2011). Yet, beyond the debate about whether coming out is critical to the development of one's identity as a sexual minority, research demonstrates both the significance and fluidity of the prioritization of multiple identities among sexual minorities—including shifts in the centrality of one's identity as a sexual minority (Diamond 2005; Kertzner 2001). For instance, in a study of gay men in midlife, Kertzner (2001) found that many of the men viewed their sexual minority identity as less important to them as they aged, with greater significance being shifted to aspects of their non-sexual identity associated with race (for men

of color), their relationship status (particularly among single men in the study), and their physical appearance (i.e., being overweight). Similarly, in a qualitative study of older lesbians, Averett et al. (2012) found that the women viewed their sexuality as less central to their identity as they aged and instead emphasized on establishing stability and a sense of security.

Multiple Dimensions of Identity and Intersectionality

Identity is a central organizing tool for understanding how human beings create and maintain a sense of self (Howard 2000). Social scientists (primarily in the fields of sociology and psychology) have been studying identity for many decades. In general, the field of inquiry has been guided by three fundamental assumptions:

1. Identities are not innate qualities, rather they are socially constructed;
2. Identities are fluid; and
3. Identities are created/recreated over and over again through processes of social interaction and meaning-making.

Utilizing these three basic building blocks, we can acknowledge that at the heart of our discussion about multiple dimensions of identity and intersectionality sits a fairly simplistic premise—each of us possesses a number of characteristics that coalesce and sometimes conflict to create the unique individuals that we become (Jones and McEwen 2000; McCall 2005). We self-identify and we are identified and labeled by others based on multiple dimensions, including our race/ethnicity, age, sexuality, sex, and social class (Hancock 2007; Roccas and Brewer 2002). While all of these characteristics constitute parts of us as unique human beings, a number of influences we encounter across time and space contribute to the salience of particular identities at any given point in time (Abes et al. 2007). By framing our understanding of the lived experiences of elder LGBT persons around the construct of multiple dimensions of identity/ multiple identities, we acknowledge and embrace this reality (Abes et al. 2007; Jones and McEwen 2000; Omi and Winant 1994; Tornstam 2005; Weber 1998).

Because our focus is on understanding and appreciating the lives of elder lesbians, gay men, bisexual men and women, and transgender persons, the fluidity of multiple identities experienced across the life course figures prominently in our discussion (Kertzner et al. 2009; Omi and Winant 1994). Although our own developmental trajectories and associated expectations and roles (i.e., becoming older, becoming a parent, partnering) certainly play a critical role in the process, the impact of embracing or being ascribed a particular identity is bigger than just knowing which predetermined box we are expected to check on a survey. In fact, given the fluidity of identity, how we self-identify may be both historically and situationally influenced (Cronin and King 2010; Deaux and Martin 2003; Howard 2000; Stirratt et al. 2007). For instance, in one's place of employment, our sexuality may seem of little relevance to us while highly relevant in others. A situation may be compounded by the fact that those around us may be prioritizing, and thus responding to, aspects of identity that we may or may not see as pertinent or primary in the moment. Or we may become a parent and come to centralize that aspect of our identity, regardless of what other aspects of our identity may remain more or less prominent as a result of our shifting priorities. In summary, as we move through various activities, interactions, and cognitive processes over the course of a given day, a month, or year(s), different aspects of our identity may be more or less salient—some of these shifts may be fleeting, while others may mark a long-term or permanent shift in our identity process (Abes et al. 2007; Fuss 1989; Kertzner 2001; McCall 2005; Roccas and Brewer 2002).

The question of which identity is primary has long been a subject of debate for many ethnic minority LGBT persons (see Chap. 6–8, 10). The politics of multiple identities, especially sexual minority status inclusion in ethnic minority communities, has become more fluid in recent decades. Moore (2010) examined strategies black LGBT persons use in black environments to proclaim a sexual minority identity that is co-occuring with a black identity. The belief is that increasing their visibility in black spaces will promote a greater understanding of minority sexuality as an identity status that can coexist rather than compete with race. One of the foci of the study was to examine the particular health and social support concerns faced by older and aging segments of this population (see Research Box 5.1).

Research Box 5.1 See Moore (2010).

Purpose: To analyze the ways black gay people who feel a sense of solidarity with the racial group experience the cross cutting issue of openly expressing a gay sexuality in black community contexts.

Method: The data for this study come from a larger project, Black Los Angeles Project, a research study examining neighborhoods, religious life, political participation, cultural production, and social justice in South Los Angeles, California. Approximately 30 months of qualitative data collection were used. This study was designed to examine the relationship that black LGBT persons have with their racial communities, the types of kin arrangements they participate in, the role religion plays in their lives, and the particular health and social support concerns faced by the older and aging segments of this population. In-depth, semi-structured interviews were conducted with self-identified LGBT African-Americans who live and/or work in predominately Black or Black and Latino neighbors. The researcher gathered data at churches, art exhibits, backyard barbeques, public forums, and other private activities.

Results: Black lesbians and gay men in LA born before 1954 tend to conceptualize black group membership as an identity status that must remain primary for the continued advancement of the race. These individuals grew up when civil rights issues began to take center stage and they experienced gay sexuality as a stigma they had to endure throughout their lives. Conversely, their younger counterparts experience gay sexuality amidst a more public discourse about LGBT sexuality.

Questions

1. Do you think that this sample is representative of black LGBT elders' attitudes about the intersection identities?
2. What are the implications of this study for larger discussions of multiple identities across diversity in the LGBT community?
3. How can this study be redesigned or replicated with multiracial LGBT elders?

Debate about whether the costs and benefits of particular identity categories can be compartmentalized or even empirically captured continues, yet indisputable evidence remains elusive. Despite this, feminist scholars have contributed some important tools to assist us in the process of inquiry. Although a large body of work in this arena exists, over the last twenty-five years Crenshaw (1993), Hooks (1984, 1990) and Collins (1990, 2000, 2005) have been central figures in the development of feminist intersectionality theory. Their work focused initially on the intersection of race and sex, with black feminist scholars arguing that despite the growing number of researchers and theorists challenging long-standing notions that supported sexist and racist structures, the complex issues associated with the intersection between the two had been largely ignored. At the heart of their critique is the argument that identities and their related opportunities for advantage/disadvantage and privilege/oppression cannot be viewed in isolation, nor can they be understood as simply additive (Bowleg 2008; Settles and Buchanan

2014; Weber and Parra-Medina 2003). Instead, the impact of oppression associated with the ageism, sexism, racism, ethnocentrism, heterosexism, and classism (among other isms) cannot be teased out into separate parts, but instead must be understood as a complex intersection of different identities (Ferguson et al. 2014; Knapp 2005; McGibbon and McPherson 2011; Meyer 2003). As a consequence of the weight of oppression being disproportionately shouldered by those who possess multiple stigmatized identities, differences in mental, physical, social, and economic well-being should be expected (Diaz et al. 2001; Kertzner et al. 2009; Meyer et al. 2008; Szymanski 2005).

The "isms" and Identity. This chapter focuses on the lives of older sexual minorities—two identity categories that are individually and collectively stigmatized and disadvantaged in myriad ways. When we examine this within the conceptualization of multiple identities as contextual in nature, we are confronted with the fact that sexual minorities spend a significant amount of their time in environments dominated by heterosexuals. In the prevailing heterosexist environment, sexual minorities experience both blatant and subtle forms of oppression and discrimination due to their sexuality. Additionally, research involving sexual minority and/or presumably (or predominantly) heterosexual samples support the endorsement of ageist views within these groups. Despite the seeming universality of ageist views, some research indicates that gay men perceive the gay community to be particularly prejudicial when it comes to older men, while many lesbians felt ageism is largely a non-issue in the lesbian community (Schope 2005). Thus, it should not be surprising that a substantial amount of discussion centers around the individual and collective impact of "isms" (e.g., racism, sexism, ethnocentrism, ageism, heterosexism) on those who are disadvantaged, with some concern over whether particular identities are being or should be privileged within that debate (Case et al. 2012). As a result, in the midst of the complexity of trying to understand the interrelatedness of diverse identities, questions arise about whether one aspect of one's identity should be considered as primary in relation to another. If we attempt to position this discourse at the intersections of identity components, we are confronted with an array of questions: Is it more challenging to be a white *gay* man, a *black* heterosexual man? an *Hispanic lesbian*? or an Asian *transgender* person? Moreover, what are the challenges of being multiracial, a sexual minority, and elderly? And, perhaps most critical for our consideration at this juncture, are these even the questions we should be asking?

As noted at the outset of this chapter, data addressing the lives of the diverse spectrum of individuals who identify as sexual minorities are limited. Despite this, research conducted in recent years offers some opportunities for glimpses into the lives of a growing number of LGBT persons from a diversity of backgrounds, and encompassing a broadening spectrum of identities (Albelda et al. 2009; Diaz et al. 2008). As a result, an examination of secondary data from three population-based studies, including the US Census, the National Survey of Family Growth (NSFG), and the California Health Interview Survey (CHIS), offers insight into a few of the ways the lives of sexual minorities converge and diverge in relation to some basic, yet influential, demographic characteristics (Albelda et al. 2009). Collectively, the information offers evidence of some of the ways that race, sex, age, and geography combine to impact the economic well-being of self-identified LGB persons. For instance, the NSFG identified higher rates of poverty for women of sexual minority status as compared to heterosexual women, yet lower rates for gay men as compared to bisexual or heterosexual men (Albelda et al. 2009). Data from the 2000 US Census revealed that lesbian couples over age 65 had a poverty rate that was twice that of heterosexual married couples. When the analysis took into consideration the possible influence of race and geographic location (more precisely, population density), the findings were even more compelling. Specifically, same-sex couples living in rural areas were twice as likely to live in poverty as those in urban areas. The

combination of race and couple status revealed that being a same-sex couple versus a different-sex couple meant significantly higher rates of poverty for African-Americans, and same-sex African-American couples had poverty rates three times that of white same-sex couples (Albelda et al. 2009). It is worth noting that limitations in the US Census Bureau's data collection process preclude examination of these relationships for single sexual minorities or those who may be part of a non-cohabiting couple. The expansion of data collection categories to include a more direct indicator of sexual minority status would offer an unprecedented opportunity to capture a meaningful picture of the number of self-identified sexual minorities living in the USA (Gates 2006). To date, while scholars and advocates have called for a change in census data collection practices as they relate to sexual minorities (Auldridge and Espinoza 2013; Brown and Grossman 2014; IOM 2011), there is no indication that the Census Bureau has plans to make this adjustment.

Research in the health and mental health fields has also exposed physical and mental well-being disparities between sexual minorities and the heterosexual majority and among LGBT persons (Auldridge and Espinoza 2013; Banks 2012; Kertzner et al. 2009), with some of these differences being linked to economic inequalities captured in the studies described above (Fredriksen-Goldsen et al. 2011; IOM 2011). In their study of LGBT persons age 50 and older, Fredriksen-Goldsen et al. (2011) found that, compared to white respondents, LGBT persons of color were more likely to experience higher rates of a number of physical and mental health problems, including HIV/AIDS, hypertension, heart disease, and diabetes, among others. These scholars go on to note that despite these elevated risks, little to no discussion focusing on addressing the specific needs of aging LGBT persons of color has occurred (Fredriksen-Goldsen et al. 2011).

Assumptions of Hierarchical Socialization. While basic demographic characteristics such as one's sex, age, race, ethnicity, and sexual orientation may be viewed simply as benign descriptive information, the way these qualities are experienced as a part of one's identity is greatly influenced by the social construction of meanings attached to those characteristics (Abes et al. 2007) and the context in which those meanings are constructed and reinforced (Jenkins 2014). Thus, the existence of prejudicial beliefs that characterize racism, sexism, ageism, and heterosexism plays a significant role in the social processes associated with identity development and identity management (Jackson III 2012; Jones 1997). As we navigate daily life, we must manage both internalized beliefs and external forces related to the socially constructed meaning assigned to various facets of our identities, and we are often challenged to do so in different environments and groups that hold varying perspectives on the "appropriate" hierarchy associated with our particular demographic profile (Raetz and Lease 2002).

Examining Multiple Oppressions

Along with multiple identities come opportunities to experience multiple oppressions (and privileges —depending on one's status location in the hierarchy). In her research examining the lives of black lesbians, Greene (1995) referred to this as "triple jeopardy," arguing that being part of three oppressed groups (i.e., women, lesbians, and blacks) resulted in the potential for black lesbians to experience a disproportionate share of the negative consequences of oppression. Following Greene's argument, we argue that elder black lesbians experience quadruple jeopardy. Similar arguments have been made by other scholars who have utilized intersectionality as a model to explore the multiplicity of identity components in LGBT-focused research (Szymanski and Gupta 2009). As suggested by the limited research available on LGBT persons, framing the potential consequences associated with possessing more than one stigmatized minority status is supported by much of our available evidence (Purdie-Vaughs and Eibach 2008; Robinson-Wood 2009).

In a study examining factors that serve as social determinants of women's health, McGibbon and McPherson (2011) argue that "the oppressions of sexism, racism, heterosexism, and ageism, to name a few, can and do happen together to produce a complex synergy of material and social disadvantage" (p. 61). As both a challenge and a reminder to social scientists and helping professionals, the authors go on to assert that this conglomerate cannot be dissected into separate parts that conveniently address the influence of one *ism* in isolation from another (McGibbon and McPherson 2011). Their assertions offer important tools to utilize when critically examining extant research, with its minimally diverse samples, and define the limits of what it may or may not be able to tell us about the lives of elderly LGBT persons.

Proceeding with this cautionary note in mind, research offers a number of insights into ways that multiple oppressions impact our lives. While stigma and discrimination often make it difficult to access study participants who are representative of the diverse population of sexual minority persons (Fish 2008; Moradi et al. 2009), a growing, albeit small, body of work exists. This research underscores the ways that members of already marginalized groups may be particularly disadvantaged as they age. For instance, in general, Black and Latino persons are disproportionately concentrated in low wage jobs that offer limited, if any, access to opportunities for advancement, health insurance, and retirement security (National Hispanic Council on Aging [NHCOA] 2014; Services and Advocacy for LGBT Elders [SAGE] 2013; Social Security Administration 2011). Limited work opportunity increases the likelihood that these individuals will experience greater health-related challenges as they age and that they will encounter these challenges with a limited spectrum of resources. While the available information is certainly limited, research suggests that this scenario may be similar, if not more problematic, for elder Black and Latino sexual minorities (Auldridge and Espinoza 2013). See Chaps. 6 and 10 for additional information on African-American/ Black and Latino LGBT elders. Against this backdrop, it is important to acknowledge that those experiencing the impact of multiple forms of oppression may be highly dependent on support from their informal care/support networks.

Diversity in Relationships

To this point, this chapter has focused on the significance of multiple identities and intersectionality in the lives of individual LGBT persons. However, given the increasing importance of social relationships as source of support as one ages, consideration of the ways sexual minority couples are impacted by intersectionality is also important. Although research on intimate relationships of sexual minorities is somewhat limited, there is an evolving body of work that speaks to the unique challenges faced by LGBT couples (Brown and Grossman 2014; Gates 2006; Jeong and Horne 2009; Kurdek 2001; Long 2008). Numerous studies of same-sex couple relationships have documented similarities in relationship quality and relationship dynamics for both same-sex and different-sex couples (e.g., Blumstein and Schwartz 1983; Kurdek 2004; Malouff et al. 2010), yet the negative consequences of minority stress in same-sex couples have also been a frequent themes. This work is guided by minority stress perspective (Meyer 1995), whereby experiences of stigmatization and discrimination, as well as differences in degree of "outness" are examined as contributing factors in relationship well-being (Green and Mitchell 2008; Otis et al. 2006). A limited body of scholarship examines the lives of older sexual minorities of color or LGBT persons who are identified in some way (e.g., race, ethnicity, SES, geographic location) that goes beyond sexuality or gender identity (L, G, B, or T) and/or sex. This dearth of information about older LGBT racial and ethnic minorities living outside urban areas was captured in Huang et al.'s (2010) content analysis of the literature,

which focused on LGB persons of color. Like the bulk of LGB research in general, their analysis found the typical profile of study participants to be young- to middle-aged living in an urban area, and relationship status is either not addressed or peripheral to the analysis.

In an effort to gain insights into the ways race, ethnicity, *and* age may impact the intimate relationships of LGBT persons, research focusing on heterosexual couples may prove useful. A case in point can be gleaned from the research that has been guided by the increasingly popular minority stress model for LGBT research (Balsam et al. 2011; Meyer 1995). Initial research using the minority stress model focused on understanding the impact of racism in the lives of African-American men and women. As Pinder-hughes (2002) discussed in her review of the literature examining African-American marital relationships, both economic conditions and sex role expectations serve to impact the stability and quality of these unions. While other factors that are unique to opposite-sex relationships were also found to be relevant in these studies, the influence of racism on economic well-being and how that intersection manifests itself as a stressor in intimate relationships is likely to traverse relationship types (NHCOA 2014; SAGE 2013). Similarly, given that members of same-sex couples are raised within the same environment as their heterosexual peers, expectations and assumptions (both positive and negative) associated with being a person of color are also potentially influential in the lives of the sexual minority couples (SAGE 2013).

Families of Choice

While the previously described complexity of the lives of LGBT persons offers a daunting array of challenges to consider when attempting to understand and appreciate the social identities of sexual minorities, the concept of "families of choice" offers yet another important element. Families of choice is a construct originally attributed to Weston (1991), who sought to understand ways that sexual minorities cope with the loss of family ties and relationships associated with rejection by their families of origin. In her qualitative study of lesbians and gay men, Weston found that many described a process of recreating many of the dynamics typically associated with traditional family models in their relationships with intimate partners and networks of friends (many of whom also identified as sexual minorities). Because Weston completed her study more than two decades ago, the role of families of choice (similar to the social anthropology concept of fictive kin) in the lives of LGBT persons holds a significant place in the sexual minority-focused literature (Cronin 2004; Grossman et al. 2000; Hughes 2007). While the development of families of choice offers both positives and negatives in the lives of elderly sexual minorities (Croghan et al. 2014), in the current context, we are particularly interested in how this socially constructed model of family relates to the multiplicity of LGBT identities and the lived experiences of elderly persons. The reader will find further discussion on the functions of families of choice in many chapters in this book.

The Convergence of Race, Gender, Sexuality, Age, and Care Networks

As we age, the quality and quantity of sources of emotional and instrumental support become increasingly relevant in our lives. This is true, regardless of one's sexuality. Despite the universality of the development of aging-related needs and concerns, for elder LGBT individuals securing access to stable supportive and affirming care networks offers unique challenges and opportunities for concern (Addis et al. 2009; Brennan-Ing et al. 2014). Care networks are constructed of both formal and informal caregivers and resources. Understanding the significance of the multiplicity of identities both within and between formal and informal care networks is highly relevant to efforts to secure positive outcomes for aging LGBT persons (Hughes and Kentlyn 2011). Thus, to better understand these relationships, below, we consider relevant aspects of informal and formal care networks separately, and then in relation to one another.

Preparing to Address the Needs of Elder LGBT Persons

In light of multiple sources of evidence indicating that sexual minorities experience myriad forms of prejudice, discrimination, and even victimization in healthcare settings, aging and LGBT advocates championed a call for action (Fredriksen-Goldsen et al. 2011). Other studies addressing the preparedness of communities of care to meet the needs of elderly LGBT persons found that only about one-third of the agencies contacted had provided their employees with any form of training related to working with LGBT persons (Knochel et al. 2011), despite indications that trainings addressing culturally competent practice with sexual minorities have been shown to be effective (Crisp et al. 2008; Porter and Krinsky 2014). An examination of the content of those trainings provides little evidence that those who are developing and/or implementing these trainings have done so with any awareness of the relevance of the intersectionality of multiple identities. Thus, despite some recognition of the needs of elder sexual minorities as a monolithic entity, any particular needs that might be associated with other aspects of elder LGBT persons' identities are treated as invisible or irrelevant.

An examination of the responses of LGBT-related educational practice in the helping professions offers a number of efforts (e.g., identification of key competencies and content, constructing comprehensive assessment, understand and articulate ways in which agency, program, and service policies marginalize and discriminate against LGBT older adults) to increase the cultural competence of future human service professionals (Fredriksen-Goldsen et al. 2014; Hardacker et al. 2014). In the process, students are learning about the unique challenges faced by sexual minorities, the essential role of families of choice, and the ways that practitioners and agencies can create a more welcoming and supportive environment and reduce barriers to access (Van Der Bergh and Crisp 2004). And, while training in being a culturally competent human service professional also challenges students to think about other marginalized and stigmatized groups (e.g., the elderly, persons of color, immigrants), similar to the bulk of extant research, this training is generally constructed based on compartmentalized identity components rather than the intersectionality of multiple identities (Eliason et al. 2010).

Clearly, formal communities of care are confronted with substantial challenges in terms of being responsive to the needs and well-being of a diverse population of elder LGBT persons. With this as a foundation, we can begin to consider ways we can develop practices, programs, and policies that are actually responsive to the needs of this heterogeneous population (Knochel et al. 2011; Leyva et al. 2014; Portz et al. 2014). A number of recent studies in various fields of the helping professions offer insight into ways to transfer this knowledge about the complexity of elder LGBT population into effective practice (Leyva et al. 2014; Porter and Krinsky 2014; Portz et al. 2014). For example, recent studies in community nursing practice have demonstrated the effectiveness of developing new programs or refining existing programs within the community through a process of active engagement with future/current program participants and service users (Fredriksen-Goldsen et al. 2014; Orel 2004). In other arenas, community-based research has given way to models of cultural competence that offer some useful techniques for increasing availability and accessibility of resources (Boulder County Aging Services 2004; Moone et al. 2014; Rainbow Train 2003).

Informal care networks. The preceding pages of this chapter offer a sampling of supportive evidence related to the relevance of various social identity factors as influences on mental and physical health and access to life-enhancing opportunities. When we consider the relevance of these factors on families of choice, we realize that LGBT elders may be particularly disadvantaged because challenges that they face may be quite similar to those experienced by members of their family of choice—a network likely to constitute their circle of informal caregivers (Brennan-Ing et al. 2014; Gabrielson 2011). Unlike their heterosexual counterparts, LGBT elders are likely to share commonalities with their informal caregivers, not the least of which may be that they are of similar ages. Whereas many heterosexuals may be more likely to have caregivers across multiple generations (e.g., children, nieces/nephews), LGBT elders' informal care networks often consist of generational peers (Brotman et al. 2007; Fitzgerald 2013; Shippy 2007).

Similarities in age may increase the likelihood that LGBT elders and their families of choice may experience concurrent increases in support and resource needs, and so additional strains may be experienced by elder LGBT persons of color (Glass and Few-Demo 2013; Lehavot et al. 2009), and sexual minorities who identify as transgender (Fredriksen-Goldsen et al. 2011; Siverskog 2014). For instance, research suggests that sexual minorities of color may be more likely to experience isolation in old age due to lower levels of integration into the LGBT community throughout their lives (Lehavot et al. 2009; Szymanski and Gupta 2009; Woody 2014). This situation may be compounded by the greater likelihood that elder LGBT persons of color are living in poverty, lacking healthcare-related resources, and experiencing higher rates of disease (Fitzgerald 2013; Fredriksen-Goldsen et al. 2011). These challenges may be particularly salient for lesbians, bisexual women, and transgender persons who may often have lived much of their lives with very limited formal and informal support networks (Fredriksen-Goldsen et al. 2011). Similarly, aging LGBT persons who are living with HIV/AIDS often have informal support networks that are largely constituted by peers who are also living with HIV/AIDS (Cantor et al. 2009). Notably, among LGBT elders living with HIV/AIDS, persons of color are disproportionately represented (Auldridge and Espinoza 2013).

Table 5.1 Suggestions for working with LGBT elders

Do not assume heterosexuality or gender identity even when you know the client is in a relationship with someone of the opposite sex, is married, or has children and grandchildren
Respect the privacy of clients you think might be LGBT
Explain and emphasize your agency's policy on confidentiality
Make sure intake forms include the category of partner or significant other. For a sex or gender question, add a category for transgender
Put LGBT-friendly language in your brochures and other program materials
Be aware transgender elders frequently face isolation, negative judgments, and ostracism from health and social service professional. Thus, educate yourself and others in your agency about gender diversity
Respect the gender that transgender clients consider themselves to be by using gender-correct pronouns
Advertise and promote your programs and services in the LGBT press

Adapted from Flaxman (2005)

Formal care networks. The availability of culturally competent formal communities of care is critical to the well-being of the diverse population of aging LGBT persons. Yet, research indicates that many LGBT minorities express great concern over needing to access aging services in environments that they either perceived to be unwelcoming or where they or their peers have already experienced prejudice and discrimination (Brotman et al. 2007; Gabrielson 2011; Hughes 2007; Johnson et al. 2005; National Senior Citizens Law Center et al. 2010). As a result, LGBT elders are more likely to forego preventive or needed treatment or care, thus increasing the likelihood of experiencing more severe physical and mental health consequences in the future (Tjepkema 2008). Unfortunately, because these concerns are not simply manifested in later life, elder lesbians, gay men, bisexual men and women, and transgender persons often enter old age having experienced a disproportionate number of health-related issues (Heck et al. 2006; IOM 2011). Research indicates that such concerns are not without merit. A collaborative study involving three prominent national organizations focused on aging (Movement Advancement Project [MAP], Services and Advocacy for Gay, Lesbian, Bisexual, and Transgender Elders [SAGE], and the Center for American Progress [CAP] 2010) documented LGBT elders' experiences of being denied services (or provided inappropriate services), and the marginalization of same-sex partners in the decision-making process. Similarly, in 2011, Fredriksen-Goldsen and colleagues reported that 13 % of their respondents (adults age 50 and over) had experienced some form of discrimination or victimization within a healthcare setting.

Intersection of informal and formal care networks. Given the centrality of families of choice in the lives of many LGBT elders, it is particularly important for human service providers and agencies to develop a comprehensive understanding of informal care networks. With studies indicating that elder sexual minorities are more likely to turn to families of choice for support, while also suggesting that a significant number of elder lesbians, gay men, and transgender persons are likely to be single and often isolated, human service professionals play a significant role in the lives of LGBT elders. Where informal networks are available, service providers and policies need to serve as a bridge connecting these critical aspects of the person's overall care network. Additionally, by being aware of the greater likelihood that LGBT elders may be less likely to have a either a traditional family network and/or family of choice network available for support, human service providers can reach out to sexual minorities to assure that they are not isolated and receive the care and support that they need as they age (Brennan-Ing et al. 2014). In addition, human service providers need to be well versed in appropriate communication strategies with LGBT elders. Flaxman

(2005) identified practical suggestions to that end (see Table 5.1).

Summary

People throughout the world have multiple and intersection identities. Other attributes include racial and gender identities, sexual orientation or gender identity, belief systems, and aging. In this chapter, we highlighted a seemingly obvious, yet often ignored, reality; elderly lesbians, gay men, bisexuals, and transgender persons are made up of a complex and fluid combination of social identities that have been influenced by their life experiences, which continue to reconfigure as they age (Abes et al. 2007; Azmitia 2014; McCall 2005). The presence of ageism, sexism, racism, ethnocentrism, classism, and heterosexism, among other sources of discrimination, has contributed to myriad inequities in the lives of LGBT elders. The consequences of those past experiences, as well as current ones, are manifested on a daily basis (Meyer 1995). As has already been documented in a number of studies, we anticipate that these consequences will continue to be manifested in differences in disease rates, life chances and opportunities, and overall quality of life across the life course. Although we are unlikely to eliminate these sources of inequity any time soon, our awareness of them should be a catalyst for change (Crisp et al. 2008; Van Den Bergh and Crisp 2004).

Intersectionality as a conceptual framework for understanding the complex identities of LGBT elders offers a useful heuristic tool with which to build a bridge between the processes of conceptualization and program development in the helping professions. Intersectionality invites us to consider not only the categories associated with different aspects of identity but also the impact associated with privileges and oppressions that correspond with those categories (Garry 2011). As a body of knowledge, extant scholarship on intersectionality reflects the influence of many disciplines. As research moves forward with the guidance of multidisciplinary teams, Bowleg (2008) argues that we will garner the benefits of creative approaches to conceptualization, measurement and analyses that better capture the complex and fluid model of social identity that is more representative LGBT lives. For example, while research is constrained by our ability to develop measures that are reliable and valid indicators of the aspects of identity we wish to consider, increasingly sophisticated statistical methods offer techniques for simultaneously considering these factors in complex ways more closely aligned with human experience (Stirratt et al. 2007). As we increase our ability to capture evidence of the intersectionality of identity, sophisticated research will offer greater insight into how we might best develop programs that avoid the compartmentalization of identity components in favor of programs that holistically embrace the complexity of LGBT elders' identities (Bowleg 2008; Weber and Parra-Medina 2003). Notably, Stirratt et al. (2007) acknowledge that while statistical analysis allows us to model a multidimensional view of the intersectionality of identities, we are still challenged to capture the contextual variation that contributes to the fluidity of identities (Deaux and Martin 2003; Stirratt et al. 2007). Environments that construct and nurture norms and values that support hierarchical views of race, ethnicity, age, sex, and sexuality, among other targets for differential treatment, contribute to the development and maintenance of social identity. Consequently, we have further evidence of the critical role that advocacy for social change can play in the elder LGBT persons lives.

Learning Activities

Self-Check Questions

1. Why is it important to understand why and how people are more than the sum of their parts?
2. What are some of the limitations of research on the LGBT population related to identity intersectionality within this population?

3. What are the fundamental assumptions used by social scientists to guide the study of identities?
4. What types of intersectionalities should be addressed when working with LGBT elders? Why are these important?
5. What are presenting problems between formal and informal care networks when working with LGBT elders?

Experiential Exercises

1. Develop a survey to determine how LGBT elders view their identities. Potential question can include how they define their identity (one vs. multiple), how they rank their identities, how elements of their identity fit with the majority or dominant group, and so forth.
2. "Walk a mile in an LGBT person's shoes"—(a) imagine yourself as an LGBT older person, (b) think of issues that you will have address because of your intersection of identities (e.g., what are the cultural concerns, what are the communication concerns), and (c) what types of strategies do you recommend to address these concerns.
3. As a human service provider, develop a protocol for your work setting that is inclusive of LGBT elders, keeping in mind that their multiple identities must be addressed.

Multiple-Choice Questions

1. An individual who is a lesbian, Latino, and age 70 is considered to be which of the following?

   (a) A triad member
   (b) Risk of triple jeopardy
   (c) Nexus of sexual orientation
   (d) Decreased risk of discrimination

2. Which of the following refers to the movement through various activities, interactions, and cognitive processes over the course of time in which different aspects of one's identity may be more or less salient?

   (a) Single identities
   (b) Compounded identities
   (c) Fluidity of identity
   (d) Particular identity

3. Which of the following is attributed to differences in mental, physical, and economic well-being due to shouldering the weight of oppression disproportionately?

   (a) Multiple stigmatized identities
   (b) Residence in certain regions of the country
   (c) Type of employment
   (d) Multiple personality disorders

4. Which of the following is at the heart of feminist intersectionality theory?

   (a) *Isms* can be understood in separate parts
   (b) *Isms* must be understood as the result of complex intersection of different identities
   (c) *Isms* can be viewed in isolation
   (d) *Isms* can best be understood as additive to other identities

5. Which of the following is particularly important for human service providers to understand in working with older sexual minorities?

   (a) The centrality of families of choice
   (b) Greater likelihood that KGBT elders may be less likely to have a traditional family network
   (c) LGBT elders are likely to be single and often isolated
   (d) All of the above
   (e) None of the above

6. Which of the following is an accurate description of identity?

   (a) Identities are innate qualities
   (b) Identities are socially constructed
   (c) Identities are fixed and static
   (d) Identities are unidimensional

7. Which of the following is a good strategy for human service providers working with LGBT elders?

   (a) It is important to share their identity with other service providers

(b) Exclude LGBT—specific language in agency brochures and materials as not to embarrass them

(c) Do not assume heterosexuality or gender identity when a client is married or have children or grandchildren

(d) Avoid using categories other than male or female sex or gender question to protect client confidentiality

8. Who is credited with construction of the concept of families of choice?

(a) Albert Ellison
(b) Vivian Cass
(c) Sigmund Freud
(d) Kath Weston

9. Which of the following is an organizing tool for understanding how human beings create and maintain a sense of self?

(a) Identity
(b) Personality
(c) Family of origin
(d) Family of choice

10. Which of the following best describe human service agencies preparedness to work with LGBT Elders?

(a) Highly qualified
(b) Inadequately qualified
(c) Interdisciplinary trained
(d) Culturally competent

Key

1-B
2-C
3-A
4-B
5-D
6-B
7-C
8-D
9-A
10-B

Resources

Center for Intersectionality & Social Policy Studies: www.intersectionality-center.org.

Lee, D., & Noble, M. (2014). *"Addressing whole identities or fragmented lives" An introductory service provision and employer guide to multiple identities and discrimination in Northern Ireland.* www.rainbow-project.org/assets/publications/addressingwholeidentitiesorfragmentedlives.pdf.

Nettles, R., & Balter, R. (eds.). (2012). *Multiple minority identities: Applications for practice, research, and training.* New York, NY: Springer.

Vakalahi, H. F. O., Simpson, G. M., & Giunta, N. (Eds.). (2014). *The collective spirit of aging across cultures.* New York, NY: Springer.

References

Abes, E. S., Jones, S. R., & McEwen, M. K. (2007). Reconceptualizing the model of multiple dimensions of identity: The role of meaning-making capacity in the construction of multiple identities. *Journal of College Student Development, 48*(1), 1–22.

Addis, S., Davies, M., Greene, G., MacBride-Stewart, S., & Shepherd, M. (2009). The health, social care and housing needs of lesbian, gay, bisexual and transgender older people: a review of the literature. *Health and Social Care in the Community, 17*(6), 647–658. doi:10.1111/j.1365-2524.2009.00866.x.

Albelda, R., Badgett, M. V. L., Schneebaum, A., & Gates, G. (2009). *Poverty in the lesbian, gay, and bisexual community.* Los Angeles, CA: The Williams Institute.

Auldridge, A., & Espinoza, R. (2013). *Health equity and LGBT elders of color: Recommendations for policy and practice.* Thousand Oaks, CA: Sage Publications Inc.

Averett, P., Yoon, I., & Jenkins, C. L. (2012). Older lesbian sexuality: Identity, sexual behavior, and the impact of aging. *The Journal of Sex Research, 49*(5), 495–507.

Azmitia, M. (2014). Reflections on the cultural lenses of identity development. In K. C. McLean & M. Syed (Eds.), *The Oxford handbook of identity development* (pp. 286–296). Oxford: Oxford University Press.

Balsam, K. F., Molina, Y., Beadnell, B., Simoni, J., & Walters, K. (2011). Measuring multiple minority stress: The LGBT people of color microaggressions scale. *Cultural Diversity and Ethnic Minority Psychology, 17*(2), 163–174.

Banks, M. E. (2012). Multiple minority identities and mental health: Social and research implications of diversity within and between groups. In R. Nettles & R. Balter (Eds.), *Multiple minority identities: Applications for practice, research, and training* (pp. 35–58). New York: NY, Springer Publishing Company.

Blumstein, P., & Schwartz, P. (1983). *American couples: Money, work, sex.* New York: William Morrow.

Boulder County Aging Services. (2004). *Project visibility: Awareness and sensitivity training manual for service providers of lesbian, gay, bisexual and transgender elders.* Boulder: CO: Author.

Bowleg, L. (2008). When Black+Lesbian+Woman ≠ Black Lesbian woman: The methodological challenges of qualitative and quantitative intersectionality research. *Sex Role, 59*, 312–325.

Bowleg, L., Huang, J., Brooks, K., Black, A., & Burkholder, G. (2003). Triple jeopardy and beyond: Multiple minority stress and resilience among black lesbians. *Journal of Lesbian Studies, 7*(4), 87–108.

Brennan-Ing, M., Seidel, L., Larson, B., & Karpiak, S. E. (2014). Social care networks and LGBT older adults: Challenges for the future. *Journal of Homosexuality, 61*(1), 21–52.

Brotman, S., Ryan, B., Collins, S., Chamberland, L., Cormier, R., Julien, D. et al. (2007). Coming out to care: Caregivers of gay and lesbian seniors in Canada. *Gerontologist, 47*(4), 490–503.

Brown, M. T., & Grossman, B. R. (2014). Same-sex sexual relationships in the national social life, health and aging project: Making as case for data collection. *Journal of Gerontological Social Work, 57*(2–4), 108–129.

Cantor, M. H., Brennan, M., & Karpiak, S. E. (2009). The social support network of older people with HIV. In M. Brennan, S. E. Karpiak, R. A. Shippy, & M. H. Cantor (Eds.), *Older adults with HIV: An in-depth examination of an emerging population* (pp. 61–74). Hauppauge, NY: Nova Science Publishers.

Case, K. A., Iuzzini, J., & Hopkins, M. (2012). Systems of privilege: Intersections, awareness, and applications. *Journal of Social Issues, 68*, 1–10. doi: 10.1111/j.1540-4560.2011.01732.x.

Collins, P. H. (1990). *Black feminist thought.* Boston: Unwin Hyman.

Collins, P. H. (2000). *Black feminist thought* (2nd ed.). New York, NY: Routledge.

Collins, P. H. (2005). An entirely different world: Rethinking the sociology of race and ethnicity. In C. Calhoun, B. Turner, & C. Rojeck (Eds.), *Handbook of sociology* (pp. 208–222). London: Sage Publications Inc.

Crenshaw, K. (1993). Mapping the margins: Intersectionality, identity politics, and violence against women of color. *Stanford Law Review, 43*(6), 1241–1279.

Crisp, C., Wayland, S., & Gordon, T. (2008). Older gay, lesbian, and bisexual adults: Tools for age-competent and gay affirmative practice. *Journal of Gay & Lesbian Social Services, 20*(1–2), 5–29.

Croghan, C. F., Moone, R. P., & Olson, A. M. (2014). Friends, family, and caregiving among midlife and older lesbian, gay, bisexual, and transgender adults. *Journal of Homosexuality, 61*(1), 79–102.

Cronin, A. (2004). Sexuality in gerontology: A heteronormative presence, a queer absence. In S. O. Daatland & S. Biggs (Eds.), *Ageing and diversity: Multiple pathways and cultural migrations* (pp. 107–122). Bristol: Policy Press.

Cronin, A., & King, A. (2010). Power, inequality, and identification: Exploring diversity and intersectionality amongst older LGB adults. *Sociology, 44*(5), 876–892.

Deaux, K., & Martin, D. (2003). Interpersonal networks and social categories: Specifying levels of context in identity processes. *Social Psychology Quarterly, 66*(2), 101–117.

DeBlaere, C., Brewster, M. E., Sarkees, A., & Moradi, B. (2010). Conducting research with LGB people of color: Methodological challenges and strategies. *The Counseling Psychologist, 38*(3), 331–362.

Diamond, L. M. (2005). A new view of lesbian subtypes: Stable versus fluid identity trajectories over an 8-year period. *Psychology of Women Quarterly, 29*(2), 119–128.

Diaz, R. M., Ayala, G., Bein, E., Jenne, J., & Marin, B. V. (2001). The impact of homophobia, poverty, and racism on the mental health of Latino gay men. *American Journal of Public Health, 91*, 927–932.

Diaz, R. M., Peterson, J. L., & Choi, K. (2008). Social discrimination and health outcomes in African American, Latino, and Asian/Pacific Islander gay men. In R. J. Wolitski, R. Stall, & R. O. Valdiserri (Eds.), *Unequal opportunity: Health disparities affecting gay and bisexual men in the United States* (pp. 327–354). New York, NY: Oxford University Press.

Eliason, M. J., Dibble, S., & DeJoseph, J. (2010). Nursing's silence on lesbian, gay, bisexual, and transgender issues: The need for emancipatory efforts. *Advances in Nursing Science, 33*(3), 206–218.

Ferguson, A. D., Carr, G., & Snitman, A. (2014). Intersections of race-ethnicity, gender, and sexual minority communities. In M. L. Miville & A. D. Ferguson (Eds.), *Handbook of race-ethnicity and gender in psychology* (pp. 45–63). New York, NY: Springer Science.

Fish, J. (2008). Navigating queer street: Researching the intersections of lesbian, gay, bisexual, and trans (LGBT) identities in health research. *Sociological Research Online, 13*(1), 12. http://www.socresonline.org.uk/13/1/12.html doi:10.5153/sro.1652.

Fitzgerald, E. (2013). *No golden years at the end of the rainbow: How a lifetime of discrimination compounds economic and health disparities for LGBT older adults.* Washington, D.C.: National Gay and Lesbian Task Force.

Flaxman, N. (2005). *Practical suggestions for working with LGBT elders*. Retrieved January 18, 2015 from www.lavenderseniors.org/wp-content/uploads/pdf/PracticalSuggestionsforWorkingwithLGBTElders.pdf.

Fredriksen-Goldsen, K. W., Hoy-Ellis, C. P., Goldsen, J., Emlet, C. A., & Hooyman, N. R. (2014). Creating a vision for the future: Key competencies and strategies for culturally competent practice with lesbian, gay, bisexual, and transgender (LGBT) older adults in the health and human services. *Journal of Gerontological Social Work, 57*(2–4), 80–107.

Fredriksen-Goldsen, K. I., Kim, H.-J., Emlet, C. A., Muraco, A., Erosheva, E. A., Hoy-Ellis, C. P., et al. (2011). *The aging and health report: Disparities and resilience among lesbian, gay, bisexual, and transgender older adults*. Seattle, WA: Institute for Multigenerational Health.

Fredriksen-Goldsen, K. I., & Muraco, A. (2010). Aging and sexual orientation: A 25-year review of the literature. *Research on Aging, 32*(3), 372–413.

Fukuyama, M. A., & Ferguson, A. D. (2000). Lesbian, gay, and bisexual people of color: Understanding cultural complexity and managing multiple oppressions. In R. M. Perez & K. A. DeBord (Eds.), *Handbook of counseling and psychotherapy with lesbian, gay, and bisexual clients* (pp. 81–105). Washington, DC: American Psychological Association.

Fuss, D. (1989). *Essentially speaking: Feminism, nature, and difference*. New York: Routledge.

Gabrielson, M. (2011). "We have to create family": Aging support issues and needs among older lesbians. *Journal of Gay and Lesbian Social Services, 23*(3), 1–13.

Garry, A. (2011). Intersectionality, metaphors, and the multiplicity of gender. *Hypatia, 26*(4), 826–850.

Gates, G. J. (2006). Same-sex couples and the gay, lesbian, bisexual population: New estimates from the American Community Survey. *The Williams Institute*. UCLA: The Williams Institute. Retrieved from: http://escholarship.org/uc/item/8h08t0zf.

Glass, V. Q., & Few-Demo, A. L. (2013). Complexities of informal social support arrangements for Black lesbian couples. *Family Relations, 62*(5), 714–726.

Green, R. J., & Mitchell, V. (2008). Gay and lesbian couples in therapy: Minority stress, relational ambiguity, and families of choice. In A. S. Gurman (Ed.), *Clinical handbook of couple therapy* (4th ed., pp. 662–680). New York, NY: Guilford Press.

Greene, B. (1995). Lesbian women of color: Triple jeopardy. In B. Greene (Ed.), *Women of color: Integrating ethnic and gender identities in psychotherapy* (pp. 389–427). New York, NY: Guilford Press.

Grossman, A. H., D'Augelli, A. R., & Hershberger, S. L. (2000). Social support networks of lesbian, gay, and bisexual adults 60 years of age and older. *The Journal of Gerontology: Psychological Sciences & Social Sciences, 55*(3), P171–P179.

Hancock, A.-M. (2007). When multiplication doesn't equal quick addition: Examining intersectionality as a research paradigm. *Perspectives on Politics, 5*(1), 63–79.

Hardacker, C. T., Rubenstein, B., Hotton, A., & Houlberg, M. (2014). Adding silver to the rainbow: the development of nurses' health education about LGBT elders (HEALE) cultural competency curriculum. *Journal of Nursing Management, 22*(2), 257–266.

Heck, J. E., Sell, R. L., & Gorin, S. S. (2006). Health care access among individuals involved in same-sex relationships. *American Journal of Public Health, 96*, 1111–1118.

Hillman, J., & Hinrichsen, G. A. (2014). Promoting an affirming, competent practice with older lesbian and gay adults. *Professional Psychology: Research and Practice, 45*(4), 269–277.

Hooks, B. (1984). *Feminist theory: From margin to center*. Cambridge, MA: South End Press.

Hooks, B. (1990). *Yearning: Race, gender, and cultural politics*. Cambridge, MA: South End Press.

Howard, J. A. (2000). Social psychology of identities. *Annual Review of Sociology, 26*, 367–393.

Huang, Y., Brewster, M. E., Moradi, B., Goodman, M. B., Wiseman, M. C., & Martin, A. (2010). Content analysis of literature about LGB people of color: 1998–2007. *The Counseling Psychologist, 38*(3), 363–396.

Hughes, M. M. (2007). Familiar theories from a new perspective: The implications of a longitudinal approach to women in politics research. *Politics & Gender, 3*(3), 370–378.

Hughes, M., & Kentlyn, S. (2011). Older LGBT people's care networks and communities of practice: A brief note. *International Social Work, 54*(3), 436–444.

Hunter, S. (2007). *Coming out and disclosure: LGBT persons across the life span*. New York: Haworth.

Institute of Medicine. (2011). *The health of lesbian, gay, bisexual and transgender people: Building a foundation for better understanding*. Washington, DC: National Academies Press.

Jackson III, B. W. (2012). Black identity development: Influences of culture and social oppression. In C. Wijeyesinghe & B. W. Jackson III (Eds.), *New perspectives on racial identity development: Integrating emerging frameworks* (2nd., pp. 33–50). New York, NY: New York University Press.

Jenkins, R. (2014). *Social identity*. New York, NY: Routledge.

Jeong, J. Y., & Horne, S. G. (2009). Relationship characteristics of women in interracial same-sex relationships. *Journal of Homosexuality, 56*(4), 443–456.

Johnson, M. J., Jackson, N. C., Arnette, J. K., & Koffman, S. D. (2005). Gay and lesbian perceptions of discrimination in retirement care facilities. *Journal of Homosexuality, 49*, 83–102.

Jones, S. R. (1997). Voices of identity and difference: A qualitative exploration of the multiple dimensions of identity development in women college students. *Journal of College Student Development, 38,* 376–386.

Jones, S. R., & McEwen, M. K. (2000). A conceptual model of multiple dimensions of identity. *Journal of College Student Development, 41*(4), 405–414.

Kertzner, R. M. (2001). The adult life course and homosexual identity in midlife gay men. *Annual Review of Sex Research, 12,* 75–92.

Kertzner, R. M., Meyer, I. H., Frost, D. M., & Stirratt, M. J. (2009). Social and psychological well-being in lesbians, gay men, and bisexuals: The effects of race, gender, age, and sexual identity. *American Journal of Orthopsychiatry, 79*(4), 500–510.

Knapp, G. A. (2005). Race, class, gender: Reclaiming baggage in fast travelling theories. *European Journal of Women's Studies, 12*(3), 249–265.

Knochel, K. A., Crogan, C. F., Moore, R. P., & Quam, J. (2011). *Ready to serve? The aging network and LGB and T older adults.* Washington, DC: National Association of Area Agencies of Aging.

Kurdek, L. A. (2001). Differences between heterosexual-nonparent couples, and gay, lesbian, and heterosexual-parent couples. *Journal of Family Issues, 22,* 727–754.

Kurdek, L. A. (2004). Gay men and lesbians: The family context. In M. Coleman & L. H. Ganong (Eds.), *Handbook of contemporary families: Considering the past, contemplating the future* (pp. 96–115). Thousand Oaks, CA: Sage.

Lehavot, K., Balsam, K. F., & Ibrahim-Wells, G. D. (2009). Redefining the American quilt: Definitions and experiences of community among ethnically diverse lesbian and bisexual women. *Journal of Community Psychology, 37,* 439–458. doi:10.1002/jcop.20305.

Leyva, V. L., Breshears, E. M., & Ringstad, R. (2014). Assessing the efficacy of LGBT cultural competency training for aging services providers in California's Central Valley. *Journal of Gerontological Social Work, 57*(2–4), 335–348.

Long, J. (2008). Interracial and intercultural lesbian couples: The incredibly true adventures of two women in love. *Couples & Relationship Therapy, 2*(2/3), 85–101.

Malouff, J. M., Thorsteinsson, E. B., Schutte, N. S., Bhullar, N., & Rooke, S. E. (2010). The five factor model of personality and relationship satisfaction of intimate partners: A meta-analysis. *Journal of Research in Personality, 44,* 124–127.

McCall, L. (2005). The complexity of intersectionality. *Signs: Journal of Women in Culture and Society, 30*(3), 1771–1800.

McGibbon, E., & McPherson, C. (2011). Applying intersectionality & complexity theory to address the social determinants of women's health. *Women's Health & Public Policy, 10*(1), 59–86.

Meyer, I. (1995). Minority stress and mental health in gay men. *Journal of Health and Social Behavior, 36*(1), 38–56.

Meyer, I. (2003). Prejudice, social stress, and mental health in lesbian, gay, and bisexual populations: Conceptual issues and research evidence. *Psychological Bulletin, 129,* 674–697.

Meyer, H., & Johnston, T. R. (2014). The National Resource Center on LGBT Aging provides critical training to aging service providers. *Journal of Gerontological Social Work, 57,* 407–412.

Meyer, I. H., Schwartz, S., & Frost, D. M. (2008). Social patterning of stress and coping: Does disadvantaged status confer excess exposure and fewer coping resources? *Social Science and Medicine, 67,* 368–379.

Moone, R. P., Cagle, J. G., Croghan, C. F., & Smith, J. (2014). Working with LGBT older adults: an assessment of employee training practices, needs, and preferences of senior service organizations in Minnesota. *Journal of Gerontological Social Work, 57* (2–4), 322–334. doi:10.1080/01634372.2013.843630.

Moore, M. R. (2010). Articulating a politics of (multiple) identities: LGBT sexuality and inclusion in Black community life. *Du Bois Review, 7*(2), 1–20.

Moradi, B., Mohr, J. J., Worthington, R. L., & Fassinger, R. E. (2009). Counseling psychology research on sexual (orientation) minority issues: Conceptual and methodological challenges and opportunities. *Journal of Counseling Psychology, 56*(1), 5–22.

Movement Advancement Project, Services & Advocacy for Gay, Lesbian, Bisexual, & Transgender Elders, & Center for American Progress. (2010) *LGBT older adults: Facts at a glance.* Can be accessed from: http://lgbtagingcenter.org/resources/resource.cfm?r= 22.

National Hispanic Council on Aging. (2014). *In their own words: A needs assessment of Hispanic OGBT older adults.* Retrieved January 18, 2015 from www.lgbtagingcenter.org/resources/pdfs/InTheirOwnWords.pdf.

National Senior Citizens Law Center et al. (2010). *Stories from the field: LGBT older adults in long-term care facilities.* Washington, DC: National Senior Citizens Law Center. Retrieved from: http://www.lgbtlongtermcare.org.

Omi, M., & Winant, H. (1994). *Racial formation in the United States from the 1960s to the 1990s.* New York, NY: Routledge.

Orel, N. A. (2004). Gay, lesbian, and bisexual elders: Expressed needs and concerns across focus groups. *Journal of Gerontological Social Work, 43*(2/3), 57–77.

Otis, M. D., Rostosky, S. S., Riggle, E. D. B., & Hamrin, R. (2006). Stress and relationship quality in same-sex couples. *Journal of Social and Personal Relationships, 23,* 81–99. doi:10.1177/0265407506060179.

Pinderhughes, E. B. (2002). African American marriage in the 20th century. *Family Process, 41*(2), 269–282.

Porter, K. E., & Krinsky, L. (2014). Do LGBT aging trainings effectuate positive change in mainstream elder service providers? *Journal of Homosexuality, 61* (1), 197–216.

Portz, J. D., Retrum, J. H., Wright, L. A., Boggs, J. M., Wilkins, S., Grimm, C., et al. (2014). Assessing capacity for providing culturally competent services to LGBT older adults. *Journal of Gerontological Social Work, 57*(2–4), 305–321.

Purdie-Vaughns, V., & Eibach, R. P. (2008). Intersectional invisibility: The distinctive advantages and disadvantages of multiple subordinate-group identities. *Sex Roles, 59*(5–6), 377–391.

Raetz, T., & Lease, J. (2002). *The construction of identity.* Unpublished manuscript. Athens: University of Georgia.

Rainbow Train. (2003). *Rainbow train: Sexual/gender minority sensitivity trainings for providers of health and social services for elders [Brochure].* Seattle, WA: Author.

Robinson-Wood, T. (2009). *The convergence of race, ethnicity, and gender: Multiple identities in counseling* (3rd ed.). Upper Saddle River, NJ: Merrill.

Roccas, S., & Brewer, M. B. (2002). Social identity complexity. *Personality and Social Psychology Review, 6*(2), 88–106.

SAGE. (2013). *Health equity and LGBT elders of color: Recommendations for policy and practice.* Retrieved January 18, 2015 from http://sageusa.org/resources/publications.cfm?ID=203.

Schope, R. (2005). Who's afraid of growing old?: Gay and lesbian perceptions of aging. *Journal of Gerontological Social Work, 45*, 23–39.

Settles, I. H. (2006). Use of an intersectional framework to understand black women's racial and gender identities. *Sex Roles, 54*, 589–601.

Settles, I. H., & Buchanan, N. T. (2014). Multiple groups, multiple identities, and intersectionality. In V. Benet-Martinez & Y. Hong (Eds.), *The Oxford handbook of multicultural identity* (pp. 160–180). Oxford: Oxford University Press.

Shippy, R. A. (2007). We cannot do it alone: The impact of informal support and stressors in older gay, lesbian and bisexual caregivers. *Journal of Gay and Lesbian Social Services, 18*(3/4), 39–51.

Siverskog, A. (2014). "They just don't have a clue": Transgender aging and implications for social work. *Journal of Gerontological Social Work, 57*(2–4), 386–406.

Social Security Administration. (2011). *Annual statistical supplement to the social security bulletin, 2010.* Retrieved January 18, 2015 from http://www.ssa.gov/policy/docs/statcomps/supplement.

Stirratt, M. J., Meyer, I. H., Ouellette, S. C., & Gara, M. A. (2007). Measuring identity multiplicity and intersectionality: Hierarchical classes analysis (HICLAS) of sexual, racial, and gender identities. *Self and Identity, 7*(1), 89–111.

Szymanski, D. M. (2005). Heterosexism and sexism as correlates of psychological distress in lesbians. *Journal of Counseling and Development, 83*, 355–360.

Szymanski, D. M., & Gupta, A. (2009). Examining the relationship between multiple internalized oppressions and African American lesbian, gay, bisexual, and questioning persons' self-esteem and psychological distress. *Journal of Counseling Psychology, 56*(1), 110–118.

Tjepkema, M. (2008). Health care use among gay, lesbian, and bisexual Canadians. *Health Reports, 19* (1), 53–64.

Tornstam, L. (2005). *Gerotranscedence: A developmental theory of positive aging.* New York, NY: Springer Publishing Company.

Van Den Bergh, N., & Crisp, C. (2004). Defining culturally competent practice with sexual minorities: Implications for social work education and practice. *Journal of Social Work Education, 40*(2), 221–238.

Van Sluytman, L. G., & Torres, D. (2014). Hidden or uninvited? A content analysis of elder LGBT of color literature in gerontology. *Journal of Gerontological Social Work, 57*(2–4), 130–160.

Weber, L. (1998). A conceptual framework for understanding race, class, gender, and sexuality. *Psychology of Women Quarterly, 22*, 13–22.

Weber, L., & Parra-Medina, D. (2003). Intersectionality and women's health: Charting a path to eliminating health disparities. *Advances in Gender Research, 7*, 181–230.

Weston, K. (1991). *Families we choose: Lesbians, gays, kinship.* New York: Columbia University Press.

Woody, I. (2014). Aging out: A qualitative exploration of ageism and heterosexism among aging African American lesbians and gay men. *Journal of Homosexuality, 61*, 145–165. doi:10.1080/00918369.2013.835603.

Young, R. M., & Meyer, I. H. (2005). The trouble with "MSM" and "WSW": Erasure of the sexual-minority person in public health discourse. *American Journal of Public Health, 95*(7), 1144–1149.

African-American and Black LGBT Elders

Debra A. Harley

Abstract

This chapter discusses issues relevant to African-American and Black LGBT elders, including historical influences that frame these issues, demographic and cultural contexts, and sociopolitical considerations that impact policy and service delivery. This chapter describes the cultural capital of the African-American community and examines Black homo–bi–transphobia, the intersection of identities is presented along with multiple oppressions and gay racism, and the ways in which historical hostilities influence help-seeking by older African-American LGBT persons are presented. Information is presented on health disparities and services. The ways in which service models nationally, cross-culturally, and multidisciplinarily work to promote effective interventions are discussed. Finally, the impact of policy on African-American LGBT elders is presented within the context in which by this population perceives services.

Keywords

African-American · Aging · Black · Health disparities · Intersectionality · LGBT

Overview

The purpose of this chapter is to discuss issues relevant to African-American and Black LGBT elders, including historical influences that frame these issues, demographic and cultural contexts, and sociopolitical considerations that impact policy and service delivery. This chapter begins with information on characteristics that comprise older African-American and Black adults. Next, relevant research is infused throughout the chapter. The chapter then describes the cultural capital of the African-American community, including perceptions about homosexuality and gender nonconformity, how elders are viewed, issues of acculturation and assimilation, and strength-based concepts. Subsequently, the chapter examines

D.A. Harley (✉)
University of Kentucky, Lexington, USA
e-mail: dharl00@email.uky.edu

© Springer International Publishing Switzerland 2016
D.A. Harley and P.B. Teaster (eds.), *Handbook of LGBT Elders*,
DOI 10.1007/978-3-319-03623-6_6

Black homophobia and other phobias and "isms" about sexual identity, including the attitudes and practices of the Black Church toward sexual minorities. Because African-American LGBT elders have multiple *positionalities* in society, the intersection of identities is presented along with multiple oppressions and gay racism. The ways in which historical hostilities influence help-seeking by older African-American LGBT persons are presented. In addition, information is presented on health service disparities of African-American LGBT elders. The chapter examines ways in which service models nationally, cross-culturally, and multidisciplinary work to promote effective interventions. Finally, given that the manner in which services are perceived is, in part, influenced by policy, the impact of policy on African-American and Black LGBT elders is presented within the context. The reader is reminded that the information in this chapter is not presented as absolute or definitive of all African-Americans or Black people. There is great intercultural, intracultural, and cross-cultural diversity within African-American, African, Caribbean, and other populations of African descent.

Learning Objectives

By the end of the chapter, the reader should be able to:

1. Identify relevant characteristics of African-American culture that influence attitudes and behaviors.
2. Discuss the concepts of homo–bi–transphobia in the African-American/Black community.
3. Describe sociocultural issues, healthcare disparities, and health-seeking patterns of African-American LGBT elders.
4. Explain service models and intervention strategies that are effective with African-American/Black LGBT elders.
5. List areas in which policy development is needed to address concerns of African-American/Black LGBT elders.

Introduction

An accurate estimate of the number of African-American and Black LGBT persons is not known, and the number of elderly LGBT among them is unknown because of an inability to determine an exact number of the total lesbian, gay, bisexual, transgender, and questioning (LGBTQ) population of all ages in the USA. Approximately 3.4 % of Americans identify LGBT and 4.6 % of African-Americans. Regardless of ethnicity, younger Americans are more likely to identify as LGBT, and among those aged 30–64, LGBT identity declines with age (Gates and Newport 2012). It is difficult to glean how many African-American or Black LGBT persons are elderly because of reasons such as the rate of non-disclosure, the limited research on sexual minorities of color, a lack of national surveys that ask about sexual orientation or gender identity, reluctance to coming out, and of variation in responses to surveys due to the methodologies used (Bostwick 2007; DeBlaere et al. 2010). However, the number of LGBT older adults is projected to more than double in size to approximately 3 million by 2050 (2009). In 2012, African-Americans made up 9 % of the older population and the African-American older population is projected to increase to 12 % by 2060 (Administration for Community Living 2012). The rapid growth of the aging population in the USA offers the opportunity to embrace diversity as it appears at all stages of life (National Hispanic Council on Aging 2013), and "understanding their differences in health and addressing disparities are critically important for improving the nation's overall health and well-being" (Today's Research on Aging 2013, p. 1).

As the reader proceeds in this chapter, one is informed that the terms African-American and Black are used sometimes interchangeably to reflect common themes across groups. At other times, the terms are used separately to reflect distinctiveness between groups. African-Americans are descended from slaves who were brought to America during the eighteenth and nineteenth centuries. The term Black is more inclusive and is comprised of diverse groups of ethnicities and cultures, including those who immigrated from Africa and the Caribbean (Welch 2003) and may include multiple heritage individuals with Black ancestry (e.g., biracial, multiracial) who experience life and development differently from monoracial minority and majority individuals (Henriksen and Paladino 2009). Persons of African descent may identify as African-American, Afro-American, Black Hispanic, Black Caribbean, Black American, and Black African (Lewis and Marshall 2012). It is not uncommon for older African-Americans to refer to themselves as *Colored*, *Negro* (both terms were used derogatorily), or *Black*, which are terms that were commonly used to refer to them for a substantial portion of their lives. These terms emphasize skin color, not cultural heritage (Paniagua 2014). In addition, while it is acceptable to use lesbian, gay, bisexual, and transgender or LGBT when referring to African-American and Black sexual minorities, it is an error to assume that all people use these terms to describe themselves. The Communities of African Descent Resource Kit (2014, http://www.glaad.org/publications.coadkit) indicates that many individuals have adopted the term "Same Gender Loving" (SGL) or other terms that are more inclusive of both sexual orientation and race, and others may not identify with any terms at all.

Elderly (age 65 and over) African-American and Black LGBT persons represent multiple classifications of minority statuses, and each of their identities dictates certain social positions in society and further relegates them to positions of marginality. For many African-American and Black LGBT elders, addressing issues of racism in general and within the LGBT community specifically, heterosexism and homophobia both internal and external to their ethnic group, emotional isolation (Kuyper and Fokkema 2010), and internalized oppression (Szymanski and Gupta 2009) have been the hallmark of their experiences. Even with the distinction of being a minority (ethnic) within a minority (sexual orientation), transgender (see Chap. 14 in this text) and bisexual (see Chap. 15 in this text) persons

are further marginalized. In fact, Dworkin (2006) refers to bisexual LGBT elders as the "invisible of the invisible minority" because as they enter into romantic relationships, they sometimes begin to identify as lesbian, gay, or heterosexual and thus become invisible as a bisexual aging person (p. 36).

Characteristics of Older African-American/Black Adults

African-American and Black older adults are heterogeneous, multidimensional, and diverse in their cultural identities and social affiliations. They represent various levels of educational attainment, socioeconomic statuses and financial stability, beliefs and values, marital status, sexual orientation and gender identity, and so forth. However, older Black adults share commonalities. Overall, older African-Americans are more highly educated than previous older generations. In 2013, 71 % of African-Americans age 65 and older had finished high school and 15 % had a bachelor's degree or higher compared to the fact that only 44 % were high school graduates and 7 % had a bachelor's degree or higher in 1998 (Administration for Community Living 2012). In employment, many were overrepresented in low-wage positions, resulting in economic insecurity in retirement. Social security benefits constitute the largest share of income of older African-Americans, but are modest in size. Many Black elders grew up in southern states during a time of legal segregation and overt discrimination, which imposed limits on their earnings, educational attainment, poor living conditions, and health outcomes (Social Security Administration 2011). A residential shift has occurred as to where the majority of older African-Americans currently live. The largest percentage of Black residents per total population in 2012 was in the District of Columbia (51.6 %) and Mississippi (28 %), with the largest total number of Black residents in New York (3.7 million) (Centers for Disease Control 2010). Table 6.1 lists the states with the largest percent of older African-Americans.

Table 6.1 States with highest percent of older African-Americans

New York	320,127
Florida	271,554
Texas	241,356
California	237,924
Georgia	236,463
North Carolina	210,772
Illinois	190,521
Maryland	166,186

Administration for Community Living (2012)

Table 6.2 Frequently occurring health conditions of older African-Americans

African-Americans	All older persons (%)
Hypertension (85 %)	72
Diagnosed arthritis (52 %)	50
Heart disease (26 %)	30
Diagnosed diabetes (40 %)	20
Cancer (17 %)	24

Adapted from Administration for Community Living (2012)

Table 6.3 Leading causes of death for African-Americans

Heart disease
Cancer
Stroke
Diabetes
Unintentional injuries
Nephritis, nephrotic syndrome and nephrosis
Chronic lower respiratory disease
Homicide
Septicemia
Alzheimer's disease

Adapted from Centers for Disease Control (2010)

In a study of self-rated health status in 2010–2012, 62 % of older African-American men and 61 % of women reported "good," "very good," or "excellent" health status compared to 78 % for White older men and 80 % for women. Positive health evaluations decline with age, with 67 % of African-American men ages 65–74 reporting "good," "very good," or "excellent" health compared with 52 % among those aged 85 or older. Similarly, 65 % of African-American women ages 65–74 reported "good" to "excellent" health, with 58 % at ages 85 or older (Administration for Community Living 2012). African-Americans have a disproportionately higher rate of chronic illnesses and lower survival rates. The most frequently occurring health issues among African-Americans include AIDS/HIV, asthma, cancer, diabetes, heart disease, hypertension, obesity, and stroke (Centers for Disease Control 2013). In addition, African-Americans have higher rates of HIV and AIDS, many of whom were infected at a younger age and who are now living longer (Baker and Krehely 2012). A combination of health inequities and financial and cultural barriers to receiving health care in later life negatively affects the health of African-American older adults. Table 6.2 compares the most frequently occurring conditions among older African-Americans compared to all other older persons. In comparison to White elders, Black elders have severe limitations in daily tasks requiring assistance with housework, personal care, and preparing meals. The life expectancy for Blacks, at any age, tends to be lower than that for Whites. In 2010,

a 65-year-old African-American male was expected to live another 15.9 years, compared with 17.7 for White males, and a Black female at age 65 was expected to live another 19.3 years, a full year less than a White woman. Comparatively, Latino males (additional 18.8 years) and Latina females (additional 22 years) are expected to liver longer than Black or White males and females (National Center for Health Statistics 2013). Interestingly, these data do not disaggregate outcomes for LGBT persons. The leading causes of death for all African-Americans are in Table 6.3.

African-American LGBT elders face challenges similar to those in both the African-American and the older adult populations as a whole. Collectively, more than 68 % of African-American elders are poor, marginally poor, or economically vulnerable, are more than one and a half times as likely as White elders to live below the poverty line, and more than one in four

African-American elders have incomes that fall below the poverty line. Some gender disparity exists among older African-American women and men with regard to living arrangement. More older African-American women are vulnerable to social isolation and economic hardship, with nearly 40 % of women ages 65 and older living alone compared to 19 % of men (Administration on Aging, n.d.). The circumstances of older LGBT African-Americans are difficult to discern and separate from the Black population at large because of their covert existence in the Black community (Harley et al. 2014). Many years of living, secretive or closeted lives often lead to a heightened sense of isolation for Black LGBT elders. Yet, as a separate group, less is known about unique challenges faced by African-American transgender persons or those who identify as queer, even though they were intricately involved in the Civil Rights Movement of the 1960s and have been active contributors to history (Roberts 2012). One of the earliest documented cases of an African-American transgender person is that of Lucy Hicks Anderson who was born in Waddy, Kentucky, in 1886, as Tobias Lawson. See Discussion Box 6.1 for information on Anderson and on Carlett Angianlee Brown, who was scheduled to become the first African-American to have sex reassignment surgery (SRS).

Discussion Box 6.1: Historical Transgender African-Americans Lucy Hicks Anderson (1886–1954): Born in Waddy, Kentucky, as Toias Lawson. When Lawson entered school she insisted on wearing dresses and began calling herself Lucy. Upon the advice of a physician, Lawson's mother raised her as a girl. After leaving school at age 15, Lucy worked as a domestic. She eventually married and then moved to California. After a divorce in 1929, she remarried in 1944 to a soldier. Eventually, when the Ventura County district attorney discovered that Lucy was biologically male, he decided to try her for perjury. Lucy was convicted of perjury and placed on probation for 10 years. Later, the federal government prosecuted Lucy and

her husband for fraud for receiving allotment checks as the wife of a member of the US Army. After her release from prison, she lived the remainder of her life in Los Angeles (http://www.blackpast.org/aaw/anderson-lucy-hicks-1886-1954).

Carlett Angianlee Brown (1927): She was born as Charles Robert Brown. In 1953, Carlett was a 26-year-old female illusionist and shake dancer from Pittsburgh. She had served in the Navy, during which time she was examined for an issue with recurring monthly bleeding through her rectal area. The medical exam revealed that she was intersex and had some female sex organs. She declined to have surgery to remove the female organs and opted for SRS instead. Her plan was to get marry after completing SRS. In order to do so, Carlett had to renounce her US citizenship because laws in countries where the surgery could be performed did not allow foreign nationals to obtain SRS. Her US passport was issued with her name as Carlett Angianlee. On July 9th, she was arrested for cross-dressing. She postponed her departure to get a feminizing face-lift in New York in August. Eventually, she was ordered not to leave the USA until $1200 in back taxes were paid. Unable to make payment, she worked as a cook at Iowa State's Pi Kappa frat house to earn money. Additional information regarding her final outcome is not found. If Carlett is still alive, she will be into her mid- to late 1970s (http://www.racialicious.com/2009/07/15/the-story-of-carlett-brown/).

Discussion Questions:

1. What sociopolitical issues are in play for Anderson and for Brown?
2. Compare and contrast the challenges facing transgender African-Americans in the 1940s, 1950s, and today.
3. How accepting was the Black community of transgender persons within the community? Civil Rights Movement?

4. Have the attitudes of the Black community changed toward transgendered persons?
5. In what ways can the Black community promote advocacy and equality for Black transgendered persons?

In 2007, a national survey of transgender and nonconforming gender populations was conducted by Trans Equality to determine discrimination experiences (www.transequality.org/PDFs/BlackTransFactsheetFINAL_090811.pdf). Of the 6456 respondents, 381 were Black or Black multiracial. While the focus of the survey was on anti-transgender bias, the results also show the complex interactions of bias with race and socioeconomic status. The survey did not identify those experiences by age. Nevertheless, "the combination of anti-transgender bias and persistent, structural and individual racism was especially devastating for Black transgender people and other people of color" (p. 1). Black transgender persons live in extreme poverty with 34 % reporting a household income of less than $10,000 per year. These data indicate that for Black transgender persons, this is more than twice the rate for transgender people of all races (15 %), four times the general Black population rate (9 %), and over eight times the general US population rate (4 %). In addition, more than half of Black respondents were HIV positive. Although African-Americans have a significantly lower suicide rate than other racial groups, nearly 49 % of Black transgender persons indicated they had attempted suicide at some point. On a more positive note, the study found that those who were "out" to their families found acceptance at a higher rate than the overall sample of transgender respondents.

Research and Practice

The National Alliance on Mental Illness (2007) acknowledges that to date, most research on LGBT populations has been done with predominately White samples and the mental health (MH) concerns and needs of LGBT of color are still largely unknown and vastly understudied. In addition, health disparities and disabilities among African-Americans are higher than their White counterparts, with women experiencing early onset of disease and disability and increased mortality (Jones 2009; Lekan 2009). LGBT older adults and LGBT elders of color deal with significant health disparities across domains related to physical and mental health, including chronic conditions and HIV/AIDS, depression, suicide, and substance abuse (Administration on Aging, 2013; Fredriksen-Goldsen et al. 2011; Institute of Medicine, 2011).

The long-term financial stability of many LGBT elders of color is shaped by employment discrimination. Many LGBT elders of color are concentrated in employment sectors with low wages, no labor unions or few labor protections, routine discrimination, and limited health and savings options. Economic security is core to the health and well-being of LGBT elders of color (Auldridge and Espinoza 2013).

Lekan (2009) emphasizes that African-American women experience more stress and health disadvantages than their White counterparts because of the interaction and multiplicative effects of race, gender, socioeconomic status, and age. Although there is a growing body of research about health concerns among African-American women in general, there exists a dearth of information on African-American lesbians (Dibble et al. 2012). Similarly, African-American gay men are rarely researched outside of a focus on HIV/AIDS. African-American transgender persons also experience many health and socioeconomic challenges including substance abuse, HIV infection, difficulty in obtaining housing and employment, and reliance on commercial sex work for survival (Clements-Nolle et al. 2001; Wilkinson, nd). Understanding bisexual Black women and men within the context of culture and community is difficult because they experience isolation from heterosexual as well as lesbian and gay communities, which may affect aspects of identity development, internalized binegativity, and access to social and psychological resources (Isarel 2007). While LGBT people of color experience the worst outcomes and receive the least institutional attention, the aging concerns of LGBT of color are virtually absent in national policy discussions on aging health and economic security (Auldridge and Espinoza 2013). Because of the limited research on LGBT elders of color, there is reliance on the literature concerning LGBT elders in general, from which information is glean about African-American LGBT elders. However, additive research for African-American LGBT should be avoided because it does not equal research applicable to this group (Bowleg 2008). As author of this chapter, I suggest that additive research may offer some comparative insight; however, should at least approached with caution.

In advancing the research of LGBT persons of African descent, Lewis and Marshall (2012) offer several considerations. First, research on Black LGBT populations should not attempt to separate the various aspects of the individual's identities into mutually exclusive categories and expect to understand their experiences. Second, research must incorporate questions of the participants that do not force them to respond to items as to which identity is more important, which identity causes more stress, or rank identities in order of concern on a daily basis. Questions such as these assume an additive value to the multiple identities, and further marginalizing as opposed to an intersecting relationship among the identities (Bowleg 2008; Lewis and Marshall). According to Wheeler (2003), researchers must realize that the intersecting identities of sexual orientation, gender, race, and ethnicity are more likely to be geometric rather than additive. Finally, Afrocentric theorizing, which has "secured its own identity among dominant Eurocentric thought" (p. 13), must stop being neglectful of prevalent sexual realities in African-American culture.

All too often, research methodologies on African-Americans and Black LGBT populations involve a comparison to White LGBT groups, with whom they share few similarities beyond sexual orientation and gender identity. Moreover, most studies on sexual minorities do not include sufficient numbers of African-American or Black participants to perform adequate or sophisticated statistical analyses. In addition, research on LGBT African-Americans focuses on urban populations and ignores those in rural setting or smaller cities (Deblaere et al. 2010). For additional information on LGBT persons in rural settings, the reader is referred to Chap. 25 in this text. LGBT persons in urban areas have the privilege of anonymity, access to more services and supports, and the opportunity to belong to an LGBT community. The language used in many research studies present another barrier to instrumentation design. Much of the terminology that is used is characteristics of the White LGBT community (e.g., "out"), which involves identification by labels, whereas in Black culture, the approach is more a use of descriptions. Researchers will need to develop measures that are consistent with indigenous structures in the Black community. Finally, limited research exists that examines African-American LGBT issues and concerns across the life span (Harley et al. 2013).

Cultural Capital

The African-American community is known as a collective society that provides support and refuge to its people. The cultural characteristics of the community consist of strong kinship bonds, valuing education, strong religious orientation, high achievement orientation, strong work ethic, self-reliance, and adaptability of family roles (Brown Wright and Fernander 2005). Table 6.4 consists of value characteristics of the African-American community. Homosexuality and nonconforming sexual identity are largely considered incompatible with values in the Black community. Lewis and Marshall (2012) suggest factors that may influence the attitudes and perceptions among Black people about LGBT persons of African descent, including racism and ancestral baggage (i.e., rejection by some in their

Table 6.4 Value characteristics of the African-American Community

Self-reliant
Oral traditions
Strong work ethic
Unity and cooperation
Flexibility in family roles
Present-time orientation
Firm child-rearing practices
Educations as a means of self-help
Strong work and achievement ethic
Strong spiritual and religious values
Respect for elders and authority figures
Collateral interpersonal relations are highly valued
Giving people status as a function of age and position
Strong kinship bonds with family, extended family, and friends
"Strong Black Woman" (pride in racial identity, self-reliance, capability in handling challenges)
Nonverbal communication patterns (body movement, postures, gestures, facial expressions)
Adapted from Robinson-Wood (2009)

own race in an attempt to project noticeable "normal" Blackness), a lack of promotion of historically accurate information on diverse Black sexuality, and selective attention bias regarding interpretations of specific biblical scriptures. Some evidence suggests that more ambivalence, tolerance, and acceptance have emerged in African-American families for LGBT family members (Hunter 2005). Hunter suggests that family instructions such as "be silent and invisible" may allow the family to accept a LGBT member without having to deal with his or her sexual orientation and the issues associated with it. In fact, the lack of disclosure increases acceptance of their sexual orientation for older LGBT Black persons. However, the circumstances for African-American LGBT elders are difficult to discern and separate from the general Black population because of their cover existence in the Black community.

Although African-American culture may be inclusive of other Black families and communities, it is a misnomer to assume that it is representative of those other diverse Black groups. There is no one description that can accommodate the various identities, behaviors, and perceptions among African-Americans (Wilson 2005). Similarly, the terms used in the African diaspora are different, with some being highly derogatory (Lewis and Marshall 2012). LGBT issues of people of color play out differently in families and communities of different backgrounds, yet many communities of color share cultural bias against homosexuality and gender nonconformity (Somjen 2009). The way in which an individual expresses his or her gender and/or sexuality may be defined by cultural values such as whether the culture focuses on the individual or the group; the level of acceptance in talking about sexuality; the degree of separation of public and private domain; the social organization and definitions of gender; the role of religion within their own culture; and the degree of assimilation into the dominate society (Rust 1996). LGBT persons of color, regardless of age, share the common experience of being a minority within a minority, which may contribute to an increased vulnerability to psychosocial issues.

African-American and Black LGBT persons have always been part of the Black community. The roles and impact of LGBT persons in the Black community was in part demonstrated through involvement in the Civil Rights Movement. On April 1, 1998, in the *Chicago Tribune*, Coretta Scott King acknowledged the role of sexual minorities stating, "gay and lesbians stood up for civil rights in Montgomery, Selma, in Albany, Georgia and St. Augustine, FL., and many other campaigns of the Civil Rights Movement. Many of these courageous men and women were fighting for my freedom at a time when they could find few voices for their own, and I salute their contributions." Although the rate of homophobia and heterosexism is high in the Black community, especially in the Black Church (which is discussed later in this chapter), most African-American LGBT persons indicate that they still find more support and refuge in the Black community, especially against the tyranny of racism in the White gay community (Boykin 1996; Green 1994; Savage and Harley 2005). For African-American LGBT people, there is "a perceived link that connects its members regardless of other differences that might also exist" (Moore 2010, p. 17). In fact, some researchers suggest that African-American lesbians, having learned to handle their ethnic minority status, have developed a great deal of resilience and personal strength and may be better equipped to also handle their status as a sexual minority (Cooper-Lewter 2007; Dibble et al. 2012; Hall and Fine 2005). Yet, gender discrimination is not equal for LGBT persons in the Black community. Lesbians often face disproportionately more ridicule in the Black community, and based on their multiple subordinate-group identities, Black lesbians have "intersectional invisibility: as targets of sexism, heterosexism, homophobia, and racism within the dominant culture and the Black community" (Purdie-Vaugns and Eibach 2008, p. 377).

Views Held About Elders. From a cultural perspective, elderly African-Americans are revered and entitled to respect within the African-American community, and a position of age carries with it a high level of cultural capital (Harley et al. 2014). Ageism is not a prevalent characteristic in the Black community; however, it is in the gay community, especially with regard to physical attractiveness. However, the reader should be aware of some generational changes within the Black community about attitudes and behaviors toward their elders. For example, elders in the Black community are increasingly targets of violence and crime, mistreatment, and assault. This shift in attitudes toward African-American elders must be placed within a culturally sensitive context and considered alongside culturally specific risk factors (Teaster et al. 2014). For example, in the African-American community, a single incidence of yelling or hitting an elder is not viewed as elder abuse, whereas physical abuse is extreme abusive behavior. Extreme abusive behavior toward elders is considered as unacceptable in the Black community (Tauriac and Scruggs 2006).

African-American elders hold the distinction of being the family historian. The elders continue the oral tradition of passing on cultural meaning, legacy, and knowledge. Within the Black community, elders are not referred to as old, but as wise, illustrating that they have reached the "age of wisdom." Although aging is associated with lived experience, chronological age is not the only criterion for ascension into the "age of wisdom." The experience that one has accumulated allows one, especially women to gain this wisdom. Experience may include emotional and spiritual support, information, advice, and service. Old age for Black women is a matter of the functions they carry out (e.g., teaching values, convening the family on certain occasions, religious role model). Thus, wise women gain prestige and power, and important matters are brought to them (Brown Wright and Fernander 2005; Peterson 1990). Peterson summarized the important role of older Black women in the family and church, "they move beyond the potential constraints of class, money and blood relationships to reinforce cultural values of the importance of children, the significance of fictive kin, the problem of clinging to possessions and the wisdom derived from lived experience" (p. 227). Given that the family and church are considered to be the two most important institutions in the Black community and a high degree of respect for elders, the question is raised, what is the role of LGBT elders within these institutions?

Deutsch (2006) suggests that through *civilized oppression* (the experience of repeated, widespread, systematic injustice), Black LGBT persons receive unequal treatment, are relegated to invisibility, and are silenced, condemned, shamed, and forbidden from participation in activities afforded to heterosexual couples.

Acculturation and Assimilation Issues. Numerous definitions of acculturation exist to explain the multifaceted ways in which changes occur at the group and individual level. Riva (2010) offers the definition of acculturation as "a dynamic process of change that individuals undergo as they interact with and adapt to a new or different cultural environment; it is an interactive process that occurs along different life domains at different rates of change" (p. 331). Inherent in the practice of acculturation is the concept of inequality and the lack of mutual respect that the dominant culture tends to project, consciously or unconsciously, on racial minorities (Wilson 2005). Assimilation is viewed more as voluntary aspiration to identify and integrate with and adapt to the ways of the dominant, Anglo-Saxon mainstream. The intent of presenting information on acculturation and assimilation is not to debate if Black LGBT elders are one or the other, but rather to illustrate that acculturation and assimilation involve changes in both values and behaviors related to identity (Schwartz et al. 2007). Cultural identity is the sense of belonging that one derives from membership in groups that provide knowledge, beliefs, values, traditions, attitudes, and ways of life (Jameson 2007). Although acculturation and cultural identity are not totally uncorrelated, an individual who is highly acculturated can have a high level of ethnic identity or a low level of ethnic identify (Moore et al. 2010). It is important to point out that race and culture are not synonymous.

For Black people in America, the assimilation model is most useful for understanding voluntary immigrants, not native-born Black who entered the USA involuntarily who were selectively incorporated through enslavement, coercion, and Jim Crow laws (Lacy 2004). Wamwara-Mbugua et al. (2006) contend "the experience of Black immigrants in the United States is different from that of other non-white groups because of the existence of a large African-American population and the complexities of race relations" (p. 428). Black immigrants may conform more to segmented assimilation (Portes and Zhou 1993) in which they take three paths of adaptation: (1) the White middle class, (2) identify with the Black underclass, and (3) carve out a path by deliberately retaining the culture and values of their immigrant community. Frequently, older Black immigrants and subsequently generations take the third path, relying on their ethnic communities for social capital, employment leads, and relief from discrimination. Segmented assimilation allows the individual to maintain an ethnic identity as an invaluable resource (Lacy).

The question of whether Black LGBT elders more acculturated because of their sexual orientation and gender identity is not known. The extent to which Black LGBT elders are acculturated or assimilated has not been studied, and, at best, one can glean from the research on acculturation of African-Americans in general. Furthermore, the reality may be that neither acculturation nor assimilation is the issue, but more one of cultural immersion in which individuals reject mainstream culture and their emotional needs are met exclusively in their ethnic or in the gay community. Where one lives may be a major determinant of cultural immersion. For example, LGBT persons who live in urban areas may immerse themselves in LGBT communities; however, this is not an option available to most LGBT people who must live in many worlds/cultures and communities.

Black Homophobia, Biphobia, Transphobia, and Heterosexism

African-American LGBT elders often face social stigma in the Black community. Historically, the Black community view homosexuality as a characteristic of European culture, and they deny, or at least overlook its existence in their own community. Many in the Black community believe that homosexuality and any form of alternative sexual identity is a strategy to destroy Black people and the Black family, is a moral sin, and goes against the values of the Black community. The Black community values privacy, which is in contrast to the White LGBT community's value of "coming out." Strong family and kinship ties stress that marriage and family always come first, and the family may present a united front against the LGBT member or disown him or her, resulting in a loss of the sense of unity that helps the LGBT member form cultural and/or race identity (Savage and Harley 2005). The National Black Justice Coalition (2009) found that while statistically African-Americans are more disapproving of marriage equality for sexual minorities, these attitudes do not arise from simple homophobia; rather, they come from their diverse experiences, opinions, and beliefs and are influenced by factors such as geographic location, age, class, and other markers of differences. Often, this moral disapprobation is linked to the pulpit and rhetoric of the conservative right that suggests that the gay rights movement has appropriated the civil rights philosophy and incorrectly equated racial oppression with oppression based on sexual orientation and gender identity (National Black Justice Coalition). As a historically oppressed group, African-Americans have placed great importance on reproductive sexuality to ensure continue existence of the group in face of racist, genocidal practices by the dominant White group (Greene and Boyd-Franklin 1996). Thus, Black LGBT individuals are seen as a threat to the social structure of the family (Battle and Bennett 2000; Boykin 1996; National Black Justice Coalition 2009).

Research suggests that homophobia is greater in the African-American community than in the European American community (National Black Justice Coalition2009; Savage and Harley 2005; Stanford 2013). The existence of homophobia among Black people in America is largely reflective of the homophobic culture in which we live (Clarke 1999). According to Clark, Black Americans assimilated the Puritan value that sex is for procreation, occurs only between men and women, and is only valid within the confines of heterosexual marriage. The result of this assimilation is that Black people have to live with the contradictions of this restricted sexual system by repressing or closeting any other sexual or erotic feelings or desires. However, the whole African-American community is not homophobic or heterosexist, and the "accusation of homophobia" directed toward the whole Black community is inaccurate (Boykin 1996, p. 185), and studies on the African-American community's attitudes and perceptions of sexual minorities continue to unfold. Nevertheless, it cannot be denied that the existence of homophobia has always been a reality in Black life (Hooks 2001). Today, the invisibility of homosexuality in the Black community remains prevalent and is synonymous with its own form of "don't ask," "don't tell." Despite the sometime disapproving attitudes and religious condemnation, the majority of Black LGBT individuals remain in predominantly Black communities and social contexts and negotiate daily with family and community. They remain because they trust in racial solidarity and racial group membership (Moore 2010), which often provide protection from racial discrimination in the larger society.

Religion and Spirituality in the Lives of Black Elders. The Black Church is recognized as the oldest and one of the most influential institutions of the Black community. Both religion and spirituality are vital components of African-American racial and cultural activities (Harley 2005a). Laderman and Leon (2003) suggest that religion supplies perhaps the best vantage point from which to describe the development of African-Americans in relationship to themselves, others, and the larger universe. National research data indicate that approximately 97 % of African-Americans identify some religious affiliation (Pew Center 2006). The church is more than a place of worship and fellowship; it is a place of advocacy, empowerment, personal and psychological support, socialization, emotional outlet, social status, political action, cultural affirmation, and connection to the community (Evans and George 2008; Loue 2014) and is essentially impossible to separate from Black life for most African-American elders. Research Box 6.1 contains a study of older African-Americans' perception of spirituality and its role in dealing with depression. The amount of support and assistance provided by the Black Church is second only to that provided by the family (Robinson-Wood 2009). In many ways, the Black Church takes on increased significance as a source of support because LGBT seniors, especially gay men, do not have children who can care for them as they age. Within the LGBT population, child rearing is much more common among racial and ethnic minority women (41 % of African-Americans) compared with White LGBT women (28 %) and less so among African-American men (14 %). However, these data include younger average ages of racial and ethnic groups in the USA (Gates and Newport 2012). In fact, lesbians and gay men are twice as likely as their heterosexual counterparts to grow old un-partnered and almost ten times more likely not to have a spouse, child, or other family member to care for them in old age (Albelda et al. 2009).

Research Box 6.1: Depression and Spirituality Wittink, M. N., Joo, J. H., Lewis, L.M., & Barg, F. K. (2009). Losing faith and using faith: Older African-Americans discuss spirituality, religious activities, and depression. *Journal of General Internal Medicine*, 24(3), 402–407.

Objective: This study aimed to understand how spirituality might play a role in the way older African-Americans conceptualize and deal with depression in order to inform possible interventions aimed at improving the acceptability and effectiveness of depression treatment.

Method: A cross-sectional qualitative interview design was used with older African-American primary care patients. Forty-seven patients were recruited from primary care practices in Baltimore, DM area, and interviews were conducted in the homes of participants.

Results: Participants in this study held a faith-based explanatory model of depression with a particular emphasis on the cause of depression. Specifically, participants described depression as being due to a "loss of faith," and faith and spiritual/religious activities were thought to be empowering in the way they can work together with medical treatments to provide the strength for healing to occur.

Conclusion: Older African-Americans are more likely to identify spirituality as important in depression care.

Questions

1. How are spiritual/religious activities facilitative of depression treatment?
2. How would you evaluate the extent to which the findings of the research represent insider versus outsider perspective?
3. What do you see as the limitations to this research methodology for Black LGBT elders?

Although reference is made to "the Black Church," the church is heterogeneous, non-monolithic, and disparate collective of churches that reflect the diversity of the Black community itself and are diversified by origin, denomination, doctrine, worship culture, spiritual ethos, class, size, and numerous other factors. Yet, Black Churches share a common history and function as a unique role in Black life, which attest to their collective identify as the Black Church (Douglas 2006). The Black Church, with its heterogeneous character, is more monolithic in its attitude toward homosexuality. The Black Church adheres to traditional religious values, which condemn homosexuality and gender nonconformity. Some Black ministers hurl condescending insults in their sermons to express distain toward non-heterosexuals (Ward 2005). African-Americans attend religious services more frequently than Whites and are less supportive of gay rights (Pew Center 2006). According to Douglas (2006), "the Black Church community, even with all of their diversity, the Black Church people are regarded as strikingly similar in their attitudes toward non-heterosexual sexualities. Black Church people are viewed as not simply homophobic but more homophobic than other populations of society" (p. 12). Although the majority of Black people in America regard themselves as Christians, growing numbers are counted among Islamists, Buddhists, Jews, and agnostics (Robinson-Wood 2009).

In a study of Black lesbian spirituality, Betts (2012) found that African-American lesbians continually strive for a sense of spiritual wholeness. While the lesbians in Betts' study had no difficulty connecting to Black culture, they did report difficulty connecting with their initial religious roots within the churches of their childhood and actively sought alternative spiritual outlets. Other studies suggest that for certain populations of Blacks, perceived religiosity is related to faith healing (Harley 2005b; Mitchem 2002; Lawson and Thomas 2007), and elderly Black women have higher religiosity (e.g., prayer, giving thanks to God, reading the Bible, going to church) than Black men (Taylor et al. 2004). Black people who may not go to church or even have a church home may still pray to the Lord when confronted with difficult times (Boyd-Franklin 2003). Even Black persons who denounce religiosity often note religious ideology as important to their moral beliefs and practices (Dyson 2003; Ward 2005). With the importance placed on religion and spirituality by African-Americans and their disapproval of homosexuality, transgender, and nonconforming gender persons, Black LGBT persons may be denied the sense of community and support afforded to others within the community when the church denies them fellowship. Many LGBT African-Americans often face the same ignorance within the very institution that has for so many been the centerpiece of their community as they face from the larger society (Harley et al. 2014). Because many LGBT persons have encountered

condemnation from churches, they often esteem personal faith in a higher power other than their religious institutions, and spirituality maintains their formal connections to religious establishments (Ward 2005). While homonegativity is not unique to Black Churches, it has dire psychosocial consequences for Black LGBT persons (Jeffries et al. 2008).

The presence of homophobia and heterosexism are persistent in the Black Church and Black community as a whole, but not in all Black Churches or all of the Black community. Clark (1983, 1999) warned that the "accusation of homophobia" should not be directed toward the whole African-American community. Nevertheless, the continual stance of many Black Churches to both condemn homosexuality and to deny fellowship to LGBT African-Americans appears to be in direct opposition to the mission of religion to be accepting of all people. Moreover, such opposition contradicts beliefs and values of the Black community as collective and communal (Harley et al. 2014). According to Greene (2000), because of the importance of family, community, and church as buffers against racism and as sources of tangible support, homophobia in the Black community often leaves LGBT persons feeling vulnerable and less likely to reveal their sexual orientation or gender identity.

Intersection of Racial/Ethnic and LGBT Identities

Frequently, Black LGBT persons are challenged to choose between their sexual and racial identities. Black LGBT persons are confronted with a dichotomy of allegiances. Meyer (2010) argues that the intersection of racial/ethnic and LGBT identities contain several basic truths. First, Blacks and other racial/ethnic minorities in the USA do not form a different culture; they are surrounded, contribute to, shape, and are affected by mainstream American culture; thus, the notion of a gay community is not alien to them. Second, many LGBT of color in the USA were raised in the same culture as their White counterparts.

Third, among immigrants to the USA, many tend to acculturate and adopt local sociocultural norms. Finally, the gay liberation movement has had a great impact globally on cultures. Although Meyer acknowledges that local cultures matter in the analysis of LGBT populations and that subculture differences and clashes with White American culture exist, a fundamental challenge to these truths is that they fail to account for social and historical contexts in which a myriad of cultural variables affect the lives of elderly African-American LGBT persons. However, this is not to say that elderly Black LGBT persons cannot have several, even seemingly, conflicting identities while maintaining a coherent sense of themselves (Meyer 2010; Singer 2004). In fact, Purdue-Vaughns and Eibach (2008) use the term *intersectional invisibility* to refer to the failure to fully recognize people with intersecting identities as members of their constituent groups. Because Black LGBT persons do not fit the prototype of their constitute group, they are likely to experience social invisibility (Lewis and Marshall 2012).

Gibson (2009) explored the behavioral and psychological strategies used by lesbians of African descent to negotiate relationships within their families of origin while simultaneously developing and maintaining an affirmative lesbian identity. The results showed that lesbians of African descent negotiated multiple identities of race, sexual orientation, disability, and gender through application of several identity management strategies (e.g., cultivate LGBT community and support systems, educate others about lesbian identity, maintain visibility, and engage in LGBT activism), including ways to manage conflicting loyalties between the community and Black community without any loss of significant relationships and cultural ties.

In a similar study, Moore (2010) examined strategies that Black LGBT people used in Black environments to proclaim a gay identity that is simultaneous with a Black identity. Moore found three distinct features: (a) Black gay protest takes on a particular form when individuals are also trying to maintain solidarity with the racial group despite the treat of distancing that occurs as a result of their sexual minority status, (b) Black sexual minorities who see their self-interests linked to those of other Blacks use cultural references to connect their struggles to historical efforts for Black equality and draw from nationalist symbols and language to frame their political work, and (c) they believe that increasing their visibility in Black spaces will promote a greater understanding of gay sexuality as an identity status that can exist alongside, rather than in competition with race. Conversely, Bates (2010) found African-American lesbians who were once married and bisexual women expressed difficulty assimilating into the African-American community since coming out. Each of these studies focused on young to middle-aged LGBT.

As is the case for any individual or group, the intermingling of identities for older Black LGBT persons represents a degree of integration. Identity models conclude with integration of sexual identity into the personality as a seamless whole, when in reality one's social circumstances change constantly and dictate priority of awareness and identity importance (Eliason and Schope 2007). For example, depending on what is occurring in society, for Black lesbians, the race may be the priority in the face of discrimination. Yet, in another situation, the murder of sexual minorities may pose greater importance than race. And still, ageism may be the salient factor. The point that Eliason and Schope make is that all people have multiple intersecting identities, and while people seek validation of all parts of their identity and not just one facet, full integration all the time is unrealistic.

Multiple Oppressions. African-American LGBT elders, unlike their younger counterparts who experience their young adult development within a dual identity or bicultural framework, experience their development through three distinct cultural perspectives: race/racism, homo-prejudice, and aging. African-American LGBT persons tend to construct their experiences in two distinct minority environments: (a) a racial minority within the dominant White culture and (b) a sexual minority within the mainstream heterosexual culture (Burlew and Serface

2006). Racial minority status appears to be a significant variable in determining the quality of life of people of color in the USA (Wilson et al. 2001). It is through the intersection oppressions of race and sexual identity that African-American and LGBT persons experience multiple oppressions. On the one hand, they are subjected to racism and oppression from mainstream society, and on the other hand, they face prejudice because of their sexual orientation from mainstream heterosexual society of all races (Burlew and Serface). In addition, African-Americans/Blacks are subjected to "colorism," a differential treatment based on skin hue, in which individuals with lighter skin color are seen as more intelligent or attractive (Kelly and Greene 2010). A lifetime of discrimination (e.g., racial inequality, anti-LGBT policies) has adversely affected African-American LGBT elders (Francis and Acey 2013).

Gay Racism. Experiences of racism by ethnic minority LGBT people in the White LGBT community are well documented in the USA and internationally (Asanti 1999; Boykin 1996; Brown 2008; Harley et al. 2013; Loiacano 1989; Plummer 2007; Stansbury et al. 2010). Smith (1999) asserts that the racism that has pervaded the mainstream gay movement only intensifies the perceived divisions between Blacks and LGBT persons. The majority of African-American LGBT persons are exposed to racist and heterosexist messages in their daily lives, and they frequently internalize these negative messages about being both a Black person and a sexual minority person (Szymanski and Gupta 2009). According to Parham et al. (1999), "irrespective of how one comes to understand the concept of racism, there is little doubt that its origins, promotion, and continuation are anchored in the context of how Whites relate to African-descent people and other people of color on individual, institutional, and cultural levels" (p. 134). It has and remains necessary to dehumanize African ancestral people and to cast them as inferior beings to enforce White, heterosexual superiority (Gibson 2009). In Cuba's LGBT community, lesbians, especially Black lesbians, continue to be one of Cuba's most socially marginalized populations (Sanders 2010). The exposure to the tri-vector of racial and sexual orientation microaggressions, and ageism are likely to manifest as health-related problems and mental health issues.

In a review of the intersections of sexual orientation, race, religion, ethnicity, and heritage languages, Van der Meide (2002) found a common theme; the assumption by developed Western nations that non-Western/non-White communities and cultures are more homophobic than the dominant Western/White communities. The basis of this assumption is not one of research, but rather one of simplistic racist and ethnophobic assumptions about the lack of sophistication or the cultural and religious backwardness of non-Western/White cultures. In this review, Van der Meide (2002, p.9) incorporates an observation by Gunnings that:

> Too often White folk in the lesbian and gay community want to latch on to statements or intimations that the Black community is more homophobic maybe because it releases them from some of the hard and painful work of dealing with their racism, personally as well as organizationally. Perhaps, it allows them to avoid becoming multicultural and multiperspectival.

The descriptive (tell how people in a group supposedly behave) and prescriptive (tells how certain groups should think, feel, and behave) beliefs (Fiske 1993) continue to shape the partnership between discrimination and prejudice, allowing them to maintain a constant course in subordinating the minority race status and preserving the majority race privileges.

World View and Historical Hostilities' Influence on Help-Seeking

African-American elders and their LGBT counterparts tend to have a high degree of suspicion of institutions and healthcare institutions because of becoming of age in the 1930s, 1940s, 1950s, and 1960s when institutional bigotry, hatred, and stigma were commonplace. They lived during an era of "forced segregation and enforced Jim Crow etiquette" (Cooper-Lewter 2007, p. 214).

Elderly Black LGBT persons may exhibit a disproportionate rate of historical hostility (Vontress and Epp 1997) relating to past dealings with Whites and systems of oppression and discrimination. For example, the Tuskegee Syphilis experiments in which Black men were infected with and untreated for syphilis and allowed to die during the 40-year study remain fresh in the minds of many African-American elders. The United States Public Health Service (USPHS) designed the Tuskegee Syphilis Study, and during its existence, the men in the study were not provided with treatment and, in some instances, were prevented from obtaining treatment (Loue 2014). The Tuskegee study is a reminder that of how Black people may be at risk from the medical community and it serves to increase distrust of health professionals and researchers, as well as decrease participation of Blacks in clinical trials. The historical devaluation of Black bodies (Lemelle 2003) continues to produce significant negative health outcomes of African-Americans. Even with social transformation, African-American LGBT elders continue to possess vivid memories of institutional and structural discrimination associated with race, gender, gender identity, socioeconomic status, and sexual orientation (Francis and Acey 2013). Like for all LGBT elders, Black LGBT elders had the additional experience of coming of age at a time of acute homophobia at every level of society (Funders for Lesbian and Gay Issues 2004) and being medically classified with a psychiatric disorder and being subject to criminal charges because of their sexual orientation (Woody 2012). Until 1973, the American Psychological Association (APA) considered homosexuality to be a mental illness.

The reaction of individuals with distrust toward an individual or group who have acted in a discriminatory way toward them is commonplace. In general, LGBT persons mistrust heterosexuals; LGBT persons of color may distrust White LGBT individuals; transgender and bisexual persons may distrust gays and lesbians; lesbians may distrust gay men; older LGBT persons may distrust young LGBT individuals; and so on. "The oppressor and the oppressed are changing social

phenomenon, dependent on context" (Eliason and Schope 2007, p. 21). The impact of dual or multiple identities of race, age, class, gender, gender identity, and sexual orientation intersects in diverse ways, which depending on rigidity of labels allows adaptations to changes in one's cultural and sexual landscape (Rust 1996).

Frequently, African-American LGBT elders are cautious about where they seek services whereas to avoid discrimination (Redman and Woody 2012). Table 6.5 identifies some concerns LGBT elders have about healthcare environments, which are magnified twofold for African-American and other ethnic minority LGBT persons. African-Americans across the age spectrum tend to underuse mental health services to the exclusion of needed mental health specialist for the following reasons: (a) reliance on personal connections such as family members, friends, and other community members, (b) reliance on primary care providers or other non-specialists, (c) dependence on emergency departments for diagnosis and treatment of mental health concerns, and (d) use of folk remedies, faith leaders, herbalists, and other nonstandard modes of care (Primm and Lawson 2010). Regardless of race, studies consistently find that LGBT persons have negative interactions with their healthcare providers and are less likely to disclose their sexual identity and behavior (Bernstein et al. 2008; Fredriksen-Goldsen et al. 2011; Funders for Lesbian and Gay Issues 2004; Mayer et al. 2008; Somjen 2009). Discrimination related to race/ethnicity and sexual orientation or gender identity can be considered a social risk for Black elderly LGBT persons' health and well-being

Research suggests that older LGBT persons are generally well adjusted (Graham 2011); however, compared to the general population, gay and bisexual men are twice as likely to have mental health concerns, and lesbian and bisexual women are three times as likely (Grant et al. 2009). However, the number of Black LGBT participants in theses studies is low. Although Black older adults have lower rates of psychiatric illness, including depression, than older White adults (Jimenez et al. 2010), substantial

Table 6.5 Concerns of behaviors from healthcare providers

Hostility
Rejection
Invisibility
Denial of care
Stigmatization
Anti-gay violence/safety
Multiple forms of discrimination
Reduction or poor quality of care
Inadequate/substandard health care
Refrain from touching a patient who is LGBT
Careless management of private information and identity disclosure
Inappropriate verbal and/or nonverbal responses from providers and office staff
Refusal of service providers and healthcare systems to recognize extended families within the gay community
Unfamiliarity of healthcare providers with the unique care needs of the LGBT population and ethnic minorities

Adapted from Auldridge and Espinoza (2013) and Hughes et al. (2011)

ethnic/racial disparities exist in the care given to Black older adults with depression (Shellman 2011). In comparison with other groups, Black older adults are less likely to seek help from mental health providers, are less likely to be identified as depressed, and often delay or fail to seek treatment until their symptoms are severe (McGuire and Miranda 2008; Neighbors et al. 2007). Nevertheless, a lower number of African-Americans in general seek mental health services. There are several explanations for lower rates of service participation, including culture-specific beliefs about the causes of mental illness, lack of awareness of mental health services, poverty, stigma, inadequate insurance coverage, lack of access to transportation, lack of culturally relevant approaches, and mistrust of service providers (Bailey et al. 2009; Connor et al. 2010; McGuire and Miranda 2008; Morrell et al. 2008). Even after entering the mental healthcare system, older Black adults are less likely to receive quality care.

Another potential explanation for underutilization of mental health services by older Black adults is the notion of "positive marginality" (Mayo 1982), which suggests that for those who exist and live in the margins of social arrangements result in strength, resilience, and vibrancy.

Mayo explains that for people who are situated at the social margins do not necessarily internalize their exclusion or devaluation, but instead embrace differences as a source of strength and sometimes as a source of empowerment. The application of positive marginality to Black LGBT elders and their tri-vector of microaggressions, one can deduce that they may demonstrate more positive psychosocial adjustment than their younger, heterosexual, and White counterparts. In fact, Hall and Fine (2005) assert that positive marginality is the cornerstone of the Black experience that provides psychological and political tools that teach survival skills for successive generations.

Healthcare and Service Disparities

Older LGBT adults in general are an at-risk population experiencing significant health disparities (Fredriksen-Goldsen 2011), which is further exacerbated for ethnic minorities. Older adults in the general population and among LGBT groups tend to be the most frequent users of healthcare services in the USA. For older LGBT adults, health concomitants of aging may be exacerbated by factors associated with gender and sexual orientation (Institute of Medicine Committee on Lesbian, Gay, Bisexual, and Transgender Health Issues 2011). Historically, disadvantaged groups (e.g., ethnic minorities, LGBT adults) within the older adult population continue to have higher levels of illness, disability, and premature death (Fredriksen-Goldsen and Muraco 2010). LGBT people of all ages are much more likely than heterosexual adults to delay or not seek medical care (Institute of Medicine Committee on Lesbian, Gay, Bisexual, and Transgender Health Issues 2011) because they usually encounter two unique obstacles in navigating healthcare, social, and human service: homophobia and heterosexism. Fear of discrimination causes LGBT elders five times less likely than non-LGBT seniors to access services (Funders for Lesbian and Gay Issues 2004). In addition, LGBT seniors of color and transgendered elders feel unwelcome even among other LGBT elders, and many view LGBT elder programs as hostile to their participation (Plumb and Associates 2003/2004). Navigating those services can be further complicated by the degree to which LGBT elders self-disclose to others (Maccio and Doueck 2002). Racial and ethnic disparities in health care exist in the broader historic and contemporary social and economic inequality and in evidence of persistent racial and ethnic discrimination in numerous sectors of American society (Institute of Medicine of the National Academies 2003). African-Americans receive necessary health care and mental health intervention at half the rate of their White counterparts (Neighbors et al. 2007). These inequities create additional barriers that do not exist for most White heterosexual older adults.

African-American and Black LGBT persons are at risk for a variety of poor physical health outcomes. Over the years, data collected have consistently demonstrated significant health disparities between minority and non-minority groups in the USA. With the passage of the Health Disparities Act, increased visibility and funding went to interventions created to address health disparities between persons of different racial/ethnic groups; however, the act neglected to place attention on the special health needs of LGBT persons. Moreover, work has been done to increase the importance of understanding and eliminating health disparities across race categories, and little work has focused specifically on the healthcare needs of ethnic minority LGBT persons (Wilson and Yoshikawa 2007). According to Wilson and Yoshikawa, "most attention to health disparities has been placed either on the needs of ethnic minorities or LGBTs, but not the needs of persons who belong to both groups" (p. 609) an, certainly not on those belonging to both groups who are elderly.

For all adults, later life is known as a period of both growth and decline, with studies overwhelmingly focused on the latter (Institute of Medicine Committee on Lesbian, Gay, Bisexual, and Transgender Health Issues and Research 2011), yet we know very little about the healthcare needs of African-American LGBT elders and health issues specific to aging, disability, health, and sexuality (Comerford et al. 2004; Dibble et al. 2012). Given the projected growth in the number of older African-Americans, numerous questions are raised about the health status, quality of life, and service delivery for Black LGBT elders. Some of the most urgent questions are as follows: Why are ethnic minority LGBT populations at heightened risk for poor health outcomes compared to other populations? Why are ethnic minority LGBT persons less likely than White LGBT persons to receive high-quality health care (Wilson and Yoshikawa 2007)? What are the long-term effects of discrimination, oppression, and homophobia on the lives of ethnic minorities?

Ethically, only culturally appropriate testing instruments and procedures should be used in the assessment of people of color. In addition, measure and scale used must be psychometrically reliable and valid and culturally sensitive within the LGBT communities. Disparities in service delivery for African-American LGBT elders may also be as a result of cultural bias or culturally insensitive assessment instrument and measures. Clinicians serving Black LGBT persons should be familiar with instruments or scales recommended to assess racial/ethnic identity, acculturation, acculturative stress, sexual identity/orientation, and internalized homophobia (Chung 2007). When assessing and treating older Black LGBT persons, circumstances that are unique to them should be part of the protocol. Consideration should be given to the impact of ageism, lifelong discrimination, and racism. In addition, the role of sexism becomes more pertinent as a covariant of ageism and racism for African-American/Black LGBT elders because of cultural gender role expectations, as well as the value (lack of) that society places on women of color.

Models for Service

The provision of services to African-American and Black LGBT elders is based on theories, concepts, and methods, which have emanated largely from Western countries and with primarily White populations, despite the fact that Afrocentric and culturally specific interventions have been recommended. Scholars from various health and human services disciplines, including psychology, counseling, gerontology, social work, medicine, public health, and others, have developed and advocated for alternate paradigms and models to understand the realities in the contexts of people of African descent. In a study of LGBT health and human services needs in New York State, one reason that high rates of barriers to care were reported is attributed to current LGBT-specific and general services that do not provide culturally sensitive services to the full range of people of color.

Great emphasis has been placed on service models being inclusive of all people. However, for LGBT populations, especially in mental health services, substantial barriers exist because of a care system that is completely unprepared to deal with their needs. In addition, LGBT persons face harassment in general and participate minimally in mental health programs, and they go off their medication, spiral down, and in a few months are back in the hospital. For these reasons, a specialized system of care is needed to

meet the needs of LGBT elders of color; thus, an ethno-specific system appears to be more appropriate. Mainstream services are not always welcoming to Black LGBT persons. It is important to recognize that treating people in the same way does not account for difference and in treating people equally may tantamount to discriminatory treatment. In essence, treating everyone in a uniform way ignores differences. The aim should be to treat every individual with the same level of dignity and respect (Social Care Institute for Excellence [SCIE] 2011). Ethno-specific programs and services do not imply an acceptance of the need for separate services for all ethnic elderly LGBT. Nevertheless, moving beyond the controversy over the pluralistic versus assimilative nature of American society, a pluralistic or multicultural model allows for inclusiveness. In the post-separate but equal era, one of the primary objections to separate programing is that if all ethnic groups subscribe to a common core of American values, it should be possible for ethnic groups to benefit from mainstream programming (Gelfand 2003). Unfortunately, this oversimplification often ignores the long-standing historical hostilities (Gelfand 2003) that have existed among LGBT Black elders, as well as mistrust and justified paranoia toward discrimination and microaggressions (Sue and Sue 2013) of which they are subjected.

According to Social Care Institute for Excellence (SCIE), LGBT persons do not necessarily feel they need special treatment, but they do not want to have to explain or justify their lives or relationships; instead, they want to be in an environment in which service providers understand issues related to LGBT persons and are competent to work in an inclusive, anti-discriminatory way. For African-American and Black LGBT elders, this sentiment becomes magnified with the addition of race and age. Thus, person-centered approaches are recommended as a means of service delivery. The multiple and intersecting identities of Black LGBT elders can come into play when designing person-centered services because they have usually experienced homophobia, transphobia, and racial discrimination in their lives and have concerns of losing choice and control over their care. For LGBT elders to have choice and control over their care and support, "they need to have accessible, sensitive mainstream services as well as the opportunity to get support from specialist services" (SCIE, p. 3).

Another emphasis of service model is on cultural competency of service providers. Too often, Black LGBT elders enter a system in which they experience the tri-vector barrier to race and ethnicity, age, and sexual orientation and gender identity. In the USA, the Affordable Care Act (ACA) may benefit LGBT populations in a variety of ways since it requires the development of a culturally competent and diverse healthcare workforce that has expertise providing care to underserved populations such as the LGBT communities. The ACA prohibits insurance companies from denying coverage based on pre-existing conditions, which would be beneficial to Black LGBT elders, of whom have many chronic conditions (Fredriksen-Goldsen et al. 2011). The ACA affords access to healthcare services, which for older Black LGBT populations may provide consistency of care (e.g., a routine annual checkup) and health outcomes (e.g., early detection, providers who are familiar with medical histories), remove barriers, and foster trust in healthcare settings (American Medical Association 2009). The reader is referred to Chap. 19 for additional information on the impact of ACA on LGBT elders.

Older adults disproportionately experience isolation. A complex set of circumstances and factors that exist at the individual, social network, community, and societal levels contribute to isolation (Elder and Retrum 2012). Elder and Retrum suggest that many disciplines, including sociology, psychology, social work, nursing, public health, gerontology, medicine, social neuroscience, public policy, and urban planning, have recognized isolation and offer approaches to isolation in older adults. There is extensive overlap across disciplines in how isolation among older adults is conceptualized (see Elder and Retrum 2012). LGBT elders have risk factors for isolation that are compounded by less support

from family members and fear of facing stigma and discrimination in the health and legal systems (Muraco and Fredriksen-Goldsen 2011). In a study of African-Americans and White older Americans, Troxel et al. (2010) found that African-Americans were the most isolated. Among older African-Americans, Black women are most likely to be socially isolated and to possess the lowest amount of social support and capital, to not to have a source of reliable transportation, to being limited in life space, to limiting activities for fear of an attack, and to not being married (Locher et al. 2005). As a marginalized group, social isolation might be intensified for African-American LGBT elders, who may be isolated from their racial community as LGBT older persons and isolated from the mainstream LGBT community as people of color (Fredriksen-Goldsen et al. 2011). In response to social isolation among LGBT elders of color, GRIOT Circle developed an intervention program called Buddy-2-Buddy. The program pairs elders who are homebound or in facilities with more active elders for visits and invites them to join in activities. The objective is to promote independence and self-reliance among LGBT elders by countering isolation and restricted mobility. Buddy-2-Buddy distinguishes itself in work with elders of color who are often reticent about discussing personal problems with strangers or outsiders (http://www.asaging.org/blog/reducing-isolation-community-engagement-service-model.pdf). In general, African-American populations, especially elders, do not share their problems with outsiders because of a high degree of distrust and privacy.

Because of multiple medical and psychosocial issues among Black LGBT elders, a team approach or collaborative model in the treatment of persons from this age, race/ethnic, and sexual orientation/gender identity group should always be used (Paniagua (2014). In addition to the clinician, physician, or mental health professional, Vazquez et al. (2010) recommend the inclusion of social workers, cultural healer, at least a family member, nursing home of care facility administrator, and the religious leader (if requested by the person and/or family as members of a multidisciplinary team. Conversely, a continuum of care is frequently used to classify services for the elder in the USA (Gelfand 2003). This continuum entails moving from placing no restrictions to becoming more restrictive. Gelfand explains that serious problems underlie the concept of the continuum of care because it does not represent the reality of American programs and services for elders. The continuum of care model is based on the faulty assumption that elderly persons have only one need at any one point-in-time. As mentioned previous in this chapter, elderly persons have multifaceted needs, and these needs may be extensive. Older persons in general and African-American LGBT elders specifically need a combination of services, and the components of these services may vary over time.

Finally, the Black community has a helping tradition and "being part of a unique community has long dominated the social consciousness of African-Americans," which emerged from a commonality of experience related to racism and oppression (Rasheed and Rasheed 2004, p. 142). Although the Black community is considered to be more homophobic than the general population, African-American LGBT persons contend to have always had more of a sense of belonging to the Black community than LGBT communities. Therefore, a consolidated approach of community-based, outreach, gatekeeper, and case-find model might offer a practical approach to identification of LGBT elders in need of services and service delivery. In fact, the Gatekeeper Model of Case Finding was created in 1978 by Raymond Raschko, a social worker in Spokane, Washington, as a community-wide system of proactive case finding to identify at-risk older adult who remain invisible to the service delivery systems created to serve them. Gatekeepers are people in the community (e.g., postal service worker, apartment manager, meter reader, code enforcement workers, emergency response teams, business owners) who come into contact with older persons through their everyday activities. They are trained to look for signs and symptoms that might indicate that an older person needs assistance (http://Spokane.wsu.edu/researchout-reach/wimhrt/A7.pdf). Using the gatekeeper model as the core of the consolidated approach offers Black LGBT elders an informal response and referral system that they may trust. The more service models that are available to deliver programming to African-American LGBT elders might increase their options to get assistance. Community-based programs have proven to be effective with in the Black community.

Policy Issues

The role of gender and sexuality is increasingly critical to policy development and implementation. The Black Racial Congress has incorporated gay rights issues as part of its agenda. One of their principles, "Gender and sexuality can no loner be viewed as a personal issue but must be a basic part of our analyses, politics, and struggles," underscores the importance and urgency to integrate gay rights into broader issues affecting the African-American community (National Black Justice Coalition 2009). Leaders in the Black community support the rights of LGBT persons as civil rights and as public policy issues. In 2005, Julian Bond as chairman of the NAACP emphasized that gay rights are civil rights, and the Rev. Al Sharpton, founder of the Harlem-based National Action Network, stated, "unless you are prepared to say gays and lesbians are not human beings, they should have the same constitutional right of any other human beings" (National Black Justice Coalition 2009, p. 4).

Health disparities among African-American elders and their LGBT counterparts are alarming, and these populations remain largely invisible in services, policies, and research (Fredriksen-Goldsen and Muraco 2010; Metlife 2010). Research suggests that knowledge of health and health disparities is crucial to inform the development and implementation of effective services and public policies (Auldridge and Espinoza 2013; Comberford et al. 2004; Fredrikson-Goldsen et al. 2011; MetLife 2010; Wilson and Yoshikawa 2007). Fredriksen-Goldsen et al. (2011) assert that in order to develop policies and effective interventions to

Table 6.6 SAGE recommendations for policy and practice for older LGBT of color

Include specific provisions for LGBT elders in the Older Americans Act (OAA), ensuring that vulnerable LGBT elders of color are able to age in good health and with broad community support

Ensure that community services and supports in the OAA are offered in a culturally and linguistically competent manner, better reaching LGBT elders of color

Increase federal funding for organizations and programmatic interventions targeting LGBT elders of color

Ensure that implementation of the Affordable Care Act engages LGBT elders of color as advocates, so that new health reform effectively reach communities of color and LGBT communities that are dealing with aging challenges

Strengthen Social Security and increase access for LGBT elders and elders of color who experience diminished economic security in their retirement years. A stronger, more inclusive Social Security will enhance the lives of millions of LGBT people of color

Improve data collection on sexual orientation and gender identity to better identify and address health disparities among LGBT elders of color

Decrease elder abuse among more vulnerable and socially isolated elders by strengthening outreach and community support to LGBT elders of color

Increase federal funding for safe and affordable senior housing and housing supports, while expanding the development of culturally and linguistically competent senior housing communities

Strengthen the federal response to HIV and aging, which includes public awareness about the issue, equipping aging, and healthcare providers with the skills to effectively serve older adults with HIV, and specifically addressing the impact of the epidemic on LGBT elders of color

Eliminate discriminatory exclusion of medically necessary transition-related care from federally funded health programs impacting LGBT older people of color

Adapted from Auldridge and Espinoza (2013)

address the needs of LGBT elders, we must first understand the conditions and factors that result in health disparities and lack of access to aging and health services. Formation of policy will continue to be compromised until we have a thorough understanding of the needs of Black LGBT elders.

Questions on sexual orientation and gender identity are rarely asked in Federal surveys or by state and local aging service providers, resulting in limited ability to understand the nature of health disparities among older Black LGBT persons. Auldridge and Espinoza (2013) recommend the federal agencies (e.g., AOA, Centers on Medicare & Medical Services) should include uniform questions on sexual orientation and gender identity in their national survey instruments and encourage state and local agencies to follow suit through their aging systems. Other recommendations by Auldridge and Espinoza on policy and practice for older LGBT persons of color are presented in Table 6.6. Equitable distribution of program resources requires consideration of the relative needs of Black LGBT elders. For example, elderly Black persons have a shorter life expectancy than White or Latino elderly. The equity argument has been put forth that because of this shorter life expectancy, African-Americans should qualify for programs and services at an earlier age (Gelfand 2003).

In the UK, the Equality Act of 2010 provides protection against discrimination for protected classes, including sexual orientation and gender identity. Comparable legislation in the USA includes Title VII of The Civil Rights Act, the Protection of Freedom Act (2012), and the Employment Nondiscrimination Act (ENDA). Some individuals will argue that the Constitution of the USA is the ultimate legislation that includes rights and protections for all persons, including LGBT persons and African-Americans. Other legislation varies state-by-state.

Barriers to effective and appropriate services for African-American LGBT elders can be eliminated through policy reform at institutional, community, and system levels. Thus, to improve healthcare access and health outcomes across the population of Black LGBT elders, we must implement policy that can reach entire communities (Wilson and Yoshikawa 2007). Policy makers should explore best practices and evidence-based practices to develop policy for African-American LGBT elders. Cost of implementation should not be the only or primary determining factor in policy development and implementation.

2002). The need and advocacy for equity in services for LGBT elders are well documented (e.g., American Society on Aging; Auldridge and Espinoza 2013; Fredriksen-Goldsen et al. 2011, 2013; Movement Advancement Project [MAP]; MetLife 2010; Services & Advocacy for Gay, Lesbian, Bisexual & Transgender Elders; Wilson and Yoshikawa 2007), and with the rapid expansion of both aging and ethnic minority populations, the time is now to increase the quality and quantity of services for those among them who are LGBT.

Summary

African-American and Black LGBT elders in the USA have been victims of a dualistic and bias system of health care and service delivery. These individuals have come to distrust service providers and the system of care that are designated for their care. Research suggests that these mistrusts, cautions, and suspicions continue to have credence. In fact, Sue and Sue (2013) refer to this mistrust as a "healthy cultural paranoia" by African-Americans that can serve as a coping strategy with respect to racism (p. 375). While various disciplines have begun to study the cultural, psychological, wellness, and resilience of elderly African-American and other LGBT persons of color, more understanding of their circumstances, life experiences, and needs is needed. Just as African-American and Black LGBT populations have differences and distinctions from White LGBT communities, there are numerous commonalities and convergences (Meyer 2010). However, recommendations for inclusion of African-American and Black LGBT elders in policy must move beyond an additive approach in which race and ethnicity are incorporated as the "other."

Healthcare and human services providers have the responsibility to make available appropriate and effective services to all consumers, regardless of minority status (Maccio and Doueck

Learning Exercises

Self-Check Questions

1. What types of challenges do African-American LGBT elders face that differ from those of their White counterparts?
2. How do historical hostilities influence help-seeking behavior of older African-American LGBT persons?
3. What type of income constitutes the largest share of income of older African-Americans?
4. Who was one of the first documented cases of an African-American transgender person?
5. Explain how the long-term financial stability of many LGBT elders of color is shaped by employment discrimination.

Experiential Exercises

1. Identify a Black Church that is accepting of LGBT persons and volunteer to help to establish a senior program and resources that is inclusive of LGBT elders.
2. Develop an anthology or documentary of older LGBT African-Americans.
3. Identify one way in which you can change the life of an LGBT African-American elder and work with him or her to implement it.

Multiple-Choice Questions

1. Which of the following African-American group is rarely researched outside of a focus on HIV/AIDS?
   a. Gay men
   b. Lesbians
   c. Bisexual men
   d. Heterosexual men

2. Which of the following increases acceptance of sexual orientation for older LGBT African-American/Blacks in their families?
   a. Coming out at an early age
   b. Strong religious ties
   c. Lack of disclosure
   d. Partial disclosure

3. In which community does the majority of older African-American/Black LGBT persons find more support and refuge?
   a. LGBT community
   b. Black community
   c. Both of the above
   d. Neither of the above

4. Which of the following is not as prevalent a characteristic in the Black community as it is in the gay community?
   a. Sexism
   b. Ageism
   c. Heterosexism
   d. Internalized homophobia

5. Unlike their younger counterparts, in which of the following cultural perspectives did African-American/Black LGBT elders experience their development?
   a. Dual identity framework
   b. Bicultural framework
   c. Racism, homo-prejudice, and aging
   d. Integration, social visibility, and aging

6. The statement, "Gender and sexuality can no longer be viewed as a personal issue but must be a basic part of our analyses, politics, and struggles," is attributed to which of the following Black organizations?
   a. Southern Christian Association
   b. National Association for the Advancement of Colored people
   c. National Black Justice Coalition
   d. Black Racial Congress

7. Which of the following are reasons as to why African-Americans underuse mental health services?
   a. Reliance on primary care providers
   b. Reliance on family members, friends, and other community members
   c. Dependence on emergency departments for diagnosis and treatment of mental health concerns
   d. All of the above
   e. None of the above

8. Which of the following approaches should be used in the treatment of African-American/Black LGBT elders?
   a. Multidisciplinary
   b. Continuum of care
   c. Selective service model
   d. Consciousness model

9. Which group among older African-American/Black adults tends to be the most economically insecure and isolated?
   a. Men
   b. Women
   c. Gay men
   d. Baby boomer

10. Which of the following is a primary barrier to quality services for African-American/Black LGBT elders?
    a. Lack of control over their care
    b. Limited transportation
    c. Lack of culturally competent service providers
    d. Prohibitions of insurance carriers

Key

1-a
2-c
3-b
4-b
5-c
6-d
7-d
8-a
9-b
10-c

Resources

BGRG (Black Gay Research Group): BGRG was developed to address the paucity of research regarding the disproportionate HIV infection rates among Black MSM. BGRB is made up of Black gay men who engage in interdisciplinary research in the fields of African diaspora studies, gender studies, sexuality studies, and public health (http://www.thebgrg.org).

Diverse Elders Coalition: The DEC advocates for policies and programs that improve aging in communities as racially and ethnically diverse people. The Coalition is made up of five national organizations representing a growing majority of millions of older people throughout the country (www.diverseelders.org).

GLAAD'S Communities of African Descent (COAD): COAD provides a Resource Kit with guidelines, terminology, and contact information for leading Black LGBT organizations and individuals as tools for more inclusive, fair, and balanced coverage of the Black LGBT community (http://www.glaad.org/publications/coadkik).

GMAD (Gay Men of African Descent): (gmad@gmad.org).

GRIOT Circle: An intergenerational and culturally diverse community-based social service organization responsive to the realities of older LGBT and two-spirit people of all colors (www.griotcircle.worldpress.com).

NBGMAC (National Black Gay Men's Advocacy Coalition): NBGMAC is committed to improving the health and well-being of Black gay men through advocacy that is focused on research, policy, education, and training (http://www.nbgmac.org).

NBJC (National Black Justice Coalition): (http://www.nbjcoalition.org).

ULOAH (United Lesbians of African Heritage): (http://www.uloah.com).

ZAMI NOBLA (*National Organization of Black Lesbians on Aging*): ZAMI is an organization for lesbians of African descent based in Atlanta, Georgia (http://www.zami.org).

ZUNA Institute: Organized in 1999, ZUNA Institute is a national nonprofit organization for Black lesbians that address issues on health, economic development, education, and public policy and strives to eliminate barriers and other forms of social discrimination (www.zunainstitute.org).

References

Administration for Community Living. (2012). *A statistical profile of older African Americans.* Retrieved June 3, 2014 from http://www.acl.gov/NewsRoom/Publications/doc/A_Statistical_Prolie_of_Older_African_Americans.pdf.

Administration on Aging. (n.d.). *AOA information for African American elders.* Retrieved June 3, 2014 from http://seniorhealth.about.com/library/news/blfa.htm.

Administration on Aging. (2013). *Older Americans behavioral health-Issue Brief 11: Reaching diverse older adult populations and engaging them in prevention services and early interventions.* Available at http://ww.aoa.gov/AoARoot/AoA_Programs?HPW/Behavioral/docs2/IssueBrief11ReachingandEngaging.PDF.

Albelda, R., Lee Badgett, M. V., Schneebaum, A., & Gates, G. J. (2009). *Poverty in the lesbian, gay and bisexual community.* Los Angeles, CA: UCLA School of Law.

American Medical Association. (2009). AMA *policy regarding sexual orientation: H-65.973 Health care disparities in same-sex partner households.* Huston, TX: Author.

Asanti, T. (1999). Racism in the 21st century: How will the lesbian & gay community respond. *Lesbian News, 24*(9), 24.

Auldridge, A., & Espinoza, R. (2013). *Health equity and LGBT elders of color: Recommendations for policy and practice.* New York: SAGE.

Bailey, R. K., Blackmon, H. L., & Stevens, F. L. (2009). Major depressive disorder in the African American population: Meeting the Challenges of stigma, misdiagnosis, and treatment disparities. *Journal of the National Medical Association, 101,* 1089–1094.

Baker, K., & Krehely, J. (2012). How health care reform will help LGBT elders. *Public Policy & Aging Report, 21*(3), 19–23.

Bates, D. D. (2010). Once-married African American lesbians and bisexual women: Identity development and coming-out process. *Journal of Homosexuality, 57,* 197–225.

Battle, J., & Bennett, M. (2000). Research on lesbian and gay populations within the African American community: What have we learned? *African American Research Perspectives, 6,* 35–46.

Betts, E. C. (2012). *Black lesbian spirituality: Hearing our stories.* Retrieved September 12, 2013 from http://www.adulterc.org/Proceedings/2012/papers/betts.pdf.

Bernstein, K. T., Liu, K. L., Begier, E. M., Koblin, B., Karpati, A., & Murrill, C. (2008). Same-sex attraction disclosure to health care providers among New York City men who have sex with men. *Archives of Internal Medicine, 168*(13), 1458–1464.

Bostwick, W. B. (2007). *Disparities in mental health treatment among GLBT populations.* Arlington, VA: National Alliance on Mental Illness.

Bowleg, L. (2008). When black + lesbian + women = black lesbian woman: The methodological challenges of qualitative and quantitative intersectionality research. *Sex Roles, 36*(2), 207–325.

Boyd-Franklin, N. (2003). Race, class, and poverty. In F. Walsh (Ed.), *Normal family process* (pp. 260–279). New York: Guilford Press.

Brown, C. E. (2008). *Racism in the gay community and homophobia in the Black community: Negotiating the gay Black male experience.* Dissertation. Blacksburg, VA: Virginia Polytechnic Institute and State University.

Brown Wright, L., & Fernander, A. (2005). The African American family. In D. A. Harley & J. M. Dillard (Eds.), *Contemporary mental health issues among African Americans* (pp. 19–34). Alexandria, VA: American Counseling Association.

Boykin, K. (1996). *One more river to cross: Black and gay in America.* New York: Anchor Books.

Burlew, L. D., & Serface, H. C. (2006). The ticultural experience of older, African American, gay men: Counseling implications. *Adultspan Journal, 5*(2), 81–90.

Centers for Disease Control. (2010). *National vital statistics system.* Retrieved June 3, 2014 from http://www.cdc.gov/minorityhealth/populations/remp/black.html.

Centers for Disease Contro. (2013). *Black and African Americn populations.* Retrieved February 20, 2015 from http://www.cdc.gov/minority/healthpopulations/REMP/black.html

Chung, Y. B. (2007). Lesbian, gay, and bisexual people of color. In M. G. Constantine (Ed.), *Clinical practice with people of color* (pp. 143–161). New York: Teachers College Press.

Clarke, C. (1983). The failure to transform: Homophobia in the Black community. In B. Smith (Ed.), *Home girls: A Black feminist anthology* (pp. 197–208). New York: Kitchen Table, Women of Color Press.

Clarke, C. (1999). In E. Brandt (Ed.), *Dangerous liaisons: Blacks, gays, and the struggle for equality* (pp. 31–44). New York: The New Press.

Clements-Nolle, K., Marx, R., Guzman, R., & Katz, M. (2001). HIV prevalence, risk behaviors, health care use, and mental health status of transgendered persons in San Francisco: Implications for public health intervention. *American Journal of Public Health, 91*(6), 915–921.

Comerford, S. A., Henson-Stroud, M. M., Sionainn, C., & Wheeler, E. (2004). Crone songs: Voices of lesbian elders on aging in a rural environment. *Affilia, 19*(4), 418–436.

Connor, K. O., Copeland, V. C., Grote, N. K., Rosen, D., Albert, S., McMurray, M. L., et al. (2010). Barriers to treatment and culturally endorsed coping strategies among depressed African American older adults. *Aging and Mental Health, 14*, 971–983.

Cooper-Lewter, N. (2007). Conceptualizing soul as a mental health resource in the Black community. In S. M. L. Logan, R. W. Denby, & P. A. Gibbson (Eds.), *Mental health care in the African American community* (pp. 213–231). New York: Haworth Press.

DeBlaere, C., Brewster, M. E., Sarkees, A., & Moradi, B. (2010). Conducting research with LGBT people of color: Methodological challenges and strategies. *The Counseling Psychologist, 38*(3), 331–362.

Deutsch, M. (2006). A framework for thinking about oppression and its change. *Social Justice Research, 19* (1), 7–41.

Dibble, S. L., Eliason, M. J., & Crawford, B. (2012). Correlated of wellbeing among African American lesbians. *Journal of Homosexuality, 59*, 820–838.

Douglas, K. B. (2006). *Black church homophobia: What to do about it.* Available at www.yale.edu/divinity/publications/reflections/spring06/12_17.pdff.

Dworkin, S. H. (2006). The aging bisexual: The invisible of the invisible minority. In D. Kimmel, T. Rose, & S. Davis (Eds.), *Lesbian, gay, bisexual, and transgender aging—Research and clinical perspectives* (pp. 36–52). New York, NY: Columbia University Press.

Dyson, M. E. (2003). *Open mike: Reflections on philosophy, race, sex, culture and religion.* New York: Basic Books.

Elder, K., & Retrum, J. (2012, May 30). *Framework for isolation in adults over 50.* AARP Foundation. Retrieved June 16, 2014 from http://www.aarpfoundation.org.

Evans, K. M., & George, R. (2008). African Americans. In G. McAuliffe (Ed.), *Culturally alert counseling: A comprehensive introduction* (pp. 146–187). Thousand Oaks, CA: Sage.

Fiske, S. T. (1993). Controlling other people: The impact of power on stereotyping. *American Psychologist, 48* (6), 621–628.

Francis, G. M., & Acey, K. (2013, February 2). *Reducing isolation: A community engagement service model.* Retrieved June 5, 2013 from http://www.asaging.org/blog/reducing-isolation-community-engagement-service-model.

Fredriksen-Goldsen, K., & Muraco, A. (2010). Aging and sexual orientation: A 25-year review of the literature. *Research on Aging, 32*(3), 372–413.

Fredriksen-Goldsen, K. I., Kim, H., Emlet, J., Muraco, A., Erosheva, E. A., Hoy-Ellis, C. P., et al. (2011). *The aging and health report: Disparities and resilience among lesbian, gay, bisexual, and transgender older adults.* Seattle: Institute for Multigenerational Health.

Fredriksen-Goldsen, K., Kim, H. J., Golsen, J., Hoy-Ellis, C. P., Emlet, C. A., Erosheva, E. A., & Muraco, A. (2013, January). *LGBT older adults in San Francisco: Health, risks, and resilience—Findings from caring and aging with pride*. Seattle: Institute for Multigenerational Health.

Funders for Lesbian and Gay Issues. (2004). *Aging in equity: LGBT elders in America*. New York: Author.

Gates, G. J., & Newport, F. (2012, October 18). Special report: 3.4 % of U.S. adults identify as LGBT. *Inaugural Gallup findings*. Retrieved May 29, 2014 from http://www.gallup.com/158066/special-report-adults-identify-as-lgbt.aspx.

Gelfand, D. E. (2003). *Aging and ethnicity: Knowledge and services*. New York: Springer.

Gibson, D. (2009). *Negotiating multiple identities: The experiences of African American lesbians. Dissertation*. New York: Seaton Hall University.

Graham, R. (2011). *The health of lesbian, gay, bisexual, and transgender people: Building a foundation for better understanding*. Institute of Medicine. Washington, DC: The National Academic Press.

Grant, J. M., Koskovich, G., Frazer, M. S., & Bjerk, S. (2009, September). *Outing age: Public policy issues affecting gay, lesbian, bisexual, and transgender elders*. Washing, DC: National Gay and Lesbian Task Force Policy Institute. Retrieved May 29, 2014 from http://www.thetaskforce.org/downloads.reports.reports/outinage_final.pdf.

Greene, B. (1994). Ethnic-minority lesbians and gay men: Mental health and treatment issues. *Journal of Consulting and Clinical Psychology, 62*, 243–251.

Greene, B. (2000). African American lesbians and bisexual women. *Journal of Social Issues, 56*, 239–249.

Greene, B., & Boyd-Franklin, N. (1996). African American lesbian couples: Ethnocultural considerations in psychotherapy. *Women & Therapy: A Feminist Quarterly, 19*(3), 49–60.

Hall, R. L., & Fine, M. (2005). The stories we tell: The lives and friendship of two older black lesbians. *Psychology of Women Quarterly, 29*, 177–187.

Harley, D. A. (2005a). The Black church: A strength-based approach in mental health. In D. A. Harley & J. M. Dillard (Eds.), *Contemporary mental health issues among African Americans* (pp. 191–203). Alexandria, VA: American Counseling Association.

Harley, D. A. (2005b). African Americans and indigenous counseling. In D. A. Harley & J. M. Dillard (Eds.), *Contemporary mental health issues among African Americans* (pp. 293–306). Alexandria, VA: American Counseling Association.

Harley, D. A., Stansbury, K. L., & Nelson, M. (2013). Sisters gone missing: The lack of focus on African American lesbians in mental health counseling and research. In H. Jackson-Lowman (Ed.), *African American women: Living at the crossroads of race, gender, class, and culture* (pp. 287–304). San Diego, CA: Cognella Academic Press.

Harley, D. A., Stansbury, K. L., Nelson, M., & Espinosa, C. T. (2014). A profile of rural elderly African American lesbians: Meeting their need. In H. F. O. Vakalahi, G. M. Simpson, & N. Giunta (Eds.), *Collective spirit of aging across cultures* (pp. 133–

155). New York: Springer Science and Business Media Publisher.

Henriksen, R. C., & Paladino, D. A. (2009). Identity development in a multiple heritage world. In R. C. Henrisken Jr & D. A. Paladino (Eds.), *Counseling multiple heritage individuals, couples, and families* (pp. 25–43). Alexandria, VA: American Counseling Association.

Hughes, A. K., Harold, R. D., & Boyer, J. M. (2011). Awareness of LGBT aging issues among aging services network providers. *Journal of Gerontological Social Work, 54*(7), 659–677.

Hunter, S. (2005). *Midlife and older LGBT adults: Knowledge and affirmative practice for the social services*. New York: Haworth Press.

Institute of Medicine (U.S.) Committee on Lesbian, Gay, Bisexual, and Transgender Health Issues. (2011). *The health of lesbian, gay, bisexual, and transgender people: Building a foundation for better understanding*. Washington, DC: National Academy of Sciences. Retrieved February 4, 2012 from http://www.ncbi.nlmnih.gov/books/NBK64806/?report=printable.

Institute for Women's Policy Research. (2011, May). *Fact sheet: Social Security and Black women* (IWPR #D496). Washington, DC: George Washington University.

Israel, T. (2007). Training counselors to work ethnically and effectively with bisexual clients. In B. A. Firestein (Ed.), *Becoming visible: Counseling bisexuals across the lifespan* (pp. 381–394). New York: Columbia University Press.

Jameson, D. (2007). Reconceptualizing cultural identity and its role in intercultural business communication. *Journal of Business Communication, 44*(3), 199–235.

Jeffries, W. L., Dodge, B., & Sandfort, T. G. M. (2008). Religion and spirituality among bisexual Black men in the USA. *Culture, Health and Sexuality, 10*(5), 463–477.

Jimenez, D. E., Alegria, M., Chen, C. N., Chan, D., & Laderman, M. (2010). Prevalence of psychiatric illnesses in older ethnic minority adults. *Journal of the American Geriatrics Society, 58*, 256–264.

Jones, D. A. (2009). Disabilities in older African American women: Understanding the current state of the literature. *Journal of National Black Nurses Association, 20*(2), 55–64.

Kelly, J. F., & Greene, B. (2010). Diversity within African American, female therapists: Variability in clients' expectations and assumptions about the therapist. *Psychotherapy: Theory Research, Practice, & Training, 47*, 186–197.

Kuyper, L., & Fokkema, T. (2010). Loneliness among older lesbian, gay, and bisexual adults: The rol of minority stress. *Archieves of Sex Behavior, 39*(5), 1171–1180.

Lacy, K. R. (2004). Black spaces, Black places: Strategic assimilation and identity construction in middle-class suburbia. *Ethnic and Racial Studies, 27*(6), 908–930.

Landerman, G., & Leon, L. (2003). *Religion and American cultures: An encyclopedia of traditions, diversity, and popular expressions* (Vol. 1). Santa Barbara, CA: ACB-CLIO.

Lawson, E., & Thomas, C. (2007). Wading in the waters: Narrative of older Katrina survivors. *Journal of the Poor and Underserved, 18,* 341–354.

Lekan, D. (2009). Sojourner syndrome and health disparities in African American women. *Annuals of Advance Nurse Science, 32*(4), 307–321.

Lemelle, Jr., A. J. (2003). *Linking the structure of African American criminalization to the spread of HIV/AIDS* (pp. 1–34). Conference papers, American Sociological Association, Annual meeting, Atlanta.

Lewis, M., & Marshall, I. (2012). *LGBT psychology: Research perspectives and people of African descent.* New York: Springer.

Locher, J. L., Ritchie, C. S., Roth, D. L., Baker, P. S., Bodner, E. V., & Allman, R. M. (2005). Social isolation, support, and capital and nutritional risk in an older sample: Ethnic and gender differences. *Social Science and Medicine, 60*(4), 747–761.

Loiacano, D. K. (1989). Gay identity issues among Black Americans: Racism, homophobia, and the need for validation. *Journal of Counseling & Development, 68,* 21–25.

Loue, S. (2014). *Understanding theology and homosexuality in African American communities.* New York: Springer.

Maccio, E. M., & Doueck, H. J. (2002). Meeting the needs of the gay and lesbian community: Outcomes in the human services. *Journal of Gay & Lesbian Social Services: Issues in Practice, Policy & Research, 14*(4), 55–73.

Mayo, C. (1982). Training for positive marginality. In C. L. Bickman (Ed.), *Applied social psychology annual* (Vol. 3, pp. 57–73). Beverly Hills, CA: Sage.

McGuire, T. C., & Miranda, J. (2008). New evidence regarding racial and ethnic disparities in mental health: Policy implications. *Health Affairs, 27,* 393–403.

MetLife. (2010, March). *Still out, still aging: The MetLife study of lesbian, gay, bisexual, and transgender baby boomers.* Westport, CT: Mature Market Institute.

Meyer, I. H. (2010). Identity, stress, and resilience in lesbians, gay men, and bisexuals of color. *The Counseling Psychologist, 38*(3), 442–454.

Meyer, K. H., Bradford, J. B., Makadon, H. J., Stall, R., Goldhammer, H., & Landers, S. (2008). Sexual and gender minority health: What we know and what needs to be done. *American Journal of Public Health, 98*(6), 989–995.

Mitchem, S. Y. (2002). "There is a balm…" Spirituality & healing among African American women. *Michigan Family Review, 7*(1), 19–33.

Moore, M. R. (2010). Articulating a politics of (multiple) identities: LGBT sexuality and inclusion in Black community life. *Du Bois Review, 7*(2), 1–20.

Moore, K. A., Weinberg, B. D., & Berger, P. D. (2010). The effect of ethnicity and acculturation on African American food purchases. *Innovative Marketing, 6*(4), 17–29.

Morrell, R. W., Echt, K. V., & Caramagno, J. (2008). *Older adults, race/ethnicity and mental health disparities: A consumer focused research agenda.* Retrieved June 11, 2014 from http://www.tapartnership.org/docs/researchAgendaOnAgingAndMHDisparities.pdf.

Muraco, A., & Fredriksen-Goldsen, K. (2011). "That's what friends do": Informal caregiving for chronically ill midlife and older lesbian, gay, and bisexual adults. *Journal of Social and Personal Relationships, 28*(8), 1073–1092.

Coalition, National Black Justice. (2009). *At the crossroads: African American same gender loving families and the freedom to marry.* Washington, DC: Author.

National Alliance on Mental Health. (2007). *Disparities in mental health treatment among GLBT populations.* Arlington, VA: Author.

National Center for Health Statistics. (2013). Deaths: Final data for 2010. *National Vital Statistics Report, 61*(4). Available at www.cdc.gov.nchs/data/dvs/deaths_2010_release.pdf.

National Hispanic Council on Aging. (2013, December). *Hispanic LGBT older adult needs assessment.* Retrieved May 29, 2014 from www.gallup.com/poll/158066/special-report-adults-identify-lgbt.aspx.

Neighbors, H. W., Caldwell, C., Williams, D. R., Neese, R., Taylor, R. J., Bullard, K., M., et al. (2007). Race, ethnicity, and the use of services for mental disorders. *Archives of General Psychiatry, 64,* 485–494.

Paniagua, F. A. (2014). *Assessing and treating culturally diverse clients: A practical guide.* Los Angeles, CA: Sage.

Parham, T. A., White, J. L., & Ajamu, A. (1999). *The psychology of Blacks: An African-centered perspective.* Upper Saddle River, NJ: Prentice Hall.

Peterson, J. W. (1990). Age of wisdom: Elderly Black women in family and church. In J. Sokolovsky (Ed.), *The cultural context of aging: Worldwide perspective* (pp. 213–227). Westport, CT: Bergin and Garvey.

Pew Center. (2006, August 3). *Pragmatic Americans liberal and conservatives on social issues: Most wan middle ground.* Retrieved September 29, 2014 from www.people-press.org/2006/08/03/pragmatic-americans-liberal-and-conservative-on-social-issues/2/.

Plumb, M. & Associates. (2003/2004). *SAGE national needs assessment: A report prepared for senior action in a gay environment.* New York: SAGE.

Plummer, M. D. (2007). *Sexual racism in gay communities: Negotiating the ethnosexual marketplace.* Thesis. University of Washington. Available at http://hdl.handle.net/1773/9181.

Portes, A., & Zhou, M. (1993). The new second generation: Segmented assimilation and its variants. *Annals of the American Academy of Political and Social Science, 530,* 74–96.

Primm, A. B., & Lawson, W. B. (2010). Disparities among ethnic groups: African Americans. In P. Ruiz & A. B. Primm (Eds.), *Disparities in psychiatric care: Clinical and cross-cultural perspectives.* Wolters

Kluwer/Lippincott Williams & Wilkins: Baltimore, MD.

Purdie-Vaugns, V., & Eibach, R. (2008). Intersectional invisibility: The distinctive advantages and disadvantages of multiple subordinate-group identities. *Sex Roles, 59*(5–6), 377.

Rasheed, M. N., & Rasheed, J. M. (2004). Rural African American older adults and the Black helping tradition. *Journal of Gerontological Social Work, 41*(1/2), 137–150.

Redman, D., & Woody, I. (2012, June 19). Creating a safe harbor for African American LGBT elders. *Aging Today.* Retrieved September 19, 2014 from http://www.asaging.org/blog/creating-safe-harbor-African American-lgbt-elders.

Riva, L. M. (2010). Acculturation: Theories, measurement, and research. In J. G. Ponterotto, J. M. Casas, L. A. Suzuky & C. M. Alexander (Eds.), *Handbook of multicultural counseling* (3rd edn., pp. 331–341). Los Angeles: Sage.

Roberts, M. (2012, March. *A look at African American trans trailblazers.* Retrieved June 3, 2014 from http://www.ebony.com/news-views/trans-trailblazers#axzz33cJowprP.

Robinson-Wood, T. (2009). *The convergence of race, ethnicity, and gender: Multiple identities in counseling* (3rd ed.). Upper Saddle River, NJ: Merrill.

Rust, P. (1996). Managing multiple identities: Diversity among bisexual women and men. In B. Firestein (Ed.), *Bisexuality: The psychology and politics of an invisible minority.* Thousand Oaks, CA: Sage.

Sanders, T. L. (2010). Black lesbians and racial identity in contemporary Cuba. *Black Women, Gender, and Families, 4*(1), 9–36.

Savage, T. A., & Harley, D. A. (2005). African American lesbian, gay, and bisexual persons. In D. A. Harley & J. M. Dillard (Eds.), *Contemporary mental health issues among African Americans* (pp. 91–105). Alexandria, VA: American Counseling Association.

Scherrer, K. S. (2009). Images of sexuality and aging in gerontological literature. *Sexuality Research & Social Policy: A Journal of the NSRC, 6*(4), 5–12.

Schwartz, S. J., Zamboanga, B. L., Rodriguez, L., & Wang, S. (2007). The structure of cultural identity in an ethnically diverse sample of emerging adults. *Basic and Applied Social Psychology, 29*(2), 159–173.

Shellman, J. (2011). Barriers to depression care for Black older adults: Practice and policy implications. *Journal of Gerontological Nursing, 37*(6), 13–17.

Singer, J. A. (2004). Narrative identity and meaning making across the adult lifespan: An introduction. *Journal of Personality, 72*(3), 437–459.

Smith, B. (1999). Blacks and gays healing the great divide. In E. Brandt (Ed.), *Dangerous liaisons: Blacks, gays and the struggle for equality* (pp. 15–24). New York: The New Press.

Social Care Institute for Excellence. (2011, April). *Implications for lesbian, gay, bisexual and transgendered (LBGT) people.* Retrieved May 30, 2014 from www.scie.org.uk.

Social Security Administration. (2011). *Annual Statistical Supplement to the Social Security Bulletin, 2010.* Retrieved January 15, 2013 from http://www.ssa.gov/policy/docs/statcomps/supplement/.

Somjen, F. M. (2009). *LGBT health and human services needs in New York state.* Albany, NY: Empire State Pride Agenda Foundation.

Stanford, A. (2013). *Homophobia in the Black church: How faith, politics, and fear divide the Black community.* Santa Barbara, CA: Praeger.

Stansbury, K., Harley, D. A., Allen, S., Nelson, N. J., & Christensen, K. (2010). African American lesbians: A selective review of the literature. *African American Research Perspective, 11*(1), 99–108.

Sue, D. W., & Sue, D. (2013). *Counseling the culturally diverse: Theory and practice* (6th ed.). Hoboken, NJ: Wiley.

Szymanski, D. M., & Gupta, A. (2009). Examining the relationship between multiple internalized oppressions and African American lesbian, gay, bisexual, and questioning persons' self-esteem and psychological distress. *Journal of Counseling Psychology, 56*(1), 110–118.

Tauriac, J. J., & Scruggs, N. (2006). Elder abuse among African Americans. *Educational Gerontology, 32*, 37–48.

Taylor, R. J., Chatters, L. M., & Levin, J. S. (2004). *Religion in the lives of African Americans: Social, psychological and health perspectives.* Newbury Park, CA: Sage.

Teaster, P. B., Harley, D. A., & Kettaneh, A. (2014). Aging and mistreatment: Victimization of older adults in the United States. In H. F. O. Vakalah, G. M. Simpson & N. Giunta (Eds.), *Collective spirit of aging across cultures* (pp. 41–64). New York, NY: Springer Science and Business Media Publisher.

Todays, Research on Aging. (2013, June). *The health and life expectancy of older Blacks and Hispanics in the United States, 28*, 1–8.

Troxel, W. M., Buysse, D. J., Hall, M., Kamarck, T. W., Strollo, P. O., Ownes, J. F., et al. (2010). Social integration, social contacts, and blood pressure dipping in African Americans and whites. *Journal of Hypertension, 28*(2), 265.

Van der Meide, W. (2002, March 15). *The intersections of sexual orientation, race, religion, ethnicity & heritage language: The state of research.* Toronto, ON: Canadian Heritage Multicultural Program.

Vasquez, L. A., Marin, M., & Garcia-Vazquez, E. (2010). Advances in multicultural assessment and counseling with culturally diverse older adults. In J. G. Ponterotto, J. M. Casas, L. A., Suzuki & C. M. Alexander (Eds.), *Handbook of multicultural counseling* (pp. 667–675). Thousand Oaks, CA: Sage.

Vontress, C. E., & Epp, L. R. (1997). Historical hostility in the African American clients: Implications for counseling. *Journal of Multicultural Counseling and Development, 45*, 170–184.

Wamwara-Mbugua, L. W., Cornwell, T. B., & Boller, G. (2006). Triple acculturation: The role of African

Americans in the consumer acculturation of Kenyan immigrants. *Advances in Consumer Research, 33,* 428.

Ward, E. G. (2005). Homophobia, hypermasculinity and the U.S. Black church. *Culture, Health and Sexuality, 7,* 493–504.

Welch, M. (2003). Care of Black and African Americans. In J. Bigby (Ed.), *Cross cultural medicine* (pp. 29–60). Washington, DC: American College of Physicians, American Society of Internal Medicine.

Wheeler, D. P. (2003). Methodological issues in conducting community-based health and social services research among urban Black and African American LGBT populations. In W. Meezan & J. I. Martin (Eds.), *Research methods with gay, lesbian, bisexual, and transgender populations* (pp. 65–78). New York: Haworth Press.

Wilson, K. B. (2005). Cultural characteristics of the African American community. In D. A. Harley & J. M. Dillard (Eds.), *Contemporary mental health issues among African Americans* (pp. 149–162). Alexandria, VA: American Counseling Association.

Wilson, P. A., & Yoshikawa, H. (2007). Improving access to health care among African American, Asian and Pacific Islander, and Latino lesbian, gay, and bisexual populations. In H. H. Meyer & M. E. Northridge (Eds.), *The health of sexual minorities: Public health perspective of lesbian, gay, bisexual, and transgender populations* (pp. 607–637). New York: Springer.

Wilson, K. B., Harley, D. A., McCormick, K., Jolivette, K., & Jackson, R. L. (2001). A literature review of vocational rehabilitation acceptance and rationales for bias in the rehabilitation process. *Journal of Applied Rehabilitation Counseling, 32*(1), 24–35.

American Indian, Alaska Native, and Canadian Aboriginal Two-Spirit/LGBT Elderly

Debra A. Harley and Reginald J. Alston

Abstract

The purpose of this chapter is to discuss the status of older two-spirit American Indian, Alaska Native, and Canadian Aboriginal two-spirit LGBT elders. Information is presented on traditional values and behaviors, two-spirit tradition and roles of elders in tribal communities, service utilization by two-spirit elders, systems of service delivery, and policy implications. The authors acknowledge the heterogeneity of these groups and do not presume uniformity across groups. Similarity, the term LGBT is used as the modern roughly equivalent of the Native term two-spirit. A brief background of two-spirit is included to provide the reader with an understanding of the history and significance of self-identity that is implicit in how two-spirit persons refer to themselves.

Keywords

American Indian · Alaska Native · Canadian Aboriginal two-spirit · LGBT elderly

Overview

Understanding the implication of health status, aging, disability, and other sociocultural and economic factors for two-spirit American Indian and Alaska Native (AIAN) and Aboriginal Peoples (AP) elders is important to investigate because little research has been done to address the extent to which disparities affect them. However, throughout the literature, historical trauma has profoundly shaped distinctive conditions of health risk and resilience of AIANs and AP, and two-spirit persons are considered to be at even greater risk for adverse health outcomes than other Natives (Fieland et al. 2007; Ristock et al. 2011). Although urban AIANs and First Nations face many of the same conditions as other urban poor, they tend to have less social support and a long history of circular migration and residential

D.A. Harley (✉) · R.J. Alston
University of Kentucky, Lexington, KY, USA
e-mail: dharl00@email.uky.edu

© Springer International Publishing Switzerland 2016
D.A. Harley and P.B. Teaster (eds.), *Handbook of LGBT Elders*,
DOI 10.1007/978-3-319-03623-6_7

mobility (i.e., regular travel between urban settings and reservations (Rhoades et al. 2005). Weaver (2012) suggests that cyclical migration is problematic, "particularly at times of illness, [it] can complicate accurate epidemiological information" (p. 477). Similar to many ethnic minority groups, AIANs and First Nations are typically overrepresented in the lower socioeconomic status; however, the reader is cautioned not to assume that all AIANs and First Nations are poor or destitute. As with any group of people, there diversity exists across demographic characteristics.

The purpose of this chapter is to discuss the status of older two-spirit AIANs and APs of Canada. Information is presented on the status of AIANs and APs, traditional values and behaviors, traditions and roles of two-spirit elders in tribal communities, service utilization by two-spirit elders, and systems of service delivery. Discussion of policy and implications for future directions are also presented. The authors acknowledge the heterogeneity of AIANs and APs in North America and do not presume to refer to the diversity of the people of tribal nations or indigenous peoples of Canada in a collectivist way. However, space prohibits discussion of each tribal nation or indigenous peoples, and so general information is presented, with specific reference to select groups. Although the term LGBT is used throughout this book to reference lesbian, gay, bisexual, and transgender persons, the term two-spirit is the preferred term of traditional American Indians and Aboriginal LGBT persons. LGBT is the modern equivalent of the Native term two-spirit (Fieland et al. 2007). Therefore, throughout this chapter, these two terms will be used interchangeably. A brief discussion of the background of two-spirit is included to explain the history and significance of self-identity implicit in how AIAN and AP two-spirit persons refer to themselves.

Learning Objectives

By the end of the chapter, the reader should be able to:

1. Identify the role of historical oppression of AIAN and AP populations.
2. Understand the traditions of two-spirit person in North American Indian culture.
3. Identify traditions and roles of elders in North American Indian culture.
4. Understand barriers to health care of North American Indians.
5. Identify health practices and disparities of North American two-spirit elders.
6. Identify policy issues and concerns affecting North American Indian two-spirit elders.

Introduction

American Indians represent a diverse population consisting of 565 tribes, including indigenous peoples of Alaska and Hawaii and more than 300 reservations that serve as indigenous homelands and seats of tribal governments (Ogunwold 2006). American Indians and Alaska Natives (AIAN) maintain a unique status as sovereign nations. As indigenous cultures, American Indians reside primarily in the West, with approximately 34 % living on-reservations and 57 % living in metropolitan areas. Urban American Indians experience significant social, health, and economic problems while having access to substantially fewer Native-specific resources than their reservation-based counterparts (Weaver 2012). American Indians (AI) comprise less than one percent of the US population, a figure the same for persons age 65 and over (Administration on Aging [AOA] 2012). The low numbers of AIs result in a relatively invisible status, which make them highly susceptible to stereotypes (Bureau of Indian Affairs 2011). The history of American Indians is complex and one of disenfranchisement and distrust of European Americans and the government. According to Walters et al. (2001), over the past century "American Indians have endured a succession of traumatic assaults on their cultural and physical well-being, and continue to disproportionately experience violence and trauma" (p. 134).

The "Aboriginal Peoples" (AP) refer to a collective name for the original peoples of North America and their descendants. Throughout this chapter, the terms Aboriginal Peoples and First Nations are used interchangeably. There are more than 50 distinct groupings among First Nations alone, with several dialects within Inuktitut. The Metis people speak a variety of First Nations languages such as Cree, Ojibwa, or Chipewyan, as well as Michif (Report of the Royal Commission on Aboriginal Peoples 1996). About 1.4 million people in Canada identify themselves as an Aboriginal person, 60.8 % of which have First Nations single identity (i.e., 45.5 % as registered or treaty Indian, 15.3 % as not a Registered or Treaty Indian), 32.3 % as Metis single identity, 4.2 % as Inuit single identity, 0.8 % as multiple Aboriginal identities, and 1.9 % as aboriginal identities not included elsewhere. The Aboriginal population increased by 20.1 % between 2006 and 2011, compared with 5.2 % for the non-Aboriginal population. The largest numbers of Aboriginal people live in Ontario and the Western provinces (Manitoba, Saskatchewan, Alberta, and British Columbia) (National Household Survey 2013). Winnipeg is home to the largest urban Aboriginal population in Canada (Ristock et al. 2011). The use of the terms Indian and Eskimo in Canada is considered pejorative. A glossary of terms for Canadian First Nations is provided in Table 7.1.

Historical trauma, the universal experience of colonization, is a shared history for two-spirit persons both within and across the heterogeneity of the tribes in North America. Ristock et al. (2011) stress that it is impossible to consider the health and well-being of Aboriginal two-spirit people without taking into account the historical impacts of colonization and its contemporary effects that interacts with socio-demographic vulnerabilities to negatively affect them. The experience of two-spirit person/LGBT is one of the dual oppressions—heterosexism from Native peoples and racism from LGBT persons (Fieland et al. 2007). Dual oppression puts two-spirit persons at compounded risk for discrimination and violent victimization (Brotman et al. 2002). Given that there is such limited research on older two-spirit persons/LGBT, information may be gleaned from studies on the general population of older Native peoples and younger two-spirit persons.

Status of AIANs and First Nations of Canada

American Indians differ in their degree of acculturation. In part, American Indians' acculturation is muddy because what actually constitutes an Indian is unclear and controversial. This controversy is heightened by several factors, for example, in the USA: (a) the United States Census relies on self-report of racial identity, (b) Congress has formulated a legal definition in which an individual must have an Indian blood quantum of at least 25 %, and (c) some tribes have developed their own criteria and specify either tribal enrollment or blood quantum levels (Sue and Sue 2013). Garret and Pichette (2000) identify levels of cultural orientation to explain the degree to which AIANs identify with native culture (see Table 7.2). In addition, urban dwellers do not have access to tribal governmental services and political decision-makers or to public housing as their counterparts on-reservations. Urban American Indians may find it difficult to exercise their rights as citizens of Native Nations and may be disenfranchised and lose their voice in tribal governance (Weaver 2012).

In Canada, AP (including Inuit and Metis) are not afforded the same privileges as other Canadians. "In 1998, a United Nation Human Rights Committee ruled that the treatment of AP within Canada stood in violation of international law and was the most pressing human rights issue facing Canadians" (Meyer-Cook and Labelle 2003, p. 36). Both the historical and current treatments of AIAN and First Nations in North America are discriminatory and oppressive. The circumstances faced by AIANs and First Nations are similar to the challenges and oppression faced by more than three million indigenous people globally. The concerns for indigenous peoples globally culminated in the United Nations Declaration on the Rights of Indigenous Peoples ("the

Table 7.1 Glossary of terms for Canadian first nation(s)

First Nation(s)—term used as a substitution for *band* or Indian, referring to any of the numerous groups formally recognized by the Canadian government under the Indian Act of 1876.

First Nation people—generally applied to both status and non-status Indians. Is not a synonym for Aboriginal peoples because it does not include Inui or Metis

First peoples—a collective term used to describe the original peoples of Canada and their descendants. It is used less frequently than terms such as Aboriginal peoples and Native peoples

Indian—collectively describes all the Indigenous People in Canada who are not Inuit or Metis. Three categories apply to Indians in Canada: (a) Status Indians—people who are entitled to have their names included on the Indian Register. Only Status Indians are recognized as Indians under the Indian Act and are entitled to certain rights and benefits under the law; (b) Non-status Indians—people who consider themselves Indians or members of a First Nation but whom the Government of Canada does not recognize as Indians under the Indian Act and are not entitled to the same rights and benefits available to Status Indians; and (c) Treaty Indians—descendants of Indians who signed treaties with Canada and who have a contemporary connection with a treaty band

Inuit—Aboriginal People of Arctic Canada

Metis—the French word for people of mixed blood. The Constitution Act of 1982 recognizes Metis as one of the three Aboriginal Peoples

Native—a collective term to describe the descendants of the original peoples of North America

Native American—commonly used term in the USA to describe the descendants of the original peoples of North America. The term has not caught on in Canada because of the apparent reference to US citizenship. Native North American has been used to identify the original peoples of

Adapted   from   http://web.archieve.org/web/201007140216555/   http://www.aidp.bc.ca/terminology_of_native_aboriginal_metis.pdf

Table 7.2 Levels of cultural orientation

Traditional—the person may speak limited English and practice traditional tribal customs and methods of worship

Marginal—the person may be bilingual but has lost touch with his or her cultural heritage, yet is not fully accepted in mainstream society

Bicultural—the person is conversant with both sets of values and can communicate in a variety of contexts

Assimilates—the person embraces only the mainstream culture's values, behaviors, and expectations

Pantraditional—the person has been exposed to and adopted mainstream values but is making a conscious effort to return to the "old ways"

Adapted from Garrett and Pichette (2000)

Declaration"), which is a framework of rights for indigenous peoples for states. Each Nation that adopts the Declaration is independently responsible for enacting domestic legislation and polices that comply with Declaration standards (Rowland 2013), though the Declaration is not legally binding for Nations that adopt it.

Cultural determinants of AIAN resistance and resilience include identity, spirituality, and traditional health practices, the very aspects of Native culture targeted by colonial persecution (Walters and Simoni 2002). For two-spirit persons in Canada, the binary concept of gender conformity that prevailed in colonial days was contrary to that of gender variance. Canadian two-spirit persons who thought in more circular ways resulted in outlawing and discrediting of any processes that that could not easily be co-opted to advance a larger agenda of profit by Europeans (Meyer-Cook and Labelle 2003). In fact, for two-spirit persons, enculturation (the process by which individuals learn or re-immerse themselves in their cultural heritage, norms, and behaviors within a contemporary context) in the form of "retraditionalization" may be a powerful process because of the denigration of their formally elevated status in many tribal communities (Fieland et al. 2007). Meyer-Cook and Labelle

(2003) suggest that for two-spirit persons to achieve a sound identity, they need to simultaneously follow two tracks of identity formation: first as Native people or people of a minority group and second as people who are differently gendered.

As a population, health statistics for American Indians reveal significant adverse outcomes (Roubideaux et al. 2004). As compared to the general US population, American Indians have alcoholism mortality rates that are more than twice as high, significantly higher obesity and diabetes rates, injury-related deaths (e.g., homicides, motor vehicle crashes, suicides), disproportionate rates of depression, and deaths from injuries and violence account for 75 % of all deaths (Centers for Disease Control [CDC] 2007; U.S. Department of Health and Human Services 2007), lower earnings, lower educational level, and higher poverty rates, violence, and depression (CDC 2011). These factors are co-occurring, which means that AIANs are simultaneously at risk for all of them, creating a potentially severe network of social and psychological risks that affect their mental well-being (Native Vision Project 2012). Rates for older AIAN or two-spirit elders are not disaggregated among the data. The Alaska Department of Labor estimates that Alaska Natives (AN) account for about 7135 ANs over age 65 and 8040 between the ages of 55 and 64, with the most rapid increase in elders between 70 and 74, followed by those 85 and older. There is a higher prevalence of chronic illnesses such as cancer and heart and lung diseases, which can lead to a higher incidence of functional disability, and a corresponding need for long-term care (Branch 2005). Table 7.3 provides priority health needs as identified by Alaska Native elders.

Currently, older single-race AIAN adults account for 0.87 % of the total US population and multiple-race AIAN for 1.53 % of the US population (Ogunwole 2006). Compared to the general population, older AIANs are less educated, have a higher divorce rate (24.0 % vs. 19.9 %), and a higher percentage has never married (11 % compared to 6.5 % of the general population) (Tamborini 2007). Several factors

Table 7.3 Priority health needs identified by Alaska Native elders

Personal care services
Comprehensive care and tracking of chronic illnesses
Medication issues
Elder abuse
Housing
Alzheimer's Disease and related disorders
Unintentional injuries (causes and prevention of falls)
Telemedicine
Elder and youth activities (sharing traditions and participating in intergenerational activities to support youth and community)
Palliative care
Traditional healing
Urban/rural differences (understand why elders are moving to town and the implications this has on service availability in urban and rural areas)

Adapted from Branch (2005)

contribute to the vulnerability of older AIANs: lower educational attainment, lower household income, greater poverty, less insurance coverage, and higher limited English proficiency. Furthermore, vulnerability might be affected by multiple contributing factors, not by a single factor (Kim et al. 2012). AIANs aged 62 and older self-reports of health status reveals that almost 46 % are in fair to poor health, compared with 33.6 % of the general population. AIANs have higher rates of work limitations at 34.3 %, compared to 15.2 for the general population (Dunaway-Knight et al. 2012). In addition, the percent of AIANs who will receive Social Security disability benefits at some point in their lives is higher than the general population (16.0 % vs. 10.8 %) (Social Security Administration 2011). Typically, the age at which a person is considered elderly in American society is 65; however, there is no such consensus among tribal nations. The Older Americans Act gives discretion to individual tribes to make this determination. The health status of AP of Canada, especially elders, is similar to that of AIANs and is substantially lower than that of average Canadians. Moreover, compared to other Canadians, AP have poorer social and economic indicators, face critical housing shortages, higher rates of unemployment, lack of access to basic health services, and lower levels of education attainment (Lafontaine 2006).

First Nations elders, including Aboriginal, Metis, and Inuit seniors, have received limited attention by researchers because as a population, Aboriginals are younger than the non-Aboriginal population (Beatty and Berdahl 2011), and a lack of epidemiological data results in pan-Aboriginal (i.e., between assimilation and traditional) evidence and approximations (Lafontaine 2006). The dire straits of Aboriginal elders is summed up thusly: they "are among the most neglected social class because of their increasing multiple physical and mental health problems and increasingly poor socioeconomic supports have forced them into even more challenging and dependent situations at an age when they should expect to be well treated and taken care of properly by both their families and governments" (Beatty and Berdahl 2011, p. 1). Metis report poorer health status than the non-Aboriginal population (Janz et al. 2009; Wilson et al. 2011) and are more likely than First Nations elders to report fair to poor health (Wilson et al. 2010, 2011). One in five Metis has arthritis or rheumatism compared to one in ten in the general Canadian population. In addition, Metis have higher rates of high blood pressure, asthma, diabetes (30 % of men vs. 14 % of non-Aboriginal men; 32 % of women vs. 11 % of non-Aboriginal women), and heart problems. First Nation elders have higher rates of disability due to injury and/or chronic disease, with 58.5 % over age 60 compared to 46.5 % of Canadian seniors (Lafontaine 2006). Aboriginal elders are more likely than non-Aboriginal elders to report daily smoking and heavy drinking; however, one in two reports not drinking at all, with the majority either never smoking or having quit smoking (Turcotte and Schellenberg 2007).

Similar to research findings in minority groups in the USA, Beatty and Berdahl (2011) identify social and economic status as the two most important determinants of health among Aboriginal elders. The prevalence of low income is higher among Aboriginal elders than non-Aboriginal elders, and Aboriginal elders are often less able to pay for private or co-funded services. Economic differences are more pronounced among First Nations who come from reservations and cannot fulfill the residency requirements and are placed at the end of long waiting lists. With the increase in the number of people receiving homecare among those without alternative income to supplement higher costs, health care beyond post-acute care is unaffordable and inaccessible to Aboriginal elders. A related issue is the underutilization of services by Aboriginal elders in cities and on-reservations. Barriers to service utilization include culture, language, affordability, jurisdiction, and problems navigating the health services system, barriers exacerbated by limited knowledge of and access to policymakers and service providers. Although some policies have helped improve competency skills and communications between service providers and minority elders, limited efforts have been made to address institutional structures, racism in gerontological settings, and access to care facilities for Aboriginal elders (Beatty and Berdahl 2011). Table 7.4 identifies health and service needs of First Nations Canadian elders.

Among other problems, Aboriginal elders encounter educational and literacy barriers, poor housing conditions, homelessness in urban areas, and elder abuse. In Canada, housing on reservations is among the poorest in the country, which means that many elders with disabilities

Table 7.4 Priority health needs of first nation elders

Culturally responsive programming and employment in healthcare systems

Coordinated elderly care funding initiative for Aboriginal caregivers

Aboriginal long-term care facilities in the major prairie cities

An integrated, coordinated, and holistic healthcare system

First Nations long-term care facilities on reservations

Palliative, respite and after hour care services

Access to all health benefits

Adapted from Beatty and Berdahl (2011)

and chronic conditions live in overcrowded and deficient homes (Health Canada 2009). Currently, federal funding policies do not allow for building of long-term care facilities on reservations (Beatty and Berdhal 2011). As a vulnerable population, medically compromised and dependent Aboriginal elders are often targets of abuse (Podneik 2008). Elder abuse occurs most frequently as physical, psychological/emotional, financial abuse, and neglect whether the elder is at home or in semi-private and public institutions. Often, elders' and families' preferences for self-determination of care are disregarded. Aboriginal elders living in Toronto identified major issues facing them including, social isolation, lack of transportation services, lack of assisted living services, lack of family peer support, lack of senior housing, poor proximity to housing services, lack of activities programming, lack of physical fitness resources, and lack of alcohol and drug abuse counseling (McCaskill et al. 2011).

Traditional Values and Behaviors

Indigenous peoples have an identity that is rooted in a particular land of origin. Cultural identity is intimately connected with and defined by traditional territories. Indigenous cultural beliefs and values (e.g., harmony, respect, generosity, courage, wisdom, humility, honesty) and spiritual practices (e.g., natural world) are inextricably linked to the land. Even when Native Peoples are displaced from their territories, with ethnic mixing, and sporadic contact with tribal homelands, the tie to core indigenous values persists (Hendry 2003; Weaver 2012). For AIAN and First Nations, family or tribe is of fundamental importance because it provides a sense of belonging and security, an extension of the tribe (Sue and Sue 2013). This sense demonstrates the persistence and resilience of the community despite change (Weaver 2012). Different families and tribes have their own cultural assets. The cultural values and behaviors presented in the remainder of this section are generalizations and their applicability should be assessed for particular clients or patients and their families. The authors acknowledge distinctiveness within and between indigenous persons in the USA and Canada, and the intent is not to obscure such distinctiveness.

Native Peoples traditionally have respected the unique individual differences (*personal differences*) among people. This respect is demonstrated through staying out of the affairs of others and expressing personal opinions only when asked. An expectation is that this courtesy will be returned. Another traditional behavior is *quietness*. The act of silence serves multiple purposes in Native life. Historically, silence contributed to survival. When angry or uncomfortable, many Native Peoples remain silent. Silence is a deeply embedded form of Native interpersonal etiquette, and Patience is a closely related value to silence. *Patience* is based on the belief that all things unfold in time. The practice of patience demonstrates respect for individuals, facilitates group consensus, and permits "the second thought" (deliberation) (http://www.nwindian.evergreen. edu/cirriculum/ValuesBehaviors.prf). In traditional Native Peoples' life, *work* is always directed toward a distinct purpose and is taken on when it needs to be done. Work is linked to accumulating only that which is needed, which reflects the nonmaterialistic orientation of many Native Peoples. *Mutualism*, as a value, attitude, and behavior, permeates everything in the traditional Native social fabric. It promotes a sense of belonging and solidarity with group members cooperating to gain group security and consensus. The traditional manner in which most Native Peoples prefer to communicate is affective (*nonverbal orientation*) rather than verbal. That is, they prefer listening rather than speaking. Talk, like work, must have a purpose, and talking for talking's sake is rarely practiced. Words have a primordial power, and when there is a reason for their expression, it is generally done carefully. Closely linked to nonverbal orientation are the highly developed and valued skills of *seeing* and *listening*. Hearing, observing, and memorizing were highly developed skills because all aspects of Native culture were transferred orally through storytelling (http://www.nwindian.evergreen.edu/curriculum/ValuesBehaviors.pdf).

For Native Peoples, traditionally life unfolds when it is time. *Time orientation* is flexible and generally not structured into compartments. Similarly, Native Peoples have an *orientation to the present* and to immediate tasks at hand. What is occurring in the present takes precedence over vague future rewards. Emphasis is placed on *being-rather-than-becoming* (however, this value has shifted significantly over the past five decades toward a more futuristic approach). Both time orientation and orientation to the present tie into the Native value of *practicality*, with a focus on approaches that are concrete and experiential. At the core of traditional Native culture is a *holistic orientation* in which every aspect of life is based on an integrated orientation to the whole. A holistic perspective is essential in Native culture and is seen in aspects ranging from healing to social organization. Likewise, *spirituality* is integrated into every part of the sociocultural fabric of traditional Native Peoples' life. Spirituality is considered a natural component of everything. Lastly, *caution* is exercised in unfamiliar personal encounters and situations. Caution is manifested as quiet behavior and placidity. In many cases, being cautious is the result of fear of how their thoughts and behavior will be perceived by those with who they are unfamiliar or in a new situation with which they have no experience (http://www.nwindian.evergreen.edu/curriculum/ValuesBehaviors.pdf).

AIAN and Aboriginal or First Nations of Canada have distinct tribal values, beliefs, and behaviors; however, as Native Peoples of North America, these groups share some common cultural practices. The extent to which two-spirit persons incorporate some or all of these practices into life is dependent upon their level of acculturation, assimilation, or pantraditional experience. The following section describes two-spirit persons of North America.

Two-Spirit People of Indigenous North America

For traditional American Indians, the terms gender roles and sexual orientation are false conceptualizations because AIANs never analyzed human sexuality in such dichotomous and categorical ways. Rather, a continuum of human sexuality and gender behavior is appropriate for different people. That is, people do what they do best (Pope 2012). From a community perspective, the major focus was on the fulfillment of social or ceremonial roles and responsibilities as a more important defining feature of gender than sexual behavior or identity (Fieland et al. 2007). American Indians have always held intersex, androgynous people, feminine males, and masculine females in high esteem. Gender is viewed as biological, whereas gender status is more culturally defined. Thus, one's gender status may be either man (masculine), woman (feminine), or not-man/not-woman. In this model, not-man is not the same as woman, and not-woman is not the same as man. Clearly, by definition women are not men; however, other social groups within a society may consist of males whose gender status is that of not-men but who are also defined as not-women. These multiple genders are part of gender role construction in American Indian societies, and service providers for such cultures must be cognizant of this contextual ambiguity (Pope 2012).

Instead of seeing two-spirit persons as transsexuals who attempt to make themselves "the opposite sex," it is more accurate to understand them as individuals who take on a gender that is different from both women and men. In essence, two-spirits "will do at least some women's work and mix together much of the behavior, dress, and social roles of women and men" (Williams 1986, p. 344). Early on the term "berdaches" was used before the term two-spirit. Berdaches refer to that scared person accepted in the native world who is said to be both female and male (two-spirited) and believed to have mystical powers (Warren 1998). The term two-spirit originated in Winnipeg,

Canada, in 1990 during the third annual Inter-tribal Native American First Nation Gay and Lesbian conference. Two-spirit was originally chosen to distance Native First Nations people from non-Native as well as from the words "berdache" and "gay" (http://www.rainbowresourcecentre.org). In 1991, the term berdache was replaced with the word two-spirit because of various negative connotations (e.g., male slaves or prostitutes) (see Williams 1986 for additional information). According to Laframbo-ise and Anhorn (2008), the term two-spirit is preferred because it emerged from Native American people, whereas the term berdache was imposed upon Native People by the colonial explorers. Table 7.5 contains various terms that have been used to describe two-spirit American Indians. One of the reasons that two-spirits received respect was out of fear because they were considered to be touched by the spirits and to have powers on the level of a shaman. Two-spirits were highly regarded as artisans, craftspeople, child-rearers, couples counselors, and tribal arbiters.

Two-spirits are considered to be a "third gender," and female two-spirits are considered to be a "fourth gender" (similar to the way that both female and male homosexuals are considered to be gay, while females are also considered to be lesbian) (http://androgyne.0catch.com/2spiritx.htm). Rather than emphasizing the homosexual-ity of two-spirits, American Indian focuses on their spiritual gifts (Williams 1986). Laframboise and Anhorn (2008) make a key distinction about

terms regarding gender-variant people, indicating that two-spirit is different from sexual orientation because such words did not exist in Native languages. As terminology referring to LGBT persons has evolved over time, gender, which "is an obligatory grammatical category in the English/French and Latin languages"… and as a linguistic term "… has no connection with biological sex or social identity of an individual" (p. 2). The relevance of the issue is where gender intersects with the Native Peoples of North America because two-spirit does not refer to people with homosexual tendencies; rather, on different genders being manifested and not on sexual preferences or practices (Lafranmoise and Anhorn). See Discussion Box 7.1 for ways in which two-spirits are honored.

It is important to point out that the term two-spirited has multiple meanings within several different contexts. For example, Aboriginal people who identify as gay or lesbian use the term because it is more culturally relevant to their identities. Aboriginal people who are transgender might also use the term two-spirit, an umbrella term for Aboriginal persons who live between socially defined male and female gender roles (Balsam et al. 2004), or they may use terms of their own Aboriginal languages (Scheim et al. 2013). Elders within Aboriginal culture teach that two-spirited people have a special place in their communities. Aboriginal culture is recognized for balance and harmony, and no one element or force dominates the others. The term two-spirit originates from the First Nations'

Table 7.5 Two-spirit American Indian gender role and sexuality terms

Tribe	Term	Meaning
Crow	bote	Two-spirit
Kamia	warharmi	Hermaphrodite spirit
Lakota Sioux	winkte	Two-soul persons
Mohave	hwame	Female-bodied person who lives as a man
Navajo	nadleehe	"The change"
Omaha	mexoga	Homosexuality
Shoshoni	tainna wa'ippe	Man–woman/woman–man
Zuni	Ihamana	Man–woman

recognition of the traditions and sacredness of people who maintain a balance by housing both female and male spirits (Wahsquonaikezhik et al. 1976). Two-spirit persons are considered a vital and necessary part of the natural world and of the community as a whole because they possess an ability to see an issue from both perspectives and can understand and help solve problems that women and men may have individually or between each other (McLeod-Shabogesic 1995).

Discussion Box 7.1

Williams (1986) describes American Indian traditionalists as seeing a person's basic character as a reflection of their spirit and emphasize it as being most important. Rather than seeing two-spirit persons as transsexuals who try to make themselves into the "opposite sex," it is more accurate to understand them as individuals who take on a **gender** status that is different from both men and women. Since everything is thought to come from the spirit world, androgynous or transgender persons are seen as doubly blessed, having both the spirit of a man and the spirit of a woman. Thus, they are honored for having two spirits and are seen as more spiritually gifted than the typical masculine male or feminine female. Many American Indian religions often look to two-spirits as religious leaders and teachers. The emphasis of American Indians is not to force every person into one box, but to allow for the reality of diversity in gender and sexual identities.

Two-spirit persons are also respected by native societies because of practical concerns. That is, they could do both the work of men and of women. They were considered hard workers and artistically gifted of great value to their extended families and community. Two-sprit persons were believed to be economically beneficial as a relative to assist with raising children, taking care of the elderly, and serving as adoptive parents for homeless children.

Questions

How does the cultural view of American Indians about two-spirit persons differ from other culture's views?
What are the similarities between the value of two-spirit persons and LGBT persons in LGBT communities?
Do two-spirit persons share characteristics with other ethnic minority groups?

Not all AIAN or First Nations who are LGBT identify as two-spirited. Those who choose to use the term two-spirit do so to reflect their sexual and gender identity and its connectedness with spirituality and traditional worldviews (Walters et al. 2006). At times, First Nation LGBT persons may choose to use the word lesbian or gay in order to be understood in Western culture. C. Thomas Edwards (1998) is cited in *We Are Part of a Tradition* and explains that American Indians do not buy into homophobia because it is a focus on sexual behavior rather than the intricate roles two-spirit persons play. In the context of gender, two-spirit people also associate with the term bi-gender, which involves having a separate male persona and a separate female one. Granted, these terms are not exactly alike; nevertheless, they are closely related in both experiences and representation of that person (http://www.rainbowresourcecentre.org). Laframboise and Anhorn (2008) suggest that it is the inner calling of contemporary two-spirited people that mix their understanding of sexuality with the perception that homosexuality was well accepted in pre-colonization instead of recognizing that these homosexual behaviors were accepted under the role of gender identity. Thus, "the modern movement of reclaiming Two-Spirit Traditions incorporates sexual orientation and sexual identity" (p. 3).

Ristock et al. (2011) interviewed Aboriginal two-spirit/LGBT persons ages 19–61 regarding migration, mobility, and health and found that most moved from First Nations communities and/or small or rural towns to metropolitan areas because doing so allowed them to find a personal identity either with their sexuality and/or gender identity and/or Aboriginal identity. Other reasons for the move were to explore the anonymity that a big city can offer when it comes to exploring the "gay lifestyle," finding others like them, for gender reassignment, and to begin a healing journey from incest and violence, they may have encountered as children. Those not actively involved in the LGBT community felt an affirmation of their identity just knowing that a large LGBT community in the city existed. Some distinction was made by two-spirit persons about the importance of having their own space because of the domination in the LGBT community by White people. A culturally specific space also allowed a place to have ceremonies.

AIAN, Aboriginal Peoples of Canada, and Two-Spirit Elders Physical and Mental Health

Individually and collectively, AIANs and AP have worse health outcomes than other ethnic minority groups and non-Hispanic Whites (NHWs). Health disparities and chronic health conditions exist with marked variation across Indian Health Service (IHS) areas and within tribes in the USA (Wright 2009) and likewise for indigenous elders in Canada (Beatty and Berdahl 2011). The disparities are especially problematic for low-income elders in indigenous communities. Older AIANs and AP have greater numbers of chronic conditions, higher rates of disease comorbidity, and higher rates of disability than do other populations of elders (Beatty and Berdahl 2011; Satter et al. 2010). Although research has focused on the physical health status of older AIANs and AP, studies pertaining to their access to healthcare service are sparse, and their mental health status has been less often documented (Kim et al. 2012). Research suggests that older

AIANs experience greater emotional and/or mental health problems compared to their peers of other racial and ethnic groups (Kim et al. 2011; Satter et al. 2010). Arguably, the impact of structural oppression including homophobia, heterosexism, and racism is likely to play a role in the physical and mental health of Aboriginal two-spirit/LGBT persons (Canadian Rainbow Health Coalition 2004; Taylor and Ristock 2011; Ristock et al. 2011). In response to the limited research on healthcare access and service, Kim et al. (2012) examined older AIANs' physical and mental health status and related healthcare use in comparison with NHWs and found that older AIANs reported poorer physical and mental health than NHWs, were less likely to see a medical doctor and to have a usual source of medical care, and were more likely to delay getting needed medical care and report difficulty understanding the doctor at their last visit. However, this study did not indicate if any of the participants were two-spirit persons.

Two-spirit persons do not have more propensity or pathology of mental illness than the general population. However, their prolonged exposure to hostile or intolerant environments can cause significant stress on LGBT persons, and having to manage stigma has far-reaching effects on their health status (Brotman et al. 2003). Although information in this section is presented on the health status of AIANs and AP with reference to two-spirit elders as applicable, the authors agree with the position of Scheim et al. (2013) that AIAN and "Aboriginal gender-diverse peoples' experiences and health statuses cannot be understood by simply summing together what is known from research on broader (AIAN), Aboriginal, or gender-diverse populations. Nevertheless, health inequities documented in studies using one or the other of these identity categories provide an important context for understanding the well-being of (AIAN) and Aboriginal gender-diverse peoples" (p. 109). Scheim et al. (2013) conducted a study to describe barriers to well-being in a sample of Aboriginal gender-diverse peoples in Ontario, Canada (see Research Box 7.1).

Research Box 7.1

Scheim, A. I., Jackson, R., James, L., Dopler, T.S., Pyne, J., & Bauer, G.R. (2013). Barriers to well-being for Aboriginal gender-diverse people: Results from the Trans PULSE Project in Ontario, Canada. *Ethnicity and Inequalities in Health and Social Care, 6*(4), 108–120.

Objective: Despite health inequities experienced by Aboriginal and transgender communities, little research has explored the well-being of Aboriginal trans people. The purpose of this study is to describe barriers to well-being in a sample of Aboriginal gender-diverse people in Ontario, Canada.

Method: Of the 433 participant in the Trans PULSE Project survey, the 32 who self-identified as First Nation, Metis, or Inuit were included in the analysis. Because of the small sample size, unweighted frequencies and proportions were calculated.

Results: The participants were almost evenly split between male-to-female and female-to-male gender spectra. The majority was under age 35, almost half were living in poverty, live in metropolitan Toronto, and none were living on a reservation. Many were homeless or unstably housed, most had experienced some form of violence due to transphobia, including physical and/or sexual violence, and life-time suicidality was high. Most had a regular family doctor but had unmet healthcare needs. Many were unable to obtain services including shelters, hormone therapy, trans-related surgery, trans-related mental health, sexual health, and addictions. However, needs were met for general health services, emergency care, and HIV or sexually transmitted infections testing. Some had seen an Elder for mental health

support and a range of family and community support for gender identity and expression were indicated.

Conclusion: Action is needed to address the social determinants of health among Aboriginal gender-diverse people. Using principles of self-determination, there is a need to increase access to health and community supports, including integration of traditional culture and healing practices. Larger study samples and qualitative research are required.

Questions

1. What implications do these findings have for including gender-diverse Elders as part of comprehensive planning healthcare services?
2. What are the limitations of this study?
3. What other research methodology and design would you recommend for this study?

Cancer is the leading cause of death for AIAN females (breast) and the third leading cause of death for males (prostate) (Paltoo and Chu 2004). Of all races, AIAN women have the lowest rates of mammogram screening (Ward et al. 2004), the youngest mean age (age 54) for breast cancer diagnosis of all racial groups (age 56–62) (Li et al. 2003) and the lowest survival rates. Ward et al. (2004) found that for all cancers combined, AIANs have lower mortality rates than the general US population, but have disproportionately lower 5-year survival rates than Whites. Of all ethnic minority groups in the USA, AIAN men have the highest rates of chronic disease (e.g., obesity, cardiovascular disease, hypertension, high cholesterol, diabetes, and smoking), and women have the highest rates of obesity, cardiovascular disease, smoking, and diabetes, and the second highest rates of hypertension and high cholesterol after African American women

(Centers for Disease Control [CDC] 2003). Again, it is supposition that older two-spirit persons are counted among these numbers.

Overall, AP has poorer health than other Canadians. The long-term health conditions that affect First Nations adults living on-reservations tend to be the same as those affecting other Canadians except for diabetes, which is more prevalent among First Nations population. Approximately, 60 % of the Aboriginal population living off-reservations has chronic conditions compared to 49.6 % of the non-Aboriginal population (Tjepkema 2002). AP living off-reservations tend to have lower prevalence of long-term conditions than those living on-reservations, with the exception for diabetes, but these rates are still typically higher than they are for other Canadian adults except for the Inuit (Galabuzi 2004). Furthermore, Aboriginal adults living off-reservations are much more likely to be obese than non-Aboriginal adults in Canada, but those living on-reservations have even higher obesity levels (Reading and Wien 2009; Tjepkema 2002). In each geographic region (urban, rural, territories) (see Table 7.6 for a list of Canada provinces and territories), the Aboriginal population living off-reservations reported higher levels of fair to poor health than their non-Aboriginal counterpart in that region and percentage did not vary significantly between regions (Tjepkema 2002). The First Nations Centre (2007) indicates a significant difference in morbidity and chronic

Table 7.6 Canada provinces and territories

Alberta
British Columbia
Manitoba
New Brunswick
Newfoundland and Labrador
Northwest Territory
Nova Scotia
Nunavut
Ontario
Prince Edward Island
Quebec
Yukon Territory

conditions for off- and on-reservation First Nations populations. For example, high blood pressure for off-reservation AP is 12 % versus 20.4 % for on-reservation, diabetes is 8.3 % for off- and 19.7 % for on-reservation, asthma is 12.5 % for off- and 9.7 % for on-reservation, and heart problem is 10.3 % for off- and 7.6 % for on-reservation. The higher rates of asthma and heart problems among off-reservation Aboriginal populations may suggest a function of lifestyle and environmental circumstances.

Aboriginal adults living off-reservations are almost twice as likely to experience a major depressive disorder compared to other Canadians (Canada Mortgage and Housing Corporation 2004). In fact, it is suspected that the rate of depression may be underdiagnosed within the Aboriginal population. Mental health consequences among AP are linked to "persistent socioeconomic inequities, intergenerational trauma, and colonial and neo-colonial processes including racialization and discrimination have taken a serious toll on the mental health of AP as reflected in alarming rates of suicide, depressions, substance abuse, and violence" (Browne et al. 2009, p. 19). Although research on Aboriginal Peoples' mental health is sparse, the First Nations Centre (2007) indicates that some evidence exists that mental health is better for Aboriginal populations living off-reservation than their on-reservation counterparts. This more favorable outcome may be credited to off-reservation AP having access to a relatively greater number of mental health services available in urban areas (Place 2012).

Rosenberg et al. (2009) report that in every age cohort, AP are more likely than non-Aboriginal people to indicate "poor/fair" health. Although chronic conditions increase with age, AP are more likely to report more chronic conditions than the comparable non-Aboriginal population. The prevalence rates of specific chronic conditions for elderly AP exceed that of non-Aboriginal people with the only exception being cancer. One possible explanation for this exception is that the lumping together of all cancers more than likely masks a number of critical differences between AP and

Table 7.7 Elderly Aboriginal peoples prevalence of specific conditions

Condition	Population	% age 65–74	% age 75+
Diabetes	Aboriginal	26	23
	Non-Aboriginal	13	13
Arthritis	Aboriginal	56	54
	Non-Aboriginal	40	47
Cancer	Aboriginal	9	5
	Non-Aboriginal	5	7
Stroke	Aboriginal	7	18
	Non-Aboriginal	3	7
Heart Disease	Aboriginal	23	36
	Non-Aboriginal	18	26
Stomach problems	Aboriginal	18	15
	Non-Aboriginal	4	5
Asthma	Aboriginal	13	11
	Non-Aboriginal	7	7
Chronic Bronchitis	Aboriginal	8	11
	Non-Aboriginal	5	6
Emphysema	Aboriginal	13	13
	Non-Aboriginal	3	4

Adapted from Rosenberg et al. (2009)

their non-Aboriginal counterparts. See Table 7.7 for prevalence of specific conditions. Presumably, elderly two-sprit Nations are included in these data. Ristock et al. (2011) found that the health concerns of Aboriginal two-spirit/LGBT persons included HIV, hepatitis C, weight issues, cancer, and diabetes. Unfortunately, no distinction of these concerns was reported based on age.

Service Utilization by Two-Spirited Elders

In a study of sexual orientation bias experiences and service needs of LGBT two-spirited American Indians, Walters et al. (2001) found that high rates of American Indians had experienced bias from the general public, ranging from 43 to 79 %. Types of biases they experienced include verbal insults, threat of attack, chased or followed, spat upon, object thrown, physical assault, assaulted with a weapon, and sexual assault. The attitudes of service providers toward AIAN were more positive than in the general population. Service providers indicated a high level of comfort working with American Indian two-spirit persons, and over 90 % of service providers indicated that they had LGBT friends and LGBT friends who are American Indian. The attitudes of service providers were consistently positive for specific subgroups of LGBT persons. However, service providers indicated a limited understanding of terminology associated with transgender, followed by homo-negativity and concepts of "passing," heterosexism, gender identity, homophobia, and sexual orientation. Research on service utilization by Aboriginal two-spirit persons in Canada is limited to nonexistent.

The problems identified facing American Indian LGBT or two-spirited ranged from HIV/AIDS epidemic to problems raising children (Walters et al. 2001) (see Table 7.8). Similar to other LGBT persons, AIAN two-spirit persons face many barriers to service utilization. Of the

Table 7.8 Problems facing American Indian two-spirit community

HIV/AIDS epidemic
Substance abuse
Homophobia in the American Indian community
Shunned by American Indian community
Homelessness
Trauma
Conflict with kin network/elders
Racism from non-American Indian LGBT
Conflict with religion
Suicide
Anti-gay violence
Conflict with Native traditions
Problems of raising children

Adapted from Walters et al. (2001)

thirteen barriers identified by Walters et al. and rated as moderate or great, nine were ranked above 50 % as a barrier (see Table 7.9). The results of the focus group study identified five main barriers for American Indian LGBT persons in accessing services: invisibility, discrimination, trauma, identity, and program planning. Walters et al. suggest that invisibility in the LGBT community stems forms the colonization process and the entrenched stereotypes that exist within

Table 7.9 Barriers to services utilization by two-spirit persons

Financial resources
Specialized programming for Native two-spirit persons
Fear of what Native community members might think
Fear of being "outed"
Stigma related being LGBT
Professionals' knowledge of Native two = spirit issues
Attitudes of Native two-spirit clients/family toward services
Staff support by non-Native LGBT agencies
Two-spirits' ability to locate services
Staff attitudes toward Native two-spirit persons
Transportation
Physical accessibility/location of services

Adapted from Walters et al. (2001)

the non-American Indian imagination that makes it difficult for two-spirit persons to identify each other for social support. In the American Indian community, invisibility is manifest as the failure to consider being LGBT as a possibility or "Native reality," which fuels homophobia within the heterosexual American Indian community. Furthermore, disclosure of one's identity as part of visibility is determined by cultural values, in which elders dictates the parameters regarding acceptable behavior. That is, it is not that the person is gay that the elder is responding to but it is how the person is behaving (Walters et al. 2001). Discrimination refers to dealing with racism in the LGBT community and homophobia in the American Indian community. A point of distinction was made between two-spirit persons on-reservations versus urban-born LGBT Indians. For those on-reservations who are required to leave because of publicly disclosing their sexual orientation, it is harder to do because of a lack of transportation, whereas urban-born two-spirit persons are able to be more open with their identity because they might be able to blend in some ways. Dealing with historical and cumulative trauma, including anti-gay violence, domestic violence, and mental and emotional abuse are the serious concerns of two-spirit persons. In addition, they fear being re-traumatized by insensitive or "homo-ignorant" service providers, including American Indians.

A critical issue for AIAN two-spirit persons is identity, or the task of integrating a healthy, positive identity both as an AIAN and as a two-spirited person. Many AIANs have lost the social and spiritual context of whom they are and are always in crisis mode in trying to hold onto traditions while dealing with the LGBT identity. Service providers find it difficult to assist two-spirit persons when struggling to develop an integrated identity because of the historical diversity in terms of tribal acceptance of two-spirit persons and the LGBT person's search for a place and identity in relation to his or her own specific tribal nation. In addition, tribal acceptance is the conflict between AIAN Christian belief systems and acceptance of two-spirit/LGBT (Pope 2012; Walters et al.

2001). Two-spirit persons declare that spirituality is extremely important in their lives and may respond to spiritual conflict with adoption of an inclusive approach to their spirituality that comprises traditional tribal, pan-Indian, and Christian influences (Balsam et al. 2004; Fieland et al. 2007).

A final theme from the focus groups was program planning, which identified four key areas. The first is the need for community-based discussion to identify culturally relevant and meaningful ways to discuss sex, sexuality, gender identity, and LGBT issues. Second was the importance of contextualizing anti-gay violence and more general two-spirited experience within the context of AIAN experience of the colonization, the historical trauma, and the cumulative effect of anti-gay victimization and resulting trauma. The third area is in-service training for all staff regardless of sexual orientation. Finally, there is a need to develop programs that focus on health and mental health issues and to create safe space for two-spirit persons, especially youths.

Another possible explanation of underutilization of services by AIAN elders is that the location of services may be a barrier. A quote from Rose Jerue in 1989, an Alaska Native elder, provides insight about the importance of elders wanting to be close to home. According to Jerue, "elders need to be near the river where they were raised" (cited in Branch 2005, p. 1). AIANs and First Nations elders do not have long-term care facilities in their communities and when requiring institutional care are often placed in facilities located great distances away. The detrimental effects of being removed from their communities may include culturally inappropriate care, language barriers, isolation from family and friends, loss of community affiliation, and loss of their social role as an elder (Lafontaine 2006).

A key issue for elderly AP is gaining access to services because generally, more services, more specialized services, and better access to them is in urban areas than in rural areas. However, access to services in urban areas does not imply more culturally sensitivity to the needs of elderly AP (Rosenberg et al. 2009). The Canadian Community Health Survey (CCHS) and

Aboriginal Peoples Survey (APS) asked three questions related to health utilization about whether in the past 12 months individuals visited a (a) physician, (b) eye doctor, and (c) nurse. The most notable difference in healthcare utilization by Aboriginal elders was a higher rate of nurse visits than non-Aboriginals, which may be due to the increased likelihood that rural and health centers on reservations are staffed by full-time nurses than physicians.

Aboriginal elders face a variety of unique issues and obstacles in the provision of healthcare services. Higher rates of Aboriginal elders are monolingual Aboriginal language-speaking, which complicates the interface between them and their largely non-Aboriginal healthcare providers. Other issues include cultural differences related to aging, medical treatment, traditional care-giving roles, the power structure inherent in Western medicine, exclusion of Aboriginal worldviews, and end-of-life (Rosenberg et al. 2009). According to Rosenberg et al., "Western medical practices are often viewed by AP as dehumanizing as they separate older AP from their communities and involve an individual-style decision making that can run contrary to traditional Aboriginal belief systems" (p. 17). These anxieties are particularly amplified for those who are monolingual and hold strongly to traditional views of health and healing. The informal caregiving is important in Aboriginal communities. Similar to AIANs and other ethnic minority groups in the USA, traditional care within Aboriginal communities is gender dependent, with women family members typically being the primary caregivers. In fact, Aboriginal households tend to have stronger gender parity in residential family size and structure, fewer women living alone, and fewer Aboriginal elders living with only their partner (Rosenberg et al. 2009).

AP, regardless of age, who move to urban areas in order to access medical services often face additional barriers, including a lack of financial and transportation support, suitable housing near medical services, type of services available, and isolation from their social support network in their home communities. The urban

Aboriginal population is fairly mobile and movement occurs both between rural and urban areas, and within urban settings (Place 2012). Access to services is only part of the equation for better health outcomes. Others are appropriateness of services and being culturally safe, to which merely living in urban areas does not overcome barriers (Adelson 2005). AP, especially Inuit and First Nations desire access to traditional healing practices, and as age and strength of Aboriginal identity increases, so does the perceived importance of access to this kind of healthcare. In fact, the *Urban Aboriginal Peoples Survey* (UAP) reveals that 72 % of Aboriginal residents in urban areas consider access to traditional healing practices to be more important than mainstream health, only 30 % have "very easy" access to them (Environics Institute 2010, p. 116). Just over half of AP in urban areas utilizes city-based Aboriginal services and organizations. Of those, Inuit (71 %) are most likely to use city-based Aboriginal services and organizations followed by off-reservation First Nations (59 %) and Metis people (48 %). Services are more likely to be accessed by those aged 45 and older and those who are of lower socioeconomic status (Environics Institute 2010).

Similar to AIANs, AP living off-reservations do not have access to the range of federally provided health services that First Nations living on-reservations and Inuit living in their communities (Place 2012). Eligibility for specific federal government programs and services for AP depends on a number of factors, including status (i.e., status vs. non-status Indians), residency, treaty, and provincial and federal legislation (Browne et al. 2009). According to Lavoie et al. (2008), every scenario of status, residency, and so forth results in a different set of benefits and services, and ambiguity of eligibility, which, eventually, leads to gaps and inconsistencies.

One other important consideration in addressing access to services for AP is the distinct issues related to women. Women make up over half of the urban Aboriginal population. Although women tend to live longer than men, they have more instances of health-related issues and are more frequent users of the healthcare system, are more likely to have low incomes, and may have been victims of violence, which is a major determinant of health and requires its own treatment (Browne et al. 2009; Native Women's Association of Canada 2007).

Systems of Service Delivery for Two-Spirited Elders

In healthcare and mental health programming, there is a need provide a cultural network that integrates the AIANs' indigenous community into treatment plans along with prevention and early intervention services (Native Vision Project 2012). Many AIANs ascribe to traditional health practices that are grounded in an indigenous worldview, which emphasizes harmony and balance. Traditional Native health practices (e.g., sweat lodge, pipe ceremony, Sun Dance, Native American Church) are ways of coping with disease and responding to adversity. Both Indians in urban areas and on reservations use traditional healing practices in conjunction with Western medicine, with traditional practices to treat the underlying cause (e.g., violation of a cultural taboo) and Western medicine to treat the symptoms (Fieland et al. 2007). Thin Elk's (2011) model combines a holistic approach with indigenous (e.g., talking circles, healers, seasonal ceremonies, and sweat lodge purification ceremonies) and mainstream approaches (e.g., one-on-one counseling) to wellness and healing. However, two-spirit persons may not be open about their identity or all their health practices because of discriminatory experiences in the American healthcare system and heterosexist attitudes among traditional healers. Among older urban AIAN patients in primary care, maltreatment and neglect are relatively common (Grant and Brown 2003).

One area of concern is the diagnosis of mental health functioning of AIANs. AIANs may conceptualize mental health differently and express emotional distress in ways that are inconsistent with the diagnostic criteria of the *Diagnostic and Statistical Manual* (DSM). For example, AIANs may express distress as ghost sickness and heartbreak syndrome. Thus, the question becomes how to elicit, understand, and incorporate such expressions of distress and responding within the assessment and treatment process of the *DSM* (Grant and Brown 2003). The most recent edition of the *DSM* contains an updated version of the Outline for Cultural Formulation (OCF), which calls for systematic assessment five categories and the Cultural Formulation Interview (CFI), which is a set of 16 questions that may be used to obtain information during a mental health assessment about the impact of culture on key aspects of an individual's clinical presentation and care (American Psychiatric Association [APA] 2013).

Although federal and state funders of behavioral health services overwhelmingly require use of evidence-based practices (EBP), of which the "gold standard" of Western-based EBP does not reflect American Indian communities with regard to cultural, linguistic, and geographical differences in prevention and early intervention, Native American cultural practices (i.e., practice-based evidence) have been increasingly used in effective service delivery (Native Vision Project 2012). There is a distinction between evidence-based practice (EBP), which is scientifically tested and validates, and practice-based evidence or community-defined evidence (CDE), which is a validated practice, which is accepted by the AIAN community but not empirically proven. EBPs are particularly challenging because they have not been tested in AIAN communities; therefore, they have not been culturally validated. Government funders mandated that behavioral health providers observe the same EBP standards in health care (Nebelkopf et al. 2011). Neblkopf et al contend that this mandate brings into question, how can Western science reconcile with indigenous knowledge to operationalize AIANs and First Nations' core values to demonstrate EBP? The suggestion is to use CDE to identify cultural adaptations to EBPs (Martinez 2011).

One approach of service delivery that has produced successful outcomes with AIANs is the Holistic System of Care (HSOC). The HSOC is a community-focused intervention that provides behavioral health care, promotes health, and prevents disease. The HSOC integrates mental health and substance abuse services with medical, dental, and HIV services and provides support for the entire family. The approach links prevention, treatment, and recovery and is based on a community strategic planning process that honors Native culture and relationships while allowing for integration of Western (EBPs) treatment modalities. The HSOC acknowledges the diversity of traditional healing beliefs among the different tribes and respects each tribe's practice of traditional medicine. This approach deals with the whole person. The emphasis is on self-help, empowerment, and building a healthy community (Native Vision Project 2012).

Although substantial fragmentation exists in many Native communities, some communities (e.g., Native community in Chicago and Portland, Oregon) have developed a strong network of human services to meet the varied needs of community members (Weaver 2012). In Canada, practices have been implemented for First Nations and Inuit elders. The First Nations and Inuit Home and Community Care (FNIACC) program has been instrumental in facilitating the development of essential programs within 606 First Nations reserves and communities and 53 Inuit communities across Canada (Cyr and Ootoova 2010). FNIHCC consists of eight regions across Canada that engage in collaborative partnerships that create sustainable change in communities and jurisdictions.

Policy Issues

Currently, health services in the USA are delivered through a system of interlocking programs made up of the IHS, tribal programs, and urban programs. The structure involves interrelationships between the federal government, tribal governments, and urban Indian groups. The IHS structure consists of three levels: headquarters, area offices, and service units including hospitals, health centers, health stations, and clinics (Tosatto et al. 2006). The IHS is based on the medical model and as such, one of the major problems is that the majority of funding goes into direct medical care (e.g., hospital and clinical care) with limited dollars available for prevention. Other challenges include a lack of resources and technical knowledge: most tribes do not have departments of public health, which "is a major contributor to the negative health disparities existing among Indian people today, on and off reservations" (Allison et al. 2007, p. 299). Another crucial problem associated with the IHS structure is the inability to bill and collect adequately for all of the services it provides.

Exponentially, Native American tribes are assuming more control of their own healthcare delivery systems and making decisions to create or plan their own departments of public health (Allison et al. 2007). Allison et al. propose three public health organizational delivery models to meet the public health needs of small, medium, and large American Indian tribes. The models become larger and more complex in the progression along the continuum. Basically, these models create an organizational structure in which services and functions are handled by specific departments and are designed with the premise that tribal governments are direct care providers. The models build on existing services provided through IHS.

In Canada, one of the greatest challenges for urban Aboriginal seniors in the healthcare system is the issue of jurisdiction, specifically for Inuit and status Indians peoples. Both Inuit and status Indian peoples face jurisdictional challenges, because while provinces and territories provide healthcare services, the federal government is responsible to pay for status Indian and Inuit health care. Although Metis and non-status peoples are declared as Aboriginal under the Constitution Act of 1982, they are not recognized as a federal responsibility. The result is that Metis and non-status Indian peoples receive the same provincial benefits as all other Canadians (Beatty and Berdahl 2011). The political jurisdiction and administrative barriers between federal, provincial, and regional authorities cause ongoing jurisdictional disputes in health regarding the provision of health services to AP (Beatty and Berdahl 2011; Cameron 2003). From a policy perspective, it is important to recognize that the off-reservation and urban Aboriginal populations in Canada are not distinct from the on-reservation and rural. They are interconnected in terms of mobility, culture, and politics (Graham and Peters 2002). AP are highly mobile between rural/reservations and urban areas, and within urban communities ("churn factor"), which has implications for policy (Place 2012).

The current policy frameworks in Canada for AP are hampered by fragmented services, judicial boundaries, and insufficient funding, which is especially challenging for elders. Understanding how two-spirit persons fit into the mix of things is still unclear. Beatty and Berdahl (2011) suggest that Canada look to Sweden, Denmark, and Iceland for alternative ways of thinking about options for elderly care in Canada. In Sweden, elderly care policy focuses on ensuring the elderly economic security, adequate housing, and good services and care. Iceland uses a model that consists of a mix of family and state involvement. Elderly care in Denmark is largely state funded. These three models contain several key components to reconcile the fragmentation of services for AP. First, they support a public push for governments to take more responsibility for long-term care with increased support for families as a means of empowering personal control among the elderly and their families. Second, they suggest more holistic Aboriginal eldercare models in Canada. Third, they advocate for inclusion of culture, community, and mixed systems. Finally, they promote community involvement as integral to proper health care (Beatty and Berdahl 2011). Presumably, specific attention is to be given to two-spirit elders in the redesign of policies and procedures.

The future brings new challenges and continuation of existing ones for development of interventions for AIANs and First Nations. One of the most substantial challenges is EBP. Since EBP is grounded in the supposition that the most effective practices are demonstrated through carefully controlled scientific experiments, which assess the causal efficacy of these practices, Nebelkopf et al. (2011) question the efficacy of EBP for measuring practices of indigenous peoples of North America. Nevertheless, a consensus in the literature is that two-spirit persons of North America and especially elders are among, if not, the most marginalized people of all in their respective country or region.

Summary

AIAN and Aboriginal elderly people are among the most vulnerable and marginalized people of North America, and two-spirits elderly are even more so. Both in the USA and Canada, these groups are recognized as disadvantaged status because of poor socioeconomic conditions on reservations and in communities, both urban and rural. Two-spirit persons among AIANs and AP of Canada are further marginalized in their communities and within the LGBT community. A combination of social and economic exclusion, barriers to health services access, ignoring culturally specific coping mechanism, ageism, and the effects of colonization converge to relegate two-spirit elders to a status of unimportance, and far worse, to that of invisibility.

Learning Exercises

Self-check Questions

1. To what extent do urban American Indians have rights as citizens to tribal government on reservations?
2. How is enculturation an empowering process for two-spirit persons?
3. How does historical trauma shape the health risk factors for Native Peoples?
4. Compared to the general population, what types of health issues are significantly higher among AIANs?
5. Among First Nations of Canada, which group has poorer health status? What health issues do they have?

Field-Based Experiential Assignments

1. Interview an AIAN or First Nations elderly LGBT persons to understand how he or she defines two-spirit identity.
2. Establish an interdisciplinary team of professionals and develop processes and procedures to work with two-spirit LGBT elders in urban areas and rural settings.
3. Construct an interdisciplinary, cross-cultural conference to address the psychological, social, health, housing, economic, education, and life-care plans of two-spirit LGBT elders. Be sure to: (a) purpose of the conference, (b) goals and objectives, (c) identify topics to be covered, (b) expert speakers, and (e) other relevant components.

Multiple Choice Questions

1. Which of the following is how American Indians analyze human sexuality?
   (a) Dichotomously and categorically
   (b) Continuum of human sexuality
   (c) Physical appearance
   (d) Biologically
2. How do American Indians define gender and gender status?
   (a) Majority and minority
   (b) Biological and ambiguous
   (c) Rite of passage
   (d) Biological and cultural
3. How are two-spirit persons viewed in First Nations' culture?
   (a) Transsexuals
   (b) People who try to make themselves the opposite sex
   (c) Individuals who take on a gender that is different from both women and men
   (d) Individuals who take on one gender identity prior to puberty, then another gender to signify adulthood
4. Why do Aboriginal Peoples view Western medical practices as dehumanizing?
   (a) They separate older Aboriginal peoples from their communities

(b) They involve individual-style decision making that can run contrary to traditional Aboriginal belief systems

(c) They exclude Aboriginal worldview

(d) All of the above

(e) None of the Above

5. Which of the following is true of two-spirit persons on reservations who are asked to leave because of publicly disclosing their sexual orientation?

(a) Lack of transportation make it harder for them to leave

(b) They are able to blend in some ways

(c) It is easier for them to integrate a positive, healthy identity

(d) Service providers' attitudes are more positive

6. Which of the following service provider is a higher rate of usage among rural Aboriginal elders than non-Aboriginal elders?

(a) Physician

(b) Specialist

(c) Nurse

(d) Eye doctor

7. Why is the diagnosis of mental health functioning of Native Peoples a concern with the way diagnostic criteria are defined in the Diagnostic and Statistical Manual?

(a) The language of the DSM is difficult to translate into many Native languages.

(b) Native Peoples conceptualize mental health differently and express emotions that are inconsistent with DSM diagnostic criteria.

(c) As a sovereign nation Native Peoples are not obligated to follow the same diagnostic criteria of the DSM.

(d) The prevalence of indigenous people is not statically significant to meet DSM diagnostic criteria.

8. With the disclosure of one's sexual identity in the American Indian community, who dictates the parameters regarding acceptable behavior?

(a) Parents

(b) Peer group

(c) Elders

(d) Tribal law

9. Which of the following is prohibited by federal policies for Aboriginal elderly in Canada?

(a) Building of long-term care facilities on reservations

(b) Staffing healthcare facilities with nurses in rural communities

(c) Renting of subsidized housing

(d) Providing healthcare services both on- and off-reservation

10. Where did the term two-spirit originate?

(a) USA

(b) Australia

(c) England

(d) Canada

Key

1—b
2—d
3—c
4—d
5—a
6—c
7—b
8—c
9—a
10—d

Resources

Indigenous Health—Australia, Canada, Aotearoa, New Zealand, and the USA—Laying claim to a future that embraces health for us all: www.who.int/healthsystems/topic/financing/healthreport/Ihno22.pdf.

NativeOut: www.nativeout.com.

The Provincial Health Services Authority of BC (training modules on Indigenous cultural competency): http://www.culturalcompetency.ca/.

Toronto-based organizations: http://www.2spirits.com/.

Tribal Equity Toolkit 2.0: Tribal Resolutions and Codes to Support Two Spirit and LBGT

Justice in Indian Country: http://graduate.
lclark.edu/live/files/15810-tribal-equity-
toolkit-20.

References

Adelson, N. (2005, March/April). The embodiment of inequity: Health disparities in Aboriginal Canada. *Canadian Journal of Public Health, 96*, S45-S-61.

Administration on Aging. (2012). *A profile of older Americans: 2012*. Washington, DC: Author.

Allison, M. T., Rivers, P. A., & Fottler, M. D. (2007). Future public health delivery models for Native American tribes. *Public Health, 121*, 296–307.

American Psychiatric Association. (2013). *Diagnostic and statistical manual of mental disorders (DSM-5)*. Washington, DC: Author.

Balsam, K. F., Huang, B., Fieland, K. C., Simoni, J. M., & Walters, K. L. (2004). Culture, trauma, and wellness: A comparison of heterosexual and lesbian, gay, bisexual, and two-spirit Native Americans. *Cultural Diversity and Ethnic Minority Psychology, 10* (3), 287–301.

Beatty, B. B., & Berdahl, L. (2011). Health care and Aboriginal seniors in urban Canada: Helping a neglected class. *The International Indigenous Policy Journal, 2*(1). Retrieved from http://ir.lib.uwo.ca/iipj/vol2.iss1/10.

Branch, K. (2005, August). Long term care needs of Alaska Native elders. U.S. Department of Health and Human Services. Retrieved July 31, 2014 from http://www.anthc.org/chs/wp/elders/upload/LTC-Report.pdf

Brotman, S., Ryan, B., & Cormier, R. (2003). The health and social service needs of gay and lesbian elders and their families in Canada. *The Gerontologist, 43*(2), 192–202.

Brotman, S., Ryan, B., Jalbert, Y., & Rowe, B. (2002). Reclaiming space-regaining health: The health care experience of two-spirit people in Canada. *Journal of Gay and Lesbian Social Services: Issues in Practice, Policy and Research, 14*, 67–87.

Browne, A. J., McDonald, H., & Elliott, D. (2009). *First Nations Urban Aboriginal Health research discussion paper*. National Aboriginal Health Organization: A Report for the First Nations Centre.

Bureau of Indian Affairs. (2011). What we do. Retrieved July 24, 2014 from http://www.bia.gov/WhatWeDo/index.htm.

Cameron, L. (2003, April). *First Nations health in Saskatchewan, 1905–2005*. Western Development Museum/Saskatchewan Indian Cultural Centre

Partnership Project. Saskatoon, SK: Saskatchewan Indian Cultural Centre and Western Development Museum.

Canada Mortgage and Housing Corporation. (2004, August). 2001 census housing series issue 6: revised Aboriginal households. *Research Highlight, Socio-economic Series 04-036*. Ottawa, ON: CMHC.

Canadian Rainbow Health Coalition. (2004). Health and wellness in the gay, lesbian, bisexual, transgendered and Two-Spirit communities: A background document. Available at http://www.rainbowhealth.ca.

Centers for Disease Control. (2003). Health status of American Indians compared with other racial/ethnic minority populations—Selected states, 2001–2002. *MMWR, Morbidity and Mortality Weekly Report, 52* (47), 1148–1152.

Centers for Disease Control. (2007). *Injuries among Native Americans: Fact sheet*. Retrieved July 24, 2014 from http://www.cdc.gov/nipc/factsheet/nativeamericans.htm.

Centers for Disease Control and Prevention. (2011). *CDC Health disparities and inequities report—United States, 2011. Morbidity and mortality Weekly report supplement* (Vol. 60). Washington, DC: Government Printing Office. Available at http://www.cdc.gov/mmwr/pdf/other/su6001.pdf.

Cyr, A., & Ootoova, E. (2010, April). *Mind body spirit: Promising practices in First Nations and Inuit home and community care*. Canada: The Canadian Home Care Association. Retrieved September 5, 2014 from www.cdnhomecare.ca.

Dunaway-Knight, A., Knoll, M. A. Z., Shoffner, D., & Whitman, K. (2012). *Measures of health and economic well-being among American Indians and Alaska Natives aged 62 or older in 2030*. Retrieved July 24, 2014 from http://www.ssa.gov/policy/docs/rsnotes/rsn2012-02.html.

Environics Institute. (2010). *Urban Aboriginal peoples study*. Toronto, ON: Author.

Fieland, K. C., Walters, K. L., & Simoni, J. M. (2007). *Determinants of health among two-spirit American Indians and Alaska Natives*. New York, NY: Springer.

First Nations Centre. (2007). *A snapshot of off-reserve First Nations health: Selected health status and determinant indicators for adults*. Ottawa, ON: National Aboriginal Health Organization.

Galabuzi, G. (2004). Social exclusion. In D. Raphael (Ed.), *Social determinants of health: Canadian perspectives* (pp. 235–252). Toronto, ON: Canadian Scholars' Press Inc.

Garrett, M. T., & Pichette, E. F. (2000). Red as an apple: Native American acculturation and counseling with or without reservation. *Journal of Counseling and Development, 78*, 3–13.

Graham, K. A. H., & Peters, E. (2002, December). Aboriginal communities and urban sustainability. Ottawa, ON: Canadian Policy Research Networks

Inc. Retrieved August 13, 2014 from http://www.urbancenter.utorontonta.ca/pdfs/clibrary/CPRNUrbanAboriginal.pdf.

Grant, J., & Brown, T. (2003). *American Indian & Alaska Native resource manual*. Retrieved July 31, 2014 from www.nami.org/Content/ContentGroups/MIO?CDResourceManual.pdf.

Health Canada. (2009). *First Nations, Inuit and Aboriginal health: Summative evaluation of the First Nations and Inuit home and community*. Ontario: Author.

Hendry, J. (2003). Mining the sacred mountain: The clash between the Western dualistic framework and Native American religions. *Multicultural Perspectives, 5*(1), 3–10.

Janz, T., Seto, J., & Turner, A. (2009). Aboriginal peoples survey, 2006: An overview of the health of the Metis population. Statistics Canada Catalogue no. 89-637-X-004. Ottawa: Minister of Industry.

Kim, G., Bryant, A. N., Goins, R. T., Worley, C. B., & Chiriboga, D. A. (2012). Disparities in health status and health care access and use among older American Indians and Alaska Natives and non-Hispanic Whites in California. *Journal of Aging and Health, 24*(5), 799–811.

Kim, G., Bryant, A. N., & Parmelee, P. (2011). Racial/ethnic differences in serious psychological distress among older adults in California. *International Journal of Geriatric Psychiatry*. doi:10.1002/gps.2825.

Lafontaine, C. (2006, November 27). Presentation to the Senate Standing Committee on Aging. Retrieved August 4, 2014 from www.naho.ca/documents/naho/publications/agingPresentation.pdf.

Laframboise, S., & Anhorn, M. (2008). *The way of the two spirited people*. Retrieved July 14, 2014 from http://www.dancingtoeaglespiritsociety.org/twospirit.php.

Lavoie, J., Forget, R., Rowe, G., & Dahl, M. (2008). *The leaving for the city project (medical relocation project phase 2): Draft report*. Winnipeg, MB: Manitoba First Nations Centre for Aboriginal Health Research (unpublished paper).

Li, C. I., Malone, K. E., & Daling, J. R. (2003). Differences in breast cancer stage, treatment, and survival by race and ethnicity. *Archives of Internal Medicine, 163*, 49–56.

Martinez, K. (2011, May). *Best practices and the elimination of disparities: The connection*. Lecture 2011 national policy summit to Address Behavioral Health Disparities within Health Care Reform, San Diego, CA.

McCaskill, D., FitzMaurice, K., & Cidro, J. (2011). *Toronto Aboriginal research project final report*. Retrieved August 8, 2014 from www.councilfire.ca/Acrobat/trarp-final-report2011.pdf.

McLeod-Shabogesic, P. (1995). *The medicine wheel: A healing journey*. Ontario: The Union of Ontario Indians.

Meyer-Cook, F., & Labelle, D. (2003). Namaji. *Journal of Gay and Lesbian Social Services, 16*(1), 29–51.

National Household Survey. (2013). Aboriginal peoples of Canada: First Nations peoples, Metis and Inuit-National Household Survey 2011. Retrieved August 4, 2014 from www.springerpub.com/instructionmaterial/9780826117977/AboriginalPeoplesinCanada-9781100222035.pdf.

Native Vision Project. (2012). *California reducing disparities Project Native American population report*. Retrieved July 31, 2014 from www.nativehealth.org/sites/dev.nh.edeloa.net/files/native_vision_report_compressed.pdf.

Native Women's Association of Canada. (2007). Social determinants of health and Canada's Aboriginal women. Ottwa, ON: Author. Retrieved August 13, 2014 from www.nwac.ca/sites/default/files/reports/NWAC_WHO-CSDH_Submission.mb.ca/.

Nebelkopf, E., King, J., Wright, S., Schweigman, K., Lucero, E., Habte-Michael, T., & Cervantes, T. (2011). Growing roots: Native American evidence-based practices. *Journal of Psychoactive Drugs, 43*(4), 263–268.

Ogunwole, S. (2006). *We the people: American Indians and Alaska Natives in the United States. Census 2000 special report CNSR-28*. Washington, DC: Census Bureau. Available at http://www.census.gov/prod/2006pubs/censr-28.pdf.

Paltoo, D. N., & Chu, K. C. (2004). Patterns in cancer incidence among American Indians/Alaska Natives, United States, 1992–1999. *Public Health Reports, 119*, 443–451.

Place, J. (2012). *The health of Aboriginal peoples residing in urban areas*. Prince George, BC: National Collaborating Centre for Aboriginal Health.

Podneik, E. (2008). Elder abuse: The Canadian experience. *Journal of Elder Abuse and Neglect, 20*(2), 126–150.

Pope, M. (2012). Native American and gay: Two spirits in one human being. In S. H. Dworkin & M. Pope (Eds.), *Casebook for counseling lesbian, gay, bisexual, and transgender persons and their families* (pp. 163–172). Alexandria, VA: American Counseling Association.

Reading, C. L., & Wien, F. (2009). Health inequalities and social determinants of Aboriginal peoples' health. Retrieved August 12, 2014 from http://www.nccah-ccnsa.ca/docs/aocialdeterminates/nccah-loppie-wein_report.dpf.

Report of the Royal Commission on Aboriginal Peoples. (1996). *Report of the Royal Commission on Aboriginal peoples* (Vol. 1, Chap. 2). From time immemorial: A demographic profile. Ottawa, Canada: Ottawa Canada Communication Group. Available at http://www.ainc-inac.gc.ca/ch/rcap/sg/sg3_e.html#9.

Rhoades, D. A., Manson, S. M., Noonan, C., & Buchwald, D. (2005). Characteristics associated with reservation travel among Native American outpatients. *Journal of Healthcare for the Poor and Underserved, 16*(3), 464–474.

Ristock, J., Zoccole, A., & Potskin, J. (2011). *Aboriginal two-spirit and LGBTQ migration, mobility, and health research project: Vancouver final report*. Manitoba, Canada: University of Manitoba.

Rosenberg, M. W., Wilson, K., Abonyi, S., Wiebe, A., Beach, K., & Lovelace, R. (2009, July). *Older Aboriginal Peoples of Canada demographics, health status and access to health care*. Social and economic dimensions of an aging population (SEDAP) research paper no. 249. Retrieved August 11, 2014 from http://socs.erv.master.ca/sedap/P/sedap249.pfd.

Roubideaux, Y., Zuckerman, M., & Zuckerman, E. (2004). A review of the quality of health care for American Indians and Alaska Natives. The Commonwealth Fund.

Rowland, J. (2013). The new legal context of Indigenous peoples' rights: The United Nations declaration on the rights of indigenous peoples. *American Indian Culture and Research Journal, 37*(4), 141–156.

Satter, D. E., Wallace, S. P., Garcia, A. N., & Smith, L. M. (2010). *Health of American Indian and Alaska Native elders in California*. Los Angles, CA: UCLA Center for Health Policy Research.

Scheim, A. I., Jackson, R., James, L., Dopler, T. S., Pyne, J., & Bauer, G. R. (2013). Barriers to well-being for Aboriginal gender-diverse people: Results from the Trans PULSE project in Ontario, Canada. *Ethnicity and Inequalities in Health and Social Care, 6*(4), 108–120.

Social Security Administration. (2011). *Disability benefits*. SSA publication no. 05-10029. Baltimore, MD: Author. Available at http://www.socialsecurity.gov/pubs/10029.html.

Sue, D. W., & Sue, D. (2013). *Counseling the culturally diverse: Theory and practice* (6th ed.). Hoboken, NJ: Wiley.

Tamborini, C. R. (2007). The never married in old-age: Projections and concerns for the near future. *Social Security Bulletin, 67*(2), 25–40.

Taylor, C., & Ristock, J. (2011). We are all treaty people: An anti-oppressive research ethics of solidarity with Indigenous Two-Spirit and LGBTQ people living with partner violence. In J. Ristock (Ed.), *Intimate partner LGBTQ people's lives* (pp. 301–320). New York: Routlege.

Thin Elk, G. (2011). *Red road approach to holistic healing*. Available at http://www.readroadapproach.com/aboutus.html.

Tjepkema, M. (2002). The health of the off-reserve Aboriginal population. *Health reports* (Vol. 13, Suppl.). Ottawa: Statistics Canada, Catalogue 82-003. Retrieved August 11, 2014 from www.statcan.gc.ca/pub/82-003-s/2002001pdf/82-003-s2002004-eng.pdf.

Tosatto, R. J., Reeves, T. C., Duncan, W. J., & Ginter, P. M. (2006). Indian health service: Creating a climate of change. In L. E. Swayne, W. J. Duncan, & P. M. Ginter (Eds.), *Strategic management of health care organizations* (pp. 626–645). Malden, MA: Blackwell Publishing.

Turcotte, M., & Schellenberg, G. (2007). A portrait of seniors in Canada, 2006. Statistics Canada catalogue no. 89-519-XIE. Ottawa: Minister of Industry.

U.S. Department of Health and Human Services. (2007). *Obesity and American Indians/Alaska Natives*. Retrieved from http://aspe.hhs.gov/hsp/07/AI-AN-obesity/report.pdf.

Wahsquonaikezhik, D., Wahsquonaikezhik, G., & Wahsquonaikezhik, S. (1976). 2-Spirited people of the 1st nation (pp. 18–31). Reprinted in We are part of a Tradition (1998). Quebec: First Nations of Quebec and Labrador Health and Social Services Commission.

Walters, K. L., Evans-Campbell, T., Simoni, J., Ronquillo, T., & Bhuyan, R. (2006). My spirit in my heart: Identity experiences and challenges among American Indian two-spirited women. *Journal of Lesbian Studies, 10*, 125–149.

Walters, K. L., Horwath, P. F., & Simoni, J. M. (2001). Sexual orientation bias experiences and service needs of gay, lesbian, bisexual, transgendered, and two-spirited American Indians. *Journal of Gay and Lesbian Social Services, 13*(1–2), 133–149.

Walyers, K. L., & Simoni, J. N. (2002). Reconceptualizing native women's health: An "indigenist" stress-coping model. *American Journal of Public Health, 92*, 520–524.

Ward, E., Jemal, A., Cokkinides, V., Singh, G. K., Cardinez, C., Ghafoor, A., & Thun, M. (2004). Cancer disparities by race/ethnicity and socioeconomic status. *Cancer Disparities, 54*(2), 78–93.

Warren, P. N. (1998). *Berdaches... and assumptions about Berdaches*. Retrieved July 24, 2014 from http://www.whosoever.org/v3i3/berdaches.html.

Weaver, H. N. (2012). Urban and indigenous: The challenges of being a Native American in the city. *Journal of Community Practice, 20*, 470–488.

Williams, W. L. (1986). *The spirit and the flesh: Sexual diversity in American Indian culture*. Boston: Beacon Press.

Wilson, K., Rosenberg, M. W., & Abonyi, S. (2011). Aboriginal peoples, health and healing approaches: The effects of age and place on health. *Social Science and Medicine, 72*, 355–364.

Wilson, K., Rosenberg, M. W., Abonyi, S., & Lovelace, R. (2010). Aging and health: An examination of differences between older Aboriginal and non-Aboriginal people. *Canadian Journal on Aging, 29*(3), 369–382.

Wright, K. N. (2009). Disparities and chronic health care needs for elderly American Indians living on or near a reservation. *American Indian Culture and Research Journal, 33*(3), 85–99.

Asian American and Native Pacific Islander LGBT Elders

Debra A. Harley

Abstract

The purpose of this chapter is to discuss issues pertaining to LGBT Asian-American and Pacific Islander (AAPI) elderly in the USA. Attention is also given to the citizenship status of foreign-born Asian-Americans. Information is presented on cultural characteristics and values of Asian culture, acknowledging that there is great heterogenerity among AAPIs. Discussion focuses on attitudes and perceptions of Asian Americans' perspectives about LGBT persons, characteristics, and issues pertinent to Asian American LGBT elders, health status and service delivery for LGBT Asian-American elders, and current health policy and practices. Whenever possible, specific reference is made to certain subgroups of persons of Asian descent.

Keywords

Asian american · Native pacific islander · LGBT elders

Overview

Given the diversity among Asian-American populations, it is not feasible to include information about all of them in this chapter. The purpose of this chapter is to discuss issues pertaining to LGBT Asian American and Pacific Islander elders in the USA. Information is presented on cultural characteristics and values of Asian culture, acknowledging that great heterogenerity exists within Asian-American and Pacific Islanders (AAPIs). The intent of presenting this information is to provide a contextual framework from which to understand attitudes and behaviors of this population. Second, research on the attitudes and perceptions of Asian-Americans' perspectives about LGBT persons is discussed. Next, the characteristics of and issues pertinent to Asian American LGBT elderly are examined. Then, health status and service delivery for LGBT Asian-American elderly is reviewed. Finally, current policy and

D.A. Harley (✉)
University of Kentucky, Lexington, USA
e-mail: dharl00@email.uky.edu

© Springer International Publishing Switzerland 2016
D.A. Harley and P.B. Teaster (eds.), *Handbook of LGBT Elders*,
DOI 10.1007/978-3-319-03623-6_8

practices pertaining to LGBT Asian American elders are examined, along with recommendations for the future. Throughout this chapter, the umbrella term Asian-Americans is used to refer to the various groups that make up this population; however, specific reference is made to certain subgroups where appropriate. In addition, efforts are made to distinguish between data that are group specific and illustrative in content through examples. Given the limited amount of research published on LGBT AAPIs, some inferences are made from AAPIs in general and generalizations are made from younger AAPI LGBT persons to older AAPI LGBT adults.

Learning Objective

By the end of this chapter, the reader will be able to:

1. Understand the role of AAPI elders in Asian communities.
2. Distinguish among cultural characteristic within AAPI cultures.
3. Distinguish between generational differences among AAPI LGBT persons.
4. Identify the attitudes and perceptions of AAPIs toward LGBT persons.
5. Identify barriers to health care and social services for AAPI LGBT elders.
6. Identify health issues and disparities of LGBT AAPI elders.
7. Understand factors contributing to resiliency among AAPI LGBT elders.

Introduction

Great diversity exists among the Asian American population, with at least 40 distinct subgroups that differ in language, religion, values, and culture. They include Chinese, Filipinos, Koreans, Asian Indians, Japanese, Vietnamese, Laotians, Cambodians, Hmongs, Hawaiians, Guamanians, and Samoans (Sue and Sue 2013). The six largest Asian American single-race subgroups are Asian Indian, Chinese, Filipino, Japanese, Korean, and Vietnamese (US Census Bureau 2012). The Asian-American population is growing rapidly and represents about five percent of the US population. Native Hawaiian and other Pacific Islanders comprise 0.4 % of the total population, with more than half reporting multiple races. Further examination reveals that over 60 % of Asian Americans are immigrants, more than two-thirds speak a language other than English at home, and approximately 40 % do not speak English well. With the exception of Japanese-Americans, Asian-American groups are now principally composed of internationally born individuals. Nearly two-thirds of AAPIs are foreign born and have arrived in the USA, since 1965. Of the Asian population in the USA, there are approximately 3.8 million Chinese, 2.8 million Asian Indians, 1.7 million Vietnamese, 1.6 million Koreans, and 1.3 million Japanese. California has the largest and most diverse AAPI population in the country (US Census Bureau 2010).

The majority of younger Asian Americans are highly educated. For Asian American and Pacific Islanders over the age of 25, over half have a bachelor's degree compared to 30 % of their White counterparts (US Census Bureau 2011a). In 2010, the median income of Asian American families was $64,308 compared to $49,445 for the US population as a whole (US Census bureau 2011b). According to Sue and Sue (2013), the presentation of Asian-Americans as the model minority is a misnomer because a closer look reveals disturbing contrasts with popular views of their success story. Specifically, Sue and Sue outline the following contrasts. First, the report of Asian American families having a higher median income than other minority groups does not take into account (a) the higher percentage of Asian American families having more than one wage earner, (b) between-group differences in education and income, and (c) a higher prevalence of poverty despite the higher median income. Second, although collectively Asian Americans show a disparate picture of extraordinarily high educational attainment, they also have a large undereducated class among certain subpopulations. Third, within Asian American communities such as Chinatowns, Manilatowns, and Japantowns exist ghetto areas with prevalent unemployment, poverty, health problems, and juvenile delinquency that people outside these communities seldom see. Fourth, Asian Americans underutilize mental health services; however, it is unclear if this is due to low rates of socioeconomic difficulties, discriminatory or culturally inappropriate mental health practices, or cultural values inhibiting self-referral (Asai and Kameoka 2005; Ting and Hwang 2009). Finally, Asian Americans have been and continue to face discrimination, racism, and anti-Asian sentiments.

Asian Americans over age 65 are among the fastest growing minority group in the USA. Between 2008 and 2030, the Asian-American elderly population is projected to grow 19 % to over 3.8 million persons (Administration on Aging, n.d.). Overwhelmingly, older Asian Americans were born outside the USA. Asian Americans immigrants comprise three distinct immigration statuses: those who voluntarily chose to come to a new country, refugees forced to leave their homeland because of war or political persecution, and decedents of immigrants. Although Asian-Americans have immigrated to the USA since the late 1800s, it was not until the 1950s that foreign-born Asian-Americans were permitted to become US citizens (Pew Research Center 2013). See Chapter "Immigrant LGBT Elders" for additional discussion on LGBT immigrants. It is safe to assume that LGBT persons are among Asian-American immigrants. As more AAPI LGBT persons come out, they continue to face invisibility, isolation, and stereotyping. Dang and Hu (2005) contend that, in particular, South Asian immigrants have come under increased scrutiny and attack after the terrorist attacks on September 11, 2001. As a result, the lives of AAPI LGBT persons "involve a complex web of issues arising from being sexual, racial/ethnic, language, gender, immigrant, and economic minorities" (p. ii).

Cultural Characteristics and Values of Asian Americans and Pacific Islanders

Collectively, AAPIs are considered as successful, law-abiding, intellectually superior than other groups, and high-achieving minorities. They are stereotyped as a resilient model minority. According to Yee et al. (2008), "this positive characterization overlooks the difficult life circumstances that some AAPI individuals experience and downplays the very real needs of those who are vulnerable to experiences of discrimination, trauma, or poverty" (p. 69). In fact, there is considerable variation in the prevalence of risk and protective factors and resiliency processes across AAPI ethnic groups (Sue and Sue 2013; Yee et al. 2008). Furthermore, generational differences exist among cultural characteristics and values of AAPIs.

Although there is substantial diversity within the board AAPI ethnic category, certain pan-AAPI values and similarities in family practices cut across AAPI subgroups. Four cultural themes are common to Chinese, Japanese, Filipino, Southeast Asian, South Asian, Hawaiian, and Samoan cultures: collectivism, a relational orientation, familism, and family obligation, all of which promote family interdependence (see Table 8.1) (Yee et al. 2008). In the USA, AAPIs create community around shared culture, their diaspora, language, and food (Alcedo 2014). Usually, elders are held in high regard within their community. Often, Asians live in an extended family. Other basic values and concepts of the modern Asian family include an emphasis on education; reserve conformity and harmony; benevolence and obligation; endurance and sacrifice; and loss of face, shame, and honor (Hu 2012). Each of these values is discussed below.

Hu (2012) suggests that the most notable aspect of the modern Asian model minority stereotype is that they are academic overachievers. Clearly, not all Asians fit this pattern. The level of achievement of Asian students can be attributed primarily to the basic notion of the family and the central role that education plays. Education is the

Table 8.1 Cultural values promote family interdependence

Collectivism: It is the tendency to place group needs and goals above the goals and desires of the individual.

Relational orientation: It is a cultural frame in which the self is defined in terms of its essential and continuing interdependence with others.

Familism: It defines a hierarchically organized extended family system as the basic social unit.

Family obligation: It includes both attitudinal and behavioral responsibilities in which children are expected to (a) show respect and affection for older family members, (b) seek their advice and accept their decisions, and (c) maintain propinquity, instrumental assistance, and emotional ties with parents across the life span.

Adapted from Yee et al. (2008)

most valued way of achieving position, and success in education is viewed as an act of filial piety (respect for parents), a highly important principle (Africa and Carrasco 2011; Hu). Another modern stereotype is that of the silent, unassertive Asian, uncomplaining, unemotional, docile, and cooperative. Because the well-being of the larger group is most important in Asian culture, great importance is placed on maintaining harmony. Thus, the greatest virtue that one can achieve is fulfilling his or her role in the whole of the family or group, and individual achievement is seen as the result of the effort of the family or group. Maintaining harmony also creates a bias against change, which is opposite of American values to encourage change. In following these principles, Asians may hesitate to initially accept invitations, may choose items of lesser value when given the choice, and may not be assertive in situations where they might speak out (Hu; Sue and Sue 2013).

Asian culture emphasizes consideration of others; thus, benevolence and obligation must be present to reinforce relationships. As a hierarchical society, Asian relationships involve a lot of obligation, which might be viewed as dependence or domination. In essence, a substantial amount of responsibility and benevolence is expected in return. For individuals of equal position, there is still the principle of reciprocity, goodness given out will come back and kindness should be paid back (Hu 2012). Overwhelmingly, Asian culture has a male-dominated power structure. Equally as important is birth order, especially for males who are expected to take on more unique responsibilities as they grow into adulthood (e.g., oldest son assists the father).

The principles of endurance and sacrifice are highly applicable to early immigrants who worked under extreme conditions in the USA and endured racism because of their willingness to work hard for so relatively little. Endurance at all costs is central to the extent to which all other Asian values are carried out and what distinguishes Asian values from values in other cultures that look at first similar. Sacrifice means that one's own situation is secondary to that of the group as a whole. Endurance is a measure of self-control and inner strength, and complaining is seen as a sign of weakness (Hu 2012). Hu believes that these values may lead to the perception of Asians as being uncomplaining and less vocal than other ethnic minority groups.

Many Americans are familiar with the concept of losing face among Asians. Maintaining good face is essential because shame and honor go far beyond the individual and reflect directly upon one's family, nation, or related group. The extent to which an individual is able to maintain good face is a kind of measurement of how well one has kept faith to traditional values and one's social standing among others. It is a strong control mechanism, which reinforces all other Asian values (Hu 2012). The act of keeping face and suppressing or not admitting embarrassing situations in the family history often manifests itself in the reluctance of Asians to seek mental health services (Sue and Sue 2013).

Many AAPIs rely on traditional health beliefs and practices (Africa and Carrasco 2011). To illustrate this point, several Native Hawaiian cultural values are presented (Mau 2010). These values are often relevant in the healthcare setting and are not intended to be an exhaustive list of

Hawaiian beliefs. First, *lokahi* (balance/harmony) sometimes referred to as "*Lokahi Triangle*" (i.e., physical body, environment, relationships with others, family members, ancestors, the Gods, and mental and emotional states) is central to understanding of health. A person's physical body cannot heal without setting right any problems within the mental or spiritual realm. Moreover, the person has to be willing to take responsibility for the healing and make amends for any wrongs that he or she might have caused in the past (Mau 2010). The second value is *ohana* (family), including the extended family or multigenerational homes, which is the primary social structure for an ethnic Native Hawaiian. Because illness affects the entire family, family members need to be involved in decision-making and treatment plans. The value of *ohana* is closely tied to the values of *laulima* (cooperation/helping) and *kuleana* (responsibility). Finally, the values of *aloha* (love, compassion) and *malama* (to care for) can influence the recipient–provider relationship because Native Hawaiians need to feel that they are being respected and cared for if they are to be willing partners in the helping relationship. Thus, a service provider must establish trust with the person. Native Hawaiians feel a strong responsibility to take care of their loved ones (Mau).

Many of the cultural characteristics of AAPIs have served them well as buffers against discrimination. However, it is important for service providers who work with AAPIs to look behind the success myth and to understand the historical and current experiences of AAPIs (Sue and Sue 2013). In fact, it is even more pressing when we realize that LGBT AAPIs underutilize healthcare and mental health services. Yet, for LGBT AAPI immigrant elders who are unprepared for the culture shock in the USA, the need for culture-specific diagnostic impressions and interventions are paramount. Efforts to assist them to integrate their different identity dimensions (e.g., race/ethnicity, sexual orientation, gender expression, culture, age) should be made with an awareness of self-perception and cultural perception.

Asian Americans and Pacific Islanders' Attitudes About LGBT Persons

Currently, limited research on the attitudes and perceptions of AAPIs toward LGBT persons exists, especially that which is both culturally relevant and linguistically appropriate (Tseng 2011). In response to this dearth of research, Tseng initiated a study of the attitudes of Asian Americans, especially Chinese-speaking Americans, toward LGBT persons using in-language interviews and using culturally specific questions. The results indicated that for Chinese-speaking Americans, gender is the most salient lens through which they define, perceive, and form their attitudes toward LGBT persons and their attitudes in relation to prominent issues including children, culture, marriage, and family. Overwhelmingly, the majority of interviewees described LGBT persons as those whose gender characteristics (e.g., appearance, gender roles in relationships, behavior) do not conform to the gender characteristics of heterosexuals. "Gender nonconformity is both the most cited definition for being LGBT and the strongest source of discomfort with LGBT persons" (Tseng, p. 4). Moreover, strict adherence to traditional gender roles manifests itself in how they conceptualize LGBT persons in relationships. When asked to describe their perceptions of LGBT persons, the majority of interviewees described GBT men. Interviewees also described LGBT persons as people who are confused about their gender identity, and some admitted extreme discomfort with LGBT persons who are neither masculine nor feminine. The interviewees expressed greater negative attitudes toward GBT men, indicating that it is worse for men to be GBT than for women.

Tseng (2011) also found that the interviewees framed the "born that way" versus "choice" in two ways. First, a majority of interviewees did not believe the causes could be narrowed down to either of the two. Second, their beliefs in either of the two concepts were not correlated with specific attitudes (i.e., acceptance versus rejection) toward LGBT persons, even for those who were certain about the causes of being LGBT. Culturally, the majority of interviewees believed that there have always been LGBT in their home countries and observed that LGBT persons are afraid to be open in their countries of birth because the culture is not accepting of them. In addition, they believe that the relatively more open and liberal nature of American and Western cultures make it possible for LGBT persons to be more open about their sexuality; consequently, the culture is an enabler of LGBT persons being open about their identities (Tseng 2011).

The attitudes of the vast majority of Chinese-speaking Americans in Tseng's (2011) study were anti-same-sex marriage. These attitudes can be categorizes as follows: (a) LGBT persons should be able to have the same rights but not to call it marriage; (b) the function of marriage is reproduction and passing down the family name; and (c) same-sex marriage is a violation of tradition, and only heterosexual marriage is recognized around the world. As parents, the interviewees indicated that they would grudgingly accept a LGBT child but not before making attempts to "correct" the child. In addition, they expressed two types of concerns. First, they were concerned about being labeled as ineffective parents who had done a poor job of raising their children. Second, they felt that it would be difficult to face close friends and relatives who may ridicule them, and they would feel a high degree of self-blame if their children turned out to be LGBT. On the question of the role that religion plays in their attitudes about LGBT person, the majority of Chinese-speaking Americans indicated that it only played a small role (Tseng). It should be noted that the majority of Chinese Americans identify as not religious (Dang and Hu 2005). Dang and Hu found that of the LGBT AAPIs in their survey, a large majority claimed to be atheist, agnostic, or without religion. Of those who did identify as having involvement in religion, on average, they said that their church or religion views being LGBT negatively and as wrong and sinful. Only 16 % said that their religion fully accepted LGBT persons. See Chapter "The Role of Religious and Faith Communities in Addressing the Needs of LGBT Elders" for further discussion of religion.

Boulden (2009) found a clash of culture between older generation and younger gay Hmong men. In this study, the researcher found that the participants described the attitudes of their parents and the older Hmong generation concerning the existence of LGBT persons as the older generation not acknowledging that lesbians and gays exists. Hmong elders have never known a Hmong who identified him or herself as gay or lesbian; thus, it was not an Asian issue, but rather a White disease and a White issue. Participants indicated that if their parents knew that they are gay, it would "break their hearts" for not having children to carry on the bloodline. Therefore, to avoid bringing shame to the family, they moved away and separated themselves. Some participants spoke of trying to manage the multifaceted conflicts and different aspects of their daily lives of being "out" at work, acting straight in public, and being and talking Hmong at home. In summary, nowhere in their multiple environments did the participants have the luxury of interacting with others while acknowledging their complete identity (Boulden 2009).

LGBT AAPIs strongly agree that homophobia and/or transphobia is a problem within the Asian-American community (Dang and Hu 2005). The perception was consistent among women, men, and transgender persons. For example, in India, being gay, the term, a recent addition to the Indian cultural dictionary, is challenged with substantial resistance. The Indian Penal Code #377 states:

> Whoever voluntarily has carnal intercourse against the order of nature with any man, woman, or animal, shall be punished with imprisonment for life, or with imprisonment of either description for a term which may extend to ten years, and shall also be liable to fine (Indian Law Info, n.d.)

The phrase, "against the order of nature," refers to any non-heterosexual relationship (Bhattar and Victoria 2007, p. 40). Clearly, alternative sexuality is defined only in terms of sexual behavior, not identity, and is compared to acts of beastiality. In both Indian tradition and pop culture, gay is still defined as abnormal and evil. LGBT persons are portrayed stereotypically in Indian society in the form of a very feminine male of *hijra*. The term *hijra* is used to define transgender, intersex, and "third gender" people who live in communities outside of society. Consequently, a fear exists among Indians that if a person identifies as gay, he will soon start to dress and act as a woman. The acceptance of the Western ideology of LGBT persons is slow among more progressive Indians, and Indian communities in the USA find it hard to accept sexual differences because sexuality is a taboo topic in India (Bhattar and Victoria).

In general, AAPIs hold negative and prejudicial attitudes toward LGBT persons. However, as with all groups, varying degrees of acceptance exist. LGBT AAPIs report experiences that are equally negative and positive within in different contexts such as family and LGBT and non-LGBT organizations (Dang and Hu 2005). One interesting result of the survey by Dang and Hu is that despite their experiences with racism in the LGBT community, LGBT AAPIs are more comfortable working in predominately White LGBT environments than they are working in predominantly straight homophobic AAPI environments.

Asian American and Pacific Islander LGBT Elderly

The US Census has numerous limitations, including but not limited to specifically asking about sexual orientation or gender identity, individuals in same-sex relationships who are not living together, and homeless LGBT persons, which does not reflect the actual full diversity of LGBT persons in the USA (Dang and Hu 2005). However, other data suggest that of the Asian and Pacific Islander population, 2.8 % of adults identify as LGBT, including 3,246,000 in the USA, 32,931 of whom are AAPIs in same-sex couples, and that 25.9 % of AAPI same-sex couples are raising children. The majority of LGBT AAPI adults live in geographic locations where there are higher proportions of AAPI

persons as opposed to areas with higher proportions of the broader LGBT population. Approximately, one-third of AAPI same-sex couples live in California, Hawaii, and New York. LGBT AAPIs are much younger than both the non-LGBT population and AAPI persons in same-sex couples. Approximately, 4 % of AAPI persons in same-sex couples are aged 65 and over (Kastanis and Gates 2013). Other characteristics of LGBT AAPIs include lower rates of college completion (42 %) as compared to AAPI non-LGBT adults (59 %); however, AAPIs in same-sex couples (58 %) have higher rates of educational attainment than their different-sex counterparts (54 %). Unemployment rates are higher for LGBT persons (11 %) compared to non-LGBT AAPIs (8 %). AAPIs in same-sex (81 %) couples are more likely to be employed than their counterparts in different-sex couples (70 %). Overall, AAPI persons in same-sex couples (40 %) are more likely to be US citizens by birth than those in different-sex couples (14 %), and same-sex couples are more likely than different-sex couples to have at least one partner with US citizenship status (Kastanis and Gates).

As with many other ethnic minority populations, not all LGBT AAPIs identify with the terms lesbian, gay, bisexual, and transgender because of cultural differences, internalized homo/bi/transphobia, and the dissociation between identity and behavior (Mangton et al. 2002). Because of cultural pressures and expectations that exist in Asian and Pacific Island cultures, lesbians and gay men and women and men who engage in same-sex behavior are required to stick to family values, marry, and have children, or place shame on their families, neighbors, and community (Boulder 2009). In fact, many Asian cultural norms render women invisible and silent. Compared to heterosexual AAPI women and both heterosexual and gay AAPI men, lesbians have a higher prevalence of tobacco use, binge drinking, marijuana, and other drug use. AAPI lesbians are less likely to adhere to traditional family-orientated gender roles, unable or unwilling to gain and receive emotional support from their families, and more likely to compete with men for masculine privileges in order to escape sexist oppression (Hahm and Adkins 2009).

In the USA, LGBT persons view "coming out" as a final revelation of their sexual orientation or gender identity. For AAPI LGBT persons, the integration of their ethnicity and their nationality as an American is known as "coming home," in which they allude to their sexuality to a family member who may not challenge it, as long as the status quo within the family is maintained (Hahm and Adkins 2009). AAPI LGBT persons tend to have a high degree of internalized biases about minority sexualities, which frequently cause them to be isolated, serve as a barrier to accessing services, and increase high-risk behavior. The internalization of homophobia by AAPI LGBT persons can serve as a direct health risk (Mangton et al. 2002). In a discussion of the LGBT Filipino community, Alcedo (2014) shared some perspectives on what LGBT elders confront with being "out" as ranging from not feeling comfortable to being forced to make connections with more people because of the need to keep healthy and being well situated in an intergenerational lesbian community. Jim Toy and George Takei are two examples that illustrate the public role of AAPI LGBT elders as activists (see Table 8.2 for their profiles).

Dang and Hu (2005) surveyed LGBT AAPIs to determine the extent to which they consider their sexual orientation and gender identity or expression as important. The results revealed that LGBT AAPIs ranked their sexual orientation or gender identity/expression as the second identity that most heavily influence their daily lives. Race/ethnicity was ranked as the most influential. Although LGBT persons often mask their sexual orientation or sexual expression and behaviors to avoid alienating their family and parents' communities, in their relationships with others, they frequently have to decide which identity will take precedence—an ethnic or sexual identity (Eng and Hom 1998). The feeling of being caught between two separate or non-integrated identities was summarized in a dialogue between two Asian American gay men as, "though we are both Asian American and gay, our surroundings rarely allow these identities to coexist" (Bhattar and Victoria 2007, p. 39). When asked to identify political issues and attitudes that are most important, LGBT AAPIs ranked immigration, hate violence/harassment, media representation, HIV/AIDS, marriage/domestic partnership, and health care as the most pressing for them compared to immigration, media representation, the economy/jobs, health care, and language barriers for Asian-Americans in general.

Table 8.2 Profile of AAPI LGBT elder activists

Jim Toy is a Chinese American activist, social worker, and a pioneer of the LGBT movement in Michigan. He is considered as the first person to come out publically as queer in Michigan, which he did at an anti-Vietnam rally in 1970. He is the founding member of several organizations, including the Ann Arbor and the Detroit Gay Liberation Movements, PFLAG/Ann Arbor, Transgender Advocacy Project, Washtenaw Rainbow Action Project, LGBT Retirement Center Task Force, and GLSEN Ann Arbor. Mr. Toy co-authored a non-discrimination policy around sexual orientation for the city and the university and the first LG Pride Week Proclamation from a governing body in the USA. He is well known for his work in establishing University of Michigan's Lesbian-Gay Male Program Office, the first LGBT center in an institution of higher learning in the USA, where he served as coordinator from 1971–1994.

George Takei is an actor, comedian, personality, and activist. He was born in Los Angeles to Japanese American parents. In 1942, he and his family were forced to move into an internment camp in Arkansas. When the war ended, he returned to California, where he completed high school and attended UCLA. He received both a bachelors and masters of art degrees in theater. He later attended the Shakespeare Institute at Stratford-upon-Avon in England and Sophia University in Tokyo. In 1959, his first professional debut as an actor on television was an episode of *Playhouse 90,* and *Ice Palace* was his first film debut. He was cast in his most well-known role, Mr. Sulu, in the Star Trek franchise, including six films. In the last 50 years, Mr. Takei has appeared in over 40 feature films and hundreds of guest-starring roles. He was presented the Order of the Rising Star and Gold Rays with Rosette for his work on USA–Japanese relations. In addition, he has an asteroid named after him, a star on Hollywood's Walk of Fame, and received an LGBT Humanist Award. Mr. Takei is well known for his community and political activism in support of the AAPI and LGBT communities.

Gay, Lesbian, and Straight Education Network (www.glsen.org)

The survey project, *A Census of Our Own*, gathered data from 364 LGBTQ Southeast Asian Americans from across the USA and found several main points (Queer Southeast Asian Census 2012). First, coming out narratives and data suggest that an alternative coming out model and culturally competent programming are needed, which addresses the unique experiences and challenged faced by LGBTQ Southeast Asians. The ability to communicate in their native language is challenging because, for example, there are no positive words within the Hmong, Khmer, Lao, or Viet languages to describe alternative sexual orientation. Second, a strict adherence to and policy of confidentiality is needed among service providers to ensure safety and garner trust of AAPI LGBT persons. In light of the role of family in the lives of elders, this may prove both difficult and necessary. Third, Southeast Asian Americans are coming out at a young age (before the age of 18). Because the process of coming out is often accompanied with psychological and emotional stress, education and safety should be essential components of any program or service. Finally, there are harsh realities of income disparities and limited economic opportunities for Southeast Asian in the USA, which adds to the pressure to contribute toward the family incomes.

While there is limited research on AAPI LGBT persons, much less research exists on transgender AAPIs. Thus, transgender (trans) and nonconforming gender (NCG) AAPIs are deserving of a closer examination within this chapter. One of the most important findings of the *National Transgender Discrimination Survey* (NTDS) of 2013 was that the combination of anti-transgender bias and structural and interpersonal racism meant that trans and NCG AAPI transgender persons of color, including AAPIs, experience particularly devastating levels of discrimination (Grant et al. 2011). Of the 6456 trans and NCG persons in the survey, 212 respondents identified themselves as Asian or Pacific Islander, or Asian or Pacific Islander and multiracial. The majority of the AAPI respondents were US citizens (84 %). The key finding of the survey revealed that AAPI transgender and NCG persons often live in extreme poverty (18 %), which is higher than the rate for trans and NCG persons of all races (15 %). It is six times the general AAPI population (3 %) and over four times the general US population rate (4 %). AAPI trans and NCG persons are affected disproportionately by HIV at a rate of 5 % compared to 2.64 % for trans and NCG persons of all races. Forty four (44 %) of AAPI trans and NCG persons have experienced significant family acceptance, with those persons being much less likely to face discrimination. Finally, 56 % of AAPI trans and NCG persons have attempted suicide due to discrimination. Other areas in which AAPI trans and NCG persons have experienced discrimination are presented in Table 8.3. In particular, discrimination in the area of health care is discussed in the following section.

Table 8.3 AAPI trans and nonconforming gender discrimination experience

Education: AAPI persons who attended school expressing a trans identity of NCG report rates of harassment (65 %), physical assault (39 %), and sexual assault (19 %) in K-12. AAPIs who were harassed and abused by teachers in K-12 settings show dramatically worse health and other outcomes compared to those who did not experience such abuse.

Employment: AAPI trans and NCG persons have an unemployment rate nearly twice that of the general population. Twenty-one percent have lost a job due to bias, and 41 % were not hired for a job due to bias. Forty-nine percent have been harasses, 8 % physically abused, and 10 % sexually assaulted at work. Twenty-three percent have been compelled to sell drugs or do sex work for income at some point in their lives.

Housing: AAPI trans and NCG persons have experienced various forms of discrimination ranging from being refused a home or apartment to being evicted due to bias. They have experienced homelessness at some point in their lives at nearly twice the rate of the general US population. AAPI trans and NCG persons are less likely than other races to own homes.

Grant et al. (2011)

Health Status, Barriers, and Service Delivery for Asian American LGBT Elderly

Several barriers prevent obtaining a full and accurate picture of access to services and service delivery for Asian American LGBT elders. First is the barrier of the omission of data reports on Asian American participants from some of the largest national health studies and surveys, along with differentiation among various ethnic subgroups in particular (Holland and Palaniappan 2012). Second, research methods for sampling respondents are often limited to persons who may have limited English proficiency and/or low socioeconomic status (SES). Finally, concerns about the validity of chosen measures for use with a particular Asian ethnic group arise because many measures are rarely validated on Asian Americans, and even fewer have been validated on the various Asian ethnic subgroups (Sorkin and Ngo-Metzger 2014). Moreover, measures have not been validated on either the Asian American elderly or LGBT population among them. Two areas in which Asian Americans consistently report low-quality care include preventive screening and detection and treatment of mental health disorders (Haviland et al. 2005). The contextual factors that impact the health of elders are influenced by the diversity within the AAPI communities with respect to health-seeking behavior and knowledge, SES, educational level, cultural traditions, and specific healthcare needs and issues (Trinh-Shervin et al. 2009).

The average life expectancy for AAPIs is 80.3 years compared to Whites at 75.1, and overall health among AAPIs as a group tends to be better than that of Whites and other ethnic groups (U.S. Office of Minority Health Resource Center 2010). Collectively, the health status of AAPIs is remarkably good; however, certain groups have high rates of illness, chronic conditions, and disability from specific health causes. As a subgroup, Asian American elders often face unique types of barriers to seeking and receiving care, including language and health literacy obstacles, culture-specific stigma around

receipt of health care, challenges with access, lack of health insurance, and immigrant status. AAPI elders are uninsured at more than double the rate of non-Hispanic White elders, and specific subgroups are uninsured at rates as high as 33 % (Sorkin and Ngo-Metzger 2014). Only 33 % of AAPIs aged 65 and over have private health insurance (Schiller et al. 2012). Although Asian Americans are less dependent on Social Security than are other groups, according to Williamson et al. (2014), without the safety net provided by Social Security, approximately 19 % of Asian elders would fall below the poverty line.

Language has been identified as the most formidable barrier for Asian American immigrants in accessing health care, especially for older adults, who are the least likely age group to be proficient in English (Jones et al. 2006; Kim and Keefe 2010). In fact, only 41 % of AAPI elders feel that they speak English "very well" (US Census 2014). AAPIs represent more than 100 languages and dialects (Africa and Carrasco 2011). Language barriers for elders have implications for both family dynamics and health care. For example, the lack of language proficiency may lead to the role disruption in Asian American families when children speak, read, and understand English better than their parents, resulting in a temporarily reversed family role. This role reversal creates awkward situations in the healthcare setting. Moreover, research suggests that even with the availability of interpreters, older AAPIs refrain from asking questions about their health (Green et al. 2005; Sue and Sue 2013).

The life expectancy of Native Hawaiian men (71.5 years) and women (77.2 years) is lower than for the state of Hawaii (75.9 years for men and 82.1 years for women) and the USA overall (Anderson et al. 2006). Mortality rates for Asian or Pacific Islander elders are lower than the rates for Whites, Blacks, or American Indians (Minino et al. 2007). However, these results are likely due to the aggregation of data from Asians, who tend to have longer life expectancies, with Native Hawaiians and other Pacific Islander racial groups, who tend to have lower life expectancies

(Braun et al. 1997). In addition, death rates for Native Hawaiians due to heart disease, cancers, stroke, accidents, and diabetes are higher than those for the state of Hawaii (Mau 2010; US Office of Minority Health Resource Center 2010). Since 2007, cardiovascular disease (CVD) has been the leading cause of death in the USA and in Hawaii. The rates of CVD vary by ethnicity and SES. Filipinos and Native Hawaiians have disproportionately higher age-adjusted mortality rates for CVD and stroke. The lowest SES groups and the rural counties of Hawaii consistently report the highest areas with CVD-risk factors (i.e., high blood pressure, smoking, obesity, physical inactivity, and diabetes). CVD is also responsible for a large portion of healthcare costs in Hawaii due to costs associated with hospitalizations (Balabis et al. 2007).

AAPI elderly people have a disproportionately high prevalence of hepatitis B. In addition, AAPI elderly people exhibit a greater prevalence of dementia than the total older population. Tuberculosis is 24 times more common among AAPIs than among Whites (Office of Minority Health, n.d.). Generally, Native Hawaiian elders were similar to their Caucasian counterparts in receiving certain preventive health care and in having healthcare coverage. In other areas of preventive care, AAPIs have lower rates of vaccination, underutilize mental health and specific health services such as cancer screening, and have poorer early detection rates compared to other ethnic groups (Reyes-Salvail et al. 2008; Salvail et al. 2003). Consistent across various ethnic groups, AAPI elders are less likely to see a primary care provider or take prescription medication for their mental health compared to non-Hispanic White older adults (Sorkin and Ngo-Metzger 2014). In an examination of frequent mental distress (FMD) prevalence rate and disparity, Reyes-Salvail et al. (2008) found the following: (a) the FMD prevalence rate in the state was 8.3 %, 8.0 % prevalence rate for lifetime anxiety, and 8.8 % for lifetime depression; (b) no significant difference in the average FDM prevalence rate between counties in the state of Hawaii; (c) adult aged 65 and over had a significantly lower prevalence rate for FMD than younger adults; (d) females had a higher FMD prevalence than males; and (e) among major ethnicities, Hawaiians (including part-Hawaiians) had the highest FMD prevalence and Japanese had the lowest; however, this disparity is an artifact of SES factor combined with age. When these factors were controlled for, the ethnic disparity disappeared. The results of this study also showed a relationship between FMD and lifestyle behaviors. Those with FMD are more likely to engage in smoking or heavy drinking than those without FMD.

Africa and Carrasco (2011) conclude that among all ethnicities, AAPIs are the least likely to seek mental health services because of a variety of factors such as, but not limited to, stigma, cultural impact of shame, language barriers, economic reasons, mind–body conceptualization, and racial discrimination (see Table 8.4 for additional barriers to seeking mental health treatments and supports). Regardless of sexual orientation and gender identity, many health disparities encountered by AAPIs have their origins in "cultural historical trauma" (Blaisdell 1996), the psychological, physical, social, and cultural aftermath of the colonialism many

Table 8.4 Barriers to AAPIs seeing mental health and healthcare services

Cultural
Health beliefs
Lack of research
Immigrant status
Avoiding shame and stigma
Access to healthcare/insurance
Fear of breach of confidentiality
Homophobia and heterosexism
Experience of prejudice and racism
Help-seeking behavior (e.g., traditional medicine)
Lack of linguistically and culturally responsive providers
Exclusion of traditional or indigenous providers by the Western system
Health literacy (ability to read and understand health content in the context of specific health situations)

Adapted from Africa and Carrasco (2011) and Kim and Keefe (2010)

indigenous people have experienced. Cultural historical trauma also refers to the cumulative emotional and psychological wounding that seems to carry forth into successive generations and affects all aspects of health (Mau 2010). According to Mau, "cultural wounding" can result in communal feelings of disruption and a sense of collective helplessness, which can in turn impact one's 'sense of self' and health-seeking behaviors (p. 21). AAPI LGBT persons identify the extent to which the underlying racism and discrimination that they experience within the mainstream, majority culture is stronger than the homophobia within the AAPI community (Boulden 2009; Mangton et al. 2002). Dang and Hu (2005) found that LGBT AAPIs overwhelmingly experience racism within the White LGBT community and transgender persons somewhat more so than lesbians or gay men. In addition, LGBT AAPIs experience some degree of racism or ethnocentrism with other AAPI LGBT persons.

As a largely immigrant and refugee population, Asian Americans face stressors related to immigration and acculturation, and confounding factors such as war experiences and abuse that make them more vulnerable to advanced depression and other mental health disorders (California Health Information Survey 2010). Takeuchi et al. (2007) indicate an individual's age at immigration adds to the complexities of immigration and the experiences of adjustment, acculturation, and assimilation when looking at the AAPI community (see Chapter "Immigrant LGBT Elders" for additional discussion on issues relevant to immigration). Specifically, Asian immigrants who arrived at age 12 or younger were at greater risk for psychiatric disorders and substance abuse, while those who arrived before age 41 also had greater risk for mood disorders, and those who came after age 41 were likely to have experienced symptom onset before immigrating to the USA. Older Asian American women have the highest suicide rate of all women over age 65 in the USA (Office of Minority Health, n.d.). Although AAPIs' use of mental health services is low, they have rates of psychological distress comparable to the general population.

Alcohol and substance abuse is increasing significantly among AAPIs, with tremendous variance among subgroups. According to the National Asian-Americans Families Against Substance Abuse (n.d.), Japanese Americans have the highest lifetime prevalence for alcohol abuse, and Vietnamese Americans are at high risk for heavy drinking. Immigrants from Japan and Korea are almost twice as likely to use alcohol than those from the Philippines, China, Vietnam, and India. Moreover, Filipino men are at greater risk than Chinese men for a lifetime substance abuse disorder. Research also suggests an association between generational status and depressive and substance abuse disorders among women, with second-and third-generation women being at increased risk.

As a subgroup, AAPI trans and NCG persons refuse medical care due to bias. In addition, they postpone care when sick or injured due to fear of discrimination. AAPI trans and NCG persons are less likely to have accessed counseling and mental health services. For AAPI trans and NCG elders, inaccessibility to mental health services in the USA is attributed often to language and cultural barriers. Thus, there are consequences for those wishing to seek certain forms of transition-related medical care that is dependent on prior counseling (Grant et al. 2011).

The role and care of AAPI elders within families vary depending on factors such as culture, filial piety values and behavior, traditionalism, and acculturation. AAPI elders serve as a family resource while they are healthy, but they may be a source of burden when their health fails. Conditions in the household and community influence how long elders are able to function independently as their health declines (Yee et al. 2008). According to Yu et al. (1993), more traditional desires such as living with one's family increased as an elder's health declined among Chinese and Korean American elders. An acculturation-related consequence for Asian American families is that they have become more accepting of the institutionalization of the elderly, but are still more reluctant to access that care than the general population (Watari and Gatz 2004). South Asian elderly women find it difficult to ask for their family's help in dealing with chronic illness or financial assistance. For these women, especially those with limited English proficiency, fear of isolation is increased disproportionately as they become less mobile due to poor health. In more traditional AAPI families, the sense of responsibility to care for their elderly members may be a barrier to seeking professional support services. In addition, the potential for elder abuse may occur when immigrant families' resources are stretched beyond their capacity to care for ill family elders (Yee et al. 2008). (see Chapters "An Overview of Aging and Mistreatment of LGBT Elders" and "Mistreatment and Victimization of LGBT Elders" for further discussion on elder mistreatment and victimization).

Among AAPI elders, the use of traditional healing practices is commonplace. Within specific subgroups of AAPIs, regardless of age, specific health questions are difficult to answer. For example, Samoans consider questions about sexual relations as distasteful. Because most Samoans are extremely private in matters about of family diseases and/or abnormalities of the genitals and consider it shameful to speak of such things, questions pertaining to these areas are usually not answered directly (Mau 2010). To illustrate this point, consider the case of Kim, a 65-year-old Samoan transgender female who is closeted and holds to traditional cultural values.

The Case of Kim Kim is a 65-year-old transgender. She has not self-disclosed her sexual identity to anyone, including her healthcare provider. At the age of 28, she went to Europe and had gender reassignment surgery, male-to-female. Kim had live in several countries after her surgery, but has lived in the UK since the age of 38. She continues to hold to the traditional values and gender role expectations of Samoan culture.

Kim has been experiencing abdominal and vaginal pain, and the pain has become severe enough that she had to go to the doctor. When asked questions about childbirth, vaginal bleeding, and other discomfort, Kim does not provide answer, responding only to say that she has past the age of such issues.

Questions

1. What other types of question can be asked of Kim before making such "highly personal and distasteful questions"?
2. How can you work with Kim to understand the purpose of disclosure as a health-related issue?
3. What might you do to reduce her fears?
4. Are there any cultural considerations that you can employ to work more effectively with Kim?

A major question arises for service providers working with AAPI LGBT elders. That is, how do we identify those who are not "out" and do not want to be identified so that they receive appropriate services? While much of the apprehension of AAPI LGBT elders to be "out" is cultural, other aspects are related to discrimination. Overall, the process to assist these elders must start, in part, with policy development and implementation.

Policy and Practice Issues

Forging a political agenda for AAPI LGBT persons is badly needed. Dang and Hu (2005) emphasize that hate crimes, police misconduct, media representation, worker exploitation, and gentrification/displacement impact AAPI LGBT persons, but their presence is absent in these campaigns. Moreover, many LGBT civil rights issues lack an Asian or immigrant analysis. Dang and Hu assert that AAPI "advocacy and social service groups must also be held accountable to the needs of all their constituents, including those of all sexual orientations, and gender identities and expressions" (p. 11). The survey, A Census of

Our Own, recommended that to counter the debilitating effects of racism, homophobia, and genderphobia, more education, resources, and systems of support are needed. In addition, mainstream LGBTQ organizations and programs fail to address the unique ways in which AAPI LGBT persons face multiple identities and multiple oppressions. Thus, there is a need for more inclusive practices, including an analysis and acknowledgment of racism, class, and genderphobia (Queer Southeast Asian Census 2012).

To improve access and quality of health care, health, and social policy, analysts need to consider several important factors that can either remove or mitigate the effects of barriers for AAPIs. First, patient characteristics such as primary language, ethnicity, culture, health literacy, insurance coverage, and immigration status must be taken into account (Kim and Keefe 2010). Africa and Carrasco (2011) emphasize that acknowledging the wide diversity of experiences within the AAPI community is critical for providing effective and efficient services responsive to particular needs and influential cultural factors. AAPI elders may exhibit a high degree of mistrust toward service providers and institutions because of past negative personal and historical experiences endured from the government (e.g., internment camps, exploitative labor practices) and racism and discrimination that have lingering impacts upon cultural groups today. The recommendation from participants in Africa and Carrasco's report is for service providers to have a "balanced approach to representation of both communities and perspectives at different levels" (p. 13).

Strength and Resiliency. AAPIs have cultural values that provide strength and resiliency and help them deal with difficult life events (Sue and Sue 2013). Enculturation or identification with racial and ethnic background can buffer prejudice and discrimination, family conflicts, and psychosocial adjustment issues (Kim 2011). Thus, both policy and practice should be geared toward promotion of cultural strengths. In addition, practitioners should maintain a distinction between identity and behavior because AAPIs participating in same-sex behavior may not always identify with the terms LGBT (Mangton

et al. 2002). Likewise, policy development and implementation will need to address potential barriers that filial piety values and behaviors may impose for service intervention.

A major barrier to effective policy development regarding AAPI families, subgroups, and LGBT AAPIs is the model minority myth stereotype. This model minority myth stereotype obstructs the examination of how AAPIs cope with normative and non-normative life span developmental hurdles that expend the resources of even the most resilient individuals and families. Furthermore, Yee et al. (2008) contend that the model minority myth stereotype, in conjunction with an overrepresentation of Asian American investigators conducting research in the biomedical and physical sciences, has reinforced the mistaken notion that there is a sufficient AAPI family research infrastructure. Similarly, the same error in reasoning may lead to such an assumption about LGBT AAPI elders. AAPIs as a population and LGBT elders in particular have been omitted from national data sets and studies. Many researchers who study AAPIs contend that since 1976, which marks the pivotal beginning in the use of data for evidence-based health policy in the USA, core issues about the lack of data persist for this population (Ponce 2011). Clearly, organizations and service providers must expand efforts to serve AAPI LGBT elders.

Summary

AAPI LGBT elders represent a unique subgroup within culturally specific populations. Their value systems are influenced by tradition, language, and a host of other factors. Many AAPI LGBT elders maintain a covert lifestyle in order to save face and to not bring shame to their families. Their multiple identities are encapsulated not only by cultural attitudinal barriers, but also by racism, discrimination, and phobias within society as a whole. All of these factors contribute to the limited research and available information on AAPI LGBT elders.

In general, AAPIs bear the burden of the stereotyped model minority, which puts them at a disadvantage for various services. AAPI LGBT elders may never exercise the option of "coming out" because they may view the risks as far too great. Thus, for both AAPI LGBT elders who are "out" and for those who are not, there is utility in using lay health workers and service providers or "cultural communicators" as facilitators for improving communication and shared decision-making (Sorkin and Ngo-Metzger 2014). In the final analysis, service providers must be able to work around many barriers that put AAPI LGBT elders at risk for poor health, social, and emotional outcomes.

Learning Exercises

Self-Check Questions

1. What is the general perception of AAPI cultures toward LGBT persons?
2. What is meant by the stereotype of Asian Americans being seen as the model minority?
3. Who are the largest Asian American single-race subgroups?
4. What are some of the often unseen challenges in Asian American communities such as Chinatowns, Manilatowns, and Japantowns?
5. Were the majority of older Asian Americans born inside or outside of the USA?

Field-Based Experiential Assignments

1. Conduct a survey of healthcare service providers or social service provider to determine their knowledge level about working with AAPI LGBT elders.
2. Interview an AAPI LGBT elder to understand issues and concerns they had about "coming out" and how they addressed them.

3. The religious view of many AAPI groups is that alternative sexuality is wrong and sinful. Develop a presentation to address their view. Be sure to include cultural concerns.

Multiple-Choice Questions

1. Which of the following Asian American cultural values creates a bias against change?
   a. Cooperation
   b. Harmony
   c. Education
   d. Benevolence
2. Which of the following means respect for parents?
   a. Ohana
   b. Uncomplaining
   c. Filial piety
   d. Emotional centeredness
3. Which of the following is a concern of AAPI parents whose child is gay?
   a. Being labeled as ineffective parents
   b. Ridicule from relatives and close friends
   c. Self-blame
   d. All of the above
   e. None of the above
4. Which of the following terms is used to define transgender, intersex, and third gender Asian Indians?
   a. Hijra
   b. Kuelna
   c. Laulima
   d. Lokahi
5. LGBT AAPI adults live in geographic locations with higher proportions of which type of populations?
   a. LGBT persons
   b. AAPI persons
   c. Diverse persons
   d. No data are available
6. What is the integration of their ethnicity and their nationality known as for AAPI LGBT persons?
   a. Coming out
   b. Assimilation

    c. Coming home

    d. Acculturation

7. What is the origin of many health disparities for both LGBT and non-LGBT AAPI persons?
   a. Hepatitis B
   b. Mental distress
   c. Cultural historical trauma
   d. Language barriers

8. Which of the following acculturation-related consequence has become more accepting for Asian American families for the elderly?
   a. Utilization of mental health services
   b. Use of substances
   c. Public assistance
   d. Institutionalization

9. Which type of health questions do Samoans find distasteful and they may not answer directly?
   a. Sexual relations
   b. Mental health
   c. Elder mistreatment
   d. Healing practices

10. Which of the following AAPI groups experience the most devastating levels of discrimination?
    a. Lesbians
    b. Gay men
    c. Bisexuals
    d. Transgender

Key

1. b
2. c
3. d
4. a
5. b
6. c
7. c
8. d
9. a
10. d

Resources

Asian Pacific American Legal Center: www.gleh.org

Asian Pacific Policy & Planning Council: www.asianpacificpolicyplanningcouncil.org

Asian and Pacific Islander Queers United for Action: www.aquadc.org

Asian and Pacific Islander Wellness Center: www.apiwellness.org

Asian Pacific Islander Resource Kit: www.glaad.org

Gay Asian Pacific Alliance: www.gapa.org

Gay Asian Pacific Support Network: www.gapsn.org

National Asian Pacific Center on Aging: www.napca.org

National Queer Asian Pacific Islander Alliance: www.noapia.org

Pacific Center for Human Growth: www.pacificcenter.org

Southeast Asia Resource Action Center: www.searac.org

References

Administration on Aging. (n.d.). *A statistical profile of Asian older Americans aged 65 and older*. Retrieved November 15, 2014 from http://www.aoa.gov/AoARoot/Aging_Statistics/Minority_Aging/Facts-on-API-Elderly2008-plain_format.aspx.

Africa, J., & Carrasco, M. (2011). *Asian American and Pacific Islander mental health: Report from a NAMI listening session*. Retrieved December 8, 2014 from www.name.org/Template.cfm?Section=Multicultural_Support1&Template=/ContentManagement/ContentDispaly.cfm&ContentID=115281.

Alcedo, M. (2014). *LGBT Filipino community*. Retrieved October 31, 2014 from http://sageusa.org/about/face/cfm?ID=22.

Anderson, I., Crengle, S., Kamaka, M. L., Chen, T. H., Palafox, N., & Jackson-Pulver, L. (2006). Indigenous health in Australia, New Zealand, and Pacific. *Lancet, 367*(9524), 1775–1785.

Asai, M. O., & Kameoka, V. A. (2005). The influence of Sekentei on family caregiving and underutilization of social services among Japanese caregivers. *Social Work, 50*, 111–118.

Balabis, J., Pobutsky, A., Baker, K. K., Tottori, C., & Salvail, F. (2007). *The burden of cardiovascular disease in Hawaii 2007*. Hawaii: Hawaii State Department of Health Retrieved November 20, 2014 form www.health.hawaii.gov/brfss/2013/11/TheBurdenofCVD.pdf.

Bhattar, R. G., & Victoria, N. A. (2007). Rainbow rice: A dialogue between two Asian American gay men in higher education and student affairs. *The Vermont Connection, 28*, 39–50.

Blaisdell, R. K. (1996). 1995 update on Kanaka Maoli (Indigenous Hawaiian) health. *Asian Pacific Islander Health, 4*(1–3), 160–165.

Boulden, W. T. (2009). Gay Hmong: A multifaceted clash of cultures. *Journal of Gay & Lesbian Social Services, 21*, 134–150.

Braun, K. L., Yang, H., Onaka, A. T., & Horiuchi, B. Y. (1997). Asian and Pacific Islander mortality differences in Hawaii. *Biodemogrphy and Social Biology, 44*(3/4), 213–226.

California Health Information Survey. (2010). *2010 survey*. Retrieved November 20, 2014 from www.chris.ucla.edu.

Dang, A., & Hu, M. (2005). *Asian Pacific American lesbian, gay, bisexual and transgender people: A community portrait. A report from New York's queer Asian Pacific Legacy Conference, 2004*. New York: National Gay and Lesbian Task Force Policy Institute.

Eng, D. L., & Hom, A. Y. (1998). *Q & A: Queer in Asian America*. Philadelphia: Temple University Press.

Grant, J. M., Mottet, L. A., Tanis, J., Harrison, J., Herman, J. L., & Keisling, M. (2011). *Injustice at every turn: A report of the National transgender discrimination survey*. Washington DC: National Center for Transgender Equality and National Gay and Lesbian Task Force. Retrieved December 5, 2014 from www.endtransdiscrimination.org/PDFs/NTDS_Report.pdf.

Green, A. R., Ngo-Metzger, Q., Legedza, A. T. R., Massagli, M. P., Phillips, S. R., & Iezzoni, L. I. (2005). Interpreter services, language concordance, and health care quality: Experiences of Asian Americans with limited English proficiency. *Journal of General Internal Medicine, 20*(11), 1050–1056.

Hahm, H. C., & Adkins, C. (2009). A model of Asian and Pacific Islander sexual minority acculturation. *Journal of LGBT Youth, 6*, 155–173.

Haviland, M. G., Morales, L. S., Dial, T. H., & Pincus, H. A. (2005). Race/ethnicity, socioeconomic status, and satisfaction with health care. *American Journal of Medical Quality, 20*(4), 195–203.

Holland, A. T., & Palaniappan, L. P. (2012). Problems with the collection and interpretation of Asian American health data: Omission, aggression, and extrapolation. *Annals of Epidemiology, 22*, 397–405.

Hu, A. (2012). *Introduction to basic Asian values*. Retrieved November 8, 2014 from http://www.asianweek.com/2012/04/28/introduction-to-basic-asian-values/.

Jones, R. S., Chow, T. W., & Gatz, M. (2006). Asian Americans and Alzheimer's disease: Assimilation, culture, and beliefs. *Journal of Aging Studies, 20*(1), 11–215.

Kastanis, A., & Gates, G. J. (2013). *LGBT Asian and Pacific Islander individuals and same-sex couples*. Los Angeles: The Williams Institute, UCLA School of Law. Retrieved November 21, 2014 from www.williamsintitute.law/ucla.edu/research/census-lgbt-demographics-studies/lgbt-api-report-sept-2013/.

Kim, B. S. K. (2011). *Counseling Asian Americans*. Belmont: Cengage.

Kim, W., & Keefe, R. H. (2010). Barriers to healthcare among Asian Americans. *Social Work in Public Health, 25*, 286–295.

Mangton, P., Carvalho, M., & Pandya, S. (2002). *Lesbian, gay, bisexual, and transgender health. A Brown Paper: The health of South Asians in the United States*. South Asian Public Health Association. Retrieved November 21, 2014 from www.sapha.org/adminkit/uploads/files/BrownPaper-LGBTHealth.pdf.

Mau, M. K. (2010). *Health and health care of Native Hawaiian & older Pacific Islander older adults*. Retrieved November 19, 2014 from http://geriatrics.stanford.edu/ethnomed/hawaiian_pacific_islander.

Minino, A. M., Heron, M. P., Murphy, S. L., & Kochankek, K. D. (2007). Deaths: Final data for 2004. *National Vital Statistics Reports, 55*(19), 1–120.

National Asian Pacific American Families Against Substance Abuse. (n.d.). *Fact sheet*. Retrieved November 20, 2014 from www.napafasa.org/resources/factsheets.htm.

Office of Minority Health. (n.d.). *Mental health and Asians*. Retrieved November 20, 2014 from http://minorityhealth.hhs.gov/tempplates/content/aspx?1v1=3&1v1IID=9&ID=6476.

Pew Research Center. (2013). *The rise of Asian Americans*. Washington DC: Author. Retrieved December 4, 2014 from www.pewsocialtrends.org/files/2013/04/Asian-Americans-new-full-report-04-2013.pdf.

Ponce, N. A. (2011). What a difference a data set and advocacy make for AAPI health. *Asian American & Pacific Islander Policy, Practice, and Community, 9*(1–2), 159–162.

Queer Southeast Asian Census. (2012). *A census of our own: The state of queer Southeast Asian America*. Retrieved December 10, 2014 from www.prysm.us/wp-content/uploads/2012/08/QSEAReportExecutiveSummary.pdf.

Reyes-Salvail, F., Liang, S., & Nguyen, D. H. (2008). Frequent mental distress prevalence and disparity: Hawaii BRFSS 2005–2007. *The Hawaii Behavioral Risk Factor Surveillance System Special Report, 6*(2). Retrieved November 20, 2014 from www.health.Hawaii.gov/brfss/files/2013/11/Frequent_Mental_Distress.pdf.

Salvail, F. R., Nguyen, D., & Huang, T. (2003). *State of Hawaii, Behavioral Risk Factor Surveillance System, From 2001 to 2003—By ethnicity, tobacco use, alcohol use*. Retrieved November 20, 2014 from http://www.hawaii.gov/health/statistics/brfss/index.html.

Schiller, J. S., Lucus, J. W., Peregoy, J. A. (2012). *Summary health statistics for U.S. adults: National Health Interview Survey 2011*. Washington DC: National Center for Health Statistics. *Vital Health Statistics, 10*(256).

Sorkin, D. A., & Ngo-Metzger, Q. (2014). The unique health status and health care experiences of older Asian Americans: Research findings and treatment recommendations. *Clinical Gerontologist, 37*, 18–32.

Sue, D. W., & Sue, D. (2013). *Counseling the culturally diverse: Theory and practice* (6th ed.). Hoboken: John Wiley & Sons.

Takeuchi, D., Alegria, M., Jackson, J., & Williams, D. (2007). Immigration and mental health: Diverse findings in Asian, Black, and Latino populations. *American Journal of Public Health, 97*(1), 11–12.

Ting, J., & Hwang, W. C. (2009). Cultural influences on help-seeking attitudes in Asian American students. *American Journal of Orthopsychiatry, 79*, 125–132.

Trinh-Shevrin, C., Islam, N. S., & Rey, M. J. (2009). *Asian American communities and health: Context, research, policy, and action*. San Francisco: Jossey-Bass.

Tseng, T. (2011). Understanding Anti-LGBT bias: An analysis of Chinese-speaking Americans' attitudes toward LGBT people in Southern California. *LGBTQ Policy Journal*. Harvard Kennedy School. Retrieved November 21, 2014 from http://isites.harvard.edu/icb/icb.do?keyword=k78405&pageeid=icb.page414494.

U.S. Census Bureau. (2010). *The 2011 statistical abstract*. Retrieved November 14, 2014 from http://www.census.gov/compendia/statab/cats/education/educational_attainment.html.

U.S. Census Bureau. (2011a). *Current population survey, annual social and economic supplement, 2010*. Retrieved November 14, 2014 from http://www.census.gov/population/www.sodemo/race/ppl-aa10.html.

U.S. Census Bureau. (2011b). *Hispanic heritage month*. Retrieved November 14, 2014 from http://www.census.gov/newsroom/release/archives/facts_for_features_special_editions/cb11-ff18.html.

U.S. Census Bureau. (2012, March). *The Asian population: 2010*. Washington DC: Author.

U.S. Census Bureau. (2014). *American community survey*. Retrieved December 11, 2014 from www.census.gov/acs/www/.

U.S. Office of Minority Health Resource Center. (2010). *Highlights in minority health and health disparities, Asian American and Pacific Islander profile*. Retrieved November 20, 2014 from www.cec.gov/omhd/highlights/2010/HMay10.html.

Watari, K. F., & Gatz, M. (2004). Pathways to care for Alzheimer's disease among Korean Americans. *Cultural Diversity & Ethnic Minority Psychology, 10*, 23–38.

Williamson, O., Gordon, F., & Pacheco, B. (2014). *Aging into poverty: Economic insecurity among older adults of color & GBT elders*. Retrieved December 4, 2014 from www.nclc.org/images/pdf/conferences_and_webinar_trainings/presentations/2013-2014/aging_into_poverty_webinar_smaller.pdf.

Yee, B. W. K., Debaryshe, B. D., Yuen, S., Kim, S. Y., & Mccubbin, H. I. (2008). *Asian American and Pacific Islander families: Resiliency and life-span socialization in a cultural context*. Retrieved November 18, 2014 from www.uhfamily.hawaii.edu/publications/journals/aapifamiliesbookchapter.pdf.

Yu, E. S., Kim, K., Liu, W. T., & Wong, S. C. (1993). Functional abilities of Chinese and Korean elder in congregate housing. In D. Barressi & D. Stull (Eds.), *Ethnic elderly and long term care* (pp. 87–100). New York: Springer.

Melanie D. Otis

Abstract

The focus of this chapter is on understanding relevant factors that may contribute to the unique experiences and challenges faced by LGBT elders of European descent. While it is often assumed that all white LGBT elders are part of a homogeneous group, the diverse cultures that can be found across the fifty countries that comprise Europe suggest that such an assumption would be misguided. In addition to the misconceptions that may result from researchers and helping professionals viewing European elders of LGBT descent as a monolithic group, is the fact that the heritage of many LGBT elders of European descent may encompass more than one country, and thus include influences from more than a single culture. This chapter considers the ways human service professionals can improve their capacity to meet the needs of all LGBT elders by considering the myriad factors that make individuals unique.

Keywords

European descent · Ethnic ambiguity · Intersectionality · Cultural competence · Families of choice

Overview

The challenges of identifying, studying, and responding to the needs and experiences of other groups generally acknowledged as representatives of the face of diversity in the LGBT community tend to ignore the heterogeneity of members of this racial majority. This chapter—which is focused on LGBT elders of European descent and presented alongside the chapters dedicated to Hispanic, Native American, and African American LGBT elders—facilitates viewing diversity in *all* its forms. The chapter clarifies what we do know and do not know about this group by integrating a discussion of LGBT elders of European descent within the

M.D. Otis (✉)
University of Kentucky, Lexington, USA
e-mail: Melanie.Otis@uky.edu

larger field of inquiry. The chapter seeks to extend our explication of what we know and what we still need to learn about the diverse lives and needs of *all* LGBT elders. This reorientation of framework permits the understanding that alongside failures to include race and ethnicity as meaningful distinctions in research and practice knowledge, we also have little awareness of what it means to live in rural areas or what it is like to be a poor or working-class LGBT elder of any race or ethnicity. A primary goal of this chapter is to dismantle counterproductive yet persistent stereotypes that the lives of all LGBT persons can be sufficiently understood through the lens of the lives of White, Anglo-Saxon, middle-class, college-educated young gay men and lesbians. To lay the foundation for a more nuanced understanding of LGBT elders of European descent, a brief discussion of the history of research and practice as it relates to this population will be articulated, and a framework will be developed to identify parameters that define LGBT elders of European descent as a unique group of individuals distinguishable from others with whom they are often grouped. This definition will lead to delineating challenges of understanding the experiences of individuals of European descent. Once the population has been defined, perspectives on coming out and self-disclosure as lesbian, gay, bisexual, or transgender at different points across the life course will be considered. The potential relevance of cohort effects (e.g., pre/post-Stonewall, Baby Boomers) on decisions about when and if one discloses his/her status as a sexual minority will be considered, along with an exploration of the difficulties that come with having the power to control the decision to disclose taken away by circumstances associated with one's own aging or the aging of one's partner, friend, or family member.

Learning Objectives

By the end of the chapter, the reader should be able to:

1. Explain reasons why it is important to consider the relevance of country of origin in the lives of LGBT elders of European descent.
2. Explain why research involving predominantly or entirely white samples should be viewed with caution even when applying the findings to persons who identify as white.
3. List steps that need to be taken to develop culturally competent practice and policies to meet the needs of LGBT elders.
4. Identify key historical events that may impact the lives of LGBT elders of European descent.

Introduction

This chapter marks a notable departure from past approaches to acknowledging the diversity and complexity of the LGBT population. The presence of a stand-alone chapter focused on LGBT elders of European descent alongside the chapters dedicated to Hispanic (e.g., Chap. 10), Native American (e.g., Chap. 7), and African American LGBT elders (e.g., Chap. 6) (among others) (e.g., Chaps. 8, 13) makes a significant statement about the importance of viewing diversity in *all* its forms. Rather than simply creating a juxtaposition of other racial and ethnic groups against the backdrop of some previously established and tacitly accepted one-dimensional, monochromatic mass labeled "Whites," this chapter represents an explicit effort to clarify what we do know and do not know about this group by integrating the discussion of LGBT elders of European descent within the larger field of inquiry in a more balanced and informative way. The challenges of identifying, studying, and responding to the experiences and needs of other groups generally acknowledged as representatives of the face of diversity in the LGBT community tend to encourage us to ignore the heterogeneity of members of this (current) racial majority. It has been suggested that the tacit acceptance of the dominance of the majority group leads members of the group to fail to see their own characteristics (e.g., race, ethnicity, social class) (Gelfand 2003). In so doing, we lose track of the reality that the white LGBT elder population consists of people from numerous countries characterized by diverse heritages and cultural norms, who self-identify across the gender spectrum and who live in different geographical corners of the USA under different economic conditions. Thus, this chapter seeks to extend our explication of what we know and what we still need to learn about the diverse lives and needs of *all* LGBT elders. It represents an effort to move scholarly inquiry, the development of best practice models, the enhancement of health and human services, and the relevant policy-related knowledge beyond crude distinctions based solely on race and ethnicity, without ignoring the reality of the importance of either (McDermott and Samson 2005). This reorientation of our framework for defining difference will allow us to see that alongside our frequent failure to include race and ethnicity as meaningful distinctions in our research and practice knowledge, we also have little awareness of what it means to live in rural areas or what it is like to be a poor or working-class LGBT elder of any race or ethnicity. In the end, a primary goal of this chapter is to move us one step closer to dismantling the counterproductive yet persistent stereotype that the lives of all LGBT persons can be sufficiently understood through the lens of the lives of white, Anglo-Saxon, middle-class, college-educated young gay men and lesbians.

To begin to lay the foundation for a more nuanced understanding of LGBT elders of European descent, a brief discussion of the history of research and practice as it relates to this population will be articulated. With this background in place, a framework will be developed to identify parameters that define LGBT elders of European descent as a unique group of individuals that can be distinguished from others with whom they are often lumped based solely on skin color. This definition will provide a platform for delineating the challenges of understanding the experiences of individuals of European descent when so much about how we view the group is based on ignoring any factors that make individuals unique and when so many of these

lesbians, gay men, bisexuals, and transgender persons have ancestral histories that encompass more than one national lineage. Once the population has been defined, perspectives on challenges associated with coming out and self-disclosure as a lesbian, gay, bisexual, or transgender at different points across the life course will be considered. The potential relevance of cohort effects (e.g., pre/post-Stonewall, Baby Boomers) on decisions about when and if one discloses his/her status as a sexual minority will be considered, along with an exploration of the difficulties that come with having the power to control the decision to disclose taken away by circumstances associated with one's own aging or the aging of one's partner, friend, or family member.

Utilizing Crenshaw's (1989) notion of intersectionality[1] will offer a framework for examining the somewhat unique way that individuals who may be viewed by many as a member of the majority (without the privileges that accompanying that position of power) become a double (and in the case of lesbians triple) minority by virtue of their immutable status associated with being elderly and their ascribed status as a result of being a sexual minority. Further distinctions among LGBT elderly of European descent will be considered in terms of the impact of geographical location, population density, and economic status. Finally, the chapter offers a look at extant service delivery models and interdisciplinary approaches currently being used in the USA and considers the influence of various disciplines on these models and programs. These models and programs will be considered in relation to efforts that are currently being

---

[1]Crenshaw's (1989) notion of the intersectionality of disadvantaged minority statuses focused on the multiple intersecting forms of oppression and discrimination that serve to compound the disadvantaged status of black women. This work was later revisited and further developed as a key part of Patricia Hill Collins's (1990) standpoint theory which offered a perspective for understanding the unique experiences of individuals who embody different minority statuses based on sex, race, ethnicity, socioeconomic status, sexual orientation, and gender identity.

undertaken in European countries, offering a foundation for identifying issues that are still in need of resolution.

History of Research and Practice Related to LGBT Elders of European Descent

Compared to that of non-LGBT persons, research on the lives of LGBT persons of any age is fairly new, with the earliest scholarly work predominantly focusing on the lives of younger gay men and, to a lesser degree, lesbians (Brown 2009). In the 1970s, however, a number of studies shifted their focus to LG elders. That early work was plagued by a variety of methodological problems, not the least of which was the reality of sampling limitations associated with barriers (e.g., fear, discrimination, victimization) that limited access to the full spectrum of persons representing the LGBT population…a challenge that continues to impact LGBT-focused research today (Bettinger 2010; Grossman 2008; Meezan and Martin 2009). With much of this early (and current) research relying on non-probability sampling techniques such as snowball sampling of friendship networks and readily accessible convenience sampling of patrons at gay and lesbian bars and LG community events, the developing images of LG lives suggested that LGBT elders simply did not exist—and if they did, they were best characterized as lonely, isolated, and depressed. Based on the dominance of gay men in much of this research, those early studies also seemed to suggest that lesbians, bisexuals, and transgender persons were also nonexistent (Shankle et al. 2003).

In 2010, Fredriksen-Goldsen and Muraco published a systematic review of 25 years of literature on LGBT elders (1984–2008). They utilized a life course perspective to examine "the interplay of the social context and historical times" to understand how both the lives of LGBT elders and the research that has attempted to illuminate our understanding of those lives are embedded in the social and historical context of the times (Fredriksen-Goldsen and Muraco 2010, p. 402). They identified a total of 58 studies that included samples of LGBT elders (50 years of age or older). Regardless of whether the work focused on gay men, lesbians, or both, much like research reported prior to 1984, samples were predominantly white and urban. For instance, 17 % involved samples that were exclusively white, and another 43 % were predominantly white (75 % or more of the sample were white). An additional 24 % of the studies either failed to collect or failed to report this information, suggesting a greater likelihood that these studies involved predominantly or exclusively white participants as well. Unlike much of the pre-1984 research, this body of work demonstrated a balance between exclusively male (21 %) and exclusively lesbian (22 %) samples, with all other samples involving both male and female participants that were represented in fairly balanced numbers within studies.[2] Approximately one-third (31 %) of the studies included some bisexual participants (ranging from 2 to 25 %[3] of the total sample); however, transgender persons were only included in two of the studies, and the study findings failed to specifically address them as a unique group. In terms of location, only 5 % of studies involved exclusively rural samples compared to 34 % involving urban samples. With 41 % failing to identify the geographical location of respondents, it is again likely that these samples were either exclusively or largely urban.

While this work had broken through the limited perspective offered by previous studies of younger lesbians and gay men, the challenges of achieving representativeness were far from overcome. This was particularly true when considering LGBT elders who were born in the early 1900s, where access can be described as difficult at best. Additionally, while some limited success may have been achieved in efforts to engage

---

[2] One study did not collect data on gender (Fredriksen-Goldsen and Muraco 2010).

[3] This study involved a snowball sampling of 16 women (75 % lesbian and 25 % bisexual) who were interviewed about their experiences as grandmothers (Orel and Fruhauf 2006).

elder lesbians and gay men in research, the inclusion of bisexual men and women in research has lagged far behind this initial research involving lesbians and gay men—and at best we can say that we are just now *beginning* to conduct meaningful focused inquiry into the lives of transgender persons of *any age* (Fredriksen-Goldsen and Muraco 2010; Grant et al. 2011; Hartzell et al. 2009).

Despite the limitations of this early research, we can say that we know a bit more about the lives of lesbian, gay, bisexual, and transgender elders today than we did in the 1970s. We know that gay and lesbian elders are more likely to be single (Brennan-Ing et al. 2014; IOM 2011; MetLife 2006, 2010), live alone (Brennan-Ing et al. 2014; Shippy et al. 2004; Wallace et al. 2011), and more likely to not have children (Fredriksen-Goldsen et al. 2011). Studies focusing on mental well-being have often identified higher levels of psychiatric disorders among LGB persons when compared with their heterosexual counterparts (Cochran et al. 2003; Meyer 2003). A variety of studies have found higher rates of disability, cardiovascular disease (Diamant and Wold 2003; Roberts et al. 2003), and certain cancers, as well as other health conditions among lesbian elders (Fredriksen-Goldsen et al. 2011). These issues may be tied to higher rates of obesity among lesbians (Boehmer et al. 2007; Clunis et al. 2005) and cigarette smoking which have been found by numerous studies (Case et al. 2004; Conron et al. 2010; Valanis et al. 2000). While gay men do not experience the same higher rates of obesity, a number of studies indicate that gay men are more likely to be dissatisfied with their bodies, which may contribute to eating disorders and concomitant health problems as they age (Kaminski et al. 2005; Russell and Keel 2002). Additionally, a significant, and growing, number of gay elders are likely to be living with HIV/AIDS (Dolcini et al. 2003; Effros et al. 2008), and their risks of contracting the virus or other STDs are elevated by the fact that they are often sexually active in the absence of using safe sex practices. The failure of medical professionals to acknowledge LGBT elders as sexual beings contributes greatly to this

problem. Exacerbating the negative impact of these physical and mental health problems, we also know that lesbians and bisexual women are more likely to live in poverty than gay men or heterosexual men or women (Albelda et al. 2009; Prokos and Keene 2010), a reality that often limits access to needed healthcare and other services as these women age (Espinoza 2011).

As previously noted, much of the extant research has failed to specifically address the experiences of bisexual men and women. Yet, the limited information we have to date suggests that the lives of bisexual men and women differ from the lives of lesbians and gay men in a number of relevant ways. For instance, elder bisexual men and women are more likely to have been married to an opposite-sex partner at some time in their lives and more likely to have children compared to lesbians and gay men (Pew Research Center 2013). While this may change for future generations, this reality in the lives of contemporary bisexual men and women offers both pluses and minuses. Bisexual men and women have been found to have a larger support network in the heterosexual community than their lesbian and gay counterparts (Grossman et al. 2000). This increases the likelihood that bisexual men and women may have additional forms of support, but it also decreases the likelihood that they will be integrated into the LGBT community and the potential sources of individual and organizational support that may be accessed there (Grossman et al. 2000).

Our understanding of the lives of transgender elders is even more limited. In general, researchers have either failed to ask whether study participants identify as transgender or, when the information is gathered, have ended up with samples of insufficient size to offer any meaningful insights that extend our understanding of their lives much beyond that of a case study (Brown and Grossman 2014). These studies do offer some important insights into the unique and difficult experiences of transgender elders, however. A notable exception to this dearth of research is the Transgender Discrimination Survey that was conducted by the National Center for Transgender Equality and the National Gay and

Lesbian Task Force (Grant et al. 2011). Family rejection was found to be a significant issue (reported by 57 % of the sample) in the lives of transgender persons in their study, thus increasing the likelihood that transgender elders live alone.

Finally, a certain irony of the limitations of much of LGBT research is particularly relevant to this discussion. Whether it be due to a lack of access or methodological issues, our knowledge of LGBT elders is dominated by information that has been gleaned predominantly from individuals who are presumably primarily of European descent. These studies offer us the best insight into the lives of LGBT elders of European descent, despite the fact that they include white people from non-European countries and may also include a small number of persons of color who are unable to be analyzed separately or comparatively. However, given the dominance of whites in these studies, they offer us a better understanding of LGBT elders of European descent than do any other group who may be marginally represented. Thus, it is noteworthy to acknowledge that research intentionally focused on studying the lives of LGBT elders of European descent does not exist by design; however, albeit by default, there is a growing body of work dominated by a well-educated, largely middle-class, urban subset of elders of European descent that continues to influence practice and policy related to all LGBT elders.

Defining the European LGBT Elder Population

Simply put, LGBT elders of European descent are those individuals whose ancestry is rooted in Europe. In the USA, this group includes individuals who may have been born in Europe and subsequently immigrated to the USA either as a child or as an adult, as well as many who represent the subsequent generations of earlier immigrants (some of whom may have US roots that span multiple generations). Their ancestral background can be traced to any one of the 50 countries that make up Europe, from the largest country—Russia (population of 142.1 million)—to the smallest—the Republic of San Marino (population of 40,000),[4] with the most substantial influence on the current US population of European descent originating from England, Ireland, Scotland, and/or Italy. The daunting numbers of distinctive heritages, and associated cultural norms, languages, religions, and perspectives, represented by the countries that constitute Europe have generally been ignored by researchers considering the relevance of ethnicity in lives of the diverse population that lives in the USA (see Table 9.1 for a list of European countries). Increasingly, however, alongside the persistent call to conduct research that allows for meaningful examination of differences that may be associated with being African America, Latino or Latina, Native American, among others, has been at least some recognition that "white" is simply an insufficient distinction to capture the meaningful differences that impact the lives of this heterogeneous group (McDermott and Samson 2005; Richmond and Guindon 2013).

Estimating the portion of the US population that can be identified as elders of European descent is equally challenging. Our most comprehensive accounting of persons in the USA comes from the US Census Bureau. Estimates from the decennial census (last completed in 2010) provide us with a fairly accurate enumeration of the number of people living in the country at the time of data collection, yet European descent is not captured as a distinct category in the census data collection process. Instead, much like other less comprehensive accountings of the population, individuals of European descent are included in the broader category labeled "White, non-Hispanic." This group consists not only of individuals of European descent, but also individuals who originate

---

[4]Technically, the smallest country in Europe is the Vatican City (population approximately 840). This sovereign city-state covers 110 acres within the city of Rome, Italy. It is the home of the Pope, with all other citizens being either clergy (the majority of the population), officials of the state, or members of the Swiss Guard (responsible for the Pope's safety).

Table 9.1 List of 50 European countries

Albania	Estonia	Lithuania	San Marino
Andorra	Finland	Luxembourg	Serbia
Armenia	France	Macedonia	Slovakia
Austria	Georgia	Malta	Slovenia
Azerbaijan	Germany	Moldova	Spain
Belarus	Greece	Monaco	Sweden
Belgium	Hungary	Montenegro	Switzerland
Bosnia and Herzegovina	Iceland	The Netherlands	Turkey
Bulgaria	Ireland	Norway	Ukraine
Croatia	Italy	Poland	UK
Cyprus	Kosovo	Portugal	Vatican City (Holy See)
The Czech Republic	Latvia	Romania	
Denmark	Liechtenstein	Russia	

from either North Africa or the Middle East. The 2010 Census estimates that there were approximately 40 million White, non-Hispanic persons who were 65 and older at that time (roughly 13 % of the total population). Of that number, around 5.5 million were 85 or older. While these estimates can be viewed as fairly accurate, the next step of attempting to estimate the number of these individuals who are LGBT elders of European descent is far more challenging and precludes creating any particularly precise parameter estimates of this group. In the face of these limitations, we must draw on our best available data as a basis for estimating this population. Based on the initial consistently cited estimates established by the Kinsey Institute (Kinsey et al. 1947) of 10 % and more recent studies which place the percentage of LGBT persons somewhere around 3.5 % of the population (Gates and Newport 2013), we can assess the current number of LGBT elders (65 and older) of European descent living in the USA to be somewhere between 1.1 and 3.4 million. Based on broader demographers' estimates for all persons in the USA, with the aging of the Baby Boomer cohort (those born between 1946 and 1964), by 2030, we can expect this number to double (Gates and Cooke 2011).

Historically, the US LGBT population has been treated as some monolithic entity that is best represented by the face of Americans of European descent. That notion has since been challenged both from within the LGBT community and by those outside the community. Today, the LGBT elder population of European descent is understood as one part of a very complex and diverse population, rather than being viewed as the gold standard for understanding all LGBT persons. While this issue is not unique to research involving sexual and gender minorities, the exposure of the color blindness of LGBT research was an important key to the development of a broader, more culturally competent approach to research focused on the lives of sexual and gender minorities (Donahue and McDonald 2005; Meezan and Martin 2009). Whereas the body of work focusing on ethnically and racially diverse samples of LGBT elders remains limited, new scholarship appears on a regular basis. We are beginning to better understand the unique impact (or at least the reality of its existence) of ethnicity and race on the lives of lesbians, gay men, bisexual men and women, and transgendered persons (Herek et al. 2010). Yet, like so many debates on intersectionality and its impact on well-being, we are challenged to find ways to avoid trading one myopic approach to scholarship and practice for another. For instance, missing in much of the extant literature is any recognition that being poor and lesbian, gay, bisexual, or transgender is different than being an L, G, B, or T person who is economically and/or socially defined as working class, middle class, or upper class. As a group of individuals of European descent may be more likely to inhabit particular socioeconomic strata in some geographical locations, economic differences impact individuals from all races and ethnicities. Thus, in many ways, we are still trying to understand the needs and experiences of poor and working-class LGBT persons of European descent. Similarly, we know relatively little about the lives of LGBT elders who live largely hidden in rural areas and small towns and cities throughout the country (Jackson et al. 2008; Otis 2009; Willging et al. 2006). See Chap. 25 for further discussion of LGBT elders in rural areas.

Cultural and Ethnic Ambiguity

Understanding what constitutes an ethnic group is an important first step in considering the challenges that are faced by elders of European descent. Ethnicity has both geographical and cultural relevance. First, ethnic groups are linked together by a common origin—no matter where one may be living today, his or her Scottish (or Irish, or Russian, or Italian, or Slovakian) ancestry offers an historic link to the past and a personal (or virtual) connection to others with whom he or she shares a common lineage. Beyond a simple geographical place on a globe, one's ethnicity can be understood in terms of the many unique cultural norms, values, beliefs, and traditions that define one's heritage as distinct from some other outwardly similar, yet unique group. Some of these cultural realities have been adopted and co-opted in myriad ways as part of US culture, while others may only endure through purposive effort on the part of group members. For instance, many of us may have food as our only insight into other ethnic groups. In larger cities, evidence of the importance of those roots is found in the contemporary presence of places like Little Italy, Chinatown, and other purposively created and sustained subcultures and ethnically homogeneous neighborhoods within the larger community. Within these areas, numerous restaurants and businesses exist that retain and celebrate the culture of origin of the inhabitants. Outside these communities and across the country, "Americanized" versions are marketed to others (often by corporations which have no connection to the represented culture), thus exposing others to the food and culture of distant places like France, Greece, Italy, or Spain. For the most part, we know little else about what makes these places unique... what makes them more than just European countries. Yet, for many who retain close connections to their heritage, culturally bound norms related to things like gender roles, sexual behavior, and religious beliefs may still have a significant impact on their personal identity.

Depending on a variety of factors, most people we encounter throughout the day to day of our lives will have little if any awareness of our ancestry. If we immigrated as a child or later in life, we might present with a slight (or pronounced) accent that leads people to wonder (or readily identify) our country of origin, but if we are US born and/or raised, the original foundation of our heritage may remain invisible to others. In research and practice, the diverse cultural backgrounds of individuals of European descent are largely ignored in favor of focusing on presumed commonalities and similarities associated with race—more specifically, white race (McDermott and Samson 2005). While it can be argued that the response of others may be dominated by assumptions that are based on the color of one's skin, this reality speaks to only one piece of what influences our life experiences and personal identities. The relevance of these cultural factors may become increasingly important as one ages and moves into a developmental stage in life where reflection on the past may be an important and valuable part of the aging process (Erikson 1982).

Historically, American culture has often been defined by a presumed universality of the meaning of being of European descent. When a critical lens was first placed on the practice of assuming that White, Anglo-Saxon people could effectively serve as informative windows into the lives of all Americans, the censure immediately focused on issues of race and ethnicity. Distinctions in race currently identified by the US Census include White (Caucasian), Black or African American, Asian, American Indian or Alaskan Native, and Native Hawaiian or Pacific Islander,[5] while ethnicity largely focuses on distinguishing between Hispanic or Latino or non-Hispanic or Latino (U.S. Census Bureau 2010). These distinctions offer no meaningful mechanism for examining potential similarities and differences between white persons of European descent and those who are not of European descent.

As various aspects of the lives of LGBT elders of European descent are considered in this chapter, it is worth noting that within Europe, the treatment of LGBT persons has been inconsistent across the continent. For instance, an LGBT person who is 85 years of age or older in 2014 would have been a teenager or young adult during the Holocaust. For older LGBT persons with German and/or Austrian heritage, the implications of Nazi Germany's treatment of homosexuals (specifically gay men) have etched a chilling image of the cost of being a sexual minority (or any minority) in a society highly invested in maintaining the power of a dominant group (Grau and Shoppmann 2013). Perhaps even more compelling, however, was the reality that Allied troops' liberation of those interned in concentration camps and prisons throughout Germany did not necessarily include imprisoned homosexuals, many of whom were required to complete their sentences before being released. Similarly, while the majority of laws created to validate Hitler's treatment of Jews and others were immediately repealed by the Allied Military Government of Germany, Paragraph 175 that prohibited homosexuality stayed on the books until 1969. This legacy speaks to the persistence of anti-LGBT sentiment in Europe at that time.

---

[5]The US Census also allows individuals to identify as "some other" race or more than one race.

Research Box 9.1: Differences in Treatment of Sexual Minorities in European Countries

European Union Agency for Fundamental Rights (2014). *European Union lesbian, gay, bisexual and transgender survey: Main results*. Author.

Objective: In 2010, the European Parliament called on the European Union to conduct a survey to examine the experiences of sexual minorities in European Member States. Specifically, the study sought to assess the prevalence of discrimination and victimization experienced by lesbians, gay men, and transgender persons.

Method: Between April 2012 and July 2012, the European Union Agency for Fundamental Rights launched an online survey to collect data from LGBT persons living in all European Member States and Croatia. The study collected data from 93,079 participants (lesbians = 16 %, gay men = 62 %, bisexual women = 7 %, bisexual men = 8 %, and transgender = 7 %). Approximately 5 % (n = 4794) of the sample was of age 55 or older.

Results: Three key findings from the study raise potential concerns. First, 47 % of the participants indicated that they had been discriminated against or harassed due to their sexual minority status. Additionally, the majority of the respondents (59 %) had been either threatened or attacked due to their perceived LGBT identity. Despite these experiences, survey respondents indicated that they rarely reported these experiences because they felt authorities would be unlikely to take any action.

Questions:

1. How might data from this study provide insight into the lives of older LGBT persons of European descent who have recently moved to the USA?

2. What does the discrepancy between the frequency of experiences of victimization and discrimination versus the frequency of reporting such events suggest about the social context in which LGBT persons live in European countries?
3. How do you think these findings might compare to data from the USA?

Finally, it is important to keep in mind that individuals of European descent may have diverse backgrounds that involve multiple European heritages. Understanding the concept of ethnic ambiguity may offer us some insight into the potential complexity of such a diverse heritage. Ethnic ambiguity refers to one possessing a mixture of ethnicity which makes it difficult for others to readily identify the person's ethnicity. As the population becomes increasingly integrated, more and more people have ethnicities that are not only ambiguous to the observer, but may also be difficult for the individual to integrate as well.

With the largest immigrant populations in the USA originating from Ireland, England, Scotland, and Germany, many of whom settled in common areas and subsequently married immigrants from other European countries, today's US population of European descent may have limited knowledge of or connection to their European heritage. Among early waves of immigrants, particularly from Western Europe, there was considerable encouragement to assimilate into a new identity as an American, thus shedding any allegiance to their European roots. In the years that followed, changes in emphasis on ethnicity would lead many immigrants to actively work to acknowledge and retain their ancestral heritage (Gelfand 2003). The challenge of integrating this heritage into their identities, when being viewed as part of a monolithic group labeled "White, non-Hispanic," has important implications for understanding how LGBT elders of European descent may view themselves and the challenges they may encounter trying to create an integrated identity that includes ethnic heritage.

Coming Out and Disclosure

Across the life course, the role of disclosure of one's status as a sexual minority retains some common threads as well as presenting some unique challenges. Regardless of one's age, coming out and the process of disclosure to others are experiences that can elicit a multiplicity of feelings, from excitement to fear—and sometimes these seemingly divergent responses across the emotional spectrum can occur concurrently (Cohen and Savin-Williams 1996). In adolescence, the process of coming out as an LGBT person is often viewed as a logical part of the developmental process that occurs as young people become aware of themselves as sexual beings and experience attractions to others (Markus and Nurius 1986). While that in no way eliminates the many concerns that are felt by the LGBT adolescent, for those to whom the youth discloses her/his sexual identity, identity development offers a seemingly natural point from which to develop a response—either positive or negative. Young people are expected to be involved in an evolving process of self-discovery and reflection. They are exposed to new ideas and are often (although usually not in terms of sexuality) encouraged to try on different ways of being in an effort to find out just who they are and who they are not. In terms of sexuality, this generally takes the form of either a reactionary response or an assumption that "this is just a phase," so there is no need to be concerned. Parents, siblings, friends, and others often assume that the self-identification as an LGBT person is a temporary stop on the way to a permanent identity as a heterosexual person. Regardless of the outcome of this process of identity development, it has been well documented that post-Stonewall generations have wrestled with the decision to disclose/not disclose in a very different environment than their predecessors. As a result, studies consistently show that individuals are identifying as sexual minorities at much younger ages and are more likely to be out to a substantial number of their family members, friends, and peers compared to their LGBT elders (Floyd and Bakeman 2006).

Research involving older LGBT persons often paints a very different picture. For instance, Grov and colleagues found that many of the participants in their study reported that they had not experienced same-sex attraction until well into adulthood or that they opted not to act on such attractions and chose a traditional path of opposite-sex marriage and children (Grov et al. 2006). Understanding the historical and social context in which these experiences unfolded is essential to understanding how older LGBT persons experience their sexual minority status today. As a point of reference, a 65-year-old in 2014 was 13-year-old in 1962—he or she experienced his or her adolescence in the 1960s. Thus, even the youngest of our older citizens experienced adolescence prior to the 1969 Stonewall Riots and came of age while homosexuality was still identified as a mental health disorder by the American Psychiatric Association (Blank et al. 2009; Floyd and Bakeman 2006). On a broader spectrum, today's LGBT elderly had front row seats either directly or via television and other media to the unrest and social change associated with the Civil Rights Movement, the Women's Rights Movement, and protests of the Vietnam War. LGBT Baby Boomers were in their thirties during the most volatile period of the AIDS crisis, a reality that means many elder gay men may have experienced the loss of partners and friends during that time. For those living in urban areas like San Francisco, New York City, Los Angeles, and Atlanta, those losses may have been numerous (Rosenfeld et al. 2012).

During this same time period, the social context surrounding sexual minorities living in European countries was quite diverse. While many European countries had never had laws that criminalized same-sex relationships, others were often quite punitive (ILGA-Europe 2014). The diversity of responses across the continent underscores many of the reasons European immigrants to the USA may hold very divergent views about their own sexuality. The recent controversy surrounding the 2014 Olympics which were held in Russia remind us that this diversity of views remains. Despite the fact that 24 European countries now recognize some form of same-sex unions, with 11 of these countries having legalized same-sex marriage, in June 2013, Russia passed a new law banning "propaganda of nontraditional sexual relations" (Herszenhorn 2013).

In 1999 Rosenfeld, a sociologist, published one of the first studies which attempted to capture the "interplay between identity, generations, and social change." The qualitative study involving 37 lesbians and gay men over the age of 65 demonstrated the importance of considering not only the timing of coming out but also the cultural and historical context in which it takes place. We know that in the midst of all of the chaos of the 1960s, there were many individuals leading secretly "out" lives within their communities and others who traveled to large urban areas for the occasional opportunity to be around other LGBT persons. Given that LGBT persons of age 65 and over grew up in the pre-Stonewall era, coming out may have been impacted by fear, practical concerns (e.g., loss of job, housing, family support), views on the appropriateness of talking about sexuality, or even the fact that they simply had never considered the possibility they might be lesbian, gay, bisexual, or transgender (Hunter 2007; Jensen 2013; Johnston and Jenkins 2003).

Does coming out matter? For those who either choose not to come out or feel unable to do so, life can often be stressful and fraught with ongoing concerns about exposure (Hunter 2007). As we age, these concerns may move from fear of losing one's job (see Chap. 28) to increasing concerns about experiencing discrimination and victimization in healthcare settings and/or senior housing (Johnson et al. 2005) (see Chap. 21). This pervasive fear of being out has been noted in a number of recent studies, with many elder LGBT persons indicating that they believe it is unsafe to be out in long-term healthcare settings (IOM 2011). A survey of service providers in those healthcare settings affirmed these fears (Johnson et al. 2005; National Senior Citizens Law Center et al. 2010). These concerns can also serve to increase the likelihood of isolation that may often accompany aging. For persons who came to acknowledge their same-sex attractions later in life (after children are grown, spouses die, retirement, etc.), the risk of experiencing isolation is even greater as long-term support systems may disappear (Brennan-Ing et al. 2014; De Vries and Hoctel 2007; Fitzgerald 2013; Kuyper and Fokkema 2010).

A number of studies have identified higher rates of mood and anxiety disorders (IOM 2011; Shippy et al. 2004), alcohol and drug use, and suicidal thoughts and attempts among LGBT persons compared to heterosexuals (D'Augelli and Grossman 2001; King et al. 2008). Juster and colleagues found the role of disclosure to be an important contributing factor to the existence of these disparities (Juster et al. 2013). Their study compared a gender-mixed sample of LGB people with a sample of heterosexuals (49 % women) to see whether there were differences in levels of psychiatric disorders, levels of stress hormones, and physiological dysregulation (allostatic load). Although the study did not involve LGBT elders, its findings have important implications for aging LGBT persons. Specifically, the study found that individuals who had completely disclosed their sexual orientation experienced lower levels of anxiety and depressive symptoms compared to LGB persons who had not fully disclosed.

Notably, other studies have supported a cohort effect related to the impact of disclosure on psychological well-being (Hunter 2007). These studies found that older cohorts of LGBT persons who indicated that they were not out to their healthcare and service providers did not necessarily display higher levels of psychological distress. A number of scholars have suggested that this is a result of the development of crisis competence, or a level of resilience, that has evolved as a result of years of navigating a homophobic environment (IOM 2011). As a result, LGBT persons develop important coping skills that serve as protective factors in daily life. While these findings are certainly a positive sign for LGBT elders who are not out, the studies are based on samples that may have experienced fairly limited needs in terms of service access. As LGBT elders have more reasons to draw upon community, social service, and healthcare systems, it is unclear how attempting to remain

invisible as a sexual minority may impact their well-being and successful aging process.

Against this backdrop, it is important to remember that while the research on coming out has documented a number of challenges for those who are not out and benefits for those who are, the bulk of this research is based on samples that are not representative of the spectrum of LGBT persons. In general, much of what we understand about coming out is based on middle-class, college-educated LGBT persons in their twenties and thirties. As a result, our understanding of the implications of a variety of factors, including cohort effects related to being out/not out, age and the timing of the decision to be out/not out, and potential cultural differences in the primacy and/or necessity to be out, is largely unexplored.

Still to be considered is the question of whether being out is an essential part of successful aging and well-being for all LGBT persons (McGarrity and Huebner 2013; Purdie-Vaughns and Eibach 2008). As previously noted, studies that account for cohort and/or cultural differences related to coming out are limited. Much of the work that has been done in the area starts from an assumption that not being out is universally problematic; thus, the subsequent inquiry is framed accordingly. The combination of this framing and the myriad of issues and barriers that challenge efforts to do population-based research contributes to the dearth of knowledge about distinct age cohorts that represent the spectrum of unique racial, ethnic, and cultural groups. Challenged by the same difficulties in terms of gaining access to representative samples, research in European countries offers little additional insight.

Of the few studies that might shed light on potential differences, some points of divergence have surfaced. For instance, in a probabilistic sample of sexual minority men (n = 372, aged 50–85 years), Rawls (2004) found that among men 60 years of age and older, level of disclosure of sexual minority status had no meaningful impact on reported levels of depression and distress. Fifteen years earlier, Adelman's (1990) study of older lesbians and gay men (born prior to 1930) living in the San Francisco area reported similar findings. This suggests that for elderly people who came of age in the 1940s and 1950s when sexuality was not a topic of public discussion, openness about one's sexual orientation may be no more relevant than openness about any individual's sexual behavior. In fact, the notion that such things are important to share publicly may be a greater source of discomfort than the experience of being a sexual minority in a heterosexist environment.

While those studies offer a modicum of insight into general age cohort differences that may exist, studies addressing cultural differences in views on coming out/being out among LGBT persons of European descent now living the USA are nonexistent. For those who were born and spent a significant part of their formative years there, research characterizing the lives of sexual minorities in various European countries does exist, albeit based on very limited samples. Since 1996, the International Lesbian, Gay, Bisexual, and Intersex Association Europe (ILGA-Europe) has been conducting studies examining issues related to social justice, inequality, and well-being associated with being a sexual minority in Europe (ILGA-Europe 2014). Additionally, the Council of Europe and the European Union collect annual data on a variety of human rights and equality issues, including numerous factors related to the treatment and protection of sexual minorities. Collectively, this information makes clear the importance of considering the specific country of origin when seeking to understand the needs and concerns of LGBT persons of European descent. As a contrasting case-in-point, consider the experiences of LGBT elders in Sweden, Georgia, and Azerbaijan. In 2014, Europe's first LGBT retirement home opened in Stockholm, Sweden—a country that legalized same-sex behavior in 1944. Just seven years prior, separate ILGA-Europe studies in Georgia (Quinn 2007) and Azerbaijan (Van der Veur 2007) found that the vast majority of sexual minorities remained closeted for fear of discrimination and/or victimization.[6] Most of the individuals who participated in the qualitative studies in Georgia and Azerbaijan were out to very few family members, and many indicated that disclosures were often accompanied by some form of hostility, violence, and/or rejection. With such divergent responses to homosexuality[7] being experienced by sexual minorities living in different European countries, it is understandable that individuals of European descent living in the USA may have very divergent views of both the necessity and the potential costs and benefits of being out.

Social and instrumental support. Although isolation and absence of social support can impact people's lives at any age, social and instrumental support can be particularly important for LGBT elders. LGBT elders tend to rely more heavily on *families of choice*, while heterosexual elders' support systems are more likely to be made up of one or more persons who are biologically or legally related. While studies indicate that many LGBT elders are satisfied with the level of support they receive from their chosen families, individuals in these constructed families of choice tend to be of similar ages and thus have/will have their own needs for support and caregiving services as they age. Over time, this leaves many LGBT elders alone and isolated as members of their support system become infirmed and subsequently die. This reality along with the fact that LGBT elders often live alone contributes to many LGBT elders expressing a fear of dying alone (Emlet 2006). Being an LGBT elder living with HIV/AIDS only serves to exacerbate these concerns (Brennan-Ing et al. 2014; McFarland and Sanders 2003; Poindexter and Shippy 2008).

---

[6]In 2009, a similar study conducted in Armenia echoed these findings (Carroll and Quinn 2009).

[7]These studies noted that most of the individuals they interviewed did not typically identify as lesbian, gay, bisexual, or transgender, but instead simply acknowledged their same-sex attractions. This finding is consistent with studies in the USA that have suggested that one barrier to reaching a diverse population of sexual minorities is the difference in researcher versus potential participant's use of language and identity-related constructs.

LGBT Elders and Being a Double Minority

Being young, White, and heterosexual has its privileges. While we may be uncomfortable acknowledging that such privilege still persists in the twenty-first century, many are also silently resistant to voluntarily relinquishing the benefits that come from inhabiting majority status (Richmond and Guindon 2013). As an LGBT elder of European descent, that place of privilege is challenged on at least two fronts (perhaps more if you are a lesbian or bisexual woman or if you identify as transgender). Most of today's elderly population came of age in a time when open hostility toward sexual minorities was the norm, and discrimination and victimization was not uncommon (Hunter 2007). For many LGBT elders of European descent, this environment made staying closeted not only an option, but often a necessity. As LGBT elders age, however, the capacity to hide one's sexuality may be increasingly difficult, thus leading some to experience a double-dose of disenfranchised minority status for the first time in their lives—being elderly and identifying as a sexual minority. For lesbians, bisexual men and women, and transgender persons, this is compounded by either gender or being a sexual minority within a sexual minority.

Responding to the Needs of LGBT Elders of European Descent

The response of various helping professionals and related systems to the needs of LGBT elders has been varied. In the USA, the limitations of efforts to encourage and train helping professionals to develop and deliver culturally competent services for LGBT elders have been consistent with the limitations identified in the scholarly literature. What knowledge has been garnered has focused on racial minorities and non-White ethnic groups, with LGBT elders of European descent being treated as homogeneous and universally privileged or challenged by factors associated with racial majority status. Against this backdrop, Fredriksen-Goldsen and colleagues have identified a number of actions that must be undertaken in our effort to train culturally competent service providers and develop and deliver services that are responsive of the needs of LGBT elderly (Fredriksen-Goldsen et al. 2014) (Table 9.2). These guidelines underscore the need for human service professionals to begin the process of becoming a culturally competent and sensitive practitioners through a process of introspection and willingness to examine and challenge potential biases.

Related Disciplines Influencing Service Delivery and Interdisciplinary Approaches

As is noted throughout this book, numerous disciplines, professions, and institutional settings play pivotal roles in the lives of elderly LGBT persons. Individual life trajectories, mental and physical health needs, economic conditions, and geographical factors coalesce to shape the nature of LGBT elders' engagement with different entities at different times in their lives, but the inevitability of aging and its concomitant needs make the institutional and systemic response critical to successful aging. Policy makers, social workers, mental health professionals, and public health officials all engage in decision making and actions that have the potential to impact the lives of LGBT elders in a multiplicity of ways—some positive, yet historically, primarily in negative ways. An effective road map to proactively working to meet the needs of LGBT elders requires an integrated, interdisciplinary response. The lives of sexual minorities are impacted by federal and state laws and regulations, institutional policies, and social norms and expectations. Addressing uneven and sometimes harsh treatment of LGBT elders living in long-term care facilities is important, but it represents only one piece of what influences quality of life for this population. Prior to living in a long-term care

Table 9.2 Recommendations for the development of culturally competent service providers and programming for LGBT elders

Critically analyze personal and professional attitudes toward sexual orientation, gender identity, and age, and understand how factors such as culture, religion, media, and health and human service systems influence attitudes and ethical decision making

Understand and articulate the ways that larger social and cultural contexts may have negatively impacted LGBT older adults as a historically disadvantage population

Distinguish similarities and differences among the subgroups of LGBT older adults, as well as their intersecting identities (such as age, gender, race, and health status) to develop tailored and responsive health strategies

Apply theories of aging and social and health perspectives and the most up-to-date knowledge available to engage in culturally competent practice with LGBT older adults

Consider the impact of larger social context and structural and environmental risks when conducting a comprehensive biopsychosocial assessment

When using empathy and sensitive interviewing skills during assessment and intervention, ensure the use of language is appropriate for working with LGBT older adults to establish and build rapport

Understand and articulate the ways in which agency, program, and service policies do or do not marginalize and discriminate against LGBT older adults

Understand and articulate the ways that local, state, and federal laws negatively and positively impact LGBT older adults, to advocate on their behalf

Provide sensitive and appropriate outreach for LGBT older adults, their families, caregivers, and other supporters to identify and address service gaps, fragmentation, and barriers that impact LGBT older adults

Enhance the capacity of LGBT older adults and their families, caregivers, and other supporters to navigate aging, social, and health services

facility, LGBT elders lived in communities where they struggled to survive economically due to persistent discrimination that reduced their lifelong earning capacity, lost homes due to the death or institutionalization of a life partner they were legally prohibited from marrying, and accelerated health decline due to delayed utilization of healthcare services and incompetent providers (Durso and Meyer 2013). Elder gay and bisexual men and transgender persons have been disproportionately impacted by the global failure of our initial response to the AIDS pandemic (Gorman and Nelson 2004). Additionally, they continue to suffer higher levels of risk due to the ongoing failure of medical professionals to address the reality of sexual behavior across the life course: an oversight that leaves many of these men at elevated risk of contracting HIV and other STDs through unprotected sex (Effros et al. 2008; Sullivan and Wolitski 2008).

A handful of studies have examined the response of various helping professionals to the needs of LGBT elders. These studies suggest the presence of homophobic and heterosexist views that influence healthcare and social service providers' views when working with sexual minorities. A recent study examined these issues in terms of long-term care facilities by asking a sample of LGBT elders and a sample of heterosexual men and women what they thought about the potential treatment LGBT elders would encounter in long-term care facilities (Jackson et al. 2008). Jackson and colleagues found that both the LGBT respondents (ranging in age from 15 to 72) and heterosexual respondents (aged 18–90) believed that LGBT persons would encounter discrimination in healthcare settings.

In response to these concerns, educational and professional development programs are focusing on the development of curricula that will increase cultural competence of current and future human service professionals working with LGBT elders (Erdley et al. 2014; Fredriksen-Goldsen et al. 2014; Hunter 2005; Leyva et al. 2014; Obedin-Maliver et al. 2011; Porter and Krinsky 2014). A survey of Area Agencies on Aging across the USA found that one-third of the 320 participating agencies had already provided training focused on the needs of LGBT elders, and the vast majority (approximately 80 %) were open to offering such trainings (Knochel et al. 2012). In guiding the efforts of human service professionals to think more expansively about what it means to be culturally aware, Hudson and Mehrotra (2014) call on us to think about both geography and migration as we seek to understand the stories of LGBT persons.

Comparison with Service Delivery Practices in Other Countries

The European Union launched its first initiative focused on the well-being of elderly people in 2010 (Age Platform Europe 2012) and has since renewed its commitment to and investment in meeting the needs of European elders. The framework for action specifically acknowledges its focus as inclusive of LGBT elders. Among the targeted areas for action are (1) the adoption of a quality framework for addressing long-term care; (2) the creation of age-friendly environments; (3) the creation of laws and policies to address discrimination in care, elder abuse, and ageism; and (4) the development of infrastructure for informal and formal support networks (Age Platform Europe 2010).

In 2008, the first LGBT-focused nursing home in Europe opened in Berlin, Germany. The opening of the 28 bed, full-care facility marked an open commitment to the elderly LGBT community in that city. Stockholm, Sweden, opened its first LGBT-focused retirement home in 2013. Most recently (2014), the first LGBT-focused retirement center in Spain opened. Beyond these examples, comprehensive assessments of the health and social service responses to the needs of LGBT elders living in Europe have not been developed. As might be expected, available research conducted in European countries shares many similarities with research conducted in the USA—it generally reflects non-probability samples of LGBT persons who are out to some degree and thus do not represent the scope of LGBT elders in Europe, nor does it offer detailed insight into the presence or absence of needed services and resources (European Union Agency for Fundamental Rights 2014; ILGA-Europe 2014).

Summary

It is safe to say that the majority of what we know about LGBT elders is based on non-Hispanic White men and women (IOM 2011). As has been noted throughout this chapter, while a substantial portion of those men and women are likely to be of European descent, few studies have explicitly addressed this population as distinct from other non-Hispanic Whites (assuming that race and ethnicity differences among study participants are acknowledged at all). Thus, cultural and ethnic differences that influence identity, physical and mental well-being, and the multiplicity of factors that influence successful aging among non-Hispanic White LGBT persons are largely ignored—the consequences of which remain unknown. Having acknowledged those limitations which exist primarily by default rather than design, we do have some insights into the lives of LGBT elders who are known to have or likely to have European heritage. In particular, we know that in addition to cohort differences that may be relevant in the lives of LGBT elders of European descent, understanding factors related to timing of immigration, country of origin, and personal allegiance to ancestral heritage may offer important insights for human service providers (ILGA-Europe 2014).

Learning Activities

Self-Check Questions

1. Why is it problematic to assume that one can understand a person's experience based on skin color?
2. Why is it so difficult to identify the portion of the U.S. population that is of European descent?
3. What types of challenges might LGBT persons with a diverse cultural heritage face?
4. In what country was the first nursing home in Europe opened?

Experiential Exercises

1. Select three countries from the list of European countries identified and Table 9.1 and compare them on several cultural factors (e.g., political structure, language, primary religions, etc.) that might influence the lives of LGBT persons living there.
2. Read the study identified in Research Box 9.1. Look for comparable data from a national study in the United States. Compare and contrast the findings of the two studies and consider similarities and differences in the factors that contribute to these findings.
3. Develop a short questionnaire that would be appropriate to use in a human services agency serving LGBT elders that would allow you to have a better understanding of service users' cultural heritage.

Multiple-Choice Questions

1. Which group is more likely to have been previously married and have children?
   (a) Gay men
   (b) Lesbians
   (c) Bisexual men or women
   (d) Transgender persons
2. Which of the following is NOT a key competency suggested by Fredriksen-Goldsen for culturally competent practice with LGBT elders?
   (a) Insisting that LGBT elders come out in healthcare settings
   (b) Distinguishing similarities and differences between subgroups of LGBT persons
   (c) Applying theory and up-to-date research on culturally competent practice when working with LGBT elders
   (d) Providing sensitive and appropriate outreach for LGBT older adults
3. Ethnic ambiguity refers to:
   (a) A person not knowing their own ethnic heritage.
   (b) A person having a diverse heritage that makes it hard for someone to tell what their ethnicity might be.
   (c) A person vaguely describing the ethnic heritage in order to avoid identifying with a particular group.
   (d) Aspects of a person's ethnic background that are irrelevant to understanding his/her experiences.
4. The census category "White, Non-Hispanic" includes individuals from which of the following countries:
   (a) Russia
   (b) Iran
   (c) Spain
   (d) All of the above
5. The first LGBT retirement home to in a European country was in:
   (a) Italy
   (b) Denmark
   (c) Sweden
   (d) Slovenia
6. Which of the following best describes what we know about the importance of coming out/disclosure for older LGBT persons?
   (a) LGBT elders need to disclose their sexual identity in order to assure good mental health.
   (b) Elder LGBT persons who do not disclose their sexual identity to others do not necessarily feel distressed or depressed.
   (c) Elder LGBT persons are more likely to come out/disclose their sexual identity than younger LGBT persons.

(d) Research has been unable to identify any age-related differences in the relevance of coming out/disclosing one's LGBT identity.

7. Kimberlé Crenshaw's model for describing the importance of considering the relevance of multiple facets of one's identity is referred to as:
   (a) Intersectionality
   (b) Multiple personalities
   (c) Symbolic interaction
   (d) Engagement

8. Compared to heterosexual elders, which of the following is *not true* of LGBT elders?
   (a) More likely to be single
   (b) More likely to have children
   (c) More likely to live alone
   (d) More likely to experience certain health conditions

9. Which of the following is most accurate to say about LGBT elders of European descent currently living in the U.S.?
   (a) LGBT elders of European descent usually have a heritage that can be traced to a single European country.
   (b) LGBT elders of European descent are primarily from Western Europe.
   (c) LGBT elders of European descent come from English-speaking countries.
   (d) Many LGBT elders of European descent have ancestral roots in England, Scotland, and/or Ireland.

10. Which of the following is most accurate to say about training/education models related cultural competence?
   (a) They teach participants to consider the experiences of LGBT elders of color.
   (b) They focus on the unique cultural experiences of white LGBT elders who come from different countries.
   (c) They are offered at the majority of agencies that provide services to LGBT elders.
   (d) They do little to improve the cultural competence of participants.

Key

1-c
2-a
3-b
4-d
5-c
6-b
7-a
8-b
9-d
10-a

Resources

American Psychological Association
   http://www.apa.org/pubs/books/4318127.aspx
Caring and Aging with Pride
   http://caringandaging.org/
Gerontological Society of America
   https://www.geron.org/
Human Rights Campaign
   http://www.hrc.org/
Movement Advance Project
   http://www.lgbtmap.org/policy-and-issue-analysis/lgbt-older-adults
National Resource Center on LGBT Aging
   http://www.lgbtagingcenter.org/resources/index.cfm?a=3
Services and Advocacy for GLBT Elders (SAGE)
   http://www.sageusa.org/about/index.cfm

References

Adelman, M. (1990). Stigma, gay lifestyles, and adjustment to aging: A study of later-life gay men and lesbians. *Journal of Homosexuality, 20*(3/4), 7–32.

Age Platform Europe. (2010, June). *European Charter of the rights and responsibilities of older people in need of long-term care and assistance.* Retrieved from http://www.age-platform.eu/images/stories/22204_AGE_charte_europeenne_EN_v4.pdf.

Age Platform Europe. (2012). *European quality framework for long-term care services: Principles and guidelines for the wellbeing and dignity of older people in need of care and assistance.* Retrieved from http://wedo.tttp.eu/system/files/24171_WeDo_brochure_A4_48p_EN_WEB.pdf.

Albelda, R., Badgett, M. V. L., Schneebaum, A., & Gates, G. J. (2009). *Poverty in the lesbian, gay, and bisexual community.* Los Angeles, CA: The Williams Institute.

Bettinger, T. V. (2010). Ethical and methodological complexities in research involving sexual minorities. *New Horizons in Adult Education and Human Resource Development, 24*(1), 43–58.

Blank, T. O., Asencio, M., Descartes, L., & Griggs, J. (2009). Intersection of older GLBT health issues: Aging, health, and GLBTQ family and community life. *Journal of GLBT Family Studies, 5*(1), 9–34.

Boehmer, U., Bowen, D. J., & Bauer, G. R. (2007). Overweight and obesity in sexual-minority women: Evidence from population-based data. *American Journal of Public Health, 97*(6), 1134–1140.

Brennan-Ing, M., Seidel, L., Larson, B., & Karpiak, S. E. (2014). Social care networks and older LGBT adults: Challenges for the future. *Journal of Homosexuality, 61*(1), 21–52.

Brown, M. T. (2009). LGBT aging and rhetorical silence. *Sexuality Research and Social Policy, 6*(4), 65–78.

Brown, M. T., & Grossman, B. R. (2014). Same-sex sexual relationships in the national social life, health and aging project: Making as case for data collection. *Journal of Gerontological Social Work, 57*(2–4), 108–129.

Carroll, A., & Quinn, S. (2009). *Forced out: LGBT people in Armenia report on ILGA-Europe/COC fact-finding mission.* Netherlands: ILGA-Europe/COC.

Case, P., Bryn Austin, S., Hunter, D. J., Manson, J. E., Malspeis, S., Willett, W. C., & Spiegelman, D. (2004). Sexual orientation, health risk factors, and physical functioning in the nurses' health study II. *Journal of Women's Health, 13*(9), 1033–1047.

Clunis, M., Fredriksen-Goldsen, K. I., Freeman, P., & Nystrom, N. (2005). *Looking back, looking forward: Lives of lesbian elders.* Binghamton, NY: Haworth.

Cochran, S. D., Sullivan, G. J., & Mays, V. M. (2003). Prevalence of mental disorders, psychological distress, and mental health services use among lesbian, gay, and bisexual adults in the United States. *Journal of Consulting and Clinical Psychology, 71*, 53–61.

Cohen, K. M., & Savin-Williams, R. C. (1996). Development perspectives on coming out to self and others. In R. C. Savin-Williams & K. M. Cohen (Eds.), *The lives of lesbians, gays, and bisexuals: Children to adults* (pp. 113–151). Orlando, FL: Harcourt Brace College Publishers.

Collins, P. H. (1990). *Black feminist thought.* Boston: Unwin Hyman.

Conron, K. J., Mimiaga, M. J., & Landers, S. J. (2010). A population-based study of sexual orientation identity and gender differences in adult health. *American Journal of Public Health, 100*, 1953–1960.

Crenshaw, K. (1989). Demarginalizing the intersection of race and sex: A Black feminist critique of antidiscrimination doctrine, feminist theory and antiracist politics. *University of Chicago Legal Forum,* 139–167.

D'Augelli, A. R., & Grossman, A. H. (2001). Disclosure of sexual orientation, victimization, and mental health among lesbian, gay, and bisexual older adults. *Journal of Interpersonal Violence, 16*, 1008–1027.

De Vries, B., & Hoctel, P. (2007). The family-friends of older gay men and lesbians. In N. Teunis & G. Herdt (Eds.), *Sexual inequalities and social justice* (pp. 213–232). Berkeley, CA: University of California Press.

Diamant, A. L., & Wold, C. (2003). Sexual orientation and variation in physical and mental health status among women. *Journal of Women's Health, 12*(1), 41–49.

Dolcini, M. M., Catania, J. A., Stall, R. D., & Pollack, L. (2003). The HIV epidemic among older men who have sex with men. *JAIDS Journal of Acquired Immune Deficiency Syndromes, 33*, S115–S121.

Donahue, P., & McDonald, L. (2005). Gay and lesbian aging: Current perspectives and future directions for social work practice and research. *Families in Society, 86*(3), 359–366.

Durso, L. E., & Meyer, I. E. (2013). Patterns and predictors of disclosure of sexual orientation to healthcare providers among lesbians, gay men, and bisexuals. *Sexuality Research and Social Policy, 10*, 35–42.

Effros, R., Fletcher, C., Gebo, K., Halter, J. B., Hazzard, W., Horne, F., & High, K. P. (2008). Workshop on HIV infection and aging: What is known and future research directions. *Clinical Infectious Diseases, 47*, 542–553.

Emlet, C. A. (2006). An examination of the social networks and social isolation of older and younger adults living with HIV/AIDS. *Health and Social Work, 31*(4), 299–308.

Erdley, S. D., Anklam, D. D., & Reardon, C. C. (2014). Breaking barriers and building bridges: Understanding the pervasive needs of older LGBT adults and the value of social work in health care. *Journal of Gerontological Social Work, 57*(2–4), 362–385.

Erikson, E. (1982). *The life cycle completed: A review.* New York: Norton.

Espinoza, R. (2011). The diverse elders coalition and LGBT aging: Connecting communities, issues and resources in a historic moment. *Public Policy and Aging Report, 21*(3), 8–11.

European Union Agency for Fundamental Rights. (2014). European Union lesbian, gay, bisexual and transgender survey: Main results.

Fitzgerald, E. (2013). *No golden years at the end of the rainbow: How a lifetime of discrimination compounds economic and health disparities for LGBT older adults.* New York: National Gay and Lesbian Task Force.

Floyd, F. J., & Bakeman, R. (2006). Coming out across the life-course: Implications of age and historical context. *Archives of Sexual Behavior, 35*, 287–296.

Fredriksen-Goldsen, K. I., & Muraco, A. (2010). Aging and sexual orientation: A 25-year review of the literature. *Research on Aging, 32*(3), 372–413.

Fredriksen-Goldsen, K. I., Kim, H. J., Emlet, C. A., Erosheva, E. A., Muraco, A., Petry, H., et al. (2011). *The health report: Resilience and disparities among lesbian, gay, bisexual, and transgender older adults.* Seattle, WA: Institute for Multigenerational Health.

Fredriksen-Goldsen, K. I., Hoy-Ellis, C. P., Goldsen, J., Emlet, C. A., & Hooyman, N. R. (2014). Creating a vision for the future: Key competencies and strategies for culturally competent practice with lesbian, gay, bisexual, and transgender (LGBT) older adults in the health and human services. *Journal of Gerontological Social Work, 57*(2–4), 80–107.

Gates, G. J., & Cooke, A. M. (2011). *United States Census Snapshot: 2010.* Los Angeles: The Williams Institute. http://williamsinstitute.law.ucla.edu/wp-content/uploads/Census2010Snapshot-US-v2.pdf3.

Gates, G. J., & Newport, F. (2013). LGBT percentage highest in DC, lowest in North Dakota. *Gallup Politics.* October 18, 2013, http://www.gallup.com/poll/160517/lgbt-percentage-highest-lowest-north-dakota.aspx.

Gelfand, D. E. (2003). *Aging and ethnicity: Knowledge and services* (2nd ed.). New York: Springer.

Gorman, E. M., & Nelson, K. (2004). From a far place: Social and cultural considerations about HIV among midlife and older gay men. In G. Herdt & B. de Vries (Eds.), *Gay and lesbian aging: Research and future directions* (pp. 73–93). New York: Springer.

Grant, J. M., Mottet, L. A., Tanis, J., Harrison, J., Herman, J. L., & Keisling, M. (2011). *Injustice at every turn: A report of the national transgender discrimination survey.* Washington.

Grau, G., & Shoppmann, C. (Eds.). (2013). *The hidden holocaust? Gay and lesbian persecution in Germany 1933–45.* New York, NY: Routledge.

Grossman, A. H. (2008). Conducting research among older lesbian, gay, and bisexual adults. *Journal of Gay and Lesbian Social Services, 20*(1–2), 51–67.

Grossman, A. H., D'Augelli, A. R., & Hershberger, S. L. (2000). Social support networks of lesbian, gay, and bisexual adults 60 years of age and older. *Journal of Gerontology Psychological Sciences, 55B*(3), 171–179.

Grov, C., Bimbi, D. S., Nanin, J. E., & Parsons, J. T. (2006). Race, ethnicity, gender, and generational factors associated with the coming-out process among gay, lesbian, and bisexual individuals. *The Journal of Sex Research, 43*(2), 115–121.

Hartzell, E., Frazer, M. S., Wertz, K., & Davis, M. (2009). *The state of transgender California: Results from the 2008 California transgender economic health survey.* San Francisco, CA: Transgender Law Center.

Herek, G. M., Norton, A., Allen, T., & Sims, C. (2010). Demographic, psychological, and social characteristics of self-identified lesbian, gay, and bisexual adults in a U.S. probability sample. *Sexuality Research and Social Policy, 7*(3), 176–200.

Herszenhorn, D. M. (2013). Gays in Russia find no haven, despite support from the west. *The New York Times.* Retrieved January 25, 2015.

Hudson, K. D., & Mehrotra, G. R. (2014). Locating queer-mixed experiences: Narratives of geography and migration. *Qualitative Social Work,.* doi:10.1177/1473325014561250.

Hunter, S. (2005). *Midlife and older LGBT adults: Knowledge and affirmative practice for social services.* New York: Haworth.

Hunter, S. (2007). *Coming out and disclosure: LGBT persons across the life span.* New York: Haworth.

Institute of Medicine. (2011). *The health of lesbian, gay, bisexual, and transgender people: Building a foundation for better understanding.* Washington, DC.: The National Academies Press.

International Lesbian, Gay, Bisexual, Trans and Intersex Association-Europe [ILGA-Europe]. (2014). *About us.* http://www.ilga-europe.org/home/about_us/what_is_ilga_europe.

Jackson, N. C., Johnson, M. J., & Roberts, R. (2008). The potential impact of discrimination fears of older gays, lesbians, bisexuals and transgender individuals living in small- to moderate-sized cities on long-term health care. *Journal of Homosexuality, 54*(3), 325–339.

Jensen, K. L. (2013). *Lesbian epiphanies: Women coming out in later life.* New York: Routledge.

Johnson, M. J., Jackson, N. C., Arnette, J. K., & Koffman, S. D. (2005). Gay and lesbian perceptions of discrimination in retirement care facilities. *Journal of Homosexuality, 49*, 83–102.

Johnston, L. B., & Jenkins, D. (2003). Coming out in mid-adulthood: Building a new identity. *Journal of Gay and Lesbian Social Services, 16*(2), 19–42.

Juster, R.-P., Smith, N. G., Ouellet, E., Sindi, S., & Lupien, S. J. (2013). Sexual orientation and disclosure in relation to psychiatric symptoms, diurnal cortisol, and allostatic load. *Psychosomatic Medicine, 75*, 1–14.

Kaminski, P. L., Chapman, B. P., Haynes, S. D., & Own, L. (2005). Body image, eating behaviors, and attitudes toward exercise among gay and straight men. *Eating Behaviors, 6*(3), 179–187.

King, M., Semlyen, J., Tai, S. S., Killaspy, H., Osborn, D., Popelyuk, D., & Nazareth, I. (2008). A systematic review of mental disorder, suicide, and deliberate self harm in lesbian, gay, and bisexual people. *BMC Psychiatry, 8*, 70.

Kinsey, A. C., Pomeroy, W. B., & Martin, C. E. (1947). *Sexual behavior in the human male.* Philadelphia, PA: W.B.

Knochel, K. A., Croghan, C. F., Moone, R. P., & Quam, J. K. (2012). Training, geography, and provision of aging services to lesbian, gay, bisexual, and transgender older adults. *Journal of Gerontological Social Work, 55*(5), 426–443. doi:10.1080/01634372.2012.665158.

Kuyper, L., & Fokkema, T. (2010). Loneliness among older lesbian, gay, and bisexual adults: The role of minority stress. *Archives of Sexual Behavior, 39*, 1171–1180.

Leyva, V. L., Breshears, E. M., & Ringstad, R. (2014). Assessing the efficacy of LGBT cultural competency training for aging services providers in California's central valley. *Journal of Gerontological Social Work, 57*, 335–348.

Markus, H., & Nurius, P. (1986). Possible selves. *American Psychologist, 41*(9), 954–969. dio:10.1037/0003-066X.41.9.954.

McDermott, M., & Sampson, F. L. (2005). White racial and ethnic identity in the United States. *Annual Review of Sociology, 31*, 245–261.

McFarland, P. L., & Sanders, S. (2003). A pilot study about the needs of older gays and lesbians: What social workers need to know. *Journal of Geronto-logical Social Work, 40*(3), 67–80.

McGarrity, L. A., & Huebner, D. M. (2013). Is being out about sexual orientation uniformly healthy? The moderating role of socioeconomic status in a prospective study of gay and bisexual men. *Annuals of Behavioral Medicine, 47*, 28–38.

Meezan, W., & Martin, J. I. (2009). Doing research on LGBT populations: Moving the field forward. In W. Meezan & J. I. Martin (Eds.), *Handbook on research with lesbian, gay, bisexual, and transgender populations* (pp. 415–427). New York, NY: Routledge.

MetLife. (2006). *Out and aging: The MetLife study of lesbian and gay baby boomers*. Westport, CT: Met-Life Mature Market Institute.

MetLife. (2010). *Still out, still aging: The MetLife study of lesbian, gay, bisexual, and transgender baby boomers*. Westport, CT: MetLife Mature Market Institute, National Center for Transgender Equality and National Gay and Lesbian Task Force.

Meyer, I. H. (2003). Prejudice, social stress, and mental health in lesbian, gay, and bisexual populations: Conceptual issues and research evidence. *Psychological Bulletin, 129*, 674–697.

Obedin-Maliver, J., Goldsmith, E. S., Stewart, L., White, W., Tran, E., Brenman, S., Lunn, M. R. (2011). Lesbian, gay, bisexual, and transgender-related content in undergraduate medical education. *Journal of the American Medical Association, 306*(9), 971–977.

Orel, N. A., & Fruhauf, C. A. (2006). Lesbian and bisexual grandmothers' perceptions of the grandparent-grandchild relationship. *Journal of GLBT Family Studies, 2*(1), 43–70.

Otis, M. D. (2009). Issues in conducting empirical research with lesbian and gay people in rural settings. In W. Meezan & J. I. Martin (Eds.), *Handbook on research with lesbian, gay, bisexual, and transgender populations* (pp. 280–299). New York: Routledge.

Pew Research Center. (2013, June 13). *A survey of LGBT Americans: Attitudes, experiences, and values in changing times*. Washington, DC: Author.

Poindexter, C., & Shippy, R. A. (2008). Networks of older New Yorkers with HIV: Fragility, resilience, and transformation. *AIDS Patient Care and STDs, 22*(9), 723–733.

Porter, K. E., & Krinsky, L. (2014). Do LGBT aging trainings effectuate positive change in mainstream elder service providers? *Journal of Homosexuality, 61*(1), 197–216.

Prokos, A. H., & Keene, J. R. (2010). Poverty among cohabitating gay and lesbian, and married and cohab-itating heterosexual families. *Journal of Family Issues, 31*, 934–959.

Purdie-Vaughns, V., & Eibach, R. P. (2008). Intersec-tional invisibility: The distinctive advantages and disadvantages of multiple subordinate group identities. *Sex Roles, 59*(5–6), 377–391.

Quinn, S. (2007). *Forced out: LGBT people in Georgia report on ILGA-Europe/COC fact-finding mission*. Netherlands: ILGA-Europe/COC.

Rawls, T. W. (2004). Disclosure and depression among older gay and homosexual men: Findings from the Urban men's health study. In G. Herdt & B. De Vries (Eds.), *Gay and lesbian aging: Research and future directions* (pp. 117–141). New York, NY: Springer.

Richmond, L. J., & Guindon, M. H. (2013). Culturally alert counseling with European Americans. In G. J. McAuliffe (Ed.), *Culturally alert counseling: A comprehensive introduction* (2nd ed., pp. 231–262). Thousand Oaks, CA: Sage.

Roberts, S. A., Dibble, S. L., Nussey, B., & Casey, K. (2003). Cardiovascular disease risk in lesbian women. *Womens Health Issues, 13*(4), 167–174.

Rosenfeld, D. (1999). Identity work among lesbian and gay elderly. *Journal of Aging Studies, 13*(2), 121–144.

Rosenfeld, D., Bartlam, B., & Smith, R. D. (2012). Out of the closet and into the trenches: Gay male baby boomers, aging, and HIV/AIDS. *The Gerontologist, 52*, 255–264.

Russell, C. J., & Keel, P. K. (2002). Homosexuality as a specific risk factor for eating disorders in men. *International Journal of Eating Disorders, 31*(3), 300–306.

Shankle, M. D., Maxwell, C. A., Katzman, E. S., & Landers, S. (2003). An invisible population: Older lesbian, bisexual, and transgender individuals. *Clinical Research and Regulatory Affairs, 20*(2), 159–182.

Shippy, R. A., Cantor, M. H., & Brennan, M. (2004). Social networks of aging gay men. *Journal of Men's Studies, 13*(1), 107–120.

Sullivan, P. S., & Wolitski, R. J. (2008). HIV infection among gay and bisexual men. In R. J. Wolitski, R. Stall, & R. O. Valdiserri (Eds.), *Unequal opportunity: Health disparities affecting gay and bisexual men in the United States* (pp. 220–247). New York: Oxford University Press.

The National Senior Citizens Law Center, The National Gay and Lesbian Task Force, Services & Advocacy for GLBT Elders (SAGE), Lambda Legal, National Center for Lesbian Rights & National Center for Transgender Equality. (2010). *LGBT older adults in long-term care facilities: Stories from the field*. Retrieved from http://www.lgbtlongtermcare.org.

U.S. Census Bureau (2010). *The older population, 2010.* Retrieved from www.census.gov/population/www/socdemo/age/.

Valanis, B. G., Bowen, D. J., Bassford, T., Whitlock, E., Charney, P., & Carter, R. A. (2000). Sexual orientation and health: Comparisons in the women's health initiative sample. *Archives of Family Medicine, 9*(9), 843–853.

Van der Veur, D. (2007). *Forced out: LGBT people in Azerbaijan report on ILGA-Europe/COC fact-finding mission.* Netherlands: ILGA-Europe/COC.

Wallace, S., Cochran, S., Durazo, E., & Ford, C. (2011). *The health of aging lesbian, gay, and bisexual adults in California.* Los Angeles: UCLA Center for Health Policy Research.

Willging, C. E., Salvador, M., & Kano, M. (2006). Unequal treatment: Mental health care for sexual and gender minority groups in a rural state. *Psychiatric Services, 57*(6), 867–870.

Debra A. Harley

Abstract

The purpose of this chapter is to understand the challenges faced by LGBT Hispanic/Latino LGBT persons in older age. In order to provide the reader with a contextual framework of Latino elders, a statistical profile is presented. Similar to other ethnic groups in the USA, Hispanics have intracultural as wells as intercultural differences. Information is presented on the Latino community's perceptions of LGBT persons, current characteristics and values and the role of acculturation, service delivery models for LGBT Hispanic elders and health policy. Attention is given to the generational difference and immigrant and US-born influences among Latinos.

Keywords

Hispanic · Latino · Elders · LGBT · Immigrant · Same-sex couples

Overview

The Hispanic/Latino population in the USA is diverse and composed of persons who are of Cuban, Mexican, Puerto Rican, Dominican, South or Central American, and Spanish genealogical origin. In the USA, the terms "Hispanic" and "Latino/a" are both used. Over four decades ago, the US government mandated the use of the terms "Hispanic" or "Latino" to categorize Americans who identify as their roots Spanish-speaking countries (Taylor et al. 2012). In this chapter, the two terms will be used interchangeably, as well as identification of Latino/a by country of origin. The Hispanic/Latino population is the fastest growing group in the USA by birth and immigration. At age 65, Latino males are expected to live, on average, an additional 18.8 years, and Latina women live an additional 22 years longer than do older whites (National Center for Health Statistics 2013). Despite having generally lower overall socioeconomic status, poorer health, and less access to health care than their non-Hispanic white counterparts, Hispanics tend to live longer than their

D.A. Harley (✉)
University of Kentucky, Lexington, USA
e-mail: dharl00@email.uky.edu

© Springer International Publishing Switzerland 2016
D.A. Harley and P.B. Teaster (eds.), *Handbook of LGBT Elders*,
DOI 10.1007/978-3-319-03623-6_10

white counterparts, with greater life expectancies at all ages. This paradox is attributed to better health habits and stronger networks of social support (Osypuk et al. 2009), which may offer protection from diseases such as heart disease, cancer, and stroke (Zhang et al. 2012). Palloni and Arias (2004) suggest that Hispanics who migrate to the USA tend to be healthier than those who remain in their home countries.

The purpose of this chapter is to present issues pertaining to LGBT Latino/a LGBT elders in the USA. Similar to other ethnic minority groups, Hispanics have been subjected to discrimination, exclusion, and inequities in employment, education, housing, health care, and access to various opportunities, all of which contextualize their experiences. First, information is presented on cultural characteristics and values and the role of acculturation. Next, research on the attitudes and perceptions of Hispanics' perspectives about LGBT persons is discussed. In order to provide the reader with a contextual framework of Latino elders, a statistical profile is presented. Information is provided on characteristics of and issues pertinent to Latino/a LGBT elders. Then, service delivery models for LGBT Hispanic elders are reviewed. Finally, current policy pertaining to LGBT Hispanic elders is examined and recommendations for the future are presented.

Learning Objectives

By the end of this chapter, the reader should be able to:

1. Identify relevant characteristics of Hispanic/Latino culture that influence attitudes and behaviors.
2. Discuss the concepts of homo–bi–transphobia in the Hispanic/Latino community.
3. Describe sociocultural issues, health disparities, and health-seeking patterns of Hispanic/Latino LGBT elders.
4. Explain service models and intervention strategies that are effective with Hispanic/Latino LGBT elders.

5. List areas in which policy development is needed to address concerns of Hispanic/Latino LGBT elders.

Introduction

There are approximately 2.3 million Hispanic elders aged 65, comprising 6.5 % of the US elderly population (US Census 2010a). By 2050, projections indicate that the population of Hispanic seniors will increase to 15 million, accounting for 17.5 % of the US elderly population (National Hispanic Council on Aging 2008). It is estimated that there are 1,419,200 (4.3 %) LGBT Latino/a adults in the USA, 146,100 in same-sex couple relationships, and 29.1 % of Latino/a same-sex couples who are raising children. Latino/a LGBT adults tend to live in geographic areas where there are higher proportions of Hispanics than that of the broader LGBT population. Almost 1/3 of Hispanic same-sex couples live in New Mexico, California, and Texas. East coast states with substantial percentages of Hispanic LGBT adults include Florida, New Jersey, and New York. The states of Nevada, Arizona, Wyoming, Colorado, and Kansas round out the top ten (Kastanis and Gates 2010). In a comparison of Latino/a same-sex couples with different-sex counterparts, same-sex couples fare better; however, socioeconomic vulnerability exists among Latina or female same-sex couples, couples raising children, and couples where one or both partners are non-citizens.

Other demographic characteristics reveal that Latino or male same-sex couples earn almost $15,000 more than Latina/female same-sex couples. In 63 % of same-sex couples, the other partner is not Latino/a compared to 32 % of different-sex couples. LGBT Latino/a adults have higher rates of unemployment than do non-LGBT Latino/a adults; among Latino/a individuals in same-sex couples, rates are similar to their different-sex counterparts. About 15 % of both LGBT and non-LGBT Latino/a adults have completed a college degree, and 26 % of Latino/a individuals in same-sex couples have completed a college degree compared to 14 % in different-sex couples. Individuals in same-sex couples are more likely to be US citizens than their counterparts in different-sex couples (80 % vs. 62 %) (Kastanis and Gates).

Elder Hispanics, LGBT and non-LGBT, face significant challenges in older age, primarily having to do with attaining financial security; maintaining good health status; accessing needed services; and having low levels of education (Administration on Aging 2010), language and communication barriers, and insufficient retirement security and other investments (Kochhar et al. 2011; US Bureau of Labor Statistics 2011). Many Hispanic elders in the USA are first-generation immigrants and are less likely to speak English as well as subsequent generations, which disadvantages them in the job market (Hakimzadeh and Cohn 2007). The majority of Hispanic elders speak Spanish at home and this linguistic isolation means that many cannot read or write well in English, and low educational attainment limits their literacy in Spanish as well (Valdez and Arce 2000).

Cultural Characteristics and Acculturation

Latinos are made up of diverse groups with varying characteristics. The majority of US Latinos assert that they have many different cultures rather than one common culture (Taylor et al. 2012). However, some common cultural values and characteristics do exist across groups. In this section, information is presented on these characteristics as they pertain to traditional Latino/a families. Interpersonal relationships are integral to the Latino/a culture, typically including respect and affection among a network of family and friends (Sue and Sue 2013). Family, religion/faith, unity, respect (respeto), and tradition are important aspects of life for Latinos that are shared across Latino groups, and regarded as cultural strengths.

Family and gender role expectations. Family is the most important social unit among Latinos, and it plays a central role in how they care for aging relatives (Cummings et al. 2011). Extended family includes relatives, close friends, and godparents. Hispanics are a collectivist group who depend on family and friends (i.e., interdependent) during the course of their everyday lives and for getting ahead (Bohorquez 2009). Each member of the family occupies a specific role and function: grandparents (wisdom), mother (self-denial), father (responsibility), godparents (resourcefulness), and children (obedience, adolescents work to help meet family financial needs) (Lopez-Baez 2006). The households of Latino families often consist of five or more members (US Census Bureau 2010b). Traditional families are hierarchical in the form, with special authority given to parents, older family members, and males–family roles are clearly delineated (Lopez-Baez 2006). The sexual behaviors of adolescent females are severely restricted, whereas male adolescents are afforded greater freedom. Marriage and parenthood tend to occur early in life and are viewed as stabilizing influences. In social activities, emphasis is placed on involving extended family and friends rather than on activities as a couple (Flores 2000).

Although Latinos with greater ethnic identity are more likely to adhere to traditional gender role expectations (males machismo, female marianismo), immigrants often experience conflict in several areas. First, Latino men may lack confidence dealing with authority figures and agencies outside of the family, which can result in feelings of inadequacy and concern about diminished authority. Second, Latino men may experience feelings of isolation and depression because of the need to be strong. They avoid talking about stressors for fear of appearing weak. Third, Latino men may have conflict over the need to be consistent in their role, and they may become more rigid in holding to traditional roles (Constantine et al. 2006). For Latina women, conflicts may involve (a) expectations associated with traditional gender roles, (b) anxiety or depression over not being able to live up to standards and roles, and (c) inability to express feelings of anger (Lopez-Baez 2006). These challenges are manifestations of Latina immigrants being socialized to feel inferior and self-sacrificing. The perception of Latinas as submissive to males often leads to a misunderstanding and omission of their influence indirectly (e.g., behind the scenes), which preserves the appearance of male control. However, with greater exposure to the dominant culture and acculturation, Latina women may question traditional expectations, and certain roles may change more than others. It is important to point out that traditional gender role expectations are not negative or restrictive. That is, the expectation of men to be good providers is part of machismo and egalitarian decision making and appears to be increasing among more acculturated Latinos (Sue and Sue 2013).

Ironically, given the importance of family in Hispanic culture, LGBT Latino elders are less likely to have social support and more likely to endure victimization and neglect than the general LGBT older adult population (Fredriksen-Goldsen et al. 2011). Many LGBT Latino elders indicate that their ties with family and the Hispanic community are often broken. Some participants in the *Hispanic LGBT Older Adult Needs Assessment* (National Hispanic Council on Aging 2013) expressed feelings of social isolation within their own families because of their identities as LGBT persons. Even LGBT Latino elders who do not face prejudice from their family or community still encounter problems of rejection, emotional and psychological abuse (including from social service organizations), and low self-esteem. These individuals felt that as painful as rejection by family members is, societal rejection is even more so because it causes a greater degree of isolation. Elders who reported a more positive experience with their families indicated that a dire need exists for more information and education for families to better understand sexual and gender diversity.

Personal quality. Respect (respeto) and dignity (dignidad) are at the core of personalism (inner quality). Personalism is a group norm emphasizing that relationship formation must be established before a task can be accomplished. In many Latino families and communities, tasks are assigned because of the relationships that have been established based on the inner respect. The "goodness" of the person determines the task he or she is assigned, especially to be trusted with loved ones and who could be given responsibility (Flores 2000).

Religion and faith values. Religion plays an important role in the lives of Latinos, is highly regarded, and is considered equally as important as family. As with other values and practices, the role of religion in the lives of Latinos has shifted among subsequent generations. In addition, the religious profile of Latinos varies by Hispanic group and nativity. For example, majorities of Hispanics (55 %) of Mexican (61 %) and Dominican (59 %) descent identify as Catholic, 49 % of Cuban Americans, 45 % of Puerto Ricans, and 42 % of those of Salvadoran descent. The remainder of the Latino population is roughly evenly divided between adherents of various Protestant traditions (22 %) and those who are religiously unaffiliated (18 %). Moreover, some Latinos take part in other forms of spiritual expressions that may encompass a mix of Christian and indigenous influences, which indicate a strong sense of the spirit world in the everyday lives of many Latinos (Pew Research Center 2014). Nevertheless, the majority of Latinos maintain some type of religious beliefs and practices. Key among these beliefs and practices is how the Church influences family life and community affairs, giving spiritual meaning to Hispanic culture, and religion as central to marriage and family life. Religion has been so much a part of Latino culture for centuries that it cannot be separated from the cultural values of the Latino people. Furthermore, even if a person does not participate in organized religion, religious beliefs are still part of family life (Pew Research Center 2014).

Bendixen & Amandi International (2010) found that the faith experience of Latinos, particularly Catholics, informs their support of fairness and equality for LGBT persons. Specifically, 69 % of Latino Christians state that their religion is accepting of all people, including

LGBT persons, and 79 % of Latino Catholics say that a person could express support for LGBT equality and still be a good Catholic. Latino Catholics are among the stronger supporters of equality. According to the Pew Hispanic Center (2007), the Catholic Church's position on homosexuality is based on a distinction between being lesbian or gay and acting on it, which allows for acceptance of being lesbian or gay while at the same time considering acting on such to be wrong and sinful. However, the message that seems to come through is that merely being gay is sinful (Human Rights Campaign, www.hrc.org/resources/entry/religion-and-coming-out-issues-for-latinas-and-lations). The impact of the demographic shift in the USA by Hispanics is becoming more evident in their influences concerning religious perceptions about LGBT persons. The Pew Hispanic Center asserts that Hispanics are changing the nation's religious landscape, especially the Catholic Church, both because of their growing numbers and because they are practicing a distinctive form of Christianity. Marianne Duddy-Burke of Dignity/USA (http://www.dignityusa.org/) reveals that "a lot of gay and lesbian Latinas and Latinos are out in English but not in their Spanish-speaking church" and some individuals choose to be only partially out.

Acculturation. Acculturation, the process of learning about the language, cultural values, and behaviors consistent with the host society, is acknowledged as a critical factor in understanding the experiences of immigrant populations (Berry 2002). The effects of acculturation are distinct among Hispanics. About half (47 %) of Hispanics indicate that they consider themselves to be very different from the "typical" American, and only 21 % say they use the term "American" most often to describe their identity. Among this group, US-born Latinos (who now make up 48 % of Hispanic adults in the USA) have a stronger sense of affinity with other Americans and America than do immigrant Hispanics (Taylor et al. 2012). The key findings of how Hispanics view their identity, language usage patterns, core values, and their views about America and their families' country of origin are presented in Table 10.1.

Acculturation is moderated by gender, age, and country of origin. For Hispanics who ascribe to traditional gender roles, it is more likely that males will have contact with non-Hispanic acculturation agents and exhibit faster language acculturation than do Hispanic females. Give the socialization difference among age groups, it would be expected that younger Latinos are more likely to acculturate faster than older Latinos. Puerto Ricans have different language usage compared to other Hispanic groups and prefer the use of English at home, work, and in social occasions (Alvarez, n.d.). Acculturation and assimilation have specific implications for Latino elders, many of whom immigrated to the USA. The immigration process and transition from country of origin to the USA has been difficult for Latino elders because of increased pressure to acculturate and assimilate, as well as how to deal with stress from hardship and poverty and a range of adverse experiences (e.g., stigma, discrimination, trauma, and abuse) (Aguilar-Gaxiola et al. 2012). Alegria et al. (2008) found that a decline in health status of immigrants (more so for Mexicans and less for Puerto Ricans) over time in the USA is associated with higher social acculturation including lifestyle, cultural practices, increased stress, and adoption of new social norms, depression and other mental health disorders, which are discussed later in this chapter.

Some research demonstrates that less acculturated older adults are more likely to experience depressive symptoms. One plausible explanation is that immigrant older adults lack the knowledge about the host culture, which creates multiple challenges in one's life, ranging from daily hassles (e.g., difficulties in maneuvering everyday activities) to chronic strains (e.g., discrimination). The result may be diminished feelings of self-worth and sense of control, which in turn may lead to elevated symptoms of depression (Chiriboga et al. 2002; Gonzales et al. 2001; Jang and Chiriboga 2010; Kwag et al. 2012). Other research suggests that acculturation may influence the experience of pain. Jimenez et al. (2013) conducted a cross-sectional study to estimate the association between acculturation and the prevalence, intensity, and functional

Table 10.1 Hispanics' views of their culture

Identity
Prefer their family's country of origin to pan-ethnic terms
Most do not have a preference for either term "Hispanic" or "Latino"; when a preference is expressed, "Hispanic" is preferred
Most do not see a shared common culture among US Hispanics
Most do not see themselves fitting into the standard racial categories used by the US Census Bureau
Latinos are split on whether they see themselves as a typical American
American experience
Their group has been at least as successful as other minority groups in the USA
See the USA as better than Latinos' countries of origin in many ways, but not in all ways.
Most immigrants say they would migrate to the USA again
Language use
Most Hispanics use Spanish, but use of English rises through the generations
Believe learning English is important
Want future US Hispanic generations to speak Spanish
Social and political attitudes
More so then the general public, believe in the efficacy of hard work
Levels of person trust are lower among Latinos than they are among the general public
On some social issues, Latinos hold views similar to the general public (e.g., homosexuality should be accepted), but are more conservative on others (e.g., abortion)
Religion is more important in the lives of immigrant Hispanics than in the lives of US–born Hispanics
Political views are more liberal than those of the general US public

Adapted from Taylor et al. (2012)

limitations of pain in older Hispanic adults in the USA and found that compared to non-Hispanic whites and English-speaking Hispanics, Spanish-speaking Hispanics had the highest prevalence and intensity of pain. However, the differences were not significant after adjusting for age, sex, years of education, immigration status (US-born vs. non-US-born), and health status (i.e., number of health conditions).

Lokpez (2010) distinguishes acculturated Hispanics as those, for whom English is the dominant language, are born in the USA or have been here for 10 or more years, live in suburban areas, conduct business in English, prefer English media, have similar purchase behaviors as the general market, and observe few or no Hispanic traditions. The transition of first- and later-generation Hispanics requires significant social and cultural adjustments, which are associated with changes in perceived health, mental

health functioning, and familial relationships (Archuleta 2012). Kwag et al. (2012) examined the correlation between acculturation, depressive symptoms, and perceived density of neighborhood characteristics in Hispanic older adults and found the impact of acculturation on depressive symptoms to be moderated by the perceived density of Hispanic neighborhoods. The researchers concluded that neighborhood characteristics are important in the lives of immigrant older adults.

Acculturation is not unidirectional, thus drawing any conclusion about its impact is complex. In a review of the literature on acculturation and Latino health in the USA and its sociopolitical context, Laea et al. (2005) concluded that "the effects of acculturation, or more accurately, assimilation to mainstream U.S. culture on Latino behaviors and health outcomes is very complex and not well understood" (p. 374).

Even with the identification of certain positive or negative trends in the subject areas reviewed about Latino acculturation, the effects are not always in the same direction and often times are mixed. The results were influenced by the subject area, measure of acculturation used, and factors such as age, gender, or other measured or unmeasured constructs. Nevertheless, acculturation is associated with several negative health-related behaviors and health outcomes in Latinos: (a) illicit drug use, (b) drinking, (c) smoking, (d) poor nutrition and diets, and (e) worse birth and perinatal outcomes (e.g., low birth weight, prematurity) as well as undesirable prenatal and postnatal behaviors (e.g., substance use during pregnancy). On the positive side, acculturation is associated with improved access to care and use of preventive health services among Latinos (Laea et al. 2005). In an examination of the role of acculturation in health behaviors of older Mexican Americans, similar results were found by Masel et al. (2006), who found that those who were proficient in English were more likely to have a history of smoking and drinking. Masel et al. concluded that this knowledge can assist health promotion programs in identifying those at-risk of engaging in negative health behaviors. The reader is referred to Laea et al. for additional information.

Hispanic Perspective Regarding LGBT Persons

Bendixen & Amandi International (2010) suggest that it is best to start from a point of shared values to understand and effectively relate to Latinos/Latinas about LGBT issues: family, respect, faith, and opposition to discrimination. Hispanics have been portrayed as particularly anti-gay and more anti-legal gay marriage than other segments of American society (Dutwin 2012). As with any population, there are varying degrees of tolerance. In fact, different from the general population, Hispanics are slightly more likely to support legal gay marriage and be open more generally toward lesbians and gay men in society (Bendixen & Amandi International 2010; Dutwin). Dutwin found that one concern with LGBT acceptance in the Hispanic community is at the "intersection of Hispanicity and religion" (p. 5). The most traditional (i.e., unacculturated) religious Latinos are the most intolerant. However, as Hispanics reside longer in the USA, the more interaction they have with other segments of society, which may potentially increase their exposure to LGBT issues and contact with LGBT persons. Thus, Dutwin hypothesizes that because generations correlate with acculturation and future generations are far more likely to comingle and be acculturated than earlier ones, over time, Hispanics will become more tolerant.

In the Pew Hispanic Center Survey (2012), 52 % of Latinos favored same-sex marriage compared to 34 % who opposed it. When asked whether sexual minorities (the term homosexuality is used in the survey) should be accepted or discouraged by society, a majority of Latinos (59 %) and 58 % of the US general population say homosexuality should be accepted, as compared to 30 and 33 %, respectfully, say it should be discouraged. Views on homosexuality vary by immigrant generation. Second-generation Hispanics (68 % vs. 24 %) and third-generation Hispanics (63 % vs. 32 %) are generally in favor of acceptance. Females (62 %) more than males (55 %) support acceptance, and younger (18- to 29-year-olds, 69 %) and middle-aged (30- to 49-year-olds, 60 %) more than older (age 50–64, 54 %, 65+, 41 %) (Taylor et al. 2012). These findings are consistent with those of an earlier poll conducted by Bendixen & Amandi International (2010), which found Latinos are broadly supportive of equality for gay people (Table 10.2).

The attitude of people toward LGBT persons is shaped, in part, by the degree to which they believe sexuality is innate, shaped by upbringing, or a matter of personal preference. In 2011, a Gallup Poll found that 42 % of Americans believe that homosexuality is due to upbringing or environment, and 40 % believe people are born homosexual. In a survey of Latinos beliefs toward lesbians and gay men, Dutwin (2012) found that 62 % believe homosexuality is due to

Table 10.2 Latino support equality for gay people

80 % believe that gay people often face discrimination
83 % support housing and employment non-discrimination protections for gay people
74 % support either marriage or marriage-like legal recognition for gay and lesbian couples
73 % sat that gay people should be allow to serve openly in the military
75 % support school policies to prevent harassment and bullying of students who are gay or perceived to be gay
55 % (and 68 % of Latino Catholics) say that being gay is morally acceptable

Adapted from Bendixen & Amandi International (2010)

biology, and 20 % to personal preference. Not surprisingly, non-religious Latinos are most likely to believe that homosexuality is biological, followed closely by Catholics compared with those who go to church, who are substantially less likely to believe that homosexuality is something with which people are born. In fact, Latinos who do not go to church at all or go infrequently are twice as likely to believe that homosexuality is biological compared to Latinos who go to church twice per week.

Research documents that LGBT persons experience a high degree of discrimination. In response to questions about beliefs of the discrimination they experience in the USA relative to other minority groups, Latinos generally believe that Latinos and gays and lesbians are discriminated against to a greater degree than are African Americans and women. Furthermore, Latinos believe that, of all minority groups, gays and lesbians experience the most discrimination (Dutwin 2012). These beliefs are linked to Latinos', especially younger Latinos, views of fairness and social justice.

A Statistical Profile of Latino Elders

The Latino population is younger than any other racial or ethnic group in the USA; thus, a small proportion of the Latino population is aged 65 and older (i.e., 7 % or 3 million) (US Census Bureau 2010a). Approximately two of three Latinos aged 65 and older live in one of four states: California, Texas, Florida, or New York. The Latino elderly population disproportionately

lives in poverty. Foreign-born Latinos elders are more likely to live in poverty than native-born Latinos. Latinos born outside the USA may be less likely to speak English, have lower levels of education, and have less access to Social Security benefits than their native counterparts (Pew Hispanic Center 2010). The median annual income for households headed by a Latino adult aged 65 and older is $22,116, compared with $29,744 for all households headed by someone aged 65 or older and $31,162 for households headed by non-Latino whites in the same age range (Bureau of labor Statistics & US Census Bureau 2009).

Latino elders have a different source of income than older adults from other racial and ethnic groups with higher income levels. The greatest source of income is from Social Security income (82 %), property (27 %), earned money from wages, salary, or self-employment (20 %) and pension (17 %). In contrast, non-Latino whites aged 65 and older have greatest income sources that include Social Security income (90 %), property (61 %), pension (33 %), and earned money (21 %) (Bureau of labor Statistics & US Census Bureau 2009). Although fewer Latino elders receive Social Security benefits, Social Security income is more important and provides at least half of their total income (National Committee to Preserve Social Security and Medicare 2008). Latinos receive Social Security at lower rates because they are less likely to have paid into the system for enough years to become eligible to receive benefits, are immigrant workers without the appropriate legal status to receive coverage, or work in the type of jobs (e.g., domestic and agricultural) in which employers tend to underreport Social Security earnings (Torres-Gil et al. 2005). The extent to which these data are applicable to LGBT Latino elders is not known.

Older Hispanic adults are vulnerable to the stresses of immigration and acculturation (National Council of La Raza 2005). Health status differs across national-origin groups. In addition, the health of US Hispanics differs by generational status. Among foreign-born Hispanics, health status and health behaviors may differ by degree of acculturation to American culture. The two leading causes of death are heart disease and cancer among Hispanics, with homicide responsible for the higher death rate among Hispanic men aged 15–24 (Tienda and Mitchell 2006). While Latinos use mental health services less than the general population, rates of usage have increased. However, bilingual patients are evaluated differently when interviewed in English as opposed to Spanish and Hispanics, who are more frequently undertreated (American Psychiatric Association 2014). Health and health behaviors of Hispanic adults are discussed in detailed later in this chapter.

Latino/LGBT Older Adults

With the growing number of Hispanic LGBT elders, a tremendous need exists for community-based organizations that serve them in a culturally and linguistically competent manner. As they age, many LGBT Hispanic elders feel excluded and isolated. Exclusion and isolation is compounded by societal prejudice and discrimination, they are as members of both a sexual minority and ethnically marginalized group. Furthermore, LGBT Hispanic elders may become estranged from family members who condemn their sexualities on religious grounds or who lack understanding. Similarly, they may experience alienation from their faith community, depending on the community's stance toward LGBT persons (National Hispanic Council on Aging 2013). An analysis of qualitative data from focus group discussions of LGBT Hispanic older adults revealed some of the following comments: (a) acceptance of LGBT persons is very difficult among Latinos because of our nature (i.e., culture); (b) family is the most important nucleus in society from which we receive understanding, love, and affections and if we do not receive that, other factors happen, such as depression or suicide; and (c) there are people who are 90 years old and have never said they are gay, they are bearing the cross because their family cannot accept that (National Hispanic Council on Aging 2013).

LGBT Hispanic elders face many of the same challenges as do older adults in the general population, such as accessing community services and benefitting fully from Medicare, Medicaid, and Social Security. However, their challenges in these areas are more difficult because of the marriage inequity for same-sex couples, which adversely affects retirement benefits and health insurance (National Hispanic Council on Aging 2013). Research on LGBT Hispanic elders is limited and based on the information from those individuals willing to acknowledge their identities and relationships. The ability of researchers to identity, recruit, and maintain contact with LGBT Hispanic elder participants for research is limited by their mistrust of unfamiliar institutions, cultural and linguistic barriers, lack of transportation, limited formal education, financial constraints, negative stigma associated with mental health problems, and lack of understanding of the purpose of the research and how it will benefit the community (Alvarez et al. 2014; Kuhns et al. 2008). In addition, transgender Hispanics tend to be excluded because of their unwillingness to self-identify or come out. Much of the information in this section consists on an overreliance on data from the *Hispanic LGBT Older Adult Needs Assessment* (National Hispanic Council on Aging 2013).

The economic status of LGBT Hispanic elders is similar to that of their non-LGBT counterparts. Hispanic male same-sex households have an average annual income of $49,800; female same-sex couples have an average yearly income of $43,000, compared to Hispanic married opposite-sex household earning $44,000 on average (Cianciotto, 2005). The lower level of economic security and being disadvantaged in the job market has implications for housing and home ownership of LGBT Latino elders. Many LGBT Hispanic elders who qualify for Section 8 housing are unable to receive it because they lack immigration status documentation of Social Security registration (National Hispanic Council on Aging 2013). Many LGBT Hispanic elders are living below the federal poverty level with insufficient funds to cover their basic living expenses. Before the US Supreme Court decision to strike down Section 3 of the Defense of Marriage Act (DOMA), which discriminated against the economic security of LGBT persons across the country, LGBT seniors of a single-income household could not claim the retirement, Social Security, or survival benefits of a deceased partner. However, the invalidation of Section 3 of DOMA only applies in states that recognize the equality of same-sex marriage.

Aging is a difficult experience in the LGBT Hispanic older community. Many LGBT Latino elders feel that, unlike Latino culture, LGBT elders are marginalized and forgotten as they age in a LGBT community that values youth and physical attractiveness. LGBT Hispanic elders feel that aging in the LGBT community is associated with loneliness, illness, and loss of economic opportunities because of being unable to advance professionally or compete in the job market, particularly for those without support of their families and do not have children to take care of them. Isolation is heightened because of the limited number of gathering places for older LGBT persons to socialize, in contrast to the number of programs and center for LGBT youth and senior centers for the elderly Spanish-speaking community. The significance of this becomes evident for LGBT elders who are rejected by their families for their sexual orientation or sexual identity (National Hispanic Council on Aging 2013).

The health status of LGBT Hispanic elders is further compromised because they are uncomfortable with sharing their sexuality with their provider. The situation is magnified for transgender Latino elders who are frequently diagnosed in advance stages of sexually transmitted diseases because they never got tested. Medical providers only pay attention to the presenting problem and do not ask or check other problems. LGBT Hispanic elders indicate that most doctors lack education about the LGBT community, are homophobic/heterosexist, and are unaware of their own insensitivity. These factors, coupled with doctors who do not speak Spanish or train in centers in Hispanic communities, further impede LGBT Hispanic elders' access to and utilization of services and may have detrimental effects on this population's health (National Hispanic Council on Aging 2013).

Social and Health Inequities of Latino and LGBT Latino Elders

Health inequities among LGBT populations of color are largely a product of unaffordable health insurance, lack of cultural competencies among healthcare providers, and prejudice about race and ethnicity (Krehely 2009). Hispanic elders have health disparities and face numerous challenges to accessing social programs and healthcare services. Adults in Latino families are more likely to be primary caregivers for elders in the home setting for extended periods of time, and without supports from professional community services, than are adults in non-Latino white families (Koerner et al. 2013). Of 65 million Americans who provide unpaid care to an adult, Hispanic households have the highest prevalence of unpaid family caregivers (National Alliance for Caregiving and AARP 2009).

Hispanic elders have a relatively high prevalence of diabetes, and 56 % of Hispanics aged more than 50 have at least one chronic health condition (National Healthcare Disparities Report 2005). Compared to non-Hispanic whites, Hispanics have higher rates of Type 2 diabetes and other manifestations of abnormal glucose metabolism. For Hispanics aged 45–74, 23.9 % of Mexican origin 15.8 % of Cuban origin, and 26.1 % of Puerto Rican origin have diabetes (Tienda and Mitchell 2006). Other prevalent health conditions include Alzheimer's disease, depression, and fatal falls. According to the National Healthcare Disparities Report, compared to the majority non-Hispanic white, elderly population, Hispanic elders have the following prominent disparities. They are less likely to: (a) achieve diabetes control (e.g., more likely to be hospitalized for diabetes), (b) receive vaccinations for pneumonia or influenza, (c) receive recommended hospital care for pneumonia, (d) receive cancer screening services, (e) have an ongoing source of care, and (f) receive counseling to increase physical activity, if overweight. In addition, Hispanic elders are more likely to fall multiple times in one year (Wallace 2006) and are less likely to receive preventive care.

Hispanic adults have lower rates of hypertension than non-Hispanic whites but are less likely to have their blood pressure controlled. Few data are available on heart disease among Hispanics; data on the incidence and prevalence of stroke are also scarce. The utility of existing data is limited because of issues of generalizability. Rates of obesity have increased among Hispanics and are higher than for non-Hispanic whites (Tienda and Mitchell 2006). Acculturated or US-born Hispanics have higher rates of obesity than immigrant counterparts because of a higher consumption of fatty foods. Park et al. (2003) found that Hispanics of Mexican origin have the highest age-adjusted prevalence of metabolic syndrome (abdominal obesity) of any racial or ethnic group. Moreover, Mexican-origin women are more likely than non-Hispanic white or black women to have metabolic syndrome, even after controlling for predisposing factors such as body mass index, alcohol consumption, physical activity, and carbohydrate intake.

Cultural (e.g., linguistic), socioeconomic (e.g., education, occupation, income), and geographical (e.g., rural) (Erving 2007) lack of awareness about services, and stigma associated with mental illness (American Psychiatric Association 2014) are barriers to health care and are main predictors of health outcomes. Bohorquez contends that while Hispanic elders share some behaviors with non-Hispanics, many traits are unique to Hispanic seniors, which dictates the

marketing and promoting of healthcare products and services to Hispanic elders. These include knowledge, access, language, education, and culture. Hispanic elders have a desire for healthy living and behavioral changes but are less aware and knowledgeable of steps to take than the general senior population. Although Hispanic elders have less access to a regular physician or insurance compared to the general population, the magnitude of access as a barrier is less than expected. The issue is that they are less likely to use services provided by healthcare professionals. This reluctance to use healthcare services may be linked to a language barrier, which makes access a daunting task and an unpleasant experience. Low educational level is related more to existing Hispanic elders than baby boomers, who are more educated and have higher earning power as they attain higher education (Bohorquez). In addition, many Latinos elders have an external locus of control related to health barrier perceptions (Valentine et al. 2008).

Bohorquez's (2009) cultural manifestations that serve as barriers to Hispanic elders receiving timely and appropriate health care include practices include interdependence, reactivity, home remedies, fear, and marianismo/machismo. In fact, Bohorquez considers culture to be "the most invisible yet powerful barrier" (p. 52). The cultural manifestations interdependence of Latino culture are not a barrier, but are introduced here as one cultural manifestation. Cultural interdependence is evident by the living arrangements of Latino elders as members of an extended household. In fact, the number of Latino elders living alone is almost half that of the general population. The family acts as a motivator for elders for maintaining good health and to be self-sufficient and to contribute to the family (Bohorquez).

The use of home remedies or natural supplements to treat illness as an alternative to Western health care is commonplace among Latinos. In some ways, the use of home remedies is linked to spirituality, and in other ways, it is linked to financial constraints, distrust of Western medicine, and lack of knowledge or awareness about health issues. Hispanics generally lack a preventive mind-set. They are more concerned about current needs as opposed to future ones. Even those with healthcare coverage will typically visit a doctor only when they are very ill. This reactive mind-set prevents detection of illness that could be treated at an earlier stage. The belief is that whatever happens is "Si Dios quiere" ("It is God's Will") (Bohorquez). Many Hispanic elders may feel that their health may be out of their control and in the hands of a "higher being," resulting in a fatalistic viewpoint (fatalism) toward their health condition (Desai et al. 2010). It is important for healthcare providers to recognize that Hispanic elders are more likely to take the advice of respected community members than the advice of their physicians. Other cultural beliefs and practices that affect Hispanic elders' response to healthcare intervention are presented in Table 10.3.

Fear is a factor that results in increased poor health status of Latino elders. Both thinking about and talking about the future health needs are seen as emotionally frightening and impractical. In part, the fear is an outcome of Latinos waiting for an illness to advance before seeking health care. As a result, their health is too poor to yield a positive outcome, consequently healthcare providers are associated with severe illness and death. Fear is also a reaction to not wanting to burden their families with healthcare costs. Finally, the ability of women (marianismo) to be successful as mother/nurturers and men (machismo) as fathers/providers does not meet these standards, and Latino elders feel diminished as individuals (Bohorquez). As a result of trying to live up to these gender role expectations, especially in light of being LGBT, Latino elders may experience depression.

Hispanic lesbians and bisexual women are at heightened risk or health disparities compared with Hispanic heterosexual women and non-Hispanic white bisexual women. Kim and Fredriksen-Goldsen (2012) suggest that although sexual minority women are at increased risk for poor health and, within-group differences among sexual minority women exist, evidence of health disparities by race/ethnicity and sexual orientation tends not to generalize to sexual minorities of color. Furthermore, the consequences of multiple stressors such as racial discrimination within sexual minority communities and anti-LGBT values within Hispanic communities may lead to an increased risk of poor physical health and mental well-being (Diaz et al. 2006; Harper et al. 2004). Kim and Fredriksen-Goldsen (2012) found that Hispanic bisexual women are more likely to experience frequent mental distress than are both non-Hispanic white bisexual women and Hispanic heterosexual women. The cumulative risk related to multiple marginalized statuses appears to lead to greater mental distress.

Research Box 10.1: Hispanic Lesbian and Bisexual Women Health Disparities

Kim, H. J., & Fredriksen-Goldsen, K. I. (2012). Hispanic lesbians and bisexual women at heightened risk or health disparities. *American Journal of Public Health, 102*(1), e9–e15.

Objective: This study investigated whether elevated risks of health disparities exist in Hispanic lesbians and bisexual women

Table 10.3 Cultural beliefs and practices affecting health care of Hispanic elders

Espiritismo—the belief in the existence of malevolent spiritual beings who may be able to negatively or positively influence the health of material beings

Prresentismo—the belief that only issues that are immediate problems should be dealt with—a belief that may cause some patients to delay seeking treatment until after complications develop

Jerarquismo—the interplay of family members in the social structure of Hispanic culture, which is predominantly a patriarchal society

Promotores—the use of trained lay persons to assist navigating the complexities of the healthcare arena

Adapted from Desai et al. (2010)

aged 18 years and older compared with non-Hispanic white lesbians and bisexual women and Hispanic heterosexual women.

Methods: Population-based data from Washington State Behavioral Risk Factor Surveillance System (2003–2009) were analyzed using adjusted logistic regression.

Results: Hispanic lesbians and bisexual women, compare with Hispanic heterosexual women, were at elevated risk for disparities in smoking, asthma, and disability. Hispanic bisexual women also showed higher odds of arthritis, acute drinking, poor general health, and frequent mental distress compared with Hispanic heterosexual women. In addition, Hispanic bisexual women were more likely to report frequent mental distress than were non-Hispanic white bisexual women. Hispanic lesbians were more likely to report asthma than were non-Hispanic white lesbians.

Conclusions: The elevated risk of health disparities in Hispanic lesbians and bisexual women is primarily associated with sexual orientation. Yet, the elevated prevalence of mental distress for Hispanic bisexual women and asthma for Hispanic lesbians appears to result from the cumulative risk of doubly disadvantaged statuses. Research is needed to address unique health concerns of diverse lesbians and bisexual women.

Questions

1. If given the opportunity, what types of qualitative would you ask of the Hispanic lesbians and bisexual participants?
2. What are the major limitations of this study?
3. Lesbians and bisexual Hispanic women in this study did not show cumulative risks in most other health indicators. What are some possible explanations?

Social support among sexual minorities is an important predictor of mental health. Given that bisexual women report stigmatization and exclusion within gay and lesbian communities, which result in distancing themselves from these communities (McLean 2008), Hispanic bisexual women likely have relatively less social support available to them than do lesbians (Herek 2002). According to Acosta (2008), Hispanic lesbians are able to construct safe environments in which they can share the challenges of being both an ethnic and sexual minority; however, bisexual Hispanic women tend to have fewer such opportunities because of a lack of social support.

LGBT Latinos are affected disproportionately by certain health issues such as mental illness, substance abuse, and addictive disorders, and HIV (especially gay men) (Cochran et al. 2007; Krehely 2009) and have the poorest self-reported status of mental health (Fredriksen-Goldsen et al. 2011). Lesbian Latinas are more likely to experience depression, and gay and bisexual Hispanics are more likely to have attempted suicide than heterosexual Hispanics (Cochran et al. 2007). Depression is prevalent among the Latino elderly population. Several studies suggest a rate between 4 and 44 % of older Latinos experience depressive symptoms, with prevalence varying by country of origin (Alvarez et al. 2014). For example, depressive symptoms for Mexicans in the USA range between 4 and 28 % (Hernandez et al. 2013) and Puerto Ricans between 17 and 44 % (Yang et al. 2008). This wide variance is attributed to how depression is defined (e.g., clinical syndrome vs. cluster of symptoms), type of measure used, whether responses were given in Spanish (or indigenous language such Quechua, Mixteco, or Triqui) or English, validity and reliability of the measure with this population, and culturally determined concepts of illness (Alvarez et al.).

Diagnosis of depression in Latino elderly people is further complicated by the relationship with cardiovascular disease, especially with cardiovascular disease being one of the most common chronic conditions and major cause of death among this population (Roger et al. 2011).

Alvarez argues that with high rates of diabetes, obesity, and hyperlipidemia in Latinos, "vascular depression" (Alexopoulous et al. 1997), which itself contributes to the development of depression in late life, it is imperative to conduct more research on these topics in Latinos. A disturbing fact is that "at present there are not randomized clinical trials that examine the efficacy of nay form of psychotherapy to treat depression in Latino older adults" (p. 39), nor are there studies evaluating which evidence-based pharmacological interventions are best suited to meet the needs of Latino elderly. However, anecdotal data suggest that cognitive behavioral therapy (CBT) may be effective. The case of Mr. Lopez (below) demonstrates issues relevant to mental illness, aging, and minority status that must be addressed for Hispanic elders.

Case Study: Mr. Lopez

Mr. Lopez is a 63-year-old Mexican immigrant to the USA. He initially came to the USA as a seasonal farm worker. Mr. Lopez has a sixth-grade education and speaks what can be considered "functional English" (i.e., can communicate well enough to meet his basic needs) but has difficulty communicating in English on a level that would allow him to interact effectively with service providers and to understand multilevel instructions. He is a single gay man who has not self-identified to his family, but is "out" among a close-knit group of friends. Mr. Lopez has lived in the USA for 18 years since being granted citizenship. He resides in a small, old, unpainted, rented house with several other individuals. He does not own a car and no public bus stop is available for 2 miles. While his standard of living is far below the poverty level, Mr. Lopez believes that compared to his life in Mexico, he is much better off.

During his last doctor's visit, Mr. Lopez appeared frightened, tense, and if the translation from the interpreter is correct, having hallucinations. As a result he was referred for a psychiatric evaluation. Mr. Lopez is uncertain of the purpose of this referral and suspects that his doctor is taking steps to have him incarcerated because of his sexual orientation.

Questions

What cultural issues can you identify that have implications for Mr. Lopez?
What assumptions did the doctor make about Mr. Lopez's symptoms?
What additional questions do you think should be investigated about Mr. Lopez?

Current disparities in mental health care for Latinos are severe and persistent, and Latinos have less access to mental health services than do whites, are less likely to receive needed care, and are more likely to receive poor-quality care when treated. Mexican Americans have more dramatic disparities in mental health care than other Latino subgroups or other ethnic minorities (Aguilar-Gaxiola et al. 2012; Alegria et al. 2007). In LGBT communities, male-to-female transgender persons are at the highest risk for mental health problems, with depression (Nemoto et al. 2011), suicidal ideations, and social isolation (Kenagy 2005; Herbst et al. 2008). The cause of these responses may be attributed to being closeted about their transgender life (De Santis 2009) and negative social interactions with others (Koken et al. 2009). Bazargan and Galvan (2012) examined the extent of perceived discrimination and depression among Latina male-to-female transgender women: participants were aged 18 and over and of the 220 women 120 (55 %) were aged 35 and over. Of the women aged 35 and over, 64 % had low severity depression, 14 % moderate severity, and 26 % high severity. However, the authors made no further distinction based on the age in reporting the results. See Research Box 10.2.

Research Box 10.2: Discrimination and Depression

Bazargan, M., & Galvan, F. (2012). Perceived discrimination and depression among low-income Latina male-to-female transgender women. *BMC Public Health*, *12*, 663–760.

Objective: This study examines exposure to perceived discrimination and its association with depression among low-income, Latina male-to-female transgender women as well as evaluates the impact of sexual partner violence and mistreatment on depression.

Method: A total of 220 Latina male-to-female transgender women in Los Angeles, California, were recruited through community-based organizations and referrals. Participants were aged 18 and older. Interviews were conducted using a structured questionnaire. Depressive symptoms were assessed using the Patient Health Questionnaire (PHQ-9). Perceived discrimination was assessed using a 15-item measure that was designed to assess the experiences of maltreatment of transgender persons. Multinomial logistic regression was used to examine the association between perceived discrimination and depression after controlling for the presence of other variables.

Results: Of the sample, 35 % reported significant depressive symptoms (PHQ-9 ≥15). Additionally, one-third of the participants indicated that in 2 weeks prior to the interviews, they had thought either of hurting themselves or that they would be better off dead. The extent of perceived discrimination in this population was extensive. Many experienced discrimination on a daily basis (14 %) or at least once to twice a week (25 %). Almost six out of ten admitted that they had been victims of sexual partner violence. Those who reported more frequent discrimination were likely to be identified with severe depression. There was also a notable association between self-report history of sexual partner violence and depression severity.

Conclusions: A significant association between depression severity and perceived discrimination was identified. The manner in which discrimination leads to increased risk of mental health problems needs further investigation. Models investigating the association between perceived discrimination and depression among transgender women should include sexual partner violence as a potential confounding variable.

Questions

1. In what ways do you think that the result could have been different if this study examined subgroups of transgender Latina older women?
2. Are these results generalizable to transgender Latina women throughout the USA?
3. How do cultural values and sexual partner violence confound these results?

Health disparities among Hispanics in general and Hispanic LGBT populations in particular are substantial compared to other groups in the USA. An understanding of social and health disparities among Hispanic LGBT elders is essential in development and implementation of culturally appropriate models of service delivery. Health disparities continue to grow among Latinos because of a lack of culturally appropriate intervention strategies and services, and mental health professional shortages (American Psychiatric Association 2014). The following section presents some effective service delivery models that have been used with Latino populations.

Models of Service Delivery

Latino-serving community-based organizations for elders are scarce. The majority of existing organizations that provide services to older Latino adults do so as part of the services that they provide to the Latino community as a whole. Of those organizations that offer services specifically to Latino elders, the most common are those related to health, social and recreational activities, housing, transportation, food security, and assistance accessing government services. Those organizations also refer their elders to other community-based organizations providing additional services such as day care at home, job training, and care management for chromic diseases. The number of national nonprofit organizations whose advocacy and service agendas focus on Latino elders is few and far between. However, two such organizations are the National Hispanic Council on Aging (NHCOA) and the National Association for Hispanic Elderly (NAHE), which have developed programs in the following areas: health promotion and disease prevention, economic security and civic engagement, leadership development, education, low-income housing, employment services, training and technical assistance, and communications and media. The majority of national Latino organizations have integrated older adults into their general initiatives even when elders are not their focus (Cummings et al. 2011).

Cummings et al. (2011) noted that the practices that are recommended for serving older adults regardless of ethnic or racial background are often valuable for Latino elders. For Latino elders, best and promising practices are often grounded in practical considerations of their unique culture, values, and familial relationships. The strong sense of family can assist service providers and the elderly Hispanic persons in achieving goals for healthcare management (Desai et al. 2010). Practices should include characteristics of Latino elders that are responsive to language, country of origin, length of time in the USA, and sexual orientation or gender

identity. In addition, distinct approaches for Latino elders should be effective, impactful, replicable, scalable, sustainable, and innovative. The "multi-service/one-stop shop" model of service provision seems to be a common and successful model among the Latino community (Cummings et al. 2011, p. 20). Outreach, the process of going into the community to find individuals who are in need of services, is an effective approach to service provision of LGBT elders. Outreach can be enhanced by prioritizing preventive health care and sending nurses or home health aides to the houses where Hispanic elders live, particularly those with disabilities and chronic conditions, to teach relative and significant others how to do a better job caring for them at home. This is especially relevant because many Latino elders prefer to live in their own homes. Cummings et al. identified several components of best and promising practices for Hispanic older adults (Table 10.4). According to Cummings et al., the use of a best and promising practices framework has two advantages. First, it provides an increased guarantee that elders are receiving the type of appropriate services they need to age successfully. Second, such a framework helps older adults feel more comfortable about asking for support and promotes their participation in programs that can enrich their quality of life.

Although lesbians and gay men are likely to experience some form of discrimination due to their sexual orientation, transgender persons are the most discriminated against. Thus, they rarely participate in community events or other programs for LGBT persons, making it difficult to provide services to them. The National Hispanic Council on Aging (2013) needs assessment of Hispanic LGBT elders suggests accommodating many transgender person's preference for nighttime appointments. Other strategies to facilitate outreach to the LGBT Hispanic community were to train LGBT persons so they can develop professionally and plan for the future, to provide sensitivity training workshops to schools, companies, and families so they would understand how to deal with the LGBT community, and to

Table 10.4 Best and promising practices

Involve family because Latinos, in general, feel more comfortable in family environments and family is highly important for this culture
Ensure that programs and services of community-based organizations are culturally competent
Ensure that community-based organizations have bilingual staff
Make information materials and resources available in both Spanish and English
Use a local church as a location to provide services to older adults because the role of religion and "God's Will" is a key factoring in shaping the lives of many Latinos
Implement community outreach strategies through local Hispanic radio and television stations
Use local Hispanic media to conduct education and outreach to older adults and their caregivers
Develop all-inclusive programs

Adapted from Cummings et al. (2011)

provide language training to overcome linguistic barriers to obtaining services. However, one of the major challenges of Latino community-based organizations is a lack of adequate funding, which directly affects their frontline staff and continuity of services. Cunnings et al. identified critical gaps in service infrastructure for Latino elders that must be addressed to ensure them better quality of care (see Table 10.5). One area in which there is a dramatic shortage is in all types of healthcare workers, especially those skilled across the spectrum on gerontology (Institute of Medicine 2008), cultural diversity (Lehman et al. 2012), and LGBT populations (Funders for Lesbian and Gay Issues 2004).

Policy

In order to meet the challenges of an increasingly older and diverse Hispanic population, the USA must set a course for a comprehensive

Table 10.5 Gaps in infrastructure for Latino elders

Civic engagement: a need for more leadership development and advocacy that empower Latinos to have a strong voice in national, state, and local policy and political debates
Affordable housing: current coordinated efforts to increase the amount of affordable housing are insufficient to adequately address the housing needs of this population. Funding is needed to improve the conditions of the private homes where many Latino elders live
Economic security: lack of economic resources to cover basic expenses—medications, medical treatments, health insurance, and home utilities—is a recurring problem. There is a critical need to increase financial literacy programs for elders and to provide legal advice about financial exploitation, consumer's rights, housing rights, age discrimination, right to work, and rights of people with disabilities
Healthcare system: the healthcare system does not prioritize the preventive healthcare needs of older adults. Prevention is the key for successful aging
Senior centers: there is a need to develop more senior centers where elders can spend their day while receiving social services and nutritious meals and engaging in intellectually stimulating social and recreational activities. Senior centers are a fundamental component of the support that families need to take care of their aging relatives
At-home care of elders with disabilities: there is a need for more homecare services for elders with disabilities. Most of the homecare services paid for by Medicare are for postsurgery care and not for older adults that have chronic illnesses, some form of dementia, issues of independent mobility, or preventive care
Transportation: the lack of adequate public transportation in rural areas is a serious problem for elders who are geographically isolated. Existing transportation services are mostly for elders with disabilities and those receiving scheduled healthcare services. Transportation is scarce for active elders to attend social and recreational activities and community-based organizations

Adapted from Cummings et al. (2011)

preparedness initiative that includes systematic attention to several factors. Cummings et al. (2011) offer recommendations for several areas of policy and/or funding challenges. First, attention must be on building a gerontology-centered educational pipeline, developing an ethnically and linguistically diverse workforce, and building the capacity of community-based organizations to serve both older adults and ethnically diverse populations. There is a clear need to increase the number of bilingual and bicultural service providers for upgrading the service capacity of Latino community-based organizations through core funding. In fact, service providers must accelerate efforts to hire bilingual staff (Rodriguez-Lopez and Tirado 2005). Second, it is critical to enhance the capacity of the existing aging service providers to serve ethnically and linguistically older adults. The general consensus of experts in the field is that there must be a significant increase in funding to agencies to provide their existing services and meet the needs of a growing population (Rodriguez-Lopez and Tirado). Third, community-based organizations should strengthen partnerships and organizational planning. Organizations should review their mission and objectives on a regular basis and explore partnerships with compatible organizations as a way to extend their mission and strengthen their programs. A key factor to building partnerships is trust. The National Hispanic Council on Aging (2013) encourages the development of partnerships that are inclusive of LGBT Hispanic elders, which allows for shared ownership of an agenda of for improving the quality of life of LGBT Hispanic older adults.

A fourth recommendation is to create Latino outreach programs. Research suggests that many Hispanic elders who do not speak English do not proactively seek services. Service providers indicate that LGBT Hispanic older adults are frequently unaware of how the "system" works, they do not know how to ask for help, do not

have access to written materials explaining availability of services, and are unaware of their rights to certain benefits (National Hispanic Council on Aging 2013). In response, organizations must develop the capacity to provide home-based assessment services, patient education, and supportive service visits (Rodriguez-Lopez and Tirado 2005). A desired outcome is to link services to those elders in need of services. Fifth, implement organizational best practices that make services more accessible. For LGBT Hispanic elders, accessibility is achieved through making sure that services are culturally appropriate, logistically appropriate, inclusive of sexual identities, and age-specific. Finally, create a LGBT Latino aging agenda (Cummings et al. 2011). Each of these recommendations is geared toward sustaining an aging infrastructure that meets the needs of Hispanic LGBT elders. It is vital that Hispanic non-English-speaking elders communicate effectively with their health and social service providers.

Policy pertaining to LGBT Hispanic elders should be grounded in both evidence-based practices and participatory research. There is a need for better data on LGBT Hispanic elders. In 2009, the report on *How to Close the LGBT Health Disparities Gap* proposed establishing an Office of LGBT Health in the US Department of Health and Human Services (HHS) (Krehely 2009). The intent of this Office is to collect and examine data on health outcomes and conditions of people based on sexual orientation, gender identity, race, and ethnicity. According to Krehely, "to improve overall public health and to use public dollars effectively and efficiently, the government must consider these factors when crafting public health programs and policies" (p. 4). Information about the LGBT health and well-being from the Department of Health and Human Services can be found at www.hhs.gov/lgbt/index.html. The 2011 (http://www.hhs.gov/lgbt/resources/reposts/health-objectives-2011.html), 2012 (http://www.hhs.gov/lgbt/resources/

reports/health-objectives-2012.html), and 2013 (http://www.hhs.gov/lgbt/resources/reposts/health-objectives-2013.html) committee reports on LGBT are also available.

In 2013, the two most compelling objectives of HHS included (a) implementation of the Supreme Court ruling invalidating Section 3 of the DOMA, and (b) engaging in broad outreach to help uninsured Americans gain access to affordable health insurance coverage through the Health Insurance Marketplaces. The impact of regulations of the Affordable Care Act remains to be seen, and the policies allowing access to partner benefits with the repeal of DOMA on health outcomes of LGBT Hispanic elders.

Summary

LGBT Hispanic elders represent a diverse group. They experience discrimination as ethnic and sexual minorities. Although family is an important part of Hispanic culture, many LGBT Latinos feel isolated from family and friends, and/or experience significant stress or problematic health behavior. Stigma and discrimination in healthcare and other services affect LGBT Hispanic elders in various ways and often lead to delays in accessing services. Often, LGBT Latinos receive poor clinical care, experience insensitivity from service providers, and face systems of services that lack knowledge about their cultural beliefs and concerns. Although LGBT Hispanic elders benefit from the types of services provided to seniors in general, they require a culturally appropriate and holistic approach to having their needs met. Their access to affordable health care, acquisition of spousal/partner benefits, behavioral health services, and adequate housing remains some of the most significant challenges. Services should involve an integrated, collaborative approach. An inclusive, broad-based research agenda is needed to learn more about the needs, life circumstances, experiences, and other challenges of LGBT Hispanic elders.

Learning Activities

Self-Check Questions

1. What are some common cultural values and characteristics that exist across Latino/Hispanic groups?
2. What are some gender role conflicts that Hispanic immigrant often experience in regard to traditional gender role expectations?
3. What are the core values of personalism among Hispanic/Latinos?
4. What are still some issues that must be addressed by Hispanic/Latino LGBT elders who do not face prejudice from their family or community?
5. What are the perceptions of LGBT Hispanic/Latino elders about aging in the LGBT community?

Experiential Exercises

1. Volunteer to work with a senior citizen center or social organization to work as a translator to explain information on outreach services to LGBT Latino elders.
2. Develop a resource manual of local services for LGBT Latino elders. Provide the manual in both Spanish and English.
3. Moderate a community forum for families of Latino LGBT elders to facilitate discussion about sexual orientation and gender identity.

Multiple-Choice Questions

1. What is the most important social unit among Latinos that plays a central role in how they care for aging relatives?
   (a) Religion
   (b) Family
   (c) Community
   (d) Country of Origin

2. Hispanics/Latinos who depend on family and friends during the course of their everyday lives and for getting ahead, are referred to as ____.
   (a) Individualist
   (b) Hierarchical
   (c) Collectivist
   (d) Independent

3. Which of the following informs Latinos/Hispanics' support of fairness and equality for LGBT persons?
   (a) Faith experience
   (b) Acculturation
   (c) Assimilation
   (d) Immigration status

4. Which of the following is the greatest source of income for Latino elders?
   (a) Earned income
   (b) Pension
   (c) Welfare assistance
   (d) Social Security

5. Which of the following is a major contributor to transgender Latinos never being tested and diagnosed in advance stages of sexually transmitted diseases?
   (a) Isolation
   (b) Lack of English proficiency
   (c) Rejection by their families
   (d) Lack of comfort with sharing their sexuality with a service provider

6. Which of the following is recommended for healthcare providers to recognize about Hispanic elders?
   (a) They are more likely to take advice of their physician
   (b) They are more likely to take advice of respected community members
   (c) They are more likely to visit a doctor on a regular basis
   (d) They are more likely to be preventive in their approach to health

7. Which of the following best reflects Latinos' attitude toward future health needs?

   (a) Talking about future health needs is seen as emotionally helpful
   (b) Talking about future health needs is seen as practical
   (c) Talking about future health needs is seen as frightening
   (d) Talking about future health needs is seen as nurturing

8. Which of the following is most likely for Hispanic bisexual women?
   (a) Less likely to have social support than lesbians
   (b) More likely to share the challenges they face of being both a sexual and ethnic minority
   (c) Less likely to have attempted suicide
   (d) More likely to self-report their mental health status

9. In which setting does Latino elders prefer to live?
   (a) Long-term care facilities
   (b) Their own home
   (c) A commune
   (d) Retirement community

10. Why is outreach programs recommended for health and social service work with Latino elders?
   (a) Latino elders response better to organized services
   (b) Latino elders frequently visit senior citizens community centers
   (c) Latino elders frequently explore partnership services
   (d) Latino elders who do not speak English do not proactively seek services

Key

1-b
2-c
3-a
4-d

5-d
6-b
7-c
8-a
9-b
10-d

Resources

Cuban American National Council: www.cnc. org

Hispanic Elders: http://www.stanford.edu/group/ ethnoger/hispaniclatino.html

National Council of La Raza: www.nclr.org

National Hispanic Council on Aging: www. hncoa.org

National Hispanic Medical Association: www. nhmamd.org

National Institute for Latino Policy: www. nilpnetwork.org

National Latino AIDS Action Network: www. latinoaidsagenda.org

National Puerto Rican Coalition, Inc.: www. bateylink.org

Working with Elderly Patients from Minority Groups: http://www.wichita.kumc.edu/fcm/ interp/elders/html

References

Acosta, K. (2008). Lesbians in the borderlands-shifting identities and imagined communities. *Gender Sociology, 22*(5), 639–659.

Administration on Aging. (2010, January). *A statistical profile of Hispanic older Americans aged 65+*. Retrieved September 29, 2014 from http://www.aoa. gov/aoaroot/aging_statistics/minority_aging/Facts-on-Hispanics-Elderly.aspx.

Aguilar-Gaxiola, S., Loera, G., Mendez, L., Sala, M., Latino Mental Health Concilio, & Nakamoto, J. (2012). *Community-defined solutions for latino mental health care disparities: California reducing disparities Project, Latino strategic planning workgroup population report*. Sacramento, CA: UC Davis. Retrieved October 20, 2014 from www.ucdmc. ucdavis.edu/newsroom/pdfLatino_mental_health_ report-6-25-2012-1.pdf.

Alegria, M., Chatterji, P., Wells, K., Cao, Z., Chen, C. N., Takeuchi, D., et al. (2008). Disparity in depression treatment among racial and ethnic minority populations in the United States. *Psychiatric Services, 59* (11), 1264–1272.

Alegria, M., Mulvaney-Day, N., Torres, M., Polo, A., Cao, Z., & Canino, G. (2007). Prevalence of psychiatric disorders across Latino subgroups in the United States. *American Journal of Public Health, 97*(1), 68–75.

Alexopoulos, G. S., Meyer, B. S., Yug, R. C., Campbell, S., Silbersweig, D., & Charlson, M. (1997). 'Vascular depression' hypothesis. *Archives of General Psychiatry, 54*, 915–922.

Alvarez, C. (n.d.). *The acculturation of middle-income Hispanic households*. Retrieved October 24, 2014 from www.revistaleadership.com/cladea/doctoral/ coloquio_ll/ALVAREZCECILIA.pdf.

Alvarez, P., Rengifo, J., Emrani, T., & Gallagher-Thompson, D. (2014). Latino older adults and mental health: A review and commentary. *Clinical Gerontologist, 37*, 33–48.

American Psychiatric Association. (2014). Mental health disparities: Hispanics/Latinos. *APA Fact Sheet*. Retrieved October 25, 2014 from www.psychiatry. org/mental-health-dispatities/Fact-Sheet/Hispanic-Latino.pdf.

Archuleta, A. J. (2012). Hispanic acculturation index: Advancing measurement in acculturation. *Journal of Human Behavior in the Social Environment, 22*, 297–318.

Bazargan, M., & Galvan, F. (2012). Perceived discrimination and depression among low-income Latina male-to-female transgender women. *BMC Public Health, 12*, 663–670.

Bendixen & Amandi International. (2010). *Talking about LGBT equality with Latinos & Hispanics*. Retrieved September 29, 2014 from www.lgbtmap.org/file/ talking-about-lgbt-equality-with-latinos-and-hispanics.pdf.

Berry, J. W. (2002). Conceptual approaches to acculturation. In K. Chun, P. Organista & G. Martin (Eds.), *Acculturation: Advances in theory, measurement, and applied research* (pp. 17–37). Washington, DC: American Psychological Association.

Bohorquez, L. (2009). Tapping in to the Hispanic senior segment. *DTC Perspective*, 51–53.

Bureau of Labor Statistics & U.S. Census Bureau. (2009). Table PINC-08. Source of income in 2008—People 15 years old and over, by income of specific type in 2008, age, race, Latino origin, and sex. *Current Population Survey, 2009 Annual Social and Economic Supplement*. Washington, DC: U.S. Census Bureau. Retrieved October 16, 2014 from http://www.census. gov/hhes/www/cpstables/032009/perinc/new08_004. htm.

Chiriboga, D. A., Black, S. A., Aranda, M., & Markides, K. (2002). Stress and depressive symptoms among Mexican American elders. *Journal of Gerontological Behavior, Psychological Science and Social Science, 57*, 559–568.

Cianciotto, J. (2005). *Hispanic and Latino same-sex couple households in the United States: A report from the 2000 census.* New York, NY: National Gay and Lesbian Task Force Policy Institute and the National Latino/a Coalition for Justice. Retrieved October 13, 2014 from http://www.lgbtracialequity.org/publications/HispanicsLatinoHouseholdsUS.pdf.

Cochran, S. D., Mays, V. M., Alegria, M., Ortega, A. N., & Takeuchi, D. (2007). Mental health and substance use disorders among Latino and Asian American lesbian, gay, and bisexual adults. *Journal of Consulting and Clinical Psychology, 75,* 785–794.

Constantine, M. G., Gloria, A. M., & Baron, A. (2006). Counseling Mexican American college students. In C. C. Lee (Ed.), *Multicultural issues in counseling* (3rd ed., pp. 207–222). Alexandria, VA: American Counseling Association.

Cummings, M. R., Hernandez, V. A., Rockeymoore, M., Shepard, M. M., & Sager, K. (2011, February). *The Latino age wave: What changing ethnic demographics mean for the future of aging in the United States.* New York, NY: Hispanics in Philanthropy. Retrieved October 16, 2014 from http://www.hiponline.org/storage/documents/HIP_LatinoAgeWave_FullReport_Web.pdf.

De Santis, J. P. (2009). HIV infection risk factors among male-to-female transgender persons: A review of the literature. *Journal of the Association of Nurses in AIDS Care, 20*(5), 362–372.

Desai, G. J., Ramar, C. N., & Kolo, G. P. (2010, August). Help for elderly Hispanic patients in managing diabetes mellitus: A practical approach. *AOA Health Watch.* Retrieved October 22, 2014 from www.cecity.com/aoa/healthwatch/aug_10/pront3.pdf.

Diaz, R., Bein, E., & Ayala, G. (2006). Homophobia, poverty, and racism: Triple oppression and mental health outcomes in Latino gay men. In A. Omoto & H. Kurtzman (Eds.), *Sexual orientation and mental health* (pp. 207–224). Washington, DC: American Psychological Association.

Dutwin, D. (2012). *LGBT acceptance and support: The Hispanic perspective.* Social Science Research Solution. Retrieved September 29, 2014 from www.ncir.org/images/uploads/publications/LGBTAS_HispanicPerspective.pdf.

Erving, C. (2007). *The health of the Hispanic elderly: Mortality, morbidity, and barriers to healthcare access.* Washington, DC: National Hispanic Council on Aging.

Flores, M. T. (2000). La familia Latina. In M. T. Flores & G. Carey (Eds.), *Family therapy with Hispanics: Toward appreciating diversity* (pp. 3–28). Boston: Allyn & Bacon.

Fredriksen-Goldsen, K. I., Kim, H., Emlet, C. A., Muraco, A., Erosheva, E. A., Hoy-Ellis, C. P., et al. (2011). *The aging and health report: Disparities and resilience among lesbian, gay, bisexual, and transgender older adults.* Seattle, WA: Institute for Multigenerational Health.

Funders for Lesbian and Gay Issues. (2004). *Aging in equity: LGBT elders in America.* New York, NY: Author.

Gonzales, H., Haan, M., & Hinton, L. (2001). Acculturation and the prevalence of depression in older Mexican Americans: Baseline results of the Sacramento Area Latino on Aging. *Journal of American Geriatric Society, 49,* 48–53.

Hakimzadeh, S., & Cohn, D. (2007, November). *English usage among Hispanics in the United States.* Washington, DC: Pew Hispanic Center. Retrieved September 29, 2014 from http://www.pewhispanic.org/files/reports/82.pdf.

Harper, G. W., Jernewall, N., & Zea, M. C. (2004). Giving voice to emerging science and theory for lesbian, gay, and bisexual people of color. *Culture of Diverse Ethnic Minority Psychology, 10*(3), 187–199.

Herbst, J. H., Jacobs, E. D., Finlayson, T. J., McKleroy, V. S., Neumann, M. S., & Crepaz, N. (2008). Estimating HIV prevalence and risk behaviors of transgender persons in the United States: A systematic review. *AIDS Behavior, 12*(1), 1–17.

Herek, G. M. (2002). Homosexuals' attitudes toward bisexual men and women in the United States. *Journal of Sex Research, 39*(4), 264–274.

Hernandez, R., Prohaska, T. R., Wang, P. C., & Sarkisian, C. A. (2013). The longitudinal relationship between depression and walking behavior in older Latinos: The "Caminemos!" study. *Journal of Aging and Health, 25,* 319–341.

Institute of Medicine. (2008). *Retooling for an aging America: Building the health care workforce.* Washington, DC: Institute of medicine of the National Academies. Retrieved October 19, 2014 from http://www.iom.edu/Reports/2008/Retooling-for-an-Aging-America-Building-the-Health-Care-Workforce.aspx.

Jang, Y., & Chiriboga, D. (2010). Living in a different world: Acculturative stress among Korean American elders. *Journal of Gerontology Series B: Psychology and the Social Sciences, 65B*(1), 14–21.

Jimenez, N., Dansie, E., Bushwald, D., & Goldberg, J. (2013). Pain among older Hispanics in the United States: Is acculturation associated with pain? *Pain Medicine, 14*(8), 1134–1139.

Kastanis, A., & Gates, G. J. (2010). *LGBT Latino/a individuals and Latino/a same-sex couples.* Los Angeles, CA: The Williams Institute. Retrieved September 29, 2014 from www.williamsinstitute.law.ucla.edu/wp-content/Census-2010-Latino-Final.pdf.

Kenagy, G. P. (2005). Transgender health: Findings from two needs assessment studies in Philadelphia. *Healing in Social Work, 30*(1), 19–26.

Kim, H. J., & Fredriksen-Goldsen, K. I. (2012). Hispanic lesbians and bisexual women at heightened risk or health disparities. *American Journal of Public Health, 102*(1), e9–e15.

Kochhar, R., Fry, R., & Taylor, P. (2011, July). *Twenty-to-one: Wealth gaps rise to record highs between Whites, Blacks, and Hispanics.* Washington,

DC: Pew Research Center. Retrieved June 19, 2014 from http://www.pewsocialtrends.org/files/2011/07/SDT-Wealth-Report_7-26-11_FINAL.pdf.

Koerner, S. S., Shirai, Y., & Pedroza, R. (2013). Role of religious/spiritual belief and practices among Latino family caregivers of Mexican descent. *Journal of Latina/o Psychology, 1*(2), 95–111.

Koken, J. A., Bimbi, D. S., & Parsons, J. T. (2009). Experiences of familial acceptance-rejection among transwomen of color. *Journal of Family Psychology, 23*(6), 853–860.

Krehely, J. (2009, December 21). How to close the LGBT health disparities gap: Disparities by race and ethnicity. *Center for American Progress*. Retrieved October 17, 2014 from http://www.amwericanprogress.org/issues/2009/12/pdf/lgbt_health_disparities_race.pdf.

Kuhns, L. M., Vazqiez, R., & Ramirez-Valles, J. (2008). Researching special populations: Retention of Latino gay and bisexual men and transgender persons in longitudinal health research. *Health Education Research, 23*, 814–825.

Kwag, K. H., Jang, Y., & Chiriboga, D. A. (2012). Acculturation and depressive symptoms in Hispanic older adults: Does perceived ethnic density moderate their relationship? *Journal of Immigrant Minority Health, 14*, 1107–1111.

Laea, M., Gamboa, C., Kahramanian, M. I., Morales, L. S., & Bautista, D. E. H. (2005). Acculturation and Latino health in the United States: A review of the literature and its sociopolitical context. *Annual Review of Public Health, 26*, 367–397.

Lehman, D., Fenza, P., & Hollinger-Smith, L. (2012). *Diversity & cultural competency in health care settings*. Retrieved October 22, 2014 from www.matherlifewaysinstituteonaging.com/wp-content/uploads/2012/03/Diversity-and-Cultural-Competency-in-Health-Care-Settings.pdf.

Lokpez, E. (2010). Reaching Hispanics: First segment by acculturation, then speak their language. *Real-World Education for Modern Marketers*. Retrieved October 24, 2014 from www.marketingproofs.com/articles/2010/3666/reaching-hispanics-first-segment-by-acculturation-then-speak-their-language.html.

Lopez-Baez, S. I. (2006). Counseling Latinas: Culturally responsive interventions. In C. C. Lee (Ed.), *Multicultural issues in counseling* (3rd ed., pp. 187–194). Alexandria, VA: American Counseling Association.

Masel, M. C., Rudkin, L. L., & Peek, M. K. (2006). Examining the role of acculturation in health behavior of older Mexican Americans. *American Journal of Health Behavior, 30*(6), 684–699.

McLean, K. (2008). Inside, outside, nowhere: Bisexual men and women in the gay and lesbian community. *Journal of Bisexuality, 8*(1–2), 63–80.

National Alliance for Caregiving and AARP. (2009, November). *Caregiving in the U.S. 2009*. Retrieved October 15, 2014 from www.caregiving.org/data/Caregiving_in_the_US_2009_full_report.pdf.

National Center for Health Statistics. (2013). Deaths: Final data for 2010. *National vital statistics report 61,*

no. 4. Retrieved September 28, 2014 from www.cdc.gov/nchs/data/dvs/deaths_2010_release.pdf.

National Committee to Preserve Social Security and Medicare. (2008). *Why Social Security is important to Latino and Latino Americans*. Washington, DC: National Center for Education Statistics. Retrieved October 16, 2014 from www.ncpssm.org/news/archive/vp_hispanics/.

National Council of La Raza. (2005). *Critical disparities in Latino mental health: Transforming research into action*. Retrieved October 25, 2014 from www.napolitano.house.gov/mhcacus/reports/Critical_Disparities_in_Latino_Mental_Health.pdf.

National Healthcare Disparities Report. (2005). *Agency for healthcare research and quality*. Rockville, MD. Retrieved October 16, 2014 from http://www.ahrq.gov/qual/nhdr05/nhdr05.htm.

National Hispanic Council on Aging. (2008). Retrieved October 15, 2014 from http://www.nhcog.org/economic_security.php.

National Hispanic Council on Aging. (2013, December). *Hispanic LGBT older adult needs assessment*. Retrieved July 7, 2014 from www.gallup.com.poll/158066/special-report-adults-idemtity-lgbt.aspx.

Nemoto, T., Bodeker, B., & Iwarmoto, M. (2011). Social support, exposure to violence and transphobia, and correlates of depression among male-to-female transgender women with a history of sex work. *American Journal of Public Health, 101*(10), 1980–1988.

Osypuk, T., et al. (2009). Are immigrant enclaves healthy places to live? The multi-ethnic study of atherosclerosis. *Social Science and Medicine, 69*(1), 110–120.

Palloni, A., & Arias, E. (2004). Paradox lost: Explaining the adult Hispanic mortality advantage. *Demography, 41*(3), 385–415.

Park, Y. W., Zhu, S., Palaniappan, L., Heshka, S., Carnethon, M. R., & Heymsfield, S. B. (2003). The metabolic syndrome: Prevalence and associated risk factor findings in the U.S. population from the Third National Health and Nutrition Examination Survey, 1988–1994. *Archives of Internal Medicine, 163*(4), 427–436.

Pew Hispanic Center. (2007). *Changing faiths: Latinos and the transformation of American religion (2006 Hispanic Religion Survey)*. Retrieved October 15, 2014 from www.pewhispanic.org/2007/04/25/changing-faiths-latinos-and-the-transformation-of-american-religion-20.

Pew Hispanic Center. (2010). *Statistical portrait of Latinos in the United States, 2008. Table 37: Poverty, by age, race and ethnicity: 2008*. Washington, DC: Author. Retrieved October 16, 2014 from http://pewLatino.org/files/factsheets/Latinos2008?Table%2037.pdf.

Pew Hispanic Center Survey. (2012). *2012 National Survey of Latinos*. Available at http://www.pewhispanic.org/2014/04/12/2012-national-survey-of-latinos/

Pew Research Center. (2014, May 14). *The shifting of religious identity of Latinos in the United States.*

Retrieved October 15, 2014 from www.pewresearch. org/religion.

Rodriguez-Lopez, L., & Tirado, C. (2005, March). Challenges to providing mental health services for Hispanic non-English speakers. *Hispanic Federation Punto De Vista Policy Brief.* Washington, DC: Hispanic Federation.

Roger, V., Go, A., Lloyd-Jones, D., Adams, R., Berry, J., Brown, T., et al. (2011). Heart disease and stoke statistics—2011 update: A report from the American Heart Association. *Circulation, 123*(4), e18–e209.

Sue, D. W., & Sue, D. (2013). *Counseling the culturally diverse: Theory and practice* (6th ed.). Hoboken, NJ: Wiley.

Taylor, P., Lopez, M. H., Martinez, J. H., & Velasco, G. (2012, April 4). *When labels don't fit: Hispanics and their views and identity.* Washington, DC: Pew Hispanic Center. Retrieved October 1, 2014 from www.pewhispanic.org/files/2012/04PHC-Hispanic-identity.pdf.

Tienda, M., & Mitchell, F. (Eds.). (2006). The health status and health behaviors of Hispanics. *Hispanics and the future of America.* Washington, DC: National Academies Press. Retrieved October 20, 2014 from http://www.ncbi.nlm.nih.gov/books/NBK199905/.

Torres-Gil, F., Greenstein, R., & Kamin, D. (2005). *The importance of Social Security to the Hispanic community.* Washington, DC: Center for Budget and Policy Priorities. Retrieved October 16, 2014 from www.cbpp.org/6-28-05socsec3.htm.

U.S. Bureau of Labor Statistics. (2011, August). *Labor force characteristics by race and ethnicity, 2010.* Report 1032. Washington, DC: Author.

U.S. Census Bureau. (2010a). Median age of the resident population by race and Latino origin for the United States and states: July 1, 2009. *Population estimates: State—Characteristics: Median age by race and Latino origin.* Washington, DC: Author. Retrieved October 16, 2014 from http://www.census.gov/popest/states/asrh/SC-EST2009-06.html.

U.S. Census Bureau. (2010b). *America's families and living arrangements: 2010.* Retrieved October 1, 2014 from http://www.census.gov/population/www/socdemo/hh-fam/cps2010html.

Valdez, R. B., & Arce, C. (2000). A profile of Hispanic elders. *Horizons Project Nationwide Demographic Report.* San Antonio, TX: Cutting Edge Communications, Inc.

Valentine, S. R., Godkin, J., & Doughty, G. P. (2008). Hispanics' locus of control, acculturation, and wellness attitudes. *Social Work in Public Health, 23*(5), 73–92.

Wallace, S. P. (2006, December 14). *Analysis of the 2003 California Health Interview Survey.* Presentation at the Academy Health on improving the health and wellbeing of Hispanic elders, Washington, DC.

Yang, F. M., Cazorla-Lancaster, Y., & Jones, R. N. (2008). Within-group differences in depression among older Hispanics living in the United States. *The Journals of gerontology Series B: Psychological Sciences and Social Sciences, 63*(1), 27–32.

Zhang, Z., Hayward, M., & Lu, C. (2012). Is there a Hispanic epidemiological paradox in later life? A closer look at chronic morbidity. *Research on Aging, 34*(5), 548–571.

Elder LGBT Veterans and Service Members

11

Thomas W. Miller

Abstract

This chapter explores the experiences and status of lesbian, gay, bisexual, and transgender (LGBT) older veterans and service members. Examined are the history and background of LGBT veterans, the efforts of the Department of Veterans Affairs to address the recognition and needs of these service members and veterans, and the creation of the VA *Office of Diversity and Inclusion* (US Department of Veterans Affairs, 2014 VA Diversity and Inclusion Strategic Plan for FY 2012–2016) and key policies and procedures that have addressed the discriminatory practices that have been a part of the military and post military experiences of LGBT individuals. A meta-analysis of elder LGBT veterans and military personnel is offered as are mental health and psychosocial adjustment issues for LGBT elder veterans. Discussed is the *Transitional Accommodation Syndrome* providing insight into understanding the process faced by LGBT veterans. Finally, clinical considerations with elderly LGBT veterans are offered as are a set of resources and references that may be beneficial for further inquiry into understanding of the issues faced by LGBT veterans across the life span.

Keywords

LGBT veterans · Military personnel · Equality · Public policy

Overview

This chapter explores the experiences and status of LGBT older veterans and service members. Examined are the history and background of lesbian, gay, bisexual, and transgender (LGBT) Veterans, the efforts of the Department of

T.W. Miller (✉)
University of Connecticut, Mansfield, USA
e-mail: tom.miller@uconn.edu

© Springer International Publishing Switzerland 2016
D.A. Harley and P.B. Teaster (eds.), *Handbook of LGBT Elders*,
DOI 10.1007/978-3-319-03623-6_11

223

Veterans Affairs to address the recognition and needs of these service members and veterans, and the creation of the VA *Office of Diversity and Inclusion* (US Department of Veterans Affairs 2014) and key policies and procedures that have addressed the discriminatory practices that have been a part of the military and post military experiences of LGBT individuals. A meta-analysis of elder LGBT veterans and military personnel is offered as are mental health and psychosocial adjustment issues for LGBT elder veterans. Discussed is the *Transitional Accommodation Syndrome* providing insight into understanding the process faced by LGBT veterans. Finally, clinical considerations with elderly LGBT veterans are offered as are a set of resources and references that may be beneficial for further inquiry into understanding of the issues faced by LGBT veterans across the life span.

Learning Objectives

By the end of the chapter, the reader should be able to:

1. Identify the transitions faced by LGBT veterans across the life span
2. Explain the history and significance of military policies regarding
3. Discuss research findings addressed in the meta-analysis
4. Present insights into understanding the discrimination faced by LGBT veterans
5. List and discuss the stages of the "Trauma Accommodation Syndrome" for LGBT veterans

Introduction

It was President Abraham Lincoln whose sensitivity to human rights etched a promise for all veterans to expect "care for all who bore the battle," as well as for all of one's family members by serving and honoring the men and women who are America's veterans. This commitment must include LGBT veterans. As human beings and as veterans, we all have a sexual orientation and a gender identity, and this shared fact means that discrimination against members of the LGBT community, based on sexual orientation and/or gender identity, is an issue that transcends that community and affects all of us.

When we speak of sexual orientation, it must be realized that this concept covers one's sexual desires, feelings, practices, and identification. Sexual orientation conceptually can be toward people of the same or different sexes. Gender identity refers to the complex relationship between sex and gender, referring to a person's experience of self-expression in relation to social categories of masculinity or femininity (gender). A person's subjectively felt gender identity may be at variance with his or her sex or physiological characteristics (Shipherd and Kauth 2014).

For many of today's older veterans, their experiences in the military was not under the auspices of Public Law 103-160, commonly known as "Don't Ask, Don't Tell" (DADT). It is important to note that transgender persons (those who have undergone gender reassignment surgery) cannot openly serve in the military and thus were not included in the DADT Repeal Act. Older lesbian veterans served at a time when their sexuality was scrutinized if they did not conform to gender stereotypes. They may have experienced lesbian baiting, "the practice of pressuring women for sex and sexually harassing them by using the threat of calling them lesbians as a means of intimidation" (Legal Policy Department of the Campaign for Military Service 1993). Furthermore, older LGBT veterans face a host of service-connected physical and mental health issues, and their partners are denied many rights and benefits, which heterosexual partners and spouses enjoy, including health benefits and family supports (Service Women's Action Network, n.d.). Similar to their nonmilitary counterparts, older transgender veterans are reluctant to seek health care and report negative experiences with healthcare institutions including thee

VA, are refused medical treatment for being transgender, and postpone or neglect to seek medical care when they are sick for fear of discrimination or maltreatment (Grant et al. 2011).

As a population, older LGBT veterans and service members represent a unique population. Estimating the number of LGBT veterans and service members is difficult for various reasons ranging from many of them being "closeted" to the current Veterans Health Administration (VHA) demographic data-collection strategies not allowing for routine identification of LGBT veterans and service members within the system. This limitation makes a population-based understanding of the health needs of LGBT veterans receiving care in VHA difficult, yet because of its patient size, the VHA is likely the largest single provider of health care for LGBT persons in the USA (Mattocks et al. 2014).

US Department of Veterans Affairs' (VA's) Office of Diversity and Inclusion (ODI)

The US Department of Veterans Affairs' (VA's) Office of Diversity and Inclusion (ODI) mission statement draws on a set of traditional core values. The VHA defines a culture and dedication involving respect, integrity, commitment, integrity, and excellence toward all veterans in their care. **Respect** involves treating all those individuals in their care and whom they employ with dignity and respect. **Integrity** refers to adhering to the highest professional standards while maintaining the trust and confidence of all with whom the Department of Veterans Affairs engage. There is also a **commitment** to serve all veterans and other beneficiaries by being "veteran-centric." **Excellence** strives for the highest quality and continuous improvement through thoughtful and decisive leadership and accountability (Department of Veterans Affairs 2015).

ODI prepares program reviews and annual accomplishment reports for such programs as Federal Equal Opportunity and Recruitment, Disabled Veterans Affirmative Action, Affirmative Employment, and People with Disabilities. The organizational structure for this office is summarized in Fig. 11.1.

The identified mission of the ODI is to build a diverse workforce and to cultivate an inclusive workplace to deliver the best services to our nation's veterans, their families, and beneficiaries.

Identified as its vision, it states that the VA is a leader in creating and sustaining a high-performing workforce by leveraging diversity and empowering employees to achieve superior results in service to our nation and its veterans (Department of Veterans Affairs 2015).

Focus on the LGBT Elder Veteran Community

It has been estimated that 9 million Americans identify as LGBT (Gates 2011). It has also been approximated that 1.5 million adults, aged 65 or

Fig. 11.1 Organizational structure

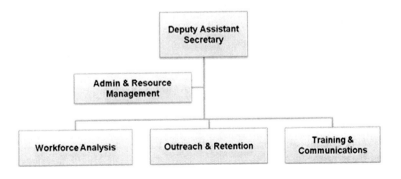

older, are LGB (no transgender estimate provided) (Movement Advancement Project) (MAP), Services and Advocacy for Gay, Lesbian, Bisexual, and Transgender Elders (SAGE), the Center for American Progress (CAP), and *LGBT Older Adults: Facts At A Glance* (National Academy on an Aging Society (GSA) and SAGE (2011). It should be noted, however, that estimates of the LGBT population may vary depending upon measurement methods and consideration of those who may not self-identify as LGBT due to societal stigma. Gates (2010) estimated in a report to the National Center for Transgender Equality that there are 70,871 LGBT individuals currently serving in the US military and over 1,000,000 veterans who are LGBT. Though the number of transgender service members and veterans is notoriously difficult to count, the *National Center for Transgender Equality* estimates that transgender individuals are twice as likely to join the US military compared to the general population.

The Department of Veterans Affairs states a commitment to a diverse workforce and an inclusive healthcare delivery environment. We understand that diversity and inclusion are essential for a high-performing organization that delivers the best service to our veterans. The LGBT community is an integral aspect of our human diversity. To that end, VA has implemented several policies and programs over the last few years that specifically address the needs and concerns of the LGBT community (Frazer 2009; Department of Veterans Affairs 2013, Movement Advancement Project 2009, 2010a, b, National Institute of Drug Abuse 2015; National Institute of Mental Health 2015). Since 2009, VA has included equal employment opportunity protections for employees on the basis of sexual orientation in the *Secretary's Annual EEO, Diversity, and No Fear Policy Statement,* which added protections based on gender identity and parental status as well. To complement this, the Department of Veterans Affairs developed and implemented an internal complaint process to provide employees with an internal avenue of redress for complaints based on these areas:

VA will not tolerate discrimination or harassment on the basis of race, color, religion, national origin, sex, pregnancy, gender identity, parental status, sexual orientation, age, disability, genetic information, or retaliation for opposing discriminatory practices or participating in the discrimination complaint process. This applies to all terms and conditions of employment, including recruitment, hiring, promotions, transfers, reassignments, training, career development, benefits, and separation.

While sexual orientation, genetic information, parental status, marital status, and political affiliation are not listed as protected bases in Title VII of the Civil Rights Act, discrimination on these bases is strictly prohibited by VA. Complaints of discrimination filed on these bases will be processed according to the aforementioned Federal EEO complaint process up to and through the investigation stage of the EEO process. The VA Office of Employment Discrimination Complaint Adjudication will issue a Final Agency Decision on the merits of the claim within 60 days of its receipt of the complaint file. Complaints filed solely on this basis will not proceed to the US Equal Employment Opportunity Commission. Other avenues of redress available to raise a claim of discrimination based on sexual orientation, gender identity, or parental status include the negotiated or administrative grievance procedure. Both permit claims of discrimination, and if otherwise appealable, raising the matter with the Office of Special Counsel and/or the Merit Systems Protection Board if the claim of discrimination is coupled with adverse impact and/or prohibited personnel practices. Although a discrimination allegation may be raised with these avenues, it does not constitute initiation of a complaint through this internal complaint process, and it does not extend the 45-day time limited to initiate such complaint with the VA Office of Resolution Management.

The *VA Office of Diversity and Inclusion* (US Department of Veterans Affairs 2014) is leading the effort to increase education and awareness of the LGBT community by establishing a formal LGBT special emphasis program. To enhance that program, an LGBT employee resource group under the auspices of the VA Diversity Council was also established. ODI holds annually nationally broadcast VA-wide LGBT Observance Program in Washington, DC, in June focusing on LGBT veterans. Additionally, we are developing cultural competency training in this area for employees, supervisors, and managers, throughout the VA system.

In the area of healthcare delivery, the VHA is committed to a patient-centered approach that organizes services around the needs and values of the LGBT veterans. To that end, in 2010, VA issued a policy statement last June providing for patient visitation rights in support of the needs of LGBT family members. Last June, VHA issued a policy directive on respectful delivery of health care to transgender and intersex individuals and is currently providing training for healthcare providers on services for transgender veterans. In 2013, VA's commitment to LGBT health care resulted in 120 VA's participating in the Human Rights Campaign (HRC) Health Equity Index (HEI) almost 80 %, which was voluntary participation. An impressive 91 of those facilities reporting or 76 % were awarded HEI 2013 Equality Leader status.

Meta-Analysis of Elder LGBT Veterans and Military Personnel

Elder LGBT must begin with understanding the incidence and prevalence rates for the presence of LGBT military and veterans in our society. The Department of Veterans Affairs' Office of Diversity and Inclusion (ODI) estimates suggest that more than 36,000 gay men and lesbians are serving in active duty, representing 2.5 % of active duty personnel (Department of Veterans Affairs 2012). When the guard and reserve are included, nearly 65,000 men and women in uniform are likely gay or lesbian accounting for 2.8 % of military personnel. Gay men and lesbians have served in all military eras in the later part of the twentieth century. In particular, military service rates for coupled lesbians far exceed rates for other women in every military era of the later twentieth century. Nearly one in 10 coupled

lesbians age 63–67 report that they served in Korea, compared with less than one in 100 of other women. Even in the most recent service period from 1990 to 2000, service rates among coupled lesbians age 18–27 are more than three times higher than rates among other women (Department of Veterans Affairs 2012).

While years of service do not differ much between coupled gay men and other men, lesbians report longer terms of service than other women. Among all women aged 18–67 who report military service, nearly 82 % of coupled lesbians and less than 74 % of other women report serving more than two years (Cáceres et al. 2008). Coupled gay men who are veterans or report training in the guard or reserve show greater racial and ethnic diversity than do other men. Among men who report guard or reserve training, the proportions of coupled gay men who are African-American and Latino exceed those of other men. Among female veterans, the pattern is the opposite of that shown with men. Coupled lesbians are more likely to be white than other female veterans and are less likely to be African-American. Coupled gay men who report guard or reserve training or who are veterans report annual incomes below that of other men, while coupled lesbians report incomes above that of other women. An exploration of employment status provides some explanation for the income gaps observed. Coupled gay men with guard or reserve training are less likely to be employed full time and more likely to not be in the labor force than other men. Conversely, coupled lesbians who are veterans or report guard or reserve training have substantially higher rates of full-time employment than other women and are less likely to report not being in the labor force.

There are five states including Dakota, Hawaii, Alaska, Virginia, and Idaho having the largest proportion of veterans among same-sex couples. Men and women in same-sex couples in North Dakota are twice as likely to be a veteran as the national average. Among metropolitan areas, Pensacola, Florida; Norfolk, Virginia; San Diego, California; Dayton, Ohio; and Santa Rosa, California, have the highest rates of veterans among same-sex couples. Pensacola's rate of 34 % is more than three times the national average. Nearly one million gay and lesbian Americans are veterans. The states with the largest population of gay and lesbian veterans include California, Florida, Texas, New York, and Georgia. Among metropolitan areas, Los Angeles, Washington, DC, San Diego, Chicago, and New York have the highest populations of gay and lesbian veterans. The District of Columbia leads all states with a rate of 10.2 gay or lesbian veterans per 1000 adults, more than double the national average. Per capita rates are also high in Vermont, Hawaii, Maine, and Washington.

LGBT Elder Veterans and Challenges of Aging

LGBT elder veterans face the typical challenges of aging, including the possibility of elder abuse or domestic violence, in combination with the threat of discrimination and abuse due to their sexual orientation or gender identity (Cook-Daniels 1998). The reader is referred to Chaps. 16 and 17 for additional information on elder abuse and mistreatment. In a 2006 study by the *Metlife Mature Market Institute*, 27 % of LGBT Baby Boomers reported that they had great concern about discrimination as they age. Cook-Daniels (1998) notes that growing up in a homophobic or transphobic environment, some LGBT elders may go to extraordinary measures to hide their sexual orientation. There may be such significant stigma for these elders that they will not label themselves. This may affect an abuse victim's willingness to seek help, out of fear of needing to "out" themselves to authorities and face possible hostility. This may also affect his or her desire to enlist home care services out of fear of abuse. LGB adults from older generations lived under severe stigmatization of their identities. Many victims of attacks due to sexual orientation do not tell others of the attacks out of fear that their sexual orientation will be disclosed or that authorities will act with hostility or indifference (D'Augelli and Grossman 2001).

Discrimination and the Don't Ask, Don't Tell Policy

The Department of Veterans Affairs' Office of Diversity and Inclusion (ODI) acknowledges that discriminatory practices have occurred toward both VHA providers and LGBT veterans. Several policies, perhaps the most significant of which was the "Don't As Don't Tell" effort, resulted in reported concerns about stigma and discrimination against LGBT veterans (Shipherd and Kauth 2014).

Among formal polices that have been cited as most discriminatory against LGBT military and veterans since its inception has been the "Don't Ask, Don't Tell" policy. Military and veterans who are lesbian, gay, bisexual, and transgender Americans have experienced historic progress over the past three years. In 2010, Congress repealed the discriminatory "Don't Ask, Don't Tell" policy, which prevented gay, lesbian, and bisexual service members from serving openly and with honesty. More recently, the Supreme Court struck down Section 3 of the Defense of Marriage Act (DOMA), which forced the federal government to deny more than 1000 federal benefits and protections to legally married same-sex couples that were freely available to different-sex couples. The Pentagon has resisted such legislation, stating that current law already grants "reasonable accommodation" of religious freedom to service members. At the same time, the White House pointed out that the amendment would actually tie the hands of commanders, who have the ultimate responsibility of ensuring good order, discipline, and unit morale and who would be helpless to stop religious bullying under the amendment. Since the successful repeal of "Don't Ask, Don't Tell," opponents of LGBT equality have made considerable efforts to undermine the effort toward inclusion and respect for both active military and for veterans. The Department of Veterans Affairs has demonstrated efforts to address this policy and correct the discriminatory impact of LGBT veterans.

Policy-Box

Don't Ask, Don't Tell (DADT) is the moniker for the former official US policy (1993–2011) regarding the service of persons who were homosexual and in the military. In 1993, Pres. Bill Clinton in 1993 signed a law (consisting of statute, regulations, and policy memoranda) directing that military personnel "don't ask, don't tell, don't pursue, and don't harass." When it was implemented in October 1, 1993, the policy theoretically lifted a ban on homosexual service that had been instituted during World War II, though, in effect, it continued a statutory ban. In December 2010, both the House of Representatives and the Senate voted to repeal the policy, and Pres. Barack Obama signed the legislation on December 22. The policy officially ended on September 20, 2011. The policy was not met with enthusiasm: Notably, military officers feared that the mere presence of homosexuals in the armed forces would undermine morale. The policy was further subverted by discrimination suits that upheld the right of gays to serve in the military without fear of discrimination. Under terms of the law, homosexuals serving in the military were not allowed to talk about their sexual orientation or engage in sexual activity, and commanding officers were not allowed to question service members about their sexual orientation. By the 15-year anniversary of the law in 2008, more than 12,000 officers had been discharged from the military for refusing to hide their homosexuality. When Barack Obama campaigned for the presidency in 2008, he pledged to overturn "Don't Ask, Don't Tell" and to allow gay men and lesbians to serve openly in the military (a stance that was, according to public opinion polls, backed by a large majority of the public). During Obama's first year in office, the Act was repealed, and the repeal took effect on September 20, 2011.

Adapted from Encyclopedia Britannica. Don't Ask, Don't Tell (DAT): http://www.britannica.com/EBchecked/topic/1553878/Dont-Ask-Dont-Tell-DADT.

Discussion Questions:

1. What was the intent of the law as Clinton passed it?
2. What were problems with the law?
3. How has repeal of the law changed the landscape for LGBT persons in the military now?

The Don't Ask, Don't Tell Policy has transitioned through a number of changes over the past decade. Summarize the key points of this policy and how it has changed for elder veterans served by the Department of Veterans Affairs.

Defense of Marriage Act

Another policy that has been cited as discriminatory is the DOMA, which has prevented the military and the Department of Veterans Affairs from extending benefits programs to the same-sex spouses of service members and veterans. As a result, same-sex spouses were denied nearly 100 military benefits that were freely available to different-sex spouses, including health care, housing allowances, and survivor benefits. On June 26, 2013, the Supreme Court struck down Section 3 of the law, clearing the way for the military to include same-sex spouses in benefits programs for the first time in our nation's history. On September 3, 2013, the Department of Defense began extending these benefits. Service members who were married before the Supreme Court ruling will receive entitlements retroactive to June 26, and those who marry in the future may start drawing benefits on the date of their marriage. Furthermore, gay and lesbian service members are eligible to receive federal spousal benefits through the military even if they are stationed in a state that does not recognize their marriages.

The military has authorized commanders to grant up to seven days of leave for stateside couples and 10 days of leave for couples overseas so they can travel to a state in America and legally wed. Although traveling to a state with marriage equality imposes a significant financial expense for military families—especially for junior enlisted members and those stationed outside the continental USA—the military's willingness to accommodate the marriage of same-sex couples despite disparate state laws is a significant step toward equality for all service members.

A concern is that the situation for veterans seeking benefits for a same-sex spouse is less clear. In an August 2013 letter to Congress, Secretary of Veterans Affairs Eric Shinseki expressed concerns about a separate statute governing veteran's benefits, which legally prevented the department from extending these benefits to the same-sex spouse of a veteran. Less than a week after that announcement, a federal judge in California overturned the statute, which arguably created a legal pathway for the Department of Veterans Affairs to recognize same-sex spouses. As a result, the Department of Justice announced that it would no longer enforce the law that restricted veteran spousal benefits to different-sex couples.

While the Department of Veterans Affairs now finds it lawful to extend veterans benefits to same-sex spouses, another factor complicates the situation. Though the Department of Defense has decided, it will judge the validity of marriages based on where a couple was married instead of where the military member is currently stationed, it is uncertain whether or not the Department of Veterans Affairs will authorize veterans in same-sex marriages eligibility for federal benefits if they reside in a state that does not recognize their marriage.

"Less than honorable discharges" for LGBT veterans have provided another area of concern for former service members. Veterans who were discharged for "homosexual conduct" under *Don't Ask, Don't Tell* received Honorable or General under Honorable discharges. Before 1993, service members who were found to have engaged in homosexual conduct were likely to receive discharges that were "Less than Honorable." This affects several elder veterans who are LGBT. A less than onorable discharge characterization can have severe consequences that follow a veteran for his or her entire life. In most states, it is legal for private employers to discriminate on the basis of a discharge characterization, and a less than honorable discharge all but disqualifies a person from working in the public sector. While there are efforts to address this issue, a *less than honorable discharge* characterization may mean forfeiture of veteran's benefits, such as G.I. Bill education benefits and healthcare coverage.

Elderly veterans who were LGBT discharged before 1993, undergo additional hurdles and a lengthy review process in efforts to obtain an upgrade for VA benefits. With the additional hurdles, advocates have called the current process "cumbersome and bureaucratic" and have noted that it could take several years for LGBT veterans to receive a response from the review board. In summary, the repeal of DADT and the Supreme Court's decision on DOMA does not mean the end of discrimination for the LGBT veterans who serve in our nation's military. It is not clear whether gay and lesbian veterans will receive spousal benefits if they do not reside in a state that recognizes same-sex marriage.

Elder LGBT Veterans

In 2012 that the VHA initiated an effort to address the specific needs of elder LGBT veterans. The *Metlife Mature Market Institute* study (2006) reveals that about one in three LGBT aging veterans did in fact report that they had great concern about discrimination as they mature and age. There are several subtle discriminatory practices facing elder LGBT veterans, but among these the most significant are regularly denied same-sex partners and restrict the most basic rights such as hospital visitation or the right to die in the same nursing home.

Many LGBT elders experience social isolation and ageism within the LGBT community itself (see Chap. 29). Also, Social Security pays survivor benefits to widows and widowers but not to the surviving same-sex life partner of someone who dies. This may cost LGBT elders $124 million a year in unassessed benefits. Married spouses are eligible for Social Security spousal benefits, which can allow them to earn half their spouse's Social Security benefit if it is larger than their own Social Security benefit. Unmarried partners in lifelong relationships are not eligible for spousal benefits. In examining the Medicaid regulations that protect the assets and homes of married spouses, when the other spouse enters a nursing home or long-term care facility, no such protections are offered to same-sex partners. Finally, tax laws and other regulations including 401(k) and pensions discriminate against same-sex partners. This often results in costing the surviving partner in a same-sex relationship financial penalties during their life. There is an extensive summary of benefits for LGBT veterans available on the Department of Veterans Affairs Web site at: http://www. benefits.va.gov/persona/lgb.asp. This resource may be beneficial in addressing benefits for LGBT veterans.

LGBT elder veterans face several challenges with respect to benefits. Summarize the key benefits to which they are entitled and how these benefits have changed for elder veterans receiving care and treatment by the Department of Veterans Affairs.

There are additional concerns faced by LGBT veterans. They often struggle with their access to adequate health care, affordable housing, or other social services that they need due to institutionalized heterosexism. Veterans who use VHA ted to be older, less educated, and unemployed than veterans who do not use VHA. Moreover, veterans who receive services from VHA have worse perceived health, use more health care, and have multiple medical comorbidities. Fore LGBT veterans being a member of both veterans and LGBT communities may contribute to a higher level of risk for poor health than membership in just one of these populations (Mattocks et al. 2014). Existing regulations and proposed policy changes in programs such as Social Security or Medicare, which impact millions of LGBT elders, are discussed without a LGBT perspective engaging the debate.

Federal programs designed to assist elderly Americans can be ineffective or even irrelevant for LGBT elders. Grant et al. (2011) and others have documented widespread homophobia among those entrusted with the care of America's LGBT seniors. Most LGBT elders do not avail themselves of services on which other seniors thrive. Many retreat back into the closet, reinforcing isolation. Several federal programs and laws blatantly treat same-sex couples differently from married heterosexual couples.

Mental Health and Psychosocial Adjustment Issues for LGBT Elder Veterans

Cook-Daniels (1998) has addressed critically important strategies necessary in the care and treatment of LGBT veterans. There are both physical and mental health issues faced by these veterans. They often face a lack of legal protections, which results in insecurity, uncertainty, and avoidance. For example, an elder male veteran who is gay with limited income has no legal right in many states to a portion of his abusive partner's income.

VA healthcare professionals are encouraged to connect and build rapport with the elder veteran who is LGBT by asking about their career/profession, friends, and personal effects. Attention is needed especially to the LGBT elder veterans' input and awareness that not all couple relationships are heterosexual. Changes are warranted to use the same terminology used by the elder (e.g., partner, roommate, friend) when referring to the other member of the couple. It is critical to ask the elder whether the partner/roommate/friend can be counted on to provide care or financial assistance to him or her, keeping in mind that a large age gap between partners in a gay couple does not necessarily imply an exploitative relationship.

Elder LGBT Veterans' Integrative Health Care

Integrative health care is the provision of coordinated care, comprehensive care, and seamless care that is accepted as a worldwide trend in healthcare provision (Miller 2012). Many LGBT elderly veterans have never heard of integrative health care, but this holistic movement has left its imprint American medicine and health care in the twenty-first century. *Treating the Whole Person* has become the standard of practice for all Americans including our veteran population. Both healthcare providers and patients alike are bonding with the philosophy of integrative healthcare provision and its whole-person approach, which is designed to treat the person, not just the disease or illness as in the past.

The physical and mental health of all veterans served through the Department of Veterans Affairs is achieved through a consumer friendly integrative approach to meeting the health and well-being of all veterans. Even before the repeal of Don't Ask, Don't Tell, the Department of Veterans Affairs launched initiatives to ensure that LGBT veterans have access to the health care and coverage they need. In 2011, the VHA released a groundbreaking policy statement on the provision of care to transgender veterans. VHA Directive 2011-024 established a policy for the department about the respectful delivery of care to transgender veterans. Directive 2011-024 affirmed VHA's zero-tolerance policy for harassment, required respectful treatment of veterans according to their self-identified gender, and clearly stated that nonsurgical transition-related care is available to transgender patients under the VA's medical benefits package. A second directive renewed these policies in 2013 and extends through February 2018.

In February 2012, the Department of Veterans Affairs extended similar protections to lesbian, gay, and bisexual veterans. A department-wide memorandum required that all VA medical centers adopt nondiscrimination and visitation policies protecting the rights of veterans, regardless of sexual orientation or gender identity. The Department of Veterans Affairs has complemented these policy directives with guidelines for implementing LGBT-inclusive care in local VA healthcare facilities. The VHA provides clinical competency training for VHA physicians to ensure that transgender veterans receive high-quality, comprehensive health care. VHA medical providers are given additional guidance on meeting the medical needs of transgender veterans through medical guidance on the use of hormone therapy. This kind of training and use of clinical standards is particularly significant because medical providers are often given insufficient training in medical school on the provision of care to transgender patients. VA medical centers have been quick to adopt these changes, and LGBT special emphasis groups may assist many of them in increasing cultural competency and conducting outreach to LGBT veterans. These significant advances in LGBT-inclusive health care have been noted by the HRC's 2013 Healthcare Equality Index. Eighty percent of VHA facilities nationwide participated in the index, and of those, more than three-quarters were awarded "Leader in LGBT Healthcare Equality" status.

Mental Health Care for Veterans Who Are LGBT

The *National Academy on an Aging Society/GSA and SAGE* (2011) identified stigmatization and its consequences along with the fear of discrimination, and its reality result in underutilization of VA healthcare services. Mental health needs are among the spectrum of health care sought by veterans who are LGBT through the Department of Veterans Affairs and other community services. The Institute of Mental Health (NIMH) and the National Institute of Drug Abuse (NIDA) report that veterans within the LGBT community have complications of depression, substance abuse, and traumatic stress disorder for which they seek treatment. In addition, LGBT Veterans face a number of transitional challenges in life. Accommodation theory (Miller 1989, 2010, 2014) has relevance for elder LGBT veterans and may aid in understanding how one cognitively processes one's understanding of self and their identity. The *Trauma Accommodation Syndrome* (1989) has aided mental health professionals in understanding and recognizing the process of coping with stressful life transitions including isolation, bullying, and stigmatization experienced by some LGBT veterans across the life span.

The *Trauma Accommodation Syndrome* (1989) identifies five sequential stages in understanding what a person goes through when he faces an environment, which is hostile discriminatory and or traumatizing as is experienced by some LGBT veterans. It is summarized in Fig. 11.2 and includes the following stages: secrecy, helplessness, avoidance, and accommodation, which many LGBT veterans and nonveterans can recognize having experienced in coping with the stigmatization they have often faced and the isolation that they have often felt.

The stage of *secrecy* involves stigmatization, isolation, and self-blame. Secrecy often occurs and is prompted by feelings of uncertainty or inadequacy, guilt, and shame. Secrecy about one's LGBT may lead to feelings of *helplessness*. The helplessness experience results in depressive

features and may show itself clinically through a limited motivational response as well as the usual signs of clinical depression.

Clinically, the *Trauma Accommodation Syndrome* (1989) is summarized through the phases, which match DSM-5 (American Psychiatric Association 2013) criteria for traumatic stress disorder and are summarized in Fig. 11.3. It reflects what any person would experience through discrimination or a hostile environment that results in traumatic stress for a human being. Discriminatory behaviors often faced by elder LGBT veterans can result in this sequence of clinical symptoms. Initially, the individual experiences a stage of secrecy and helplessness. During this stage, the person may develop characteristic symptoms of anxiety and stress that is not easily managed. Often this may lead to psychological reactivity, a sense of fear or feelings of helplessness. At the same time, it may lead to physiological reactivity as realized through somatization. Such reactivity, whether physical or psychological, often results in individuals revisiting the life transition they are facing both consciously and unconsciously. The revisiting process is often cyclical for the individual, which leads to ineffective coping strategies such as avoidance, detachment, irritability, numbing, hyper-vigilance, marked by cognitive disorganization, sleep difficulty, and recurrent distress. For an elder LGBT veteran, these symptoms may result in a functional depressive reaction to the thoughts and feelings they experience. Eventually, this leads the individual to accommodate the trauma and learn to cope with the discrimination resulting in adjusting or adapting to the discrimination.

Fig. 11.2 Stages of the "Trauma Accommodation Syndrome" for LGBT veterans

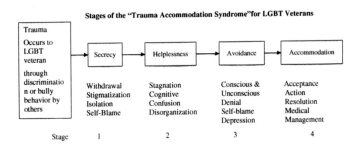

Stages of the "Trauma Accommodation Syndrome" for LGBT Veterans

Trauma Occurs to LGBT veteran through discrimination or bully behavior by others	Secrecy	Helplessness	Avoidance	Accommodation
	Withdrawal Stigmatization Isolation Self-Blame	Stagnation Cognitive Confusion Disorganization	Conscious & Unconscious Denial Self-blame Depression	Acceptance Action Resolution Medical Management
Stage	1	2	3	4

The Five Phases of the "Trauma Accommodation Syndrome"

Adapted For LGBT Elderly Veterans

Thomas W. Miller Ph.D.

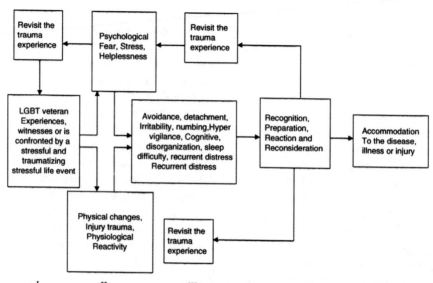

| I | II | III | IV | V |

Fig. 11.3 The five phases of the "Trauma Accommodation Syndrome" adapted for LGBT elderly veterans

The impact of discrimination experienced by LGBT elder veterans has led to mental health issues. Explain how the *Transitional Accommodation Syndrome* provides insight into understanding the process faced by these veterans. Summarize the key stages of accommodation for some elder LGBT veterans.

Clinical Considerations with Elderly LGBT Veterans

There has been a growing literature on clinical care and treatment interventions that are directly relevant to elderly veterans who are LGBT (Israel et al. 2008; Riggle et al. 2008; Shelton and Delgado-Romero 2013; Gonzalez et al. 2013; Simmons and White 2014). Most seek professional assistance, care, and treatment for supportive identity affirming counseling, along with negotiating new, contextual understanding of self. There is also often the need for guidance and brainstorming ways to navigate various social systems and locating resources such as mentors and community support. Issues related to self-image, coming out, managing identities in different environments, alcohol and substance abuse and anxiety, depression, and other typical mental health concerns.

Summary

The Department of Veterans Affairs has made inroads in the care and treatment of elderly LGBT veterans since the joint memorandum on LGBT inclusion was sent to Veterans Integrated Service Network VISN and VA Medical Centers Directors by the Principal Deputy Under Secretary for Health and the Deputy Under Secretary for Health for Operations and Management. That memorandum directed VA medical facilities to undertake at least three specific initiatives in Fiscal Year 2013 to "help build a welcoming and inclusive environment for LGBT Veterans within their facility." Among the suggested initiatives was participation in the Healthcare Equality Index

(HEI) survey for 2013. The HEI, a quality improvement tool created by the HRC in collaboration with the Gay and Lesbian Medical Association, benchmarks best practice and policy for equal treatment of LGBT patients and families within US healthcare systems. The Office of Health Equity (OHE) served as the VHA program coordinator for the 2013 HEI and a resource to facilities pursuing HEI endorsement. In 2013, 121 VA facilities participated in the HEI, with 92 achieving leadership status. Information about this achievement and the 570 projects undertaken in FY 2013 is available on the OHE SharePoint site (see paragraph 8.d.) dated July 1, 2014 IL 10-2014-14 5. For elder veterans who are LGBT, equality post military and in later life is not just an issue of fairness; it is also about facing the reality that LGBT Americans serve in uniform and make sacrifices on our behalf, just like their heterosexual counterparts. It is the explicit duty of members of Congress and the commander in chief to support our military and to ensure that the men and women in uniform are able to perform to the best of their abilities, particularly to support the FY 2014 National Defense Authorization Act —the single-most critical bill to ensuring the functioning of our nation's veterans so that there is appropriate care for our veterans and LGBT equality for all service members who are honored LGBT elder veterans.

Acknowledgments The author wishes to acknowledge the guidance and assistance of James C. Holsinger MD PhD, University of Kentucky and former Chief Medical Director Department of Veterans Affairs; Monica Roy PhD VA medical Center and NE VA HealthCare, Boston MA; Katie Miller, Research Assistant for the LGBT Research and Communications Project at the Center for American Progress; Andrew Cray, Policy Analyst for the LGBT Research and Communications Project. Special appreciation is extended to Jillian C. Shipherd, PhD National Center for PTSD, Women's Health Sciences Division, VA Boston Healthcare System, Boston, Massachusetts, and Boston University School of Medicine, Boston, Massachusetts, and Michael R. Kauth, PhD with the VHA South Central (VISN 16) Mental Illness Research, Education, and Clinical Center (MIRECC), and Michael E. DeBakey VA Medical Center, Houston, TX; and Baylor College of Medicine, Houston, for their guidance and resources in the completion of this chapter.

Resources

US Department of Veterans Affairs' (VA's) Office of Diversity and Inclusion (ODI)
Jillian C. Shipherd, PhD Michael R. Kauth, PhD. Lesbian, Gay, Bisexual, and Transgender (LGBT) Program Coordinators Office of Patient Care Services (10P4Y) at VA Central Office, Washington, DC
VHA Office of Health Equity, Washington, DC
Case-Based Transgender E-Consultation with Department of Veterans Affairs
Three regional Transgender E-Consultation programs: Loma Linda, CA (VISN 22), Minneapolis, MN (VISN 23), Tucson, AZ (VISN 18)
VHA Transgender & LGB Education SharePoints: Contact: Michael.Kauth@va.gov or Jillian.Shipherd@va.gov
American Psychological Association: www.apa.org/pi/lgbt/resources/
World Professional Association for Transgender Health: www.wpath.org
Healthy People 2020 available at: http://www.healthypeople.gov/2020/topicsobjectives2020/overview.aspx?topicid=25
Gay, Lesbian Medical Association: www.glma.org

Learning Exercises

Self-Check Questions (5 questions)

1. What are transitions that LGBT veterans face that are not faced by those elders who are not veterans?
2. Explain the significance of the "Don't Ask, Don't Tell" policy.
3. Discuss discrimination faced by LGBT elder veterans.
4. Discuss and explain the "Trauma Accommodation syndrome.
5. What are particular challenges of aging faced by LGBT veterans?

Experiential Assignments

1. Visit a VA medical Center and request an appointment with the Director of the facility to discuss policies and procedures in addressing the healthcare needs of LGBT veterans
2. Vet Centers provide community outreach. Meet with one of the counselors in the Vet Centers in your area to discuss screening and treatment interventions offered through the Vet Center program
3. Contact the VA Office of Diversity and Inclusion (ODI) and ask for information about their annual report and how they are addressing their mission and vision statement.

Multiple-Choice Questions (10)

1. What is not a key feature of the mission statement of the US Department of Veterans Affairs' Office of Diversity and Inclusion?
   a. Silence
   b. Respect
   c. Integrity
   d. Commitment
2. The population of LGBT elder veterans is
   a. Nonexistent
   b. Totally unknown
   c. Easily identifiable
   d. Identified somewhat
3. Coupled gay men who are veterans or report training in the guard or reserve, when compared to heterosexual veterans
   a. Similar
   b. Predominantly Asian
   c. More often African-American and Hispanic
   d. More often from urban areas
4. Coupled gay women who are veterans or report training in the guard or reserve, when compared to heterosexual veterans
   a. More often white
   b. Predominantly Asian
   c. More often African-American and Hispanic
   d. More often from urban areas

5. Challenges that LGBT elders face include all these except
   a. Isolation
   b. Threat of discrimination
   c. Adequate social services
   d. Fear of abuse
6. The policy regarded as the most discriminatory for LGBT veterans was
   a. Social Security
   b. Don't Ask, Don't Tell
   c. Medicare
   d. Elder Justice Act
7. What are ways that the Veterans Administration is working to help LGBT elders?
   a. Training of the workforce
   b. Training the military
   c. Adapting clinical standards for treatment
   d. All of the above
8. In the past, mental health care for LGBT veterans has been
   a. Excellent
   b. Fairly adequate
   c. Good
   d. Poor
9. Historically, LGBT Elder veterans have been treated _____ by the Veterans Administration:
   a. Fairly
   b. Unfairly
   c. Adequately
   d. Appropriately
10. Stages of the "Trauma Accommodation Syndrome" for LGBT Veterans include all the following except:
    a. Secrecy
    b. Helplessness
    c. Accommodation
    d. Reimbursement

Key (For Multiple-Choice Questions)

1-a
2-d
3-c
4-a
5-c
6-b

7-d
8-d
9-b
10-d

References

American Psychiatric Association. (2013). *Diagnostic and statistical manual of mental disorders* (Vol. 5). Washington, D.C: American Psychiatric Association. (Text Revision).

Cáceres, C.F., Konda, K., Segura, E.R., & Lyerla, R. (2008, Aug). Epidemiology of male same-sex behavior and associated sexual health indicators in low- and middle-income countries: 2003–2007 estimates. *Sexually Transmitted Infections, 84*(1), i49–i56. doi: 10.1136/sti.2008.030569.

Cook-Daniels, L. (1998). Lesbian, gay male, bisexual and transgendered elders: Elder abuse and neglect issues. *Journal of Elder Abuse & Neglect, 9*(2), 35-49. Available at: http://www.tandfonline.com/doi/abs/10.1300/J084v09n02_04

D'Augelli, A., & Grossman, A. (2001). Disclosure of sexual orientation, victimization, and mental health among lesbian, gay, and bisexual older adults. *Journal of Interpersonal Violence, 16*(10), 1008–1027. Available at: http://jiv.sagepub.com/content/16/10/1008

Department of Veterans Affairs. (2014). *VA Diversity and Inclusion Strategic Plan for FY 2012–2016.* Washington, D.C. Available at: http://www.diversity.va.gov/products/diar.aspx

Department of Veterans Affairs. (2015). *Office of Diversity and Inclusion* (ODI). Washington, D.C. Available at: http://www.diversity.va.gov/programs/lgbt.aspx

Department of Veterans Affairs. (2013). *Federally mandated reports: DVA Reports Achieves.* Washington, D. C. Available at: http://www.diversity.va.gov/products/reports.aspx

Department of Veterans Affairs. (2012). *VA benefits for elderly veterans.* Washington, D.C. Available at: http://www.benefits.va.gov/persona/veteran-elderly.asp

Frazer, S. (2009). *LGBT Health and Human Services needs in New York State.* Albany, NY: Empire State Pride Agenda Foundation. Available at: http://www.prideagenda.org/Portals/0/pdfs/LGBT%20Health%20and%20Human%20Services%20Needs%20in%20New%20York%20State.pdf

Grant, J.M., Mottet, L.A., Tanis, J., Harrison, J., Herman, J.L., & Keisling, M. (2011). *Injustice at every turn: A report of the national transgender discrimination survey.* Washington, D.C.: National Center for Transgender Equality and National Gay and Lesbian Task Force.

Gates, M.A. (2010). Post-traumatic stress disorder in veterans and military personnel: Epidemiology, screening, and case recognition. *Psychological Services, 9*(4), 361–382.

Gates, G. (2011). *How many people are lesbian, gay, bisexual, and transgender?* Williams Institute: UCLA School of Law. Available at: http://williamsinstitute.law.ucla.edu/wp-content/uploads/Gates-How-Many-People-LGBT-Apr-2011.pdf

Gonzalez, K. A., Rostosky, S. S., Odom, R. D., & Riggle, E. D. B. (2013). The positive aspects of being a parent of an LGBTQ child. *Family Process, 52*(2), 325–337.

Israel, T., Gorcheva, R., Burnes, T. R., & Walther, W. A. (2008). Helpful and unhelpful therapy experiences of LGBT clients. *Psychotherapy Research, 18*(3), 294–305.

Legal Policy Department of the Campaign for Military Service. (1993).

Mattocks, K. M., Kauth, M. R., Sandfort, T., Matza, A. R., Sullivan, J. C., & Shipherd, J. C. (2014). Understanding health-care needs of sexual and gender minority veterans: How targeted research and policy can improve health. *LGBT Health, 1*(1), 50–57.

Miller, T. W. (1989). *Stressful life events.* New York: International Universities Press Inc.

Miller, T. W. (Ed.). (2010). *Handbook of stressful transitions across the life span.* New York: Springer Publishers Incorporated.

Miller, T.W. (Ed.). (2012). Praeger handbook of Veterans' Health: Volume III: *Mental health: Treatment and rehabilitation.* Santa Barbara, California: Praeger ABC-CLIO Publishers. ISBN 978-0-313-38349-6; eISBN 978-0-313-38350-2.

Movement Advancement Project. (2009). Snapshot advancing gender equality. Available at: http://www.lgbtagingcenter.org/resources/resource.cfm?r=501

Movement Advancement Project, Services and Advocacy for Gay, Lesbian, Bisexual, and Transgender Elders, & Center for American Progress. (2010a). *LGBT older adults and inhospitable health care environments.* Available at: http://sageusa.org/uploads/lgbt_environments.pdf

Movement Advancement Project, Services and Advocacy for Gay, Lesbian, Bisexual, and Transgender Elders, & Center for American Progress. (2010b). *LGBT older adults: Facts at a Glance.* Available at: http://lgbtagingcenter.org/resources/resource.cfm?r=22

MetLife Mature Market Institute, Lesbian and Gay Aging Issues Network (ASA), & Zogby International. (2006). *Out and aging: The MetLife study of lesbian and gay baby boomers.* MetLife: New York. Available at: http://www.metlife.com/assets/cao/mmi/publications/studies/mmi-out-aging-lesbian-gayretirement.pdf

National Academy on an Aging Society (GSA), & SAGE. (2011). Integrating lesbian, gay, bisexual, and transgender older adults' into aging policy and practice. *Public Policy and Aging Report, 21*(3), 1–36.

Available at: http://www.sageusa.org/uploads/PPAR%20Summer20111.pdf

National Institute of Mental Health (NIMH). (2015). Transforming the understanding and treatment of mental illnesses. Bethesda, Maryland. Available at: http://www.nimh.nih.gov/index.shtml

National Institute of Drug Abuse (NIDA). (2015). The science of drug abuse and addiction. Bethesda, Maryland. Available at: http://www.drugabuse.gov/

Riggle, E. D. B., Whitman, J. S., Olson, A., Rostosky, S. S., & Strong, S. (2008). The positive aspects of being a lesbian or gay man. *Professional Psychology: Research and Practice, 39*(2), 210–217.

Service Women's Action Network. (n.d.). *After repeal: LGBT service members and veterans—The facts*. New York, NY: Author.

Shelton, K., & Delgado-Romero, E.A. (2013). Sexual orientation microaggressions: The experience of lesbian, gay, bisexual and queer clients in psychotherapy. *Psychology of Sexual Orientation and Gender Diversity, 1*(S), 59–70.

Simmons, H., & White, F. (2014). Our many selves. In L. Erickson-Schroth (Ed.), *Trans bodies, trans selves: A resource for the transgender community* (pp. 3–23). New York: Oxford.

Shipherd, J.C., & Kauth, M.R. (2014, August 8). *LGBT Veteran health care is coming out of the closet*. Washington, D.C: American Psychological Association.

LGBT Elders and the Criminal Justice System

12

Tina Maschi, Jo Rees, Eileen Klein and Ron Levine

Abstract

This chapter explores LGBT elders with histories of incarceration. Due to the paucity of the literature available on this population, this chapter provides new data from a qualitative study of ten formerly incarcerated LGBT elders' experiences prior to, during, and after release from prison. Consistent with intersectionality theory, a core theme of self and the social mirror emerged from the data that represented LGBT elders' ongoing coming out process of unearthing their 'true selves' despite managing multiple intersectional stigmatized identities, such as being LGBT, elderly, HIV positive, Reverse order, a member of a racial/ethnic minority, and being formerly incarcerated. These exploratory findings further our awareness of an overlooked population of LGBT elders involved in the criminal justice system. The implications for interprofessional and interdisciplinary policy and practice that incorporate suggestions from the formerly incarcerated LGBT elders for systemic reform are presented.

Keywords

Aging · Older Adults · Elders · Minority issues · Public health · LGBT issues · Intersectionality · Prisons · Community reentry · Community reintegration · Social integration

T. Maschi (✉) · R. Levine
Fordham University, New York, USA
e-mail: tmaschi@fordham.edu

J. Rees
Department of Social Work, Long Island University,
New York, USA

E. Klein
Department of Social Work, Ramapo College,
New York, USA

R. Levine
Be the Evidence and Prisoners of Age,
New York, USA

Overview

The purpose of this chapter is to explore lesbian, gay, bisexual, and transgender (LGBT) elders with histories of incarceration. This chapter reviews the history of research and practice in this area, major issues and relevant policies, new

© Springer International Publishing Switzerland 2016
D.A. Harley and P.B. Teaster (eds.), *Handbook of LGBT Elders*,
DOI 10.1007/978-3-319-03623-6_12

research that is critical to understanding LGBT elder in the criminal justice system, and the role of interdisciplinary practice in improving service delivery for this population. Due to the paucity of the literature available on this population, this chapter provides new data from a qualitative study of ten formerly incarcerated LGBT elders' experiences prior to, during, and after release from prison. Consistent with intersectionality theory, a core theme of self and the social mirror emerged from the data that represented LGBT elders' ongoing coming out process of unearthing their 'true selves' despite managing multiple intersectional stigmatized identities, such as being LGBT, elderly, HIV positive, formerly incarcerated, and a racial/ethnic minority. These exploratory findings further our awareness of an overlooked population of LGBT elders involved in the criminal justice system. The implications for interprofessional and interdisciplinary policy and practice that incorporate suggestions from the formerly incarcerated suggestions for systemic reform are discussed.

Learning Objectives

By the end of the chapter, the reader should be able to:

1. Articulate some of the common experiences of LGBT elders involved in the criminal justice system, especially related to prison and community reintegration.
2. Identify intersectional social locations or identities of LGBT elders with criminal justice histories.
3. Describe the sources of trauma, stress, and oppression and resilience among this population.
4. Identify service and justice gaps on how to improve the interprofessional response to LGBT elders involved in the criminal justice system.

Introduction

The steady growth of a graying of the global prison population is perhaps most challenging in the United States (USA). The USA has the highest rate of incarceration in the world (Walmsley 2013). As of 2013, prisoner population rates per 100,000 were 716 in the USA compared to 475 for Russia, 148 in the UK, 121 in China, and 118 in Canada (Walmsley 2013). In 2012, one of every 35 adult residents in the USA (2.9 %) was in jail, prison, or on parole or probation (Glaze and Herberman 2012). Of the estimated 1.5 million persons in the state and federal prison in the USA in 2013, 18 % ($n = 270,000$) are aged 50 and older (Carson 2014).

A profile of older adults in USA prisons portrays a diverse population that disproportionally affects vulnerable populations based on characteristics such as age, race/ethnicity, gender, and disability (Maschi et al. 2014). For example, in the US prison population aged 50 and older, the vast majority are men (96 %) compared to women (4 %) and are disproportionately racial ethnic groups (black = 45 %, Latino = 11 %, 10 % = other) compared to whites (43 %; Guerino et al. 2011). Health status varies; some individuals have functional capacity, while others suffer from disabilities or serious, chronic, and terminal illnesses such as HIV/AIDS, cancer, and dementia or mental health (e.g., depression, anxiety, psychosis) and substance abuse problems (36 %; BJS 2006; Maschi et al. 2012a, b). The majority report a history of victimization, grief and loss, and chronic stress prior to and during prison and varying levels of coping and social support (Maschi et al. 2012c, 2013b).

Despite this knowledge, there is a dearth of research that examines the experiences of LGBT elders involved in the criminal justice system. The pathways to prison for older adults in prison may include one or more cumulative inequalities (Maschi and Aday 2014), such as social disadvantage based on age, race, education, socioeconomic status, gender, disability, legal or immigration status, and sexual minority status (Maschi et al. 2014). These accumulated inequalities can influence access to health and social services, economic resources, and justice across the life course. This is uniquely applicable because of their criminal justice history, which is largely not addressed in intersectionality theory.

History of Research and Practice Pertinent to This Topic

Civil and human rights advocacy groups that respect an inherent dignity of older and LGBT persons are gaining momentum. The United Nations has designated a number of special needs populations that are subject to special protections. These special populations include lesbian, gay, bisexual, and transgender (LGBT) prisoners and older prisoners in addition to prisoners with mental health care needs, disabilities, racial and ethnic minorities, women, foreign-born nationals, and prisoners with terminal illness or under a death sentence (United Nations Office on Drugs and Crime [UNODC] 2009). Given that many people in prison have complex needs, the likelihood is quite high that incarcerated people who are LGBT would also be represented in one or more of these vulnerable care populations.

Yet, the little information available on LGBT people in prison is mostly based on younger as opposed to older persons. In a US Department of Justice report on sexual victimization in jails and prisons (Beck et al. 2013), inmates identifying their sexual orientation as gay, lesbian, and bisexual were among those with the highest rates: 12.2 % of prisoners and 8.5 % of jail inmates reported sexual victimization from other inmates, and 5.4 % of prisoners and 4.3 % of jail inmates reported victimization by staff. It is of concern that inmates with mental health needs who were identified as non-heterosexual reported the highest rates of inmate-on-inmate sexual victimization (i.e., 14.7 % of jail inmates and 21 % of prison inmates). In a study of violence in California prisons, transgender women in men's prisons were 13 times as likely to experience sexual violence than were other prisoners (Jenness et al. 2007). Incarcerated LGBT persons also have health care concerns that include sexually transmitted diseases (STDs), including HIV/AIDS, and mental health and substance use disorders. The health care of transgender prisoners is often an administrative issue versus a health care issue due to institutional policies preventing hormone and/or transition-related care (Marksamer and Tobin 2014).

LGBT persons are also at high risk of family rejection, homelessness, and unemployment due to bias and discrimination based on their LGBT status. LGBT persons may reject (lack) access to prison-based rehabilitative services for fear of being assaulted by other incarcerated persons or correctional staff. Incarcerated LGBT people have special considerations pre- and post-release because they may not have ready access to family supports or therapeutic services, especially if they have experienced trauma during their incarceration (UNODC 2009). These scant findings suggest that LGBT elders released from prison, especially those with complex issues, such as being HIV positive with comorbid health and mental health issues, may also experience the collateral consequences of incarceration, ageism, and homophobia. The complexity of their situation may create additional barriers for (LGBT) them to gain access to culturally responsive healthcare, housing, employment, and social welfare benefits (Maschi et al. 2012c). Additional research is needed to further our knowledge of public health issues, especially as it relates to diverse elders who are at a heightened risk of health and justice disparities. Therefore, in this next section, we present new findings on the experiences of LGBT elders before, during, and after prison and service providers that were used to identify research, practice, and policy gaps.

Discussion Box 12.1
The current literature finds that there are scant findings that suggest that LGBT elders released from prison, especially those with complex issues, such as being HIV positive with comorbid health and

mental health issues, may experience the collateral consequences of incarceration, ageism, and homophobia.

The complexity of their situation may create additional barriers for them to gain access to culturally responsive healthcare, housing, employment, and social welfare benefits. In an essay form or in a small group discussion, please answer the following questions:

1. What do you think accounts for the lack of research or information on LGBT elder involved in the criminal justice system compared to other LGBT issues?
2. Based on existing cross-disciplinary theories or your own thoughts, what do you think accounts for the interpersonal social and structural barriers for LGBT to access services and justice?
3. How do you think access to services or justice can be achieved for LGBT elder in the criminal justice system?

Major Issues of Chapter Topic and the Relevant Policies

Due to the lack of research on LGBT elders involved in the criminal justice system, the following two-phase qualitative study was conducted to explore the experiences of formerly incarcerated LGBT elders before, during, and after prison. Research in this area has important implications for developing an intersectional LGBT aging sensitive and social and public care approach to prevention and intervention that target diverse elders' pathways to prison and community reintegration, including care transitions. The number of diverse elders behind bars has increased more than 1300 % since the early 1980s and is projected to increase four times by 2030 (Human Rights Watch [HRW] 2012).

Correctional service providers are ill-prepared to address the specialized long-term health and social care needs of an older special needs population (Maschi et al. 2013a, b). In the USA, federal and state governments spend a combined $77 billion annually to operate correctional facilities (ACLU 2012). A coordinated public health practice and policy response can assist with improving access to health and justice for an all-too-often group of minority elders (Maschi et al. 2012c, 2014).

Research Box 12.1

Title of Research: LGBT Elder and the Criminal Justice System

Research Question: What do LGBT elders report about their experiences before, during, and after prison?

Methods: This qualitative study participatory translation research methods is featured in this chapter. The study was conducted in two phases. Phase one consisted of in-depth interviews with 10 LGBT elders released from prison. Phase two consisted of a photograph and film documentary project.

Results: Participants commonly reported experiences of discrimination and victimization. A core theme of self and the social mirror emerged from the data that represented LGBT elders' ongoing coming out process of unearthing their 'true selves' despite managing multiple intersectional stigmatized identities, such as being LGBT, elderly, HIV positive, formerly incarcerated, and a racial/ethnic minority.

Conclusion: These exploratory findings further our awareness of an overlooked population of LGBT elders involved in the criminal justice system. The implications for interprofessional and interdisciplinary policy and practice that incorporate suggestions from the formerly incarcerated suggestions for systemic reform are discussed.

Discussion Questions (essay or small or large group discussion)

1. What are your thoughts on participatory action research in which the faces and personal background of participants are known?
2. How does this differs from traditional research methods in which anonymity or confidentiality is a core research ethic?
3. If you were to design a study of LGBT elders in the criminal justice system, what would be the purpose and rationale of your study, your research question, and the methods used?

Methods

Research Design

Phase One: The authors used a research design that they refer to as 'participatory translational research,' which was conducted in two phases. In phase one, LGBT elder adults aged 50 and older released from prison within the past five years were recruited to participate in the project. The research team posted an announcement and invitation that described the study on the bulletin boards of regional correctional community service providers and parole offices. Handouts were available directly below the posted study announcement and an invitation for potential participants to review and voluntarily respond to the research team by phone or mail. Snowball sampling methods also were used to recruit participants in Brooklyn, New York, which had a high concentration of LGBT persons in the community and an LGBT psychosocial program.

Ten participants who responded to the announcement and invitation met with the members of the research team to find out more about the study and provided their informed consent to participate in the study. First, two ninety-minute focus groups were conducted with formerly

incarcerated LGBT elders, with five participants persons per group. The focus group interview schedule consisted of ten open-ended questions that asked attendees about their experiences before, during, and after prison. One week later, each participated in a one-on-one 90 minute, semi-structured in-depth interview. All interviews were held in a private room at the principal investigator's office building that was at a central location and easily accessible by public transportation. All interviews were administered by the principal investigators and two trained MSW students with personal histories of incarceration. The one-on-one interview schedule was divided into three parts that asked participants detailed questions about their experiences of self and community before, during, and after prison. The interviews were recorded using a digital audio recorder and were transcribed verbatim. Participants were offered a thirty-dollar gift card for their participation for each interview completed.

The qualitative data from service providers and formerly incarcerated older adults were analyzed using Tutty et al.'s (1996) qualitative data analysis coding scheme. The first step involved identifying 'meaning units' (similar to in vivo codes) from the data, that is, the first-level codes were assigned to the data to accurately reflect the writer's exact words (e.g., true self, homo-thug). Next, second-level coding and first-level 'meaning units' were sorted and placed in their respective categories (e.g., 'going in' or 'coming out' of prison). A constant comparative strategy was used to ensure that meaning unit codes were classified by similarities and differences and carefully analyzed for relationships, themes, and patterns. The categories were examined for meaning and interpretation. A conceptually clustered diagram was constructed to detect patterns and themes and develop a process model (Miles and Huberman 1994).

Phase Two: Phase two was a participatory action documentary project. A collaborative partnership was formed by the research team and formerly incarcerated LGBT volunteers to design and implement the project to increase public awareness and combat societal stigma. The LGBT elders were especially concerned about the invisibility and lack of culturally responsive services for incarcerated and formerly incarcerated LGBT elders. Ron Levine, a social documentary photographer and creator of the 'Prisoners of Age' project, was recruited to be a part of the team. The 'Prisoners of Age' project has been an ongoing is a series of photographs and interviews with elderly inmates and corrections personnel conducted in prisons both in the USA and Canada since 1996. A photograph of an elder transgender person in prison can be found in the chapter appendix (See Image 12.1). The exhibit is designed to play a role in stimulating social and institutional change by addressing the issues of social justice and human dignity through images and interviews. The photograph exhibits have been shown internationally.

For the first round of recruitment, three formerly incarcerated LGBT elders agreed to participate in a short documentary project. The participants signed a release form for their photographs and interview excerpts to be used for the documentary project. The 90-min interviews were shot with a Canon 5D mark II camera and 50- and 85-mm lenses. Sound was direct to film using a RODE shotgun microphone attached to the flash plate. During the shooting, the filmmaker asked the participants to describe their past and current experiences, and future goals. The footage was edited to be a 5-min documentary short.

Self and the Social Mirror

Phase One Qualitative Results

An overarching theme 'self and the social mirror,' emerged from data about that described their lifelong process of managing the 'visible' and 'invisible' prisons of oppression, social stigma, and criminal justice involvement. Self in the social mirror was defined as a dynamic personal, interpersonal, and historical process that involved the mutual reflection (or deflection) of participants' diverse selves with family and friends and society. Many participants described a lifelong process of integrating aspects of their social identities or location that were commonly subject to bias, discrimination, and violence. Many participants viewed themselves by one or more of following identities (or social location): being a racial/ethnic minority, older, HIV positive, LGBT, formerly incarcerated with a mental health and/or substance diagnosis, occupational

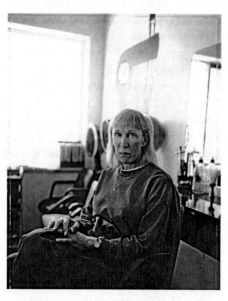

Christine White, 53
Grand Valley Institution, Ontario
31 bank robberies across Canada dressed as a man,

I am a trans-gender person. I was incarcerated November 8th of 1998. I have spent about 3 years and 7 months in segregated custody. Cells you wouldn't put dogs into for longer than a day.

I was quite successful in my domain of work which was Industrial Construction Manager and Engineering Services Manager. But when I had the gender change things certainly changed to the negative.

When I went through the change, I basically hid-out for a few years. The satirical part is that I get ostracized by society and then by my family and I guess, in retrospect, I should have probably sought the post-gender surgery counseling to deal with these issues...

I'm not a typical inmate. I've had, you know, a long dark road and I've had a different culture than most of these people so, at this stage I've applied for the position of grievance coordinator. I'm probably the first one of first in the female jails who is actually pursuing the interests of women.

Image 12.1 Prisoners of age photograph of Christine White. *Photo* © Ron Levine. Reprinted with permission status and income, and geographic location. Participants shared their views on how they multiple social identities or locations, such as race/ethnicity, sexual orientation, or their serious mental health status. When asked to 'tell me about yourself,' participants commonly identified themselves as LGBT and then added one or more other aspects of themselves.

> I am an African-American female, 55, um, what else do I want to say. Um, I'm presently unemployed. I was incarcerated for like six years on a drug charge. Um, and um, it wasn't easy, but I'm okay now.

> I'm a lesbian um, presently. I'm not in any committed relationship or anything like that and um, well. I'm presently doing, I'm focusing on my recovery you know and just trying to stay in the community.

> Um, Latino and I'm LGBT, GQ. And I did sixteen years in prison for manslaughter and I learned a lot in prison. It took me time to learn about myself. I was a closet gay person, didn't want nobody to know who I was, and I'm learning how to live life, and I'm in a relationship for six years, and I love myself today.

> I did ten years, six months in prison. I am a gay male. I'm in a committed relationship for the last six years. Um, I'm presently working in the mental health field in a psychosocial club and advocacy program for LGBT members. Um, helping to be a liaison between their therapist and the support they receive. Um, one of the things that um, I'm trying to do after coming out of prison for so long is to establish a working relationship um, and being a productive person.

Building 'Immunity' to Social Stigma

Participants commonly reported that they faced challenges to developing a strong sense of self and a relationship to their families and communities. Social stigma was described as a communicable disease in which some participants developed immunity to external oppressive attitudes and practices. Some feedbacks seemed to accurately mirror and support the expression of their 'true selves.' Other feedback was potentially obstructive to that expression. Many participants described a multi-dimensional 'coming

out' and self-acceptance process, which included being LGBT. Social and historical circumstances influenced how they negotiated this identity before, during, and after prison. One 55-year-old formerly incarcerated woman shared the following:

> Well, no, well I don't know if it's me, but I personally don't care how a person feels about me. You understand what I'm saying. My attitude is that if you don't like what I represent, don't, don't, you know, don't say nothing to me. I can keep it moving and that's it and that's all so nobody, I never got approached on that but I'm quite sure you know, it would whatever but I never personally got approached about it so as far as me being LGBT and being incarcerated, it wasn't a problem for me.

Another participant described how he was always prepared to protect himself and vocalize his rights, especially to culturally incompetent community professionals and service providers.

> You have to put your guards up in every way possible that's going to help you to get ahead, being gay for me, HIV positive, black, you know, a whole lot of stuff, you know. So, you have to set up certain things that are going to defend you along the way. Otherwise you're going to get swallowed up. I'm not just accepting anything but capable of advocating for myself, especially when I need affirming program services. If you can't advocate, that becomes a stumbling block.

Many participants shared their earlier life experiences in which mirroring from families, peers, and communities varied concerning how they chose to share one or more of their 'intersectional' aspects of self. It is important to understand that identity is comprised of many different facets, including, but not limited to, our biological sex, gender identity and expression, sexual identity, class, race, and age. We make choices throughout our lives to express or hide these aspects of ourselves. Ward (2008) has shown that race, class, gender, and sexuality are important in structuring our identity and that examining our sexuality is integral to viewing the intersectionality of the many facets of self. Being HIV positive, having a serious mental health illness, or being LGBT and engaging in criminal behavior are often selectively disclosed to families, peers, and other social circles.

Being HIV Positive: By immediate family, like my mother, father, sister, and brother, I know and they all know my HIV status. Uh, my father, I haven't really told my status, you know, um. You know, even though I know he would love me because I'm his son and, and he would just, I mean, he wouldn't have a choice, but I just don't feel comfortable coming out telling him that I'm HIV positive. I brought it to my mother's attention, and my mother, she's like, she says, no, don't tell him, you know, and I don't know why, but I just keep, we're just keeping that a secret. But everybody else knows. My brother knows. My sister knows. My aunt knows, you know.

Being Diagnosed with a Mental Illness: Growing up, my family wasn't really cool with being mentally ill so I couldn't be mentally ill. I was not able to go to a psychiatrist. I was not able to take medication, and I was damn sure not able to talk about how I felt or what was going on. So, I self-medicated with drugs. The voices were getting loud, drink a little bit more, smoke a little bit more.

Most of the time voluntary um, but a lot of the times involuntary because my mother had to put me there. I can't even count. Let's say 30 times from the age of 26 to 35. I think I went to the psych hospital, about two or three times a year for like 10 to 12 years.

Being Gay and Engaging in Violent Behavior: That they all knew my name in jail. One guard, her name was R, said yo, R's back. I used to stay in the lock up a lot and she would ask, 'Like are you sure you are a homo?' The officers used to tease me like how could a homo be doing all this. Homos don't do this.

'Inside' Prison

The legal system itself may have imposed discrimination prior to actually being sentenced and entering prison. Individuals may be exposed to the personal feelings or biases of the police, lawyer, or judge who impacts their treatment and sentencing. Participants described prison as a mixed experience of self in their social mirror. All participants acknowledged the cruelty of prison, especially for LGBT persons. Yet, despite the conditions of confinement, participants also acknowledged that they could use their time to gain greater insight and clarity about themselves and take accountability for their crimes. Many participants provided a thick description of the grave and dangerous social conditions of confinement,

especially for gay men and transgender persons in men's prisons compared to lesbian, bisexual, or transgender person in a women's prison. As participants described below, the culture of prison was full of systemic bias and discrimination that limited their access to rehabilitative services and basic safety and protections.

It was like this in jail, if you are male and gay so you should like it, you know. So um, it was really hard to go through that and try to deal with the day, you know, and days were long, you know. You were up at 7, you know, and even your time locked in your cell wasn't a safe time, because if they wanted you, they could tell a CO to crack your cell and they would run in on you. You know it was really frightening. It was hard to get yourself mentally ready for the morning because you never knew what was going to happen that day, and that's a real terrible feeling like, what's going to happen to me today. Every day was like, I got to keep up. I got to keep up. I got to look left. I got to look right because people were just being abused all throughout my stay, and the LGBT was just assaulted so many times on a regular basis. Everyone got it, but the LGBT men, they just you know, they were washing and underwears and anything their parents sent them or friends sent them, they would take them you know and they would make them cook for them and wash their pots. It was just frightening.

The CO's didn't care about anything. They watched gay people get raped. They would walk the tier and see you being raped in your cell or being beaten in your cell, and they would keep on walking, you know. Um, they would see you get beat and raped in the shower room, and they wouldn't say anything, and when you needed help to cry out to the CO, it was like crying out to air, you know, because they weren't going to do anything.

'Gay' Coping in Prison

When it came to negotiating their sexual and gender identity, participants described choosing among one of three 'gay' coping strategies: fight (i.e., defending the right to be openly gay), flight (i.e., complete distancing from one's LGBT identity in prison often out of fear of safety), or keeping it out of 'sight' (i.e., selectively disclosing one's LGBT identity). The choice to use one of these coping strategies influenced their level of access to health, mental health, and rehabilitative services, including education.

Flight: Well, nobody, nobody, nobody knew I was gay. Only a few guys I let know, but other people, I just say no, I'm not gay. I'm old man. Having sex in prison is not acceptable. No, if you get caught, they send a letter to your house, or they tell your family over the phone, you know. You go to the box. Some, some officer, some CO, some correctional officer, they'll let you be with your lover in, in the other cell. Some people you just paid the officer off, be kind of cigarette or with drugs.

Out of Sight: Um, it was a hard life in jail because you had to walk around like on pins on needles. It wasn't that good especially if you was gay or bisexual. I wasn't the type of person to walk around and? Advertise, and only a few people knew. I wasn't the type of person that wanted to be taken advantage of and being raped, so I had to learn how to defend myself in jail. I went through a lot of, lot of tough times. It wasn't that easy for me. But I'm easy to get along with so I guess my uh, word of mouth got me by. I was able to get along with everybody. I wasn't selfish. You know, try to stick with this one, that one. I stuck with who I needed to stick with to get by in jail if it helped me that way.

Fight: How did I cope with being gay in prison? I did when in Rome, do as Romans. When in Rome, do as Romans. I was in jail I did what jail people do. So I hung out with a crew that were crazy. I was hearing voices, I was crazy so we did the same thing and the only reason they accepted me is because I was just as dangerous as they were. I was always gay all my life so when I got in jail um, I never went into you know, segregation or into the gay quarters. I always went into general population and um, I made myself deal with what was going on and I became one of the people that were there. Fighting was just, I don't know if it was more because I was LGBT or because it's just what you do in jail, but I know that I went through a lot being an openly gay person in jail because the attacks and things that happen to uh, that I had observed happen to gay people were really frightening, and I just made it a way of my dealing in jail that it wouldn't happen to me so I became a really, really wild person um, they have a name for gays like me in jail and it's homo thug. I became like one of the fearless gay people in jail um, I just didn't want to be raped.

'Coming Out' of Prison

Return to Community. Participants' perceptions of self in the social mirror continued to evolve after they 'came out' of prison. Many participants, especially those with long-term prison sentences, described feeling fear if correctional or community program staff did not help prepare them for impending release. Preparation for reentry is essential for individuals to reintegrate into the community successfully. Aside from challenges of returning to the community with the stigma of having served time, there may be essential skills that have to be mastered for them to manage in the community, such as budgeting, meal preparation, and accessing essential social services for medical and mental health needs. Some of those returning to the community have been 'in the system' for so long that they have lost their ability to care for themselves independently and have become 'institutionalized.' Since entering prison, they have been told when to get up; had their meals prepared; and were provided with shelter, medical care, and direction for most of their daily activities.

Isolation in Community. Entering the community and relearning self care, managing the demands of maintaining housing in terms of cleaning, shopping, and cooking, and interacting with others in a socially acceptable way are critical to remain outside of incarceration. For some, life outside of prison is isolating, and they have very little left of family, friends or social supports.

There was nothing for me out there, which made coming home a little more frightening, and for the LGBT it's like that. Why leave prison, I'm getting three hots and a cot. I don't have to fight for the food, you know. Some of us don't want to come out, and it was a feel like, what am I going to do at this late age. I think I came out at, I've been out almost four years. I came out at 46 years old. I didn't know what, what am I going to do, where am I going. I knew I didn't want to go to a program and stay at a program you know, like programs and, you know, it pushes us out to the street.

Other participants reported adopting a positive attitude of success on their road to recovery despite anticipated challenges posed by the culturally destructive social mirroring and practices. One participant described how he prepared himself psychologically, emotionally, and spiritually to triumph over challenges, especially bias and discrimination, he believed he would face being older and gay and serving a 15 year sentence for attempted murders.

Everything's been beautiful. I just don't allow it to be any other way. Every day I wake up, I'm so appreciative to not be behind bars. Nothing that comes up, no weather conditions or anything, and my partner says, baby, you are up at 6 o'clock no matter what goes on. I praise God in the morning, and just like yeah, it's time to go. I think I was given a second chance. My second chance. A second chance at life, and I just don't want to mess it up. I can't say there has been any difficulties. There's been situations, and I just take them in stride. Because all of it is a work in progress. I went into mainstream, I didn't wait for the housing because I was in a relationship that I wanted to do, and they had informed me that any of the housing that I got would not allow me and my partner to merge. And as I said, I'm 50. I'm not going to be living alone. And going to see my partner who lives in the Bronx and I'm over here, you know. They are not recognizing LGBT relationships. That's an issue.

Access to Services. Some participants talked about the advantages of having a stigmatized label that comes with legal protections and services, which include having an HIV positive status or diagnosed with a serious mental illness.

And you were talking about like supports coming out of prison, you know, being LGBT and be labeled HIV, you get a lot of stigma but you get a lot of support on your transition out. Otherwise, we don't get anything. Um, we don't even get the assistance to try to get housing. You have to find a social worker and tell her look, can you start the paperwork, because I heard it could be done from here, and then she be like, well I don't know about that. Will you look it up while the paperwork's here, you know, and be on them like I know something that you could do for me. But if you don't, you know what I'm saying, but for us coming out and you're not HIV positive, then you

don't find something for yourself, you're going to the street.

Referral for services to assist with mental health, health, housing vocational and/or educational services is very important in community reentry. Having the dual stigma of being incarcerated, having a medical or psychiatric diagnosis, and needing social and financial supports upon release are critical for most individuals released from a forensic setting. Participants shared how reentry or housing supports and services that were not LGBT and aging friendly influenced their ability to express to be open about themselves and receive adequate peer, family, professional, and/or community support.

The housing that I was in was lovely, but I was with people that weren't LG affirming and weren't as mentally equipped as I was so I was having to live in. Sometime in the environment that wasn't safe for me, and sometime wasn't healthy for me.

Well, when I came out um, there was a reentry program, I worked with them very well. They helped me out in a lot of ways. I went to school with them um, I went through their training program, and I even got jobs through them so they helped me out a long way until I was able to get on my feet again at a reentry program. But they did not have LGBT and aging services. That right there if it was it was kept in the closet. I didn't see too many open gay people there you know saying just straight thugs, you know, from the street and stuff like that from locked up, but it wasn't really, if it was it was under the cover, it was in the closet, but it wasn't brought out in the open like that, it was just mostly thugs.

Housing. Another important consideration in housing is the restrictions placed on certain types of offenders. There may be restrictions on where they can reside, such as not within a certain distance of a school, park, or public housing. This may make returning to family or their prior residence impossible. Being relocated after serving time to an unfamiliar, or unsafe area, has obvious implications. There may be curfews or required appearances that make finding employment, or attending a program, difficult. One participant described the drawbacks for not having services that integrate LGBT, aging, and criminal justice services:

I don't think like, when you get out if you are LGBT they have a few things but you age out at 24 and those are the couple of things that they have right now but for our age 40 and 50 there are no specific services. They don't even have housing where they can sufficiently put you. Yeah, they got one LGBT elder program now, but I don't seem them helping people coming out of jail. That's support for, you know, people on the street for LGBT but coming out for senior citizens like if you are LGBT in jail and you're getting out, they going are going to push you over there at the LGBT youth center. But for anybody over that age, there's nothing. And then when you get 40, it's like you're on your own, we're letting you go, but where you going is on you. They don't have no kind of referrals. They have no kind of support so everything is really on you to be strong and look for, but people get discouraged really quickly because it's like next to no that you are going to find services. And the services that they have, they may not be able to accept you because they are at their quota with LGBT but 40–50+. We have to depend on our family and most of us don't have that.

Rainbow Heights: A Pocket of Hope. All of the participants were members of the Rainbow Heights Club, which is an LGBT affirmative psychosocial service provider in Brooklyn, New York. Their staff has been trained to work with LGBT-identified clients with multiple problems related to their mental health, past history, and skill set. The participants described their experiences there:

> There's not a lot for the LGBT. I thank God for Rainbow Heights and being a person that can provide service for people that have nowhere to go to be themselves, to be safe, to eat a meal. To get support and referral to a lot of things that they may need in their life but we are only one and we're the only one in the whole United States, Rainbow Club so more.

Phase Two Results

For phase two, the first filming took place in Bedford-Stuyvesant in April 2014. The three volunteers, Randy, Mark, and Dwon, identified themselves as formerly incarcerated LGBT elders who had spent most of their recent prison sentences at Sing-Sing Correctional Facilitate in upstate New York. Recently, Randy and Mark were legally married under New York State law. The photograph and interview session lasted about an hour and a half. An excerpt of the interview transcript can be found in Table 12.1 in the chapter appendix, and photographs can be found in Images 12.2 and 12.3 in the appendix. The final short documentary was edited down to 5 minutes by Mr. Levine. In the interviews, Randy spoke about his life before prison and his life within the penitentiary, emphasizing his experiences as a gay man within the prison system. He talked generally about survival in prison and specifically about his survival techniques as a member of the LGBT community in prison, his coping skills, and his own personal experiences. Mark appeared to be shy and spoke minimally about his experiences. Dwon discussed his experiences living his life on the 'down low,' and about hiding his homosexual identity by dating both men and women in the past. He emphasized his wish to find a life mate like Randy and Mark have done. The five-minute short documentary can be found on the Prisoners of Age Facebook page at the following link: https://www. facebook.com/photo.php?v=1020421799903883 4&set=vb.1493049016&type=2&theater.

Research Critical to Issues Discussed in This Chapter

This qualitative study explored the experiences of formerly incarcerated LGBT elders. A central theme of self and the social mirror-emerged participants described a process in which they built a strong sense of self and pride, often in response to bias, prejudice, discrimination, and violence due to the nature of their multiple minority identities, which included being LGBT, HIV positive, racial/ethnic minority, formerly incarcerated, and being diagnosed with a serious mental illness. Despite the many challenges, most of the participants described resilient coping strategies that helped them navigate oppressive attitudes and practices that were pervasive in community and institutional settings.

Table 12.1 Excerpt from interview transcript prisoners of age documentary on formerly incarcerated LGBT elders

RE: My name is Duwan. I'm 55-years old. I was born in Brooklyn, New York. I was on the down low. You know, I didn't really start coming out into—well I came out when I was young. But, I mean, it was just really hard for me to accept that, you know, and I went through men and women, because I was trying to find myself, you know

RE: I'm Randy Killings, and I'm 49. Well I was originated in Brooklyn, and my mom had me in Jamaica and came back to New York

RE: My name is Mark. I'm 44-years old. I was born in Manhattan. Went to prison for a while. And now I'm here enjoying my life

IN: So tell me, I want to hear the love story

RE: Well, actually we met on the medication line going to medication that one night. And one of our mutual friends had brought Mark down. I think he had just got transferred here

RE: Yeah, I got transferred here

RE: He said I got somebody I want you to meet, and he told him the same thing. And when we met I just was attracted instantly, which was unusual for me, because I don't usually deal with any kind of activity in jail. But when I saw him I said you're going to be my husband. And he laughed. And the next day we started a relationship

RE: I grew up always gay, but I was so boisterous and strong with it I didn't get a lot of abuse or stigmas or things that most gays go through

RE: Everywhere I went everyone would be like, you know, that's Randy, he's gay, but you all don't mess with him. He ain't dealing with that, you know

RE: We were in something called maximum prison. Maximum prison, people who are not actually coming home for a very long time if they're coming home. So the mindset is like this is mine, this is how I'm going to run it, and that's how it was, and there was no changing it

RE: Because you have to get stronger in jail, you really do, because there's such a closed in community where if you're not strong enough you'll get sucked under

RE: Yes, you get sucked under

RE: You'll be devoured

RE: I was always a good person, but the reason I was in jail this time was because at that time I was into a lifestyle where it was a lot of money. I hung out with a lot of guys, it was a stick up crew. And we wore a lot of jewelry and stuff. And I smoked crack. As I was leaving the guy tried to rob me outside of the crack house, and we were fighting, and I punched him hard, and he fell backwards onto the Johnny pump, and it went through his head. In the time it took for me to be released they told me, they gave me a CRD to get out. I immediately just laid down everything. I stopped using, which was predominately my problem. I transferred to another side of **, which was called the Core Program, which helped people integrate back into society and give them an option. And I knew that if I went back to where I was from that it would be really, really hard for me. I signed for Project Renewal PTS Program. It was Transition Housing for Parolees. Right there I prayed that God would take the taste out of my mouth not to get high, because I got clean, but it was a different feeling when I was in the free air, you know. So I had to go to a program for a year, which I completed very, very quickly. I graduated in like four months. And my director said, you know, you have a gift, because I was always helping people and connecting with them. And he said maybe you need to think about counseling

RE: I look at them, and I see these two how their relationship, you know, I mean, they're married and stuff like that, and that's what I want to be. Right now, you know, I'm looking. I'm hoping to find somebody nice that, you know, I could grow old with, you know, spend the rest of my time with

Link to 5 min documentary: https://www.facebook.com/photo.php?v=10204217999038834&set=vb.1493049016&type=2&theater

These findings build upon the existing literature on marginalized LGBT elders. Similar to Addis et al. (2009), review of the literature on the needs of LGBT older people, these findings also showed that discrimination based on a LGBT sexual orientation has a major impact on meeting their needs in health and social services. The narratives from the current study of formerly incarcerated older adults underscore their struggle to be recognized for their true selves, which

Image 12.2 Randy and
Mark. *Photo* © Ron
Levine. Reprinted with
permission

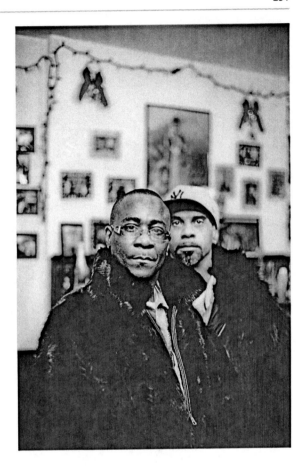

consisted of multiple intersectional identities and
striving for individual and collective empowerment. Many participants expressed the strong
desire to engage in the dialogue about what are
the problems and solutions for LGBT minority
elders. In recognition of this request, the recommendations for system reform are taken
directly from formerly incarcerated LGBT elders.
As shown in Table 12.2 of the chapter appendix,
participants recommended the adoption of more
compassionate and affirming practice and policy
approaches, non-discrimination and special population considerations, post-prison release access
to culturally responsive safe and affordable
housing, services, family and peer supports, and
leadership and justice and advocacy opportunities. These recommendations have implications
for interprofessional and interdisciplinary service
delivery and approaches.

Policy Box 12.1 Review Table 12.2 of
the chapter appendix provides policy
recommendations by and for LGBT elders
to improve service systems and organizational and legislative policies that impact
LGBT persons in prison and after their
release. Choose one of the theme areas:
(1) adoption of more compassionate and
affirming practice and policy approaches,
(2) non-discrimination and special population considerations, (3) post-prison
release access to culturally responsive
safe and affordable housing services,
(4) family and peer supports, and (5) justice and advocacy opportunities. Provide at
least 1–2 recommendations on how organizational and/or legislative policies can be
improved at the local, state, federal, and/or

Image 12.3 Dwon. *Photo* © Ron Levine. Reprinted with permission

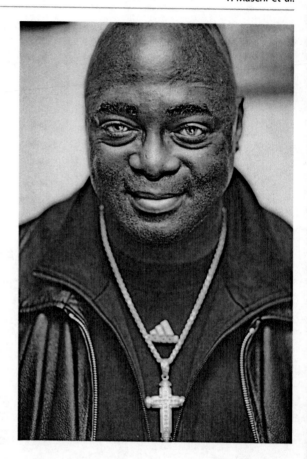

international level to help improve access to services and justice for LGBT elders in prison or after their release. Develop an action plan on how to realize these recommendations (e.g., building coalitions, advocacy campaigns, contacting legislators).

Related Disciplines Influencing Service Delivery and Interdisciplinary Approaches

Based on the existing literature and the current study findings, we recommend a holistic and comprehensive social and public care response that targets primary (prevention), secondary (at

risk), and tertiary (targeted population) assessments and intervention with LGBT elders at risk of criminalization or current or past criminal justice involvement. As illustrated in the first-hand accounts of formerly incarcerated LGBT elders, they have had adverse experiences in service delivery systems that include health care, mental health care, social services, and the criminal justice system. Implicated in the narratives of elders is the often less-than-adequate services and sometime abusive treatment of law enforcement (e.g., police or correctional officers), social workers and psychologists (in or out of the prison), medical doctors and nurses, educators, and lawyers. There are many factors that seem to account for the lack of culturally responsive treatment of LGBT elder with criminal justice histories, which include the fragmentation of services, lack of communication between service

Table 12.2 Formerly incarcerated LGBT elders recommendations for system reform

1. **Adoption of more compassionate and affirming practice and policy approaches**

We need to reform the whole criminal justice process. Like the intake process in prison. I don't know if they do it like that as some type of scare tactic or what. The way they the intake is like they can give you like a very negative outlook on, on, on, on life in prison. And if you're not an open-minded person, you can go through your whole sentence being in fear. I think they need to be a little bit more compassionate on intake because if you're full of fear, you're not open to anything, you know. So you go in jail or prison and you think you got to fight or you got to do this. It's just not true. You don't have to fight your way through jail. It's like anything in life. If you're not educated about the situation, it can be bad

We need a special unit in prison for only the -LGBT. Some, some of them can't be in population. They're scared to go to population to get raped or get stabbed. They could separate the LGBT person from population, you know, put another jail for them only. I seen lot of LGBT people in prison got beat up, stabbed, all, all type of worse things happen to them

I think they need to start hiring more LGBT more correction officers. Like LGBT, you can't be a part of the LGBT community and be a corrections officer, did you know that. Not be openly gay. You can be an openly lesbian but you can't be an openly gay man and they let women, they put in areas where they are not going to do any good. They put the women in non-visiting room. They need to let female correctional officers to be up on the tiers or in the dorms. They put the men up there and that is all corrupt. They think it's cute to see if the homo get beat up because they don't like

I believe that if people had better, like if there was better planning for people that's coming out, out of prison system, a lot of them wouldn't be going back to jail. A lot of them would change their ways, and they would become productive members of society, LGBT or not

2. **Nondiscrimination and special population considerations**

And one of the things you were talking about in jail that really needs to change, gays in prison should be able to safely go to school. Right now they can't. They'd be attacked. In prison, they need to separate the jobs for older and people that's younger. I worked in a mess hall, and that's a hard job, and, you know, if you're up in age and you got your, you know, the older you get, the more aches and pains you have, you know, and working in the mess hall, I don't see it being good for somebody that's 55 or 60

They need to have senior citizen things up there in prison for people that are senior citizens, I mean, because when you're old, I mean, everybody gets old. I mean, already you're forgetful in the mind and stuff like that. You get senile and stuff like that, you know. Um, they should have just a, I can't say, um, a certain place, but, I mean, they should have something for seniors too, you know, because - How can you put a 60-something year-old man in with the regular population of 15 and 16-year-old kids. I wish they would have places for people who are of that age, something to do for them and something to keep their mind on the right thing, you know, where they won't get into trouble or get hurt

3. **Post reentry access to culturally responsive safe and affordable housing and social services**

Cheaper housing, housing, affordable housing, connected to a therapist, connection to treatment. All these things— Affordable treatment because now, safe housing is essential in being able to successfully adjust back into the community. Living in a high crime area, that has a majority of unemployed or underemployed residents that may be socially stigmatized will reduce the ability to manage. In addition, some of these areas have high rates of victimization of residents, and easy access to illegal activities and drugs. Adding identification as LGBT can exacerbate community discrimination and oppression

Housing is a big issue. Let's say you're coming out of jail, and, and you're eligible for SSI or whatever, right? They should have some type of housing program that will meet like the budget of a person that's on SSI. I think that's another reason why a lot of people go back to jail because they feel safer there, because at least they know that when the night comes, they got somewhere to sleep. They got some food and they're comfortable with it, for some people

One thing that was really hard and I found a couple of things when I got out of jail that were LGBT and the housing situation. There was some terrible housing. And that's not just for the LGBT over 50, it's the housing situation but it harder for an LGBT person because like I said we are pushed into mainstream and they're not friendly. So having something housing where it could be more LG affirm and I'm not saying build a big house for only LGBT but at least let it be affirming where I can go there and be okay and not go shopping and my neighbor come busting my door because I'm gay and take my food because that happens

We need intergenerational services for LGBT people. I work in a LGBT program and I think we're from age 21 to I think closer to 60. I see the age integration of the people. I think we need to learn to live together even age differences because that makes a community. To be able to respect or the, I know when I grew up how I respected the older people. And I like to be around the older people. And, and I help the older people and that's one of the things we need to get back into what a community is integration of LGBT people of all ages

Specific services for people who are at least age 50 or older, LGBT, and formerly incarcerated. For programs, we need them more affirming. See everyone says we need something for the gays, something for the, no, we need a firm thing so we can integrate and learn to live

(continued)

Table 12.2 (continued)

I would like them to have more places for people that's on the down low, or they're not on the down low, just gay. They just ready to come out or for the LGBT and stuff like that, they need to have a lot more places for them, you know, places where they could go and like TV and stuff like that, but I don't know how true, I never really, when I always went, I never said I was gay, you know, so I didn't get put with a gay guy. I got put in the regular population, you now

For release programs, they really got to somewhere to put people, aging LGBT people. Lesbian and gay people, aging people they are just throwing them back in the street or putting them in a house where there are mostly either sitting there drinking or drugging or mourning themselves to death because they are left in a room and they have nothing to do

4. Mental health and social needs

More activities, more sponsoring of something for the LGBT seniors. We don't have anything. Even if they go into regular senior citizen. Senior citizens are just like kids. They are just bias as kids so, you know, just more resources for us

We need a lot with diabetes because a lot of our seniors are coming down with it, especially the black and Puerto Ricans, because we are limited to our resources of eating you know.

So if it is something that is available for a closeted gay person, maybe his therapist or the counselor or someone they have seen hears that or you suspect somebody, well you know, they have housing for LGBT, here's some information. I don't know if that applies for you, let me make that decision and then tell you, you know what this is who I am and I like to keep it between me and you so sign me up. But there should be some way that it can get out because it is really stigmatized in jail. So most of the men who are out there trying to be the biggest are the most gay. But they are not going to say, you know, but then again they don't need the services because they going back to having a sexual life and perform their self as a heterosexual person but there are people that are in that are so, I think, I think there would be a response because people, first of all, they will get this information when they were out. Second of all, it will give them some hope that I'm going to come out but I'm coming out for the right reasons and I'm going to get some support and direction

5. Family and peer and mentoring supports

To be able to integrate, you are going to somewhere and have the same thing happen to you in jail going into some of these program and housing and one of the things that I wish they would offer more is support for LGBT coming out of jail because if you can't go home and most of them have been thrown out, disowned, or, you know, families don't associate with us and we wind up going back to the streets doing what we did to get us back in jail. If you identify, your family first of all if they are not loving and caring to you like they should be, they are going to put you out and once you get in jail, they don't really have specials cops to say okay don't mess with the LGBT leave them alone. We are not going to let you rape them. They don't care

Start to have something for LGBT specific, you know, supports. Okay and starting in prison. Yes because we need to have that hope and have an LG person come to prison and say hey, I'm out here, look at me. And I think that's great when you probably come up with a way to craft it. My only thought is does it then put, if you have an LGBT person coming in, does that put people at danger, people then become to know if they are LGBT

We need more coming out of jail for people to know that there is hope like a role model thing. Like guys I've been where you at but we can still get here. Don't let your past keep you suppressed. Look forward. Look up. Because we don't get that hope. We don't get someone from the LGBT coming in jail saying hey, guy I'm out there and I'm doing it. It's not anything and there's no hope in jail saying that hey guy I got this place for you that you can go to that's just for you. We don't get that. Now they come in here and tell everybody that's straight, we've got this, this, this but we don't have anything in jail coming out saying well, we got some support lined up for you. Not yet and that's what needed because it's frightening, like I said it's a revolving door. They don't have this support, what are you doing, you're not equipping them to go out there and survive. You're equipping them to go back and come back

6. Justice and policy advocacy opportunities

For policies, I would change stop and frisk of course. And there is no law but their treatment of gays. They have no respect for gays. There's nothing in line that they can say they are breaking and not doing, it's just their treatments toward especially the gay men, and I can't even say lesbians. There's very few cops that will be angry with lesbians but all cops are angry in treatment of gay people or trans people. It's just horrible

One of the things that we should always have is someone in the LGBT, in like on the returning is access to a lawyer. They should have an LGBT person, affirming person to defend us because we get no defense by regular attorneys. Now, I mean that's one time that will probably predict some things and coming out we can work on that end but going in, I need somebody like, they don't even want to talk to you. We need yeah, LGBT representation of lawyers, otherwise they may not want to talk to you or really understand or help you

We need to have the opportunity to be more visible and have our voices heard. What better way to let people and professionals know what needs to change for LGBT elders providers, and lack for training to work with LGBT elders that have multiple intersectional identities that may include race and ethnicity, gender, HIV/AIDS history, serious mental illness, substance use issues, and criminal offense histories.

In general, there is a significant need for affirming services in health and mental health, law, social services, education and vocational training to help people in the prison and community reintegration process. A comprehensive response is needed to address the pervasive and multisystemic biases, prejudice, and discrimination experiences of LGBT minorities across the life course that places them at risk of criminalization and/or involvement in the criminal justice system. When LGBT elders feel that they cannot reveal their true identity to access services they need in prison or in the community, it leads to a disregard of their unique challenges by health, mental health, and other service providers that would be instrumental in accessing housing and financial resources. Fear of discrimination and exclusion may lead to an avoidance of disclosure, and therefore, a true evaluation of service is needed. This group tends to remain marginalized and invisible to heterosexual social service providers (Addis et al. 2009).

In the prior literature and current study findings, access to education in prison or after prison release is important. Both in prison and in the community, LGBT people experience discrimination in accessing education. However, in prison, this is even more so because many LGBT people in prison did not attend or were not allowed to attend educational classes because of personal safety and prison management issues. In the current study highlighted in this chapter, clients who attend the Rainbow Heights psychosocial club clearly described facing discrimination from other service providers, such as medical professionals, therapists, and social service providers, especially with housing. In fact, many of the narratives suggest the visible and invisible 'prisons' in which society attempts to place them. One participant described how discrimination on the basis of LGBT identities

creates a 'prison in the community' and asked, 'what's the difference from being in jail?'

A recovery approach is recommended to assist LGBT elders being released from the criminal justice system to feel more comfortable in accessing services for their mental health, health, housing, and other important 'social, legal' and other supports. Engagement without exacerbating stigmas of their LGBT identity and criminal history is essential to begin establishing a helping relationship. It is important to provide services that consider diverse needs including, vocational, educational, financial, clinical and housing services. The Substance Abuse and Mental Health Services Administration (SAMSHA 2012) has estimated that 12 percent of male offenders and 24 % of female offenders have a mental health and/or substance use disorder. Many researchers indicate that this may be even higher in the LGBT population (Brown and Pantalone 2011; Mustanski et al. 2010).

For any treatment to have efficacy, it must treat the whole individual, not only the presenting disorder. Best practices include addressing and integrating services with culturally responsive providers. These services may include supported employment, family education, peer support, case management, and advocacy services. Organizations like The Rainbow Heights Club, a self-help and advocacy program specifically designed to provide services to LGBT individuals, may be a key component in community reintegration (Hellman and Klein 2004). Places for socialization and acceptance are crucial as one reenters the community from prison. Isolation, discrimination, and lack of stable supports can only have a negative outcome.

Mental health and other educational and service providers need to provide trauma-informed care for those reentering from the criminal justice system. To adequately adjust to the community, people have to be taught strategies to address traumas they have experienced and to overcome some of the detrimental coping mechanisms they may have employed in the past, which may include substance abuse. Partnering with criminal justice professionals and working on a comprehensive culturally competent unified plan is a first step in the process of managing complex issues in reintegration. Entering the community without adequate funds for food, shelter, and medical needs creates a barrier to success, as does a lack of social support.

Lastly, consistent with Ka'Opua et al. (2012), we recommend the need for returning prisoners to have timely access to social service programs and services as well as trauma-informed care to help cope past trauma histories as well as the trauma of incarceration. For more details on a trauma-informed approach, please see the Substance Abuse and Mental Health Services Administration's (2010) recommendations on trauma-informed care at: http://beta.samhsa.gov/nctic/trauma-interventions.

Summary

This chapter reviewed the experiences of LGBT elders' experiences prior to, during, and after incarceration. The information that is available, including the current study findings described in this chapter, suggests that biases, discrimination, violence, and criminalization are common experiences reported by LGBT elders. Intersectionality theory 'that incorporates incarceration history as a social identity or location, is an important consideration for developing interprofessional and interdisciplinary practices across service settings. As described throughout the chapter, many of these diverse elders were not only LGBT but racial ethnic minorities with histories of HIV/AIDs, serious mental illness and substance abuse, trauma, and/or committed drug or serious violent offenses. A holistic comprehensive approach is recommended that involves interprofessional and intersectoral collaboration to address service and policy gaps that are commonly experienced by LGBT elders in prior to prison, during prison, and after release from prison. Promising practices, such as the Rainbow Heights psychosocial club in Brooklyn, New York, are highlighted as a LGBT-affirming service provider that is helpful for LGBT elders released from the criminal justice system.

Appendix

Images of Incarcerated and Formerly Incarcerated LGBT Elders

See Images 12.1, 12.2 and 12.3.

Learning Exercises

Self-Check Questions

1. Race, class, gender, and sexuality are important in structuring our identity and that examining our sexuality is integral to viewing the _____ of the many facets of self. (Answer: intersectionality)
2. LGBT persons, especially elders, are at high risk of direct violence in the form of _____ and/or _____victimization. (Answer: sexual or physical)
3. _____ research after gather narrative data from participants to gain a in-depth portrait of their lives. (Answer: qualitative)
4. For LGBT survivors of trauma, _____ is a recommended intervention strategy. (Answer: trauma-informed care)
5. For LGBT elders with serious mental illness and substance use problems, a _____ approach is recommended. (Answer: recovery)

Field-Based Experiential Assignments

1. Visit a LGBT elder center or service provider in your geographic location or attend a LGBT event, and write about your experiences, especially as it relates to your impressions of the LGBT community prior to the visit and after it.
2. Visit the United Nations-Free and Equal Campaign located at and join the campaign: https://www.unfe.org/en. Review the

materials, including the fact sheets to learn more about the human rights challenges facing lesbian, gay, bisexual and transgender (LGBT) people everywhere and the actions that can be taken to tackle violence and discrimination and protect the rights of LGBT people everywhere. In essay form or in small group discussion, choose one of the problems and the solutions to write about or discuss: (1) LGBT Rights: Frequently Asked Questions, (2) International Human Rights Law, (3) Equality and Non-Discrimination. (4) Criminalization, (5) Violence, or (5) Refuge and Asylum.

3. View the short documentary on LGBT elders released from prison short at: https://www.facebook.com/photo.php?v=10204217999038834&set=vb.1493049016&type=2&theater.

In essay form or group discussion, describe your thought and feelings having watched this videos. Did any of your viewpoints change after watching the video? If so, please share in essay form or group discussion.

Multiple-Choice Questions

1. Which country has the most number of incarcerated people in the world?
   (A) Russia
   (B) China
   (C) India
   (D) USA

2. LGBT elders are at high risk of what types of discrimination and oppression?
   (A) Housing
   (B) Employment
   (C) Violence
   (D) All of the above

3. Research that actively involves participants voice in the research project is commonly referred to as:
   (A) Quantitative research
   (B) Chi-Square Analysis
   (C) Participatory Action Research
   (D) Descriptive Research

4. What percentage of incarcerated LGBT people in US prisons report being raped:
   (A) 75 %
   (B) 35 %
   (C) 12 %
   (D) 64 %

5. The USA spend about how much annually to operate correctional facilities?
   (A) One million
   (B) Two and a half million
   (C) 15 billion
   (D) 77 billion

6. Social documentary often is used to:
   (A) Foster dialogue
   (B) Stimulate debate
   (C) Stimulate social and institutional change
   (D) All of the above

7. Social Stigma among LGBT elders involved in the criminal justice system can be experienced:
   (A) As a result of negative attitudes about their LGBT identity and/or criminal justice involvement
   (B) Internally in the form of self hatred and low self worth
   (C) Is not an issue
   (D) Both A and B

8. Comprehensive services for LGBT elders released from prison may included:
   (A) Housing and Employment
   (B) Access to health, mental health, and social services
   (C) Histories of Trauma
   (D) A and B only
   (E) All of the Above

9. For treatment to be effective with LGBT elders with mental health issues released from prison:
   (A) Medication must be prescribed
   (B) It must treat the whole individual, not just the mental disorder
   (C) Be GLBT affirming
   (D) B and C only

10. An essential element or elements of treatment with LGBT elder released from prison is the following:
    (A) Engagement without exacerbating stigma
    (B) Child care availability
    (C) Offering space for socialization and acceptance
    (D) Both A and C

Key

1–2-D
3-C
4-C
5-D
6-D
7-D
8-E
9-D
10-D

Resources

Be the Evidence International-Rainbow Justice Project: http://www.betheevidence.org/rainbow-justice-project/

Equal Rights Center: http://www.equalrightscenter.org/site/PageServer?pagename=issues_lgbt

Huffington Post Op-Ed on Prison Rape and Gay Rights: http://www.huffingtonpost.com/rodney-smith/prison-rape-gay-rights_b_4504331.html

Just Detention International: http://www.justdetention.org

Lamba Legal-Criminal Justice: http://www.lambdalegal.org/blog/topic/criminal-justice

Prison Rape Elimination Act (PREA) Resources Center: http://www.prearesourcecenter.org/about (Resources on LGBT persons in prison)

Prisoners of Age: http://www.prisonersofage.com/home

Rainbow Heights Club: http://www.rainbowheights.org

Sero Project: http://seroproject.com

Services and Advocacy for Gay, Lesbian, Bisexual Elders (SAGE): http://sageusa.org/index.cfm

Transgender Law Center: http://transgenderlawcenter.org/issues/prisons

Transequality-Jails Prison Resource: http://transequality.org/PDFs/JailPrisons_Resource_FINAL.pdf

United Nations Office on Drugs and Crime: http://www.unodc.org

United Nations Office on Drugs and Crime Handbook on Prisoners with Special Needs: http://www.unodc.org/documents/justice-and-prison-reform/Prisoners-with-special-needs.pdf

United Nations-Free and Equal Campaign: https://www.unfe.org/en

References

Addis, S., Davies, M., Greene, G., MacBride-Stewart, S. & Shepherd, M. (2009). The health, social care and housing needs of lesbian, gay, bisexual and transgender older people: A review of the literature. *Health and Social Care in the Community, 17*(6), 647–656. doi:10.111/j.1365-2524.2009.00866.x

American Civil Liberties Union [ACLU]. (2012). *At America's expense: The mass incarceration of the elderly*. Washington, DC: Author.

Beck, A. J., Berzofsky, M., Caspar, R., & Krebs, C. (2013). *Sexual victimization in prisons and jails reported by inmates, 2011–2012*. Retrieved September 18, 2014, from http://www.bjs.gov/content/pub/pdf/svpjri1112.pdf

Brown, L., & Pantalone, D. (2011). Lesbian, gay, bisexual and transgender issues in trauma psychology: A topic comes out of the closet. *Traumatology, 17*(2), 1–3. doi:10.1177/1534765611417763.

Bureau of Justice Statistics [BJS]. (2006). *Mental health problems of prison and jail*. Retrieved November 4, 2012, from http://bjs.ojp.usdoj.gov/index.cfm?typbdetail&iid789

Carson, E. A. (2014). *Prisoners in 2013*. Retrieved September 18, 2014, from http://www.bjs.gov/content/pub/pdf/p13.pdf

Glaze, L. E., & Herberman, E. J. (2012). Correctional populations in the United States, 2012. Retrieved September 18, 2014, from http://www.bjs.gov/index.cfm?ty=pbdetail&iid=4843

Guerino, P., Harrison, P., & Sabol, W. (2011). *Prisoners in 2010*. Retrieved June 1, 2012, from http://bjs.ojp.usdoj.gov/content/pub/pdf/p10.pdf

Hellman, R., & Klein, E. (2004). A program for lesbian, gay, bisexual and transgender individuals with major mental illness. *Journal of Gay and Lesbian Mental Health, 8*(3–4), 67–82.

Human Rights Watch [HRW]. (2012). Old behind bars. Retrieved January 31, 2012, from http://www.hrw.org/reports/2012/01/27/old-behind-bars

Jenness, V., Maxon, C. L., Matsuda, K. N., & Sumner, J. M. (2007). *Violence in California correctional facilities: An empirical examination of sexual assault* (Center for Evidence-Based Corrections). Retrieved September 18, 2014, from http://www.wcl.american.edu/endsilence/documents/ViolenceinCaliforniaCorrectionalFacilities.pdf

Ka'Opua, L. S., Petteruti, A., Takushi, R. N., Spencer, J. H., Park, S. H., Diaz, T. P., et al. (2012). The lived experience of native Hawaiians exiting prison and reentering the community: How do you really decriminalize someone who's consistently being called a criminal? *Journal of Forensic Social Work, 2,* 141–161.

Marksamer, J., & Tobin, H. J. (2014). *Standing with LGBT prisoners: An advocate's guide to ending abuse and combatting injustice.* National Center for Transgender Equality. Retrieved September 18, 2014, from http://transequality.org/PDFs/JailPrisons_Resource_FINAL.pdf

Maschi, T., & Aday, R. (2014). The social determinants of health and justice and the aging in prison crisis: A call to action. *International Journal of Social Work, 1,* 1–15.

Maschi, T., Kwak, J., Ko, E. J., & Morrissey, M. (2012a). Forget me not: Dementia in prisons. *The Gerontologist,*. doi:10.1093/geront/gnr131.

Maschi, T., Sutfin, S., & O'Connell, B. (2012b). Aging, mental health, and the criminal justice system: A content analysis of the literature. *Journal of Forensic Social Work, 2,* 162–185.

Maschi, T., Viola, D., & Sun, F. (2012c). The high cost of the international aging prisoner crisis: Well-being as the common denominator for action. Gerontologist.

doi:10.1093/geront/gns125. (First published on October 4, 2012.)

Maschi, T., Viola, D., & Morgen, K. (2013a). Trauma and coping among older adults in prison: Linking empirical evidence to practice. *Gerontologist.* doi:10.1093/geront/gnt069. (First published online July 19, 2013.)

Maschi, T., Viola, D., Morgen, K., & Koskinen, L. (2013b). Trauma, stress, grief, loss, and separation among older adults in prison: the protective role of coping resources on physical and mental wellbeing. *Journal of Crime and Justice,.* doi:10.1080/0735648X.2013.808853.

Maschi, T., Viola, D., Harrison, M., Harrison, W., Koskinen, L., & Bellusa, S. (2014). Bridging community and prison for older adults and their families: Invoking human rights and intergenerational family justice. *International Journal of Prisoner Health, 19* (1), 1–19.

Miles, M. B., & Huberman, A. M. (1994). *Qualitative data analysis.* Thousand Oaks, CA: Sage Publications.

Mustanski, B. S., Garafalo, R., & Emerson, E. M. (2010). Mental health disorder, psychological distress and suicidality in a diverse sample of lesbian, gay, bisexual and transgender youths. *American Journal of Public Health, 100*(12), 2426–2432.

SAMSHA Einstein Expert Panel Report. (2012). http://www.samhsa.gov/traumaJustice/pdf/Final%20CoOccurring_Disorders_Report_031014_508.pdf

Tutty, L. M., Rothery, M., & Grinnell, R. M. (1996). *Qualitative research for social workers.* Needham Heights, MA: Allyn and Bacon.

United Nations Office on Drugs and Crime [UNODC]. (2009). *Handbook for prisoners with special needs.* Vienna, Austria: Author.

Walmsley, R. (2013). World prison population list (10th Ed.). Retrieved September 18, 2014, from http://www.prisonstudies.org/sites/prisonstudies.org/files/resources/downloads/wppl_10.pdf

Ward, J. (2008). *Respectably queer: Diversity culture in LGBT activist organizations.* Nashville, TN: Vanderbilt University Press.

Immigrant LGBT Elders

Amanda E. Sokan and Tracy Davis

Abstract

LGBT immigrant elders suffer multiple jeopardy by virtue of being members of disadvantaged groups (i.e., elders, LGBT, immigrant). Although it is invisible to many, immigration is an important issue for LGBT populations due to its impact on the individuals who may be seeking refuge, same-sex couples, and their families. Immigration status can determine a lifetime of opportunity or disadvantage. The striking down of Section 3 of DOMA is a much-needed step in the right direction, but there is much more that needs to be done. Comprehensive immigration reform is critical to address the needs and concerns of this vulnerable population.

Keywords

Immigrant/immigrant population · Undocumented · Life course · Multiple jeopardy · Cumulative advantage/disadvantage

Overview

This chapter focuses on immigrant LGBT elders. It reviews their status as legally and socially disadvantaged minorities and presents unique barriers and inequities, resultant from their status. The combination of age, immigrant status, and sexual orientation can result in a "multiple jeopardy" or increased vulnerability that creates unique barriers and inequities (Stoller and Gibson 1999b). In this chapter, the authors explore factors that contribute to some of these barriers and inequities, explore policies and practices that affect this population and provide strategies for individuals who work with LGBT elders. We begin the chapter by defining the immigrant population; we review their status and provide a comparison of natives/non-immigrants using US data. Next, we will examine major issues that affect immigrant LGBT elders, including

A.E. Sokan (✉)
University of Kentucky, Lexington, KY, USA
e-mail: ausoka2@uky.edu

T. Davis
Rutgers University, Stratford, NJ, USA
e-mail: ted58@shrp.rutgers.edu

© Springer International Publishing Switzerland 2016
D.A. Harley and P.B. Teaster (eds.), *Handbook of LGBT Elders*,
DOI 10.1007/978-3-319-03623-6_13

immigration reform and recent legal developments on same-sex marriage. This section also reviews implications for service delivery from an interdisciplinary perspective. Research implications and future directions are also discussed.

Learning Objectives

1. Define immigrant populations.
2. Differentiate immigrant versus non-immigrant status.
3. Describe the impact of LGBT immigration rights and implications for elders.
4. Critically evaluate the challenges posed by current immigration policy and status to the rights of LGBT elders.
5. Explain how the intersection of sexual orientation/gender identity, immigration status, and age creates multiple jeopardy.
6. Discuss the importance of immigration reform and benefits for LGBT elders.
7. Explain why immigration reform is an LGBT issue.
8. Discuss factors which enhance optimal service delivery to immigrant LGBT elders.
9. Identify major immigration issues encountered by immigrant LGBT elders.
10. Identify countries that recognize same-sex relationships for immigration purposes and implications for LGBT elders.
11. Identify challenges faced by LGBT couples that include a foreign-born spouse or partner.
12. Explore the implications of the trend toward changing legal and public opinion on the rights of immigrant LGBT elders.

Key terms

DOMA 1996	LGBT	Multiple jeopardy
Cumulative advantage/ disadvantage	Immigrant/ Immigrant population	Undocumented
Foreign-born/ Native-born/Citizen/ non-citizen	Marital equality/ parity	Life Course

Introduction

In the USA, many LGBT immigrants, both documented and undocumented, are part of a same-sex couple or relationship. As members of multiple minority groups, LGBT immigrants face numerous sociocultural, political, and legal challenges. Among immigrant detainees, LGBT persons face a unique set of issues, with transgender persons being at greater risk because the Department of Homeland Security (DHS) and Immigration and Customs Enforcement (ICE) do not recognize detainees by their gender identity, but by their gender at birth (Gruberg 2013a, b, c). LGBT immigrants who immigrated to the USA at a young age and aged here present with different characteristics and challenges than those who immigrated at an older age. For example, those who immigrated as children tended to have an easier path to citizenship than older more recent immigrants.

In this chapter, we present issues that affect LGBT elders who are immigrants. The time line or period of their immigration to the USA and their countries of origin also influences their perceptions and experiences as immigrants. LGBT immigrants may be privileged or disadvantaged depending on their country of origin, race, and age. For LGBT older immigrants, the intersection of identities and the sum of all of their identities influence their interactions within their ethnic community, LGBT community, and the broader community. In this chapter, we offer the reader insight into relevant issues for LGBT immigrants, especially as they age. It is not our intent to categorize or characterize LGBT immigrants, rather to assist the reader to gain an understanding of disparities and inequalities faced by this population across multiple domains.

Defining Immigration Population and Status

Who is an immigrant? Who are the immigrant populations? What does it mean to be part of an immigrant population? Does membership confer a status, and if so, how does it compare to the status of non-immigrant populations? In order to explore these questions, important immigration-related concepts must be identified and defined, such as immigrant populations, documented versus undocumented, naturalized versus non-citizens.

Immigrant Populations—Definitions

Definitions of immigrant populations, as well as the criteria that determine these definitions, differ from one country to another. However, according to the Organisation for Economic Co-operation and Development (OECD), the most commonly used definitions are based upon country of birth and nationality (OECD 2013). Using *country of birth criteria*, immigrant populations are defined as those who live in a country (known as host country) different from that in which they were born. Where *nationality criteria* are used, immigrant populations are defined as those holding a nationality different from the host country. Under this scenario, a person may be considered an immigrant even if he or she was born in the host country. The criteria used can also reflect the host country's view of how citizenship may be acquired (OECD 2013). For instance, country of birth criteria reflects *jus soli* —the right of the soil by which citizenship is automatically linked to place of birth, while nationality reflects *jus sanguinis*—the right of blood, wherein citizenship is derived from the nationality of the parents. Generally, countries have self-determined paths from "immigrant" to "national" status. Variations exist and depend upon or are influenced by each country's rules governing how citizenship may be acquired by non-nationals, however defined. Foreign-born persons may acquire citizenship through a *naturalization* process, while those who do not do so remain *non-citizens*.

Countries also prescribe the manner in which immigrants may reside legally in the host country. For instance, in the USA, those who follow established rules for migration are known as documented immigrants, while those who do so without legal authorization are considered *undocumented immigrants*.

According to the US Census Bureau's American Community Survey (ACS), in the USA, the term *foreign born* refers to persons who are not US citizens at birth, including naturalized citizens, legal permanent residents, and other classes of migrants such as the temporary (e.g., students), humanitarian (e.g., refugees), as well as undocumented migrants (US Census Bureau: American Community Survey Report 2012b). *Native born* refers to those born in the US, Puerto Rico, or the US Island Area, or those born abroad to at least one parent who is a US citizen (ACS 2012b). In 2012, the total US population was 313,914 million (Census Bureau 2012a, b; OECD 2013a). According to the 2010 ACS, about 13 % of US population (40 million) is foreign born. Department of Homeland Security estimates indicate that approximately 11.5 million are undocumented (Hoefer et al. 2011). OECD data reflect a growing trend in immigrant populations, with higher immigrant numbers for countries such as Canada, Australia, Israel, and New Zealand that range from 20 to 40 % of their total populations (OECD 2013b).

In sum, immigrant populations include foreign-born persons or persons who still hold a nationality other than that of the host country; they may be documented or undocumented, and their numbers continue to increase (OECD 2013b).

Immigrant Populations—Status

Immigrant populations often exhibit demographic and socioeconomic differences when compared to their native-born counterparts. Status differences within immigrant populations exist, for instance, by race, country of origin, length of stay in the host country (recent or earlier immigrants), and whether they are documented or undocumented aliens (OECD 2013). The vast majority (about 2/3rds) of immigrants have come to the USA since 1990. Generally, compared to native-born populations, immigrants are more likely to be at a disadvantage socioeconomically: with lower levels of education, higher levels of labor force participation, lower income, and a higher likelihood of living in poverty (ACS 2010).

Immigrant LGBT Elders

The growth in both the aging and immigrant segments of the US population give credence to an increased interest in LGBT elders. As both segments grow as a percentage of the overall population, we can expect a parallel increase in the LGBT population. For those involved, the key issues that affect immigrant populations and aging populations join those affecting LGBT populations. Consequently, immigrant LGBT elders are likely to face multiple jeopardy owing to disadvantages due to age, immigrant status, and sexual orientation.

Elders, persons aged 65 and over, comprise approximately 13 % of the US population (US Census Bureau 2012). In the absence of precise data about the number of foreign-born LGBT persons in the USA, the Williams Institute on Sexual Orientation and Gender Identity Law and Public Policy at UCLA School of Law (Williams Institute) conducted an analysis of data from multiple sources including the Pew Research Hispanic Center, Gallup Daily Tracking Survey data, and the US Census Bureau's 2011 American Community Survey. As reported by Gates (2013), this analysis estimates that there are approximately 804,000 foreign-born LGBT in the USA, of which about 70 % (637,000) are documented and 30 % (267,000) are undocumented. Of that number, it is estimated that persons 55 and over make up about 22 % of immigrants who self-identify as LGBT, while among the undocumented, the number is about 4 % (Gates 2013). Because many LGBT individuals are reluctant to identify as such, these estimates may be undercounts. LGBT elder immigrants (both self-identified and otherwise) can be broadly divided into two groups—recently arrived immigrants and earlier cohorts of

immigrants who have aged in place within their host country. Together, they make up a significant segment of the US population. This fact, coupled with the fact that there are currently a large number of younger LGBT immigrants who will likely age in place over time, makes a focus on this group pertinent and timely.

Immigrant LGBT Elders—Status

Similar to other immigrants, LGBT elders exhibit differences when compared to native-born populations. In presenting the data on population estimates and other demographic information, the Williams Institute reviews a number of socioeconomic factors associated with LGBT adult immigrants (individuals and same-sex couples) including race, gender, labor force participation, levels of employment, and annual income (Gates 2013). Some key findings are presented below:

- About 150,800 people are LGBT immigrants aged 55 and over. Of this number, an estimated 140,800 are documented, while 10,000 are undocumented.
- LGBT immigrant elders are more likely to be Hispanic, Asian, or Pacific Islander.
- Fourteen percent (14 %) of same-sex couples include a foreign-born partner or spouse. Same-sex couples include an estimated 113,300 foreign-born individuals (naturalized or non-citizens). Among same-sex couples, 54,600 are non-US citizens; 24,700 are bi-national; and for 11,700, both partners were non-citizens.
- Among same-sex couples aged 55 and older, 23 % (13,800) include a foreign-born person who acquired naturalization status, while 10 % (5,600) include a person who is a non-citizen.
- Non-citizens in same-sex couples are more likely to be economically disadvantaged.
- Male same-sex couples have lower median annual personal incomes despite higher

Table 13.1 Median annual personal income by sex, couple type, and citizenship status

		Same sex			Different sex		
		Non-citizens	Naturalized	Native born	Non-citizens	Naturalized	Native born
In labor force	Men	14,000	40,000	48,500	26,000	45,000	50,000
	Women	22,400	45,000	38,500	16,800	30,000	31,500
Not in labor force	Men	0	13,000	14,000	7800	15,600	24,000
	Women	1500	28,000	11,500	0	3,100	6600

Source Gates (2013), LGBT adult immigrants in the USA, Williams Institute

educational levels, regardless of labor force participation.

- Female same-sex couples report higher median annual personal incomes compared to those in different-sex couples, regardless of labor force participation or citizenship status.
- Among LGBT couples, both male and female have higher labor force participation rates (Table 13.1).

Countries that Recognize Same-Sex Relationships for Immigration Purposes

Like other migrants, LGBT individuals migrate for many reasons: personal, political, religious, and economic. LGBT individuals may also migrate to avoid persecution from their family, community, and even government because of their sexual orientation or gender identity (Tabak and Levitan 2013).

Although there are no international legal instruments tailored to offer protection for LGBT human rights, there has been an increasing trend toward recognition of the necessity and importance of assuring that human rights extend to LGBT populations. In a paper discussing global human rights and LGBT migrants, Tabak and Levitan (2013) state that this increased awareness can be seen in the actions of international and regional legal bodies who have sought to extend the application of human rights principles to LGBT populations. For instance, Tabak and

Levitan (2013) cite the example of the United Nations Human Rights Committee that extended the principles of the International Covenant on Civil and Political Rights (ICCPR) to LGBT persons by expanding the reference to "sex" in Article 26 to include sexual orientation. They argue that such actions are important because of their potential to impact states that are parties to these treaties, and as such are required to be compliant with their provisions.

Protecting the human rights of LGBT immigrants is important because even when they leave their home countries, they may still face discrimination and disadvantage in host countries. In many countries, including those with conducive environments, LGBT persons may face discrimination and persecution especially from immigration laws, policies, and practices.

Discussion Box 1

How have human rights agencies/bodies attempted to extend their provisions to cover LGBT populations? Look up the agencies or bodies provided below. What do you think?

(a) Committee on Economic, Social and Cultural Rights http://www.ohchr.org/EN/HRBodies/CESCR/Pages/CESCRIndex.aspx

(b) European Court of Human Rights http://www.echr.coe.int/Pages/home.aspx?p=home

(c) Inter-American Commission on Human Rights

http://www.oas.org/en/iachr/mandate/what.asp

(d) The Yogyakarta Principles
http://www.yogyakartaprinciples.org/principles_en.htm

Immigration laws and their application to LGBT populations vary across countries in terms of their nature, scope, and recognition of same-sex relationships. These laws run the gamut from non-recognition of same-sex relationships to the creation of special legal status to marriage equality provisions (Human Rights Watch: Immigration Equality (HRWIE) 2006). According to Human Rights Watch: Immigration Equality data (2006), only nineteen countries recognize lesbian and gay relationships for immigration purposes. These recognitions came about in these countries in a variety of ways, including legislative action, court-mandated changes, national referendum, and immigration policy reform (HRWIE 2006).

Until 2013, the USA was not one of the nineteen countries that recognized same-sex couples. However, recent challenges to the Defense of Marriage Act (DOMA 1996), and the Supreme Court decision upholding the unconstitutionality of Section 3, have opened the door to reviewing the treatment of same-sex unions to ensure parity with opposite-sex unions for immigration purposes. In a statement on July 1, 2013, Secretary of Homeland Security Janet Napolitano stated,

> "... I have directed U.S. Citizenship and Immigration Services (USCIS) to review immigration visa petitions filed on behalf of a same-sex spouse in the same manner as those filed on behalf of an opposite-sex spouse." Thus, at the time of this writing, the US now recognizes "marital unions" including those legally valid in other jurisdictions, for immigration purposes.

Table 13.2 presents a list of countries that recognize same-sex relationships for immigration purposes, rights conferred, and some of the criteria required to do so.

Discussion Box 2: A Tale of Two Same-Sex Couples

Review the following cases:

(a) Richard Adams and Anthony Sullivan—Parties in the first federal lawsuit seeking equal treatment for a same-sex marriage in US history.

(b) United States v. Windsor (2013)—Supreme Court decision on Section 3, Defense of Marriage Act, 1999.

In what ways were these cases similar or different? What was the outcome in each case, and what do you think explains the difference? Analyze the impact of these decisions.

History of Research and Practice—LGBT Immigrant Elders

The history of research and practice pertinent to the topic of immigrant LGBT elders is an extremely abbreviated one. This should perhaps not be unexpected, given that the history of research and practice in relation to LGBT elders in general is relatively truncated. In the USA, LGBT baby boomers, who are reaching retirement age, are in effect the first generation of elders who have "come out" in our history (Insight Center for Community Economic Development 2012). As a result of the lack of coming-out among LGBT individuals, particularly among elders who grew up in a time when being LGBT was unheard of, the opportunities for research have been relatively limited. However, we are now experiencing a tremendous increase in the number of "out" LGBT elders. By the year 2030, it is expected that the number of LGBT older adults in the USA will increase to more than four million (Fredriksen-Goldsen et al. 2011).

Table 13.2 Countries that recognize same-sex relationships for immigration purposes

	Country	Who	Status	Rights	Criteria (examples)
1.	Australia	Lesbian or gay partner	Interdependency visa	Same as for heterosexual common-law spouses	Exclusive relationship; 12-month duration
2.	Belgium	Legal marriage/spouse; Partnerships (includes other countries)	Visa Type D; Type C (with view to marry)	Extended stay for more than 90 days; Same for heterosexual relationships	Stable relationship; Family unification
3.	Brazil	Partners	Visas: – temporary – permanent – concubine	No comprehensive national-level acknowledgment; Some rights recognized by the federal government (e.g., rights to social security and pension)	Legal/formal relationship; Proof of stable relationship; Certificate of concubinage
4.	Canada	Spouses, common-law partner, conjugal partner	Broad immigration rights	Same as for different-sex couples	Marriage in Canada; Partner age = 16 or older; Cohabitation for at least a year to establish conjugal status
5.	Denmark	Registered partner, spouse or cohabiting partner	Typically residence permit in either foreign partner's country, or Denmark depending on individual's circumstances	Same general immigration policies apply	At least 24 years old; Ability of resident to provide support; Attachment to Denmark more than any other country
6.	Finland	Spouse (includes registered partner), cohabitant	Residence permit, fixed term or permanent, depending on individual's circumstances	Residence permit; Migration benefits	Family ties; 18 years old; Proof of marriage, partnership, or cohabitation
7.	France	All unmarried couples (same or different sex)	Legal status, with some rights of marriage	Residence: - Temporary (post-I year wait period, renew yearly) – Permanent (after 5 years; renewable every 10 years)	Civil Solidarity Pact; Personal connections to France
8.	Germany	Registered life partner	Residence permit Long-stay visa	Most rights enjoyed by heterosexual couples; Equal immigration rights	Sponsor must be citizen or permanent resident; Able to provide financial support
9.	Iceland	Registered partnerships; Cohabiting partner; Spouses	Permit to stay; Permanent residence (spouses)	Same immigration rights as married spouses	18 years old; Cohabitation for at least 2 years, plus intent to continue if unmarried
10.	Israel	Partners	No national-level legal status	1-year work permit; Temporary residence (yearly renewal); Permanent residence after 7 years	Evidence of sincere, genuine relationship

(continued)

Table 13.2 (continued)

	Country	Who	Status	Rights	Criteria (examples)
11.	The Netherlands	Partner through civil marriage, registered partnership, cohabitant agreement	Broad immigration rights	Provisional residence permit (first step); Full residence permit	Both at least 18 years old; Sponsor must be Dutch citizen, permanent or legal resident; Provide financial support
12.	New Zealand	Partner through civil union, marriage, or de facto union	Same as for married couples	Work visa; Residence visa; Residence permit	Age 18 (16 with legal consent of parents/guardians); Genuine, stable, committed relationship; 12-month cohabitation. Citizen/resident as sponsor
13.	Norway	Spouse, registered partner (at least 3 years), cohabiting partner	Most rights enjoyed by heterosexual couples	Immigration rights available	Over 18 at time of marriage/registered partnership; Proof of intent to/live in Norway; Sponsor can support financially; 2 years of permanent and established relationship (for cohabitation)
14.	Portugal	Partners in de facto unions Cohabitants (more than 2 years)	Same status as common-law spouses (less than heterosexual marriage); Relationship recognized for immigration purposes	Temporary authorization for residence (2 years, renewable); Permanent residence (post-5 or 8 years depending on partner's nationality)	Sponsor must be citizen or permanent resident; Proof of unmarried status; Common-law partnership for more than 2 years
15.	South Africa	Spouse (marriage/civil union); Permanent cohabitation	Full title and rights of marriage under the law; Parity under immigration law	Same immigration rights as married persons	Permanent relationship; Cohabitation; Mutual financial and emotional support; Proof via affidavit and notarial contract
16.	Spain	Spouses	Civil marriage code includes same-sex couples	Same rights as married couples	Valid marriage with Spaniard, or between two resident foreigners
17.	Sweden	Spouses, registered partners, cohabiting partners	Recognizes same-sex relationships; Same rights as married opposite-sex couples	Residence permits (yearly, first 2 years); Permanent residence permit	Family ties; Proof of relationship
18.	Switzerland	Spouses (marriages, civil unions); Registered partners	Immigration laws apply.	3-month visa (to obtain registered partnership); Type B residence permit (annual renewal if relationship persists); Type C resident permit (after 5 years)	Proof of union (Recognizes unions valid in other countries)

(continued)

Table 13.2 (continued)

	Country	Who	Status	Rights	Criteria (examples)
19.	UK	Civil partners; Spouses	Eligible for immigration same as heterosexual marriage	Entry clearance (for proposed civil partnership); 2-year residence (post-partnership registration); Indefinite Leave to Remain; Temporary residents can apply for permanent residence with civil partners	Civil partnership (plus those formalized in other jurisdictions); At least 16 years old; Not in partnership or marriage to another; Genuine/ongoing relationship; No reliance on public funds
20.	USA	Partners in marital unions; Fiancés/fiancées	Treat same as opposite-sex marriages	Immigration laws apply with equal effect; Recognizes marriages/unions legally valid in other jurisdictions	Marital unions; Sponsor must be citizen or legal permanent resident

Source Appendix B: Countries Protecting Same-Sex Couples' Immigration Rights, Human Rights Watch and Immigration Equality (2006). http://www.hrw.org/reports/2006/us0506/10.htm

Despite the recent recognition of the increasing number of LGBT elders, some of whom are immigrants, research efforts have lagged behind. Of the available research on LGBT elders, immigrant LGBT elders have rarely been included. Surprisingly, organizations that are designed to provide resources and conduct research with LGBT elders rarely have information for or about immigrant LGBT elders. However, several do provide information on best practices in working with LGBT elders, some of which can be used for working with immigrant LGBT elders. There are still many, many unanswered questions that require immediate attention.

In light of several recent policy changes regarding immigration, concerns surrounding immigrant LGBT elders are making their way to the forefront, thus the impetus for this chapter within this handbook and future research. The remainder of this chapter will highlight what is known about immigrant LGBT elders, address some of the major concerns surrounding this population, and propose suggestions for future research and practice.

Research Box 1

As mentioned in the chapter, there is a paucity of scholarly research regarding LGBT immigrant elders. Within this chapter, there are references to many issues that are worthy of research. Select a topic specific to LGBT immigrant elders and develop potential research projects. Think about the title of the research project, the objectives, research questions, methods, potential participants, and recruitment of participants, as well as the type of results you would anticipate. Also, think about any potential service delivery implications that your research project may have.

LGBT Immigration Issues

LGBT individuals face many issues as they age; for those who are immigrants, there are additional unique issues. Further compounding issues that LGBT elders may face, many federal, state, or local agencies that provide services for older adults are not designed to address the specific concerns of LGBT elders. In fact, several studies have found that widespread homophobia exists among individuals and organizations entrusted to care for America's older adults (National Gay and Lesbian Task Force Foundation 2011).

Prior to 2013, the immigration system in the USA did not recognize same-sex marriages. In June of 2013, the United States Supreme Court ruled Section 3 of DOMA unconstitutional, requiring the US immigration system to recognize same-sex relationships for immigration purposes (US Citizenship and Immigration Services 2014a, b). While this is a major milestone the issues with immigration for LGBT individuals have not been eliminated. With the striking down of Section 3 of DOMA, there are more opportunities for immigration to the USA for LGBT individuals; however, a strong infrastructure for supporting immigrant LGBT elders does not yet exist in the USA. For example, LGBT elders often face economic challenges, such as finding and maintaining employment due to discrimination and anti-LGBT bias (Services and Advocacy for Gay, Lesbian, Bisexual, and Transgender Elders; National Hispanic Council on Aging; and Diverse Elders Coalition 2014). Furthermore, some states within the USA maintain bans on same-sex marriages; thus, same-sex couples in those states are not recognized as surviving spouses or dependents, which precludes them from receiving surviving spouse benefits if their partner dies, further exacerbating economic challenges.

Economic realities may pose challenges to basic survival, because they affect other issues such as housing. Of the LGBT elders who qualify financially for Section 8 housing, many are ineligible due to lack of immigration status documentation or social security registration (Services and Advocacy for Gay, Lesbian, Bisexual and Transgender Elders; National Hispanic Council on Aging; and Diverse Elders Coalition 2014). In addition to housing challenges, immigrant LGBT elders may have issues

accessing health care for a number of reasons including, language barriers, unfamiliarity with the health care system, lack of immigration status documentation, and lack of health insurance. Undocumented LGBT immigrants are barred from accessing federal health care benefits, including the exchanges established through the 2010 Affordable Care Act (Wasem 2012). This lack of coverage is why many undocumented LGBT individuals forgo medical treatment, and when they do attempt to access care, many times they are unable to afford the care (Baker and Krehely 2011).

Invisibility of LGBT in the Immigration Debate

The LGBT population has long had a history of exclusion in society generally, often born out of fear, ignorance, negative stereotypes, or prejudice about LGBT sexual orientation or gender identity. Especially where prejudice exists or attitudes to LGBT sexual orientation and gender identity is negative, there often exists at best, a paucity of, or at worst, a total lack of awareness and sensitivity to LGBT issues, needs, and concerns. To the extent that these go unnoticed, LGBT populations are effectively rendered invisible and therefore marginalized.

Invisibility also occurs because of the reluctance, reticence, or inability of many in the LGBT population to self-identify as LGBT or publicly acknowledge their sexual orientation or gender identity, due to fear of retribution, stigma, or otherwise. As members of a legally and socially disfavored minority group (Services and Advocacy for Gay, Lesbian, Bisexual, and Transgender Elders (SAGE), and Movement Advancement Project (MAP) 2010), exclusion can occur at personal and societal levels, with the latter being more systematic. For instance, historically, non-inclusive laws, policies, or practices have placed LGBT individuals at a disadvantage in various spheres including access to jobs, housing, and social services (Burns et al.

2013). Also, damaging has been exclusion from public discourse on issues with salience for the LGBT population, an example being immigration and immigration reform.

Immigration reform has been a hot topic in recent years, generating a lot of discussion across all sectors of society. Such discussion often centers on the need for reform of the existing law to address challenges posed by an estimated 11 million undocumented immigrants in the USA (Gates 2013). Public opinion and discourse often center on issues such as refugees, and illegal or undocumented immigrants from Latin, Asian, and African countries; in particular, the influx of Latinos from Mexico, migrant labor, and status of the so called "DREAMers"—children brought to the USA illegally by their parents. Debate also focuses on high visibility cases such as the 1999 Elian Gonzalez case, illegal border crossings, and issues of territorial or homeland security, as well as foreign nationals seeking the "American Dream." However, issues of concern to gay and lesbian populations do not garner the same level of discourse or awareness and so are invisible in the immigration debate.

Notwithstanding the silence on the issue, immigration reform is an LGBT issue for a number of reasons. First, about 267,000 of the 11 million undocumented elders in USA are LGBT (Gates, 2013). Second, Hispanics, who make up a large percentage of the undocumented population, constitute the largest segment of LGBT populations, making immigration reform doubly pertinent for those who fall within these two categories—(i.e., both a Latino and LGBT issue). Third, and most importantly, the major challenge under the current immigration system is the lack of parity in status and recognition afforded to same-sex relationships as compared to opposite-sex relationships. For instance, this lack of parity creates problems for binational couples, whereas the US citizen or legal resident is unable to sponsor a partner or spouse for legal residence. Immigration inequality for LGBT couples has created a number of hardships, including the forced separation of families, threat of or actual deportation of foreign-born/non-citizen partners, as well as exclusion from benefits (e.g. legal,

social, employment/work, health, economic), enjoyed by opposite-sex couples in similar circumstances (Burns, et al. 2013). Misinformation, misconceptions, and lack of awareness of the application and effect of immigration law and system increase LGBT vulnerability to discrimination and disadvantage. An article entitled, *Not Just an "Issue"—Invisibility in the Immigration Debate Hurts Real People*, by Brian Pacheco and published in the Huffington Post on May 7, 2013, reflects this position.

Discussion Box 3

In the news media:

Separately, both LGBT rights and immigration reform have been topical issues recently, receiving a significant amount of news coverage. When these issues overlap, they raise pertinent questions and concerns for LGBT elders. Conduct an online search for news items and/or find news articles on the intersection of LGBT rights and immigration law/reform, such as *Not Just an "Issue"—Invisibility in the Immigration Debate Hurts Real People* by Brian Pacheco and published in the Huffington Post on May 7, 2013.

What issues of relevance to LGBT elders are raised when these areas overlap?

In what way, if at all, does this overlap increase LGBT vulnerability to discrimination and disadvantage?

How might this affect well-being in later life?

Immigration Reform as an LGBT Issue

As a result of the events of September 11, 2001, concerns around citizenship and immigration have risen to the forefront of political discussions in the USA. Some argue that in the wake of the events of 9–11, anti-immigration policies were put into place making it more challenging or impossible for some to immigrate to the USA

(Lewis 2010–2011). Though some of the policies were put into place subsequent to September 11, 2001, some policies were in place prior to September 11, 2001. A lot of these policies were enforcement immigration policies rather than immigration reform policies. Many believed that enforcement immigration policies would lead to reductions in illegal immigration and produce positive outcomes in the future (Giovagnoli 2013). Regardless of when the policies were implemented, certain groups are more vulnerable to the anti-immigration policies, such as LGBT individuals seeking asylum in the USA from Middle Eastern countries (Lewis 2010–2011). Enforcement immigration policies led to increased spending on immigration in the USA, increased numbers of deportation, additional state implemented anti-immigration laws, increased separation of families, and increased discrimination (Lewis 2010–2011). In 2012, federal election results indicated that voters were not satisfied with enforcement immigration and sought a shift toward immigration reform (Giovagnoli 2013), hence the proposal of bills such as the Border Security, Economic Opportunity, and Immigration Modernization Act of 2013, which is still pending.

Currently, about 11 million undocumented immigrants are living in the USA of which hundreds of thousands identify as LGBT. Unfortunately, little is known about undocumented elder LGBT individuals. This subgroup (i.e., undocumented LGBT individuals, including elders) is in desperate need of immigration reform. LGBT undocumented elders find themselves at the intersection of three marginalized groups: the LGBT population, the undocumented population, and the elderly population, thus making them one of society's most vulnerable populations. Immigration reform would assist undocumented LGBT immigrants in four ways: (1) create a path to citizenship; (2) improve the treatment of immigrants held in detention centers; (3) improve the health, safety, and well-being of LGBT immigrants; and (4) improve the US asylum system for LGBT applications.

First, immigration reform has the potential to create paths to citizenship that do not include

unrealistic requirements, which in turn could lead to increased wages and job security, preservation of family unity, greater access to social services (Burns et al. 2013), increased opportunities to pursue higher education, and the chance to live without the constant threat of deportation (Gruberg 2013a, b, c). Second, reforms need to include serious changes to detention center standards to ensure the protection, dignity, and privacy of those detained who are frequently victimized. Unfortunately, LGBT immigrants who are detained while awaiting deportation or trial are often sexually assaulted and harassed by guards or other detainees (see Chap. 12), subjected to prolonged periods in solitary confinement, denied necessary medical care, and/or denied proper hormonal therapy for transgendered individuals (Gruberg 2013a, b, c). Typically, solitary confinement is used for punishment; however, in the case of many LGBT individuals, it is used to "protect" them from assault. Thus, many LGBT individuals are in essence being punished for their sexual orientation. One potential solution to this problem is to utilize alternative detention programs in an effort to decrease the number of LGBT immigrants in detention centers, which may be a more cost-effective strategy (Gruberg 2013a, b, c). Third, immigration reform has the potential to positively influence well-being and increase immigrants' access to health care and social services, including culturally competent care for LGBT immigrants. Finally, reforms should improve the US asylum programs, specifically by lifting the one-year ban for submitting asylum claims (National Immigrant Justice Center 2010). One in five refugees seeking protection in the USA is denied asylum claims because he or she misses the one-year deadline for filing such claims (National Immigrant Justice Center, 2010). Since the deadline for filing was initiated in 1996, over 79,000 cases have been denied simply based on the deadline (Gruberg 2013a, b, c). While this deadline and unfortunate denial of asylum cases affect all immigrants, it disproportionately affects LGBT immigrants who are seeking asylum from countries that criminalize homosexuality (Gruberg 2013a, b, c). Additionally, immigration reform would significantly increase the number of immigration judges and legal personnel assigned to these asylum cases (Gruberg 2013a, b, c). If the current immigration reform bill is passed, LGBT immigrant elders could significantly benefit from the aforementioned changes. Immigration is and will continue to be one of the most critical components of US public policy. Moving forward, it will be important to specifically include elder LGBT immigrants in immigration reform discussions, so that bills that are passed are inclusive of the needs of all immigrants.

Policy Box 1

Toward equity for same-sex relationships DOMA—To be or not to be?

In light of the 2013 court decision to strike down Section 3 of the Defense of Marriage Act, (DOMA, 1996) do you think that DOMA should be repealed? What recourse is there for same-sex relationships especially in states which currently ban unions? How would passage of the proposed bill—Uniting American Families Act—redress the situation?

As an advocate for immigrant LGBT elders, you have been invited to address the Judicial Committee on this issue. How would you frame your argument, and what would be your rationale for doing so?

Immigration Rights and Implications for Elders

LGBT elders are in a particularly vulnerable position. They simultaneously face the challenges of aging, plus legal inequity, social stigma and discrimination because of their sexual orientation or gender identity, as well as disadvantage because of immigration status. This multiple jeopardy creates a unique intersection of disadvantage that further marginalizes this population, especially because these disadvantages and experiences have accumulated over time. The Life course perspective and the theory of cumulative advantage/disadvantage help us understand the potential impact these disadvantages can inflict in later life. The life course perspective is a conceptual approach which explains that historical events, experiences, and actions which occur over the life span shape an individual's aging experience (Stoller and Gibson 1999), while according to the theory of cumulative advantage/disadvantage, benefits and burdens encountered by individuals or groups have a tendency to accumulate and thus compound, as time passes (Dannefer 2003).

Current immigration laws and policies provide very few protections for LGBT populations and in fact have negative implications for many LGBT. Calls for immigration reform that is inclusive, fair, and reasonable have focused on a number of issues, such as (a) the recognition of same-sex relationships, and marriage equality for binational unions; (b) alternatives to detention for undocumented immigrants being held in detention facilities; (c) ending deportations; and (d) provision of asylum for LGBT seeking protection from persecution in their home countries, as mentioned previously.

For LGBT elders, a major reform issue relates to establishing parity with opposite-sex relationships. Marriage equality and recognition of permanent relationships, as some countries have done through processes like the "registered partnerships" designation, is a key right because of its impact on access to many other rights, benefits, and protections. It would allow a US citizen/legal resident sponsor a partner for legal residency in the USA. Residency would confer rights and benefits such as family reunification by reducing separations, as well as assure access to benefits enjoyed by heterosexual couples like access to social services and programs, and taxation related benefits. In addition, legal residency would improve opportunities for employment, job security, and better wages, thus enhancing financial security and well-being in later life.

Implications for LGBT elders vary. Forced separation, deportations, and self-exile by LGBT due to exclusive immigration policies and practices contribute to social isolation in old age for those who find themselves separated either from their partners or from their family of origin. For LGBT elders, this is critical because it reduces their social convoy or networks, which is a source of social support, especially if they suffer stigma and lack of acceptance within the community. In the absence of familial caregivers, they may have to live in residential facilities where they may be exposed to stigma, prejudicial treatment, or hostile environments (SAGE and MAP 2010).

Living in long-term care institutions may also create other challenges. Non-inclusive polices or homophobia may cause facilities to indulge in practices that abrade individual rights. For instance, a nursing home may not allow cohabitation or support the individual's expression of gender identity. Also, giving priority to biological families or families based upon opposite-sex unions exposes LGBT elders to unequal treatment under immigration laws and other programs and services. The implication is pertinent especially for health matters. Lack of legal status can bar LGBT elders from health care benefits, visitation rights, as well as medical and end-of-life decision making. Its effect on employment, job security, and income over the life course affects financial welfare in later life and during retirement. The 2010 multi-agency report, "*Improving the Lives of LGBT Older Adults,*" provides illustrative examples of the implications of exclusion on same-sex couples. According to the report,

> Most Americans and their elected leaders are unaware of the many ways in which unequal treatment and ongoing social stigma can hurt and impoverish LGBT elders. Consider the older gay man who loses the family home when his partner requires long-term institutional care; a heterosexual spouse would be protected from the same fate under Medicaid rules. Or consider the lesbian elder who is forced to spend her last days alone in the hospital because the federal government will not grant family medical leave to a close friend who would otherwise take care of her at home (SAGE and MAP 2010).

Advocates for immigration reform for LGBT immigrants continue to draw attention to these and other concerns. Even the stalled Border Security, Economic Opportunity and Immigration Modernization Act of 2013, which sought to address some of these challenges by providing a pathway to citizenship for undocumented immigrants, needs to go further. In a report for the Center for American Progress, authors Burns, Garcia, and Wolgin (2013) note issues that reform must address. Burns et al. state that the law needs to eliminate discrimination against binational same-sex couples and afford them rights and protections given to heterosexual couples by recognizing same-sex unions and committed partnerships for those in jurisdictions that ban same-sex marriages. These changes or amendments would help promote family unity and reduce the number of deportations, or those who live under the threat of deportation.

If passed by Congress, such a bill will open the way to equality for LGBT immigrants. For example, the right to sponsor a same-sex partner or spouse would allow the sponsored individual to obtain the legal right to live and work in the US. This in turn would allow such individuals to invest and save for the future, be engaged in the community, and live openly and with dignity with loved ones—all of which benefits both present and future cohorts of LGBT elders. We have begun to see a trend in changing public opinion and in the judiciary about same-sex couples, which may bode well for immigration reform.

Case Discussion 1: What would you do?

You are the Administrator-in-Training at Rest-A-while Acres, a 30-bed nursing home. You have a recently arrived resident Kevin (Kay) A. Scrunchman. Kay's birth certificate and records show that she was born 70 years ago, a male child. For the past 45 years or so, Kay has lived her life as a female. She intends to continue to do so and has requested a room with a female roommate. The Director of Nursing and staff insist on placing Kay with a male roommate, and assistants report discomfort with helping her wear dresses and apply makeup. You do not have any single rooms in your facility.

What if any are Kay's rights?

What, if any, are your responsibilities?

What would you advise?

Immigration Benefits

As previously mentioned, the US Supreme Court struck down Section 3 of the DOMA in June of 2013. Prior to striking down Section 3, US Citizenship and Immigration Services and other federal agencies had to define marriage as the union of a man and a woman, precluding same-sex couples from access to more than 1000 federal programs and benefits available to heterosexual spouses (Gruberg 2013a, b, c), including the right of a US citizen to sponsor a spouse for legal immigration. As a result of the striking down of Section 3 of DOMA, additional benefits became available to same-sex married couples. The repeal allows US Citizenship and Immigration Services to recognize same-sex marriages between a US citizen or legal permanent resident and a non-citizen, as long as the marriage is valid (i.e., took place in a state where same-sex marriage is legal), to be sufficient for immigration benefits (Gruberg 2013a, b, c). In addition to being able to sponsor a same-sex spouse for legal immigration, the repeal of Section 3 of DOMA has led to additional benefits now available to same-sex binational couples, including sponsoring stepchildren, protecting domestic violence survivors from deportation, admitting fiancé(e)s of US citizens and their children, recognizing follow-to-join benefits, reducing barriers for transgender individuals in heterosexual marriages, and allowing undocumented spouses to apply for a hardship waiver.

US immigration law provides preferential treatment to those considered immediate family of the US citizen. For immigration purposes, this includes spouses, children, and parents. US citizens and legal permanent residents are eligible to bring their unmarried children under 21 years of age to the USA. The immigration law defines the parent–child relationship using terms such as "born in wedlock," "adoption," and "stepchild" (USCIS 2014a, b). Prior to June 2013, LGBT binational families were at risk of separation because the law did not allow recognition of their marriage, thus preventing access to sponsorship benefits provided to other families (Gruberg

2013a, b, c). Before the removal of Section 3, definitions used in the immigration law were based on the assumption that all families were comprised of heterosexual married couples raising biological or adopted children. However, LGBT families are formed in a variety of ways, for instance the children may be adopted, the biological child of only one spouse, or born via artificial insemination or surrogacy (Gruberg 2013a, b, c). Prior to June 2013, if the US citizen or legal permanent resident was not biologically related to the child or on the adoption paperwork, then the relationship to the child was not recognized because the marriage was not recognized by the federal government (Gruberg 2013a, b, c). Family reunification provisions are extremely important for many LGBT binational couples, including some elders. Now that Section 3 has been repealed, same-sex marriages can be recognized, and married LGBT binational couples have access to the same family reunification benefits as other families. US citizens and legal permanent residents who can apply for immigration benefits for their same-sex spouse can also do so for their spouse's children, as their own stepchildren.

There are programs like those under the Violence Against Women Act (VAWA), which offer services to aid in protecting immigrants who are victims of violence. The VAWA permits certain categories of abused immigrant spouses and their children to self-petition for permanent residency in the USA and receive employment authorization and public benefits (Immigration Center for Women and Children [ICWC] 2014). VAWA was put in place to assist immigrants without legal immigration status to leave an abusive spouse without fear of deportation. Essentially, VAWA provides a means of escaping violence and establishing safe and independent lives. Prior to 2013, LGBT individuals without legal immigration status were not included in the VAWA provisions, despite the fact that they are not immune from partner violence. After the striking down of Section 3 of DOMA, the protections afforded by VAWA are now available to spouses in same-sex relationships (ICWC 2014). Additionally, the non-abused same-sex spouse of a US citizen or legal permanent resident whose children are abused by the citizen may qualify as well (Gruberg 2013a, b, c).

Same-sex couples can now access the K visa, which allows fiancé(s) and the unmarried minor children of US citizens to legally enter the USA so that they can be married within 90 days of entrance. It also allows the fiancé to immediately apply for work authorization. Once the couple is married, the foreign citizen can then apply for permanent legal resident status and can remain in the country until the application is processed (USCIS 2014a, b).

Some LGBT legal permanent residents who were married or had children before becoming legal permanent residents and whose spouses or children did not initially accompany them to the USA are now eligible for the follow-to-join benefits. Follow-to-join benefits mean that the spouse or children who did not physically accompany the legal permanent residents to the USA do not have to wait until a visa number becomes available. Instead, the legal permanent resident is required to notify the US consulate that he or she is a legal permanent resident, and the spouse can then apply for an immigrant visa (USCIS 2012).

Individuals who illegally enter the USA must first leave the country before becoming eligible to apply for a green card. Typically, spouses and children of a US citizen who entered illegally have to wait 3 or 10 years depending on how long they were in the USA before leaving voluntarily or being deported, before they can gain authorization to apply for legal permanent resident status. However, if the immigrant is able to obtain a hardship waiver, he or she may not have to wait for 3 or 10 years before applying for a green card. Hardship waivers reduce the amount of time an undocumented immigrant must wait before applying to be a legal permanent resident. Hardship waivers are only available to spouses and children of US citizens.

Transgender individuals in heterosexual marriages should no longer be subjected to any special requirements or conditions in order to prove that their marriage is a heterosexual marriage due to the repeal of Section 3 of DOMA (Immigrant Legal Resource Center 2013). Prior to June 2013, these benefits were not available to same-sex partners, as they were not recognized by the federal government. With the repeal of Section 3, significant strides have been made in affording same-sex couples the same benefits as others. However, there is still a long way to go. For instance, there are thousands of undocumented LGBT immigrants and unmarried immigrants who await immigration reform, so that they can have a clear-cut pathway to citizenship in the USA.

LGBT Couples that Include a Foreign-Born Spouse

In 2013, there were an estimated 113,300 foreign-born individuals, including naturalized citizens and non-citizens who are part of a same-sex couple (Gates, 2013). Approximately, 54,600 of these individuals are not US citizens (Gates 2013). Additionally, there are an estimated 24,700 same-sex couples that are binational (i.e., one US citizen and one non-citizen) and approximately 11,700 same-sex couples comprised of two non-citizens (Gates 2013). In total, 87,900 same-sex couples residing in the USA include a foreign-born spouse or partner (Gates, 2013). When compared to foreign-born individuals in heterosexual relationships, foreign-born individuals in same-sex couples are more likely to be male and younger (Gates 2013). Non-citizens in both same-sex and heterosexual couples are economically disadvantaged (Gates 2013). Naturalized citizens who are in same-sex couples are more likely to be Hispanic (37 % vs. 31 %, respectively) and White (30 % vs. 26 %) and less likely to be Asian, as compared to their heterosexual counterparts (Gates 2013). Regarding non-citizens, individuals in same-sex couples are also more likely than those in heterosexual couples to be White (28 % vs. 16 %, respectively) but less likely to be Hispanic (46 % vs. 58 %) and Asian (16 % vs. 20 %)

(Gates 2013). Regardless of citizenship status, the majority of men and women in same-sex couples have higher levels of education as compared to their counterparts, with the exception of non-citizen same-sex women (Gates 2013). The aforementioned data, while not specific to LGBT elders, provide an overview of LGBT couples that are comprised of a foreign-born spouse or partner.

Specifically, focusing on older adults, approximately 10,000 undocumented LGBT immigrants are 55 years of age or older, while approximately 140,800 of documented LGBT immigrants are 55 years of age or older (Gates 2013). Adults 55 and older account for 23 % of naturalized citizens who are foreign born and living in the USA, and 10 % of non-citizens (Gates 2013). In general, there is very little demographic data available regarding LGBT immigrants and even less regarding LGBT elder immigrants. With the striking down of Section 3 of DOMA, there are more opportunities for LGBT couples that include a foreign-born spouse or partner—with that change may come more opportunities to learn more about LGBT elders in binational couples.

Implications for Service Delivery from an Interdisciplinary Perspective

In this chapter, we have introduced and discussed some of the major issues that affect immigrant LGBT elders and how current immigration policies and practices act to disadvantage and marginalize immigrant LGBT elders through unfair and unreasonable treatment. People are a product of their life course and the events, challenges, and opportunities, which shape them to create patterns of accumulated advantage and/or disadvantage over time. These cumulative advantages or disadvantages impact later life in terms of both experiences and expectations, and ultimately affect well-being and adjustment in old age. Bearing this in mind, it is important for those who work, provide care, or otherwise interact with LGBT elders to be cognizant of these issues and their implications for clients. These service

and care providers span a broad range of disciplines, including social work, health care-including mental health, financial planning, geriatric services management, legal services (elder law), as well as advocacy groups. Each professional or service provider must begin by asking at least these two salient questions:

(1) In order to optimally identify and address my client's needs and maximize benefits, what challenges and opportunities are posed by being an immigrant LGBT elder? and (2) Understanding these, how can I best assure, promote, or protect his/her interests?

Potential implications for service delivery are many and will vary depending on the disciplinary area and individual client circumstances. However, there are some general guidelines that are helpful to consider when providing care and service to immigrant LGBT elders, regardless of status and situation. These general guidelines have been articulated by a number of advocacy and research groups with expertise in and knowledge of LGBT population, such as the National Center for Lesbian Rights, Transgender Law Center; American Immigration Council Legal Action Center; and Services and Advocacy for Gay, Lesbian, Bisexual and Transgender Elders (SAGE). According to these groups, in order to provide competent care and services to immigrant LGBT elders, service and care providers must do the following:

- **Be tolerant and comfortable with LGBT people and issues**
  It is important to examine personal attitudes and their effect on how one perceives, thinks, and treats LGBT people, in order to overcome or address disinterest, discomfort or apathy which may have a negative impact on service delivery.
- **Be knowledgeable and aware**
  Knowledge and awareness of the challenges faced by LGBT populations pave the way to understanding and empathy. Knowledge can be acquired by getting to know and building relationships with LGBT individuals, community, advocates, and organizations, as well as through training and education. It is important to learn about myths regarding

LGBT, and to develop familiarity with and/or obtain access to local, regional, and national resources for LGBT populations. In addition, exposure to positive imagery and portrayal of LGBT people can also help improve knowledge, sensitivity, and awareness.

- **Create an LGBT-friendly work environment**

  As with other minority/disadvantaged groups, providing staff education and sensitivity training, as well as instituting LGBT-friendly policies are useful strategies. Resources or materials for clients should be inclusive and diverse. Hiring LGBT personnel not only ensures inclusion of LGBT views, but also promotes overall diversity in the organization or workplace. Providing LGBT cultural competency training can enhance the creation of a culture of inclusivity and a safe environment where clients feel able to discuss sensitive issues.

- **Language**

  Language is often a barometer for attitude, understanding, and expertise. Inclusive language treats all clients fairly and reasonably and avoids assumptions about sexual orientation and gender identity. For instance, in a practice advisory entitled *"Tips for legal advocates working with lesbian, gay, bisexual and transgender clients,"* the National Center for Lesbian Rights (NCLR) and its partners California Rural Legal Association(CLRA) and Legal Services for Children (LSC) recommend asking clients questions such as "are you in a relationship" rather than "do you have a boyfriend?" (NCLR, CLRA, and LSC 2013). It is also important to consider each individual client, and their unique circumstance(s) as far as practicable. Avoid generalizations and assumptions about LGBT clients, by using language used by the client to define him/herself. This avoids using language which may imply judgment, e.g., words such as "lifestyle" or "sexual preference" (NCLR, CLRA, and LSC 2013).

- **Be sensitive and astute in approach**

  Acknowledge the client's use or choice of name, pronoun especially in transgender cases, and request clarification if in doubt. Privacy and confidentiality should always be respected. Also be aware of the implications of past history on LGBT elders. For example, consider the potential for social isolation due to past issues with family separation, the possibility of a definition of "family" which may be different, likelihood of poverty or financial challenges due to unfavorable work experience or inability to work because of immigration status, and other consequences of marginalization.

- **Recognize that not all issues are about LGBT status**

  LGBT elders may face concerns or challenges that do not pertain to sexual orientation and gender and should be treated accordingly. In so doing, it is important to be aware of the potential effect of a history of prejudice, discrimination, and stigma both on LGBT elders' self-perception and their response to others. Being an advocate for clients may involve confronting prejudice, stereotypes, and discrimination in others.

- **Be mindful of available resources**

  Know where and how to contact LGBT organizations and advocacy groups as needed and to keep information current. This is especially important as the LGBT landscape undergoes legal and public opinion changes. These organizations have access to and offer valuable information, research, and counsel to help inform effective strategies.

- **Know your limitations**

  Be self-aware. Know when to seek outside help and to make referrals for service, advocacy, resource needs, support groups, and the like if appropriate and as necessary.

In sum, always consider the client's needs. Make him or her comfortable, follow her lead, or let her set the tone and build trust. Avoid a "one size fits all" approach. Try to understand the unique issues, problems, situations, and factual circumstances faced by the client. Keep abreast of changes in the law, educate staff, and be cognizant of the various avenues for help, information, or other resources.

Finally, consider how best to optimize service delivery using an interdisciplinary approach because of the benefits that seamless delivery and a continuum of care offer to older adults. Ultimately, the best approach is one within which professionals understand not just how to address the issues they confront in a way that shows cultural competence in LGBT issues, but also how best to do so in order to support the work of others so as to provide seamless and optimal service to clients. Immigrant LGBT elders face disadvantage on three fronts—ageism on account of old age, immigrant status (both documented and undocumented) and because of sexual orientation or gender identity. Multiple jeopardy and its implications for well-being and adaptation in later life must be considered in service delivery.

Implications for Future Research and Summary

In early 2015, as we complete this chapter, immigration reform is topical and in a state of flux. We are currently awaiting action from Congress. Although recent changes to immigration policies have been beneficial for LGBT immigrants, immigration reform is still a major issue for the LGBT immigrant population and its non-immigrant partners. There is a paucity of data on LGBT populations in general and, more specifically, LGBT elder immigrants, despite the amount of fragmented information from advocacy groups, Web sites, and other publications. While there are inherent challenges to collecting data on undocumented people, especially undocumented LGBT individuals due to fear and stigma, we are sorely in need of systematically and rigorously conducted quantitative and qualitative research data that can support policy reform and practice. Because of the many issues that affect LGBT elders and their non-immigrant partners, there is a wide open vista for research—we suggest several areas. We need a better idea of the demographic scope of documented and undocumented immigrant LGBT elders and their partners. We must assess the needs and challenges of LGBT elders and their partners in order to develop policies and practices that will address their service needs. Additionally, there are more specific research questions, for instance, the role and meaning of marriage in same-sex relationships in terms of access to, preference for, and feasibility of marriage among LGBT individuals compared to heterosexual relationships. This is an important question in light of the recent Supreme Court ruling. That decision created marriage equality for same-sex couples, but is it sufficient? Do we need to address other forms of commitment among those in same-sex relationships, such as civil unions or registered partnerships? If so, what are the implications for immigration? Are there barriers to being married, and if so, how should these be considered or addressed? Should those who show commitment be considered similar to spouses, for immigration purposes and benefit? This is important because we have seen how immigration status contributes to socioeconomic disadvantages, which accumulate across the life course and ultimately determine well-being and adaptation in old age.

Public attitudes are changing toward LGBT individuals, toward immigration issues, and specifically relating to immigrants who are undocumented; these changes will likely impact immigration reform. As the numbers of LGBT elder immigrants and their partners increase, the issues that confront this demographic are only going to become more salient. Thus, developments in this arena need to be monitored and understood if we are to promote policies and practices, which work to optimize service delivery to this population.

This chapter has emphasized that LGBT immigrant elders suffer multiple jeopardy by virtue of being members of disadvantaged groups (i.e., elders, LGBT, immigrant). Although invisible to many, immigration is an important issue for LGBT populations due to its impact on the individuals who may be seeking refuge, same-sex couples, and their families. Immigration status can determine a lifetime of opportunity or disadvantage. The striking down of Section 3 of DOMA is a much-needed step in the right direction, but there is much more that needs to be done. Comprehensive immigration reform is critical to address the needs and concerns of this vulnerable population.

Learning Exercises

Word Search

Find the words below and make sure that you know what they mean.

```
T N E M T A E R T L A U Q E N U S P
Z Q W F B Y N O S T P P B Y O E N I
W D S I D I Y O N T V E O K X F A H
M B N J N D N A I L I G E U C B T S
N R M E O D R A C N Y G A N R K I N
R G O M G G S S T A U L M S K Q V E
O V A F I A M O K I O L T A Z O E Z
B E Y M E Z I A R R O H I I Q Q B I
N D M S I R R R I R G N J V S N O T
G I K Z Q T N E R I U Z A P I Q R I
I G T V A X N O R A X L O L D C N C
E T U T I T S N I S M A I L L I W O
R W L V A Z A N Z T Z X R N K L Z T
O H Y T K M T U B B A V E U G G A H
F W I J U S S O L I S R V S A B W T
V O P H T N N Q O S E I G U E T D A
N T R A N S G E N D E R X I G M W P
G E N D E R I D E N T I T Y M R A T
T R O P P U S L A I C O S L W M S S
M U L T I P L E J E O P A R D Y I Z
```

BINATIONAL
CIVIL UNION
DOMA
FOREIGN BORN
GENDER IDENTITY
HUMAN RIGHTS
IMMIGRANT
IMMIGRATION REFORM
JUS SOLIS
LGBT
MARRIAGE EQUALITY
MULTIPLE JEOPARDY
NATIVE BORN
PATH TO CITIZENSHIP
SAME SEX MARRIAGE
SEXUAL ORIENTATION
SOCIAL SUPPORT
STIGMA
TRANSGENDER
UNDOCUMENTED MIGRANTS
UNEQUAL TREATMENT
WILLIAMS INSTITUTE
WINDSOR RULING
YOGYAKARTA

24 of 30 words were placed into the puzzle.

```
T N E M T A E R T L A U Q E N U S P
+ + W + B + N + S T + + + Y + E N I
+ + + I + I + O N T + + O + X + A H
M + + + N D N A I + I G + U + + T S
N R + E O D R A + N Y G A + + + I N
R + O M G G S + T A U L M S + + V E
O + A F I A + O K I O L T A + + E Z
B + + M E + I A R R O H I + + + B I
N + M + + R R R I R G N + V + + O T
G I + + + T N E R I U + A + I + R I
I + + + A + N O R A + L + L + C N C
E T U T I T S N I S M A I L L I W O
R + + + A + A + + T + X + N + L + T
O + + T + M + + + + A + E + G G + H
F + I J U S S O L I S R + S + B + T
+ O + H + + + + + + + + G + E T + A
N T R A N S G E N D E R + I + M + P
G E N D E R I D E N T I T Y M + A +
T R O P P U S L A I C O S + + M + S
M U L T I P L E J E O P A R D Y I +
```

(Over, Down, Direction)
BINATIONAL(5,2,SE)
CIVILUNION(16,11,NW)
DOMA(6,4,SW)
FOREIGNBORN(1,15,N)
GENDERIDENTITY(1,18,E)
HUMANRIGHTS(4,16,NE)
IMMIGRANT(2,10,NE)
IMMIGRATIONREFORM(17,20,NW)
JUSSOLIS(4,15,E)
LGBT(16,13,S)
MARRIAGEEQUALITY(19,1,S)
MULTIPLEJEOPARDY(1,20,E)
NATIVEBORN(17,2,S)
PATHTOCITIZENSHIP(18,17,N)
SAMESEXMARRIAGE(18,19,NW)
SEXUALORIENTATION(17,1,SW)
SOCIALSUPPORT(13,19,W)
STIGMA(9,2,SE)
TRANSGENDER(2,17,E)
UNDOCUMENTEDMIGRANTS(20,1,S)
UNEQUALTREATMENT(16,1,W)
WILLIAMSINSTITUTE(17,12,W)
WINDSORRULING(3,2,SE)
YOGYAKARTA(14,2,SW)

Self-Check Questions

1. How did the striking down of Section 3 of DOMA impact same-sex couples in the USA and abroad?
2. Explain why immigration reform is an LGBT issue.
3. Describe how immigration reform would assist undocumented LGBT individuals.
4. List and describe several of the benefits afforded to LGBT couples since the striking down of Section 3 of DOMA
5. List and describe strategies for service delivery for LGBT elders.

Multiple-Choice Questions

1. In the USA, *Native Born* refers to individuals born where?
   (a) Continental USA and US Islands
   (b) Puerto Rico
   (c) Anywhere as long as one parent is a US citizen
   (d) All of the above
2. LGBT elders are considered to be more susceptible to vulnerabilities due to:
   (a) Age
   (b) Sexual orientation
   (c) Immigrant status
   (d) All of the above
3. Approximately what percentage of the 55 and older documented immigrant population identifies as LGBT?
   (a) 5 %
   (b) 53 %
   (c) 72 %
   (d) 22 %
4. With the striking down of Section 3 of DOMA, same-sex couples regardless of where they reside within the USA have the same rights as heterosexual couples?
   (a) True
   (b) False

5. Same-sex marriages in the USA are valid for immigration purposes as long as
   (a) The couple has been married for a minimum of 2 years
   (b) The couple was married in a location where same-sex marriage is legal
   (c) The couple has no children
   (d) None of the above
6. Currently, undocumented immigrants have how long to file asylum claims:
   (a) 2 years
   (b) 3 years
   (c) 10 years
   (d) 1 year
7. An estimated _____ percent of LGBT immigrant are over age 55 are undocumented.
   (a) 10
   (b) 20
   (c) 4
   (d) 50
8. Section 3 of DOMA was struck by the US Supreme Court in:
   (a) June 2013
   (b) June 2006
   (c) June 2014
   (d) June 1999
9. Since the striking down of Section 3 of DOMA, immigrant LGBT are now afforded several benefits including all of the following, except:
   (a) Access to the K visa
   (b) Follow-to-join benefits
   (c) Inclusion in VAWA provisions
   (d) Tax deferments
10. LGBT immigrants are more likely to be Hispanic, Asian, or Pacific Islander.
   (a) True
   (b) False

Key For Multiple-Choice Questions

1. (a)
2. (d)

3. (d)
4. (b)
5. (b)
6. (d)
7. (c)
8. (a)
9. (a)
10. (a)

Resources

A. **Useful organizations**:

Services and Advocacy for GLBT Elders (SAGE)
305 Seventh Ave, 15th Floor
New York, NY 10001
Tel. 212-741-2247
Fax. 212-366-1947
Email: info@sageusa.org
Web site: http://www.sageusa.org/
The Lesbian, Gay, Bisexual and Transgender Community Center
(Largest LGBT multi-service organization on the East Coast; second-largest LGBT center in the world)
208 W 13 St New York, NY 10011
Tel. 212-620-7310
Email: info@gaycenter.org
Web site: https://gaycenter.org/
National Resource Center on LGBT Aging
National Headquarters
C/o Services and Advocacy for GLBT Elders (SAGE)
305 Seventh Avenue
6th Floor
New York, NY 10001
Tel. 212-741-2247
Fax. 212-366-1947
Email: info@lgbtagingcenter.org
Web site: http://www.lgbtagingcenter.org/

B. **Other Organizational Links/websites**

The US Administration on Aging: http://www.aoa.gov/

Center for American Progress: http://www.americanprogress.org/

FORGE/Transgender Aging Network: http://forge-forward.org/aging/

Immigration and Citizenship: http://www.usa.gov/Citizen/Defense/Citizenship.shtml

Immigration Equality: https://immigrationequality.org/

Immigrant Legal Resource Center: http://www.ilrc.org/

National Center for Transgender Equality: http://transequality.org/

National Gay and Lesbian Task Force: http://www.thetaskforce.org/

National Senior Citizens Law Center: http://www.nsclc.org/

Old Lesbians Organizing for Change: http://www.oloc.org/

Southerners on New Ground: southernersonnewground.org

Transgender Individuals Living Their Truth, Inc.: http://tiltt.org/

US Citizenship and Immigration Services: http://www.uscis.gov/

US Immigration and Customs Enforcement: http://www.ice.gov/

ZAMINOBLA (National Organization of Black Lesbians on Aging): http://zami.org/

C. **Audio–visual (Video) Resource**

LGBT Older Adults in Long-Term Care Facilities: Video Stories from the Field
http://www.nsclc.org/index.php/health/long-term-care/lgbt-older-adults-in-long-term-care-facilities-video-stories-from-the-field/
National Citizen Law Center
1444 Eye Street, NW Suite 1100
Washington, DC 20005
Tel. 202-289-6976
Web site: http://www.nsclc.org/

References

Baker, K., & Krehely, J. (2011). *Changing the game: What health care reform means for gay, lesbian, bisexual, and transgender Americans.* Washington:

Center for American Progress and the National Coalition for LGBT Health. Available at http://www.american-progress.org/wp-content/uploads/issues/2011/03/pdf/acalgbtexec_summ.pdf.

Burns, C., Garcia, A., & Wolgin, P.E. (2013). *Living in dual shadows: LGBT undocumented immigrants.* Washington: Center for American Progress. Available at http://cdn.americanprogress.org/wp-content/uploads/2013/03/LGBTUndocumentedReport-6.pdf.

Burns, C. & Garcia, A. (2013). *Infographic: The LGBT Undocumented: By the Numbers.* "Centers for American Progress, March 8, 2013, available at http://www.americanprogress.org/issues/immigration/news/2013/03/08/55676/infographic-the-lgbt-undocumented-by-the-numbers/.

Dannefer, D. (2003). Cumulative advantage/disadvantage and the life course: Cross-fertilizing age and social science theory. *Journal of Gerontology: Social Science, 58B*(6), 327–337.

Fredriksen-Goldsen, K. I., Hyun-Jun, K., Emlet, C. A., Muraco, A., Erosheva, E. A., Hoy-Ellis, C.P., & Goldsen, J. et al. (2011). *Aging and Health Report-Disparities and Resilience among lesbian, gay, bisexual, and transgender Older Adults.* Institute for Multigenerational Health.

Gates, G. J. (2013). *LGBT Adult Immigrants in the United States.* The Williams Institute. Retrieved from http://williamsinstitute.law.ucla.edu/wp-content/uploads/LGBTImmigrants-Gates-Mar-2013.pdf.

Giovagnoli, M. (2013). *Overhauling immigration law: A brief history and basic principles of reform.* Retrieved from http://www.immigrationpolicy.org/perspectives/overhauling-immigration-law-brief-history-and-basic-principles-reform.

Gruberg, S. (2013a, November). *Dignity denied: LGBT immigrants in U.S. immigration detention.* Retrieved February 13, 2015 from http://cdn.americcanprogress.org/wp-content/uploads/2013/11/immigrationEnforcement.pdf.

Gruberg, S. (2013b). *Additional immigration benefits are available for same-sex couples after DOMA repeal.* Retrieved from http://www.americanprogress.org/issues/lgbt/news/2013/07/17/69826/additional-immigration-benefits-are-available-for-same-sex-couples-after-doma-repeal/.

Gruberg, S. (2013c). *What immigration reform means for the LGBT community.* Retrieved From http://www.americanprogress.org/issues/immigration/news/2013/06/11/65942/what-immigration-reform-means-for-the-lgbt-community/.

Hoefer, M., Rytina, N., & Baker, B. (2011). *Estimates of the unauthorized immigrant population residing in the United States: January 2011.* Retrieved from http://www.dhs.gov/xlibrary/assets/statistics/publications/ois_ill_pe_2011.pdf.

Human Rights Watch: Immigration Equality (HRWIE). (2006). *Family, unvalued discrimination, denial, and the fate of binational same-sex couples under U.S. Law.* Retrieved from http://www.hrw.org/reports/2006/us0506/FamilyUnvalued.pdf.

Immigration Center for Women and Children. (2014). *Violence Against Women Act.* Retrieved from http://icwclaw.org/services-available/violence-against-women-act-vawa/.

Immigrant Legal Resource Center. (2013). *Marriage equality in immigration law: Immigration benefits for same-sex married couples.* Retrieved from http://www.ilrc.org/files/documents/marriage_equality_in_immigration_law_-_immigration_benefits_for_same-sex_married_couples.pdf.

Insight Center for Community Economic Development. (2012). *Securing our future: Advancing economic security for diverse elders.* Diverse Elders Coalition. Retrieved from: http://www.diverseelders.org/wp-content/uploads/2012/08/Diverse_Elders_Report_2012_FINAL.pdf.

Lewis, R. (2010–2011). Lesbians under surveillance: Same-sex immigration reform, gay rights, and the problem of queer liberalism. *Social Justice, 37*(1), 90-106.

National Center for Lesbian Rights, California Rural Legal Association & Legal Services for Children. (2013). *Tips for legal advocates working with lesbian, gay, bisexual and transgender clients.* Available at http://www.nclrights.org/wp-content/uploads/2013/07/Proyecto_Poderoso_Flyer_cd.pdf.

National Gay and Lesbian Task Force. (2011). *Challenges facing LGBT elders.* Retrieved from http://www.thetaskforce.org/issues/aging/challenges.

National Immigrant Justice Center. (2010). *The one-year asylum deadline and the BIA.* Human Rights First, and Penn State Law.

Organisation for Economic Co-operation and Development. (2013a). *OECD Factbook 2013: Economic and social statistics.* OECD Publishing. DOI: 10.1787/factbook-2013-en.

Organisation for Economic Co-operation and Development. (2013b). *Migration-stocks of immigrants.* Retrieved from http://www.oecd.org/publications/factbook/38336539.pdf.

Services & Advocacy for Gay, Lesbian, Bisexual & Transgender Elders, National Hispanic Council on Aging, & Diverse Elders Coalition. (2014). *In their own words: A needs assessment of hispanic LGBT older adults.* Retrieved from http://issuu.com/lgbtagingcenter/docs/intheirownwords/1?e=2766558/6779269.

Services & Advocacy for Gay, Lesbian, Bisexual, & Transgender Elders (SAGE) & Movement Advancement Project (MAP). (2010). *Improving the lives of LGBT older adults.* Retrieved from http://www.lgbtmap.org/file/improving-the-lives-of-lgbt-older-adults.pdf.

Stoller, E. P., & Gibson, R. C. (1999a). Part 1: The life course perspective: Aging in individual, sociocultural and historical contexts. *Worlds of difference: Inequality in the aging experience* (pp. 18–28). SAGE: Thousand Oaks, CA.

Stoller, E. P., & Gibson, R. C. (1999b). Introduction: Different worlds in aging: Gender, race and Class.

Worlds of difference: Inequality in the aging experi-ence (pp. 4–7). SAGE: Thousand Oaks, CA.

Tabak, S., & Levitan, R. (2013). LGBT imigrants in immigration detention. *Forced Migration Review, 42,* 48–50.   http://www.fmreview.org/en/sogi/tabak-levitan-detention.pdf.

U.S. Census Bureau. (2012a). State and County Quick-Facts. *Data derived from Population Estimates, American Community Survey, Census of Population and Housing, State and County Housing Unit Esti-mates, County Business Patterns, Nonemployer Sta-tistics, Economic Census, Survey of Business Owners, Building Permits.* Retrieved from http://quickfacts. census.gov/qfd/states/00000.html.

U.S. Census Bureau. (2012b). *The foreign-born popula-tion in the United States: 2010. American Community Survey Reports.* By E. M. Grieco, Y. D. Acosta, G. P. de la Cruz, C. Gambino, T. Gryn, L. J. Larsen, E. N. Trevelyan, and N. P. Walters. Retrieved from http://www.census.gov/prod/2012pubs/acs-19.pdf.

U.S. Citizenship and Immigration Services. (2014a). *Chapter 2: Definition of child for citizenship and naturalization.* Retrieved from http://www.uscis.gov/ policymanual/HTML/PolicyManual-Volume12-PartH-Chapter2.html#S-A.

U.S. Citizenship and Immigration Services (2014b). *Same-sex marriages.* Retrieved from http://www. uscis.gov/family/same-sex-marriages.

Wasem, R. E. (2012). *Noncitizen eligibility for federal public assistance: Policy overview and trends.* Wash-ington Congressional Research Service, 2012. Avail-able at https:www.fas.org/sgp/crs/misc/RL33809.pdf.

Loree Cook-Daniels

Abstract

No stigmatized group in U.S. history has seen as much progress as quickly as transgender people. Current transgender elders represent virtually the full history of the transgender experience; this chapter explores how this history has impacted language, generational rifts within the community, and trans elders' self-image. It discusses what is known about trans-specific health care (hormone use and gender-related surgery), including trans older adults' experiences of health care discrimination. It covers the two primary approaches to trans health care—the Standards of Care and the informed consent models—and why identification documents are so important to trans people. General health, mental health, and violence issues are covered, along with "stages of emergence" of trans identity and social relationship issues. Sexuality and safer sex comes next. It closes with recent policy changes, including developments related to marriage, Social Security, veterans, employment, housing, long-term care facilities, and services for victims of violence.

Keywords

Transgender · LGBT · Aging · Health disparities · Standards of care · Violence

Overview

No stigmatized group in U.S. history has benefited from as many policy and social attitude improvements as quickly as have transgender people. The current generations of transgender people. The current generations of transgender elders represent virtually the full history of the transgender experience, ranging from days when there was no word for their identity to today, when "transgender" has become a word even the U.S. President feels comfortable using on nationwide television (Obama 2015). That unprecedented diversity makes generalizations about this population beyond impossible; the goal of this chapter is therefore to explore just some of the major conundrums, challenges, and joys facing those who serve, research, make

L. Cook-Daniels (✉)
FORGE, Milwaukee, USA
e-mail: LoreeCD@aol.com

© Springer International Publishing Switzerland 2016
D.A. Harley and P.B. Teaster (eds.), *Handbook of LGBT Elders*,
DOI 10.1007/978-3-319-03623-6_14

policy for, make community with, befriend, and love transgender elders.

The chapter starts with terms and definitions by focusing on how much change there has been around transgender issues during the lifetimes of current trans elders. This discussion should explain why a variety of terms will be used throughout this chapter: it is critical that those working with the transgender community not become wedded to any particular term or definition, as they are in constant flux and vary from individual to individual. (We do the same with pronouns, including using "they" as a personal pronoun, for the same reasons: to help the reader get used to recognizing that a variety of pronouns are currently being used within the trans community.) We next move on to explore generational issues affecting the trans community, including those that cause intra-community strife. After reviewing the limitations of existing research on trans elders, the chapter discusses what is known about trans-specific health care (hormone use and gender-related surgery), including trans older adults' experiences of discrimination within the health care system. One of the ways the experience of trans people differs from their LGB peers is their dependence on professionals for health care and identification papers. The chapter covers the two primary approaches to trans health care—the Standards of Care and the informed consent models—and why identification documents are so important to trans people. General health, mental health, and violence issues are tackled together to reflect emerging research on the effects trauma has on physical as well as mental health. The section on therapy includes one expert's "stages of emergence" of trans identity. The chapter then addresses social relationships, covering some of the issues with which SOFFAs (Significant Others, Friends, Family and Allies) may struggle. Sexuality and safe sex comes next, with brief discussions of sexual orientation and libido changes, how trans elders handle dating disclosure, and how religion has affected some trans elders' sexuality. We end with an overview of recent policy changes in the lives of American trans elders, including developments related to marriage, Social Security, veterans, employment, housing, long-term care facilities, and services for victims of domestic violence, sexual assault, dating violence and stalking.

Learning Objectives

By the end of this chapter, the reader should be able to:

1. Discuss some reasons for the existing diversity of terms and beliefs among trans elders.
2. Give possible reasons for the dearth of research on transgender elders.
3. Describe some of the unique ways in which professionals of various sorts influence trans people's identities and lives.
4. Explain how violence and discrimination might affect a trans elder's life circumstances.
5. List some of the concerns SOFFAs—Significant Others, Friends, Family, and Allies—of trans elders might have.
6. Discuss some of the ways in which federal government policies might impact trans elders' lives.

Introduction

Development of Terms, Identities, and Communities

Unlike some other cultures, Western industrialized nations such as the U.S. have had no traditional role for people who do not spend their lives fully identifying with the "boy" or "girl" label they were given at birth (Feinberg 1997). That does not mean the people we now call transgender or trans did not exist; it does mean that they had no common term for themselves and, for the most part, no or few role models.

Some, like jazz musician Billy Tipton (1914–1989), succeeded in living as their preferred gender for years or even decades, often without anyone else knowing their gender history (Middlebrook 1999). Others found more or less comfortable homes in gay male or lesbian communities, which have been more tolerant of cross-dressing, masculine women, and feminine men. People who were assigned male at birth and who were attracted to women often married women and dressed in women's clothing in secret or with their wives' consent. The stories of how people who were assigned female at birth, had a masculine identity, and were attracted to men before the modern transgender concept emerged have, for the most part, not been told.

The lack of both role models and language began to change when Christine Jorgensen's "sex change" was widely publicized in 1952. This "ancient history" is, in fact, within the lifespan of current trans elders: if Jorgensen had not died of cancer in 1989, she would now be entering her 90s. Indeed, many current trans elders start their "coming out" stories by recounting how they first ran into an article about her (Brevard 2001; Feinberg 1997; Sanchez 2015).

The publicity about Jorgensen did not mean that everyone who had a gender identity different from the sex they were assigned at birth ran out and had a sex change (which was still very hard to procure). Even if they do not talk about their gender identity or show "cross-gender" behaviors, trans people pick up society's message: if you were "born a boy," you will always be male and vice versa: anyone who believes differently is not just mistaken, but possibly sinful, dangerous, perverted, and/or mentally ill. It could also be illegal. Beginning in the mid-1800s, many jurisdictions passed laws forbidding cross-dressing. Some laws specified how many pieces of clothing must belong to the person's assigned sex in order to be legal (Brevard 2001; Meyerowitz 2002). Consequently, most current trans elders spent decades trying to fit into their assigned roles (sometimes by entering "hyper-masculine" careers such as the military or construction or striving to be the most "feminine" person on the block) and/or denying or suppressing their feelings. The timing of when any given person realizes that these attempts to fit in are failing differs for each individual. Therefore, current trans elders could have

"transitioned" (begun living publicly as a gender different from the sex they were assigned at birth) anytime from their 20s through their 70s.

The point at which this transition occurs is critical. As we just discussed, families and society do their best to teach trans people how *not* to be trans. (Contrast this with an African-American or Catholic person who is taught by their parents and others how people of their race or religion are expected to act, believe, and survive.) Instead, trans people learn "how to be trans" from other trans people once they make contact with them.

"How to be trans" has been under constant and rapid change since Christine Jorgensen came to public awareness. The time period in which a trans elder first made contact with the trans community therefore will significantly influence both how he or she thinks of himself or herself and gender identity, and the terms they use.

In the 1950s and 60s, Virginia Prince worked to create an identity that was neither homosexual nor "transsexual" (a term that had been coined in 1949). She called heterosexual men who wore women's clothing (part-time or full-time) "transvestites" or "transgenderists" and sought to delineate the differences between the various categories so that the male cross-dressers were not "made to bear stigma they do not deserve." (Meyerowitz 2002, p. 181). Prince's careful parsing of "types," accompanied by disdain for those in other categories, remains sadly common. The trans community to this day still has often-vicious arguments over who belongs and which groups are more "real" or "deserving" than others. We will return to the implications of these divisions later.

Some did find their way to helping professionals, although this was not always a pleasant experience. In 1962 professional entertainer Aleshia Brevard felt the surgeon she found was "twisted and disgusting," but he was willing to perform surgery when no one else would (Brevard 2001, p. 10). Unfortunately, she had to castrate herself first because U.S. law otherwise required her surgeon to place her testicles— which would have continued to produce testosterone—inside her body.

Case Study 1: Aleshia Brevard

Ten years after Christine Jorgensen introduced herself to America, Aleshia Brevard transitioned at age 23.

Although even then male-to-female (MTF) transsexuals were expected to live publicly as women for "several years" before they had gender reassignment surgery, Brevard's surgeon waived that requirement because she had been performing professionally as a drag queen. But in San Francisco in the 60s, drag queens were forbidden by law from appearing on the streets in female clothing. "Ultimately," Brevard said, "his decision to waive my daily, comprehensive experience as a woman made my transition much more difficult." Brevard had grown up totally entranced by glamorous Hollywood movies, and it was Hollywood's vision of femininity that formed her view of womanhood. She said, "'Passing' for female was not my dilemma. Ensuring a comfortable passage into the real world of women could only come with exposure to their daily experiences." The world of most genetic women is made up of the little things, not the glamour. While my daytime 'real girl' sisters toiled for unequal pay, rocked society's cradle, and struggled for complete emancipation, I waited impatiently for twilight hours when I could pose and preen."

As with many other women of her time, Brevard's primary goal was to snag a man to put a ring on her finger. She dated many men and won the brass (or gold) ring 3 times. At least two of those times, she never told her husband of her transsexual history.

Keeping stealth didn't protect her from violence; many husbands and boyfriends as well as strangers were abusive. After one attempted rape she wrote, "I did not file charges. I had not been sexually assaulted, and should I accuse my attacker,

a strong possibility existed that the police would discover my transsexual identity. Even genetically-born female victims of physical rape are required to defend themselves in court. I feared the police more than I hated my assailant. They might consider my attacker's actions reasonable. With my history, I didn't dare take the risk." In the last chapter of her book she summarizes, "My need for love and acceptance, when coupled with an overwhelming lack of self-esteem, made me a willing victim."

Twice she had to prove her "womanly worth" by submitting to a genital examination: once by police when a person who had tried to rape her reported her to police, and once when an employer was tipped off that she was "really a man."

In her autobiography, *The Woman I Was Not Born to Be: A Transsexual Journey,* she said: "At the time of my surgery, the prevailing professional and personal advice for a transsexual was for her to totally turn her back on the past. As in a witness-protection program, to create a new life, everything and everyone you'd known must cease to exist." She writes, "'Do you have children, Aleshia?' was an invariable first-date question. I didn't always meet it head on. The minute my boyfriend asked about children, I pulled out a tear-stained portrait of my mythical late son, Jason. I carried a picture of a beautiful four-year-old boy in my wallet. 'Jason' was my protection. I shared the lie of his drowning so often that I started to wonder if it wasn't true."

One of the first U.S. professionals openly linked with trans people was endocrinologist Harry Benjamin, who had begun treating what we would now call transgender patients in the 1920s and 1930s (Meyerowitz 2002). He consulted with Dr. Alfred Kinsey on several patients and met and befriended Christine Jorgensen at a dinner party in 1953. Although Benjamin had published papers and spoken to professional audiences for years, the publishing of his 1966 book, *The Transsexual Phenomenon,* is viewed as seminal. The year 1966 also saw the establishment of John Hopkins Hospital's sex-reassignment surgery program. Other, usually university-based, sex reassignment clinics soon followed. These clinics often had onerous requirements for their applicants. For one thing, all those seeking to move from MTF were required to be attracted to men and FTM had to profess attraction to women, as the surgery was in part viewed as a cure to homosexuality. Applicants were also expected to have similar life histories, which led to trans people counseling each other on "what to say." Interestingly, the professionals drew a different conclusion about what was happening: one wrote, "These patients are simply awful liars. They lie when there is no need for it whatsoever." (Meyerowitz 2002, p. 164). Even with coaching from other trans people, most applicants "failed": of the more than 2000 people who applied to John Hopkins' clinic in its first two and a half years, only 24 got the surgery they sought. (Meyerowitz 2002).

Another major milestone occurred in 1979 when the first professional organization devoted to the subject emerged: the Harry Benjamin International Gender Dysphoria Association (Meyerowitz 2002). One of its first acts was issuance of "Standards of Care" (SOC), which it recommended that all professionals follow. (In 2007, the organization changed its name to the World Professional Association for Transgender Health, or WPATH.) The SOC included such protocols as requiring trans people to have had extensive psychological counseling and a "real life test" of living for a prescribed period of time in their target gender before accessing hormones and/or surgery (WPATH 2015). Although many of the requirements followed what the university clinics had previously mandated, the SOC did permit and encourage independent therapists and health care providers to provide care to trans people, making it easier for trans people to access care.

Not every development could be considered progress. In 1980, the American Psychiatric Association (APA) took its first official notice of trans people with the new mental health diagnosis of Gender Identity Disorder (GID) (APA 1980). Despite the removal of homosexuality from the Diagnostic and Statistical Manual (DSM) in 1973, being transgender remains a mental illness, although the name of the diagnosis was softened in 2013 to Gender Dysphoria (APA, 2013). Trans social and advocacy groups began organizing in the late 1960s and early 1970s, but the '70s was also when many feminist groups split over whether transwomen should be treated like other women (Meyerowitz 2002; Stryker 2008).

Case Study 2: Lou Sullivan

In the 1980s, Louis Sullivan illustrated the possible interrelationships among figuring out one's own identity, matching that with and against the surrounding institutions, and leading social change. Lou originally thought he was a "female transvestite." Later he heard about a female-to-male (FTM) transsexual, and began to believe he, too, could be a man. The sex change clinic at Stanford University disagreed; Lou was attracted to men and, while lesbian transwomen had by then been reported on, the professionals were not yet ready to "create" a gay transman. Lou increased his efforts to find and help other FTMs, in the process publishing "Information for the FTM Crossdresser and Transsexual," the first FTM-specific resource document, in 1980–1981, and in 1986 founding what became FTM International. He also embarked on what was ultimately a successful educational and advocacy campaign to convince the powers-that-be that gender identity and sexual orientation are separate aspects of a person's identity and should not be the basis of discrimination by health care professionals.

Lou ultimately did secure the surgeries he wanted. He also contracted AIDS. Before his death in 1991, Lou said of himself: "I have never regretted changing my sex, even for a second, despite my AIDS diagnosis, and in some twisted way feel that my condition is proof that I really attained my goal of being a gay man—even to the finish, I am with my gay brothers."

The emergence of the Internet in the late 1980s and 1990s impacted the trans community in ways that cannot be overemphasized. For the first time, people could privately search for and find information on other people who did not feel like the sex everyone told them they were. Being able to find similar others and, more importantly, learn from them that there were social and medical steps they could take to ease their pain, transformed countless lives. The number of open and visible trans people exploded, allowing for the creation of many more conferences and organizations. One of those was the Transgender Aging Network (TAN), which was founded in 1998. Originally designed to network professionals interested in trans aging issues, the listserv was soon swamped by older trans people seeking personal advice. TAN quickly spun off the listserv ElderTG, which has provided peer support and advice to trans people age 50+ (and their close Significant Others, Friends, Family, and Allies [SOFFAs]) ever since.

Both terms referring to the trans community and its size have continued to change rapidly. In the 2000s, more and more people began identifying as neither female nor male, but something else. Until very recently, such individuals were often described as "genderqueer" or "gender non-conforming" and typically used uncommon non-gendered pronouns. In the last few years the term "gender non-binary" has emerged and use of "they" as a personal pronoun has exploded. Although "MTF" and "FTM" used to be extremely common terms used to describe trans people, many now object to them as making the sex-assigned-at-birth seem at least as (if not more) important than the person's true gender identity. Some people abhor the term "transgendered" for grammatical or other reasons, while others defend its continued use. As the number and conceptual sophistication of the community increase even more, more terminology change is inevitable. So is how the community is organized. With growing numbers have come further divisions of the trans community based on other demographics: the first FTM-specific national conference was in 1995, and the Trans People of Color Coalition formed in 2010, for example.

As this chapter goes to press, the new Amazon-sponsored television show *Transparent* is winning awards for its groundbreaking portrayal of a parent and her three adult children as they navigate her gender transition at age 70 (Amazon 2015). Like the Internet, the new availability of public, detailed depictions of trans people's lives may well change the future of the trans community. No longer will trans people of any age be as dependent on finding the trans community to learn "how to be trans": the lessons will be accessible to everyone, right on their television screen or computer monitor.

Diversity Implications for Services, Groups, and Communities

What all these variations—in terms, concepts, timing, demographic-based organizing, etc.—mean for trans elders is that saying anything about them as a group is nearly impossible. Even defining terms is problematic, because what "transsexual" means to one person may well be different from what it means to another person who also uses the label. That is why FORGE Transgender Aging Network teaches that what is most important to know about labels for trans people is the Terms Paradox. The Terms Paradox explains that it is critical for people to learn what term trans persons use for themselves and then reflect that term back to them in conversation. Using the same term affirms respect for trans persons' right to their own identity. The paradox is that the term by itself is not meaningful without further discussion: two individuals who refer to themselves with the same label may have very different experiences and expectations. The only way to know what those experiences or expectations are is to ask that particular individual (FORGE 2012).

This lack of an agreed-upon history and culture can be problematic. One trans elder may harbor negative prejudices about another "type" of trans elder, and changes made to please some may upset others. At the 2014 Transgender Spectrum conference held in St. Louis, Missouri, the organizers proudly announced that all bathrooms had been made gender neutral. One trans elder, who had transitioned in mid-life, complained to organizers: "I wanted all my life to get out of men's bathrooms, and now you're saying it's progress to have me go to a bathroom with a urinal in it?" (Anonymous, personal communication, November 21, 2014). Another trans elder wrote about an effort in her town, "There is an effort here to make bathrooms gender-neutral. To me that is the epitome of stupidness. I do not want to be in the same bathroom as a male or 'gender-neutral' person!" (Anonymous, personal communication, August 25, 2014).

The tension between trans elders and younger peers may also increase as completely different paths open to the younger population. In 2012, Riki Wilchins, a trans activist and author now in her 60s, published a very controversial essay called "Transgender Dinosaurs and the Rise of the Genderqueers." In it, Wilchins wrote, "My political identity for 30 years has been built on the foundation of my being visibly transgender.... [W]hat if all that were wiped away? Who would I be? What would I have become? With [out] all the activism and writing that identity forced on me during the birth of transgender liberation, would I even be writing this today?"

Discussion Box 1
Elders who need assistance are usually cared for by younger people. Young people are coming out as trans earlier than past generations and are increasingly being supported by parents, school-based groups like Gay/Straight Alliances, and health care providers, who may even supply them with

hormone blockers that enable them to skip developing unwanted "other gender" physical features like breasts or a deep voice. Trans elders, on the other hand, often have long, hard histories of being discriminated against and having to fight for respect.

- What kind of conflicts might occur within aging services or in other service settings between younger and older trans people?
- What commonalities exist between the two populations and their disparate histories?
- In what ways can compassion and understanding between the generations be fostered?

Her point is that trans life has changed drastically. Rather than spending decades trying to fight who they are, an increasing number of children are not only publicly declaring their transgender identity, but also finding acceptance and support. Wilchins notes,

With adolescents increasingly taking androgen blockers [which will save many young transwomen from growing up with larger frames, deeper voices, and Adam's apples and young transmen from growing breasts and menstruating] with the support of a generation of more protective, nurturing parents, public transsexuality is fading out. And I don't mean only that in a generation or two we may become invisible in the public space. I mean rather that in 10 years, the entire experience we understand today as constituting transgender – along with the political advocacy, support groups, literature, theory and books that have come to define it since transgender burst from the closet in the early 1990s to become part of the LGB-and-now-T movement – all that may be vanishing right in front of us. In 50 years it might be as if we never existed. Our memories, our accomplishments, our political movement, will all seem to only be historic. Feeling transgender will not so much become more acceptable, as gayness is now doing, but logically impossible.

Although this view of the "generational" cracks in the trans community is extreme, it does point to a key truth: being a trans elder now is different than it ever was before, or ever will be again.

A Dearth of Research

Research on trans elders is sparse. The first problem is defining who is under the "trans umbrella." Does one include people who identify as the sex they were assigned at birth, but who dress in the "other" gender's clothing? Are "genderqueers" who may present to the world as "typical" men or women but who have a different internal identity included? Or are we just talking about people who are living full-time in a gender not congruent with the sex they were assigned at birth?

Until very recently, there have been no nationally representative studies that have included questions around gender identity, and so no way to draw any conclusions about trans people as a whole. Instead, what research exists has been based on "snowball" or convenience sampling, in which trans elders are identified through organized trans or LGBT groups and/or by one trans elder connecting researchers to another. These research methods have many drawbacks in general, but the problems are intensified because of the unique way trans elders connect (or not!) with other trans people.

Policy Box 1

Trans people are invisible in most research simply because researchers have not asked about gender identity. When advocates began pushing to change this practice, questions arose about what, exactly, to ask. One study of university students found that twice as many trans people were identified when a two-step question was asked compared to one question that gave four response options: female, male, transgender, other (Tate 2012). This occurs in part because many trans people identify themselves simply as female or male and not as transgender.

The Williams Institute convened a panel of experts who now recommend this two-step question for determining whether respondents are trans (Herman 2014). Note that this recommendation would likely NOT pick up people who cross-dress (whose gender identity may still match the sex they were assigned at birth).

Recommended measures for the "two-step" approach:

Assigned sex at birth

What sex were you assigned at birth, on your original birth certificate?
Male
Female

Current gender identity

How do you describe yourself? (check one)
Male
Female
Transgender
Do not identify as female, male, or transgender

We discussed earlier the generational divide between current trans elders and today's generation of trans youth, many of whom will be able to grow up without visible physical traces suggesting they were born a different sex. Another type of "generational" divide is less tied to age than to when a given trans elder "came out" as trans. Some who are now in their 70s and 80s transitioned in their 20s and 30s and have lived most of their lives simply viewing themselves (and being viewed by others) as "male" or "female." Many others struggled to fit into their assigned roles for decades and "came out" only when they learned about trans people from the Internet (or, now, from shows like *Transparent*). Still others "come out" when a major life event occurs. Mid- or late-life transitions can occur when certain people are no longer in the picture due to death, retirement, or an empty nest. They can also occur when an individual has a heart attack or cancer diagnosis and realizes that time for living authentically may be running out. Some reach a point of sacrifice fatigue and decide that they have devoted enough of their life to being what other people want them to be. Still others remain comfortable with early compromises, such as making a living as a man but socializing as a woman.

How involved any given trans elder is with the larger trans community obviously varies from person to person. In general, however, many try to connect with other trans people in local support groups and/or online in order to "learn the ropes" and find referrals to trans-friendly professionals such as therapists and doctors. Once they have successfully transitioned, however, many prefer to live their lives as any other man or woman would, and so they sever their ties to the trans community. This is one reason why it is so difficult to research trans elders: many are not connected to any trans group or even to other trans individuals.

A vivid example of the results of this "woodworking" or "going stealth" phenomenon comes from the groundbreaking 2011 survey of more than 6400 trans people, *Injustice at Every Turn* (Grant et al. 2011a). Although its authors—the National Center for Transgender Equality and what was then the National Gay and Lesbian Task Force—issued additional analyses of multiple sub-populations, they were reluctant to publish separate findings on trans elders because that data seemed so "off." It took careful cross-walking of the data to understand what had happened: barely 2 % of the *Injustice at Every Turn* respondents age 55+ had been living in their current gender for more than 10 years. In other words, virtually all of them were mid- or late-life transitioners (Grant et al. 2011b). Because nearly 80 % of them were also MTFs, that means that most had likely had successful careers as men and faced anti-trans discrimination only late in life. They therefore had higher incomes, higher educational levels, higher home ownership rates, better health, and fewer discrimination experiences than their younger trans peers.

In contrast, the *Aging and Health Report*, which also published its first wave of data in 2011, recruited trans elders primarily through local LGBT aging groups (Fredriksen-Goldsen et al.). We can imagine that trans elders who connect with such groups do so because they are more isolated and/or have higher social and practical needs that they are trying to fill. The *Aging and Health Report* trans respondents produced data more in line with having experienced decades of discrimination, violence, and stigma.

The third primary source of data on trans elders comes from various FORGE studies, in particular ones focused on sexuality, sexual violence, and elder abuse (Cook-Daniels and Munson 2010). Although these were national, online studies aimed at all ages of trans people, our Transgender Aging Network and ElderTG programs led to much higher than usual elder participation. These three sources provide most of what we now know about current generations of trans elders, which we will review next.

Each of these studies recruited anyone who defined themselves as "transgender", and so may include a wide variety of identities, physical presentations, and histories. FORGE surveys may also include SOFFAs speaking about their trans loved one's experience.

Trans-specific Health Issues

The first health concern many people think of when they think of trans people is, "what are the health effects of long-term hormone use?" Most of the long-term prescription medications that Americans take—including anti-depressants, statins, beta-blockers, and pain-killers as well as hormones—have not been around long enough to show what happens when taking them for 30 years. However, a 2014 Medscape article, "Largest Study to Date: Transgender Hormone Treatment Safe," reported that very few side effects were found among 2000 trans people who had taken hormones for an average of 5.6 years for the MTFs and 4.5 years for the FTMs (Louden 2014). The most common serious side effect was venous thromboembolism, which affected approximately 1 % of those taking estrogen, causing blood clots that can be serious or even fatal. Not all trans people take hormones, and dosages vary based on the prescribing physician, whether the person's body is still producing its own hormones (which may need to be countered), and, in some cases, how old the person is or what other medical problems they have. Among the *Injustice at Every Turn* respondents, 76 % of the 55–64 year olds and 82 % of the 65+ respondents had had hormone therapy (Grant et al. 2011b).

What is actually a bigger issue for the health of trans elders is their surgical status. Until very recently, virtually no private health insurance company or public health care program would cover gender affirmation surgeries. Consequently, few elders have been able to afford to have genital surgery. *Injustice at Every Turn* found that only 21–23 % of MTFs and *none* of the FTMs age 55+ reported having had genital surgery (Grant et al. 2011b). The reason that this is a health issue is that without genital surgery, FTM and MTF elders cannot hope to "pass" when they are naked on the examination table: their transgender history is literally visible. This may well contribute to the reluctance of many trans elders to access health care. It may also cause trans elders to refuse recommended services such as home health care and nursing home placement.

Field-Based Experiential Assignment Box 1

One of the areas of trans policy that is changing the fastest is health care coverage of trans-related health care. For many years, nearly every health insurance policy contained a "transgender exclusion" that said the company would not cover any costs related to a sex change. Although these provisions were generally intended to exclude coverage of hormones and surgery, in practice they were sometimes used to deny trans people care for injuries and illnesses that were totally unrelated, such as a broken arm. These policies are falling like dominoes. The Affordable Care Act has been interpreted to make such trans exclusions illegal, and at press time, 9 states and the District of Columbia have

agreed and required insurers in their states to eliminate all such exclusions. In 2014, one third of Fortune 500 companies offered coverage of trans-related health care (including surgeries).[1] 2014 was also the year in which Medicare reversed its long-standing trans exclusion, permitting enrollees to petition for coverage of their sex-related surgeries.

- Research the current state of health insurance and public programs' trans health exclusions. How much change has there been since this book was written?
- Where did you find updated information? From trans advocacy organizations, the government, or others?
- If you have access to one or more trans elders, ask them about their experiences with trans health care exclusions.

Also contributing to underutilization of health care are discrimination and fear. Although most elders are eligible for Medicare or Medicaid, previous employment discrimination may well leave retirees with insufficient funds for co-pays and the like: 21 % of those 65+ and 35 % of those 55–64 told the *Injustice at Every Turn* researchers they had postponed medical care when they were sick or injured because they could not afford it (Grant et al. 2011b); 22 % of the trans elders in the *Aging and Health Report* said the same (Fredriksen-Goldsen et al. 2011). More importantly, trans people often experience discrimination by health care professionals: 40 % of the trans elders in the *Health and Aging Report* study said they had been denied or provided inferior health care because they were trans (Fredriksen-Goldsen et al. 2011). One trans elder

---

[1] http://hrc-assets.s3-website-us-east-1.amazonaws.com//files/documents/CEI-2015-rev.pdf#__utma=149406063.688421561.1384098938.1416873933.1422635387.23&__utmb=149406063.2.10.1422635387&__utmc=149406063&__utmx=-&__utmz=149406063.1422635387.23.22.utmcsr=google|utmccn=(organic)|utmcmd=organic|utmctr=(not%20provided)&__utmv=-&__utmk=260347149, p. 6.

told FORGE Transgender Aging Network: "One Navy doctor refused me care when a suture site related to my sex reassignment surgery became infected" (Cook-Daniels and Munson 2010, p. 156). Another said, "I have decided not to have any life-extending surgery because of past mistreatment by nurses at [the Veterans Administration hospital]" (Cook-Daniels and Munson 2010, p. 153).

One of the most important differences between being lesbian, gay, or bisexual and being transgender is that transgender is a status that often can be obtained only through interaction with and even cooperation from professionals. Medical professionals are required to prescribe medications or conduct surgery (unless a person accesses "black market" drugs or silicone injections, for example, with their attendant health and legal risks). However, many medical professionals will not provide gender-related services to transgender individuals unless those individuals have met what is now called the World Professional Association for Transgender Health (WPATH)'s Standards of Care requirements, which many trans people view as "hoop jumping" (Susan's Place 2011). Although more recently many professionals have moved to an "informed consent" model that eliminates many of the previous "gatekeepers," some trans elders remain wary of physical and mental health care providers in general (FORGE 2011).

Identification Documents

Another way trans people differ from their non-trans LGB peers is in their reliance on other types of professionals and bureaucrats to help them change identification documents. These changes may require going to court, producing letters from health care and/or mental health care professionals, paying fees, and tracking down historical documents. In a (thankfully lessening) number of cases, trans people must prove they have had surgery on their genitals before their documents can be reissued. Most people have multiple documents that identify who they are,

and so this process can be costly in both time and money. When trans people do not change all of those documents, they run the risk of everything from intrusive questions to outright violence when their normal course of business requires them to produce a document such as a driver's license or health insurance card.

How big of a problem is this? The *Injustice at Every Turn* study found that more than 50 % of their older respondents had either not tried to update the name and/or gender marker on their driver's license or state identification card or had been denied the requested changes (Grant et al. 2011b). More than 60 % had not updated (or were denied the right to update) their Social Security records. Indeed, only 21 % of those aged 55–64 and 28 % of those aged 65+ said that "all" of their identification had been changed. That means nearly 80 % of transgender elders are at risk of being involuntarily outed, depending on which forms of identification are demanded by a service provider, police officer, or even a retail clerk (Grant et al. 2011b).

Field-Based Experiential Assignment Box 2

The next time you have to fill out a personal information form for a health care professional or agency, examine it carefully. Where would a trans person share the information they are trans? Is there a checkbox or question that the trans person can just check or answer? Or would a trans person have to "bring the topic up" by making a note somewhere? If they do need to write a note, under what section could it go? Does the name of that section suggest stigma? Now look around the room and/or examine the way the professional or agency describes themselves in brochures or websites: do they give any indication they know trans people exist? What evidence might a trans client see that would suggest whether or not this professional or agency is likely to be trans-friendly? If you were trans, would you declare your identity or history on this form? If not, why not?

> Would you wait until you could talk to someone personally? If so, how would you bring the topic up?

General Physical and Mental Health Issues

The Adverse Childhood Experiences (ACE) study (Centers for Disease Control 2006) has established that early experiences of trauma and discrimination can have life-long negative health effects not just for mental and emotional well-being, but also when it comes to physical illness (U.S. Centers for Disease Control and Prevention 2014). One pathway to these health problems likely develops when trauma survivors engage in risky behaviors to manage post-trauma symptoms such as depression and anxiety. Trans older adults in the *Aging and Health Report* study were more likely than their LGB age peers to smoke (15 % vs. 9 %), drink to excess (12 % vs. 8 %), use drugs ("other than those required for medical reasons") (14 % vs. 11.5 %), and engage in HIV risk behavior (20 % vs. 18 %) (Fredriksen-Goldsen et al. 2011). They were also less likely to regularly engage in moderate physical exercise (74 % vs. 82 %). Consistent with the ACE causation theory, the *Aging and Health Report* also found that transgender older adults were roughly twice as likely to experience suicidal ideation as the non-transgender LGB respondents (71 % vs. 36 %), and were more than twice as likely to experience depression (48 % vs. 29 %) (Fredriksen-Goldsen et al. 2011). Even further down the trauma/health pathway were the *Aging and Health Report* physical health findings: the trans elders had higher rates of congestive heart disease (20 % vs. 12 %), diabetes (33 % vs. 14 %), obesity (40 % vs. 25 %), and asthma (33 % vs. 15 %), despite the fact that the transgender cohort in this study was on average younger than the non-trans sample [The cohorts had roughly the same rates of high blood pressure and arthritis, while the transgender cohort had lower rates of HIV/AIDS (4 % vs. 9 %) and cancer (16 % vs. 19 %).]. Overall, 33 % of the trans elders in this study reported their health as "poor", compared to 22 % of their LGB peers (Fredriksen-Goldsen et al. 2011). Disability rates were also higher: 62 % of the trans respondents said they had a disability, compared to 46 % of the non-transgender LGB sample (Fredriksen-Goldsen et al. 2011).

Also consistent with this trauma-to-health-problem theory is how much violence, discrimination, and trauma that trans elders have experienced. The trans respondents in the *Aging and Health Report* had nearly twice as many lifetime "negative events" (e.g., job loss, housing or health care discrimination, police misconduct, verbal or physical violence, etc.) as did their LGB peers: 11–6. They were more than twice as likely to have experienced domestic violence in the past year (16 % compared to 7 %) (Fredriksen-Goldsen et al. 2011).

Of particular concern is sexual violence, which multiple studies have found is inflicted on roughly half of all trans people (Cook-Daniels and Munson 2010; Kenagy 2005; Kenagy and Bostwick 2005). Fifty-three of the more than 300 respondents to FORGE's 2004 survey of transgender sexual violence survivors were age 50–64. Most of these trans older adults had been assaulted for the first time before they were 19. Twenty-three percent (23 %) were first assaulted between 19 and 40, and 18 % were first assaulted between the ages 41 and 60 (Cook-Daniels and Munson 2010). We emphasize "first" assaulted because only about a third (37 %) experienced only one sexual assault; the rest were victimized multiple times, sometimes by multiple perpetrators on multiple occasions. Sixteen percent (16 %) of the perpetrators were female, and 2 % were themselves trans. About a third of the victims said that at the time of the assault their perpetrator perceived them to be male, a third said they were perceived to be female, and 14 % said they were "visibly transgender" or (7 %) androgynous. Thirteen percent (13 %) did not know how their perpetrator perceived their gender. About half (55 %), however, thought their gender was a contributing factor to why their perpetrator chose to sexually assault them. Nineteen percent (19 %) said their gender was not a factor in the assault (one said, "*My uncle wasn't picky*"), with the rest saying they did not remember, were unsure, or gave another answer (Cook-Daniels and Munson 2010). Many of these statistics, it should be noted, counter common myths about who is victimized by sexual assault and who does the victimizing.

Few of the victims reported their assaults to anyone. While some of the victims may have been too young at the time to fully understand what had happened or been reluctant to talk to adults, some didn't report for other reasons. One trans older adult said,

> My ex[-wife] had me convinced she could turn everyone against me and take my kids and eventually my grandkids away from me and that no one would want to deal with a queer (of whatever stripe I was) like me (Cook-Daniels and Munson 2010, p. 149).

Another said, "*I was considered a male at the time; no one would have believed I was raped by a female*" (Cook-Daniels and Munson 2010, p. 149).

Transgender sexual assault survivors often bear lifelong scars. One trans older adult survivor noted,

> [I could use] social support, and therapy to help me develop the missing social skills that are a consequence of my childhood abuse, and my years and years of cognitive dissociation…. (Cook-Daniels and Munson 2010, p. 150).

Although many trans survivors worry that therapists and others will (erroneously) think they are trans because they were sexually assaulted, there are survivors who feel the two are connected:

> I understand that my gender dysphoria arises from the childhood abuse. I had researched this area fairly carefully, and if useful, I have literature suggesting abuse as a possible cause of gender dysphoria (Cook-Daniels and Munson 2010, p. 151).

Mental Health Counseling and Therapy

Trans people tend to have extremely high rates of contact with mental health professionals. Eighty-five percent (85 %) of the older respondents in *Injustice at Every Turn* had had counseling, as had 77 % of the respondents to FORGE's 2004 sexual violence survey (Grant et al. 2011b; FORGE 2004). Undoubtedly, some of what drives trans people to counseling is "simply" needing to figure out what to do when what they feel about themselves is different from what everyone else tells them that they should feel. Another large percentage go to therapy only because that's what the Standards of Care have required: in order to access hormones and/or surgery, physicians have often required trans patients to first produce letters from one or even two mental health professionals. Other trans people use counselors to help them cope with "minority stress" (the microaggressions and other daily hassles that come from being part of a stigmatized minority) or the long-term effects of trauma.

For those counseling a transgender person through a gender transition, the most-recommended guide is Arlene Istar Lev's 2004 *Transgender Emergence: Therapeutic Guidelines for Working with Gender-Variant People and Their Families*. In it, she sets out a 6-stage "States of Emergence" that trans people go through:

1. *Awareness*—In the first stage, gender-variant people are often in great distress. The therapeutic task is the normalization of the experiences involved in emerging transgendered.
2. *Seeking information/reaching out*—In the second stage, gender-variant people seek to gain education and support about transgenderism. The therapeutic task is to facilitate linkages and encourage outreach.
3. *Disclosure to significant others*—The third stage involves the disclosure of

transgenderism to significant others—spouses, partners, family members, and friends. The therapeutic task involves supporting the transgendered person's integration in the family system.

4. *Exploration*: *Identity and self-labeling*—The fourth stage involves the exploration of various (transgender) identities. The therapeutic task is to support the articulation and comfort with one's gendered identity.

5. *Exploration*: *Transition issues/possible body modification*—The fifth stage involves exploring options for transition regarding identity, presentation, and body modification. The therapeutic task is the resolution of the decisions and advocacy toward their manifestation.

6. *Integration*: *Acceptance and post-transition issues*—In the sixth stage the gender-variant person is able to integrate and synthesize (transgender) identity. The therapeutic task is to support adaptation to transition-related issues (Lev 2004, p. 235).

Because of therapists' role as "gatekeepers" to hormones and surgery for those professionals who follow the Standards of Care, many trans people do not reveal other issues such as mental health problems or past trauma to the therapists they are seeing in order to sidestep the possibility the therapist will use this information as a reason not to recommend transition-related health care (FORGE 2004). Not surprisingly, this conundrum leads many in the trans community to have ambivalent feelings about accessing professional counseling.

Identification Documents

In addition to health care professionals, many trans people must rely on other types of professionals and bureaucrats to help them change identification documents. These changes may require going to court, producing letters from health care and/or mental health care professionals, paying fees, and tracking down historical documents. In a (thankfully lessening) number of cases, trans people must prove that they have had surgery on their genitals before their documents can be reissued. Most people have multiple documents that identify who they are, so this process can be costly in both time and money. When trans people do not change all of those documents, they run the risk of everything from intrusive questions to outright violence when their normal course of business requires them to produce a document such as a driver's license or health insurance card.

How big of a problem is this? The *Injustice at Every Turn* study found that more than 50 % of older respondents had either not tried to update the name and/or gender marker on their driver's license or state identification card or had been denied the requested changes. More than 60 % had not updated (or were denied the right to update) their Social Security records. Indeed, only 21 % of those aged 55–64 and 28 % of those aged 65+ said that "all" of their identification had been changed (Grant et al. 2011b). That means nearly 80 % of transgender elders are at risk of being involuntarily outed, depending on which forms of identification are demanded by a service provider, police officer, or even a retail clerk.

Family and Social Relationships

In the western world, family and social relationships are completely bound up with gender. It is even hard to describe your family relationships with words that don't reveal the person's gender (ex: wife, father, sister, uncle, grandmother). When someone transitions from one gender to another, they typically change their name and what pronoun they prefer. Changing long-standing mental habits like a person's name can be surprisingly difficult, a process that is made even more painful if the trans person sees errors as evidence of disrespect or non-acceptance. But it is not just words that must be changed: if your mother becomes your father, do you treat him differently? If grandpa puts on a dress, are you supposed to open the door for him when the two of you are out in public? If a store clerk mistakenly calls your older companion "he" when she's really a "she," does not correcting the clerk mean you are disrespecting your companion, or protecting both of you? How are you supposed to tell your favorite stories if the person you are talking about is no longer the gender they were then?

Field-Based Experiential Assignment Box 3

Tell someone about a recent experience you had with another person, but avoid all mention of your companion's gender. That will likely mean avoiding their name, gendered pronouns, and gender-related relationship words like wife, grandfather, and daughter.

How easy or hard was it to do? If it was relatively easy, what do you think made it easier for you?

Ask someone who is much older than you to do the same exercise. How easy or hard was it for them?

For partners, the challenge is much greater. Everyone assumes everyone else's sexual orientation based on with whom they partner. (This is one of the reasons bisexuals are so "invisible": unless they are known to have both a female partner and a male partner, most observers "forget" they are bisexual and therefore label them according to whether their current partner is same- or "opposite"-sex.) A spouse's or partner's transition from one gender to another may help the world recognize their gender identity, but it will obscure their partner's sexual orientation. Thus, a long-term lesbian may lose her community and be treated as heterosexual when her partner transitions female-to-male, and the wife of a MTF may find herself being treated like a lesbian when she's out with her spouse. Although the ongoing reduction of anti-LGBT discrimination, stigma, and stereotyping will continue to make transition easier for partners,

they will still have to cope with one of the central questions the trans person has likely been grappling with for years or even decades: is it ok for the world to see me differently than I know myself to be?

Discussion Box 2

Although "LGBT" is a common acronym, in practice many people think about this population only in terms of people with same-sex attractions. In addition, many "LGBT" organizations and events are—unconsciously or deliberately—built around an oppositional model: what makes them LGBT is that heterosexuals are not present. Many trans people, however, are partnered with people who appear to be the "opposite" sex, and some partners still identify as heterosexual even if their partner has transitioned and they now appear to be a same-sex couple.

- What are the ways in which individuals or an organization may (perhaps unconsciously) send a message that they do not welcome heterosexuals?
- If a group is used to thinking of heterosexual people as "the others," what might need to happen to make that group safe and welcoming for heterosexual trans elders and their partners?
- What language would you use in publicity materials to ensure heterosexual trans elders and their partners know they are welcome?
- What might need to happen to ensure other LGBT participants do not discriminate against or accidentally offend heterosexual-identified participants?

Depending on their predilections, the significant others, friends, family, and allies (SOFFAs) of a transitioning trans person may also struggle with much deeper questions. If they believed what society has said—that sex and gender are the same thing, binary, and unchangeable—they may wonder if other things they believe are actually false. Facing new evidence that people can change something as seemingly permanent as their sex or gender, they may wonder if what they have personally accepted as permanent is, in fact, changeable. Their minds may play "what if" games with them: Did they do anything that might have caused their loved one to be trans? Could they have changed the outcome? More personally, what would their life be like now if they had not abandoned their dream because of their parents' opposition? (Boenke 2003).

Unfortunately, many trans people and professionals believe that what SOFFAs need to do is "understand what being trans is." All too often people respond to SOFFAs' concerns with explanations and books instead of listening to them and partnering with them as they work through the various issues. Some SOFFAs do not get that far: facing just the first layer of adjustments, they make a cut-and-run decision. This seems particularly likely to happen when there are young grandchildren involved: the adult child may say they do not want the grandchild "exposed" to the trans person, and so cut all family ties. One trans elder told FORGE Transgender Aging Network:

> My son and daughter-in-law will not let me see my grandson. They think I will do something to him. I don't even know him now. It breaks my heart not to see him (Cook-Daniels and Munson 2010, p. 156).

Ironically, young children are likely to be unfazed by a gender change. Although children learn the difference between males and females early on, it is only in later childhood that people learn that people are not supposed to change from one to the other. As long as the grandparent (or other older person) still loves and plays with them, most young children adapt to a gender change quickly and easily (Haines et al. 2014).

Some SOFFAs even fight back against their trans loved one—literally. The wife of one trans elder used to throw the windows open and yell to the neighbors about the "titted freak" she lived with. Another elder reported that her wife had always been abusive:

> My ex would get drunk and demand sex, starting with our 'wedding night.' She required me to do stuff outside, in the pool, on the deck, and sometimes in the kitchen with the children or grandchildren out and about in the next room.... My ex liked to try to rip my penis off or cut it off with her nails, and verbally abused me while we had sex (FORGE 2004).

A service provider reported what happened to one trans elder she was working with: "I am currently working with a trans victim who was assaulted and threatened at the church she has belonged to for more than 35 years. She was told, 'I will beat you like the man you are,' and as the perpetrator was saying this, he was hitting her and telling her to leave the church" (Cook-Daniels and Munson 2010, p. 155).

Whether it is easier or harder for SOFFAs to cope when a trans person transitions at mid-life or later is still to be determined. The *Injustice at Every Turn* study does give us some preliminary data, however. For example, 56–59 % of the older respondents had lost their partnership because of their transgender identity, compared to 45 % of the whole sample. The older group was slightly less likely to agree that their family was as "strong today as before I came out," but slightly more likely to say their family relationships are improving over time. They were also slightly less likely to have their relationship with their children blocked by their ex-partner, although that happened to 22 % of those ages 55–64 and 27 % of those 65+ (compared to 29 % of the full sample). Their children, however, were far more likely to choose not to speak to or spend time with them: 40–41 % of the older cohort said they had experienced this, as compared to 30 % of the whole sample (Grant et al. 2011b).

Older trans people also reported a great deal of friend loss, with 64 % of those age 55–64 and 60 % of those 65+ (compared to 58 % of the overall sample) reporting in the *Injustice at Every Turn* study that they had lost close friends due to their trans status or history (Grant et al. 2011b). One trans elder told FORGE, *"My closest friend of over 30 years finally said, 'I just can't handle this [trans stuff].' No contact in years"* (Cook-Daniels and Munson, p. 156).

In some cases, SOFFAs do not know they have a trans person in their life. This usually happens because a trans person has taken no steps to change their gender presentation and has not told anyone their actual gender identity. In rare cases, post-transition elders have succeeded in keeping their trans history a secret even from children and partners. In one such case, hospital personnel successfully treated a woman for prostate cancer without her husband ever learning the specific type of cancer she had (Hopwood, personal communication 2012).

Sexuality

In 2007–2008, FORGE conducted a national, online survey about sexuality issues of trans people and their partners Nearly 300 of the respondents were age 50 and over; only their answers are reflected here.

Respondents had a wide variety of thoughts about how their transness affected their sexuality. Twenty-two percent (22 %) said their transness "completely" shaped their (or their partner's) sexuality, while 48 % said it "somewhat" shaped it. Only 29 % said their transness had "no affect" on their sexuality (Cook-Daniels and Munson 2010). Here is how some respondents explained the connection:

Before T[estosterone], I couldn't see myself being with a man in the context of being female. Once I began to see myself as physically masculinized, the context changed.

I've had [sexual reassignment surgery] and my sexuality changed from one based on sensuality to an emotions based one.

Before I admitted to myself that I was trans, I was almost convinced I was asexual, because the thought of sex was disgusting, even though I found myself attracted to people.

I am not physically capable of any sexual activity I would really want to do. I am a eunuch. I have no desire to display that particular deformity to another human being. All attempts to work around it have thus far been miserable humiliating failures.

Well, it has meant I'm a lifelong virgin.

Laughing…it doesn't. Trans is an umbrella term that goes, and goes, and goes…on for ever, ever, ever, ever, ever, ever, ever. Who I am is not a

medical condition. Does your root canal affect your sexuality and identity? (Cook-Daniels and Munson 2010, pp. 160–161, 169).

Partners of older trans adults also commented on how their sexuality had changed:

I had no idea how much change there would be for me (non-trans) and how difficult it would be to find what works for us [sexually] over the long term.

I was femme and queer identified before I began to seriously date transmen, but my experience dating FTM(s) has created new particularities of my desire and identification (Cook-Daniels and Munson 2010, p. 161).

Asked if their sexual orientation had changed over time, 54 % said yes (9 % didn't know) (Cook-Daniels and Munson 2010). Their narrative responses indicated that the primary reasons for the change included becoming more comfortable in their body, finally discovering their "true" orientation, hormones changing their feelings, and curiosity about other genders' bodies and sexualities. Eighty percent (80 %) said their libido had been affected by being trans, with 57 % saying it had increased and 22 % saying it had decreased. Testosterone use tended to increase libido, but both MTFs and FTMs reported an increase in libido due to an increased comfort with their body and/or less shame. Estrogen use tended to decrease libido, but respondents of all genders also reported an unwillingness to expose their body to another person and/or disappointment or shame about their body (Cook-Daniels and Munson 2010). One respondent illustrated the complex interplay that can happen within couples that are together before and after transition:

My cisgender [non-transgender] partner's libido has diminished due in part to menopause but prior to that, it was because she had 'shut it down' prior to my getting surgery because I had denied her sex back when I had a lot of shame and lack of comfort in my body. Now that I'm in a very good place about my sexuality and physical state, she is having a hard time thinking of herself as a sexual being again. I feel very badly about this and take much of the responsibility for where we currently find ourselves. (Cook-Daniels and Munson 2010, p. 166).

Only a few respondents had body parts that were sexually "off-limits," but some of those who did have no-touch zones noted they had them for gender related as well as trauma related reasons:

> Vaginal penetration is painful and not something a man wants done to him.
> It is off limits to play with trans-person's boobs because he does not enjoy admitting that he has them (Cook-Daniels and Munson 2010, p. 162).

Many people renamed their "gendered" body parts. Created names included bonus hole, chesticles, and trannycock.

One dilemma trans people face when dating—particularly if they have not had genital reconstruction surgery—is if, when, and how to disclose their trans status. Four percent (4 %) of survey respondents *never* told their sexual partners they were trans. One transmasculine person said, "*I have casual sex with men at an adult bookstore once in a while and don't reveal I'm trans and for the most part hide that I have a female body.*" Another 3 % told only when they were in bed: one person said she told, "*When he asks, 'What's THAT?'*" (Cook-Daniels and Munson 2010, p. 166). Most—41 %—said they discussed it "only at the point when we might become sexually involved." Twenty percent (20 %) told on the first date, and 32 % wouldn't set up a date until they had come out to the person. Disclosure did cause the potential partner to back out a third of the time, but 40 % of the time disclosure did not change the interaction and in 27 % of the cases, it actually increased the person's interest or attraction (Cook-Daniels and Munson 2010, p. 167).

A particular concern for trans older adults is HIV and other sexually transmitted infections. Even now HIV-related safer sex materials have largely been marketed to gay men, leaving many heterosexuals and those in the lesbian community feeling like they do not need to be concerned with safer sex issues. That means that because even coupled mid- or late-life transitioners may want to "try out" their new bodies or appearances with new sexual partners, they may enter the dating pool with little awareness of how to manage risks. Ironically, both surgically constructed vaginas and vaginas exposed to testosterone are thought to be more fragile and susceptible to tears, increasing risk (Kenagy 2002). Of additional concern is the fact that most safer sex materials focus only on condom use, which does not adequately address the body parts, sexuality, or psychology of trans people.

FORGE found that 33 % of the older trans adults it surveyed were practicing safer sex, 25 % were celibate or not in a relationship, and 19 % were "fluid bonded." Another 13 % "sometimes" practiced safer sex, and 10 % "never" did (Cook-Daniels and Munson 2010). Some respondents appeared unclear on what safer sex is: "*I'm sterile and my spouse also is*" (Cook-Daniels and Munson 2010, p. 165). Some noted that their gender role beliefs precluded safer sex: "*Mostly I do what my partner wants (he is the man, I am the woman).*" "*I am a sex slave to my male partners, doing whatever they want to please them*" (Cook-Daniels and Munson 2010, p. 164).

One gave more detail:

> I only negotiate for BDSM play in the beginning to find someone who will allow me to serve and submit myself to them. I negotiate safer sex opposite maybe what I should but actually I want a man to cum in me and not use condoms as I feel a great need and desire for the seed of a man I guess much like a woman desiring to get pregnant. Once I have a partner I do whatever pleases Him (Cook-Daniels and Munson 2010, p. 164).

Some trans older adults' sexuality was affected by their religious beliefs:

> I am a born again Christian. God gives me the power not to do anything that causes me to act as a transgendered person. My faith is on Jesus Christ.
> All sexual activities are off limits. Prior to transitioning I believed I was a heterosexual male. Now I am a lesbian and I am having conflicts with my walk with Christ and homosexuality (Cook-Daniels and Munson 2010, p. 163).

In the Public World

Although public perceptions about trans people are changing rapidly—*Time* magazine put trans actress Laverne Cox on its cover in 2014 with the headline "The Transgender Tipping Point"—most trans people have experienced a lot of stigma and discrimination. The *Injustice at Every Turn* report starts this way:

> Transgender and gender non-conforming people face injustice at every turn: in childhood homes, in school systems that promise to shelter and educate, in harsh and exclusionary workplaces, at the grocery store, the hotel front desk, in doctors' offices and emergency rooms, before judges and at the hands of landlords, police officers, health care workers and other service providers (Grant et al. 2011a, p. 2).

Ninety percent of respondents had experienced harassment, mistreatment, or discrimination on the job, with 26 % losing a job because they were trans. Fifty-three percent (53 %) reported being verbally harassed or disrespected in a place of public accommodation, and (19 %) had experienced homelessness at some point due to being trans. Those who had interacted with police said that 22 % of the time, they were harassed rather than helped. On nearly all questions, trans people of color reported experiencing more discrimination, disrespect, and violence than did trans people who were perceived to be white (Grant et al. 2011a).

Policy Advances

Many recent public policy advances are trying to address these issues. The spread of legal same-sex marriage has eliminated some of the problems trans couples have faced when courts were asked to determine the trans person's sex in order to rule on whether their marriage was valid (opposite-sex) or not (same-sex). Even so, this battle is still being fought. In 2014, 92-year-old World War II veteran Robina Asti had to get legal help to force Social Security to give her the survivors' benefits her husband had earned. Social Security has since issued a memo clarifying how it makes decisions involving such marriages (see policy resources box).

Discussion Box 3

Advocacy for trans elders can require a delicate balancing act. Many times advocates seek to literally put a face on the issue by presenting how it affects one individual. This approach requires sensitivity. How do you present what needs to be changed without making the person look like a victim? How do you explain what makes the trans person different while still promoting within the audience a sense of identification and shared humanity?

A well-done example of such an advocacy piece around trans aging issues is the 7:40-min video Lambda Legal did for their 92-year-old client Robina Asti. Watch the video at http://www.lambdalegal.org/blog/20140129_robina-asti-92-year-old-transgender-widow and consider the following questions.

1. What was the primary image and fact about Asti that the video was built around?
2. What techniques were used to "humanize" Asti's story?
3. How did Asti tie what she had learned from her profession into her decision to transition?
4. Which typical questions about trans people did Asti's video address?

Studies have consistently found that trans people are more likely to be military veterans than are their lesbian, gay, and bisexual peers or even non-trans heterosexuals, even though open transgender people are still not allowed to be active military. Thirteen percent of Americans of all ages are military veterans (Newport 2012). *Injustice at Every Turn* found that 20 % of all trans people are veterans, but that rate rises to 40 % of 55–64 year olds and 54 % of those 65+ (Grant et al. 2011b). The *Aging and Health Report* found that while 26 % of their LGB older adults were veterans, 41 % of the trans elders were (Fredriksen-Goldsen et al. 2011). The Veterans Administration has responded to the large number of trans vets by issuing two national directives on how they should be cared for (see policy resources box).

Employment discrimination against transgender people has been widespread, leading to overall low incomes. *Injustice at Every Turn* found that 27 % of trans respondents had annual incomes below $20,000 (Grant et al. 2011a). Because of discrimination, many trans people are forced into sex work or other forms of the underground economy. This issue affects older trans people as well as younger ones. One older adult told FORGE:

> I prostitute myself at age 55 because even though I'm a [post-operative transsexual] and passable [as a woman], no one passes 100 % of the time. NO ONE. Job discrimination is bad because you're stuck with fellow employees 8 hours a day, 40 hours a week. That much harassment is bad for one's mental health (Cook-Daniels and Munson 2010, p. 159).

Low-income workers (especially if they have been working outside the Social Security system) obviously have lower retirement incomes, as well, which suggests financial precariousness for many trans elders. However, the *Injustice at Every Turn* study also demonstrated that when in life a person transitions has a lot to do with income. Only 2 % of people age 55 + in that study had transitioned more than 10 years earlier, so overall incomes were relatively high: half made $50,000 a year or above (Grant et al. 2011b).

Employment discrimination against trans people is being actively addressed at the federal and many state levels. In 2012 the Department of Justice issued a memo officially declaring that employment discrimination against trans workers is illegal under Title VII's ban on sex discrimination (see policy resources box). The Obama Administration has issued multiple Executive Orders and other guidance protecting trans people who are federal workers or who work for federal contractors (see policy resources box).

Housing discrimination is also a problem. Even the mid- to late-transitioners in the *Injustice*

at Every Turn study reported having become homeless as a result of their trans identity or history, with 10 % of those age 55–64 having experienced that, and 8 % of those 65+ (Grant et al. 2011b). In 2012 the U.S. Department of Housing and Urban Development (HUD) issued final rules specifying that any federally-funded or federally-insured housing could no longer discriminate against anyone on the basis of gender identity or sexual orientation (see policy resources box).

The HUD rule covers many congregate living facilities for elders, but a remaining area of need is around long-term care. At press time the most that had been done for trans residents of nursing homes and other long-term care facilities was the Administration on Community Living's 2014 issuance of an online training tool for personnel of such facilities on how to appropriately and respectfully treat LGBT residents (see policy resources box). Further guidance on behalf of trans residents of long-term care facilities is still needed, although the federally-funded National Resource Center on LGBT Aging has issued some useful documents, such as "I Have a New Trans Client…Now What?" (see policy resources box A).

One last recent policy improvement deserves mention here. In 2013, Congress passed the Violence Against Women Reauthorization Act (VAWA) with a non-discrimination provision that, for the first time in any federal program, explicitly protected beneficiaries from being discriminated against on the basis of both gender identity and sexual orientation. Since trans people experience such high rates of sexual assault and domestic violence (the Act also provides services for victims of stalking and dating violence), this protection may well affect many trans elders (see policy resources box).

Summary

Deep down, every elder—indeed, every human—wishes for the same thing: see me for who I am and love me for who I am. That wish cannot be fulfilled by people who bring stereotypes of any kind to the table, as those stereotypes will obscure who is really sitting before them. That insight may be especially true of trans elders, who by definition spent at least part of their lives struggling to make the world see something very basic about them that was NOT being seen: their gender identity. Our task as service providers, caregivers, and advocates is two-fold: 1) to counter stereotypes and prejudices wherever we find them, particularly when they fuel the denial of rights and/or respect; and 2) to bring to each trans elder we work with a clean slate so that together, we can write and affirm their unique journey.

Learning Exercises

Multiple Choice Questions

1. What is the Terms Paradox?
   (a) It is critical to know the definitions of all trans-related terms.
   (b) It is critical to use the same terms the trans elder you are working with uses.
   (c) Trans-related terms tell you nothing about someone's experiences or expectations.
   (d) Answers (b) and (c).

2. Why is Christine Jorgensen important to many trans elders?
   (a) The publicity around her was when they first realized changing your sex was possible.
   (b) She was an early organizer of trans support groups.
   (c) She was the surgeon many trans elders went to for genital reconstruction surgery.

3. Which of the following might affect what words trans elders use to label themselves?
   (a) Their age
   (b) The years in which they transitioned
   (c) Their beliefs about whether they deserve stigmatization
   (d) All of the above
   (e) None of the above

4. Which of the following is NOT a reason many trans people transition in mid- to late-life?
   (a) A health scare makes them realize they have limited time left
   (b) They lose their youthful attractiveness and decide it would be better to be the other sex
   (c) Family members die or move out
   (d) They retire
   (e) They experience sacrifice fatigue

5. To "transition" and live as another gender a transgender person MUST:
   (a) Use hormones
   (b) Have surgery
   (c) Change their identification papers
   (d) All of the above
   (e) None of the above

6. Trans people have the following sexual orientations:
   (a) Lesbian/gay
   (b) Bisexual or pansexual
   (c) Transgender
   (d) Heterosexual
   (e) All of the above
   (f) (a), (b), and (d)

7. Which of the following is used as an alternative to the WPATH Standards of Care?
   (a) Informed consent model
   (b) The American Psychiatric Association's Diagnostic and Statistical Manual (DSM)
   (c) Christine Jorgensen's biography
   (d) All of the above
   (e) None of the above

8. Which of the following have been proven to be side effects of long-term hormone use?
   (a) Hot flashes
   (b) Heart disease
   (c) Dementia
   (d) All of the above
   (e) None of the above

9. A person who was assigned female at birth has a male gender identity and lives as a man. Which term would he NOT use to describe himself?
   (a) FTM
   (b) Transsexual

(c) Trans woman

(d) Male

10. Federal policies have recently been improved for transgender people in what areas?
    (a) Employment
    (b) Housing
    (c) Social Security
    (d) Marriage
    (e) Services for victims of domestic violence and sexual assault
    (f) All of the above
    (g) None of the above

Key

1-d

2-a

3-d

4-b

5-e

6-e

7-a

8-e

9-c

10-f

Self-check Questions

1. How do trans people "learn to be trans"? How have historical and cultural changes impacted how people "learn to be trans"?
2. What are some of the conflicts within the trans community?
3. In what ways might discrimination and violence affect a trans elder's health?
4. Trans elders may feel dependent on non-trans professionals in ways LGB elders are not. What are some of those ways?
5. What are some of the issues SOFFAs of trans people may face as the result of having a trans person in their life?
6. What are some of the ways in which transgender people say their gender identity and/or transition have impacted their sexuality?
7. What are some of the public policies affecting trans people that have changed in recent years?

Resources

Key Policy Resources for Trans Elders Box A

U.S. DOJ memo specifying that Title VII (employment non-discrimination law) covers transgender employees http://www.justice.gov/opa/pr/attorney-general-holder-directs-department-include-gender-identity-under-sex-discrimination

Executive Order protecting LGBT employees of federal contractors http://big.assets.huffington post.com/LGBTEO.pdf

Guidance Regarding the Employment of Transgender Individuals in the Federal Workplace http://www.opm.gov/policy-data-oversight/diversity-and-inclusion/reference-materials/gender-identity-guidance/

Veterans Administration memo on providing healthcare to transgender and intersex veterans http://www.va.gov/vhapublications/ViewPublication.asp?pub_ID=2863

Equal Access to Housing in HUD programs—final rule covering sexual orientation and gender identity http://portal.hud.gov/hudportal/documents/huddoc?id=12lgbtfinalrule.pdf

Social Security memo on determining legality of marriages involving trans people https://secure.ssa.gov/poms.nsf/lnx/0200305005

Social Security memo on changing the gender marker on Social Security records https://secure.ssa.gov/poms.nsf/lnx/0110212200

Frequently Asked Questions about the nondiscrimination grant condition in the Violence Against Women Act Reauthorization Act of 2013 http://ojp.gov/about/ocr/pdfs/vawafaqs.pdf

Organization Resources Box B

FORGE Transgender Aging Network and ElderTG http://forge-forward.org/aging

National Resource Center on LGBT Aging http://lgbtagingcenter.org

National Center for Transgender Equality http://transequality.org/

World Professional Association for Transgender Health http://www.wpath.org/
Transgender American Veterans Association http://tavausa.org/

Document Resources Box C

Hot, Safe Sex for Transmasculine Folks and Partners http://forge-forward.org/wp-content/docs/HIV-FTM-web1.pdf
Hot, Safe Sex for Transfeminine Folks and Partners http://forge-forward.org/wp-content/docs/HIV-MTF-web1.pdf
Professional organization statements supporting transgender health care http://www.lambdalegal.org/sites/default/files/publications/downloads/fs_professional-org-statements-supporting-trans-health_4.pdf
Building Respect for LGBT Older Adults (online training for long-term care facility staff) http://lgbtagingcenter.org/training/buildingRespect.cfm
Creating End-of-Life Documents for Trans Individuals: An Advocate's Guide http://www.lgbtagingcenter.org/resources/pdfs/End-of-Life%20PlanningArticle.pdf
Improving the Lives of Transgender Older Adults: Recommendations for Policy and Practice http://www.lgbtagingcenter.org/resources/pdfs/TransAgingPolicyReportFull.pdf
I Have a New Transgender Client...Now What? http://www.lgbtagingcenter.org/resources/pdfs/newTransClientFactSheet.pdf

References

Amazon. (2015). *Transparent: Awards*. Retrieved from http://www.imdb.com/title/tt3502262/awards.

American Psychiatric Association. (1980). *Diagnostic and statistical manual of mental disorders* (3rd ed.). Washington, DC: Author.

American Psychiatric Association. (2013). *Diagnostic and statistical manual of mental disorders* (5th ed.). Washington, DC: Author.

Boenke, M. (ed.). (2003). *Trans forming families: Real stories about transgendered loved ones* (2nd ed., expanded). Hardy, VA: Oak Knoll Press.

Brevard, A. (2001). *The woman I was not born to be: A transsexual journey*. Philadelphia, PA: Temple University Press.

Cook-Daniels, L., & Munson, M. (2010). Sexual violence, elder abuse, and sexuality of transgender adults age 60+: Results of three surveys. *Journal of GLBT Family Studies. 6*(2), 142–177. Available from: http://forge-forward.org/wp-content/docs/trans-aging-3-surveys.pdf.

Feinberg, L. (1997). *Transgender warriors: Making history from Joan of Arc to Dennis Rodman*. Boston, MA: Beacon Press.

FORGE. (2004). Responses from "Sexual violence in the tansgender community" survey (Unpublished raw data).

FORGE. (2011). Responses from "Transgender peoples' access to sexual assault services" survey (Unpublished raw data).

FORGE. (2012). *FAQ: The terms paradox*. Milwaukee, WI: Author. Available at http://forge-forward.org/wp-content/docs/FAQ-06-2012-terms-paradox.pdf.

Fredriksen-Goldsen, K. L., Kim, H.-J., Emlet, C. A., Muraco, A., Erosheva, E. A., Hoy-Ellis, C. P., & Goldsen, J. (2011). *The aging and health report: Disparities and resilience among lesbian, gay, bisexual and transgender older adults*. Retrieved from: http://caringandaging.org/wordpress/wp-content/uploads/2011/05/Full-Report-FINAL-11-16-11.pdf.

Grant, J. M., Mottet, L. A., Tanis, J., Harrison, J., Herman, J. L., & Keisling, M. (2011a). *Injustice at every turn: A report of the national transgender discrimination survey*. Washington, D.C.: The National Center for Transgender Equality and the National Gay and Lesbian Task Force.

Grant, J. M., Mottet, L. A., Tanis, J., Harrison, J., Herman, J. L., & Keisling, M. (2011b). Responses from respondents age 55+ (Unpublished raw data).

Haines, B. A., Ajayi, A. A., & Boyd, H. (2014). Making trans parents visible: Intersectionality of trans and parenting identities. *Feminism & Psychology, 24*, 238–247.

Herman, J. L. (Ed.). (2014). Best practices for asking questions to identify transgender and other gender minority respondents on populationbasedsurveys. Los Angeles, CA: The Williams Institute.

Kenagy, G. (2002). HIV among transgendered people. *AIDS Care, 14*(1), 127–134.

Kenagy, G. (2005). The health and social service needs of transgender people in Philadelphia. *International Journal of Transgenderism, 8*(2/3), 49–56.

Kenagy, G., & Bostwick, W. (2005). Health and social service needs of transgendered people in Chicago. *International Journal of Transgenderism, 8*(2/3), 57–66.

Lev, A. I. (2004). *Transgender emergence: Therapeutic guidelines for working with gender-variant people and their families*. New York, NY: Haworth Clinical Practice Press.

Louden, K. (2014, July 2). Largest study to date: Transgender hormone treatment safe. *Medscape Family Medicine*. Retrieved from http://www.medscape.com/viewarticle/827713.

Meyerowitz, J. (2002). *How sex changed: A history of transsexuality in the United States*. Cambridge, MA: Harvard University Press.

Middlebrook, D. W. (1999). *Suits me: The double life of Billy Tipton*. London: Virago Press.

Newport, F. (2012, November 12). In US, 24 % of men, 2 % of women are veterans. *Gallup Press*. Retrieved from http://www.gallup.com/poll/158729/men-women-veterans.aspx.

Obama, B. (2015, January 20). *State of the union* (speech). Washington, D.C.

Sanchez, D. M. (2015, January 26). Trans allies and my treaty of the heart. *The Bilerico Project*. Retrieved from http://www.bilerico.com/2015/01/trans_allies_and_my_treaty_of_the_heart.php#I3Kl1G6lekm6eEb2.99.

Stryker, S. (2008). *Transgender history*. Berkeley, CA: Seal Press.

Susan's Place. (2011). *Re: Would the SOC be any better if run by post-op trans people?* [Online forum discussion]. Retrieved from http://www.susans.org/forums/index.php?topic=105988.0.

Tate, C. C., Ledbetter, J. N., & Youssef, C. P. (2012). A two-question method for assessing gender categories in the social and medical sciences. *Journal of Sex Research, 50*(8), 767–776.

U.S. Centers for Disease Control and Prevention. (2014). *Adverse childhood experiences study*. Multiple documents available. Retrieved from http://www.cdc.gov/violenceprevention/acestudy/.

Wilchins, R. (2012, December 6). Transgender dinosaurs and the rise of the genderqueers. *Advocate*. Retrieved from http://www.advocate.com/commentary/riki-wilchins/2012/12/06/transgender-dinosaurs-and-rise-genderqueers.

World Professional Association for Transgender Health (WPATH). (2015). *Standards of care* (all versions available at http://www.wpath.org/site_page.cfm?pk_association_webpage_menu=1351&pk_association_webpage=4655).

Bisexuality: An Invisible Community Among LGBT Elders

15

William E. Burleson

Abstract

This chapter discusses issues relevant to bisexual elders, including invisibility, homophobia and biphobia, lack of understanding, and a scarcity of research and resources. Bisexual elders face the same issues as all elders, such as the need for financial planning, health care, assisted living, estate planning, and more, not to mention isolation, feelings of loss, depression, and ageism. Bisexual elders also face the additional issues that lesbian and gay elders must navigate such as invisibility, coming out, and marginalization and discrimination due to homophobia. In addition, bisexual elders also face issues that are either amplified—such as a lack of supportive social networks—or uniquely theirs—such as biphobia and a lack of bi-specific research, support, and services. As a consequence, it is critical for people who offer services to elders to avoid judgment and assumptions.

Keywords

Bisexual · Aging · Health disparities · LGBT · Queer theory

Overview

While bisexuality is common, it is often misunderstood, dismissed, and ignored by both mainstream culture and the lesbian and gay communities, adding a new layer of challenges for seniors. Bisexual elders face the same issues as all elders, such as the need for financial planning, health care, assisted living, estate planning, and more, plus isolation, feelings of loss, depression, and ageism. Bisexual elders must also navigate the additional issues that many lesbian and gay elders face such as coming out, marginalization, and discrimination due to homophobia. Adding to these challenges is that bisexuals typically enjoy few if any bisexual-specific social networks, support, and services. Service providers may be well-intentioned, but scant research, lack of cultural competency training, and few relevant

W.E. Burleson (✉)
Minneapolis, Minnesota, USA
e-mail: billburl1@gmail.com

resources often result in increased isolation and marginalization for the seniors in their care. The result is measured in health disparities and stress for bisexual elders.

Learning Objectives

By the end of this chapter, the reader should be able to:

- Describe how bisexuals elders' experience differs from straight and gay and lesbian elders,
- Communicate how health disparities affect bisexuals,
- Articulate the different service needs of bisexual elders, and
- Offer possible solutions to the problem of isolation and a lack of community support.

Introduction

I found it not really upsetting, but more unsettling. Whoa, what just happened? Or, more accurately, when? I had to laugh, if just a little. It felt like the day my AARP invite arrived in the mail or the first time a clerk offered me a senior discount.

I've given many talks about bisexuality, the bisexual experience, and the bi community at various venues including colleges, bookstores, community centers, and conferences. It's a patter I've got down so pat that one time, working without notes, I somehow flipped back to an earlier part of the talk and repeated ten minutes, I'm told, quite verbatim. Not a failing memory—I'm only fifty-five as I write this—more stuck in a rut and time for a fresh speech.

Therefore, when I was invited to participate in a panel discussion about bi history, I did not think much about it. The generally hidden, often forgotten, and always interesting cultural history of my community is something I am quite comfortable talking about and lending a little context to.

It is a small world and an even smaller one when you are on stage with other LGBT speakers, and I knew everyone on the panel quite well. We sat on the riser, in simple hard chairs, in front of a room arranged classroom style. People filed in. When the room was full and the panel moderator began to introduce us, I had an overwhelming feeling of being one part in a "what do these things have in common" test.

- We were old. Or, no, not really—we were old compared to the youthful audience.
- Then I knew: I was to be the bisexual elder.
- I WAS the history. They wanted to hear from me firsthand about my experiences in the ancient days of the seventies, eighties, and nineties.

Since that presentation I have come to expect to play that role, and when presenting on bisexuality, I make sure to talk about the good old days. I have even come to enjoy it.

For me, aging is an interesting social experiment: I have found people treat me with increasing respect as I grow older. I am also seemingly less threatening to young men and increasingly invisible to women. I assume this trend will only increase, with watersheds like the first time someone offers me their seat on the bus and the first time someone talks loudly to me.

Those moments I will not enjoy.

The point is:

- I, as well as many of my peers, are getting older.
- LGBT activism is a mature movement, with the first waves of people coming out in the 1970s now gray, retiring, and needing services, services that may at times differ from the general population, services that may need to be delivered in ways that are new.
- The Bi piece of the LBGT puzzle is no different, with the first groups of 1970s bisexuals going gray, a group who well remember a time before "LGBT" or even "GLBT," a group having no intention of accepting any less than cultural competence among service providers.

Therefore, it is critical that service providers become educated on the issues affecting not only lesbians and gays, but also bisexuals (Kimmel et al. 2006).

Challenges to a Complete Definition

How bisexuals and bisexuality fits into a discussion of aging depends on how we choose to define bisexuality. One would think defining bisexuality to be easy and the purview of the Oxford English Dictionary. In fact, defining bisexuality is fraught with challenges, mired in culture, and in flux in our changing times.

In *Bisexuality, Not Homosexuality*: *Counseling Issues and Treatment Approaches* Horowitz and Newcomb (1999, p. 148) state: "Bisexuality is difficult to define. Must one engage in sexual activity with both sexes to assume a bisexual identity? What if a person has sexual or affectional desires for both sexes but does not act on them? What if a person is involved in a monogamous, long-term same-sex relationship but has had previous satisfactory heterosexual relationships?"

Researchers have often looked at behavior as the test, and many people see the gender of one's sexual partners as proof of one's sexual orientation. If we define "bisexual behavior" as having been sexual with women and men or with more than one gender, then we are talking about the needs of a huge part of society. For example, Alfred Kinsey's studies done in the 1940s and 1950s found that 37 % of men had had at least one sexual experience with another man at one time in their lives (Kinsey et al. 1948). This number is usually considered an overestimate, having been taken from a convenience sample in not typical circumstances such as in prisons and with male prostitutes. Accordingly, published in 1994, the *National Health and Social Life Survey* (NHSLS) found very different results. It utilized face-to-face interviews of 3432 people to find that approximately 9 % of men and 4 % of women had ever had any same-gender sex partners (Michael et al. 1994).

These data are about behavior and not identity. Just because a person identifies as straight does not mean that they have not had or do not still have sex with people of the same gender. Conversely, many gay men have had or do have sex with women, and many lesbians have had or do have sex with men. For example, in a 2000 survey conducted by the *Advocate* about 75 % of lesbian respondents reported having had sex in the past with at least once with a man, and 6 % said they have had sex with a man in the last year (Remez 2000). Meanwhile, the *Annual Review of Sex Research* in 1997 reported that 62–79 % of gay identified men report a history of "heterosexual contact" (Doll et al. 1997).

We must think of sexual orientation as something different—and more culturally significant—than behavior. Being straight, lesbian, gay, or bisexual is about feelings and attractions, not confined to actions alone. Indeed, we see self-identified bisexuals with all varieties of partner choices. Vernallis (1999, p. 349) reports in the *Journal of Social Philosophy*, "Some people identify as bisexuals although they have only experienced sex with one gender, perhaps because they have sexual desires for and fantasies about both genders." Bisexuals may or may not have had lovers of different genders. They may or may not be monogamous. They may or may not ever have had sex in their entire lives. Take, for example, a catholic priest who has been celibate his entire life, yet this person has a sexual orientation, and he may identify as straight, or bi, or gay.

That bisexuality is not defined by behavior is a very important point for bisexuals because many people believe bisexuals need both a man and a woman as a sexual partner. For example, if a self-identified bisexual woman is in a monogamous relationship with, say, another woman, she is now assumed to be lesbian.

Therefore, it is ironic that focusing on behavior means that the number of people identified as bisexual is inflated (counting people who have been sexual with more than one gender regardless of how they feel or identify) while erasing them as well (no longer considering a person's attractions and self-identity, defining them by their partners).

It should be noted that psychological research has provided us with many measures for orientation, from the Kinsey Scale (Kinsey et al. 1948) to the Klein Sexual Orientation Grid

(Klein 1993) to M. D. Storms in Sexual Orientation and Self-Perception (1978), and all have some descriptive value as well as challenges, none of which we will discuss here. Instead, the focus for our purposes will be on self-perception and self-identification, and less on diagnosis. If we are to look at the common challenges and solutions that bisexuals face in aging, measuring, or questioning people's identity labels is less useful than acknowledging and embracing an older person's choice of orientation label and community and looking at the cultural commonalities that these monikers connote.

Bisexuality Defined

For the purposes, of this chapter, we will look to the San Francisco Human Right Commission (2011) LBGT Advisory Committee (date unknown) for a good working definition: "...bisexual is the term that is most widely understood as describing those whose attractions fall outside an either/or paradigm." In other words, bisexuals are people who are neither straight nor gay or lesbian.

Also, we will use the most quoted definition for "bisexual" within the community itself, from Robyn Ochs (taken from http://robynochs.com/bisexual/) long time bi activist from Boston: "I call myself bisexual because I acknowledge that I have in myself the potential to be attracted—romantically and/or sexually—to people of more than one sex and/or gender, not necessarily at the same time, not necessarily in the same way, and not necessarily to the same degree."

How Many People Identify as Bisexual?

For the sake of this discussion of bisexuals and aging, we will limit ourselves to people who identify as bisexual, a more definable group with many issues in common. According to several studies, people who identify as bisexual are the largest single part of the LGBT community in the USA, with more women identifying as bisexual

than lesbian, and fewer men identifying as bisexual than gay (San Francisco Human Right Commission, date unknown). For example,

- 2002 National Survey of Family Growth reported that among men, 2.3 % identified as gay and 1.8 % as bisexual, while among adult females, 1.3 % identified as lesbian and 2.8 % as bisexual (Mosher et al. 2005).
- In *The Journal of Sexual Medicine* (Herbenick et al. 2010) reports that among adult males 4.2 % identified as gay and 2.6 % as bisexual, while among adult females, 0.9 % identified as lesbian and 3.6 % as bisexual.
- In 2007, a survey found that among LGBT identified individuals, 68.4 % of men identified as gay and 31.6 % as bisexual, while 34.7 % of women identified as lesbian and 65.3 % as bisexual (Egan et al. 2008).

Although we will be using self-identity to discuss bisexuality, it is safe to assume that many people who otherwise would do not identify as bisexual because of social barriers. It is difficult to estimate the proportion of the population that remains "in the closet," as it is no easy decision to call oneself bisexual. Plus, "being closeted" goes both ways: while many bisexuals identify publically—and presumably to people doing surveys—as straight, many bisexuals may publically identify as gay or lesbian (Keppel 2006) for a host of reasons that will be discussed below. Further reducing the number of people potentially identifying as bisexual is that many elders may not even have the word "bisexual" in their tool kit (Keppel 2006).

Common Questions Asked About Bisexual Persons

With scant public acknowledgment and awareness of bisexuals in the USA, it is little wonder that many people have questions and misconceptions about bisexuality. The following are common questions that bisexuals are asked.

- **Are bisexuals mentally ill?** Bisexuality is not classified as a mental illness. However, it is worth mentioning that bisexuals, like many out-groups, face stress from discrimination and isolation and may show increases in health—including mental health—disparities (Healthy People 2020 2010).
- **Is being bisexual a choice?** This question assumes that people who identify as bisexual should "pick a side" or are actually closeted lesbians and gays. As previously discussed, recognizing bisexuality as not defined by behavior. Acknowledging bisexuality as an orientation helps us see being bisexual as not a choice, just as being gay or straight is not a choice (Hayes 2001).
- **Are all bisexuals non-monogamous?** Bisexuals may or may not be monogamous (Kimmel et al. 2006). Many bisexuals are in long-term monogamous relationships, many are single and not sexual with anyone, many travel in the polyamorous community (which we will discuss below), and many are fans of the swinger community. In other words, bisexuals are just like straights, gays, and lesbians, and knowing that someone is bisexual tells us nothing about the person's relationship status or whether or not the person is monogamous.
- **Are bisexual men all married guys cheating on their wives?** As with the last question, there certainly are a number of bisexual men who cheat on their wives. But again, many bisexual men live quiet lives with their same-gender or different gender partners and would not think of cheating. Some bisexual men are non-monogamous by agreement with their partners, something far different from "cheating."
- **Is bisexuality just a phase on the way to being lesbian or gay?** Senior service providers, given the age and experience of their clients, will likely work with many LGBT people who are very firm in self-identity. That said, this stereotype knows no age. Though many gays and lesbians at one time considered the possibility that they may be bisexual, this experience cannot be generalized to all people who identify as bisexual. In fact, one-third of bisexuals previously identified as gay or lesbian before identifying as bisexual (Fox 2004).

The Intersection of Bisexuality and Transgenderism

> Bisexuality and transgender identities both resist simplification, both cannot be reducible to some simple formula.—Bedecarre in the journal *Hypatia* (2001)
>
> My transsexuality and my bisexuality are inextricably linked. Since the transsexuality has been there since the earliest times I can remember, that was the beginning of the journey. Realizing I was bisexual came much, much later.—A guest on the Bi Cities! Show (Burleson 2005)

In most places around the country, there is a strong connection between the transgender and the bisexual communities. Indeed, the two communities have been strong allies.

Why is this? One reason certainly is because they both have a natural affinity born of living in the gray areas. Both are neither one thing nor the other; both confound the people who view the world in simple either/or dualist manner. Both communities get it, and they both are more likely to get it about each other than people who do not have a personal relationship to this ambiguity.

Another reason the two communities work well together is that there are a lot of people who are both bisexual and transgender. For example, a female to male transgender (FTM) who previously only considered men for partners might well re-evaluate that stand now that he is living as a man. For many, the challenges and changes involved in coming to terms with being transgender inevitably leads to re-evaluating much of one's life, including sexuality.

Plus, many bisexuals express that they are attracted to people as individuals and not according to their genitalia; therefore, some bi's may embrace gender ambiguity in a way that leaves more room for friendships and relationships with transgender people.

One obvious and important reason is the two communities have been allies by virtue of their exclusion from the lesbian and gay communities, and for very similar reasons. The transgender community is a thorn in the side of many lesbian and gay people who wish to claim, "We are just like straight people." Many gay and lesbian people, and bi people, too, carry around their share of trans-phobia. Simply because someone is not straight does not mean they automatically get a masters in human sexuality or that all their prejudices magically disappear. As bisexuals fight to be included in gay and lesbian events and in the names of organizations, it is natural for the bisexual community to support the transgender community in their parallel and simultaneous struggles for recognition and inclusion. Perhaps it is an alliance of convenience, but I prefer to think of it as an alliance of understanding.

Bisexuality and Health

It is critical that bisexual health issues be addressed in the USA and addressed at their root causes. According to *Bisexual Invisibility: Impacts and Recommendations* from the San Francisco Human Right Commission, LGBT Advisory Committee (date unknown),

> One area where we see the effects of biphobia and bi-invisibility is in the health and well-being of bisexuals, [men who have sex with men and women] and [women who have sex with men and women]. This is because, as confirmed by the available research, these groups experience greater health disparities compared to the broader population, and they continue to experience biphobia and bi-invisibility from healthcare providers, including providers who may be gay or lesbian, or are knowledgeable about homosexuality and accepting of their gay and lesbian clients.

Bisexuals on average tend to suffer health disparities due to the continued marginalization of the community, minority stress, and inadequate culturally competent services. According to the *Healthy People 2020 Bisexual Health Fact Sheet* (2010), bisexual women and men have the lower emotional well-being than heterosexuals, gays or lesbians. Bisexual women report lower levels of social support than heterosexual women and lower or similar levels to lesbians, and bisexual and gay men have lower social support levels when compared with heterosexual men

(Dobinson, Healthy People 2020 2010). Bisexuals report higher cholesterol than do heterosexuals (New Mexico Department of Health, Healthy People 2020 2010), high rates of smoking (American Lung Association, Healthy People 2020 2010) (New Mexico Department of Health, Healthy People 2020 2010), and higher rates of current asthma than heterosexuals (New Mexico Department of Health, Healthy People 2020 2010). Bisexual adults report nearly three times the rate of intimate partner violence as heterosexuals (New Mexico Department of Health, Healthy People 2020 2010).

Bisexual women were less likely to be insured or be underinsured and have difficulty obtaining medical care (Diamant et al., Healthy People 2020 2000). Bisexual women have higher rates of all types of cancer (Dobinson, Healthy People 2020) and higher rates of heart disease than heterosexual women. This should be expected, because bisexual women reported higher rates of risk factors for both cancer and heart disease, such as the previously mentioned higher rates of smoking and high cholesterol, plus high blood pressure, and higher average BMI (but lower than for lesbians) (Dobinson, Healthy People 2020 2010). Adding to the problem is that bisexual women have the higher rate of never having a pap test than lesbians and straight women (Dobinson, Healthy People 2020 2010) and were less likely than heterosexual women to have had a mammography (Koh, Healthy People 2020 2000).

Bisexuals show higher rates of binge drinking than do their heterosexual counterparts (Healthy People 2020 2010), bisexual women report the high rates of alcohol use, heavy drinking, and alcohol-related problems when compared to heterosexual and lesbian women and higher rates of drug use than heterosexual women (Dobinson, Healthy People 2020 2010). According to *Healthy People 2020*, bisexual adults report twice the rate of depression, higher levels of anxiety, and nearly three times the suicidal ideation compared to heterosexual adults. Bisexual men and women report high levels of self-harm, suicide attempts, and thoughts of suicide (Healthy People 2020 2010).

Although these numbers reflect ongoing health disparities across age groups, the implications for service providers to seniors are clear: when it comes to bisexuals and health, it is critical to be aware and watchful, offer culturally competent care, and to studiously avoid the stigma and isolation that many bisexuals experience.

What do we know about the bisexual community and HIV? Unfortunately, there is little research, with bisexuals usually a subset of a study of homosexuals. For example, over a decade into the epidemic one researcher (Doll et al. 1997) found that, in 166 articles mentioning bisexual men over a ten-year time period, only twenty-one pointed out any differences between bisexual men and gay men, and only eight gave information exclusively about bisexual men. In the same ten years, the researchers found only sixty-one articles mentioning bisexual women, twenty-two of which compared bisexuals with lesbians. Only three concerned bisexual women exclusively. In fact, even today, the prevalence of HIV in the bisexual community is unknown. Even though 76,075 men with AIDS (21 % of AIDS cases in men who have reported sex with men) through 1996 report a history of "bisexual behavior," as previously discussed, this does not mean they were bisexual. We know even less about bisexual women.

And yet, according to *Bisexual Invisibility: Impacts and Recommendations* from the San Francisco Human Right Commission, LGBT Advisory Committee (date unknown),

> In the 1980s and 1990s, bisexuals were vociferously blamed for the spread of HIV (even though the virus is spread by unprotected sex, not a bisexual identity). However, a 1994 study of data from San Francisco is also worth noting: it found that at that time, bisexually identified [men who have sex with men and women] weren't a common vector or "bridge" for spreading HIV from male partners to female partners due to high rates of using barrier protection and extremely low rates of risky behavior.

These data reveal that there are more assumptions about the role of bisexuals in the HIV/AIDS epidemic than there are facts, so once again, people should be cautious making assumptions about HIV status or risk.

Identity Issues Bisexual Elders May Face

Bisexuals face the same barrier as all parts of the LGBT community: homophobia. LGBT people have long been deterred from embracing their sexual orientation because they are under the threat of social ostracism, employment and other discrimination, and violence. Considering the legal sanctions and physical and psychological abuse that many bisexuals must identify as bisexually at all. This situation has improved greatly since Stonewall (the 1969 riot in New York that for many marks the beginning of the LGBT movement), and tolerance has made extraordinary gains in much of the USA. However, the growing acceptance of gays and lesbians—and, perhaps, bisexuals as well—should not be assumed to be the experience of older bisexuals, who may live in communities or associate with peers who they fear—rightly or wrongly—would be less than accepting.

Biphobia

However, bisexuals also face their own unique brand of discrimination. Commonly referred to as "Biphobia," bisexuals—despite their greater numbers—may be thought of as representing an inferior position to lesbians and gays in the LGBT community (Kimmel et al. 2006). Straight homophobes seldom bother with nuances between the L, G, B, and T, and many gay and lesbian people dismiss bisexuals as pretenders, straight swingers, confused, mentally ill, immoral, disease vectors, traitors, and more. When seeking bisexual supportive services, gay or lesbian, even supposedly "LGBT" services, can constitute a "bait and switch," promising understanding and delivering its own variety of discrimination.

This active discrimination is facilitated by the defining issue facing bisexuals of all ages: invisibility. Being gay or lesbian offers role models and a narrative that is well-defined, however, often inaccurate and problematic in its own right. Not so for bisexuals. The reason for the invisibility is obvious. Consider this hypothetical: Shirley and Ruth have been together for thirty years and now live in assisted living. The other residents know them as a lesbian couple. Yet, is that accurate? One or both could be bi. Some fellow residents might know them well enough to know their orientation accurately, or they could metaphorically or literally, fly a big flag saying, "We're Bi." Short of these two situations, a large majority of people would identify them as lesbian. Most people make assumptions about other people's orientation according to the gender of their partner, an easy and it's practical assumption because it is often correct. Sometimes, however, as previously discussed, it is inaccurate; a situation that makes bisexuals invisible (Burleson 2005).

As a result, many bisexuals feel isolated and may think there is nothing for them or even that they are alone. Most bisexuals have little knowledge of services available to them (should they be so lucky as to have services available to them), instead encountering and perhaps even internalizing the previously discussed plethora of myths and stereotypes. This is true for bisexuals of all ages, but may be especially true for elders. Elder bisexuals may know no one else who is bisexual (or, more likely, know who around them IS bisexual). They may not even have the words to describe their feelings. Also, while younger bisexuals may be coming out and finding support in colleges and in various organizations, current elders grew up in a time that did not allow space for bisexuals (Keppel 2006).

Thus bi-invisibility has significant repercussions for locating a supportive community. According to Kimmel et al. (2006, p. 45), "Community support is important for everyone no matter what their sexual identity is." The vast majority of bisexuals in the USA cannot find a community gathering of any kind anywhere within a reasonable distance. Similarly, bisexual invisibility is an added challenge in locating services, whether its supportive healthcare professionals or counseling services, both because they may not exist because of a lack of understanding the need in provider communities and difficulty accessing services that do exist.

What do bisexual elders who find community encounter? There is at present a great deal of discussion in the bisexual community regarding the suitability of the term "bisexual," especially among younger people and at colleges. Indeed, in a recent needs assessment I authored (Burleson 2013) on behalf of a Minnesota bisexual advocacy group, the Bisexual Organizing Project, I identified an uneasy relationship in the bisexual community between those embracing "bisexual" and a growing number of people who reject the bisexual identity in favor of "fluid," "pansexual," "omni-sexual," "queer," and other new labels. Many people self-identifying as one of these new labels expressed how they see "bisexual" as implying there to be only two genders and thus not recognizing the spectrum of gender identity. On the other hand, some reject these new labels as faddish or hurtful in themselves: with non-bisexuals once again defining what it means to be bisexual. For the elder having grown up at a time when bisexuality was not discussed or was discussed and deeply stigmatized, embracing "bisexual" often took taken great courage (Keppel 2006), and rejection of the identity as somehow flawed may be understandably unwelcome and painful.

A good example of how generational differences color identity labels is the term "Queer." Queer as an insult from the past remains hurtful to many, especially those who are older and may have grown up with the term as only a pejorative one. Meanwhile, for nearly two decades now the word has enjoyed varying degrees of success as a reclaimed disparagement that is now embracing of all parts of the LGBT family. Many bisexuals embraced this term for its inclusiveness and perhaps the term that many bisexuals have long sought, uniting the LGBT community under one label. However, queer also has the additional connotation of "Otherness," of embracing queer people's separation from the norm (Burleson 2005), a separation that many LGBT people may not feel, and a separation that many elders may not embrace as they search for their identity in a world offering them so little guidance.

A proliferation of new identity labels only adds to the burden of "coming out" for people who are barely embracing or even understanding their own feelings of multiple attractions, especially a person whose life journey may have been a long. It is hard to guess how this issue will settle out—fad or sea change—but it would seem that this issue will likely continue to challenge, and perhaps even redefine, bi activism into the future.

Aging as Bisexual

In their search for a supportive community, bisexual elders can be seen as whipsawed by two competing forces. First, they may suffer the same lack of community that most bisexuals experience, plus more. Finding community has been greatly facilitated by the Internet, either a face to face community or a virtual one. Not long ago, if there was a bisexual meeting, support group, or social event, one might call a social service hotline for referrals (if one was savvy enough to locate the number), count on word of mouth, or hope to be lucky enough to spot a flyer somewhere. The Internet has changed that, and now for anyone—including elders—who are online, if there is a gathering within a reasonable distance, it is as easy to locate as a good sushi restaurant. And for those who live in a place where there are no opportunities for physical meetings, one can always find a virtual community online. However, not all have benefited equally. In 2012, while 97 % of 18- to 29-year-olds used the Internet, only 57 % of those sixty-five and older did (Zickuhr and Madden 2012). Therefore, many elders are left behind.

Second, should they find a "bricks and mortar" local community of regularly scheduled meetings, social nights, and perhaps even an organization of some sort, older bisexual people may not feel included by virtue of their age. As one of our case studies suggests, older adult bisexual people may feel that activities are designed for young people, or, at least, dominated by a younger generation.

In fact, should they locate a community—virtual or in person—it may not be the community they were looking for. As discussed previously, this is an exciting time in LBGT history. In many places, the bi community of conferences and tents at Pride Festivals represents a dynamic culture of younger bisexuals on the cutting edge of redefining what bisexuality means, if and where the bisexual community fits into a GBT narrative, and even if "bisexual" as a term is to be embraced or discarded. This may not be the discussion for which older bisexuals are seeking.

For all parts of the LGBT community support services are critical, but bisexual elders may face additional challenges when accessing those. Should they be in the process of coming out to family and friends, bisexual elders face the same challenges that older lesbians and gays face, including the reactions of adult children and even spouses. Service providers to people who are elderly may be called upon to help a family deal with a coming out crisis (Kimmel et al. 2006). However, the service provider should not assume that people coming out bisexual to their partners want to end their relationships. The person may be more hoping to live an authentic life with those they love.

The above was a common situation I found when I facilitated a group for married men as part of an HIV prevention program. The men who attended were often older and many were retired, with nearly all identifying as bisexual, many in the closet, as well as many having been out for decades. The isolation from mainstream LGBT organizations and services (other than our little circle) was nearly universal, and in this group, the men finally found their community. What may surprise some is that, generally, these men were not looking to end their marriages, and instead often talked of their love and physical attraction to their wives.

LGBT elders may or may not be "out" to a therapist or service provider, and bisexual elders even less than gays or lesbians (Keppel 2006). Bisexual elders may want to access heterosexual support rather than LGBT services (Kimmel et al. 2006) for many reasons. Bisexuals who have been out for many years may or may not be connected to community or services and may or may not want to be. They may be single or have a partner/spouse of many years. They may be monogamous or not. If not monogamous, they may be public about it, keep it private between their families or partners, or they may be secretive. If not monogamous, they may have a primary relationship and occasional more casual relationships or they may have long-term relationships with more than one person (Kimmel et al. 2006).

However, this latter group deserves further discussion. In the USA, there is a thriving subculture called the polyamorous community. "Polyamorous," or "many loves," is defined by the Polyamory Society (2012) as "The non-possessive, honest, responsible and ethical philosophy and practice of loving multiple people simultaneously" (Author unknown, www. polyamorysociety.org). The polyamorous community parallels the bisexual community in organization, with clubs, non-profits, groups, and conferences in many major cities. Though people of all orientations may identify as polyamorous, most would agree that bisexuals are over represented. As one member of a poly group said to me, "You don't have to be bisexual to be poly, but it sure helps."

How do polyamorous bisexuals experience aging differently, if at all? Given a lack of data on this topic, it would need to be a question that warrants further investigation. However, it is imperative that service providers avoid judgment and biases (Keppel 2006; Kimmel et al. 2006) while being accepting and supportive of alternative relationships, and whenever possible, make accommodations for the bisexual elder's needs.

Implications of Service Delivery for Bisexual Elders

The chief implication for people offering services to bisexual elders is the need to avoid assumptions. For example, regardless of sexual orientation, healthcare providers need to individually assess the need for pap smears and breast exams for women and provide information on HIV and

STDs for bisexuals of all genders (Kimmel et al. 2006). Service providers should allow for alternative relationship models, including polyamorous relationships, both in their support and in accommodations, if they are to effectively serve bisexuals (and polyamorous people of all orientations). Lastly, it is important not to assume the nature of someone's self-identity. Bisexuals are rendered invisible by a culture that says they are all straight, gay, or lesbian. Assuming people's orientation from their appearance, habits or relationships are a sure route to poor services.

Becoming more knowledgeable about resources available in the community (e.g., support groups, bisexual friendly churches, community organizations, and social events) is critical to offering needed services as well as demonstrating one's competence (Keppel 2006). For example, in the group of married men's mentioned earlier, one man in his seventies (who had been out to for decades) lost his wife. This man benefited greatly from support and understanding from the other men in the group who understood him in a way non-bisexuals may struggle to do. Groups such as this may be critical to a person's well-being, and the elder in need of face-to-face support services and desire help in locating one.

Lastly, continuing education for service providers is also critical. I would argue that the best education, however, is not from a book but instead from talking to and getting to know the needs individuals. Listening, understanding, and meeting people where they are may be both the best education one can obtain and the best service one can provide.

Summary

This chapter on bisexual elders is merely start of a conversation about how to offer quality services to bisexual seniors. There is much work to be done in understanding this unique population. For example, little has been written regarding the rich ethnic, racial, cultural, and economic diversity within the bisexual community and its implications for services (Kimmel et al. 2006).

As Lady Bird Johnson said, "Getting old is not for the faint of heart." It is the charge of service providers to bisexual elders to make the process as smooth as possible.

Research Box

In the framework of a constructionist approach, a life-course point of view, and traditional concepts borrowed from identity theory, the authors report on a study of fifty-six San Francisco bisexuals. The data show that by midlife, changing life commitments among the participants were associated with a decrease in sexual involvement, a move toward sexual activity with just one sex, a decrease in contact with the bisexual subculture, and a decrease in the salience of a bisexual identity. Given these changes, the data reveal the opposite of what might be expected—an increase rather than a decrease in the certainty about and stability of the bisexual identity. The authors show that this was due to the continuation of dual attractions that were positively regarded even as there was a move away from a bisexual lifestyle. In explaining these findings, they discuss the interplay between sexual communities, relationships, selves, and sexuality.

Abstract from Weinberg, M. S., Williams, C. J., & Pryor, D. W. (2001). Bisexuals at midlife commitment, salience, and identity. *Journal of Contemporary Ethnography*, *30*(2), 180-208.

Discussion Questions:

1. What are other reasons that contribute to changes toward sexual activity with just one sex?
2. What other changes as adults age could contribute to the authors' findings?

3. What appears to be the strongest influences on the tendency discussed in the literature?

Learning Exercises

Self-Check Questions

1. What does it means to be a bisexual elder?
2. What are healthcare disparities facing bisexual elders?
3. Discuss discrimination faced by bisexual elders.
4. What are unique service needs for bisexual elders?
5. What are solutions for decreasing isolation of bisexual elders?

Experiential Assignments

1. Go on the Internet and search for a story of the experience of a bisexual elders. Write your impressions of what it is like.
2. Look on the Internet to find about services targeted to bisexual elders.
3. Write down your reactions to the author's reflections on being a bisexual elder.

Multiple-Choice Questions (10)

1. A bisexual person is?
   (a) Really gay
   (b) Really lesbian
   (c) Conflicted
   (d) A person who is attracted to more than one gender
2. Challenges that bisexual elders face include
   (a) Isolation
   (b) Few target social services

(c) Invisibility

(d) All of the above

3. The single largest part of the LGBT community is
   (a) Lesbian
   (b) Gay
   (c) Bisexual
   (d) Transgender

4. What two members of the LGBT community have been strong allies for advocacy?
   (a) Gays and Lesbians
   (b) Gays and transgender persons
   (c) Gays and bisexual persons
   (d) Bisexual persons and transgender persons

5. Which LGBT groups identify more strongly with ambiguity?
   (a) Gays
   (b) Transgender
   (c) Bisexuals
   (d) (b) and (c)
   (e) (a) and (c)

6. Which of the following has the highest reported rates of binge drinking?
   (a) Gay men
   (b) Lesbians
   (c) Transgender persons
   (d) Bisexuals

7. Which of the below is not a health problem for older bisexual persons?
   (a) Overweight
   (b) Underweight
   (c) High cholesterol
   (d) Intimate partner violence

8. Bisexual women have rates higher than their heterosexual counterparts of the following:
   (a) Cancer
   (b) Underinsurance
   (c) Difficulty obtaining medical care
   (d) All of the above

9. What identify issues do bisexuals face?
   (a) Homophobia
   (b) Employment discrimination
   (c) Social ostracism
   (d) All of the above

10. What one word best describe the community of bisexual elders?
    (a) Invisible
    (b) Well-recognized
    (c) Well organized
    (d) Protected under the law

Key (for multiple-choice questions)

1-d
2-d
3-c
4-d
5-d
6-b
7-d
8-d
9-b
10-a

Resources

- Bi Resource Center http://www.biresource.net/
- BiNet USA http://www.binetusa.org/
- American Institute of Bisexuality http://www.americaninstituteofbisexuality.org/
- Bisexual Organizing Project http://www.bisexualorganizingproject.org/
- *Bisexual Community Needs Assessment 2012* http://www.bisexualorganizingproject.net/Bi-Needs-Assessment.html
- *Bisexual invisibility: impacts and recommendations*, San Francisco Human Right Commission LBGT Advisory Committee http://www.birequest.org/docstore/2011-SF_HRC-Bi_Iinvisibility_Report.pdf
- *Healthy People 2020* http://www.healthy people.gov/
- *The bisexuality report: Bisexual inclusion in LGBT equality and diversity* http://bisexual research.wordpress.com/reportsguidance/reports/thebisexualityreport/

References

American Lung Association. (2010). Smoking out a deadly threat: Tobacco use in the LGBT community. Taken from *Healthy people 2020 bisexual health fact sheet, healthy people 2020 revised: November 2010.* Retrieved July 1, 2014, from http://www.lgbttobacco.org/files/HP2020BisexualPeople.pdf.

Bedecarre, C. (2001). Swear by the moon. *Hypatia, 2*(3), 2001.

Burleson, W. E. (2005). *Bi America: Myths, truths, and struggles of an invisible community.* New York: Routledge.

Burleson, W. E. (2013). *Bisexual community needs assessment 2012.* Minneapolis: Bisexual Organizing Project.

Diamant, A. L., Wold, C., Spritzer, K., Gelberg, L. (2000). Health behaviors, health status, and access to and use of health care: A population-based study of lesbian, bisexual and heterosexual women. *Family Medicine, 9* (10), 1043–1051. Taken from *Healthy people 2020 bisexual health fact sheet, healthy people 2020 revised: November 2010.* Retrieved July 1, 2014, from http://www.lgbttobacco.org/files/HP2020BisexualPeople.pdf.

Dobinson, C. (2010). Top ten bisexual health issues. Sherbourne Health Center, Toronto. Appendix A. *Healthy people 2020 bisexual health fact sheet, healthy people 2020* taken from http://www.healthypeople.gov/2020/topicsobjectives2020/overview.aspx?topicid=25.

Doll, L., Myers, T., et al. (1997). Bisexuality and HIV risk: Experiences in Canada and the United States, annual review of sex research, 8, pp. 102. Taken from the *Healthy people 2020 bisexual health fact sheet, healthy people 2020* Revised: November 2010. Retrieved July 1, 2014, from http://www.lgbttobacco.org/files/HP2020BisexualPeople.pdf.

Egan, P. J., Edelman, M. S., & Sherrill, K. (2008). *Findings from the hunter college poll of lesbians, gays, and bisexuals: New discoveries about identity, political attitudes, and civic engagement.* New York: Hunter College, City University of New York.

Fox, R. (2004). *Current research on bisexuality.* Binghamton: Harrington Park Press.

Hayes, B. G. (2001). Working with the bisexual client: How far have we progressed? *Journal of Humanistic Counseling, Education & Development, 40*(1), 11–20.

Herbenick, D., Reece, M., Schick, V., Sanders, S. A., Dodge, B., & Fortenberry, J. D. (2010). Sexual behavior in the United States: Results from a national probability sample of men and women aged 14–94. *Journal of Sexual Medicine, 7*(suppl 5), 255–265.

Horowitz, J., & Newcomb, M. (1999). Bisexuality, not homosexuality: Counseling issues and treatment approaches. *Journal of College Counseling, 2*(2), 148–163.

Keppel, B., (2006). Affirmative psychotherapy with older bisexual women and men. Co-published simultaneously in *Journal of Bisexuality, 6,* 1/2. In R. C. Fox (Ed.), *Affirmative psychotherapy with older bisexual women and men* (pp. 67–102). Binghamton, NY: Harrington Park Press, an imprint of The Haworth Press.

Kimmel, D., Rose, T., & David, S. (2006). *Lesbian, gay, bisexual, and transgender aging: Research and clinical perspectives.* New York: Columbia University Press.

Kinsey, A. C., Pomeroy, W. B., & Martin, C. E. (1948). *Sexual behavior in the human male.* Philadelphia: W. B. Saunders.

Klein, F. (1993). *The bisexual option* (2nd ed.). New York: Haworth Press.

Koh, A.S. (2000). Use of preventive health behaviors by lesbian, bisexual, and heterosexual women: questionnaire survey. *Western Journal of Medicine, 172*(6), 379–384. Taken from *Healthy people 2020 bisexual health fact sheet, healthy people 2020 revised: November 2010.* Retrieved July 1, 2014, from http://www.lgbttobacco.org/files/HP2020BisexualPeople.pdf.

Michael, R. T., Gagnon, J. H., Laumann, E. O., & Kolata, G. (1994). *Sex in America: A definitive survey.* Boston: Little, Brown and Company.

Mosher, W. D., Chandra, A., & Jones, J. (2005). Sexual behavior and selected health measures: men and women 15–44 years of age, United States, 2002. In *Advance data from vital and health statistics, 362.* Hyattsville, MD: National Center for Health Statistics.

New Mexico Department of Health. (April 2010). New Mexico's progress in collecting lesbian, gay, bisexual, and transgender health data and its implications for addressing health disparities. Retrieved from *Healthy people 2020 bisexual health fact sheet, healthy people 2020 revised: November 2010.* Retrieved July 1, 2014, from http://www.lgbttobacco.org/files/HP2020Bisexual People.pdf.

Ochs, R. (2014). *A few quotes from Robyn Ochs.* Retrieved July 12, 2014, from http://robynochs.com/bisexual/.

Polyamory Society. (2012). Retrieved June 23, 2014 from www.polyamorysociety.org.

Remez, L. (2000). As many lesbians have had sex with men, taking a full sexual history is important. *Family Planning Perspectives, 32*(2), 2730–2736.

San Francisco Human Right Commission LBGT Advisory Committee. (2011). *Bisexual invisibility: Impacts and recommendations,* San Francisco, CA.

Storms, M. D. (1978). Sexual orientation and self-perception. *Perception of emotion in self and others, advances in the study of communication and affect* (pp. 165–180). New York: Plenum.

Vernallis, K. (Winter 1999). Bisexual monogamy: Twice the temptation but half the fun? *Journal of Social Philosophy, 30*(3), 347–368.

Zickuhr, K., Madden, M. (2012). *Older adults and internet use, pew research internet project.* Retrieved July 12, 2014 from http://www.pewinternet.org/2012/06/06/older-adults-and-internet-use/.

Part III

Mistreatment and Victimization of Older LGBT Persons

An Overview of Aging and Mistreatment of LGBT Elders

16

Amanda E. Sokan and Pamela B. Teaster

Abstract

Many older adults experience their later life as a time when they may be able to enjoy the company of family and friends to an extent not possible during their working years. Most older adults, including those who are LGBT, remain in their homes as they age; most enjoy good and appropriate treatment by their family members, their extended family, and their services providers. However, for some older adults, old age is marred by unhealthy dependencies of families, friends, and others to the point that the older adult may experience abuse, neglect, and exploitation discretely or in escalation. Such harsh and life-threatening treatment of individuals in later life can occur in community as well as facility settings, as a single occurrence or over a protracted period of time. Elder mistreatment is thought to affect one in nine older adults, with 23.5 instances of mistreatment going unreported for each one reported to authorities.

Keywords

Elder mistreatment · Elder abuse · Policies · Services · LGBT

Overview

Many older adults experience their later life as a time when they may be able to enjoy the company of family and friends to an extent not possible during their working years. Most older adults, including those who are LGBT, remain in their homes as they age; most enjoy good and appropriate treatment by their family members, their extended family, and their services providers. However, for some older adults, old age is marred by unhealthy dependencies of families, friends, and others to the point that the older adult may experience abuse, neglect, and exploitation discretely or in escalation. Such harsh and life-threatening treatment of individuals in later life can occur in community as well as facility settings, as a single occurrence or over a protracted period of time. Elder mistreatment is thought to affect one in nine older adults

P.B. Teaster
Virginia Tech, Blacksburg, VA, USA
e-mail: pteaster@vt.edu

A.E. Sokan (✉)
University of Kentucky, Lexington, KY, USA
e-mail: ausoka2@uky.edu

© Springer International Publishing Switzerland 2016
D.A. Harley and P.B. Teaster (eds.), *Handbook of LGBT Elders*,
DOI 10.1007/978-3-319-03623-6_16

(Acierno et al. 2010), with 23.5 instances of mistreatment going unreported for each one reported to authorities.

Learning Objectives

By the end of the chapter, the reader should be able to:

1. Identify the types of elder mistreatment.
2. Understand the scope of elder mistreatment.
3. Explain the settings of abuse.
4. Identify policies and services for LBGT elders who are abused.

Introduction

For many people, aging is accompanied by an increased reliance on family members, caregivers, and friends. Reliance on others, especially caregivers, can cause enormous stress for LGBT elders because of their vulnerability to those who may discriminate against and abuse them (Balsam and D'Augelli 2006). Every year, one in nine older adults are reported to experience mistreatment at the hands of a trusted other, and, in most instances, at the hands of a family member (Acierno et al. 2010). The most recent prevalence study conducted in the state of New York indicates that for one report to an agency, a staggering 23.5 go unreported (Lachs et al. 2011). A population of older adults, set to rise to 20 % of the population by 2030, portends that the problem will only increase unabated unless current efforts improve and escalate. Despite zealous advocacy efforts to staunch the problem, elder mistreatment remains highly underfunded. According to Teaster et al. (2006b), for Adult Protective Services there were 253,421 reports of abuse of adults age 60 and over or 832.6 reports for every 100,000 people over the age of 60. Although LGBT elders face the same types of abuse, violence, and neglectful situations as their heterosexual counterparts, they also encounter exploitation because of their sexual identity (Teaster et al. 2014).

Research suggests that because of their sexual orientation and gender identity, LGBT elders experience victimization in the form of verbal abuse, threat of violence, physical assault, sexual assault, threat of orientation disclosure, discrimination, and physical attack. Among LGBT elders, men experience physical attack nearly three times more often. LGBT elders are less likely to seek help for abuse (National Center on Elder Abuse 2013). Social isolation is also a risk factor for elder abuse. LGBT elders are more likely to age alone than their heterosexual counterparts (Frazer 2009). Because of living in isolation and fear of discrimination, many LGBT elders are at high risk for elder abuse, neglect, and various forms of exploitation (National Academy on an Aging Society, GSA & SAGE 2011) See Chap. 30 for additional discussion of the impact of isolation for LGBT elders.

The purpose of this chapter is twofold. First, this chapter provides insights into the topic of elder mistreatment in general. Second, although issues of elder mistreatment of LGBT elders is discussed in detail in Chap. 17, the information presented in this chapter is intended to assist the reader to better understand the deeper and more nuanced issue of elder mistreatment as it concerns adult persons who are LGBT. In one respect, this chapter is a prelude to discussion of LGBT elders as a vulnerable population for mistreatment. Material presented in this chapter helps readers understand issues surrounding elder mistreatment in general and LGBT elder mistreatment in particular so that the reader can identify the problem and its context as well as mechanisms and systems in place for its amelioration and prevention. Discussed in this chapter are definitions of elder abuse, federal legislation regarding elder abuse, organizations that address elder abuse, and information concerning the impact of elder mistreatment at federal, state, local, and individual levels.

Elder Abuse and Its Definitions

The issue of elder mistreatment has been plagued by definitional ambiguity in the United States because, when it is considered a crime as it is in many instances, its definition is one established by state statutes or regulations. Statutory definitions have plagued the progress of research, as collection of elder abuse data did not comport to the language of the law or of public administration. For nearly three decades, the field of elder abuse has wrestled with this incongruity, with most researchers ceding to statutory definitions because of their overwhelming influence on how state governments collected the administrative data upon which they often relied (e.g., Teaster et al. 2006a, b; Bonnie and Wallace 2003; Nerenberg 2008).

The problem of elder abuse and its definition is hardly unique to the United States. Both developed and developing countries around the world have grappled with the same definitional problem. An international study of elder abuse by Podnieks et al. (2010), involving a total of 53 countries (362 respondents) from the six WHO world regions revealed an inadequate knowledge of laws and services about the issue and that barriers to addressing the problem included language issues and literacy.

A watershed document, *Elder Mistreatment: Abuse, Neglect, And Exploitation in An Aging America*, was produced by the National Academy of Sciences (NAS) in 2003, which has been highly influential in subsequent research and has even gained prominence worldwide (Podnieks et al. 2010). The document describes elder mistreatment as "(a) intentional actions that cause harm or create a serious risk of harm (whether or not harm is intended) to a vulnerable elder by a caregiver or other person who stands in a trust relationship to the elder or (b) failure by a caregiver to satisfy the elder's basic needs or to protect the elder from harm" (Bonnie and Wallace 2003, p. 40). The NAS definition made the important distinction and demarcation that abuse was to be perpetrated by a trusted other. Thus, the issue of self-neglect, the mainstay issue of

Adult Protective Services (see explanation below) caseloads, was considered elder abuse but not elder mistreatment. Also, abuse not committed by a trusted other was considered simply a crime with the elder as the victim.

Another important definition, also well received throughout the world is that promulgated by the World Health Organization (WHO), which indicates that elder abuse is "a single, or repeated act, or lack of appropriate action, occurring within any relationship where there is an expectation of trust which causes harm or distress to an older person". It is important to point out that, under the World Health Organization definition, elder mistreatment can take on multiple forms or repeated acts of abuse, a term referred to as *polyvictimization* (Ramsey-Klawsnik and Heisler 2014). Regardless of whether the abuse is a one-time occurrence or happens multiple times, the broad definition encompasses a variety of settings and a number of types, which are discussed below.

Settings of Abuse

Elder abuse occurs in two main settings, in community settings and in facility settings. Community settings can and do include an elder's own home or the home of an individual or individuals with whom the elder lives, typically that of a family member. Family members and friends with whom the elder may cohabitate, typically are the predominant abusers (Acierno et al. 2010). It is estimated that 90 % of all elder abuse occurs in community settings. These settings are difficult to permeate because there are fewer eyes and ears that witness the abuse first-hand than in facility settings (Teaster and Roberto 2004; Teaster et al. 2006b).

Elders are also abused in facility settings. These include a range of locations that provide long-term care, including adult congregate living, assisted living facilities, group homes, mental hospitals, and nursing homes. According to Hawes (2003), on an average day, approximately

1.6 million people live in a about 17,000 licensed nursing homes, and another estimated 900,000 to 1 million live in about 45,000 residential care facilities. Research suggests that the 2.5 million vulnerable individuals in these settings may well be at higher risk for abuse and neglect than older persons who live at home, as discussed below. Less is known about the prevalence of abuse in skilled nursing facilities than in other long-term care facilities. For example, elders living in skilled nursing facilities are among the most vulnerable members of society, precisely because they are often dependent on those employed by it for total care.

Typologies of Elder Mistreatment

As context for the global definitions presented earlier are the various types of elder abuse that may happen to an elder once or co-occur, these being physical, sexual, verbal/emotional, neglect (both active and passive), and financial abuse/exploitation. Self-neglect is another type of abuse that is also discussed within this chapter because of its implications for the LGBT community, and a topic that is discussed in greater detail in Chap. 17.

Physical Abuse According to the abuse typologies provided by the National Center on Elder Abuse (n.d.), *physical abuse* is characterized by the use of physical force that may result in bodily injury, physical pain, or impairment. Physical abuse may include but is not limited to acts of violence including striking (with or without an object), hitting, beating, pushing, shoving, shaking, slapping, kicking, pinching, and burning. In addition, inappropriate use of drugs and physical restraints, force-feeding, and physical punishment of any kind also are examples of physical abuse (Table 16.1).

From research on adults in community settings only and conducted by Acierno et al. (2010) the prevalence of physical abuse was 1.6 %. Similar studies of abuse by family members of community dwelling elders by Laumann et al.

(2008) reveal its prevalence to be 0.02 %, and Lachs et al. (2011) found 22.4 per thousand. The most recent national study of elder abuse reporting to APS (Teaster et al. 2006b) revealed 10.7 % of reports of physical abuse substantiated over a year's time.

Sexual Abuse Sexual abuse, thought to be the most hidden of the abuses (Ramsey-Klawsnik and Teaster 2012; Teaster and Roberto 2004) is defined by the NCEA (n.d.) as "non-consensual sexual contact of any kind with an elderly person. Sexual contact with any person incapable of giving consent is also considered sexual abuse. It includes, but is not limited to, unwanted touching, all types of sexual assault or battery, such as rape, sodomy, coerced nudity, and sexually explicit photographing." Acierno et al. found its prevalence to be 0.06 %, Lachs et al. found 0.03 per thousand for a documented case study, and Teaster et al. (2006b) found 1.0 substantiated reports to APS. Occurring in community and facility settings, sexual abuse is difficult to prove when an allegation is not followed up on immediately. For example, Ramsey-Klawsnik and Teaster et al. (2007) found that very few allegations involved a physical examination, let alone an examination by a Sexual Abuse Nurse Examiner (SANE).

Emotional Abuse/Psychological Abuse According to the National Center on Elder Abuse (n.d.), emotional or psychological abuse involves infliction of anguish, pain, or distress through verbal or nonverbal acts. This form of abuse includes but is not limited to verbal assaults, insults, threats, intimidation, humiliation, and harassment. Infantilizing an older person; isolating elders from family, friends, or regular activities; giving elders the "silent treatment;" and social isolation are examples of emotional/psychological abuse. In the Acierno et al. study (2010), its prevalence was 4.6 %, in Laumann's study, it was 9 %, and in the Lachs study (2011), it was found to be 16.4 % per thousand. In the Teaster et al. (2006b) study, there were 14.8 % substantiated reports of neglect in one year's time.

Table 16.1 Signs of elder mistreatment by type

Type	Signs and symptoms
Physical	• Injuries, scars, or other signs of physical trauma: e.g. Old or new bruises, lacerations, abrasions, black eyes, welts, sprains, dislocations, fractures of bone or skull, broken bones; internal injuries and/or bleeding • Untreated/unexplained or inadequately explained injuries in different stages of healing: e.g. Open wounds, cuts, punctures • Physical signs of being punished: e.g. Broken eye glasses/frames or other medical aid, burns • Signs of being restrained: e.g. Rope marks, pressure or imprint marks • Evidence of prescription drugs/medication underuse or overdose based on laboratory results • Sudden change in elder's behavior or ability to walk or sit • Caregiver refuses/is reluctant to allow visits with elder alone • Report by elder of being hit, kicked, harmed or mistreated
Sexual	• New or old bruises around breasts or genital area • Unexplained genital infections, sexually transmitted disease, or vaginal or anal bleeding/pain • Presence of bloody, stained or torn underwear/clothing • Flinching from touch • Report of sexual assault or rape made by an elder
Emotional/psychological	• Emotional agitation, upset, or unexplained fear • Extreme withdrawal, non-responsive or non-communicative behavior • Isolation • Exhibiting behavior such as biting, sucking, rocking, or other behavior usually attributed to dementia • Report of verbal or emotional mistreatment made by an elder
Neglect	• Dehydration: e.g. Dizziness, dry mouth, skin, or eyes; little or no urination • Unattended or untreated health problems: e.g. bed sores, depression • Malnutrition: e.g. Weight loss, lack of food • Poor personal hygiene and care: e.g. Looking unkempt, dirty, clothing that is soiled, torn, or inadequate for the weather • Unclean and unsanitary environment/living conditions: e.g. Evidence of dirt, garbage; insect/rodent/pest infestation, soiled bedding, fecal/urine smell, spoiled food • Unsafe or hazardous environment/living condition: e.g. Lack of amenities (electricity, heat, water), faulty wiring or fire hazards • Report of neglect or mistreatment made by an elder
Financial or material exploitation	• Sudden or unexplained changes in bank account or banking practice: e.g. a person accompanying an elder makes an unexpected/unexplained withdrawal of large sums of money • Financial mismanagement or poor financial stewardship: e.g. Using an elder's ATM card to make an unauthorized withdrawal of funds; presence of unpaid bills despite the sufficiency of financial resources • Unexpected changes to legal or financial documents: e.g. Changes to a Will; inclusion of additional names as signatories on an elder's bank account/card • Provision of services that are not necessary or substandard care: e.g. Making payment for unneeded services; overpayment for care; unnecessary or unauthorized purchases • Sudden appearance of unknown or previously uninvolved relatives or "new" friends: e.g. Person claiming rights to an elder's affairs and possessions; unanticipated or unexplained transfer of assets to a family member or someone outside the family; giving generous "gifts" • Fraud: e.g. Unexplained disappearance or misuse of funds or valuable possessions; forgery of an elder's signature for financial transactions or to obtain title to possessions • Report of financial exploitation made by an elder

(continued)

Table 16.1 (continued)

Type	Signs and symptoms
Self-neglect	• Dehydration: e.g. Dry eyes, mouth, skin; infrequent or no urination • Malnutrition: e.g. Lack of food, weight concerns • Untreated or poorly addressed medical conditions: e.g. Non-compliance with or refusing medication • Unsanitary or unclean environment/living quarters: e.g. Hoarding, garbage, animal/insect infestation, lack of working bathing/toilet facilities, smell of feces or urine • Poor personal hygiene: e.g. Unkempt appearance, dirty skin and nails; soiled or torn clothing • Poor personal care: e.g. Inadequate or inappropriate clothing; lack of required medical devices or supports such as dentures, hearing aids, eye glasses, cane/walker; drug/alcohol dependence • Challenging living arrangements: e.g. Inadequate housing, homelessness, lack of social support, isolation • Unsafe or hazardous environment /living conditions: e.g. Absence of light, heating, plumbing, running water; fire risks or other dangers, home in state of disrepair

Source National Center on Elder Abuse (NCEA) (n.d)

Neglect Neglect, which can be either active or passive, is defined by the NCEA "as the refusal or failure to fulfill any part of a person's obligations or duties to an elder. Neglect may also include failure of a person who has fiduciary responsibilities to provide care for an elder (e.g., pay for necessary home care services) or the failure on the part of an in-home service provider to provide necessary care. Neglect typically means the refusal or failure to provide an elderly person with such life necessities as food, water, clothing, shelter, personal hygiene, medicine, comfort, personal safety, and other essentials included in an implied or agreed-upon responsibility to an elder." For neglect, Acierno et al. (2010) found a prevalence of 5.1 %, in the Lachs study (2011), it was found to be 18.3 % per thousand, and in the Teaster et al. (2006b) study, there were 20.4 % substantiated reports of neglect in one year's time.

Exploitation This form of abuse is much the object of study in recent years because of its association with other forms of abuse. Financial or material exploitation is defined as the illegal or improper use of an elder's funds, property, or assets. Examples include, but are not limited to, cashing an elderly person's checks without authorization or permission; forging an older person's signature; misusing or stealing an older

person's money or possessions; coercing or deceiving an older person into signing any document (e.g., contracts or will); and the improper use of conservatorship, guardianship, or power of attorney. Concerning exploitation, Acierno et al. (2010) found a prevalence of 5.2 % by a family member, in the Lachs study (2011), it was found to be 42.1 % per thousand, in the Laumann et al. study 3.5 %, and in the Teaster et al. (2006b) study, there were 14.7 % substantiated reports of exploitation in a year's time.

The Context of Exploitation For the first time, a study conducted by the MetLife Mature Market Institute (2009) revealed that exploitation that was captured by the news media cost $2.6 billion a year. A follow-up study in 2011 revealed that the dollar amount had escalated to $2.9 billion per annum. When financial exploitation occurs in community settings, it usually involves a family member who has mental health or substance abuse problems or both. Other forms of exploitation can involve persons designated as an elder's power of attorney or court-appointed guardian. When the exploitation occurs in facility settings, about which less has been studied than in community settings, it can also involve residents of the facility or staff members, in addition to family members. Less examined exploitation by individuals and entities include magazine subscription scams, paving scams, telephone scams, Internet scams, and religious scams.

One way to differentiate the types of exploitation was conceived by the authors of the Met-Life Mature Market Institute study (2011): crimes of occasion, desperation and predation. Crimes of occasion or opportunity occur when a victim is merely a barrier in the way of what the perpetrator wants. For instance, an elder has money, assets, and the like, and an occasion presents itself for the perpetrator to access the resource. An occasion scenario was seen in the case of the holiday crime in which a woman was electrocuted with a stun gun and robbed after allowing someone into her home whom she thought was a pharmacist delivering medications. The occasion was the open door and a person whom she thought she could trust.

Crimes of desperation are typically those in which perpetrators are so desperate for money that they will do whatever it takes to get it. Many perpetrators are dependent on an elder parent for housing and for income. The desire for more money may be heightened due to the need for drugs, alcohol, and their gender, or some combination. The exploiter comes to believe that, in return for care, he or she is due compensation (money or possessions), and often on a continuing basis.

Finally, crimes of predation or occupation occur when trust is established for the purpose of financially abusing later. A relationship is built, either through a bond of trust created though developing a relationship (romantic or otherwise) or as a trusted professional advisor. Taking assets is accomplished by stealth and cunning.

Self-neglect Though not regarded as elder mistreatment because it does not involve abuse by a trusted other, elder self-neglect is one of the most vexing of the abuses encountered, precisely because its origin is difficult to pinpoint and because, in its most extreme form, the problem devolves into a public health risk and can result in removal of the elder from his or her home and concomitant loss of the individual's civil rights. According to NCEA (n.d.), self-neglect occurs when the behavior of an elder threatens his or her own health or safety and manifests itself as a refusal or failure to provide himself/herself with adequate food, water, clothing, shelter, personal hygiene, medication (when indicated), and safety precautions. An elder is not self-neglecting if he or she is mentally competent, understands the consequences of decisions, and makes a conscious and voluntary decision to engage in acts that threaten his/her health or safety as a matter of personal choice.

Self-neglect is reported to be the bulk of APS caseloads (Teaster et al. 2006b). When self-neglect of a community member is purported to occur, some of the thorniest of problems emerge. This situation could be an example of triple jeopardy for an LGBT elder who may become isolated due to his or her age, his or her sexual minority status, and because of fears about coming out to those who might help the situation. Because LGBT elders may have reduced social networks as they age, they may be susceptible to self-neglectful situations. The following scenario is emblematic: on the one hand, the LGBT elder and his or her deplorable situation is revealed and he or she, including all the animals and putrid food, stacks of newspaper and boxes are removed and given appropriate care (the appreciative community scenario). Alternately, the elder is forced, by the heavy hand of government, to do something that is abhorrent to him or her, and due to being LGBT, may suffer more intrusions because she is lesbian, old, and vulnerable. The long and intrusive arm of the state has interfered, once again, with a helpless citizen, and he or she is powerless in the face of this unique form of government intrusion (the elder/community as victim of government intervention).

Federal Legislation that Addresses Elder Abuse

The Older Americans Act

The Older Americans Act (1965) was the first federal level initiative aimed at providing comprehensive services for older adults. Based on a model of active aging, the Act created the National Aging Network, which is composed of Administration on Aging (now, the Administration for Community Living (federal level), State Units on Aging (state level), and Area Agencies on Aging (local level). The Act must be continually reauthorized by Congress, which has never allocated funding commensurate with its lofty aspirations. Though services are supposed to be provided based on age of the recipients (generally 60 years of age and older), they have become more and more focused due to historically flat or slight increases in funding. Notably, the Act has funded nutrition and supportive home and community-based services, disease prevention/health promotion services, training for employment, the National Family Caregiver Support Program and the Native American Caregiver Support Program, and elder rights programs (Title VII or the Vulnerable Elder Rights Protection Title). The purpose of Title VII was to strengthen and coordinate the Long-Term Care Ombudsman Program; Programs for the Prevention of Abuse, Neglect and Exploitation; State Elder Rights and Legal Assistance Development Programs; and Insurance/Benefits Outreach, Counseling and Assistance Programs. Two of the programs are discussed below in greater detail: the National Center on Elder Abuse and the Long-Term Care Ombudsman Program, predominantly local programs that are usually housed in Area Agencies on Aging.

The National Center on Elder Abuse

Directed by the U.S. Administration on Aging, the National Center on Elder Abuse (NCEA) is a resource for policy makers, social service and health care practitioners, the justice system, researchers, advocates, and families (National Center on Elder Abuse, n.d.). Operated under the Department of Health and Human Services, it provides such resources as training, advocacy information, research findings, interpretation of elder abuse statutes, a hotline, and celebration of

World Elder Abuse Awareness Day (WEEAD). The Center is re-established through a competitive request for proposals every four years. The newest iteration of the NCEA was awarded to the Keck School of Medicine of the University of Southern California, along with the USC Davis School of Gerontology, the American Bar Association and other organizations dedicated to supporting the aging in America. Through these organizations, the NCEA will provide technical assistance and training to states and community-based organizations to develop effective prevention, intervention and response efforts addressing elder abuse as well as conduct research and advocate for policy changes on behalf of older adults (Snelling 2014).

Long-Term Care Ombudsmen

Area Agencies on Aging (AAA) are a nationwide network of state and local programs that help older people plan and care for their needs. Area Agencies on Aging receive funds through the Administration for Community Living (ACL) and were established by the Older Americans Act, with their goal being to keep elders living independently in their own homes for as long as possible. Over 600 AAAs exist nationwide and provide social services and nutrition services for elders, as well as support for caregivers of elders. In addition, AAA is a useful resource for professionals and practitioners who care for or provide services for elders. AAAs typically house the long-term care ombudsman, which is discussed in greater detail below (Smith 2010; Stupp 2000).

Existing in all states, Long-Term Care Ombudsmen (LTCO), are advocates for residents of nursing homes, board and care homes, assisted living facilities and similar adult care facilities. They work to resolve problems of individual residents and to bring about changes at the local, state and national levels that will improve residents' care and quality of life. The Long-Term Care Ombudsman Program is authorized and funded under Title VII, Chapter 2,

Table 16.2 Responsibilities of the Long-Term care Ombudsman

Educate and inform	Provision of education and information on long-term care related issues and concerns
	Facilitation of public comment on laws, regulations, policies, and actions
	Provision of information to residents about long-term care services
Represent and protect	Representation of residents' interests before governmental agencies
	Protection of residents by seeking administrative, legal, and other remedies as appropriate
	Identification, investigation, and resolution of complaints made by or on behalf of residents
	Promotion of development of citizen organizations to participate in the program
Advocate and support	Advocating for changes to improve quality of life and care for residents
	Provision of analysis, commentary, and recommendations on which affect residents' rights, health, safety and welfare
	Provision of technical support and assistance to develop resident and family councils to protect the well-being and rights of residents

Source Older Americans Act, Title VII, Chapter 2, Sections 711/712

Sections 711/712 of the Older Americans Act, as well as other federal, state, and local sources (Administration for Community Living, n.d.). Each state has an Office of the State Long-Term Care Ombudsman headed by a full-time state ombudsman. Local ombudsman staff and volunteers work in communities throughout the country as part of statewide ombudsman programs, assisting residents and their families and providing a voice for those unable to speak for themselves. The Administration for Community Living funds the National Long-Term Care Ombudsman Resource Center, which is operated by the National Consumers' Voice for Quality Long-Term Care (or Consumer Voice), in conjunction with the National Association of States Agencies on Aging United for Aging and Disabilities (NASUAD), and which provides training and technical assistance to state and local ombudsmen. Program data for FY 2013 provide a flavor of the activities by LTCO: services to residents were provided by 1,233 full-time equivalent staff and 8,290 volunteers, trained and certified to investigate and resolve complaints who helped resolve 190, 592 complaints, initiated by residents, their families, and other concerned individuals, provided 335,088 consultations to individuals, visited 70 % of all nursing homes and 29 % of all board and care, assisted living and similar homes at least quarterly, and conducted 5,417 training sessions in facilities on such topics as residents' rights. In addition the LTCO provided 129,718 consultations to long-term care facility managers and staff

and participated in 21,812 resident council and 2,371 family council meetings (Administration for Community Living, n.d.). Ombudsmen help residents and their families and friends understand and exercise rights guaranteed by law, both at the Federal level for nursing homes and for States that provide rights and protections in board and care, assisted living and similar homes. Table 16.2 lists the responsibilities of the long-term care ombudsman.

Other Federal Legislation to Address Elder Mistreatment

In addition to the Older Americans Act mentioned above, there are two other important pieces of federal legislation that address elder mistreatment. These are the Social Security Block Grants and the Elder Justice Act (EJA).

Social Security Block Grants

Language in Title XX of the Social Security Act of 1974 gave permission for states to use Social Services Block Grant (SSBG) funds for the protection of adults as well as children (Mixson 1995). By the early 1980s, all states had created an office with the responsibility for providing protective services to some segment of the population, including services to the needy despite the absence of authorizing legislation (NAPSA 2014; U.S. Congress 1981). SSBG funds proved helpful in the establishment of programs to address elder mistreatment, especially Adult Protective Services (discussed below), but the funds are inadequate and diminishing even though reports of elder mistreatment are increasing.

The Elder Justice Act

The Elder Justice Act (EJA) was passed in 2010 as part of the Patient Protection and Affordable Care Act. Although passage of the EJA was truly a victory for the field of elder mistreatment, as of yet, the victory has been somewhat pyrrhic, as the EJA never received funding for its many outstanding provisions and it is set for reauthorization in 2015. Importantly, components of the Act have been undertaken, most notably the formation of the Elder Justice Coordinating Committee, composed of representatives from such agencies as the Administration for Community Living (ACL), the National Institute of Justice (DOJ), and the Social Security Administration. The EJA requires that the Department of Health and Human Services oversee the development and management of federal resources for protecting older adults from elder abuse, including establishing, enhancing, or funding:

- The Elder Justice Coordinating Council
- An Advisory Board on Elder Abuse
- Elder Abuse, Neglect, and Exploitation Forensic Centers
- Long-Term Care
- State and local adult protective service offices
- Grants to long-term care ombudsmen programs and for the valuation of programs
- Programs to provide training
- Grants to state agencies to perform surveys of care and nursing facilities

The EJA also includes directives for the U.S. Department of Justice (DOJ) for the prevention of elder abuse, which include:

- Developing objectives, priorities, policies and long-term plans for elder justice programs
- Conducting a study of state laws and practices relating to elder abuse, neglect and exploitation
- Making available grants to develop training and support programs for law enforcement and other first responders, prosecutors, judges, court personnel and victim advocates
- Ensuring that DOJ dedicates sufficient resources to the investigation and prosecution of cases relating to elder justice

A final feature of the EJA is the creation of a nationwide database and program for background checks for employees of care facilities. The EJA stipulates that elder abuse perpetrated in a long-term care facility must be reported immediately to law enforcement (EJC Fact Sheet 2014). (See Policy Box 16.1 on The Elder Justice Act).

Policy Box 16.1
The Elder Justice Act

Elder abuse is a complex issue demanding a multifaceted policy response that combines public health interventions, social services programs, and criminal law enforcement for abusive behavior. To address this problem, the Elder Justice Act was enacted as part of the Patient Protection and Affordable Care Act (ACA, P.L. 111-148, as amended). Provisions of the Act attempt to provide a coordinated federal response by emphasizing various public health and social service approaches to the prevention, detection, and treatment of elder abuse. The Elder Justice Act is the first national, comprehensive legislation to address abuse, neglect, and exploitation of elders. To date, most activities and programs authorized under the Elder Justice Act have not received federal funding through the appropriations process. Moreover, the authorizations of appropriations for most provisions under the act expire on September 30, 2014. Because of inadequate funding, the federal government has not fulfilled its role to address the prevention, detection, and treatment of elder abuse. Despite the paucity of discretionary appropriations, select elder justice activities have received mandatory funding appropriated through the ACA Prevention and Public Health Fund (PPHF). First, in FY2012, the Secretary of the Department of Health and Human Services (HHS) transferred $6.0 million to the Administration for Community Living (ACL) from the PPHF for new grants to states and tribes to test elder abuse prevention strategies. In FY2013, $2.0 million was transferred to ACL from the PPHF for elder justice activities, to fund the development of the National Adult Protective Services Data Reporting System Project. No other PPHF funds were transferred to ACL for elder justice activities for FY2014.

Source: Colello, K.J. (3 September 2014). The Elder Justice Act: Background and issues for Congress. Washington, D. C.: The Congressional Research Service.

Questions

1. Why has the Act received inadequate funding?
2. What types of initiatives have been funded?
3. What are the implications for the issue of elder mistreatment should the Act expire?

Organizations and Entities that Address Elder Mistreatment

A number of programs and organizations have evolved to address the different types of elder mistreatment delineated earlier. It is not within the scope of this chapter to explain them all, and so the topics presented below represent some of the more notable efforts operating on federal, state, and local levels.

Adult Protective Services

"*Adult Protective Services* (APS) are those services provided to older people and people with disabilities who are in danger of being mistreated or neglected, are unable to protect themselves, and have no one to assist them" (NAPSA 2001, p. 1). In most states, APS programs are the first responders to reports of the abuse, neglect, and exploitation of vulnerable adults. A vulnerable adult is regarded as a person being mistreated or in danger of being mistreated and who, due to age and/or disability, is unable to protect himself or herself. Though most APS programs serve vulnerable adults regardless of age, some serve only older persons (based either on their age or incapacity). A few programs serve only adults ages 18–59 who have disabilities that keep them from protecting themselves. Interventions provided by APS include, but are not limited to receiving reports of adult abuse, neglect, or exploitation; investigating the reports; assessing risk; developing and implementing case plans, service monitoring, and evaluation. Further, Adult Protection may provide or arrange for a wide selection of medical, social, economic, legal, housing, law enforcement, or other protective emergency or supportive services (NAPSA 2001).

Most APS programs have statutory and program coverage that includes both younger and older adults (68.5 % with statutes and 63.0 % with programs). According to Teaster et al. (2003) the state administering body responsible for its elder/adult services program was most typically the state human services agency and separate from the State Unit on Aging (SUA) (54.0 %). Forty percent (40.0 %) of programs were administratively housed under the SUA.

Over half of APS programs investigate in community and facility settings, with all authorized to investigate in domestic settings

(100.0 %), and over in institutional settings (68.5 %). Approximately sixty-five percent (64.8 %) had the authority to investigate in mental health/mental retardation settings. Some form of reporting laws exist for all APS programs. Most states and territories named health care professionals (e.g., licensed and registered nurses, physicians, and nurse aids) as mandated reporters (Teaster et al. 2003).

Multidisciplinary Teams

Multidisciplinary Teams (MDTs) typically operate on the local level and are composed of professionals from diverse disciplines who work together to address community-identified issues related to elder abuse (Anetzberger et al. 2004; Brandl et al. 2007; Nerenberg 2006; Teaster et al. 2003; Wiglesworth et al. 2006; Navarro et al. 2013). Over the past three decades, MDTs have evolved as increasingly viable groups to address elder mistreatment prevention and intervention due to the recognition that no single discipline or agency could adequately or appropriately address the problem. See Research Box 16.1 for a study on multidisciplinary teams in California.

Research Box 16.1
Outcomes of an Elder Abuse Forensic Center Navarro et al. (2013). Holding abusers accountable:

An elder abuse forensic center increases criminal prosecution of financial exploitation. *The Gerontologist, 53*(2), 303–312.
Purpose: Despite growing awareness of elder abuse, cases are rarely prosecuted. The aim of this study was to examine the effectiveness of an elder abuse forensic center compared with usual care to increase prosecution of elder financial abuse.
Design and Methods: Using one-to-one propensity score matching, cases referred to the Los Angeles County Elder Abuse Forensic Center (the Forensic Center)

between April 2007 and December 2009 for financial exploitation of adults aged 65 and older ($n = 237$) were matched to a population of 33,650 cases that received usual care from Adult Protective Services (APS).

Results: Significantly, more Forensic Center cases were submitted to the District Attorney's office (DA) for review (22 %, $n = 51$ versus 3 %, $n = 7$ usual care, $p < 0.001$). Among the cases submitted, charges were filed by the DA at similar rates, as was the proportion of resultant pleas and convictions. Using logistic regression, the strongest predictor of case review and ultimate filing and conviction was whether the case was presented at the Forensic Center, with 10 times greater odds of submission to the DA (Odds ratio = 11.00, confidence interval = 4.66–25.98).

Implications: Previous studies have not demonstrated that elder abuse interventions impact outcomes; this study breaks new ground by showing that an elder abuse multidisciplinary team increases rates of prosecution for financial exploitation. The elder abuse forensic center model facilitates cooperation and group problem solving among key professionals, including APS, law enforcement, and the DA and provides additional resources such as neuropsychological testing, medical record review, and direct access to the Office of the Public Guardian.
Questions

1. What is an elder abuse forensic center?
2. What are other desired outcomes of MDTs?
3. What do you see as the limitations to this research methodology?

Purposes of MDTs are to help resolve difficult cases, enable service coordination and identify gaps in services (Teaster et al. 2003; Teaster and

Wangmo 2010). The proliferation of MDTs has been accompanied by a growing demand for highly specialized expertise in such areas as financial abuse, forensic evidence, and evidence-based practice (Teaster et al. 2003; Nerenberg et al. 2012). An example of one state mandating the establishment of MDTs is featured in Discussion Box 16.1.

Discussion Box 16.1

Kentucky's Local Coordinating Councils on Elder Abuse

In the Commonwealth of Kentucky, under the aegis of the Area Agencies on Aging, local Adult Protective Services (APS), and the Kentucky Cabinet for Health and Family Services (CHFS), Local Coordinating Councils on Elder Abuse (LCCEA) were established in each Area Development District (ADD). The organization of each LCCEA reflects the needs of the region or county that it represents. Membership is drawn from different communities such as social services, health, legal, law enforcement, civic and banking. As a result, LCCEA members include a diverse group made up of APS personnel, local law enforcement officers and state police, judges and prosecutors, care providers, long-term care ombudsmen, academics, bankers, and other advocates for the elderly.

The goals for LCCEAs can be found on the CHFS website. LCCEAs are charged to:

(a) Develop and build an effective communitywide system of prevention and intervention that is responsive to the need of victims, perpetrators, family members and formal or informal caretakers.

(b) Identify and coordinate the roles and services of local agencies that work with elder abused, neglected or exploited victims and to investigate or prosecute elder abuse cases.

(c) Monitor, evaluate, and promote the quality and effectiveness of services and protection in the community.

(d) Promote a clear understanding of elder abuse, current laws, elder rights and resources available in the community.

(e) Serve as a clearinghouse for information on elder issues.

Additional information about the development and work of LCCEAS can be found online on the CHFS Website: http://chfs.ky.gov/dcbs/dpp/eaa/talkaboutit.htm

To Do:

Visit the CHFS website listed above and review the information on LCCEAs. Also look at the Model Protocol for Local Coordination Councils on Elder Abuse, as well as the case histories of suspected elder abuse or neglect that were investigated by the Kentucky Cabinet for Health and Family Services and or law enforcement authorities.

Discussion Questions:

1. How are the Councils coordinated at the local level? At the state level?
2. What are recent activities in which the Councils have participated?
3. What kind of MDT is associated with the Councils? Do these differ by region?
4. How would you go about setting up a local coordinating council in your county or region?

Summary

This chapter has provided overview information on elder mistreatment and the programs and services that have evolved to address the needs of this vulnerable population, a vulnerability exacerbated when sexual minority status is an additional factor. While much has been done to address the problem, there is still a tremendous need for greater excellence in research and practice (and the two working in concert). It is critical that higher levels of attention and funding be dedicated to this growing issue and problem, particularly because, that in the near future, the issue and problem of elder mistreatment will only increase in scope and severity.

Resources

Selected Annotated Resources Related to Elder Mistreatment

CANE: The Clearinghouse on Abuse and Neglect of the Elderly.

The Clearinghouse on Abuse and Neglect of the Elderly (CANE), located at the University of Delaware Center for Community Research and Service, is the nation's largest computerized catalog of elder abuse literature.

Website: http://www.cane.udel.edu/

National Committee for the Prevention of Elder Abuse (NCPEA): www.preventelderabuse.org

NCPEA is an association of researchers, practitioners, educators, and advocates working to protect the safety, security, and dignity of America's most vulnerable citizens. Established in 1988 to achieve a clearer understanding of abuse and provide direction and leadership to prevent it. NCPEA is a partner with the National Center on Elder Abuse.

National Clearinghouse on Abuse in Later Life (*NCALL*):

Website: http://ncall.us/

Through advocacy and education, the National Clearinghouse on Abuse in Later Life (NCALL) works everyday to improve victim safety, increase abuser accountability, expand coordinated community response, and ultimately, put an end to abuse in later life.

National Center on Elder Abuse (NCEA) http://www.ncea.aoa.gov/about/index.aspx)

The NCEA is one of 27 Administration on Aging-funded Resource Centers. The NCEA is the place to turn to for up-to-date information regarding research, training, best practices, news and resources on elder abuse, neglect and exploitation. The Center provides information to policy makers, professionals in the elder justice field, and the public.

National Consumer Voice for Quality Long Term Care

Website: http://healthfinder.gov/FindServices/Organizations/Organization.aspx?code=HR1872

The National Consumer Voice for Quality Long-Term Care is a 501(c)(3) nonprofit organization founded as the National Citizens' Coalition for Nursing Home Reform (NCCNHR) in 1975 by Elma Holder. The organization represents the consumer voice at the national level for quality long-term care, services and supports by advocating for public policies that support quality care and quality of life responsive to consumers' needs in all long-term care settings; empowering and educating consumers and families with the knowledge and tools they need to advocate for themselves; training and supporting individuals and groups that empower and advocate for consumers of long-term care; and promoting the critical role of direct-care workers and best practices in quality care delivery.

Safe Horizon

Website: http://www.safehorizon.org/

Safe Horizon is the largest victims' services agency in the United States. Safe Horizon offers assistance and support to children, adults, and families affected by crime and abuse throughout New York City, through 57 program locations, including shelter, in-person counseling, legal services, and more.

Other Resources

Websites

Administration on Aging (AoA—http://www.aoa.gov)

Administration for Community Living (ACL—www.acl.gov)

Elder Justice Coalition (www.elderjusticecoalition.com)

National Adult Protective Services Association (NAPSA—www.napsa-now.org)

National Committee for the Prevention of Elder Abuse (NCPEA—www.preventelderabuse.org)

National Association of Area Agencies on Aging (N4A—www.n4a.org)

National Association of States Agencies on Aging United for Aging and Disabilities (NASUAD—www.nasuad.org)

National Center on Elder Abuse (NCEA—www.ncea.aoa.gov)

National Consumers' Voice for Quality Long-Term Care (or Consumer Voice—http://theconsumervoice.org)

National Institute of Justice (NIJ—www.nij.gov)

National Long-Term Care Ombudsman Resource Center (NORC—www.ltcombudsman.org/)

Social Security Administration (www.ssa.gov)

World Health Organization (http://www.who.int/ageing/projects/elder_abuse/en/)

Learning Exercises

Self-Check Questions

1. Explain what is meant by physical abuse.
2. Explain what is meant by neglect by a caregiver.
3. Discuss differences between elder abuse in community versus facility settings.
4. Characterize who are most often the victims of elder abuse.
5. What services are available for those elders who have been abused in community settings? In facility settings?

Experimental Exercises

1. Interview an APS staff member about a case of exploitation that he or she has worked recently.
2. Interview Long-Term Care Ombudsman about a case of exploitation that he or she has worked recently.
3. List ways that you could prevent elder abuse.

Multiple-Choice Questions

1. In what setting do we think elder mistreatment occurs most often?
   (a) Community settings
   (b) Facility settings
2. What type of abuse is not considered mistreatment?
   (a) Physical abuse
   (b) Neglect
   (c) Exploitation
   (d) Self-neglect
3. All of the below are examples of a trusted other except:
   (a) Banker
   (b) Family member
   (c) Stranger
   (d) Home health worker
4. Who are most likely perpetrators in community settings?
   (a) Repair persons
   (b) Housecleaners
   (c) Bankers
   (d) Family members
5. A holiday crime occurred when a woman was electrocuted with a stun gun and robbed after allowing someone into her home whom she thought was a pharmacist delivering medications. Is this a crime of:
   (a) Predation
   (b) Desperation
   (c) Occasion
   (d) None of the above
6. What type of abuse constitutes the bulk of APS caseloads?
   (a) Abuse

(b) Neglect

(c) Exploitation

(d) Self-neglect

7. Which of the entities below does not address elder mistreatment?

(a) Police

(b) Long-term care ombudsman

(c) Adult Protective Services

(d) None of the above

(e) All of the above

8. Which of the entities below is the most frequent program of first report when there is an allegation of the abuse of an elder?

(a) Police

(b) Long-term care ombudsman

(c) Adult Protective Services

(d) None of the above

(e) All of the above

9. Which piece of legislation most directly affects the issue of elder mistreatment?

(a) Social Security Act

(b) Medicare

(c) The Elder Justice Act

(d) Age Discrimination in Employment Act

10. What is the most hidden form of elder mistreatment?

(a) Sexual abuse

(b) Physical abuse

(c) Psychological abuse

(d) Self-neglect

Key for multiple-choice questions

1-a

2-d

3-c

4-d

5-c

6-d

7-e

8-e

9-c

10-d

References

Acierno, R., Hernandez, M. A., Amstadter, A. B., Resnick, H. S., Steve, K., Muzzy, W., & Kilpatrick, D. G. (2010). Prevalence and correlates of emotional, physical, sexual, and financial abuse and potential neglect in the United States: The National Elder Mistreatment Study. *American Journal of Public Health, 100,* 292–297. doi:10.2105/ajph.2009.163089.

Administration for Community Living, n.d. Long-Term Care Ombudsman Program (OAA, Title VII, Chapter 2, Sections 711/712). Retrieved on December 17, 2014 at http://www.aoa.acl.gov/AoA_Programs/Elder_Rights/Ombudsman/index.aspx.

Anetzberger, G. J., Dayton, C., Miller, C. A., McGreevey, J. F., & Schimer, M. (2004). Multidisciplinary teams in the clinical management of elder abuse. *Clinical Gerontologist, 28,* 157–171.

Balsam, K. F., & D'Augelli, A. R. (2006). The victimization of older LGBT adults: Patterns, impact and implications for intervention. In D. Kimmel, T. Rose, & S. David (Eds.), *Lesbian, gay, bisexual, and transgender aging: Research and clinical perspectives* (pp. 110–130). New York, NY: Columbia University Press.

Bonnie, R. J., & Wallace, R. B. (Eds.). (2003). *Elder mistreatment: Abuse, neglect, and exploitation in an aging America.* Washington, D.C.: National Academies Press.

Brandl, B., Dyer, C. B., Heisler, G. J., Otto, J. M., Stiegel, L. A., & Thomas, R. W. (2007). *Elder abuse detection and intervention: A collaborative approach.* New York: Springer Publishing.

Elder Justice Coalition (2014). *Fact sheet—summary of the elder justice act and status.* Retrieved December 7, 2014 from http://elderjusticecoalition.com/factsheets.

Frazer, S. (2009). *LGBT health and human services needs in New York state.* Empire State Pride Agenda Foundation. Albany, NY. Retrieved December 27, 2014 from http:www.prideagenda.org/Portals?0?pdfs/LGBT%20 and %20Human%20Services%20Needs%20in%20New%20York%20State.pdf.

Hawes, C. (2003). Elder abuse in residential long-term care settings: What is known and what information is needed. In R. J. Bonnie & R. B. Wallace (Eds.), *Elder mistreatment: Abuse, neglect, and exploitation in an aging America* (pp. 446–500). Washington, D.C.: National Academies Press.

Laumann, E. O., Leitsch, S. A., & Waite, L. J. (2008). Elder mistreatment in the United States: Prevalence estimates from a nationally representative study. *The Journals of Gerontology Series B: Psychological Sciences and Social Sciences, 63,* S248–S254.

Lachs et al. (2011). Elder abuse: Under the radar. Lifespan of Greater Rochester Inc. Retrieved December 10, 2014 from http://www.lifespan-roch.org/documents/ElderAbusePrevalenceStudyRelease.pdf.

MetLife Mature Market Institute. (2009). *Broken trust: A report on the financial abuse of elders*. Westport, CT: Metlife Mature Market Institute.

Mature Market Institute (2011). *The MetLife study of elder financial abuse: Crimes of occasion, desperation, and predation against America's elders*. Westport, CT: Metlife Mature Market Institute.

Mixson, P. M. (1995). An adult protective services perspective. *Journal of Elder Abuse & Neglect, 7*(2–3), 69–87.

NAPSA (May 2001). *History of adult protective services.* Retrieved on December 2, 2014 at http://www.napsa-now.org/about-napsa/history/history-of-adult-protective-services/.

National Center on Elder Abuse (n.d.). *15 Questions & Answers About Elder Abuse*. Retrieved December 5, 2014 from http://www.ncea.aoa.gov/Resources/Publication/docs/FINAL%206-06-05%203-18-0512-10-04qa.pdf.

National Center on Elder Abuse. (2013). *Mistreatment of lesbian, gay, bisexual, and transgender (LGBT) elders*. Retrieved December 27, 2014 from www.ncea.aoa.gov/Resources/Publication/doc/NCEA_LGBT_ResearchBrief_2013.pdf.

Navarro, A. E., Gassoumis, Z. D., & Wilbur, K. H. (2013). Holding abusers accountable: An elder abuse forensic center increases criminal prosecution of financial exploitation. *The Gerontologist, 53*, 303–312.

Nerenberg, L. (2006). Communities respond to elder abuse. *Journal of Gerontological Social Work, 46*, 5–33.

Nerenberg, L. (2008). *Elder abuse prevention: Emerging trends and promising strategies*. New York: Springer Publishing Company.

Nerenberg, L., Davies, M., & Navarro, A. E. (2012). In pursuit of a useful framework to champion elder justice. *Generations, 36*, 89–96.

Podnieks, E., Anetzberger, G. J., Teaster, P. B., Wangmo, T., & Wilson, S. (2010). Worldview on elder abuse: An environmental scan. *Journal of Elder Abuse and Neglect, 22*, 164–179.

Ramsey-Klawsnik, H., & Heisler, C. (2014). Polyvictimization in later life. *Victimization of the Elderly and Disabled, 17*(1), 3–6.

Ramsey-Klawsnik, H., Teaster, P. B., Mendiondo, M. S., Abner, E. L., Cecil, K. A., & Tooms, M. R. (2007). Sexual abuse of vulnerable adults in care facilities: Clinical findings and a research initiative. *Journal of the American Psychiatric Nurses Association, 12*, 332–339.

Ramsey-Klawsnik, H., & Teaster, P. B. (2012). Sexual abuse of health care facility residents: Adult Protective Services and facility policy and practice implications. *Generations, 36*, 53–59.

Smith, J. (2010). Area agencies on aging: A community resource for patients and families. *Home Healthcare Nurse, 28*(7), 416–422.

Snelling, S. (2014, September 29). Keck School of Medicine to house National Center on Elder Abuse. *USC News*. Retrieved from https://news.usc.edu/69159/keck-school-of-medicine-to-house-national-center-on-elder-abuse/.

Stupp, H. W. (2000). Area agencies on aging. A network of services to maintain elderly in their communities. *Care Management Journal, 2(1)*, 54–62.

Teaster, P. B., Harley, D. A., & Kettaneh, A. (2014). Aging and mistreatment: Victimization of older adults in the United States. In H. F. O. Vakalahi, G. M. Simpson, & N. Giunta (Eds.), *The collective collective spirit of aging across cultures* (pp. 41–64). New York, NY: Springer.

Teaster, P. B., Nerenberg, L., & Stansbury, K. (2003). A national study of multidisciplinary teams. *The Journal of Elder Abuse and Neglect, 15*, 91–108.

Teaster, P. B., & Roberto, K. A. (2004). The sexual abuse of older adults: APS cases and outcomes. *The Gerontologist, 44*, 788–796.

Teaster, P. B., Roberto, K. A., & Dugar, T. D. (2006a). Intimate partner violence of rural aging women. *Family Relations, 55*, 636–648.

Teaster, P., Dugar, T., Mendiondo, M., Abner, A., Cecil, K., and Otto, J., (2006b). *The 2004 survey of state adult protective services: Abuse of adults 60 years of age and older*. Washington D.C.: National Center on Elder Abuse.

Teaster, P. B., & Wangmo, T. (2010). Kentucky's local elder abuse coordinating councils: A model for other states. *Journal of Elder Abuse and Neglect, 22*, 191–206.

U.S. House Select Committee on Aging. (1981). Elder abuse: An examination of a hidden problem. *All U.S. Government Documents (Utah Regional Depository)*. paper 136. Retrieved on December 1, 2014 at http://digitalcommons.usu.edu/govdocs/136.

Wiglesworth, A., Mosqueda, L., Burnight, K., Younglove, T., & Jeske, D. (2006). Findings from an elder abuse forensic center. *The Gerontologist, 46*, 277–283.

Mistreatment and Victimization of LGBT Elders

Pamela B. Teaster and Amanda E. Sokan

Abstract

The mistreatment and victimization of older LGBT adults is slowly coming to light in both practice and research. However, at this point, few studies examine this phenomenon. What is certain is that being LGBT may place elders at increased risk for mistreatment due to factors such as isolation, previous exposure to a traumatic event, and reticence to seek assistance from informal and formal networks. Penalties for elder mistreatment must be utilized by law enforcement more frequently, and statues that explore elder mistreatment as a hate crime also explored. It is critical that advocates, practitioners, researchers, and policy makers understand, intervene in, and prevent the mistreatment of LGBT elders.

Keywords

Mistreatment · Victimization · LGBT elders · Social isolation · Elder abuse

Overview

The purpose of this chapter is to explore the scope of the problem of the mistreatment of LGBT elders. In the first part of this chapter, we look closely at those who are characterized as

mistreated. Second, we discuss possible remedies to the problem of mistreatment and victimization. Next, we suggest future research on the topic. Finally, we examine model programs and approaches for prevention and intervention. Chapter 17 provides an important adjunct to Chap. 16 and provides information concerning who is mistreated, how they are mistreated, and why they are mistreated. Elder mistreatment and victimization are recognized as both a national and international health crisis. Research suggests that elder mistreatment and victimization occur across all ethnicities, in various settings, and within cultures that once held elders in high

P.B. Teaster (✉)
Virginia Tech, Blacksburg, VA, USA
e-mail: pteaster@vt.edu

A.E. Sokan
University of Kentucky, Lexington, KY, USA
e-mail: ausoka2@uky.edu

regard. Although LGBT elders often experience the same types of mistreatment and victimization as elders in general, LGBT elders have their experiences within the context of being sexual minorities. This additional *positionality* not only sets LGBT elders apart from their non-LGBT counterparts, it also necessitates specific and unique approaches to addressing the problem of elder mistreatment and victimization. Given this context, it is our intent to highlight discrimination by practice and policy against LGBT elders and to focus on disparities in response to mistreatment and victimization of LGBT elders as a culturally diverse population that is already marginalized by age, socioeconomic status, and a host of other demographic characteristics.

Learning Objectives

By the end of the chapter, the reader should be able to:

1. Identify the incidence and prevalence of elder mistreatment.
2. Characterize victims and perpetrators of LGBT elder mistreatment.
3. Discuss risk factors for LGBT elder mistreatment.
4. Explain possible remedies for LGBT elder mistreatment.
5. Discuss future research on LGBT elder mistreatment.
6. Identify select programs and approaches on LGBT elder mistreatment.

Introduction

According to Gates (2011), approximately nine million Americans identify as lesbian, gay, bisexual, or transgender (LGBT). Of that population, the Movement Advancement Project (MAP), Services and Advocacy for Gay, Lesbian, Bisexual, and Transgender Elders (SAGE), and the Center for American Progress

(CAP) (2010) estimate that 1.5 million adults aged 65 and over are LGB, with no reliable estimates for elders who identify as transgender. All estimates are likely undercounts due to the as yet considerable stigma associated with "coming out" at any age. "Coming out" for elders may be even more problematic than for their younger counterparts (e.g., historical mistreatment of those who identify as LGBT, decreased desirability being older and LGBT, increased possibility of being dependent on others). Elders who identify as LGBT face yet another challenge, which is that of experiencing elder mistreatment. Some LGBT elders must often contend with abusing, neglecting, or exploiting family members, including intimate partner violence that can result in social isolation and low help-seeking behaviors (National Center on Elder Abuse 2013).

The Scope of the Problem

It is necessary to emphasize at the outset of this chapter that the information available on the mistreatment of LGBT elders is, at best, only a rough estimate or extrapolation from extant data sources. Furthermore, information on transgender elder mistreatment is even more limited. Stated in earlier chapters, many elders are highly reticent to "come out" or stay out because of the treatments and attitudes that they have witnessed: the AIDS epidemic, various court cases concerning same-sex marriages, and individual treatment and classification of LBGT persons that, despite apparent greater acceptance, are still pervasive today. According to the MetLife Mature Market Institute LGBT elders study (2006), 27 % of baby boomers reported that discrimination was a great concern for them.

D'Augelli and Grossman (2001) surveyed 416 LGB elders aged 60 and over to explore lifetime victimization based on their sexual orientation. Nearly two-thirds reported experiencing some form of sexual orientation victimization, with males reporting more overall victimization than their female counterparts. Of that group, the authors went on to say that 29 % had been physically assaulted. Similarly, Frazer (2009) surveyed 3500 LGBT elders aged 55 and older and found that 8.3 % reported being abused or neglected by a caregiver due to homophobia; 8.9 % reported being financially exploited for the same reason. Persons who identify as transgender reported that 42 % experienced some type of physical violence or abuse and that 80 % experienced verbal abuse or harassment (MAP 2009). Fredrikson-Goldsen et al. (2011) found, in a study of 2560 LGBT elders, that due to the perception of being LGBT, 82 % of elders had been victimized once in their lives, with 64 % being victimized at least three times.

One area almost never considered in the elder mistreatment literature is that of transgendered elders (Cook-Daniels 2002) (see Chap. 14). Research is bearing out that the social intolerance of transgendered people may be even more intense than that of LGB persons (Lombardi et al. 2002). Violence is caused both by those who are intimate and by those who are distant to him or her. Such maltreatment serves to decrease help-seeking and increase isolation, which in turn make transgendered individuals even more at risk for abuse (e.g., little social support and a history of experiencing a traumatic event) (Acierno et al. 2010).

Although research is continually refining estimates of the incidence and prevalence of elder mistreatment, major national studies of elder mistreatment have, in the main, neglected to include variables that identify elders who are LGBT (Chap. 16). However, it is possible, by extension, to develop a rudimentary understanding of elder mistreatment as it affects LGBT victims, whose unique and individual experiences are discussed below.

LGBT Victims of Elder Abuse

LGBT victims of elder abuse are victimized in several ways. First, as Cook-Daniels stressed (2002) the society in which LGBT elders aged was extremely homophobic. For example, gay men were routinely fired from their positions, rejected by their families, targets of police brutality and harassment, and, until present times, denied the right to marry and its associated rights. Further,

> Social condemnation of people who have relationships or sex with persons of their own gender is so strong that even those who do not identify themselves as gay or lesbian, those who do not associate with other known Gays or Lesbians, and those who 'come out' late in life nevertheless adopt many of the same protective behaviors and social adaptations as those who have long labeled themselves as Gay (Cook-Daniels 2002, p. 3).

Although some protective behaviors may safeguard elders from abuse (e.g., larger friend networks in later life), other behaviors result in becoming more isolated over time and consequently make the elder more vulnerable to abuse, neglect, and exploitation (Acierno et al. 2010). A number of factors, including being LGBT, as well as age-related changes, can make an LGBT elder at risk for abuse.

LGBT elders are particularly vulnerable to abuse for a variety of reasons. These individuals are more likely to be estranged from family members or to be childless, which decrease access to children or family members for support when they need care. Another reason LGBT elders are at risk for mistreatment and victimization is discrimination in healthcare, human services, and some long-term care (LTC) facilities. Too often the forms of discrimination in LTC facilities are dismissed or ignored. Examples of mistreatment and victimization include harassment, limits on visitors, prohibiting same-sex couples from sharing a room, or refusal to recognize a person's gender identity.

Characteristics of Victims. In a national prevalence study by Acierno et al. (2010), in which self-report data were collected from 5777 older adults, average age of 71.5 years, 60.2 % (3477) were female and 39.8 % (2300) were male. As of yet, no information on sexual orientation of the men and women has been discussed in peer-reviewed publications. Respondents indicated that 56.8 % were married or cohabitating, 11.8 % (677) were separated or divorced, 25.1 %

(1450) were widowed, and 5.2 % (303) had never married. Also, and by self-report, 87.5 % (4876) of respondents were White, 6.7 % were African American, 2.3 % were American Indian or Alaskan Native, 0.8 % (49) were Asian, and 0.2 % (13) were Pacific Islanders.

Similarly, in the New York State Prevalence study by Life span of Greater Rochester (2011), which surveyed 4136 adults aged 60 years of age and older and which also did not provide information on sexual preference, respondents' self-reports revealed the following victims' characteristics: 20.3 % were between 60 and 64 years of age, 38.0 % were between ages 65 and 74, 29.1 % were ages 75 and 84, and 12.7 % were aged 85+. The self-reported gender breakdown was 35.8 % male and 64.2 % female. Respondents self-reported being 65.5 % were Caucasians, 26.3 % were African Americans; 1.6 % were Asian/Pacific Islanders; 7.6 % were Hispanic/Latino; 1.9 % were American/Aleut Eskimos; and 2.9 % were "other" races.

A much smaller and national study, which also did not collect data on LGBT elders, examined 26 cases reported and screened in for investigation concerning the alleged sexual abuse of older men (aged 50 and older) residing in nursing homes. Cases occurred in five states within a six-month time period. Of these, six were confirmed upon investigation by Adult Protective Services (APS) or other regulatory agencies. Victims tended to be predominately white males with cognitive and physical deficits that limited their ability for self-care. The most typical sexual abuse alleged and substantiated was fondling. Residents were more often substantiated as the abuser than other perpetrators. The sexual abuse of older men in nursing homes crossed gender, cultural, and role boundaries.

Victims' Risk Factors. Age may well be a risk factor for mistreatment, although studies regarding its significance are ambivalent. State agencies (e.g., APS; Teaster et al. 2006) and empirical studies concentrating on specific types of abuse (e.g., sexual, financial) have identified adults aged 75 and older as being particularly susceptible to mistreatment (Burgess et al. 2000; Met-Life Mature Market Institute2011). National community-based studies by Acierno et al. (2010) and Laumann et al. (2008) revealed that young-old individuals (60–69) were more prone to abuse than their older counterparts, especially emotional and physical abuse. The linkage between age and risk of mistreatment or abuse may be related to the increasing numbers in the population of old–old and oldest–old elders, many of whom may experience a decline in health results in greater dependence on others for self-care than for the general population of older adults.

Lack of social support. Elders at advanced ages may also experience reduced interactions with members of their social network than those of their younger counterparts, which may be a protective factor for mistreatment. According to Charles and Carstensen (2010), older adults have a propensity to judge the trustworthiness of others more favorably than do their younger counterparts and, consequently, may exacerbate their vulnerability for financial exploitation. Castle et al. (2012) examined age differences in perceived trust using neuroimaging methodology and posited that "older adults might have a lower visceral warning signal in response to cues of untrustworthiness, which could make deciding whom to trust difficult" (p. 20851).

Both Acierno et al. (2010) and Amstadter et al. (2011) stress that low levels of social support are correlated with the occurrence of all types of elder abuse. Elders who are lonely or isolated are significantly more vulnerable to elder mistreatment than are elders with strong support systems. According to Acierno et al. (2010), low social support was associated with more than triple the propensity for mistreatment of any form to be reported by elders. Further, Amstadter et al. (2011) found that low levels of social support significantly predicted the likelihood of older adults experiencing emotional and physical mistreatment (see Chap. 30 for further discussion of social isolation).

Gender. In the general older adult population, older women are more likely to be victimized than older men (Hightower 2004; Wisconsin Coalition Against Domestic Violence 2009; Krienert et al. 2009). Higher rates of older women who experience mistreatment may be attributed to their longer life span (and the associated vulnerabilities mentioned above), which may provide the occasion to be in contact with potential abusers (Krienert 2009). Women are subjected to higher rates of family violence across their life span than men. This fact, together with research by Acierno et al. (2010) revealing that previous exposure to a traumatic life event (e.g., interpersonal and domestic violence) increases an elder's risk of late life mistreatment, may explain how vulnerabilities related to gender and power dynamics create a component of risk for elder abuse (Wisconsin Coalition Against Domestic Violence 2009).

Race. In addition to gender, Lachs et al. (1997) found that race was a risk factor for mistreatment: more black elders appeared at risk for mistreatment than their white counterparts. However, the authors acknowledged that a limitation of their findings was their use of APS cases as the unit of analysis. Similarly, Tatara (1999) found that black and Hispanic elders were overrepresented in data on elder abuse victims (31 state APS systems), whereas nearly one in three victims known to authorities was a minority elder. Different cultures and how they define and approach elder mistreatment may serve to protect or promote the occurrence of a minority elder's risk for mistreatment (DeLiema et al. 2012; Horsford et al. 2010).

Physical health. Poor overall health and disabilities that impair an elder's ability to self-care may exacerbate his or her risk for abuse. According to Laumann et al. (2008), older adults who reported any type of physical vulnerability were 13 % more likely to report verbal mistreatment than study participants who reported none. Similarly, Acierno et al. (2010) reported that the likelihood of financial exploitation by both family members and strangers increased for older adults with more severe physical disabilities and that poor health predicted neglect. Further analysis of these data by Amstadter et al. (2011) revealed that the need for assistance with activities of daily living and poor health status were significant correlates of emotional abuse,

physical abuse, neglect, and financial abuse and exploitation of older adults (see Chap. 33 for additional information on LGBT elders and disabilities).

Cognitive Impairment. Changes in cognitive functioning also have been associated with increased risk of physical abuse, emotional abuse, caregiver neglect, and financial exploitation. In a study of 8932 older adults in Chicago, of which 238 were identified as victims of elder abuse by social service professionals, Dong et al. (2011) noted that several types of age-related cognitive changes contributed to elder abuse risk. After controlling for other known risk factors (e.g., medical conditions, depressive symptoms, and little social support), lower levels of global cognition, higher dementia severity, lower levels of episodic memory, and slower perceptual speed were all independently associated with an increased risk of abuse. Cognitive impairment increases exponentially with age and is perhaps the most pervasive and salient risk factor for financial abuse and exploitation (Sherod et al. 2009).

Other risk factors. Additional risk factors for the general population of elders were examined by Acierno et al. (2010) who found that 45.7 % (2262) of respondents self-reported low household incomes, 80.9 % (5174) were unemployed or retired, 22.3 % reported poor health, 62.0 % had experienced a previous traumatic event, 43.6 % perceived their social support as low, 40.8 % used some form of social services, and 37.8 % needed some assistance with activities of daily living.

In the Lifespan of Greater Rochester study (2011), for victims for whom respondent agency/programs reported about living arrangements, 45.8 % lived alone, 16.9 % lived with spouses or partners, 17.3 % lived with adult children, 7 % lived with sons-in-law or daughters-in-law, 6.3 % lived with grandchildren, 4.7 % lived with other relatives, and 8.8 % lived with other non-relatives. Over three-fourths of agencies were unable to provide incomes of reported victims; however, for the 17.4 % who could report this information, 59.3 % of victims were living at or below the poverty threshold.

Discussion Box 17.1: Victim Characteristics
Discussion Questions:

1. How might abuse victims who are LGBT elders differ from those of the majority population?
2. Discuss the challenges related to service provision facing LGBT elder victims seeking help.
3. Discuss the challenges related to confronting perpetrators of the abuse of LGBT elder victims.
4. Examine one resource in detail and how it might be of help to elder LGBT victims.

LGBT Elders and Risk Factors

Findings from the research literature on heterosexual adults suggest that many factors—demographic, social, cultural, historical, behavioral and psychological—singularly or in concert, may exacerbate, moderate, or reduce the risk for LGBT elder abuse. In addition to conditions shared with their heterosexual counterparts, older LGBT adults have different healthcare needs by virtue of their sexual minority status. Such needs include diets that may be too rich and exercise that is too infrequent, stresses from unhealthy or violent relationships, and sexually transmitted diseases that are ignored or poorly diagnosed because of societal stigma (Institute of Medicine [IOM] 2011). A 2012 CDC report on HIV among gay, bisexual, and men who have sex with men (MSM) revealed that health challenges for this population include higher risk factors and incidence of health disorders among lesbian and gay elders (see Chap. 20). By extrapolation, these healthcare needs create the potential for LGBT elders to be dependent upon others for care in ways different from their heterosexual counterparts, and in addition to these disparities, their sexual minority status may exacerbate their

vulnerability, and hence, their potential to be abused in old age. Reticence to ask for help may increase their susceptibility to episodic and prolonged periods of abuse, as evident from the MetLife Mature Market Institute study (2006) revealing that more than 50 % of LGBT baby boomers believed they would receive disrespectful and undignified treatment from healthcare professionals.

A recent cross-sectional study by Fredriksen-Goldsen et al. (2014) of 2560 LGBT adults aged 50 and older investigated the relationship between physical and mental health-related quality of life. The study revealed that physical and mental health quality of life was negatively associated with discrimination and chronic conditions and positively associated with social support and being male. The authors found that mental health was positively associated with positive sense of sexual identity and negatively with sexual identity disclosure. The influence of discrimination on the 80+ group affected them more than other age groups.

Though in no way all, some LGBT elders may be disproportionately victims of intimate partner violence (Cook-Daniels 2002). Similar to the experiences of younger victims, issues of power and control are pervasive when considering this form of elder abuse (Brandl 2004; Nelson et al. 2004; Pillemer and Finkelhor 1988; Podnieks 1992). Though little data exist, some older LGBT persons possess a "perfect storm" of risk factors for intimate partner violence: societal homophobia, reduced social networks, previous exposure to a traumatic event, reticence to help-seek, low self-esteem, and fear of being outed and being placed in a facility.

The interaction between discrimination and physical and mental health quality of life requires a consideration of LGBT elders in LTC facilities. Like their non-LGBT counterparts, more elders are using the broad spectrum of services offered by the LTC industry including nursing homes, continuing care retirement communities, skilled nursing facilities, and boarding homes to name a few. LGBT elders are, however, more likely to rely on LTC facilities because of fractured or unavailable traditional systems of support (SAGE

2010). Often, as stated earlier, many LGBT elders conceal their sexual orientation and gender identity for fear of discrimination or victimization. Between October 2009 and June 2010, a national online survey conducted by the National Senior Citizens Law Center (NSCLC) in collaboration with Lambda Legal, National Center for Lesbian Rights, National Center for Transgender Equality, National Gay and Lesbian Task Force, and Services and Advocacy for GLBT Elders (SAGE), sought to identify issues facing LGBT elders in LTC. Of the 769 respondents that included family members, friends, and social as well as legal service providers, 284 self-identified as LGBT elders. Survey data indicated that over 40 % (328) of the respondents reported 853 incidents of elder mistreatment in various LTC facilities, with verbal and physical harm caused by residents and staff being the most common form of mistreatment. Survey results also showed that more than 50 % of LGBT elders surveyed believed that they would suffer neglect or abuse by staff of the LTC facility, with a majority believing that disclosing one's sexual orientation or gender identity would attract discrimination from LTC facility staff and residents alike.

It is clear that little work has been conducted on LGBT victims of elder mistreatment. At the same time, it is also clear that elder LGBT victims do experience elder mistreatment and, in some respects, may be even more vulnerable to it than those of the majority population. This vulnerability is compounded by the fact that interventions for the abuse and its effects on LGBT individuals, both mentally and physically, are woefully lacking. Thus, the victimization of such elders may be either a re-victimization at a later age or a new victimization altogether. Also, LGBT elders may more likely be polyvictims (see Chap. 16) than their heterosexual counterparts. Suggested in earlier chapters, one way of addressing such problems is to understand and be sensitive to the needs of LGBT elders. Another is to understand those who perpetrate this type of elder mistreatment and in this way, to both intervene in and prevent the problem from occurring in the first place.

Characteristics of Perpetrators

If there is little known about LGBT victims of elder mistreatment, even less is known about abusers of LGBT elders. This paucity of information is understandable in light of the fact that there is so little known about LGBT victims and that there is so little known about elder abusers in the general population as well. As with the section above, at this time, it is only possible to characterize the perpetrators of elder mistreatment and then, by extrapolation, understand some of the characteristics of those who abuse LGBT elders.

Amstadter et al. (2010) examined perpetrator and incident characteristics of the mistreatment of older adults (age 60+) in a national sample of 5777 older men and women. The sample revealed that perpetrators of physical mistreatment against men had more "pathological" characteristics as compared to perpetrators of physical mistreatment against women. Perpetrators of physical mistreatment (compared to emotional and sexual mistreatment) evidenced increased likelihood of legal problems, psychological treatment, substance use during the abuse incident, living with the victim, and being related to the victim.

The Lifespan study of mistreatment (2011) revealed that, for the two-thirds of agencies able to report age information for abusers, 7.7 % of reported abusers were in the younger than age 18-year category; 44.8 % were in the 18–45 age category; 25.6 % were in the age 46–59 age category; and 22 % were in the 60 years and older category. For those agencies able to report some information on gender of the abuser, 66.3 % were male abusers and 33.7 % were female abusers. For agency/programs able to provide information on the relationship between victim and abuser, 26 % were spouses or partners, 39.7 % were the victims own adult children, 2 % were sons or daughters-in-law, 9.5 %; were grandchildren, 9.5 %; 3.5 % were friends or neighbors, 0.65 % were paid home care workers, 13.1 % other relatives; and 5.6 % were other non-relatives.

Research Box 17.1: Caregivers of LGBT Elders

Brotman, S., Ryan, B., Collins, S., Chamberland, L., Cormier, R., Julien, D., ... & Richard, B. (2007). Coming out to care: Caregivers of gay and lesbian seniors in Canada. *The Gerontologist, 47*(4), 490–503.

Purpose: This article reports on the findings of a study whose purpose was to explore the experiences of caregivers of gay and lesbian seniors living in the community and to identify issues that emerged from an exploration of access to and equity in health care services for these populations.

Design and Methods: The study used a qualitative methodology based upon the principles of grounded theory in which open-ended interviews were undertaken with 17 caregivers living in three different cities across Canada.

Results: Findings indicated several critical themes, including the impact of felt and anticipated discrimination, complex processes of coming out, the role of caregivers, self-identification as a caregiver, and support.

Implications: We consider several recommendations for change in light of emerging themes, including expanding the definition of caregivers to be more inclusive of gay and lesbian realities, developing specialized services, and advocating to eliminate discrimination faced by these populations.

Questions

1. What is it like to "come out" in late life? Why would one do so in late life?
2. Describe what it is like to be a caregiver of an LGBT elder.
3. What do you see as the limitations to this research methodology?

Discussion Box 17.2: Abuse, re-victimization, or prejudice continued?

Consider the following scenarios:

Scenario I

Hans and Joe have lived together as committed partners for almost 45 years. Because of the homophobic attitude of their families, they have maintained respectful but distant relations with family members, especially Hans'. Five years ago, Hans' health began to fail, and since that time Joe has taken care of Hans in their home. Unfortunately, just before the holidays, things took a turn for the worst, and despite medical intervention and care, Hans died from complications of his disease. He was 78 years old. After the funeral, Joe went out of town to visit with mutual friends so he would not be home alone for the holidays. When he returned a week later, he found that his home was locked up, locks changed, and his personal belongings stashed in boxes and stacked beside the garage. Hans' brother and sister informed Joe that following Hans' demise, he no longer had any right to live in the house, or have any access to Hans' property. Joe is 74 years old.

• Is this abuse, re-victimization, or prejudice continued?

Scenario II

When Agatha's aunt could no longer afford to pay for her residence at DunRoamin' Glen, a seniors-only independent living and retirement community, she decided to bring her into her home. Agatha's family is looking forward to meet the new addition to the family. Agatha, however, has failed to tell her family that "Aunt Maud," who is now 65, has spent the last 20 years as "Michael."

- How might everyone involved be prepared?

In a national study of APS by Teaster et al. (2006), with data from eleven states, 52.7 % of perpetrators were female. For the seven states reporting ages for alleged perpetrators, 4.3 % were under 18 years of age, 10.6 % were 18–29, 16.1 % were 30–39, 25.6 % were 40–49, 18.5 % were 50–59, and 11.2 % were 60–69. Among those that provided information on the relationship of the perpetrator to the victim, the most common was that of adult child (32.6 %), followed by other family member (21.5 %), unknown relationship (16.3 %), and spouse/intimate partner (11.3 %).

Ramsey-Klawsnik et al. (2008) discussed research findings concerning 119 alleged sexual perpetrators reported to state authorities for abusing elderly individuals residing in care facilities. The largest group of accused was employees of the facilities, followed by facility residents, followed by victims' family members and visitors to the facilities. Upon investigation by APS and regulatory staff, 32 individuals were confirmed as sexual perpetrators against vulnerable elders. Male and female alleged and confirmed sexual perpetrators were identified as well as both male and female elderly sexual abuse victims.

In a study of APS in the state of Kentucky in press found that no differences existed between number of male and female perpetrators when the sex of the perpetrator was identified. For the 96 victims (excluding self-neglect and guardianship), 37.0 % of perpetrators were adult children, 30.4 % were staff members in facilities, and 14.1 % were spouses or a significant other. Other less frequently occurring perpetrators were siblings (5.4 %), niece/nephews and grandchildren (3.2 %, each), and other perpetrators (6.5 %). Though as yet highly infrequently utilized by the justice system, states are continuing to develop remedies for the crime of mistreatment of elders, which are discussed in the following section.

Remedies

Legal Remedies. LGBT elders who are victims of mistreatment have some remedies available to them; however, they are not without real costs. For mistreatment that is criminal in nature, a court case could be protracted, and upon all the information presented, the result could be that the perpetrator receives little or no punishment. Courts may be reticent to execute restraining orders for the harassment of LGBT elders in IPV cases. Furthermore, for those elders hitherto in the closet, pursuing a legal remedy may result in more exposure of the victim's status as LGBT, and consequently to further discrimination and unequal treatment. In the USA, states have laws that address the mistreatment or abuse of elders, both community dwelling and those who reside in institutions. These laws are varied and may be statutes, which are part of APS laws, or distinct laws criminalizing elder mistreatment. In addition, basic or general criminal laws such as those relating to assault, battery, manslaughter, or murder may be used to prosecute acts against older adult victims (Heisler and Stiegel 2002; AARP 2012). Elder victims may also bring civil suits against perpetrators. Remedies available to elder mistreatment victims include restraining orders, punitive damages, compensation, and restitution for losses incurred and/or damages suffered (National Center for Victims of Crime 1999).

In some states, special laws exist that provide enhanced penalties for crimes against older adults, including mistreatment, designed to deter such crimes. For instance, in Nevada, the term of imprisonment for a crime against a person aged 60+ may be double the prescribed term for the offense; in Louisiana, the minimum sentence for any violent crime against an older adult is five years without parole, and in Georgia, enhanced penalties exist such as recovery of punitive in addition to actual damages suffered, for those found guilty of deceptive business practices involving elders (National Center for Victims of Crime 1999).

Other than laws regarding elder abuse and mistreatment, certain general criminal laws, such as laws against hate crimes or "bias crimes," are applicable to victimized LGBT elders (Morrow 2001). Hate crimes are defined as crimes where the perpetrator's conduct was driven by bias, prejudice, or hatred on the basis of actual or perceived notions of an individual or group's status regarding race, color, religion, national origin, ethnicity, gender, or sexual orientation (US Congress 1992). Clearly, LGBT elders fall within this definition, subject as they often are to heterosexism and homophobia that may place them in environments that may be fearsome, dangerous, or hostile (Cahill and Smith 2002). States with bias crime laws often have enhanced penalties, such as harsher sentencing for these crimes, because bias/hate crimes cause harm to and/or increase vulnerability of already disadvantaged individuals or groups, as well as to discourage hate and bias or prevent such crimes (Lawrence 2002). Although all states in the USA have some form of hate or bias law, with a majority including enhanced penalties, as Table 17.1 shows, less than one-third have laws that deal with bias or hate crimes based on the sexual orientation and gender identity (Human Rights Campaign 2013; Leiberman 2010; Leadership Conference on Civil Rights Education Fund (LCCREF) 2009).

In these states, laws with enhanced penalties may provide remedies to LGBT elders including right to pursue civil action in addition to criminal penalty and harsher sentencing for offenders (Lawrence 2002). Although the remedies identified above may provide some relief for elder LGBT victims of mistreatment, whether under mistreatment laws, general criminal laws, or hate/bias crime laws, more still needs to be done. In order to provide appropriate protection from harm as well as to redress or ameliorate harm if and when it does occur, the development of policy initiatives and strategies will be necessary. Such initiatives and strategies will need to address increasing the number of states with laws against sexual orientation or gender identity-related hate crimes, imposing stiffer or

Table 17.1 States with laws addressing hate or bias crimes based on sexual orientation and gender identity

California	Colorado	Connecticut	Delaware
District of Columbia	Hawaii	Maryland	Massachusetts
Minnesota	Missouri	Nevada	New Jersey
New Mexico	Oregon	Vermont	Washington

Source Human Rights Campaign (2013). Available at www.hrc.org/statelaws

tougher penalties and consequences on convicted offenders, increasing requirements for mandatory reporting of offenses, providing training for professionals—legal, social, health, criminal justice, and law enforcement to help enhance prosecution (National Center for Victims of Crime 1999). In addition, it is important to increase public awareness and sensitivity about the vulnerability of LGBT elders as victims of abuse and mistreatment, both by virtue of age and LGBT status.

Policy Box: Commission for LGBT Senior Affairs

Your local county and city government recently set up a commission for senior affairs as part of a broader initiative to make the area a livable community and address the needs of its aging population. As a long-term care ombudsman, you are aware of many of the concerns faced by older adults in facilities within the county. One such challenge relates to the safety and well-being of elderly LGBT residents who suffer discrimination and abuse in LTC facilities from staff and residents. You would like to craft a policy for consideration by the seniors' commission, requiring LTC facilities to consider the unique needs of LGBT residents.

- What factors should be considered in creating this policy? Why?
- Explain your rationale for targeting LGBT elders specifically.

Programs and Approaches

**Services and Advocacy for GLBT Elders
(SAGE).** SAGE is the country's largest and
oldest organization dedicated to improving the
lives of LGBT elders. With its headquarters
located in New York City, its mission is to
address issues related to LGBT aging. SAGE
offers services and programs to LGBT older
people throughout New York City and via its
national affiliate program, SAGENet, which
includes 27 affiliates located in 20 states across
every region of the country. Affiliates provide
services and programs to LGBT elders living in
the community. Affiliates serve as advocates for
the support of LBGT elders on the city and state
policies that affect them (http://www.sageusa.
org/advocacy/sagenet.cfm). SAGE offers a variety of services and programs (e.g., the arts and
culture and health and wellness). Another service
offered by SAGE, AGEWorks, is an employment
program for LGBT elders that, like SAGENet,
has sites around the country. SAGE conducts
advocacy for public policies affecting LGBT
elders at federal, state, and local levels in order to
improve LGBT elders' economic security, community support, and health and wellness. SAGE
also trains aging providers and LGBT organizations on concerning how to support LGBT older
elders in LTC settings. The organization offers
cultural competence training as part of its
National Resource Center on LGBT Aging and
retains a training corps of nearly 40 cultural
competence experts throughout the USA (http://
sageusa.org/about/what.cfm).

National Resource Center on LGBT Aging.
Established in 2010 through a federal grant from
the US Department of Health and Human Services, the National Resource Center on LGBT
Aging is the only technical assistance resource
center and clearinghouse in the country devoted
exclusively to improving the quality of services
and supports offered to LGBT elders. The Center
provides training, technical assistance, and educational resources to aging providers, LGBT
organizations, and LGBT elders. SAGE, discussed above, leads the Center and collaborates

with 18 leading organizations throughout the
USA (http://www.lgbtagingcenter.org/).

Other Organizations and Resources. As of
this writing, the number of resources that address
LGBT elders is proliferating rapidly. There are
now assisted living facilities and nursing homes
that openly cater to elders who are LGBT.
Innovative programs targeted at LGBT elders
and designed to provide a continuum of health,
wellness, and social services to community
dwelling LGBT elders are emerging in various
communities across the USA. An example is the
Chicago Elder Project at Howard Brown Center.
This program is offered in conjunction with
community partners (including Rush University
Medical Center, CJE-Senior Life, Heartland
Alliance, and Midwest Palliative and Hospice
Care) to serve LGBT elders by providing culturally competent and sensitive care (Howard
Brown Health Center, http://www.howardbrown.
org). Advocates for the rights of elders, such as
the Long-Term Care Ombudsman (see Chap. 16
), The NSCLC, Lambda Legal, the National
Center for Lesbian Rights, the National Center
for Transgender Equality, and he National Gay
and Lesbian Task Force, are helping raise to the
visibility and ensure the rights of elders who are
LGBT.

Conclusion

Readily apparent from this chapter on mistreatment of LGBT elders is that few studies on elder
mistreatment collect information on LGBT elder
abuse. Also readily apparent is that the time has
come for inclusion of this variable or variables in
these datasets. LGBT elders who are mistreated
are victims (polyvictims) in a multiplicity of
ways—for their sexual orientation, gender identify, historic trauma either felt or experienced and
the abuse or abuses (e.g., physical abuse, neglect,
or exploitation) that they experience when they
are abused. Seeking redress for elder mistreatment is also fraught with peril. Should an elder
disclose what was previously undisclosed, the

old issues of being ostracized or mistreated solely because of one's sexual preference could be less tolerable than enduring the abuse. Even if an elder discloses what was previously disclosed, many service systems and providers are, as yet, untrained and unsympathetic for the elder's plight and thus the intervention offered may do more harm than good. These authors stress that it is high time to include LGBT issues in research on elder abuse in order to understand incidence and prevalence of the problem in this community, to characterize victims and perpetrators, to delineate and bolster available remedies, to conduct meaningful research and advocacy, and, most importantly, to improve the quality of life of present and future LGBT elders.

Summary

The mistreatment and victimization of older LGBT adults are slowly coming to light in both practice and research. However, at this point, few studies examine this phenomenon. What is certain is that being LGBT may place elders at increased risk for mistreatment due to factors such as isolation, previous exposure to a traumatic event, and reticence to seek assistance from informal and formal networks. Penalties for elder mistreatment must be utilized by law enforcement more frequently, and statues that explore elder mistreatment as a hate crime also explored. It is critical that advocates, practitioners, researchers, and policy makers understand, intervene in, and prevent the mistreatment of LGBT elders.

Learning Exercises

Self-Check Questions

1. Why is there so little information available on victims of mistreatment who are LGBT elders? How might researchers go about researching this issue?

2. How might agencies and programs better intervene in the abuse of LGBT elders?
3. What are risk factors for elder mistreatment? How might these differ for LGBT elders?
4. What are the differences between LBGT elder mistreatment in community settings and facility settings?

Experiential Exercise

Arrange a group screening of GenSilent, a documentary on LGBT elders available from http://stumaddux.com/GEN_SILENT.html.

1. What issues or concerns are raised in this documentary?
2. Identify factors which may increase or trigger elder abuse/mistreatment potential.
3. What strategies would you recommend to ameliorate the situation? Explain?

Resources

AARP's Pride Homepage: This is AARP's online home for the lesbian, gay, bisexual, and transgender (LGBT) community. The page is designed to spotlight articles on news, personal finance, relationships, travel, and other topics of concern to older gay Americans, and their family and friends (http://www.aarp.org/relationships/friends-family/aarp-pride.html?cmp=RDRCT-PRID_MAY10_011).

CenterLink: The Community of LGBT Centers: This is the community of LGBT centers exists to support the development of strong, sustainable LGBT community centers and to build a unified center movement (www.lgbtcenters.org).

Eldercare Locator: Searchable database from the Administration on Aging on issues such as Alzheimer's, caregiving, elder abuse, Financial Assistance, Food and Nutrition, Health Insurance, Healthy Aging, Home Repair and Modification, Housing, In-Home Services, Legal

Assistance, Long-Term Care, Nursing Home, Transportation, Volunteerism (www.eldercare.gov/).

Family Equality Council: The Family Equality Council is America's foremost national advocate dedicated to family equality for lesbian, gay, bisexual, and transgender (LGBT) parents, guardians and allies. It has grown into the leading policy advocate on federal and state issues that impact today's modern families, including foster care and adoption, safe schools, family medical leave, parenting protections, domestic partnership, and marriage (www.familyequality.org/).

LGBT Aging Issues Network: American Society on Aging's constituent group who are professionals working to raise awareness about the concerns of lesbian, gay, bisexual, and transgender (LGBT) elders (www.asaging.org/lain).

The National Center on Elder Abuse: The National Center on Elder Abuse (NCEA) serves as a national resource center dedicated to the prevention of elder mistreatment. NCEA serves as a national clearinghouse of information for elder rights advocates, law enforcement, legal professionals, public policy leaders, researchers, and others working to ensure that all older Americans will live with dignity, integrity, independence, and without abuse, neglect, and exploitation (www.ncea.aoa.gov).

National Gay and Lesbian Task Force: Aging Issues: The mission of the National Gay and Lesbian Task Force is to build the grassroots power of the lesbian, gay, bisexual, and transgender (LGBT) community. The Task Force focuses on aging as one of their delineated issue areas (http://www.thetaskforce.org).

Old Lesbian Organizing for Change (OLOC): Provides old lesbians with the chance to meet like-minded women in our common struggle to confront ageism, to share mutual interests, and to experience the joy and warmth of playing and working together (http://www.oloc.org).

Parents, Families and Friends of Lesbians and Gays (PFLAG): Parents, Families and Friends of Lesbians and Gays provides opportunity for dialogue about sexual orientation and gender identity, and acts to create a society that is healthy and respectful of human diversity (www.community.pflag.org/).

Prime Timers Worldwide: The Prime Timers is a social organization that provides older gay and bisexual men the opportunity to enrich their lives. Prime Timers are older gay or bisexual men (and younger men who admire mature men). Their members are men who choose to have their social lives enriched by the diverse activities in which our members engage. No single definition can describe Prime Timers, as they come from all walks of life. Prime Timers involve themselves in their community with volunteerism, politics, gay issues, arts, entertainment, and every other facet of healthy living (www.primetimersww.org).

References

AARP. (2012). *Personal and legal rights in policy book, 2011–2012* (Chap. 12). Retrieved January 16, 2015 from http://www.aarp.org/content/dam/aarp/about_aarp/aarp_policies/2011_04/pdf/Chapter12.pdf

Acierno, R., Hernandez, M. A., Amstadter, A. B., Resnick, H. S., Steve, K., Muzzy, W., & Kilpatrick, D. G. (2010). Prevalence and correlates of emotional, physical, sexual, and financial abuse and potential neglect in the United States: The National Elder Mistreatment Study. *American Journal of Public Health, 100*, 292–297. doi:10.2105/ajph.2009.163089.

Amstadter, A. B., Cisler, J. M., McCauley, J. L., Hernandez, M. A., Muzzy, W., & Acierno, R. (2011). Do incident and perpetrator characteristics of elder mistreatment differ by gender of the victim? Results from the National Elder Mistreatment Study. *Journal of Elder Abuse and Neglect, 23*(1), 43–57.

Brandl, B. (2004). Assessing for abuse in later life. *National clearinghouse on abuse in later life (NCALL): A project of the Wisconsin coalition against domestic violence.* Retrieved March 01, 2015 from http://ncall.us/sites/ncall.us/files/resources/Assessing%20and%20Responding%20to%20ALL.pdf

Burgess, A., Dowdell, E., & Prentky, R. (2000). Sexual abuse of nursing home residents. *Journal of Psychosocial Nursing, 38*(6), 10–18.

Cahill, S., & South, K. (2002). Policy issues affecting lesbian, gay, bisexual, and transgender people in retirement. *Generations, 26*(2), 49–54.

Castle, E., Eisenberger, N. I., Seeman, T. E., Moons, W. G., Boggero, I. A., Grinblatt, M. S., & Taylor, S. E. (2012). Neural and behavioral bases of age differences in perceptions of trust. *Proceedings of the National Academy of Sciences, 109*, 20848–20852.

Charles, S. T., & Carstensen, L. L. (2010). Social and emotional aging. *Annual Review of Psychology, 61*, 383–409. doi:10.1146/annurev.psych.093008.100448.

Cook-Daniels, L. (2002). *Lesbian, gay male, bisexual and transgendered elders: Elder abuse and neglect issues* (pp. 1–11). FORGE. Retrieved from http://forge-forward.org/wp-content/docs/LGBT-Elder-abuse.pdf

D'Augelli, A., & Grossman, A. (2001). Disclosure of sexual orientation, victimization, and mental health among lesbian, gay, and bisexual older adults. *Journal of Interpersonal Violence, 16*(10), 1008–1027. Retrieved December 27, 2014 from http://jiv.sagepub.com/content/16/10/1008

DeLiema, M., Gassoumis, Z. D., Homeier, D. C., & Wilber, K. H. (2012). Determining prevalence and correlates of elder abuse using promotores: Low-income immigrant Latinos report high rates of abuse and neglect. *Journal of the American Geriatrics Society, 60*, 1333–1339. doi:10.1111/j.1532-5415.2012.04025.x.

Dong, X., Simon, M., Rajan, K., & Evans, D. A. (2011). Association of cognitive function and risk for elder abuse in a community-dwelling population. *Dementia and Geriatric Cognitive Disorders, 32*, 209–215. doi:10.1159/000334047.

Frazer, S. (2009). *LGBT health and human services needs in New York State*. Albany, NY: Empire State Pride Agenda Foundation. Retrieved December 27, 2014 from http://www.prideagenda.org/Portals?0?pdfs/LGBT%20and%20Human%20Services%20Needs%20in%20New%20York%20State.pdf

Fredriksen-Goldsen, K. I., Kim, H.-J., Emlet, C. A., Muraco, A., Erosheva, E. A., Hoy-Ellis, C. P. et al. (2011). *The aging and health report: Disparities and resilience among lesbian, gay, bisexual, and transgender older adults—key findings fact sheet*. Seattle: Institute for Multigenerational Health. Retrieved from https://depts.washington.edu/agepride/wordpress/wp-content/uploads/2012/10/factsheet-keyfindings10-25-12.pdf

Fredriksen-Goldsen, K. I., Kim, H. J, Shiu, C., Goldsen, J., & Emlet, C. A. (2014). Successful aging among LGBT older adults: physical and mental health-related quality of life by age group. *The Gerontologist*, 1–15. doi:10.1093/geront/gnu081

Gates, G. (2011). *How many people are lesbian, gay, bisexual, and transgender?* Williams Institute, UCLA School of Law. Retrieved December 27, 2014 from http://williamsinstitute.law.ucla.edu/wp-content/uploads/Gates-How-Many-People-LGBT-Apr-2011.pdf

Heisler, C. I., & Stiegel, L. A. (2002). Enhancing the justice system's response to elder abuse: Discussions and recommendations of the "improving prosecution" working group of The National Policy Summit on elder abuse. *Journal of Elder Abuse and Neglect, 14* (4), 31–54.

Hightower, J. (2004). Age, gender and violence: Abuse against older women. *Geriatrics and Aging, 7*(3), 60–63.

Horsford, S. R., Parra-Cardona, J. R., Post, L. A., & Schiamberg, L. (2010). Elder abuse and neglect in African American families: Informing practice based on ecological and cultural frameworks. *Journal of Elder Abuse and Neglect, 23*(1), 75–88. doi:10.1080/08946566.2011.534709.

Human Rights Campaign. (2013). State hate crimes laws. Available at http://hrc-assets.s3-website-us-east-1.amazonaws.com//files/assets/resources/hate_crimes_laws_022014.pdf

Institute of Medicine. (2011). *The health of lesbian, gay, bisexual and transgender people: Building a foundation for better understanding*. Washington, DC: The National Academies Press.

Krienert, J. L., Walsh, J. A., & Turner, M. (2009). Elderly in America: A descriptive study of elder abuse examining national incident-based reporting system (NIBRS) data, 2000–2005. *Journal of Elder Abuse and Neglect, 21*(4), 325–345. doi:10.1080/08946560903005042.

Lachs, M. S., Williams, C., O'Brien, S., Hurst, L., & Horwitz, R. (1997). Risk factors for reported elder abuse and neglect: A nine-year observational cohort study. *The Gerontologist, 37*, 469–474. doi:10.1093/geront/37.4.469.

Laumann, E. O., Leitsch, S. A., & Waite, L. J. (2008). Elder mistreatment in the United States: Prevalence estimates from a nationally representative study. *The Journals of Gerontology Series B: Psychological Sciences and Social Sciences, 63*, S248–S254.

Lawrence, F. M. (2002). Hate crimes. *Encyclopedia of Crime and Justice*. Retrieved January 17, 2015 from Encyclopedia.com: http://www.encyclopedia.com/doc/1G2-3403000136.html

Leadership Conference on Civil Rights Education Fund (LCCREF). (2009). *Confronting the new faces of hate: Hate crimes in America*. Retrieved January 17, 2015 from http://www.protectcivilrights.org/pdf/reports/hatecrimes/lccref_hate_crimes_report.pdf

Lieberman, M. (2010). *Hate crime laws: Punishment to fit the crime (Op.Ed.)*. The Anti-Defamation League. Available at http://www.adl.org/press-center/c/hate-crime-laws-punishment-to-fit-the-crime.html#.VLpfJBs5DIU

Lifespan of Greater Rochester, Inc., Weill Cornell Medical Center of Cornell University, & New York City Department for the Aging. (2011). *Under the radar: New York State elder abuse prevalence study—self-reported prevalence and documented case surveys* (pp. 1–134). Retrieved from http://www.lifespan-roch.org/documents/UndertheRadar051211.pdf

Lombardi, E. L., Wilchins, R. A., Priesing, D., & Malouf, D. (2002). Gender violence: Transgender experiences with violence and discrimination. *Journal of Homosexuality, 42*(1), 89–101.

MetLife Mature Market Institute. (2006). *Out and aging: The MetLife study of lesbian and gay baby boomers*. New York: MetLife Mature Market Institute.

Institute, Met Life Mature Market. (2011). *The MetLife study of elder financial abuse: Crimes of occasion, desperation, and predation against America's elders*. Westport, CT: Metlife Mature Market Institute.

Morrow, D. (2001). Older gays and lesbians: Surviving a generation of hate and violence. *Journal of Gay and Lesbian Social Services, 13*(1/2), 151–169.

Movement Advancement Project. (2009). *Snapshot advancing gender equality*. Retrieved December 27, 2014 from http://www.lgbtagingcenter.org/resources/resource.cfm?r=501

Movement Advancement Project, Services & Advocacy for Gay, Lesbian, Bisexual, & Transgender Elders, & Center for American Progress. (2010). *LGBT older adults: Facts at a glance*. Retrieved December 27, 2014 from http://lgbtagingcenter.org/resources/resource.cfm?r=22

National Center for Victims of Crime (1999). New York City Alliance Against Sexual Assault: *Factsheets: Elder abuse and the law*. Retrieved from http://www.svfreenyc.org/survivors_factsheet_74.html

National Center on Elder Abuse. (2013). Mistreatment of lesbian, gay, bisexual, and transgender (LGBT) Elders. *Research brief*. Retrieved January 24, 2015 from www.ncea.aoa.gov/.../docs/NCEA_LGBT_Researchbrief_2013.pdf

Nelson, H. D., Nygren, P., McInerney, Y., & Klein, J. (2004). Screening women and elderly adults for family and intimate partner violence: A review of the evidence for the U.S. Preventive Services Task Force. *Annals of Internal Medicine, 140*, 387–396.

Podnieks, E. (1992). National survey on abuse of the elderly in Canada. *Journal of Elder Abuse and Neglect, 4*, 5–58.

Pillemer, K., & Finkelhor, D. (1988). The prevalence of elder abuse: A random sample survey. *The Gerontologist, 28*, 51–57.

Ramsey-Klawsnik, H., Teaster, P. B., Mendiondo, M. S., Marcum, J. L., & Abner, E. L. (2008). Sexual predators who target elders: Findings from the first national study of sexual abuse in care facilities. *Journal of Elder Abuse and Neglect, 20*(4), 353–376.

Sherod, M. G., Griffith, H. R., Copeland, J., Belue, K., Krzywansky, S., Zamrini, E. Y., et al. (2009). Neurocognitive predictors of financial capacity across the dementia spectrum: Normal aging, mild cognitive impairment, and Alzheimer's disease. *Journal of the International Neuropsychological Society, 15*, 258–267. doi:10.1017/S1355617709090365.

Tatara, T. (1999). Introduction. In T. Tatara (Ed.), *Understanding elder abuse in minority populations* (pp. 1–9). Philadelphia: Taylor & Francis.

Teaster, P. B., Dugar, T., Mendiondo, M., Abner, A., Cecil, K., & Otto, J. (2006). *The 2004 survey of state adult protective services: Abuse of adults 60 years of age and older*. Washington, D.C.: National Center on Elder Abuse.

U.S. Congress. (1992). H.R. 4797. 102nd Congress, 2nd Session.

Wangmo, T., Teaster, P. B., Mendiondo, M., Grace, J., Blandford, C., Fisher, S., Wong, W., & Fardo, D. (2014). An ecological systems examination of elder abuse: A week in the life of adult protective services. *The Journal of Elder Abuse and Neglect, 26*(5), 440–457.

Wisconsin Coalition against Domestic Violence. (2009). *Elder abuse, neglect, and family violence: A guide for health care professionals*. Madison, WI: Wisconsin Coalition against Domestic Violence and Wisconsin Bureau of Aging and Disability Resources.

The Prevalence of Elder Bullying and Impact on LGBT Elders

Robin P. Bonifas

Abstract

This chapter reviews bullying and relational aggression among LGBT older adults. The intent of this chapter is to define and characterize late-life bullying in general and discuss unique manifestations of this phenomenon for LGBT elders. Special attention is given to peer victimization associated with intersectionality and microaggressions for this population, as well as common types of bullying and the impact bullying experiences have on emotional well-being and quality of life. Promising interventions to minimize bullying related to sexual orientation and gender identity in senior living environments are discussed and include civility training, bystander intervention, and policies and procedures that guide respectful social interactions and prohibit discriminatory actions.

Keywords

Bullying · Relational aggression · Peer victimization · Micro aggression · Organizational intervention

Overview

Bullying and relational aggression are typically viewed as challenges faced by children and youth in school settings, yet this phenomenon extends across the life span and includes older adults as well. Studies estimate that anywhere from 10 to 20 percent of older adults living in communal settings, such as assisted living facilities and nursing homes, are exposed to peers' bullying behaviors (Bonifas and Kramer 2011; Pillemer et al. 2014). These experiences are associated with negative outcomes including social isolation, reduced self-esteem, exacerbation of preexisting mental health conditions, and disruptive feelings of fear, anxiety, and worry (Bonifas 2011). Although no research studies to date have specifically examined bullying among lesbian, gay, bisexual, or transgender (LGBT) elders, individuals participating in diverse samples report experiencing bullying and other forms of victimization based on their sexual

Author's note: I would like to thank Sherri Shimansky for her review of earlier versions of this chapter and her thoughtful recommendations for strengthening it.

R.P. Bonifas (✉)
Arizona State University, Phoenix, USA
e-mail: robin.bonifas@asu.edu

orientation (Bonifas 2011; Fredriksen-Goldsen et al. 2011). Because individuals who are perceived as different from the dominant population often become targets for bullying, it is likely that LGBT older adults experience negative peer interactions on a regular basis and face associated negative outcomes. The purpose of this chapter is to orient readers to the current state of knowledge regarding bullying and relational aggression as it applies to LGBT elders, with emphasis on understanding the phenomenon itself and relevant points of intervention. The chapter begins with a definition of bullying and relational aggression, continues with a review of the characteristics of these phenomena among older adults, and follows with a discussion of bullying and relational aggression in the context of intersectional LGBT aging, drawing on extant research to illustrate prevalence, incident characteristics, and negative outcomes. The chapter concludes by presenting a promising framework to guide intervention and service delivery to this population.

Learning Objectives

By the end of the chapter, the reader should be able to:

1. Understand the definitions and characteristics of elder bullying.
2. Identify bullying tactics used against LGBT elders.
3. Describe promising interventions to minimize bullying of LGBT older adults.

Introduction

Conceptually, bullying is an act of cruelty, intimidation, and aggression from one person toward another. Bullying is intentional in nature and a behavior that is often repeated and habitual.

The act of bullying may involve but is not limited to force, threat, insult, coercion, gossip, or abuse. Although bullying may involve abuse, it is distinctly different in several ways. An important difference between the two is who is engaging in the negative behavior or aggressive act and who is on the receiving end of it. With elder abuse, the victim is a vulnerable adult, typically in a position of dependency on a non-vulnerable abuser for some type of personal care or instrumental assistance, such as bathing or financial management. With bullying, both the bully and the target of bullying are vulnerable adults, and the victim is not dependent on the bully for any type of care or assistance. See Chaps. 16 and 17 for a comprehensive discussion of elder abuse and mistreatment.

Bullying of and by elders is a growing problem, especially for LGBT elders. For example, studies suggest that approximately 20 % of older adults in community living settings report experiencing some type of bullying since moving in (Bonifas 2011; Trompetter et al. 2011). While there are no exact statistics on the number of LGBT elders who are bullied, rates of overall victimization are high (Fredrikson-Goldsen et al. 2011). For example, in long-term care settings, 38 % of individuals who experienced some type of mistreatment were LGBT; the most common type of mistreatment was verbal or physical harassment by other residents (National Senior Citizens Law Center 2011). Bullying can have serious consequences for LGBT elders, including problems with sleeping, reduced sense of safety, social isolation, fearfulness, anxiety, and depression.

Background: Understanding Late-Life Bullying and Its Impact on Older Adults

Bullying is defined as intentional repetitive aggressive behavior that involves an imbalance of power or strength (Hazelden Foundation 2011). Associated peer victimization extends beyond this definition to include the experience of "persistent negative interpersonal behavior" (Rayner and Keashly 2005, p. 271) that is directed at a specific individual or a group of individuals. Within these intersecting definitions, three specific types of bullying are recognized: verbal, antisocial or relational, and physical.

Verbal Bullying. Verbal bullying refers to the use of words to intimidate or otherwise usurp another's power. Example behaviors include name-calling, malicious teasing, hurling insults, taunting, threatening, or making sarcastic remarks or pointed jokes. For example, George, a resident of an assisted living facility, described threatening remarks he regularly endured from a co-resident: "There's one that tries to be the number one tough guy. [He comes up] to me [and says] 'One of these days, I'm gonna smack you with a hammer'" (Bonifas 2011). While it was unclear as to whether the aggressor actually possessed a hammer and intended to use it, nevertheless, the threat alone contributed to considerable emotional distress for George.

Antisocial or Relational Bullying. Antisocial or relational bullying involves behaviors that are intended to hinder another's social relationships or limit their social connections; it can either be verbal or nonverbal. During late-life, bullying often takes this form (Trompetter et al. 2011; Hawker and Boulton 2000). Example behaviors include shunning, excluding, or ignoring; gossiping; spreading rumors; and using negative nonverbal body language, such as mimicking someone's walk or disability, making offensive gestures or facial expressions; purposefully turning one's head or body away when the target speaks, using threatening body language, or purposefully encroaching on personal space. John's experience provides an example of shunning behavior: after relocating to senior housing in another state following the loss of his home during Hurricane Katrina, several residents of his senior apartment complex began spreading rumors that he was a longtime homeless man and was the first in a deluge of formerly homeless people who were going to be "dumped" into their building. As a result, other residents began to avoid him (Bonifas and Frankel 2012).

Physical bullying. Physical bullying includes actual bodily contact with the target or the target's belongings, including pets. Example behaviors include pushing, hitting, kicking, destroying property, or stealing. Hitting can be with a hand, a closed fist, or a mobility aid, such as a cane. An example of this type of bullying is described in Reese's (2012) article for *ABC News*, which reports 71-year-old Bernadine Jones'[1] bullying experiences as instigated by her 87-year-old neighbor, Maria Zuravinski. A resident of a senior housing community, Ms. Jones stated that she was working in the community's garden when "Zuravinski approached her one day and accused her of disturbing some of her personal plants…the confrontation escalated when Zuravinski began yelling at her, calling her names, hit her with her cane and then spit on her" (p. 2). Reese goes on to explain that Ms. Jones continued to be subjected to similar behaviors from her neighbor; at one point, Ms. Zuravinski even attempted to strike Ms. Jones' dog with her cane.

Peer behaviors older adults find most problematic. In a study of negative social relationships and bullying in assisted living settings, residents described the types of peer behaviors and interaction patterns they found most distressing; results are listed in Table 18.1 (Bonifas and Kramer 2011).

What is noteworthy about the peer behaviors and interaction patterns identified as most problematic is that some fit the definition of bullying and victimization described above (i.e., name-calling, gossiping, and physical aggression), while others align with the concept of microaggression described by Sue (2010): "brief and commonplace daily verbal, behavioral, and environmental indignities, whether intentional or unintentional, that communicate hostile, derogatory, or negative racial, gender, sexual orientation, and religious slights and insults to the target person or group" (p. 5). This definition certainly fits negative social interactions such as exposure

---

[1]Throughout this chapter, when first names are used, the name is fictitious; when full or last names are used, the name is actually the individual's name as reported in a publically accessible resource.

Table 18.1 Peer social interaction patterns older adults report as the most distressing

1. Exposure to loud arguments in communal areas
2. Being the focus of name-calling and disparaging remarks
3. Being the focus of gossiping and rumor-spreading
4. Being bossed around or told what to do
5. Negotiating value differences, especially related to diversity of beliefs stemming from differences in culture, spirituality, or socioeconomic status
6. Competing for scarce resources, especially seating, television programming in communal areas, and staff attention
7. Being harassed to loan money, cigarettes, or other commodities
8. Not being able to avoid listening to others complain
9. Experiencing physical aggression
10. Witnessing psychiatric symptoms that are frightening or disruptive

Table 18.2 Examples of the emotional impact of late-life bullying

1. Anger/annoyance
2. Intense frustration
3. Fearfulness
4. Anxiety/tension/worry
5. Retaliation followed by shame
6. Self-isolation
7. Exacerbation of mental health conditions
8. Reduced self-esteem
9. Overall feelings of rejection
10. Depressive symptoms, including changes in eating and sleeping
11. Increased physical complaints
12. Functional changes, such as decreased ability to manage activities of daily living
13. Increased talk of moving out
14. Suicidal ideation

to loud arguments (#1), listening to others complain (#8), and witnessing disruptive psychiatric symptoms (#10). Microaggressions contribute to harm when no harm is intended, particularly related to negative emotional outcomes such as reduced self-esteem and lowered self-worth (Sue 2010). In addition, microaggressions reflect the overall milieu of an environment, including pervasive negativity and bias toward certain individuals and groups. This is relevant for older LGBT individuals who are often faced with subtle heterosexism and homophobia (Erdley et al. 2014). As such, microaggressions are considered as a type of bullying throughout this chapter.

The emotional impact of late-life bullying. Contrary to the childhood adage "sticks and stones may break my bones, but names will never hurt me," older individuals who are the targets of bullying are significantly impacted by their peers' negative behaviors. Verbal and antisocial behaviors are more common than physical violence, but all types of bullying negatively affect those who experience them. Mrs. Jones, mentioned in the Reese (2012) news article above, reported feeling so distressed by her neighbor's behavior that she was "afraid to go out [her] door." She explained, "I have to look out before I leave" (p. 2). Even

individuals who are exposed to the bullying experiences of others, but who are not victimized themselves report deleterious outcomes. For example, one assisted living resident described how co-residents' yelling at one another kept him awake at night, not only because of the noise disruption, but also because of his fears of potential escalating violence. He stated, "It is the uncertainty of what [they] are going to do that I find most unsettling" (Bonifas 2011). Fearfulness and self-isolation are only two examples of the negative ramifications of bullying; Table 18.2 depicts additional common reactions. Items 1 through 7 are from research conducted by Bonifas (2011), and items 8 through 14 where identified by Frankel (2012) during her practice experience of working with a senior care organization to address bullying among older adults.

The Impact of Bullying and Relational Aggression on LGBT Elders

As noted above, no research to date has focused exclusively on the bullying experiences of LGBT older adults; however, research on victimization among this population and on late-life bullying in general provides a framework for considering the likely impact this phenomenon has on the older LGBT community. Furthermore, the literature on discrimination and oppression in the context of intersectionality sheds additional light on the negative social interactions this population is exposed to and can help estimate both the potential for and prevalence of bullying among LGBT older adults. Based on what is currently known, three hypotheses about older LGBT bullying can be postulated: first, it exists; second, it occurs frequently; and third, it has a negative impact on well-being. This section reviews research findings that support these three hypotheses beginning with a discussion of intersectionality.

Intersectionality and LGBT older adults. Intersectionality, or being a member of more than one marginalized group, is associated with greater risk of negative outcomes (Barker 2008). For example, LGBT older adults have higher rates of poor physical health, chronic disability, and mental health conditions when compared to the older adult population in general (Adelman et al. 2006; Fredriksen-Goldsen et al. 2011). Greater incidence of negative outcomes, in turn, contributes to additional levels of intersectionality because individuals with poor health, disability, and mental illness are also stigmatized. As such, LGBT older adults may have three or more marginalized identities by simultaneously belonging to the following groups: older adults; sexual and/or gender minorities; and persons with a disability, health, and/or mental health condition. This multi-intersectionality further heightens their vulnerability, which has relevance for bullying—individuals who are vulnerable are at the highest risk to be targeted. For example, older adults with more depressive symptoms and lower self-esteem—both states of vulnerability—report they experience more peer victimization relative to their counterparts with fewer depressive symptoms and higher self-esteem (Bonifas and Kramer 2011). Given the vulnerability associated with multiple areas of intersectionality, LGBT older adults likely experience similar, if not higher, levels of risk.

Generational differences in acceptance of sexual and gender diversity. Many of today's LGBT older adults lived through the McCarthy era (i.e., Lavender scare) when homosexuality and gender minority status were criminalized and highly stigmatized at a societal and political level. Although homophobia and heterosexism remain present in American society, there is a greater acceptance and inclusion of LGBT people when compared to earlier times, especially among younger age groups (see Chap. 30 for further discussion on inclusion). However, older adults may retain strongly negative views about LGBT individuals consistent with their generational cohort. As a result, many LGBT older adults are reluctant to relocate to retirement or long-term care settings due to fear of non-acceptance by heterosexual peers (Sullivan 2014). Evidence supports that such fears are not unfounded: assisted living residents voice difficulty adjusting to communal environments with co-residents who hold opposing views and divergence life experiences (Bonifas and Kramer 2011). For example, one resident said, "For me, the hardest part [of being in assisted living] has been living with people I have never associated with in my life" (Bonifas 2011). Another individual stated, "I'm being forced to associate with people that I have nothing in common with and I don't even like…I was not prepared for this" (Bonifas 2011). While most participants in the corresponding study were discussing the challenges associated with living with individuals who were struggling with mental illness, substance abuse, and who had different value systems based on socioeconomic status, it is not unlikely that sexual orientation and gender identity minority status might be a point of contention for some senior housing residents. Given such values, the potential for microaggresions toward LGBT older adults in communal living settings is extensive.

Microaggression. The experience of one assisted living resident, Glen, attests to the heterosexist attitudes among his co-residents and to the presence of microaggressions. As an older gay man who participated in Bonifas and Kramer's (2011) study of negative social relationships in assisted living, he noted that other residents viewed homosexuality with "a lot of personal hate and fear" and surmised generational differences played a role in such biases, explaining "It's a generational thing...younger people accept gay people and lesbians; people my age don't" (Bonifas 2011). Exposure to pervasive homophobia in the overall living environment took its toll on Glen. For example, several straight men in the study reported bullying experiences that involved being taunted with accusations of being gay; these accusations were viewed as highly insulting and the topic of angry debate in communal areas. Glen described what it was like to regularly hear the outrage of peers who felt the ultimate insult was an insinuation that they were like him. "I got down, really down...it was really, really unfair to say something like that to be mean, it was awful" (Bonifas 2011).

The characteristics and prevalence of bullying among LGBT older adults. While the number of LGBT older adults who experience bullying and other forms of peer victimization is unknown, *Caring and Aging with Pride: The National Health, Aging and Sexuality Study* (CAP) provides evidence for the existence and extent of bullying experiences among older LGBT people (Fredriksen-Goldsen et al. 2011). Study participants reported high rates of victimization stemming from their actual or perceived sexual orientation or gender identity. Indeed, among the national sample of 2560 LGBT older adults, 82 % indicated they had experienced victimization at least once, and 64 % reported numerous incidents of victimization (Fredriksen-Goldsen et al. 2011). Victimization included behaviors associated with bullying: physical assault, property damage, threats of being outed,[2] threats of physical violence, and verbal assault.

The impact of bullying among LGBT older adults. A small-scaled study of negative social relationships in assisted living facilities provides additional evidence of LGBT bullying and

illustrates the emotional impact of bullying experiences. Among 28 assisted living residents in the sample, one participant self-identified himself as a gay man. He shared his experiences of co-residents' verbal harassment associated with his sexual orientation and the emotional pain stemming from repeatedly being referred to as a "fag" by his peers (Bonifas 2011). He stated, "It really hurt, like being stabbed in the heart." The verbally abusive comments and pervasive negativity directed toward his sexual orientation contributed to difficulties managing underlying mental health issues; he believed that subsequent emotional distress fostered behavioral decompensation, especially related to depression associated with a bipolar condition (Bonifas 2011). The impact of negativity toward homosexuality cannot be underestimated. For example, as noted above, fears related to the possibility of an intolerant and homophobic environment contribute to LGBT elders' reluctance to enter senior housing and long-term care facilities (Stein et al. 2010). Many LGBT seniors are concerned with having to return to the closet in order to be accepted by peers, which is a prospect they wish to avoid (Sullivan 2014). Similarly, LGBT elders may experience involuntary outing as a form of bullying; this can lead to significant distress, especially for individuals who prefer not to disclose their sexual orientation due to fear of discrimination or biased treatment in health and social services settings (Erdley et al. 2014).

Policy implications of bullying among LGBT older adults. As readers may surmise from the limited research on bullying among LGBT elders, at this writing there is no legislation that addresses bullying prevention for this population group. What is more, there is no legislation that addresses late-life bullying for any segment of the older adult population! However, elder abuse laws, regulations for nursing home resident rights, and anti-discrimination legislation do provide some level of protection. For example, the following behaviors are addressed by legislation prohibiting elder abuse: physical abuse, emotional abuse, sexual abuse, and financial exploitation (National Center on Elder Abuse, n. d.). Federal legislation

---

[2]Having their sexual orientation or gender identity revealed to others against their will.

outlining the rights of individuals living in nursing homes specifies that residents' autonomy and choice must be promoted and staff must strive to create "an environment that maintains or enhances each resident's dignity and respect in full recognition of his or her individuality" (American Health Care Association 2006, pp. 77). As such, sexual orientation and gender identity are elements of individuality that must be protected, at least in nursing home settings. In addition, the Fair Housing Act, which governs senior living organizations, prohibits discrimination based on gender, so any mistreatment related to gender identity may violate this legislation (National Senior Citizens Law Center 2011). In spite of these basic levels of protection, senior advocates are endeavoring to create legislation that is specific to bullying because some behaviors, such as relational aggression, may not meet the criteria for abuse or discrimination under existing laws. Many of these efforts are similar to those that have helped prevent and minimize bullying among children and youth in school settings.

For example, Jerome Halberstadt and his colleagues from the Stop Bullying Coalition (www. StopBullyingCoalition.org) in the greater Boston area have worked tirelessly over the past few years to draw legislators' attention to bullying of older adults and persons with disabilities living in multifamily subsidized housing. This group recently introduced two bills focused on bullying prevention to the Massachusetts legislature that focused on bullying prevention. According to Mr. Halberstadt, HD3228/SD442 would "require landlords and managers to act to prevent and remedy bullying in the residential environment... and to work with residents to develop plans, to train and educate staff and residents, to receive and act on reports of bullying, and to discipline transgressors for infractions" (Personal communication, January 17, 2014).

At the present time, bullying prevention policy exists primarily at the organizational level. For example, some senior centers require attendees to sign oaths of agreement that they will refrain from making disparaging comments

Table 18.3 Civility Pledge

1. View everyone in positive terms
2. Work on building common knowledge
3. Build strong relationships of trust
4. Remember our shared humanity
5. Value both the process and the results
6. Look both inside and outside for guidance (Personal communication, May 13, 2013).

during their visits to the center (Reese 2012). Some senior housing organizations ask tenants to strive for civility in their daily interactions with co-residents and to publically commit such intentions. For example, Diane Benson, a resident service coordinator for a senior apartment complex in the Midwest, encourages tenants to sign a *Civility Pledge* (Forni 2002) (Table 18.3) conveying a commitment to do the following daily:

Critical Research on LGBT Elders and Bullying

As the dearth of research on the bullying experience of LGBT elders suggests, research is sorely needed in this area. Descriptive studies are necessary to categorize the types of bullying, including relational aggression and microaggressions that members of the LGBT community experience and the extent to which they are exposed to such incidents. Although gossiping, name-calling, bossiness, and harassment for monetary loans and other valued commodities were perceived as highly problematic among a majority sample of heterosexual individuals (Bonifas and Kramer 2011), LGBT individuals may perceive other peer behaviors as more distressing. In addition, extant research indicates LGBT individuals are significantly diverse (Fredriksen-Goldsen et al. 2011); as such, attention to the specific experiences of lesbians, gays, bisexuals, and transgender individuals is also imperative.

Table 18.4 Assisted living residents' suggestions to address late-life bullying

1. Offer residents or tenants onsite anger management classes

2. Set limits with people who bully or "pick on" others

3. Hold regular meetings to promote resident communication

4. Develop rules and expectations that guide acceptable resident behaviors

5. Foster partnerships between residents and facility management for prevention and problem resolution

Outcome studies are also needed to determine the impact bullying experiences have on LGBT elders' emotional well-being and quality of life. While bullying is consistently associated with negative outcomes across the life course, differentiating outcomes that are unique to LGBT elders is warranted given that their life experiences diverge from their heterosexual counterparts (Sullivan 2014). The intersectionality of LGBT aging further supports the necessity of outcome research whereby LGBT seniors may experience disporportionally deleterious effects from bullying due to the conjoint vulnerabilities of age, sexual orientation, chronic illness, and disability (Barker 2008; Fredriksen-Goldsen et al. 2011).

Findings from both descriptive and outcomes studies can subsequently inform the development of interventions to prevent bullying of older LGBT individuals and minimize the potential for negative outcomes when it does occur. Small-scale intervention testing is currently underway to evaluate the effectiveness of approaches to minimize late-life bullying for older adults in general. See the following section for a brief review of the work of Marsha Frankel and colleagues to promote bystander intervention among older adults and Alyse November's work to prevent bullying in retirement settings. As similar intervention research expands to larger samples, a specific focus on effectiveness for LGBT individuals will help identify modification strategies that can tailor approach to individualized needs.

Assisted living residents have given their input into the types of organizational-level policies that are most important to them in addressing bullying in their living environments; their valuable suggestions are listed in Table 18.4.

An Intervention Framework to Reduce Late-Life Bullying Among LGBT Elders

In this author's experience, many people view the individual who bullies as the primary problem requiring a solution to prevent bullying incidents. However, intervention at the organizational level is the most crucial. Bullying behavior is less likely to occur in settings where it is not tolerated and where active steps are taken to both prevent and minimize it. This section reviews promising interventions to address LGBT bullying using senior housing organizations such as retirement apartments, assisted living facilities, and nursing homes as a backdrop.

Organizational interventions. Interventions at the organizational level emphasize approaches that will foster the creation of a caring community. As identified by Sullivan (2014), acceptance from others in the communal environment is paramount to LGBT elders' emotional well-being. At this level, both residents of the setting and employees of the setting need to work together to promote a pervasive climate of equality and respect; all disciplines from management to direct care staff to maintenance workers can contribute to an organizational milieu that promotes a feeling of safety and belonging. Key elements for creating a caring community include policies and procedures that guide behavioral and social interactions, tenant/resident and employee training that fosters inclusiveness and empathy, and environmental elements, such as signage, that reflect respect for diversity.

Policies and procedures guiding social interactions. Policies and procedures guiding appropriate social interactions are the most useful when conjointly developed by tenants/residents and management. To ensure that identified behaviors reflect LGBT elders' needs, active

Table 18.5 Exemplary behaviors to include in policy and procedure statements (DSACF, n. d.)

1. Pay attention
2. Listen
3. Be inclusive
4. Avoid gossip
5. Show respect
6. Be agreeable
7. Apologize
8. Give constructive criticism
9. Take responsibility

efforts need to be made to include their voices in explicitly stating what types of social interaction patterns are prohibited. Statements that promote respect for diversity should specifically mention sexual orientation and gender identity as examples. In tandem with prohibited behaviors, a list of corresponding behaviors that are encouraged is helpful to inform tenant/residents and employees as to what is acceptable. Table 18.5 lists some examples of positive behaviors suggested by *Speak Your Peace: The Civility Project* sponsored by the Duluth Superior Area Community Foundation (DSACF).

Tenant/resident and employee training. In addition to policies and procedures that govern respectful social interactions, both tenants/residents and employees require training in how to effectively adhere to the policies. Just because a policy statement dictates that everyone in the community should be treated with respect does not mean that people comply! Important elements of a bullying prevention training program include (1) an overview of the bullying and its characteristics in late-life with emphasis on uniqueness of diverse groups including LGBT elders; (2) understanding organizational policies and procedures for addressing bullying and relational aggression between tenants/residents; (3) responding to tenants/residents who bully without violating individual rights, for example, limit-setting, nonviolent communication, and promoting strategies that retain power in healthy ways; (4) how and when to make a report regarding problematic behavior; (5) assurances

of an overall caring community approach that protects residents and staff, including those who are LGBT; and (6) bystander intervention skills.

Bystander intervention training involves teaching people who witness bullying incidents how to effectively intervene to stop the behavior. Alcon et al. (2014) developed a training program to help older adults take action to reduce social bullying that occurs in their housing communities. Building on the idea that most bullying occurs in the presence of peer witnesses, this 60- to 75-min training aims to enable older adults to understand what social bullying is, differentiate it from everyday negative behaviors, and learn steps they can personally take to minimize bullying directed at them or at their peers.

The training intervention has three components: (1) an overview of late-life bullying, (2) discussion of the cycle of bullying and the role of bystanders in prevention, and (3) learning and practicing skills to thwart bullying. The overview component first engages participants by asking them to reflect on the question "What do you think of when you hear the term 'bullying?'" Facilitators then formally define bullying, detail the nature of bullying among older adults, including the characteristics of bullies and targets, and describe how bullying impacts seniors and their living communities. The cycle of bullying is then explained, as depicted in Table 18.6, and emphasis is placed on how both bystanders and victims can intervene to disrupt the cycle.

Intervention involves standing up to the individual who bullies by first recognizing that the problem resides with him or her, then making direct eye contact, responding calmly in a manner that defends the victim, challenges the bully's behavior, or redirects his or her negative

Table 18.6 The cycle of bullying (Alcon et al. 2014)

1. Bully targets victim or victims
2. Supporters and followers participate in the bullying
3. Victim and onlookers do not intervene
4. Bully is empowered to continue his or her behavior
5. Onlookers do not intervene
6. Cycle of bullying continues to repeat

behavior, and then disengaging. The workshop involves role-play demonstrations of thwarting bullying using these strategies and offers participants the opportunity to practice new skills. To specifically address bullying among LGBT older adults, the model by Alcon et al. (2014) could be modified to involve employees as well as tenant/residents and include a role-play scenario that features bullying involving sexual orientation or gender identity minority status. Preparatory content that sensitizes participants to this population's needs would also be necessary.

Environmental elements that respect diversity and promote inclusiveness. This type of organizational intervention addresses the overall milieu of the organization and includes specific attention to environmental features that promote inclusiveness and safe spaces for LGBT older adults. Such elements include some photos and artwork that include positive images of same-sex couples or transgender individuals, books and magazines that cater to the LGBT community, and pamphlets and marketing materials for inclusive health and social services organizations in the community. To promote LGBT elders' feelings of acceptance, Sullivan (2014) draws attention to the importance of "reflecting LGBT seniors in published materials, including important dates and events such as PRIDE month on agency calendars, [and] ensuring in-take forms are inclusive" (p. 244). Even basic symbols of inclusion and acceptance can create feelings of comfort for LGBT older adults, such as rainbow stickers posted in offices (Erdley et al. 2014).

Along with making the physical environment safe and inclusive, it is critical to incorporate strategies that increase caring and empathetic behaviors throughout the organization. As positive behaviors increase, problematic interactions will naturally diminish. Interventions can be fairly simple; for example, potential approaches might include (1) acknowledging members of the community that go out of their way to welcome new tenants/residents and anyone who is perceived as "different," including sexual orientation and gender identity minorities; (2) institute a "Caring Squad" whose job is to notice acts of kindness and reward them, and (3) nominate

"Empathy Leaders" each month to recognize tenants/residents and staff who have been especially compassionate to vulnerable individuals and groups. Such activities send the message that caring and empathy are effective ways to achieve recognition, which aid in creating a feeling of acceptance and safety for LGBT older adults.

At the same time, it is important to understand that developing a caring community is a process and organizational change may be slow. Improvements will not happen overnight, and gains can only be made over time. Indeed, in one assisted living facility, after beginning a community culture change effort it was several months before residents began to report feeling more respect for diversity and for one another's perspectives (Personal communication, Dr. Jay Hedgpeth, June 07, 2012).

Summary

This chapter presented an overview of the current state of knowledge regarding bullying and relational aggression related to LGBT elders, with emphasis on understanding the phenomena itself and potential points of intervention. Bullying and relational aggression were defined; bullying was characterized as repetitive aggressive behavior involving an imbalance of power between the bully and the target of bullying, and relational aggression was characterized as a type of bullying that involves nonviolent relationship-based aggression. The chapter discussed how bullying manifests among older adults in general and how it is specifically exhibited among LGBT elders given this population's multi-intersectional experiences. The negative impact of being bullied in late-life was examined, with evidence of reduced emotional well-being stemming from bullying experiences, with example outcomes including social isolation, anxiety, depressed mood, and pervasive fearfulness. For LGBT elders, relational aggression based on sexual orientation and gender identity and fears of potential discrimination and bias were especially salient to the felt need to return to the closet upon entering primarily heterosexual senior housing environments. The chapter concluded with a description of a promising framework to minimize bullying and relational aggression aimed at LGBT elders. Suggested interventions focused on organizational change and included the following: (1) developing policies and procedures that promote caring communities; (2) commitments to civil social interaction by both older consumers and staff; (3) bystander intervention training; and (4) the addition of environmental elements that foster inclusiveness.

event; what are some other potential strategies for increasing power that would not violate the rights of others?

4. The chapter addresses bullying interventions at the organizational level; what interventions might be appropriate to change the behaviors of individuals who bully? What about strategies to minimize negative outcomes for victims?

Appendix Items Developed with Sherri Shimansky, MSW, MPA

Discussion Box 18.1

Discussion Questions:

1. The chapter explains that one of the differences between late-life bullying and elder abuse is that with bullying, the victim is not dependent on the bully for care or services, whereas with abuse, the victim is dependent on the abuser in some capacity? What other differences exist between bullying and abuse?

2. Much attention has been given to bullying among children and youth in contrast to bullying among older adults; why do you think disparities exist between these two age groups in perceptions of the seriousness of the problem? How can we raise awareness of both the existence of late-life bullying and its negative impact on elder well-being?

3. One of the interventions suggested in the chapter is to offer older adults who bully healthy alternatives for obtaining power or a sense of control, for example, by leading a group or organizing an

Learning Exercises

1. Read more about the disparities and resilience among lesbian, gay, bisexual, and transgender older adults in Fredrikson-Goldsen et al. 2011 full report available at: http://caringandaging. org/wordpress/wp-content/uploads/2011/05/ Full-Report-FINAL-11-16-11.pdf

2. Read "LGBT Older Adults in Long-Term Care Facilities: Stories from the Field"—the collaboration of six organizations seeking to better understand these experiences is available at: http://www.lgbtagingcenter.org/ resources/resource.cfm?r=%2054

3. Research the term "Lavender Scare" online to learn more about the historical perspectives on sexual orientation and gender identity that influenced LGBT elders' earlier life experiences.

4. Read the 2012 SAGE (Services and Advocacy for GLBT Elders) and National Center for Transgender Equality report "Improving the Lives of Transgender Older Adults" to learn more about the specific social, economic, and service barriers facing gender non-conforming elders available at: http:// transequality.org/sites/default/files/docs/ resources/TransAgingPolicyReportFull.pdf

5. Learn more about LGBT rights under the Federal Nursing Home Reform Act from Natalie Chin of Lambda Legal. Video available on YouTube and at: http://www.sageusa. org/resources/videos.cfm?ID=153

6. Read how lesbian, gay, bisexual and transgender aging issues are becoming federal concerns by Loree Cook-Daniels (2011) available at: http://forge-forward.org/wp-content/docs/LGBT-federal-policy-changes.pdf

Self-Check Questions

1. What are the three types of bullying discussed in the chapter?
2. What is relational aggression?
3. How is bullying distinguished from abuse?
4. What are examples of 'intersectionality'?
5. What anti-LGBT bullying tactics were used in the chapter?
6. How can peers or onlookers intervene to disrupt the bullying cycle?

Experiential Exercises

1. Explore anti-discrimination laws in your own state; the 2010 document "Our Maturing Movement: State-by-State LGBT Aging Policy and Recommendations" is a good starting resource. What previous recommendations have been met? What recommendations still exist? It is available at: http://nwnetwork.org/wp-content/uploads/2012/08/2010-NGLTF-Our-Maturing-Movement_State-by-State-LGBT-Aging-Policy-Recommendations3.pdf
2. Contact the Ombudsman's office in your state to learn about efforts to protect LGBT older adults living in nursing homes; a good resource is National Long-Term Care Ombudsman Resource Center at http://www.theconsumervoice.org
3. Contact LGBT advocacy groups to explore efforts to improve quality of life for older adults in your local area; suggested advocacy groups include the following: Gay and Lesbian Medical Association http://www.glma.

org; Equality Federation http://equalityfederation.org; and PFLAG http://community.pflag.org

Multiple-Choice Questions

1. Bullying and relational aggression are associated with which negative outcomes?
   (a) Social isolation
   (b) Increase in teen pregnancy
   (c) Reduced self-esteem
   (d) Answers (a) and (c) only
   (e) All of the above
2. Assisted living residents find which of the following most distressing?
   (a) Being the focus of gossiping and rumor-spreading
   (b) Being harassed to loan money, cigarettes, or other commodities
   (c) Exposure to loud in communal areas
   (d) Being bossed around or told what to do
   (e) All of the above.
3. Microagressions
   (a) Contribute to harm when none was intended
   (b) Are considered misdemeanors
   (c) Are acts of physical violence
   (d) All of the above
4. Some basic levels of protections for LGBT elders include
   (a) Prohibition of physical, emotional, sexual, and financial abuse
   (b) Promoting autonomy, respect, and dignity in nursing homes
   (c) Housing discrimination based on gender
   (d) All of the above
5. Promising interventions to address bullying at an organizational level include
   (a) Providing LGBT training to all employees
   (b) Using signage that reflects diversity acceptance

(c) Creating an exclusive community house LGBT wing

(d) All of the above

(e) Answers (a) and (b) only

6. Which of the following represents a primary difference between late-life bullying and elder abuse?

(a) Abuse causes physical harm to the victim, but bullying does not.

(b) Abuse has a long-lasting negative impact, whereas bullying does not.

(c) Abuse is most often perpetrated against someone who is dependent on the aggressor for care or instrumental assistance; with bullying, this is typically not the case.

(d) Abuse most commonly occurs in nursing home settings, but bullying occurs in virtually all senior living environments.

7. Bystander intervention involves which of the following elements:

(a) Teaching the targets of bullying how to defend themselves against bullies.

(b) Teaching individuals who witness bullying how to effectively intercede to stop its occurrence.

(c) Developing policies and procedures that guide civil behavior in senior living organizations.

(d) All of the above.

8. Which of the following represents the most accurate definition of bullying?

(a) Intentional repetitive aggressive behavior that involves an imbalance of power or strength.

(b) Nonviolent behavior designed to hinder social relationships and connectedness.

(c) Intentional behavior intended to cause physical or psychological harm toward someone dependent on the aggressor.

(d) Ridiculing or teasing someone in public.

9. About how many older adults living in senior housing organizations experience peer bullying?

(a) 50 %

(b) 5 %

(c) 30 %

(d) 20 %

10. A type of bullying unique to LGBT older adults is

(a) Relational aggression

(b) Gossiping

(c) Outing

(d) Stealing

Answer Key

1. d
2. e
3. a
4. d
5. e
6. c
7. b
8. a
9. d
10. c

Resources

Gender Public Advocacy Organization (genderPAC): www.gpac.org

Tolerence.org: www.tolerence.org

The Consumer Voice http://theconsumervoice.org

Assisted Living Consumer Alliance http://www.assistedlivingconsumers.org

National Resource Center on LGBT Aging http://www.lgbtagingcenter.org/

References

Adelman, M., Gurevitch, J., deVries, B., & Blando, J. (2006). Openhouse: Community building and research in the LGBT aging population. In D. Kimmel, T. Rose, & S. David (Eds.), *Lesbian, gay, bisexual, and transgender aging: Research and clinical perspectives* (pp. 247–264). New York, NY: Columbia University Press.

Alcon, A., Burnes, K., & Frankel, M. (March, 2014). *Social bullying: Training older adults to make a positive difference*. Workshop presentation at the American Society on Aging, Aging in American Conference, San Diego, California.

Association, American Health Care. (2006). *The long term care survey*. Washington, D. C.: Author.

Barker, R. M. (2008). Gay and lesbian health disparities: Evidence and recommendation for elimination. *Journal of Health Disparities Research and Practice, 2*, 91–120.

Bonifas, R. P. (2011). *Understanding challenging social relationships in senior housing communities*. Phoenix, Arizona: Unpublished raw data; Arizona State University.

Bonifas, R. P., & Frankel, M. (March, 2012). *Is it bullying? Strategies for assessing and intervening with older adults*. Workshop presentation at the Aging in America Conference of the American Society on Aging, Washington, D. C.

Bonifas, R. P., & Kramer, C. (November, 2011). *Senior bullying in assisted living: Residents' perspectives*. In Poster presentation at the 64th annual scientific meeting of the gerontological society of America, Boston, Massachusetts.

Cook-Daniels, L. (2011). *Lesbian, gay, bisexual and transgender aging issues become federal concerns*. Available at http://forge-forward.org/wp-content/docs/LGBT-federal-policy-changes.pdf.

Erdley, S. D., Anklam, D. D., & Reardon, C. C. (2014). Breaking barriers and building bridges: Understanding the pervasive needs of older LGBT adults and the value of social work in health care. *Journal of Gerontological Social Work, 57*(204), 362–385.

Forni, P. M. (2002). *Choosing civility: Twenty-five tools of considerate conduct*. New York: Saint Martin's Press.

Fredriksen-Goldsen, K. I., Kim, H. J., Emlet, C. A., Muraco, A., Erosheva, E. A., Hoy-Ellis, C. P., & Petry, H. (2011). *The aging and health report: Disparities and resilience among lesbian, gay, bisexual, and transgender older adults*. Seattle, WA: Institute for Multigenerational Health.

Hawker, S. S. J., & Boulton, M. J. (2000). Twenty years' research on peer victimization and psychosocial maladjustment: A meta-analytic review of cross-sectional studies. *Journal of Child Psychology and Psychiatry, 41*, 441–455.

Hazelden Foundation. (2011). *Bullying is a serious issue*. Available at http://www.violencepreventionworks.org/public/bullying.page.

National Center on Elder Abuse. (n. d.). *What is elder abuse?* Retrieved from http://www.ncea.aoa.gov/faq/index.aspx.

National Senior Citizens Law Center in collaboration with Lambda Legal, National Center for Lesbian Rights, National Center for Transgender Equality, National Gay and Lesbian Task Force and Services and Advocacy for GLBT Elders (SAGE). (2011). *LGBT Older Adults in long-term care facilities: Stories from the field*. Retrieved from http://www.lgbtagingcenter.org/resources/resource.cfm?r= 54.

Pillemer, K., Mosqueda, L., & Castle, N. (November, 2014). *Resident to resident elder mistreatment: Findings from a large scale prevalence study*. Symposium presentation at the 67th annual scientific meeting of the gerontological society of American, Washington D. C.

Rayner, C., & Keashly, L. (2005). Bullying at work: A perspective from Britain and North America. In S. Fox & P. E. Spector (Eds.), *Counterproductive work behavior: Investigations of actors and targets* (pp. 271–296). Washington, DC: American Psychological Association.

Reese, R. (March 22, 2012). Georgia woman, 87, accused of bullying neighbor. *ABC News*. Available at http://abcnews.go.com/blogs/headlines/2012/03/georgia-woman-87-accused-of-bullying-neighbor/.

Stein, G., Beckerman, N., & Sherman, P. (2010). Lesbian and gay elders and long-term care: Identifying the unique psychosocial perspectives and challenges. *Journal of Gerontological Social Work, 53*, 42–435.

Sue, D. W. (2010). *Microaggressions in everyday life: Race, gender, and sexual orientation*. Hoboken, NJ: Wiley.

Sullivan, K. M. (2014). Acceptance in the domestic environment: The experience of senior housing for lesbian, gay, bisexual, and transgender seniors. *Journal of Gerontological Social Work, 57*(2–4), 235–250.

Trompetter, H., Scholte, R., & Westerhof, G. (2011). Resident-to-resident relational aggression and subjective well-being in assisted living facilities. *Aging and Mental Health, 15*, 59–67.

Debra A. Harley

Abstract

The purpose of this chapter was to examine the impact of healthcare reform in the USA on LGBT elders, especially the Affordable Care Act (ACA). Attention is given to health disparities and coming out risk factors for LGBT elders, health systems challenges for LGBT elders, advantages and disadvantages of healthcare reform on LGBT elders, and future directions of healthcare reform in the USA. Where appropriate, discussion from an international perspective is included, especially Canada and the UK. It is not the intent of this chapter to endorse any point of view over the other or to be advisory about healthcare issues. The intent is to present multiple perspectives concerning the benefits and debates of healthcare reform on seniors, especially LGBT elders.

Keywords

Healthcare reform · LGBT elders' health · LGBT health disparities

Overview

Health policy is a set of decisions taken by governments or healthcare organizations to achieve a desired health outcome (Cherry and Trotter Betts 2005). Navarro (2007) contends that the scope of health policy is beyond medical care and extends to any action that affects health.

Health policy planning and reform can be achieved at the international level through regulations that guide communities in preventing and responding to acute public health risks that have the potential to threaten people worldwide, at national levels with legislation, or on local levels with internal guidelines for patient caseloads in local clinics (An et al. 2015). An et al. suggest that it is necessary to consider the context in which policies are made or implemented because the setting often includes policy challenges. These challenges include but are not limited to (a) a dearth of societal resources, (b) different needs and competing interests from consumers

D.A. Harley (✉)
SAGE, New York, USA
e-mail: respinoza@sageusa.org

© Springer International Publishing Switzerland 2016
D.A. Harley and P.B. Teaster (eds.), *Handbook of LGBT Elders*,
DOI 10.1007/978-3-319-03623-6_19

and stakeholders, (c) conflict between efficiency and fairness, (d) deep uncertainty about the future, and (e) political, social, and cultural issues with regard to policy design and implementation (An et al. 2015). In the USA, healthcare reform has an extensive history with limited change and impact until recently. In 2010, two major federal statutes became law, the Patient Protection and Affordable Care Act (PPACA) and the Health Care and Education Reconciliation Act of 2010 (H.R. 4872), which amended the PPACA. The purpose of this chapter was to examine the impact of healthcare reform in the USA, especially PPACA (more commonly referred to as the Affordable Care Act [ACA]) on LGBT elders. In this discussion of the ACA, the term "Obama care" is not used due to its negative political and bipartisan connotation, because it detracts from an examination of what is both beneficial and challenging about this legislation. Attention is given to health disparities and coming out risk factors for LGBT elders, health systems challenges for LGBT elders, advantages and disadvantages of healthcare reform on LGBT elders, and future directions of healthcare reform for LGBT elders. Although the primary focus of this chapter is on healthcare reform in the USA, whenever possible, discussion from an international perspective, especially Canada and the United Kingdom, is also included. In addition, this author does not intend to endorse any particular point of view or to be advisory about healthcare issues, but rather to present multiple perspectives concerning the benefits and debates of healthcare reform on older adults, especially those who are LGBT.

Learning Objectives

By the end of the chapter, the reader should be able to:

1. Identify health risk and challenges for LGBT elders.
2. Understand the advantages and disadvantages of healthcare reform legislation for LGBT elders.
3. Identify gaps in healthcare reform for LGBT elders.
4. Identify future areas of need in healthcare reform and implementation for LGBT elders.

Introduction

Although the focus of this chapter is on healthcare reform, some discussion of healthcare concerns and disparities of LGBT elders is referenced throughout. LGBT elders are at risk of health disparities from several perspectives, including minority stress as a sexual minority; a life course perspective in which events at each stage of life influence subsequent stages; legal, political, and social issues; an intersectionality perspective because of multiple identities and the ways in which they interact; and the social–ecological perspective in which older adults are surrounded by spheres of influence such as families, communities, and society (Ard and Makadon 2012; Institute of Medicine [IOM] 2011). Overall, research on the LGBT population and its health status throughout the life course is limited, with more research focusing on gay men and lesbians than on bisexual and transgender persons, to a lesser extent on racial and ethnic minority groups, and even less attention on LGBT elders (IOM). In 2012, Health and Human Services Secretary Kathleen Sebelius applauded the ACA as "the strongest foundation we have ever created to begin to closing LGBT health disparities." There is a consensus in the literature that LGBT populations have unique health experiences and needs; however, in the USA, we have not quantified the experiences and needs to know exactly what they are (IOM; SAGE 2012). Nevertheless, we do know that LGBT persons are more likely than their heterosexual counterparts to experience difficulty in accessing health care (Ard and Makadon 2012).

Before the passage of the ACA, the healthcare system in the USA was the most expensive in the world, yet delivered lower quality outcomes than systems of other industrialized countries (Saul 2009). The US counterpart, Canada, has the second most expensive healthcare system among industrialized countries with universal health care (Barua and Clemens 2014). Once the majority of the provisions of the ACA are implemented, it is estimated that approximately thirty million previously uninsured Americans will have access to health care (Congressional Budget Office 2012). A key component of the ACA, the Community Living Assistance Services and Supports (CLASS) Act, was designed to provide public voluntary long-term care insurance, which could have helped to shield elderly people from catastrophic out-of-pocket costs, but was dropped in 2011. The primary reason for discontinuing CLASS was challenges about financial viability (Kelley et al. 2013).

The healthcare reform debate includes arguments representing the benefits and disadvantages as well as mixed implications of healthcare reform legislation. The view of those who espouse mixed implications suggests that one has to expect negative aspects to any plan that takes monies out of Medicare and that such a plan will invariably going to cut some people's benefits. In addition, the claim that ACA will close the "doughnut hole" in Medicare Part D is not as generous as originally portrayed (Kaplan 2011). In essence, ACA lowers a patient's cost obligation for co-payment (i.e., the benefit), but it is not the same as saying that individuals will not have any cost exposure whatsoever (Kaplan). Kaplan stresses that enrollees in managed care (MC) plans are likely to be less satisfied with the new law because MC plans will raise premiums or may discontinue their participation in the program altogether. In either case, the result will likely be higher costs, reduced benefits, and fewer options for enrollees in Medicare managed care plans.

Health Disparities and Coming Out Risk Factors for LGBT Elders

This section examines **implications** of health disparities for LGBT elders. Overwhelmingly, the literature confirms the existence of health disparities for LGBT elders and adverse consequences in healthcare services and other sociocultural aspects. The first step in addressing LGBT Americans' health disparities is ensuring that policymakers, medical professionals, healthcare workers, and social service providers have a clear understanding of those disparities. Federal health surveys are an essential tool in determining how disparities and differences are recognized and addressed in subpopulations (Rosenthal 2009). Healthcare reform legislation contains a number of provisions to address healthcare disparities (e.g., advisory councils, prioritize the elimination of health disparities, develop a public health insurance option, expand health data collection). Rosenthal stresses that LGBT health disparities in each of these areas should be considered along with racial, ethnic, and geographic disparities.

Health disparities are increased with revealing one's sexual orientation and sexual identity to healthcare providers because of discrimination, stigma, and poor quality of care. LGBT elders and their caregivers have faced discrimination in the healthcare system for most of their lives. Both historical hostilities and current prejudices against LGBT populations have resulted in many LGBT elders not revealing their identities to healthcare providers or delaying or avoiding seeking medical or mental health intervention (Ard and Makadon 2012). Chapter 20 further discusses the risk factors associated with both disclosure and non-disclosure of sexual orientation and gender identity in the USA.

According to Baker and Krehely (2012), governments and service providers rarely track health data on LGBT persons, resulting in its limited availability, which suggests that later life carries unique health challenges for LGBT persons, particularly in areas that have a high concentration of HIV/AIDS, mental health, and chronic health conditions. See Chaps. 20, 23, and 32 for further discussion on healthcare and sexual practices, mental health counseling, and disabilities among LGBT elders. In the study and discussion of LGBT health disparities, the specific needs of transgender persons are seldom explored separately. From the 2011 *National Healthcare Disparities Report* findings, transgender persons (a) are more likely to be uninsured and less likely to have employer-based health insurance than the general population; (b) postpone care when sick or injured and postpone preventive health care due to cost, discrimination, and disrespect by providers, with female-to-male transgender persons being most likely to postpone care due to discrimination; and (c) one in five has been denied services by a doctor or other provider due to their gender, with racial and ethnic minority transgender persons being more likely to be denied services (Agency for Healthcare Research and Quality 2012). Of LGBT populations, transgender persons are at greater risk of receiving inferior health care or being denied health care because of their sexual identity (Fredriksen-Goldsen et al. 2011). In addition, the number of clinicians who have had knowledge or have received training about health issues pertinent to transgender persons further exacerbates their risk factors (Kaufman 2010). Healthcare practitioners, for example, may not realize that physical examinations or intimate care are sources of extreme anxiety to transgender adults, be unfamiliar with the outcomes of less refined surgical techniques, which may result in appearance of genitalia that are "abnormal," and may not understand that physical examinations and screening tests should be predicated on the organs actually presented instead of the appearance of the person (Feldman 2010; Kaufman 2010).

LGBT elders and their caregivers face discrimination in the healthcare system, and heterosexism effectively works to create obstacles to achieving full equality for LGBT persons (Brotman et al. 2006). Greenesmith et al. (2013) offer a guide to understanding the benefits of ACA and LGBT families. The guide provides a basic overview of the ACA, a review of how the act helps LGBT persons and their families, and an explanation of how the person and his or her family can access affordable health insurance (see the "Resources" section of this chapter under the Center for American Progress for the location of the guide). In Canada, two notable organizations that are run by lesbian and gay community groups are the 519 Community Centre in Toronto and The Centre in Vancouver that have highly organized and advanced programs for gay and lesbian elders and their caregivers (Brotman et al. 2007). Brotman et al. (2007) acknowledge that even with the efforts, policies, and practices of these organizations in addressing issues facing gay and lesbian elders in Canada, they remain marginalized within mainstream health and social service agencies. The result is isolation and invisibility of both LGBT persons and caregivers in environments often marked by intolerance and avoidance.

Health Systems Challenges for LGBT Elders

Over 50 years ago, both the USA and Canadian healthcare systems were similar. Over time, Canada moved toward a universal single-payer system that covers the majority of expenditures and without co-payment or user fees for all medically necessary hospital and physician care for all fully insured persons as required by the Canada Health Act. Over 90 % of hospital expenditures and almost 100 % of total physician services are funded by the public sector (Library of Parliament Research, n.d.). It is important to note that the Canadian system provides pubic coverage from a combination of public and private delivery and is not a system of socialized medicine, but rather one of universal health care (Barua and Esmail 2013). The USA and Turkey are the only two members of the Organization for Economic Cooperation and Development (OECD) without some form of formal universal health coverage. The OECD is an organization that acts as a meeting ground for 30 countries that believe in the free market system. The OECD provides a forum for discussing issues and reaching agreements (www.oecd.org).

One of the major challenges the Canadian healthcare system facing is lengthy wait times for treatment, often months long and sometimes stretching over a year (Barua and Esmail 2013). Wait times are not a characteristic of universal healthcare countries. Other countries with universal health care (e.g., Belgium, France, Germany, Japan, Luxembourg, Korea, Switzerland, the Netherlands) typically report few problems with wait times (Barua and Clemens 2014). Canadians faced with long periods of wait times have resorted to seeking non-emergency treatment outside of Canada. Among the 12 major medical specialties surveyed by the Fraser Institute, the most patients receiving care outside Canada were in urology, general surgery, and ophthalmology, and the least likely were in cardiovascular surgeries, radiation treatment for cancer, and chemotherapy for cancer (Barua and Esmail 2013). Unfortunately, the survey did not distinguish the age cohorts of these patients.

In addition to concerns and challenges that confront individuals as they age, LGBT elders face at least three unique barriers and inequities that impact their health and access to health care, positive engagement with their communities, and psychosocial adjustment. These barriers include (a) social stigma and prejudice, past and present; (b) reliance on informal families of choice for social connections, care, and support; and (c) laws and programs that fail to address or create barriers to better health and well-being for LGBT elders (Baker and Krehely 2012). Although there are no LGBT-specific diseases, numerous health disparities affect LGBT persons, especially older adults. For example, LGBT persons have higher rates of depression, anxiety, suicidal ideation, and substance abuse than their heterosexual counterparts (IOM 2011; Ruble and Forstein 2008; see Chaps. 23, 24). These higher rates of pathology are attributed to the minority stress they experience on the basis of sexual orientation and gender identity, and when these identities intersect with the inequalities associated with race, ethnicity, and social class, their trauma is magnified (see Chaps. 5–10). In addition, the lack of knowledge and cultural competency about LGBT populations in the healthcare system further discourage LGBT elders from seeking care. See Chap. 20 for further discussion about cultural competency of healthcare providers.

In both the USA and Canada, the inclusion of LGBT persons in health and well-being initiatives has been overwhelmingly from the perspective of an illness-based focus, such as HIV/AIDS, and from an oppressive and one-dimensional analysis (Berkelman 2012; Mule et al. 2009). A similar approach is seen throughout the world (World Health Organization 2012). Mule et al. make several observations about similarities in public health between the USA and Canada. First, although both the USA and Canada recognize health determinants that comprise four health fields: biology, lifestyle, environments, and health care, they downplay the impact of social structures in health while focusing on individual relational action and responsibility. Second, in the case of LGBT persons, a microlevel or individualized lifestyle approach continues to dominate health promotion by targeting high-risk populations through large-scale campaigns in which interventions promote risk reduction through behavior change (Mule et al. 2009). Finally, illness and behavior remain the primary focus and sexual orientation and gender identity, as social locations in the broader social health structures, simply do not register. In Canada, LGBT persons are included in human rights protection, inclusive of healthcare services, but for the most part, they have not been recognized as an identifiable population within the healthcare sector (Mule 2007), and gender identity is absent from most human rights legislation across Canada with the exception of the Northwest Territories and the City of Toronto (Rainbow Health Network 2008).

In Uganda, health workers could become the frontline enforcers of the newly passed Anti-Homosexuality Act of 2014. The *Draft Guidelines for Health Workers Regarding Health Services for Homosexuals* suggests that healthcare facilities would be made more dangerous for LGBT persons. The guidelines specify that health workers could break confidentiality of gay and lesbian patients, even when not required by law in cases when a person has been sodomized or in cases of "aggravated homosexuality" (i.e., same-sex intercourse repeatedly, same-sex intercourse with a minor or persons with a disability or a persons who has HIV) as defined by the Anti-Homosexuality Act (Feder 2014). In addition, under the provisions of the draft guidelines,

Table 19.1 Practices by nurses to improve quality of care of LGBT patients

Realize that they already have LGBT patients or residents
Change the way information is gathered from the patient
Ask questions about sexual orientation and gender identity separately
Questions such as marital status may need to be amended
If an adult identifies as transgender, the nurse must ask how the client wishes to be addressed
Ask what surgeries have been completed, as it may directly affect the care needed

Adapted from Jablonski et al. (2013)

healthcare workers might be in a vulnerable position of being charged with promoting homosexuality, even in cases where they have been approved to provide services or conduct research with lesbian and gay persons. Researchers, health workers, or health facilities are solely responsible to ensure that no acts of promotion or recruitment of subjects into acts of homosexuality, as stipulated by the Anti-Homosexuality Act, occurs. In fact, one clause of the act reads, "In the event of promotion or recruitment, they shall be held accountable" (Feder 2014).

In the healthcare system, nurses are typically the first point of contact for patients, and as the front line of care, they can directly impact the quality of care of LGBT elders' experience (Jablonski et al. 2013). Jablonski et al. recommend practices that nurses can follow to improve the quality of care they provide to LGBT patients (see Table 19.1). Although all clinicians and service providers should be trained in culturally appropriate knowledge and skills in working with LGBT elders, it is essential for those who initially have contact with patients.

Rosenthal (2009) indicates that health information technology will significantly reduce costs and increase coordinated care, but it can also put LGBT persons at risk. For example, comprehensive care requires that a primary care provider to know about a patient's sexual behavior, gender history, and other sensitive information. However, not all providers need access to all information (e.g., there is not need for an orthopedist to know that a person is gay). The result might be the exposure of too much information, which in turn could expose LGBT persons to discrimination by healthcare providers (Rosenthal 2009).

Impact of Healthcare Legislation on LGBT Elders

Healthcare legislation for older adults in the USA has its origins in the passage of the Medicare legislation enacted in 1965. At that time, President Lyndon Johnson signed the legislation, declaring that no longer will older Americans loose their life savings due to illness (Beschloss 2006). The intent of Medicare was to provide healthcare coverage to persons aged 65 and older and to protect elders from financial risks. However, Medicare does not cover the full financial cost of poor health among elders, requiring many enrollees to pay significant out-of-pocket co-payments and deductibles. In addition, Medicare does not cover a variety of services particularly valuable for those with chronic diseases or a lifelong illness (Kelley et al. 2013). Alternatives to ACA have focused on voucher plans with greater cost sharing; however, such plans would most likely increase, not decrease, out-of-pocket medical expenditures for Medicare recipients (e.g., the bipartisan options for the future, *Choices to Strengthen Medicare and Health Security for All*, by Senator Ron Wyden of Oregon and Senator Paul Ryan of Wisconsin, www.budget.house.gov/uploadedfiles/wydenryan.pdf). The primary goal of this plan was "to strengthen traditional Medicare by permanently maintaining it as a guaranteed and viable option for all of the nation's retirees" and simultaneously "expanding choice for seniors by allowing the private sector to compete with Medicare in an effort to offer seniors better quality and more affordable healthcare choice" (p. 1). The plan included the following components: (a) choice, (b) affordability, (c) protecting the guarantee, (d) protecting seniors, (e) protecting the safety net, and

(f) lifelong choices. The Wyden–Ryan plan seek to respond to the fast-paced growth of Medicare spending, which is growing more than twice as fast as the economy.

Throughout the twentieth century, healthcare coverage was too expensive and difficult to obtain for many Americans and more so for LGBT persons. Michael Adams, Executive Director of SAGE, in 2009 described the lack of attention of federal policy on LGBT issues in the past eight years (i.e., President George W. Bush's administration) as a "wasteland" (SAGE Matters 2009, p. 3). Kerry Eleveld, Senior Political Correspondent for The Advocate magazine, added, with the attempt of President Obama and the Congress "to overhaul our health care system and bring more Americans into the fold, older Americans will undoubtedly be a high-priority constituency" (SAGE Matters 2009, p. 5). Moreover, SAGE (2012) asserts that health reform has dramatically improved healthcare coverage for LGBT elders who face health disparities, aggravated by a lifetime of discrimination and higher economic insecurity, in several ways (a) by expanding coverage, (b) strengthening consumer rights and protections, and (c) improving data collection efforts and a host of other benefits.

In general, most people agree that healthcare reform is a step in the right direction in equalizing access to and improving the quality of health care for LGBT persons. The point of division or disagreement is about the extent to which reform is effective beyond access. On the one hand, Baker and Krehely (2012) consider the Affordable Care Act (ACA) as "the most significant and far-reaching reform of America's health system since the creation of Medicare and Medicaid in the 1960s" (p. 21). Baker and Krehely espouse two major advantages of the ACA to include (a) the introduction of new protections and options for patients in the private health insurance market and (b) expansion of access to more comprehensive benefits and services that focus on improving our nation's health and lowering healthcare cost by investing in keeping people healthy in the first place. The ACA also includes provisions such as

expanding cultural competency in the healthcare workforce to include LGBT issues, improving data collection to better identify and address health disparities, and recognizing the increasing diversity of America's families (Baker and Krehely 2011). The ACA has implications for LGBT elders from an intersectionality perspective as well: Sexual minorities, elderly, and persons overrepresented with HIV (SAGE 2014).

According to SAGE, for older LGBT persons, poor health represents the cumulative effect of a lifetime of discrimination, and the ACA prevents health insurers from denying coverage or charging higher premiums based on preexisting conditions, or a person's sexual orientation or gender identity. The significance of this provision is that access to care is expanded for transgender persons and those living with HIV/AIDS, who often face life-threatening discrimination in healthcare coverage. For older persons who already have coverage through Medicare, the ACA has provisions that improve the benefits available through adding free wellness checkups and prevention services. For persons with HIV, the benefits include prescription drug coverage, laboratory services, and chronic disease management. The ACA ended lifetime dollar limits on essential health benefits, cracked down on frivolous cancellations of policies, and made it illegal to arbitrarily cancel health insurance simply because the policyholder got sick (SAGE 2014). See Table 19.2 for ways in which ACA impact on elders.

Chance (2013) acknowledges that the ACA's reformatory focus on increasing access to care will likely work to remedy some of the discrimination that results in the LGBT community's disparate access to care. However, Chance believes that the ACA "fails to comprehensively combat the broader LGBT healthcare discrimination because it will do nothing to remedy the stigma that results in lower quality care" (p. 376). Chance identifies the major disadvantages of the ACA, which result in gaps in access to quality medical services that include failure to address the social stigma associated with a patient's LGBT status and failure to address specific needs of the LGBT community. The recommended

Table 19.2 Affordable Care Act's impact on elders

Reduce prescription drug cost in Medicare Part D
Provide a free annual wellness visit for all Medicare beneficiaries
Provide free Medicare coverage of vital preventive services
Encourage better care coordination
Expand coverage for seniors under age 65
Protect patent rights and lower costs in the private health insurance market
Provide new options for long-term care
Increase access to home-based care
Nursing home transparency
Protecting seniors from abuse and neglect
Implement the Elder Justice Act

Adapted from Baker and Krehely (2012), Medicare.org (2013)

reforms include a national legislative and regulatory effort for training competent providers for LGBT patients. Chance recommends "amending the ACA to include provisions requiring applicable agencies to issue rules aimed at increasing implementation and utilization of LGBT-specific cultural competence training provides a convenient vehicle for such reform" (p. 399). In addition, Congress should amend the ACA to require agencies that administer research funding to place a condition on receipt of those funds to treat disadvantaged persons such as those who LGBT (e.g., medical schools). Finally, although not directly related to the ACA, LGBT-specific cultural competence can also be achieved at the state level, stipulating that licensing boards require a certain number of hours of LGBT cultural competence training as a condition of renewed licensure. Chance suggests amending the ACA to address discriminatory attitudes is a better choice for such reform than other avenues.

Those who argue that healthcare reform legislation may have potential negative consequences for seniors suggest several disadvantages. First, health reform will not shore up Medicare's financing, despite claims to the contrary (The Senior Citizen League [TSCL] www.seniorsleague.org). The assurance by lawmakers that healthcare reform would keep the Medicare trust in the black for several additional years is challenged by the Congressional Budget office (CBO), which claims the government is "double counting." In 2009, a CBO memo stated that "the saving to the health insurance trust would be received by the government only once, thus they cannot be set aside to pay for future Medicare spending and, at the same time, pay for current spending on other parts of the legislation or on other programs" (http://www.cbo.gob/publications/25017). Second, as providers experience cuts and go out of business, seniors may have reduced access to medical care (TSCL). To support this notion of the long-term assumption for Medicare and aggregate national health expenditures, reference is made to the Chief Actuary of the government's Centers for Medicare and Medicaid services who connotes that providers for whom Medicare constitutes is a substantive portion of their business could find it difficult to remain profitable, and without legislation intervention, might end their participation in the program, possibly jeopardizing access to care for beneficiaries (www.cms.gov/Research-Statistics-Data-and-System/Statistics-Trend-and-reports/ReportsTrustFunds/downloads/2010TR AlternativeScenario.pdf).

Many LGBT elders are classified as having low socioeconomic status and limited resources and, as such, may be eligible for the Medicaid program. For persons who are eligible for full Medicaid coverage, Medicare healthcare coverage is supplemented by services (e.g., nursing facility care beyond the 100-day limited covered by Medicare, eyeglasses, hearing aids) that are available under their state's Medicaid program. For persons enrolled in both programs, any services covered by Medicare are paid for by the Medicare program before any payments are made by the Medicaid program because Medicaid is always the payer of last resort (Annual Statistical Supplement 2011). Even so, Medicare does not cover all of a senior's medical expenses.

Older adults who qualify for the federal government program have several options to purchase additional health insurance called Medicare

Advantage plans, which is classified into three basic categories: Private-Fee-for-Service, Health Maintenance Organization (HMO), or Preferred Provider Organization (PPO). According to the Centers for Medicare and Medicaid Services, the most recent addition to the lineup to help manage the health care of senior Americans is the Accountable Care Organizations (ACO). ACO is a collection of healthcare providers who come together and assume responsibility for the care, quality, and cost of healthcare services for a specified group of people. ACO is not an insurance plan. The ACO model is designed to (a) deliver accountable care, (b) emphasize quality of care (a point that Chance (2013) argues is a shortcoming of ACA), (c) coordinate care for patients, and (d) reduce costs by reducing waste (Botek 2015).

Future Directions of Healthcare Reform

The future direction of healthcare reform is uncertain. It is also uncertain whether healthcare reform will regress to something previously known and tried or to something innovative and exploratory. However, several certainties do exist. First, there will continue to be opponents to whatever type of healthcare reform and healthcare legislation is proposed, and second, increases in health care spending along with fiscal pressures created by an aging population and increasing prevalence of debility and chronic conditions make it likely that out-of-pocket expense will continue to rise (Kelley et al. 2013). In addition, an ongoing challenge for healthcare delivery and healthcare reform is related to increasing costs and the ability of the government to continue to fund Medicare and Medicaid in the USA and universal health care in Canada, the ability of individuals to be able to afford health insurance, and the quality of care for LGBT elders. According to Kelley et al., the "average" elder will pay approximately $39,000 in out-of-pocket medical cost during the final five years of life, and a "typical" elder in the top 25 %

of medical expenditures will pay about $101,791 in the five years preceding their death (see Research Box 19.1).

Research Box 19.1 Out-of-Pocket Medical Costs

Keyyey, A. S., McGarry, K., Fahle, S., Marshall, S. M., Du, Q., & Skinner, J. S. (2013). Out-of-pocket spending in the last five years of life. *Journal of General Internal Medicine, 28*(2), 304–309.

Objective: To determine the cumulative financial risks arising from out-of-pocket healthcare expenditures faced by older adults, particularly near the end of life.

Method: Retrospective analyses of Medicare beneficiaries' total out-of-pocket healthcare expenditures over the last five years of life were conducted using the nationally representative Health and retirement Study (HRS) cohort. The subjects were HRS decedents between 2002 and 2008, using each subject's date of death to define a 5-year study period and excluding those without Medicare coverage at the beginning of this period (n = 3209). The total out-of-pocket healthcare expenditures in the last 5 years of life and expenditures as a percentage of baseline household assets were examined. Then, stratified results by marital status and cause of death. All measurements were adjusted for inflation to 2008 US dollars.

Results: Average out-of-pocket expenditures in the 5 years prior to death were $38,688 (95 % confidence interval $36,868, $40,508) for individuals and $51,030 (95 % CI $47,649, $54,412) for couples in which one spouse/partner dies. Spending was skewed, with the median and 90th percentile equal to $22,885 and $89,106, respectively, for individuals, and $39,759 and $94,823, respectively, for couples. Overall, 25 % of subjects' expenditures exceeded baseline total household assets and 43 % of subjects' spending surpassed their non-housing assets. Among those survived by a spouse, 10 % exceeded total baseline assets and 24 % exceeded non-housing assets. By cause of death, average spending ranged from $31,069 for gastrointestinal disease to $66,155 for Alzheimer's disease.

Conclusion: Even with Medicare coverage, elderly households face considerable financial risk from out-of-pocket healthcare expenses at the end of life. Disease-related differences in this risk complicate efforts to anticipate or plan for health-related expenditures in the last 5 years of life.

Questions

1. What are the limitations to this study?
2. Overall, what does this study demonstrate about health-related financial costs?
3. What does this study suggest about out-of-pocket expenditures for an aging population and increasing prevalence of chronic illness?

As the USA discusses, debates, and determines the next steps for healthcare reform, Barua and Clemens (2014) suggest consulting the Canadian model in terms of what to avoid rather than as a model for reform or replication. In reality, the Canadian healthcare model "is comparatively expensive and imposes enormous costs on Canadians in the form of waiting for services, and limited access to physicians and medical technology" (p. 2). Moreover, evidence indicates that excessive wait times lead to poorer health outcomes and, in some cases, death. Arguably, for many LGBT persons who frequently delay receiving health care, increased wait times further comprise their health outcomes. Conversely, Friedman (2013) argues that a Canadian-style, single-payer health plan would reap huge savings realized from reduced paperwork and negotiated drug prices that will pay for quality coverage for all and at less cost to families and businesses. Friedman advocates for The

Table 19.3 Ways single-payer program would improve health system

Extend coverage to all uninsured Americans
Reduce barriers to access for the currently insured by eliminating burdensome co-payments, deductibles, and other out-of-pocket spending for medical care
Improve benefits by covering services such as dental and long-term care
Eliminate inequity in the treatment of less affluent patients by paying providers the same fee for each patient regardless of income or employment
No financial barriers or financial harm resulting from seeking care
Patients have their choice of physicians, providers, hospitals, clinics, and practices

Adapted from Friedman (2013), Physicians for a National Health Program (2011)

Expanded & Improved Medicare For All Act (H. R. 676) as progressive taxation to "replace regressive and obsolete funding sources including federal, state, and local government spending on private health insurance for government employees, and state and local government spending on Medicaid and other health programs" (p. 1). See Table 19.3 for ways in which a single-payer program would improve the healthcare system in the USA.

The goal of The Expanded and Improved Medicare For All Act is to ensure that all Americans will have access, guaranteed by law, to the highest quality and most cost-effective healthcare services regardless of their employment, income, or healthcare status. Essentially, health care becomes a fundamental human right without financial barriers or hardship resulting from obtaining care (Physicians for a National Health Program 2011). Clearly, the focus of H.R. 676 aligns with the needs of and respect and dignity for LGBT elders in the healthcare system. Its intent is to provide every person living or visiting in the USA and the US Territories with a Medicare For All Card and identification number once they enroll at the appropriate location. H.R. 676 will cover all medically necessary services (see Table 19.4) (Physicians for a National Health Program 2011).

Table 19.4 Medically necessary service covered by H. R. 676

Primary care
Medically approved diet and nutrition services
Inpatient care
Outpatient care
Emergency care
Prescription drugs
Durable medical equipment
Hearing services
Oral surgery
Eye care
Chiropractic
Long-term care
Palliative care
Podiatric care
Mental health services
Dentistry
Substance abuse treatment

Adapted from Physicians for a National Health Program (2011)

Since 2003, H.R. 676 has been introduced in every Congressional session. The bill, if adopted, would usher the USA into a single-payer model for healthcare financing, mirroring the rest of the industrialized world. Supporters of the bill see it as the only way to guarantee quality care and sustainably cut costs (Federal Information & News Dispatch 2015). This view is consistent with that of Chance's (2013) position for amending the ACA to ensure the quality of care, not only access for LGBT persons. Ironically, reintroduction of H.R. 676 came on the same day as House Republicans voted for the 56th time to repeal the ACA (Federal Information & News Dispatch 2015).

The future of healthcare policy will need to address health disparities of LGBT elders. Importantly, LGBT elders themselves are emerging as active participants in the debate on reform—they are forging ahead with their own healthcare planning and are increasingly vocal about LGBT-specific and appropriate services. Just as policy and legislation have changed to include legal protections for LGBT elders that prohibit discrimination based on sexual orientation and gender identity by hospital participating in Medicare and Medicaid (Fredriksen-Goldsen et al. 2012), the future of healthcare reform must follow suit.

Summary

Health care is becoming increasingly expensive, particularly for persons with chronic conditions, which disproportionately affects LGBT elders. Decisions about financing strategies for the health care of all persons in the USA rests in the hands of political forces divided not only along party lines, but also along judgments about the rights of LGBT persons. Regardless of the direction that healthcare reform takes, cost containment, access to care, and quality of care should be the hallmark. Many LGBT elders have been and continue to be victimized by inadequacies in the present healthcare system, all the more problematic because the USA spends more per person on health care as any other country, yet lags behind on key indicators such as life expectancy and preventable deaths.

Learning Activities

Self-Check Questions

1. What is the relationship between Medicaid and Medicare for LGBT elders?
2. What are the reasons for LGBT elders' health disparities?
3. What are the advantages and disadvantages of the Affordable Care Act for LGBT persons?
4. What are some of the challenges to policy implementation of healthcare reform?
5. How are health disparities for LGBT populations consistent across different countries?

Experiential Exercises

1. Interview a healthcare provider to discover their knowledge level in working with LGBT elders. In addition, ask questions to determine the service providers' comfort working with LGBT population. See whether they are more or less comfortable working with a particular subgroup of LGBT persons.
2. Imagine yourself as an LGBT elder who now has to decide upon a health insurance plan. What are some questions would you ask?
3. Volunteer to work with LGBT elders to develop a personalized self-advocacy health strategy.

Multiple-Choice Questions

1. Which of the following is the payer of last resort for individuals enrolled in both Medicare and Medicaid?
   (a) Medicare
   (b) Medicaid
   (c) Supplemental Security Income
   (d) Social Security Disability Income
2. Which key component was dropped from the Affordable Care Act?
   (a) Elder Care Assistance
   (b) Independent Living Assurance
   (c) Community Living Assistance Services and Supports
   (d) Fairness Assurance and Community-Based Supports
3. Which of the following is considered the strongest foundation in closing health disparities for LGBT persons?
   (a) Medicare
   (b) Medicaid
   (c) Americans With Disabilities Act
   (d) Affordable Care Act
4. Which of the following is the most recent addition to the options for managing health care for older Americans?
   (a) Private-Fee-for-Service
   (b) Preferred Provider Organizations
   (c) Accountable Care Organizations
   (d) Health Maintenance Organizations

5. Which of the following law can hold healthcare workers, their facilities, or researchers accountable for "promoting homosexuality"?
   (a) Ugandan Anti-Homosexuality Act
   (b) International Gay Protection Act
   (c) Canadian Anti-Sodomy Law
   (d) Universal Human Rights Law
6. What is a disadvantage of health information technology for LGBT persons?
   (a) May expose too much information about a person's sexual identity to providers who do not need to know
   (b) May expose an LGBT person to discrimination by healthcare providers in certain situations
   (c) All of the above
   (d) None of the above
7. Canada has which of the following type of healthcare system?
   (a) Socialized
   (b) Universal
   (c) Medicare
   (d) Medicaid
8. From which type of perspective in most parts of the world has been the inclusion of LGBT persons in health and well-being initiatives?
   (a) Illness based
   (b) One-dimensional
   (c) Oppressive analysis
   (d) All of the above
   (e) None of the above
9. Which of the following is a criticism of the comprehensiveness of the Affordable Care Act for LGBT persons?
   (a) Fails to remedy the stigma that results in lower quality care
   (b) Discourages improved data collection to better identify and address health disparities
   (c) Decreases access to free wellness checkups and prevention services
   (d) Fails to crack down on frivolous cancellations of policies
10. Which of the following statements most accurately reflect the government and service providers' data collection on the health of LGBT persons?

(a) They collect data every 10 years with the Census
(b) They rarely track health data
(c) They will violate HIPPA in so doing
(d) They prioritize type of data collected

Key

1-b
2-c
3-d
4-c
5-a
6-c
7-b
8-d
9-a
10-b

Resources

Advancing Effective Communication, Cultural Competence, and patient-and-Family-Centered Care for the Lesbian, Gay, Bisexual, and Transgender (LGBT) Community: A Field Guide (The Joint Commission): http://www.jointcommission.org/assets/1/18/LGBTFieldGuide.pdf

Affirmative Care for Transgender and Gender Non-Conforming People: Best Practices for Front-line Health Care staff: http://www.lgbthealtheducation.org/wp-content/uploads.13-017_TransBestPracticesforFrontlineStaff_v9_04-30-13.pdf

Agency for Healthcare Research and Quality: www.ahrq.gov/

Center for American Progress- The Affordable Care Act and LGBT Families: Everything You Need to Know: www.fafilyequality.org/_asset/5gqpft/FEC-CAP-LGBT-AVA-Families-Guide.pdf

Do Ask, Do Tell: Talking to your provider about being LGBT: http://www.lgbthealtheducation.org/wp-content/uploads/COM13-067_LGBT HAWbrochure_v4.pdf

Fenway Health/National LGBT Health Education Center: www.lgbthealtheducation.org

LGBT Training Curricula for Behavioral Health and Primary Care Practitioners: www.hrsa.gov/LGBT/lgbtcurricula.pdf

Medicare.org: www.medicare.org

National Resource Center on LGBT Aging: www.lgbtagingcenter.org

Optimizing LGBT Health Under the Affordable Care Act: Strategies for Health Centers: http://www.lgbthealtheducation.org/wp-content/uploads/Brief-Optimizing-LGBT-Health-Under-ACA-FINAL-12-06-2013.pdf

Rainbow Health Ontario (RHO): www.rainbowhealthontario.ca

The ACA and LGBT Older Adults Discussion Guide: www.issues.com/lgbtagingcenter/doc/affordablecareactandlgbtolderadults

References

Annual Statistical Supplement. (2011). *Medicaid program description and legislative history*. Retrieved February 5, 2015 from http://www.ssa.gov/policy/docs/statcomps/supplement/2011/medicaid.html.

An, R., Huang, C., & Baghbabian, A. (2015). Health policy analysis. In E. Mpofu (Ed.), *Community-oriented health services: Practices across disciplines* (pp. 17–40). New York, NY: Springer.

Ard, K. L., & Makadon, H. J. (2012). *Improving the health care of lesbian, gay, bisexual, and transgender (LGBT) people: Understanding and eliminating health disparities*. Boston: The Fenway Institute. Retrieved January 30, 2015 from www.lgbthealtheducation.org/wp-content/uploads/12-054_LGBTHealtharticle_v3_07-09-12.pdf.

Baker, K., & Krehely, J. (2011). *Changing the game: What health care reform means for gay, lesbian, bisexual, and transgender Americans*. Washington, DC: Center for American Progress. Retrieved January 29, 2015 from http://www.americanprogress.org/issues/2011/03/aca_lgbt.html.

Baker, K., & Krehely, J. (2012). How health care reform will help LGBT elders. *Public Policy and Aging Report, 21*(3), 19–23.

Barua, B., & Clemens, J. (2014, June 13). *Canada not a good example of universal health care*. Retrieved February 10, 2015 from http://www.fraserinstitute.org/research-news/news/display.aspx?id=21499#.

Barua, B., & Esmail, N. (2013, December 20). *Seeking relief outside Canada's borders*. Retrieved February 10, 2015 from http://www.fraserinstitute.org/research-news/news/display.aspx?id=20716#.

Berkleman, R. (2012). The United States government's response to HIV/AIDS today: 'Test and Treat' as prevention. *Journal of Public Health Policy, 33*(3), 337–343.

Beschloss, M. (2006). *Our documents: 100 milestone documents from the National Archives.* New York, NY: Oxford University Press.

Botek, A. M. (2015). *For seniors, a new model to deliver "accountable care".* Retrieved February 5, 2015 from http://www.agingcare.com/Articles/accountable-care-organization-help-seniro-health-care-150489.htm.

Brotman, S., Ryan, B., & Meyer, E. (2006). *The health and social service needs of gay and lesbian elders: Final report.* Montreal, Canada: McGill University School of Social Work.

Brotman, S., Ryan, B., Collins, S., Chamberland, L., Comier, R., Julien, D., et al. (2007). Coming out to care: Caregivers of gay and lesbian seniors in Canada. *The Gerontologist, 47*(4), 490–503.

Chance, T. F. (2013). "Going to pieces" over LGBT health disparities: How an amended Affordable Care Act could cure the discrimination that ails the LGBT community. *Journal of Health Care Law and Policy, 15*(2), 375–402.

Cherry, B., & Trotter Betts, V. (2005). Health policy and politics: Get involved. In B. Cherry & S. Jacobs (Eds.), *Contemporary nursing: Issues, trends, and management* (pp. 211–233). St. Louis, MO: Elsevier.

Congressional Budget Office. (2012). *Updated estimates for the insurance coverage provisions of the Affordable Care Act, Updated for the recent Supreme Court Decision 13.* Retrieved January 30, 2015 from http://www.cbo.gov/sites/default/files/cbofiles/attachments/43472-07-24-2012-CoverageEstimates.pdf.

Feder, J. L. (2014, April 22). *Ugandan health workers could become front-line enforcers of Anti-homosexuality Act.* Retrieved February 9, 2015 from http://www.buzzfeed.com/lesterfeder/updated-ugandan-guidelines-could-make-health-workers-front-l#.ul51yZP3n.

Federal Information & News Dispatch. (2015, February 5). *Rep. Conyers and 44 House democrats reintroduced "The Expanded and Improved Medicare For All Act".* Retrieved February 10, 2015 from http://www.insurancenewsnet.com/oarticle/2015/05/rep-conyers-and-44-house-democrats-reintroduce-the-expanded-and-improved-medi-a-591393.html#.VNrmm8bysk.

Feldman, J. (2010). Medical and surgical management of the transgender patient: What the primary care clinician needs to know. In H. J. Makadon, L. Mayer, J. Potter, & H. Goldhammer (Eds.), *The Fenway guide to lesbian, gay, bisexual, and transgender health.* Philadelphia, PA: American College of Physicians.

Fredriksen-Goldsen, K. I., Kim, H. J., Emlet, C. A., Muraco, A., Erosheva, E. A., Hoy-Ellis, C. P. et al. (2011). *The aging and health report: Disparities and resilience among lesbian, gay, bisexual, and transgender older adults.* Retrieved January 1, 2015 from http://caringandaging.org/wordpress/wp-content/uploads.2011/05/Full-ReportOFINAL-11-16-11.pdf.

Friedman, G. (2013, July 31). *Funding HR 676: The expanded and improved Medicare for All Act—How we can afford a national single-payer health plan.* Retrieved February 10, 2015 from www.pnhp.org/sites/default/files/FundingHR676_Friedman_7.31.13.pdf.

Greenesmith, H., Cray, A., & Baker, K. (2013, May 23). *The Affordable Care Act and LGBT families: Everything you need to know.* Retrieved January 23, 2015 from www.familyequality.org/_asset/5gqpft/FEC-CAP-LGBT-ACA-Families-Guide.pdf.

Institute of Medicine. (2011, March). The health of lesbian, gay, bisexual, an transgender people: Building a foundation for better understanding. *Report Brief.* Washington, DC: Author.

Kaplan, R. L. (2011, February 8). *Elder law expert: Health care reform act a mixed bag for seniors.* Retrieved February 5, 2015 from http://phys.org.news/2011-02-elder-law-expert-health-reform-html.

Kaufman, R. (2010). Introduction to transgender identity and health. In H. J. Makadon, K. H. Mayer, J. Potter, & H. Goldhammer (Eds.), *The Fenway guide to lesbian, gay, bisexual, and transgender health.* Philadelphia, PA: American College of Physicians.

Kelley, A. S., McGarry, K., Fahle, S., Marshall, S. M., Du, Q., & Skinner, J. S. (2013). Out-of-pocket spending in the last five years of life. *Journal of General Medicine, 28*(2), 304–309.

Library of Parliament Research. (n.d.). Retrieved February 8, 2015 from www.parl.gc.ca/information/library/PRBpublis/944-e.htm.

Mule, N. J. (2007). Sexual orientation discrimination in health care and social service policy: A comparative analysis of Canada, the UK, and USA. In L. Badgett & J. Frank (Eds.), *Sexual orientation discrimination: An international perspective* (pp. 306–322). New York, NY: Routledge.

Mule, N. J., Ross, L. E., Deeprose, B., Jackson, B. E., Daley, A., Travers, A. et al. (2009). Promoting LGBT health and wellbeing through inclusive policy development. *International Journal for Equity in Health, 8* (18). doi:10.1186/1475-9276-8-18.

National Healthcare Disparities Report. (2012). *Lesbian, gay, bisexual, and transgender populations in the 2011 National Healthcare Disparities Report* (AHRQ Publication No: 12-M030). Rockville, MD: Agency for Healthcare Research and Quality. Available at http://www.ahrq.gov/qual/qrdr11.htmm.

Navarro, V. (2007). What is a national health policy? *International Journal of Health Services, 37*(1), 1–14.

Physicians for a National Health Program. (2011). *Summary: H.R. 676, The Expanded & Improved Medicare For All Act.* Retrieved February 10, 2015 from http://www.pnhp.org/news/2011/february/summary-hr-676-the-expanded-improved-medicare-for-all-act.

Rainbow Health Network. (2008). Trans rights are human rights: Canadian Human Rights Act Amendment (gender identity). Toronto: Rainbow Health Network-Trans Health Lobby Group. Retrieved

February 9, 2015 from http://www.rainbow healthnetwork.ca/files/CHRA%20Trans%20Human% 20Rights%20Fact%20Sheet.doc.

Rosenthal, J. (2009, July 27). *LGBT issues in health reform: Issues brief on making health reform work for all Americans*. Retrieved February 9, 2015 from https://cdn.americanprogress.org/wp-content/uploads/ issues/2009/07/pdf/lgbthealth.pdf.

Ruble, M. W., & Forstein, M. (2008). Mental health, epidemiology, assessment, and treatment. In H. J. Makadon, K. H. Mayer, J. Potter, & H. Goldhammer (Eds.), *The Fenway guide to lesbian, gay, bisexual, and transgender health* (pp. 187–208). Philadelphia: ACP.

SAGE Matters. (2009). How will the Obama administration affect the issues facing LGBT elders? *SAGE matters: The source for news on LGBT aging*. New York, NY: Author.

SAGE. (2012). *SAGE health reform issues*. Retrieved January 20, 2015 from http://www.sageusa.org/issues/ reform.cfm?&print=1.

SAGE. (2014, May). *LGBT older adults, HIV and the Affordable Care Act*. New York, NY: Author. Retrieved January 31, 2015 from www. lgbtagingcenter.org/resources/pdfs/SAGEIssuesBrief-HIVACAandLGBTOlderPeoplke-May2014.pdf.

Saul, M. (2009, August 23). Expensive without the results: Health care in the U.S. Costs the most, not the best in the world. *New York Daily News*. Retrieved January 29, 2015 from http://aticles.nydailynew.com/ 2009-08-23/news/17930526_1_health-care-universal-coverage-primary-care.

World Health Organization. (2012). Global health sector strategy on HIV/AIDS 2011-2015. Available at www. who.int/hiv/pub/hiv_stragegy/en/.

Healthcare, Sexual Practices, and Cultural Competence with LGBT Elders

Tracy Davis and Amanda E. Sokan

Abstract

Research on the health of LGBT elders is limited. However, we do know that LGBT older adults often have poorer health status as a result of a combination of factors including health challenges such as sexual orientation, gender identity issues, as well as a history of marginalization, prejudice, and the effects of non disclosure in health care encounters. Additionally, commonly held misconceptions regarding the sexual practices of older adults contribute to the poorer health outcomes experienced by some LGBT individuals. LGBT older adults, like others, are entitled to quality health care. This chapter introduces and discusses some of the major issues that affect the health of LGBT elders and explores opportunities to begin addressing these issues. Additionally, it reviews implications for improving service delivery from an interdisciplinary perspective and future research directions.

Keywords

Cultural competence · HIV/AIDS · Health disparities · Minority stress · Non-disclosure

Overview

This chapter focuses on healthcare practices with lesbian, gay, bisexual, and transgender (LGBT) elders. Attention is given to the current state of

T. Davis (✉)
Rutgers University, Stratford, NJ, USA
e-mail: ted58@shrp.rutgers.edu

A.E. Sokan
University of Kentucky, Lexington, KY, USA
e-mail: ausoka2@uky.edu

healthcare practices with LGBT elders and the challenges and opportunities they present. Further, this chapter explores methods for best practices for healthcare professionals who provide care for this population.

We begin this chapter by reviewing the history and healthcare practices with LGBT elders. Next, we explore major issues surrounding healthcare practices with LGBT elders, for instance common misconceptions about sexuality of patients, training needs of staff, (e.g., cultural competency), data collection and clinical interviews, sexual intimacy, and HIV/AIDS. This chapter

© Springer International Publishing Switzerland 2016
D.A. Harley and P.B. Teaster (eds.), *Handbook of LGBT Elders*,
DOI 10.1007/978-3-319-03623-6_20

also reviews implications for improving service delivery from an interdisciplinary perspective.

Learning Objectives

1. Identify the training needs of staff who work with LGBT elders.
2. Describe the obstacles in providing optimal health care to LGBT elders.
3. Identify misconceptions regarding the sexuality of patients.
4. Describe the need for sexual intimacy among older adults.
5. Explain LGBT elders' risk factors for HIV/AIDS.
6. Understand the importance of LGBT cultural competency in healthcare settings.
7. Describe the major goals and components of LGBT cultural competency training program.
8. Understand the impact of non-disclosure of sexual orientation and gender identity on the care of LGBT older adults.

Introduction

LGBT elders represent an extremely marginalized population, as a result of age and sexual orientation or gender identity. The number of older adults in the USA is increasing rapidly; in fact approximately 10,000 individuals turn 65 every day. Healthcare needs often increase with age, for instance Medicare beneficiaries on average have at least three chronic conditions (Center for Medicare and Medicaid Service [CMS] 2012). Among Medicare enrollees, physician visits and consultations increased from 11,395 per 1000 in 1999 to 15,437 per 1000 in 2009 (Federal Interagency Forum on Aging-Related Statistics [FIFAR] 2012). The LGBT population is not exempt from this reality. This rapid population aging will significantly impact the lives of LGBT individuals who often grow old without sufficient support, including health

care. In fact, it may be compounded by healthcare needs that are unique to the LGBT population, such as sexual orientation, gender identity, and a history of marginalization. In recent years, we have seen cultural shifts that have allowed segments of the LGBT population to achieve legal rights making it easier for some to live openly as LGBT individuals. Some of the recent changes have brought the barriers and needs of LGBT elders more visibility; however, there are still many issues to be addressed including the healthcare practices of LGBT elders.

History and Practice

The history and practice relating to health care with LGBT elders is relatively short. In recent years, there has been recognition of the importance of conducting research in order to better understand the needs of LGBT individuals and establishing the best practices in order to increase the quality of health care for LGBT individuals. However, research efforts specifically regarding healthcare practices with LGBT elders have lagged behind. In the USA, we are experiencing a tremendous increase in the number of "out" LGBT elders, which is very different from what has been seen, in the past there were relatively small numbers of "out" LGBT elders; however, by the year 2030, it is expected that the number of LGBT older adults in the USA will increase to more than 4 million (Fredriksen-Goldsen et al. 2011).

The available research on healthcare practices with LGBT elders has focused on the provision and awareness of services specifically for LGBT elders (Knochel et al. 2012; Hughes et al. 2011), promoting awareness of LGBT aging issues in nursing programs (Lim and Bernstein 2012), and surveying the training of healthcare providers and nursing home social service directors (Bell et al. 2010; Rogers et al. 2013; Porter and Krinsky 2013). Services and Advocacy for GLBT Elders (SAGE) has released several publicly available documents with recommendations for policy and practice. Furthermore, the National Resource Center on LGBT Aging published a document on collecting health-related data from LGBT elders. Unfortunately, very few practices have implemented the recommendations provided by these organizations. While there is a limited amount of available research specifically regarding LGBT elders, some of the available research on LGBT individuals in general can be applied to older adults. For instance, The Fenway Institute's (2012) publication on gathering data on sexual orientation and gender identity in clinical settings can be used with older adults.

In light of the growing number of LGBT older adults in the USA and elsewhere, there is a definite need for more research aimed at understanding the needs and desires of LGBT elders regarding their interaction with health care and for the development of best practices for healthcare providers. An initial step in developing best practices for providers should be striving to eliminate commonly held misconceptions about the sexuality of patients.

Common Misconceptions About Sexuality of Patients

Within our society, there is an extremely prevalent misconception that older adults are not sexual beings and that the desire to engage in sexual activity diminishes with age; research does not support this misconception (Lindau et al. 2007; Trompeter et al. 2012). All existing literature suggests the desire to engage in sexual activity is present among all human beings and continues into later life. In fact, many older people continue to have satisfying sex lives into their seventies, eighties, and even nineties (Vann 2014). Unfortunately, many healthcare providers also hold these common misconceptions and therefore potentially miss opportunities to discuss sexuality with their older patients. Discussions surrounding sexuality with older patients are extremely important because older adults maintain an interest in and desire to engage in

sexual activity, but may face challenges that may then cause them to miss opportunities for sexual activity and/or to place themselves at risk for contracting sexually transmitted infections and diseases. The number of older adults being diagnosed with HIV is increasing. In 2010, individuals aged 50 and older accounted for approximately one-fifth of those living with HIV infection (CDC 2013a). The number of older adults infected with other sexually transmitted infections is also increasing. For example, the number of individuals aged 55 and over diagnosed with chlamydia increased from 4,311 in 2009 to 6,801 in 2013, those diagnosed with Gonorrhea increased from 2,766 in 2009 to 4,327 in 2013, and those diagnosed with syphilis increased from 607 in 2009 to 912 in 2013 (CDC 2014b). Oftentimes, healthcare providers make assumptions regarding older adult's sexual orientation, assuming that the majority of older adults are heterosexual (National Resource Center for LGBT Aging, n.d.). The possibility that an older patient is lesbian, gay, bisexual, or transgendered is rarely considered.

Another common misconception regarding older adults and sexuality is that due to their advanced age, they should know how to protect themselves from sexually transmitted infections and diseases when in fact the opposite is true (Centers for Disease Control and Prevention [CDC] 2013a). The current generation of older adults grew up in a time when sexual health education was not a part of general education and thus never learned how to properly protect themselves.

Misconceptions surrounding drug use among older adults also exist and impact their sexuality. Many healthcare practitioners, as well as other members of society, generally believe that older adults do not use illicit drugs and thus are less likely to ask older patients questions about illicit drug use. While research does suggest that illicit drug use declines with age, research now shows that the baby-boom generation (individuals born between 1946 and 1964) has relatively higher rates of illicit drug use than previous generations (Wu and Blazer 2010). Illicit drug use can increase the risk of transmitting sexually transmitted diseases and infections—particularly among older adults who may be unaware of how to protect themselves against disease and infection (CDC 2013a). In addition to illicit drugs, the sharing of equipment (e.g., needles) for non-illicit drugs can increase one's risk for diseases and infections. For example, if two older adults share diabetic injection medication, there is the potential to spread sexually transmitted diseases and infections. Many older adults internalize these common misconceptions and in turn feel embarrassed or ashamed that they have a continued interest in sexual activity. Thus, many older adults are unwilling to bring the subject of sexuality up to their healthcare provider. Older adults should not be embarrassed or ashamed to ask their healthcare provider questions regarding their sexuality. Sexual contact is correlated with better health, higher relationship satisfaction, and better stress management (American Association of Retired Persons [AARP] 2011). There is a great need to increase the training and preparedness of healthcare providers who see older adults, so that they inquire about older patients' sexuality and are able to field questions about their sexuality.

Sexual Intimacy

Adults maintain the need for intimacy as they age. Most need to feel close to others as they grow older (National Institute on Aging [NIA] 2013). The type of intimacy that an adult seeks may change with age; for instance, holding hands, touching, and kissing may be sought by more older adults as opposed to having sexual intercourse.

There are normal age-related changes that affect both men and women. These changes can sometimes affect the ability to have and enjoy sex (NIA 2013). As women age, the vagina can shorten and narrow, and the vaginal walls can become thinner and stiffer (NIA 2013). Women may also have less vaginal lubrication (NIA 2013). These changes can affect the ability to enjoy sex and can increase a women's risk for

contracting sexually transmitted infections and diseases. The thinning and reduced lubrication of the vagina can lead to increased risk of a vaginal tear, thus increasing the susceptibility to sexually transmitted infections and diseases. As men age, erectile dysfunction (ED) becomes more common (NIA 2013). ED is the loss of ability to achieve and maintain an erection suitable for sexual intercourse (NIA 2013). It may take a man a longer time to achieve an erection, and the erection may not be as firm or as large as it used to be in a man's earlier years (NIA 2013). The loss of the erection after an orgasm may take less time, and the time in between erection may become longer (NIA 2013). An occasional problem with erection is not a problem, but if it occurs regularly, then medical attention should be sought. Healthcare providers should be willing and able to aid older adults in addressing concerns with sexual intimacy.

In addition to normal age-related changes that can affect the sexual lives of both older men and women, several chronic conditions also affect the sexual lives of older adult. Older adults who suffer from joint pain associated with arthritis can experience pain and discomfort during sex. The National Institute on Aging (NIA 2013) suggests that exercise, drugs, and possibly joint replacement surgery may relieve some of the arthritic pain. Rest, warm baths, and changing the position or timing of sexual activity can be helpful in reducing arthritic pain that may interfere with sexual activity (NIA 2013). Chronic pain can interfere with intimacy, it is not a normal part of aging, and can often be treated with medications. However, some pain medicines can interfere with sexual function. Some people with dementia show increased interest in sex and physical closeness and may have difficulty determining appropriate sexual contact (NIA 2013). Furthermore, individuals with severe dementia may not recognize their spouse or partner but may still have sexual desires and exhibit sexual behavior (NIA 2013). This can cause some discomfort for the spouse or partner. Working with a healthcare professional who has training in dementia care can be very helpful. Diabetes is one of the illnesses that can cause ED in some men (NIA

2013). Women with diabetes are more likely to have yeast infections, which can cause sexual activity to be uncomfortable or undesirable (NIA 2013). Medications can help with the side effects of diabetes on sexual intimacy for both men and women. Heart disease can affect both men and women in regard to sexual intimacy due to narrowing and hardening of the arteries, which can change the blood vessels, so that the blood does not flow freely. Thus, men and women with heart disease may have problems with orgasm (NIA 2013). Heart disease may also cause problems with obtaining and maintaining erections for men (NIA 2013). Loss of bladder control or leakage of urine can be problematic for many older adults, especially in women. Extra pressure on the stomach during sex can cause bladder leakage, which may cause some individuals to avoid sex (NIA 2013). Changing positions during sex or seeking treatment for incontinence can help the problem. Also, depression can affect both men and women's desire for sexual intimacy. Depression is fairly common among older adults and should be treated appropriately. A 2011 national study on LGBT older adults found that more than half of LGBT elders had been told by their doctor that they had depression, approximately 39 % had seriously considered suicide, and approximately 53 % felt isolated from others (Fredriksen-Goldsen et al. 2011).

Sexual intimacy can be problematic in certain environments such as nursing care facilities. The desire for sexual intimacy does not go away with age, and this is true for those in nursing and assisted living facilities, as well. Unfortunately, conditions in nursing and assisted living facilities may hamper the ability to satisfy a need for sexual intimacy. Personal barriers (e.g., physical disabilities, the adverse effects of prescribed medications, cognitive impairment, and lack of partners) inhibit sexual intimacy (Katz 2013). In addition, residents also lack privacy, as they are often encouraged to leave their doors open and unlocked, and staff members often come in and out frequently. The attitudes of staff and families often cause significant barriers to sexual expression in nursing facilities (Katz 2013). Due to the fact that many nursing facilities lack policies

designed to help guide and support staff responses, much is left up to personal interpretation of the staff (Katz 2013). Nursing facilities should be encouraged to develop policies surrounding sexual expression by residents. Such policies may help provide guidance for the safe expression of sexual desire and provide training for staff in how to handle these situations. Specifically, staff training on LGBT older adult's needs should be mandated. It should be made clear that anti-LGBT discrimination will not be tolerated. Advocates should push for laws mandating training for nursing home personnel and residents (Redman 2011). For example, in 2008, California passed a law requiring the Department of Public Health to design and implement regular cultural competency training on LGBT issues (Redman 2011). Furthermore, Ombudsman programs must take a stronger advocacy role in protecting LGBT residents from bullying and discrimination (Redman 2011). Further research and data collection is needed to uncover additional problems LGBT residents face in nursing homes.

It is important for healthcare providers to remember that older adults maintain desires for sexual intimacy. It is important for healthcare providers to work with older adults to maintain their sexual health and to help them meet their intimacy goals and to avoid the transmission of diseases.

Policy Box #1

In conjunction with management at your local senior center, you recently provided an educational workshop that addressed sexuality and health in aging, including intimacy, safe practices, sexual orientation, and gender identity issues to clients and staff. Because of the enthusiasm and positive feedback received from attendees and the potential benefits of such a program, you would like to solicit your state department of Aging's support in making this a required annual program in senior centers statewide. Write a policy paper to the head of the state department of aging, in which you present your argument for the need and benefit of adopting this educational program.

HIV/AIDS

On June 5, 1981, the CDC first published a report about the occurrence of a disease later referred to as acquired immune deficiency syndrome (AIDS). This report is often referred to as the "beginning of AIDS" in the USA, as it described the symptoms of five homosexual men with what are now known as "opportunistic infections" (US Health and Human Services [HHS], n.d.). Initially, the disease was thought to affect only homosexual men, and so by 1982, the disease had acquired the name gay-related immune deficiency syndrome (GRID).

However, by mid-1982, the disease was reported among injection drug users, and soon hemophiliacs presented with the disease. By 1983, the retrovirus that causes AIDS was identified and given the name it has today, human immunodeficiency virus (HIV). In 1985, the identification of HIV prompted researchers to develop a test for the disease. A few years later, the first anti-HIV drug, AZT (Zidovudine), was approved by the Food and Drug Administration (FDA). With the ability to test for the virus and to provide medications for it, prevention efforts commenced. While there have been major advancements in regards to HIV/AIDS over the past 33 years, there is currently no cure or effective vaccine for HIV/AIDS. Prevention remains the best and most effective strategy for reducing incidences of HIV/AIDS among older adults (Powderly and Mayer 2003). A comprehensive prevention program should include the provision of education, screening/testing for HIV/AIDS, and the prompt treatment of those who are infected.

Currently, more than 35 million people worldwide are living with HIV (The Joint United Nations Programme on HIV/AIDS [UNAIDS]

2014). In the USA, approximately 1.1 million individuals are living with HIV (UNAIDS 2014); furthermore, it is estimated that one in five individuals with HIV/AIDS are unaware that he or she is infected (UNAIDS 2014). A growing number of people aged 50 and older are living with HIV infection; older adults accounted for approximately 19 % or 217,300 of the estimated 1.1 million cases of HIV in the USA (CDC 2013a). Of the estimated 47,500 new HIV infections in 2010, older adults aged 55 and over accounted for approximately 2,500 (5 %) of the new infections (CDC 2013a) and is expected to increase. In 2010, 44 % of the estimated 2,500 new HIV infections among people aged 55 and older were among gay, bisexual, or other men who have sex with men (MSM) (CDC 2013a). Research suggests that the LGBT population has been disproportionately affected by the AIDS epidemic, marginalizing particular subgroups within LGBT older adult populations (i.e., men who have sex with men, transgender elders, and older lesbians) (Services and Advocacy for Gay, Lesbian, Bisexual and Transgender Elders [SAGE] 2010). Older adults of color are disproportionately affected by HIV. The CDC (2013a) reports that older African Americans and Latinos were 12 and 5 times, respectively, more likely to contract HIV as compared to their white counterparts. Because the risk of female-to-female transmission of HIV is relatively low; oftentimes, lesbian and bisexual women are overlooked regarding their risk for HIV by themselves and by healthcare providers. However, lesbian and bisexual women can engage in high-risk behaviors just like anyone else. For example, lesbians can increase their risk for HIV by having oral sex without a protective barrier, sharing sex toys without disinfecting them or using a barrier, and sexual play that involves the exchange of vaginal fluids or blood (SAGE 2010). Also, lesbian and bisexual women can have unprotected sex with male partners and inject drugs and share needles.

The risk factors for HIV are the same for everyone. HIV is transmitted through blood, semen, pre-seminal fluid, rectal fluids, vaginal fluids, and breast milk from an HIV-infected person. The fluids must come in contact with a mucous membrane found inside the rectum, the vagina, the opening of the penis or the mouth or damaged tissues or be directly injected into the bloodstream in order for transmission to occur (CDC 2014a). These risk factors are the same for everyone regardless of race, sexual orientation, gender identity, sex, or age. Older adults are often considered to be at greater risk for HIV due to lack of awareness about HIV and how to prevent transmission, and as a direct result, unknowingly place themselves at risk for HIV and other sexually transmitted infections. For example, many widowed and divorced people are dating again and are less likely to protect themselves because of their lack of awareness of how the disease is transmitted. Again, as mentioned in the previous section, there are physiological changes among older men and women that can increase their risk for contracting HIV. Due to older adults' increased risk for HIV, it is extremely important to increase educational efforts aimed at increasing older adults' knowledge about HIV and to screen older adults for HIV (Davis 2013). Early detection improves infected persons' chances of living longer, particularly for older adults.

Unfortunately, older adults are more likely to receive a late diagnosis and to have a short progression between HIV and AIDS. Older adults are more likely to have a delayed diagnosis because symptoms of HIV resemble symptoms of other chronic illness common among many older adults or normal aging. For example, loss of energy, short-term memory loss, and weight loss are all symptoms of HIV, but they also may be associated with normal aging or associated with other common conditions among older adults (SAGE 2010). A late diagnosis means a late start to treatment and possibly more damage to an already weakened immune system (CDC 2013a).

Despite the fact that we know that early detection is essential to improving older adults' chances of survival, many healthcare providers still fail to acknowledge older adults risk for HIV and do not ask questions about sexual partners or drug use (SAGE 2010). Additionally, many LGBT elders fear discrimination from healthcare providers because they are not open and honest about their needs. Between the lack of recognition of older adults' HIV risk factors among many providers and the fears of many elders, HIV screening rarely occurs and early detection is minimal (SAGE 2010). Again, as with previously discussed issues (e.g., sexual orientation or sexual intimacy) in older adults there is a great need to increase the training and preparedness of healthcare providers who see older adults, so that they better prepared to inquire and address questions about older patients sexuality.

Profile of LGBT Elders
Donald

Donald is a 56-year-old white man who was married for 24 years, a relationship he entered into right out of college. He contracted HIV from an affair with a young man he met at a work-related conference. He says they used condoms, but when one "came off" the young man assured him he was HIV negative. Donald did not think he had reason to doubt the man, given his healthy appearance. Once Donald received his HIV diagnosis, he disclosed to his wife that he was gay. They stayed together until "the kids were out of the house."

Discussion Questions

What new insights did you gain from reading a little bit about Donald? Were you surprised about his "coming out" so late in life?

Ramón

Ramón is a 50-year-old bisexual Latino who has been sexually active since 18. Finding out he had HIV brought up feelings of being punished. He also has had to cope with homophobia in Latino culture. He knows of many youth who ran away from home to escape their parents' rejection. Consequently, some found themselves engaging in high-risk sexual activities that left them infected with any number of STIs. He strongly encourages everyone to use protection and take care of themselves.

Discussion Questions

Were you surprised by Jorge's story? Do you agree or disagree with his depiction of the Latino community as very homophobic?

These profiles were taken directly from *older and wiser: the many faces of HIV* a publication by ACRIA (2012). https://www.dropbox.com/s/oc041bhfd5w1orl/ACRIA_OAW_EN.pdf.

Disclosure and Non-disclosure as Obstacles to Adequate Health care

In comparison to their heterosexual counterparts, LGBT people exhibit more risky behaviors and have worse health outcomes (IOM, Institute of Medicine 2011; US Department of Health and Human Services [DHHS], Health Resources and Services Administration 2011). The health of this population, including older adults, is made more challenging because of the unique needs and concerns related to their sexual minority status, and which contribute to health disparities with some variations within subgroups. For instance,

within the LGBT population, there are higher rates of risky behaviors such as smoking, higher levels of breast cancer and obesity among lesbian women; anal cancer in gay and bisexual men, and violence/abuse in personal relationships (IOM 2011; Barbara et al. 2007). Additionally, LGBT people when compared to their heterosexual counterparts exhibit higher rates of mental health problems such as suicidal ideation/attempts, anxiety and mood disorders, and higher rates of substance abuse (Durso and Meyer 2012). See Chaps. 23 and 24 for further discussion on mental health and substance abuse. Table 20.1 provides a breakdown by condition and subgroup.

The overall tendency toward poor health status has been attributed to a number of factors that act as barriers to health. Major contributory factors include lack of or inadequate training of healthcare professionals on how to address LGBT healthcare needs, minority stress, and disclosure or non-disclosure of LGBT sexual orientation or gender identity to healthcare providers. Inadequate training is a barrier against optimum health because it inhibits professionals who are uninformed about the unique healthcare needs of LGBT patients. Minority stress theory posits that members of disadvantaged groups suffer stress—for instance, the discrimination, stigma, and homophobia experienced by LGBT as a disadvantaged minority cause them to suffer chronic stress, which contributes to poor health (Durso and Meyer 2012). Below, we consider how a patient's non-disclosure and/or disclosure of sexual minority status (i.e., sexual orientation or gender identity) can act as a barrier or obstacle to health care.

Table 20.1 Health disparities: sample conditions and variations by LGBT subgroups

Health condition	Lesbian (%)	Gay (%)	Bisexual (%)		Transgender (%)
			Men	Women	
Depression	27	29	35	36	48
Anxiety	22	22	24	34	39
Suicidal ideation	35	37	39	40	71
Disability	50	41	50	50	66
Obesity	34	19	18	34	40

Source Fredriksen-Goldsen et al. (2011)

Disclosure as an Obstacle to Adequate Health care

In light of the unique challenges posed by being lesbian, gay, bisexual, or transgender to the health of the individual, it is important to ask whether LGBT older adults disclose their sexual orientation or gender identity to their healthcare providers. Disclosure is important because it promotes honesty in the healthcare encounter, which in turn leads to improved care (Lambda Legal 2010; Durso and Meyer 2012). Disclosure allows the healthcare provider access to information necessary for the development and provision of appropriate interventions, patient education, as well as mechanisms to support and manage optimal health. The ability of healthcare providers to work with patients to facilitate disclosure is recognized as an integral part of providing culturally competent care (The Joint Commission 2011). Generally, LGBT patients would prefer that their healthcare providers are aware of their sexual orientation (Stein and Bonuck 2001). However, according to a 2010 report on a study conducted by Lambda Legal, many LGBT felt that disclosure was an obstacle to care. In the report entitled *When Health Care Isn't Caring: Lambda Legal's Survey on Discrimination against LGBT People and People Living with HIV* (2010), over 50 % of the study's 4916 respondents felt that disclosure of sexual orientation or gender identity had negative consequences. Also, respondents cited increases in discriminatory treatment; exposure to practices and policies that were prejudicial, derogatory or inflexible; abusive behaviors; substandard care; and refusal of care (Lambda Legal 2010). The Lambda Legal study and report found that the type and frequency of negative response post-disclosure varied among LGBT subgroups, with transgender and gender non-conforming persons suffering the most impact. Similarly, Durso and Meyer (2012) found that the negative impact of disclosure was the greatest for transgender persons and LGBT who were also racial or ethnic minorities (Lamda Legal 2010; Durso and Meyer 2012). Table 20.2 provides examples

Table 20.2 Examples of respondent's experiences after disclosure to healthcare providers

Types of discrimination in care	
More than 50 % of respondents reported at least one of the following:	
• Refusal of needed care	
• Healthcare professionals refusal to touch patient	
• Using excessive precautions	
• Healthcare professionals using harsh or abusive language	
• Being blamed for their health status	
• Healthcare professionals being physically rough or abusive	
Percentage by subgroup	
Respondent	%
Lesbian, gay, or bisexual (LGB) respondents	56
Transgender and gender-nonconforming respondents	70
Respondents living with HIV	63

Source Lambda Legal (2010). Available at www.lambdalegal.org/health-care-report

of respondent's experiences after disclosure to healthcare providers.

Overall, the perception that disclosure creates more vulnerability prevents LGBT older adults from having open honest discussions with their care providers. This, in turn, exacerbates the already negative health status and poorer outcomes that they suffer. In order to ensure that LGBT older adults receive quality care, it is critical to promote disclosure on the part of patients, as well as to evoke appropriate and professional responses by health providers and staff.

Non-disclosure as an Obstacle to Health care

The preceding section showed that for many in the LGBT population, disclosure to health and other service or care providers concerning sexual orientation or non-conforming gender identity may lead to undesired consequences. These undesired consequences which run the gamut from discrimination, reprisals, abuse, substandard treatment to refusal to treat, understandably create fear, mistrust, and reluctance or refusal to disclose sexual minority status among LGBT older adults (Fredriksen-Goldsen et al. 2011).

Beyond fear (of mistreatment), or the desire to avoid the negative consequences of disclosure, other factors also contribute to non-disclosure. Durso and Meyer (2012) identified privacy concerns as another reason for non-disclosure, the presumption of heterosexuality by healthcare workers, as well as a perception that sexual orientation is irrelevant to health care. For these reasons, non-disclosure may be even higher in healthcare settings (Petroll and Mosack 2011; Bernstein et al. 2008). There is some support for the notion that non-disclosure to providers occurs even where the LGBT patient has come out to family, coworkers, and heterosexual and LGBT friends (Durso and Meyer 2012). This situation should be of concern to all, especially in light of the acknowledged poor health status of LGBT older adults. Studies have found variations in patterns of non-disclosure among LGBT subgroups as well as factors likely to predict disclosure or non-disclosure in healthcare encounters or settings. For instance, when compared to gay men, higher rates of non-disclosure were found among bisexual men (Bernstein et al. 2008; Durso and Meyer 2012), while factors such as health status, relationship status, and level of internalized homophobia were found to predict disclosure versus non-disclosure among lesbians (St. Pierre 2012). Socioeconomic factors are also relevant. Ethnic/racial minorities within the LGBT population have higher rates of non-disclosure (Bernstein et al. 2008; Petroll and Mosack 2011), as do those with lower income or financial status (Petroll and Mosack 2011; St. Pierre 2012). Other patient characteristics such as immigrant status, health history, gender, and parenthood status have also been found to influence disclosure (Durso and Meyer 2012). Non-disclosure is also more likely among those with lower levels of education as well as LGBT who live in rural areas (Petroll and Mosack 2011). Thus, it is critical that healthcare providers recognize the heterogeneity that exists within the LGBT population, and distinguish between

Table 20.3 Example of factors influencing non-disclosure

Socioeconomic	Race/ethnicity; education level; gender; financial status/income
Patient characteristics	Health history; immigration status; parenthood status; color; personal identity as LGBT
Minority stress	Degree of: internalized homophobia; connection to LGBT community; discrimination history and experience; expectations of stigma; multiple jeopardy—e.g., heterosexism/racism/sexism/ageism

issues that are specific to or shared among subgroups (Durso and Meyer 2012).

Generally, the likelihood that an LGBT patient will disclose his or her sexual orientation or gender identity has been found to be influenced by (a) degree or strength of connection to the LGBT community and (b) sense of LGBT identity (Durso and Meyer 2012). Those with a lower sense of LGBT identity or poor connection to the LGBT community are more likely to practice non-disclosure. This finding is important to bear in mind when dealing with older adult LGBT patients who may have a long history of struggle with their sexual orientation, gender identity or are isolated from the LGBT community. Table 20.3 provides examples of factors influencing non-disclosure.

Regardless of the reason for non-disclosure, it is important to facilitate disclosure, especially in healthcare encounters, because of the potential of non-disclosure to contribute to poor health and poorer health outcomes. For instance, Durso and Meyer (2012) found that non-disclosure related to poorer psychological health at follow-up a year after. Providers who are unaware of the older adult's LGBT identity are less likely to provide appropriate patient education on pertinent issues, relevant advice or recommendations regarding preventive care, such as screenings, vaccines, and testings (Petroll and Mossack 2011; Durso and Meyer 2012). They are also less likely to recognize the need to connect these patients to available support, care, service, and other LGBT resources within the community.

Also, such providers may be less likely to seek out information, knowledge and training on LGBT issues and concerns because they assume that their patient base does not require these skills. Non-disclosure inadvertently contributes to the "invisibility" of LGBT older adults, their issues, needs, and concerns (Jablonski et al. 2013) and exacerbates health disparities. Ultimately, non-disclosure negatively affects the ability of providers to identify unmet needs and deliver quality and appropriate care to LGBT older adult patients, thereby increasing patient stress, contributing to poor health outcomes and overall poor health status.

Promoting Disclosure and Reducing Non-disclosure

Healthcare and other service providers to LGBT older adults need to remove barriers to disclosure within healthcare settings and other environments. To do so, providers must eliminate the presumption of heterosexuality when dealing with patients and include questions on sexual orientation and gender identity as key elements of care for all patients (Durso and Meyer 2012). It is also important to recognize the heterogeneity of the LGBT population to avoid generalizations that may obfuscate within-group variations in experiences and healthcare needs. In addition, providers must be sensitive to the increased barriers faced by LGBT patients who are also simultaneously members of other disadvantaged groups. Taking into account how individual patient characteristics, mediate or influence LGBT experiences when they seek, access, or use health care, may help increase patient comfort. Strategies which are based upon, and, enhance the development of awareness and understanding of LGBT issues are critical and necessary. Such strategies open the door to increased trust, reduced fear, and anxiety and the establishment of safe environments, in which patient/provider encounters can optimize health outcomes and improve overall health status for LGBT older adults. Providing appropriate cultural competence training to staff and personnel who work with

LGBT older adults will better equip them to encourage and facilitate disclosure of sexual orientation and gender identity by LGBT patients.

Discussion Box #1

You have been scheduled for a repeat appointment with a patient whom you think might be a member of the LGBT population. You think that obtaining this information is important to help you provide quality care. Explain your rationale for thinking so. How would you go about facilitating a conversation on this issue? What questions might you ask? What concerns, if any, do you have?

Discussion Box #2

According to the National Resource Center on LGBT Aging (2012), most aging service providers and LGBT organizations seeking information on how best to *support and serve* LGBT elders often ask the following questions:

(a) How is aging as an older lesbian, gay, bisexual and/or transgender adult different than aging as a heterosexual and/or non-transgender adult?

(b) How can agencies reflect and honor these differences?

What do you think? How would you answer these questions?

Training Needs of Staff

The Centers for Disease Control and Prevention's (CDC) report, The *State of Aging and Health in America 2013*, provides "a snapshot of the health and aging landscape in the United States" (CDC 2013b, p. 2). According to this report and as mentioned earlier, longevity and the aging of the baby boomers, one of the largest cohorts in history has resulted in an unprecedented growth in the size of the population aged 65 and over. Of this segment of the population, two-thirds live with multiple chronic conditions and account for 66 % of US healthcare expenditures (CDC 2013b).

Generally, older adults consume a disproportionate amount of healthcare and long-term care services, as the demand for these services tend to increase as age increases, requiring the skills of a variety of staff and personnel in mental health, physical health, long-term care, and other aging services (McGinnis and Moore 2006). According to a report by the LGBT advocacy group, Services and Advocacy for Gay, Lesbian, Bisexual and Transgender Elders (SAGE), healthcare settings can be challenging environments for LGBT elders (SAGE 2010). Factors that create barriers and/or influence the care received by LGBT elders are often driven by heterosexism and homophobia. These factors include open discrimination by staff which may create a hostile environment, lack of familiarity with the needs of LGBT elders, as well as, LGBT elders' own reluctance to engage because of past negative experience. For instance, in a report about how inhospitable the healthcare environment is for LGBT people, the organization Services and Advocacy for Gay, Lesbian, Bisexual and Transgender Elder (SAGE) cites a 2006 study by MetLife Mature Market Institute that indicates that more than 50 % of LGBT baby boomers believed they would not receive respectful and dignified treatment from healthcare professionals (SAGE 2010).

The level of provider/staff knowledge, awareness, and comfort when dealing with LGBT elders and the issues they present is a key factor. Research indicates that many providers or staff who work in the aging industry (e.g., healthcare organizations, long-term care facilities, and other aging services) lack the education or training to enable them to care for LGBT elders because of LGBT issues in education and training curricula. For instance, a study that examined LGBT-related content in 150 undergraduate medical education programs in USA and Canada between 2009 and 2010 concluded that on average, five hours were devoted to LGBT issues. In addition, a large degree of variation existed across programs in terms of quantity and content covered, as well as perceptions regarding the quality of instruction received (Obedin-Maliver et al. 2011). In another study of social services in Michigan, Hughes et al. (2011) found that "perceptions of invisibility" make it difficult to recognize the concerns of LGBT elders and provide culturally appropriate services. These barriers have implications for the health of LGBT elders because they increase the likelihood of failure or delay in seeking health care, which in turn adversely affects overall health status and may result in poorer or negative health outcomes, as well as increased rates of premature need for institutional care. Institutionalized LGBT elders suffer additional challenges because many LTC staff such as social services directors, certified nursing assistants, and other caregivers lack adequate training in LGBT issues and concerns, in addition to homophobia and heterosexism (Bell et al. 2010).

Staff Training. LGBT older adults constitute a community despite the variations across these subgroups, as discussed previously. The increasing recognition that the needs of this community and its unique challenges must be addressed is evidenced by the statement attributed to Kathy Greenlee, Assistant Secretary of Aging, during the award of $900,000 for the development of a national resource center on LGBT aging in 2010 (SAGE 2010). In the same vein of recognition, reporting on the state of aging and health in the USA in 2013, the CDC issued a series of calls to action that included a call for communities, professionals, and individuals to address aging and health issues that affect the LGBT community (*CDC—The State of Aging and Health in America* 2013b). LGBT older adults have a shared culture that reflects their sexual minority status, history of marginalization, bias, prejudice and stigma, as well as health, social and economic disparities. This shared culture must be understood in order to appropriately address LGBT needs generally and is essential to ensuring that LGBT older adults have access to and receive relevant, quality health services in an inclusive, non-discriminatory fashion (National Resource Center on LGBT Aging 2012). To do so, professionals and staff of service agencies and organizations who work with LGBT older adults must learn to provide culturally competent care. Proper training of staff can help reduce or eliminate these barriers by providing sensitivity awareness to combat discrimination, as well as useful education and information to increase awareness of the particular health care and related social needs of LGBT elders.

According to the National Resource Center on LGBT Aging, cultural competence occurs when an organization has established systems and has trained staff members to identify and address the needs of LGBT elders (Meyer 2011). A variety of formats can be used for increasing awareness such as incorporation into medical school/training curricula, inclusion in licensure board examinations, on-the-job training using webinars, online self-paced learning with evaluations, as well as through continuing medical education (CMEs). In order to effectively care for LGBT elders, personnel in HCOs, LTC facilities, and other caregivers require cultural competency training.

Cultural Competency Training—Components

According to the National Resource Center on LGBT Aging (2012) cultural competency training needs to address the following:

1. Cultural awareness—Knowledge
   Improving knowledge about LGBT older adult history and experience regarding access and utilization of services.
2. Cultural humility—Attitude
   Recognizing that each LGBT older adult is the expert of his/her own experience, regardless of the knowledge of the provider or staff.
3. Cultural responsiveness—Behavior
   Learning and putting into practice new patterns of behavior for dealing with LGBT older adults, and effectively applying these new behaviors both in individual and organizational settings.

Cultural competence increases awareness, promotes visibility of LGBT aging issues, and enhances the quality of services delivered (National Resource Center on LGBT Aging 2012). The overall goal of cultural competence training is to ensure that the attitudes, actions, and practices of health and other care providers contribute to the creation of healthcare environments that augur well for the safety, inclusion, and welfare of LGBT older adults. Table 20.4 provides a suggested list of topic areas to be addressed in cultural competency training.

Research Box #1
Successful Aging
Title of Research: Successful Aging Among LGBT Older Adults: Physical and Mental Health-Related Quality of Life by Age Group.

Objective: To investigate the relationship between physical and mental health-related quality of life and covariates by age group. Design and Methods: This study used a cross-sectional research design to survey LGBT adults aged 50 and older ($N = 2560$). The survey was conducted by Caring and Aging with Pride: The National Health, Aging, and Sexuality Study via collaborations with 11 sites across the US linear regression analyses was used to test specific relationships and moderating effects of age groups (aged 50–64, 65–79; and 80 +).

Results: Physical and mental health quality of life was found to be negatively associated with discrimination and chronic conditions, but positively associated with social support, social network size, physical and leisure activities, substance nonuse, employment, income, and being male when controlling for age and other factors. Mental health quality of life was also positively associated with positive sense of sexual identity and negatively with sexual identity disclosure. For the 80 + group, the influence of discrimination was particularly salient.

Table 20.4 Cultural competency training—suggested components

Knowledge (cultural awareness)	Attitude (cultural humility)	Behavior (cultural responsiveness)
Definitions Key terms, concepts, e.g., relationships, descriptions, and self-identity. *History/culture/experience* Prejudice, discrimination, fear; impact—distrust, delayed access to care, avoidance, health disparities *LGBT/LGBT Aging* (issues, concerns, needs—health/health conditions, legal, social) *Health disparities* Differences and similarities among subgroups *Barriers to care and origin* For (a) LGBT older adults (b) staff, (c) community/environment Access to care and services *Language* Appropriate use, terminology, impact; assumption avoidance *Practices* Identify evidence-based/best practices	*Supportive* *Confidential* *No assumptions* *Understanding* *Service* *Respect* *Professionalism* *Fairness and equity* *Sensitivity* *Deference* Honor individual's perspective as expert of own experience	*Inclusive practices and policies* Non-homophobic; non-heterosexist—forms, materials, procedures, practices, marketing etc. *Respectful, advocate* Trust building, continuity *Safe culture/environment* Focus/create safe environment; fair compassionate services. Provide feedback, address bias in others *Commitment* Outreach, ongoing training, measure effectiveness *Systems approach* Embrace diversity—business as usual; data collection to inform practice and procedures *Embed training in culture*—orient, refresh, update

Source Adapted from National Resource Center on LGBT Aging (2012)

Conclusions: This is the first study to examine physical and mental health quality of life as an indicator of successful aging, among LGBT older adults. Thus, this is considered a first to better understand successful aging in regard to physical and mental health in this understudied population. It is critical to continue to investigate factors that contribute to good health among this population in order to develop appropriate interventions to increase good health among this population and to address challenges they may face.

Fredriksen-Goldsen, K. I., Kim, H. J, Shiu, C., Goldsen, J., & Emlet, C. A. (2014). Successful Aging among LGBT Older Adults: Physical and Mental Health-Related Quality of Life by Age Group. *The Gerontologist*, 1–15.

Questions:

1. In addition to physical and mental health, what other factors should be considered when thinking about successful aging?
2. What research should be conducted as a follow-up to this research?

Does cultural competency training make a difference? There is research evidence to support the notion that it does. In a study about the effectiveness of cultural competence training, Knochel et al. (2010) found that agencies that provided training to staff performed better with their LGBT clients were twice as likely to receive requests for assistance from lesbian, gay and bisexual clients and were three times as likely to receive requests of assistance from transgender clients than agencies that did not provide cultural competence training. In other studies, cultural competency trainings have been found to produce at least a short-term impact on recipients' knowledge, attitudes, and behavior intentions (Porter and Krinsky 2013). Repetition and reinforcement through training updates or refresher courses, and the establishment of best practices for the care of LGBT elders can extend these short-term benefits. Other studies indicate that repeated opportunities for interaction also improve sensitivity and awareness of LGBT elder issues and concerns. For instance, a study by Sanchez et al. (2006) found that medical students who had repeated clinical encounters with LGBT patients were more knowledgeable about their health concerns, had more positive attitudes, and provided better care than those who did not.

Ultimately, the application of a systems approach, which recognizes that elements within a unit or entity are often interactive, interdependent, and exert influence on each other, may yield the best results (Bronfenbrenner 1979). Healthcare organizations and long-term care institutions can help improve staff/LGBT elder encounters by providing LGBT cultural competency training, incorporating LGBT curricula into ongoing educational offerings, and providing refresher courses. Providing opportunities for staff to interact with LGBT elders will boost comfort and understanding, as will providing less experienced staff with mentors who have a track record of working well with this population. HCOs and LTC institutions should also revise organization-wide regulations, forms, and processes to be inclusive and respectful of the LGBT population. In addition, rewarding staff for participation in training, recognitions, awards, or incentives for desired behaviors also reinforce learning and practice (Knochel et al. 2012). Such practices help reduce health disparities by creating environments in which LGBT elders may feel safe and validated (Hughes et al. 2011). Effective, timely, and ongoing training and education of staff who work with LGBT elders is a necessary first step and will go a long way toward reducing the potential effect of multiple jeopardy arising out of aging and sexual orientation in later life.

Caveat

A final word (of caution) about cultural competency trainings: there are some limitations to the effectiveness of cultural competency training. For instance, staff training does not cover other potential players in the environment such as vendors or other patients or residents in LTC facilities. An important component of cultural competency training should thus be how to provide feedback and address bias displayed by others (Meyer 2011). It is also crucial to recognize that the effectiveness of cultural competency training is dependent on ensuring that all staff, providers, or personnel receive timely and updated training. However, the reality of organizations, staff turnover, and scheduling constraints may result in the presence of untrained staff. It is important to schedule regular, as well as makeup or catch-up sessions, periodic updates, and refresher sessions. Finally, embedding cultural competency in the organization's culture allows inclusion and respect for diversity to be the usual way of business in the organization, consequently ensuring that the healthcare environment is a safe place for all, and especially LGBT older adults (Meyer 2011; National Resource Center on LGBT Aging and SAGE n.d.). Table 20.5 provides a list of tips that can be applied to promote success in cultural competence training.

See Experiential Learning Activity #1 in Appendix.

Discussion Box #3

You are the administrator of Restoration Acres, a medium-sized skilled nursing facility. You recently became aware of a CMS memo that requires that LTC facilities notify residents of their rights to have visitors, including same-sex relationships in the definition of spouses and domestic partners, as well as to ensure full and equal

Table 20.5 Cultural competence training—tips for success

- Train all staff, at all levels

- Address how to identify and address the needs of LGBT older adults

- Use trusted and credible trainers

- Enhance knowledge and skills about LGBT older adults, and their intersecting identities of race, ethnicity, and culture

- Make cultural competency training a mandatory part of all on-the-job/in-service training

- Tailor training to provide knowledge useful for the role/job performed by the employee

- Become familiar or investigate training resources developed by and/or available at advocacy and research organizations such as SAGE and the National Resource Center for LGBT Aging

- Evaluate the options available and select the programs that best fit your need.

- Remember that inclusion is an ongoing process— establish processes, measure, evaluate, retool if necessary

Adapted from SAGE (2012) and the National Resource Center on LGBT Aging (n.d.)

---

visitation privileges to all visitors. To your knowledge, there are at least three LGBT elders in your facility, and you want to be sure that you provide a supportive environment.

Is compliance with this memo enough? Why or why not?
What if anything else would you recommend? Why?

See Discussion Box #2

Policy Box #2 What effect, if any will the striking down of Section 3 of the Defense of Marriage Act (DOMA), by the Supreme Court have on LGBT elders in the health arena? Why?

Data Collection and Clinical Interview

The need for cultural competency extends to research (i.e., data collection) and to the clinical interview. Healthcare providers, researchers, and other individuals must be culturally competent when collecting data and conducting clinical interviews. Collecting LGBT data in clinical settings is extremely important step toward understanding the healthcare needs of LGBT persons and working toward reducing health disparities among this population, thus promoting health equity (Bradford et al. 2011). Unfortunately, patient information regarding sexual orientation and gender identity is often not collected or discussed with providers. The majority of providers do not know how to have discussions about sexual orientation and gender identity with their patients, which further contributes to the invisibility of LGBT patients in clinical settings and contributes to the lack of LGBT-inclusive cultural competency and clinical training for providers (Bradford et al. 2011).

Many societal and structural barriers still exist that prohibits the collection of data on sexual orientation and gender identity. For instance, structural barriers include poverty in LGBT communities (Badgett et al. 2013), lack of provider training to address the specific healthcare needs of LGBT people (Obedin-Maliver et al. 2011), low rates of health insurance coverage for LGBT individuals, and lack of access to culturally appropriate health care (Mayer et al. 2008). Anti-LGBT discrimination still continues to occur in healthcare settings, thus creating additional barriers to care. Surveys of both providers and patients indicate that LGBT people experience prejudicial treatment in clinical settings and that some providers maintain anti-LGBT attitudes (Lambda Legal 2010; Smith and Matthews 2007). Consequently, many LGBT individuals report culturally incompetent care, and as a result fail to seek health care because of fear of poor treatment (Bradford et al. 2011).

The Fenway Institute in Boston, Massachusetts, has suggested that information regarding sexual orientation and gender identity be collected in two ways: on the patient registration forms with demographic information and by having providers gather the information directly from patients (Bradford et al. 2011). LGBT individuals can be hesitant to provide information about the sexual orientation or gender identity due to fears about privacy and confidentiality. These fears are only made worse with the recent computerization of health information and highly publicized cases of breaches in confidentiality (Forsyth 2011). With proper techniques and standards, these threats are manageable. Providers should ask permission to include information about patients' sexual orientation and gender identity in their medical record (Bradford et al. 2011). Patients should be assured that all information will be kept confidential and that the information will allow healthcare practitioners to provide comprehensive care.

The Fenway Institute has developed several suggestions on how to collect the necessary data. For example, the Fenway Institute suggests including the following question on intake forms: "Do you think of yourself as: lesbian, gay, or homosexual, straight or heterosexual, bisexual, something else, or do not know." The Institute also suggests that providers ask questions directly of patients about sexual orientation, behavior, and gender identity during initial patient visits. Providers should start with open-ended questions, such as "Tell me a little bit about yourself" (Bradford et al. 2011). While sharing information about themselves, patients may bring up information about issues related to sexual orientation or gender identity, which may open the door for discussions. Healthcare settings can create an environment in which individuals might feel more comfortable discussing issues of sexual orientation and gender identity by conveying the message that LGBT people are welcome in the clinical setting (Bradford et al. 2011). For instance, posting a rainbow flag, the logo of the Gay and Lesbian Medical Association (Cahill and Valadez 2013), or including brochures and advertisements specifically for LGBT individuals can help to convey the messages that LGBT people are welcomed in a healthcare setting.

It is important to acknowledge that there is still a long way to go in improving the collection of data from LGBT individuals in healthcare settings. It is inevitable that some patients will not disclose information about sexual orientation or gender identity in clinical settings. However, collecting this information can improve health outcomes of LGBT patients, will help in advancing the understanding of LGBT health (Bradford et al. 2011), and enhance the delivery of culturally competent care.

Discussion Box #4

Practice asking questions about sexual orientation and gender identity by partnering with a classmate or coworker and asking each other the questions presented below. Upon completion, discuss the exercise.

Questions regarding Sexual Orientation

1. Do you have any concerns or questions about your sexuality, sexual orientation, or sexual desires?[a]

Or, preface the questions with a statement. Some patients will be more receptive to that approach. For instance, "I am going to ask you some questions about your sexual health and sexuality that I ask all of my patients". The answers to these questions are important for me to know how to help keep you healthy. Like the rest of this visit, this information is strictly confidential.[a]

2. "Do you have a partner or spouse"? or "Are you currently in a relationship"?[b]

3. "Are you sexually active"?[b]

4. "When was the last time you had sex"?[b]

5. "When you have sex, do you do so with men, women, or both"?[b]

6. "How many sexual partners have you had during the last year"?[b]

7. "Do you have any desires regarding sexual intimacy that you would like to discuss"?[b]

Questions regarding Gender Identity

(continued)

1. Because gender issues affect so many people, I ask patients if they have any relevant concerns. Anything you say will be kept confidential. If this topic isn't relevant to you, tell me and I will move on.[b]

2. "What is your gender"?[c]

3. "Do you consider yourself to be transgender"?[c]

Adapted from the following sources: [a]Makadon (2011), [b]Bradford et al. (2011), [c]The National Resource Center on LGBT Aging and SAGE, n.d.

See Experiential Learning Activity #2 in Appendix.

Health Assessment

Health assessment procedures provide a useful mechanism for collecting data to help increase knowledge about issues, which affect the health of LGBT older adults. Appropriately designed and administered assessments provide data necessary to inform evidence-based practices that support the delivery of quality, patient-centered care. Such data are useful both to improve patient care as well as to improve our knowledge and understanding of factors that influence or impact the health status of LGBT older adults such as needs, disparities, barriers, both across the life course and as they age.

As discussed earlier, the fact that LGBT older adults have added health challenges and disparities related to their sexual minority status, obtaining information regarding the individual's sexual orientation and gender identity, must be a key component of every health assessment conducted on all older adults. The importance of such data collection has been recognized by a number of entities such as the Institute of Medicine, which recommends that these data be included on electronic health records (IOM 2011). In *Healthy People 2020*, The US Department of Health and Human Services

advocated that healthcare providers ask questions about and support the sexual orientation of patients in order to improve patient–provider interactions and enhance LGBT health (HHS 2010). In addition, Section 4302 of the Patient Protection and Affordable Care Act (ACA) encourages collection of this information in healthcare encounters (SAGE n.d. [c]).

Beyond demographic questions about sexual orientation and gender identity, health assessments should also cover other issues found to affect the health status and overall well-being of LGBT older adults. For example, providers should assess mental health and psychological well-being, with questions which address depression, anxiety, and substance abuse, as well as factors such as isolation, the presence of social supports, and delays or other barriers to seeking care or accessing services (Fredriksen-Goldsen et al. 2011). Collating this information will help document, elucidate, and develop best practices for enhancing the health of LGBT older adults (Gay and Lesbian Medical Association [GMLA] 2001). In addition to being a mechanism for data collection, the health assessment sets the stage for a healthcare encounter where LGBT older adults can be their "authentic selves" in an inclusive, safe, and supportive environment (National Resource Center on LGBT Aging n.d.).

See Experiential Learning Activity #3 in Appendix.

Research Implications and Future Directions

Globally, some countries are making great strides to recognizing same-sex couples, while other countries seem to be going in the opposite direction. In the USA, we are beginning to see a change, as evidenced by the number of states supporting same-sex unions. However, extreme challenges for same-sex couples remain. Regardless, the LGBT population is increasing as more individuals are coming out. As the aging population increases in number, we can expect a parallel increase in the number of LGBT older adults. The current paucity of LGBT research has negative implications for health care and services, hence the push for cultural competency training for healthcare providers. Obviously, research must catch up with LGBT aging issues. Research has to repsond to the demand for knowledge, as well as document current realities of LGBT older adults and project future needs. To begin, we need a better idea of the demographic scope of LGBT older adults and the perceived needs among this population. In addition, rather than treating LGBT as a homogenous group, we need research on the health disparities and needs of various subgroups within this population. Additionally, we should use the life course perspective to examine cohort differences among older adults in health care, particularly in light of current political shifts. In terms of research, we need research aimed at designing culturally appropriate preventative care for this population based on the information from current generations. Among healthcare providers, interventions should be developed and tested to increase knowledge regarding providing care to the LGBT population and the various subgroups and to increase cultural competence among providers.

Summary

In this chapter, we have introduced and discussed some of the major issues that affect the health of LGBT elders and how current healthcare practices and policies act to disadvantage and marginalize LGBT elders through unfair and unreasonable treatment. One thing is clear—any attempt to mitigate the problems and improve health for LGBT older adults must begin with a healthcare environment built on trust, honesty, and openness between the healthcare provider and the care recipient. We need for LGBT older adults to be able to openly discuss their sexual orientation and gender identity and health issues when they seek health care. Healthcare providers

in turn must bear the responsibility for creating an environment in which discussions about sexual orientation and gender identity are welcome by their knowledge, attitudes, and behaviors.

Unfortunately, the history of marginalization among LGBT older adults in all segments of society also contributes to health status. For instance, the social context and lived experience of LGBT older adults might include challenges in relationships such as partner violence, poverty, stigma, and socioeconomic status might affect access to quality health care. So, too, does the legal context of LGBT older adults, for instance, immigration status, same-sex unions, access to social security affects access to quality health care. Beyond healthcare provider, all disciplines with the potential to provide care to this population would benefit from understanding the need to be culturally competent when providing services to LGBT older adults. Ultimately, health status for LGBT older adults is best achieved through a multidisciplinary team of care and service providers working together to provide culturally competent and seamless care in all sectors.

LGBT older adults have poorer health status as a result of a combination of factors including health challenges as a result of sexual orientation, gender identity issues, as well as a history of marginalization, prejudice, and the effects of non-disclosure in healthcare encounters. LGBT older adults, like others, are entitled to quality health care. A critical step in reducing healthcare disparities and improving health and well-being for LGBT older adults requires the creation of inclusive healthcare environment. An inclusive healthcare environment is one in which system-wide policies and practices acknowledge LGBT individuals and all staff and personnel are culturally competent in LGBT issues. Furthermore, staff and personnel's knowledge, attitude, and behavior indicate sensitivity about LGBT aging needs which encourages trust and disclosure among LGBT older adults. Comprehensive review of policies and practice in the healthcare environment is needed to address the needs and concerns of this vulnerable population.

Learning Exercises

Experiential Assignment #1

Visit your local Long-Term Care Ombudsman's Office or an advocacy group for LGBT older adults in long-term care facilities. Ask for de-identified information or case review for one or two incidents involving staff/residents/family and a LGBT older adult relating to health.

Review the incident: What were the issues? What were the implications for the LGBT older adult? How was the matter resolved? What if anything could have been done to avoid the situation, or address the problem in the first case? If you were to create a cultural competence training workshop to prevent these sorts of problems in the future, what would that workshop look like? Explain your rationale.

Experiential Assignment #2

Interview two older adults of whom one must be a member of the LGBT population, about their health concerns as they age. Your questions should include health status, access to care, delivery of services, and quality of care. Compare the responses. How are they similar or different? Why? What implications if any emerge for their health? How do these interviews add to what you are learning about LGBT older adults and health?

Experiential Assignment #3

Challenging beliefs and feelings about LGBT aging through self-examination using role-play, through which students explore their beliefs, feelings, and attitudes about LGBT older adult sexuality, roles, identity, and orientation. Role-play occurs in the context of a healthcare encounter. One student plays the role of the healthcare provider, while another student plays the role of a lesbian, or gay, or bisexual, or transgender older adult. Roles can then be reversed if desired.

Suggested scenarios:

(A) Older adult comes out as gay to the healthcare professional,

(B) LGBT older adult encounters a homophobic healthcare provider, and

(C) Healthcare encounter in which provider is trying to conduct a health assessment of an older adult believed to be LGBT.

Script should provide opportunities for the following:

1. Explore or showcase negative versus positive interventions with LGBT older adult patients and
2. Opportunities for introspection and self-examination of personal beliefs, feelings, attitudes, and expectations

Process:

1. Review and encourage open discussion about the issues raised and/or addressed.
2. Encourage students to discuss their observations, feelings, and discomforts if any.
3. Address any myths or stereotypes which come up.
4. Provide feedback and clarification as necessary.

Self-Check Questions

1. Explain how common misconceptions about patients sexuality impacts LGBT elders overall health.
2. Describe several of the age-related changes that could influence an older adult's participation in sexual intimacy.
3. List and describe barriers to data collection among LGBT individuals in healthcare settings.
4. What obstacles impede the delivery of optimal health care to LGBT elders?
5. Discuss the effect of non-disclosure of sexual orientation or gender identity by LGBT elders on healthcare delivery. How can this issue be addressed from the perspective of the:
   (a) LGBT older adult and
   (b) healthcare provider.

6. What are the training needs of staff who work with LGBT older adults?
7. Identify the risk factors for HIV/AIDS among LGBT older adults.
8. Explain the importance of having LGBT cultural competency in healthcare personnel and settings.
9. Identify the three dimensions of cultural competency.
10. You are creating a LGBT cultural competence training program/workshop for healthcare providers in your county. Discuss the goals and components required to make it an effective program.
11. Explain why it is necessary not to treat the LGBT population as monolithic group, especially in relation to health and health care.

Multiple Choice Questions

1. Oftentimes, healthcare providers assume that older adults are as follows:
   (a) Homosexual
   (b) Transgender
   (c) Heterosexual
   (d) Asexual
2. Compared to previous generations, rates of illicit drug abuse among baby boomers are relatively/have relatively higher rates of illicit drug use as opposed to previous generations:
   (a) Lower
   (b) Higher
   (c) Similar
   (d) Nonexistent
3. Many older adults do not bring up the topic of sexuality with their healthcare providers because:
   (a) They do not desire to be sexually active.
   (b) They do not believe that their healthcare provider will have the answers to their questions.
   (c) The healthcare provider often brings the topic up before the older adult has a chance to.

(d) They feel embarrassed or ashamed because they have internalized misconceptions regarding older adults and sexuality.
4. Structural barriers to obtaining health-related data from LGBT elder patients include the following:
   (a) Poverty in the LGBT community
   (b) Lack of provider training to address the specific health needs of the LGBT population
   (c) Low rates of health insurance among LGBT individuals
   (d) Lack of access to culturally appropriate health care
   (e) All of the above
5. Which of the following statements is NOT true?
   (a) HIV is not a concern among older adults
   (b) Symptoms of HIV are often confused with symptoms of other chronic conditions that often affect elders.
   (c) Making a diagnosis of HIV among older adults can be more challenging.
   (d) Older adults get HIV the same way that young people do.
6. A person's gender identity if different from sex at birth should:
   (a) Always be honored
   (b) Never be honored
   (c) Be honored only if you are comfortable doing so
   (d) Be honored only if the person has undergone particular medical interventions and a legal name change
7. The terms "sexual orientation and gender identity"….
   (a) Mean the same thing
   (b) Can be used interchangeably
   (c) Have different meanings and are not interchangeable
   (d) Can be used interchangeably when referring to lesbians only
8. Which of the following statements is correct? In order to assure better care experience and positive outcomes,

(a) LGBT elders should be treated like all other older adults.

(b) It is not enough to treat LGBT elders like the general older adult patient.

(c) Sexual orientation or gender identity is not a relevant consideration.

(d) Providers and practitioners should avoid embarrassing LGBT elders by bringing up sexual orientation or gender identity.

9. In order to be effective, cultural competence training should address:

(a) Knowledge

(b) Behavior

(c) Attitude

(d) A, B, & C

(e) Knowledge and behavior

10. You are the staff responsible for administering or arranging for certain sex-linked preventive care for the clinic's patients. This week, you have a management intern shadowing your office. You are meeting with Janet Doe, a transgendered person who is in the clinic for her annual health check. You need to schedule some tests including mammogram and Pap smear. Which of the following constitutes best practices in order to ensure that Ms. Doe received appropriate care?

(a) The intern asks Ms. Doe what surgeries she has had as a transgender person.

(b) You ask Ms. Doe what surgeries she has had as a transgender person, while the intern takes notes.

(c) You provide privacy for Ms. Doe to answer the questions about what surgeries she has had as a transgender person.

(d) Ms. Doe is not asked any questions about any surgeries she has had as a transgender person.

Key

1. d
2. b
3. d
4. e
5. a
6. a
7. c
8. b
9. d
10. c

Resources

The National Resource Center on LGBT Aging
http://www.lgbtagingcenter.org/resources/index.cfm

Centers for Disease Control and Prevention-HIV among Older Adults
http://www.cdc.gov/hiv/risk/age/olderamericans/

Health Equity and LGBT Elders of Color
http://www.lgbtagingcenter.org/resources/pdfs/Sage_PolicyBrief_HealthEquity.pdf

LGBT Health
http://www.hrsa.gov/lgbt/

Stanford LGBT Medical Education Group
http://med.stanford.edu/lgbt/resources/

The Fenway Institute
http://www.fenwayhealth.org/site/PageServer

Services and Advocacy for Gay, Lesbian, Bisexual and Transgender Elders (SAGE)
http://www.sageusa.org/

Lambda Legal—National organization committed to achieving full recognition of the civil rights of lesbians, gay men, bisexuals, transgender people and those with HIV through impact litigation, education and public policy work.
www.lambdalegal.org/health-care-fairness.

References

AIDS Community Research Initiative of America (ACRIA). (2012). older and wiser: many faces of HIV. Retrieved from https://www.dropbox.com/s/oc041bhfd5w1orl/ACRIA_OAW_EN.pdf.

American Association of Retired Persons (AARP). (2011). *8 Reasons sex improves your health*. Retrieved from http://www.aarp.org/relationships/love-sex/info-06-2011/sex-improves-men-health.2.html.

Badgett, L., Durso, L., & Schneebaum, S. (2013). *New patterns of poverty in the lesbian, gay, and bisexual community*. Los Angeles: The Williams Institute. Retrieved from http://williamsinstitute.law.ucla.edu/wp-content/uploads/LGB-Poverty-Update-Jun-2013.pdf.

Barbara, A. M., Doctor, F., & Chaim, G. (2007). *Asking the right questions 2: Talking with clients about sexual orientation and gender identity in mental health, counselling and addiction settings*. Toronto: Center for Addiction and Mental Health. Retrieved from https://knowledgex.camh.net/amhspecialists/Screening_Assessment/assessment/ARQ2/Documents/arq2.pdf.

Bell, S. A., Bern-Klug, M., Kramer, K. W. O., & Saunders, J. B. (2010). Most nursing home social service directors lack training in working with lesbian, gay, and bisexual residents. *Social Work in Health Care, 49*(9), 814–831.

Bernstein, K. T., Liu, K., Begier, E. M., Koblin, B., Karpati, A., & Murrill, C. (2008). Same-sex attraction disclosure to health care providers among New York City men who have sex with men: Implications for HIV testing approaches. *Archives of Internal Medicine, 168*, 1458–1464.

Bradford, J. B., Cahill, S., Grasso, C., & Makadon, H. J. (2011). *Policy focus: How to gather data on sexual orientation and gender identity in clinical settings*. The Fenway Institute. Retrieved from http://thefenwayinstitute.org/documents/Policy_Brief_HowtoGather..._v3_01.09.12.pdf.

Bronfenbrenner, U. (1979). *The ecology of human development: Experiments by nature and design*. Cambridge, MA: Harvard University Press.

Cahill, S., & Valadez, R. (2013). Community-based approaches to HIV prevention that address anti-gay stigma. *Psychology and AIDS Exchange, 34*, 69–81. doi:10.1057/jphp.2012.59

Center for Addiction and Mental Health (CAMH). (2007). *Asking the right questions: Talking with clients about sexual orientation and gender identity in mental health, counseling and addition settings*. Retrieved from https://knowledgex.camh.net/amhspecialists/Screening_Assessment/assessment/ARQ2/Documents/arq2.pdf.

Centers for Disease Control and Prevention (CDC). (2013a). *HIV among older Americans*. Retrieved from http://www.cdc.gov/hiv/risk/age/olderamericans/.

Centers for Disease Control and Prevention (CDC). (2013b). *The state of aging and health in America 2013*. Atlanta, GA: Centers for Disease Control and Prevention, US Department of Health and Human Services. Retrieved from http://www.cdc.gov/features/agingandhealth/state_of_aging_and_health_in_america_2013.pdf.

Centers for Disease Control and Prevention (CDC). (2014a). *HIV transmission*. Retrieved from http://www.cdc.gov/hiv/basics/transmission.html#panel0.

Centers for Disease Control and Prevention (CDC). (2014b). *2013 Sexually transmitted disease surveillance*. Retrieved from http://www.cdc.gov/std/stats13/default.htm.

Centers for Medicare and Medicaid Services (CMS). (2012). *Chronic conditions among medicare beneficiaries*. Retrieved from http://www.cms.gov/Research-Statistics-Data-and-Systems/Statistics-Trends-and-Reports/Chronic-Conditions/Downloads/2012Chartbook.pdf.

Committee on Lesbian, Gay, Bisexual, and Transgender Health Issues and Research Gaps and Opportunities. Board on the health of select populations, Institute of Medicine. (2011). *The health of lesbian, gay, bisexual, and transgender people: Building a foundation for better understanding*. Washington DC: Institute of Medicine. Retrieved from http://www.iom.edu/Reports/2011/The-Health-of-Lesbian-Gay-Bisexual-and-Transgender-People.aspx.

Davis, T. (2013). *An exploratory study of primary care providers' HIV prevention practices among older adults*. Unpublished doctoral dissertation, University of Kentucky, Lexington, Kentucky.

Durso, L. E., & Meyer, I. H. (2012). *Patterns and predictors of disclosure of sexual orientation to healthcare providers among lesbians, gay men, and bisexuals*. Sexuality Research and Social Policy, 1. UCLA: The Williams Institute. Retrieved from http://escholarship.org/uc/item/08b546b6.

Federal Interagency Forum on Aging-Related Statistics (FIFAR). (2012). *Older Americans 2012: Key indicators of well-being*. Retrieved from http://www.agingstats.gov/agingstatsdotnet/Main_Site/Data/2012_Documents/Docs/EntireChartbook.pdf.

Forsyth, J. (2011). Medical records of 4.9 million exposed in Texas data breach. *Reuters*. www.reuters.com/assets/print?aid=USTRE78S5JG20110929. Accessed September 29, 2011.

Fredriksen-Goldsen, K. I., Kim, H.-J., Emlet, C. A., Muraco, A., Erosheva, E. A., Hoy-Ellis, C. P. et al. (2011). *The aging and health report: Disparities and resilience among lesbian, gay, bisexual, and transgender older adults—key findings fact sheet*. Seattle: Institute for Multigenerational Health. Retrieved from https://depts.washington.edu/agepride/wordpress/wp-content/uploads/2012/10/factsheet-keyfindings10-25-12.pdf.

Fredriksen-Goldsen, K. I., Kim, H. J, Shiu, C., Goldsen, J., & Emlet, C. A. (2014). Successful aging among LGBT older adults: physical and mental health-related quality of life by age group. *The Gerontologist*, 1–15.

Gay and Lesbian Medical Association (GMLA). (2001). *Healthy people 2010: A companion document for LGBT health*. San Francisco: GMLA, 2001 April. Retrieved from https://www.nalgap.org/PDF/Resources/HP2010CDLGBTHealth.pdf.

Hughes, A. K., Harold, R. D., & Boyer, J. M. (2011). Awareness of LGBT aging issues among aging services network providers. *Journal of Gerontological Social Work, 54*(7), 659–677.

Institute of Medicine. (2011). *The health of lesbian, gay, bisexual, and transgender people: Building a foundation for better understanding.* Washington, DC: The National Academies Press.

Jablonski, R. A., Vance, D. E., & Beattie, E. (2013). The invisible elderly: Lesbian, gay, bisexual, and transgender older adults. *Journal of Gerontological Nursing, 39*(11), 46–52.

Katz, A. (2013). Sexuality in nursing care facilities: A personal choice or a problem? *American Journal of Nursing, 113*(3), 53–55.

Knochel, K. A., Croghan, C. F., Moone, R. P., & Quam, J. K. (2010). *Ready to serve? The aging network and LGB and T older adults.* Washington, DC: National Association of Area Agencies on Aging. Retrieved from http://issuu.com/lgbtagingcenter/docs/readytoserve.

Knochel, K. A., Croghan, C. F., Moone, R. P., & Quam, J. K. (2012). Training geography, and provision of aging services to lesbian, gay, bisexual, and transgender older adults. *Journal of Gerontological Social Work, 55*(5), 426–443.

The Fenway Institute. (2012). *How to gather data about sexual orientation and gender identity in clinical settings.* Retrieved from http://www.fenwayhealth.org/site/DocServer/Policy_Brief_WhyGather..._v6_01.09.12.pdf?docID=9141.

The Joint Commission. (2011). Advancing effective communication, cultural competence, and patient- and family-centered care for the lesbian, gay, bisexual, and transgender (LGBT) community: A field guide, Oak Brook, IL

The Joint United Nations Programme on HIV/AIDS (UNAIDS). (2014). *Fact Sheet 2014.* Retrieved from http://www.unaids.org/en/media/unaids/contentassets/documents/factsheet/2014/20140716_FactSheet_en.pdf.

Lamda Legal. (2010). *When health care isn't caring: Lamda legal's survey of discrimination against LGBT people and people with HIV.* New York: Lamda Legal

Lim, F. A., & Bernstein, I. (2012) Promoting awareness of LGBT issues in aging in a baccalaureate nursing program. *Nursing Education Perspectives, 33*(3), 170–175.

Lindau, S. T., Schumm, L. P., Laumann, E. O., Levinson, W., O'Muircheartaigh, C. A., & Waite, L. J. (2007). A study of sexuality and health among older adults in the United State. *New England Journal of Medicine, 357*, 762–774.

Makadon, H. J. (2011). Ending LGBT invisibility in health care: The first step in ensuring equitable care. *Cleveland Clinic Journal of Medicine, 78*(4), 220–224. doi:10.3949/ccjm.78gr.10006

Mayer, K. H., Bradford, J. B., Makadon, H. J., Stall, R., Goldhammer, H., & Landers, S. (2008). Sexual and gender minority health: what we know and what needs to be done. *American Journal of Public Health, 98*(6), 989–995.

McGinnis, S. L., & Moore, J. (2006). *The impact of the aging population on the health workforce in the United States: A summary of key findings.* Rensselaer,

NY: Center for Health Workforce Studies, School of Public Health, SUNY Albany.

Meyer, H. (2011). Safe spaces? The need for LGBT cultural competency in aging services. *Public Policy and Aging Report, 21*(3), 24–27.

National Resource Center on LGBT Aging and SAGE. (n. d.). *Inclusive questions for older adults: A practical guide to collecting data on sexual orientation and gender identity.* Retrieved from http://www.lgbtagingcenter.org/resources/resource.cfm?r=601.

National Institute on Aging. (2013). *Sexuality in later life.* Retrieved from http://www.nia.nih.gov/health/publication/sexuality-later-life.

National Resource Center on LGBT Aging. (2012). *Inclusive services for LGBT older adults: A practical guide to creating welcoming agencies.* New York: National Resource Center on LGBT Aging, SAGE. Retrieved from http://www.lgbtagingcenter.org/resources/resource.cfm?r=487.

Obedin-Maliver, J., Goldsmith, E. S., Stewart, L., White, W., Tran, E., Brenman, S., et al. (2011). Lesbian, gay, bisexual, and transgender-related content in undergraduate medical education. *JAMA, 306*(9), 971–977.

Petroll, A. E., & Mosack, K. E. (2011). Physician awareness of sexual orientation and preventive health recommendations to men who have sex with men. *Sexually Transmitted Diseases, 38*, 63–67.

Porter, K. E., & Krinsky, L. (2013). Do LGBT aging trainings effectuate positive change in mainstream elder service providers? *Journal of Homosexuality, 61* (1), 197–216. doi:10.1080/00918369.2013.835618.

Powderly, W. G., & Mayer, K. H. (2003). Centers for disease control and prevention revised guidelines for human immunodeficiency virus (HIV) counseling, testing, and referral: Targeting HIV specialist. *HIV/AIDS, 37*(15), 813–819.

Redman, D. (2011). *LGBT long-term care issues.* Retrieved from http://www.lgbtagingcenter.org/resources/resource.cfm?r=64.

Rogers, A., Rebbe, R., Gardella, C., Worlein, M., & Chamberlin, M. (2013). Older LGBT adult training panels: An opportunity to education about issues faced by the older LGBT community. *Journal of Gerontological Social Work, 56*(7), 580–595.

Sanchez, N. F., Rabatin, J., Sanchez, J. P., Hubbard, S., & Kalet, A. (2006). Medical students ability to care for lesbian, gay, bisexual and transgendered patients. *Journal of Family Medicine, 38*(1), 21–27.

Services and Advocacy for GLBT Elders (SAGE). (n.d. [a]). *Aging programs and services.* Retrieved from http://www.sageusa.org/issues/aging.cfm.

Services and Advocacy for GLBT Elders (SAGE). (n.d. [b]). *Ten things every LGBT older adult should know about HIV/AIDS.* Retrieved from http://www.lgbtagingcenter.org/resources/pdfs/TenThingsHIV.pdf.

Services and Advocacy Gay, Lesbian, Bisexual and Transgender Elders (SAGE). (n.d.[c]). *Health and health care.* Retrieved from http://sageusa.org/issues/health.cfm

Services and Advocacy for GLBT Elders. (2010). *SAGE awarded $900 K federal grant.* Retrieved from http://www.lgbtagingcenter.org/newsevents/newsArticle.cfm?n=1.

Services and Advocacy for GLBT Elders (SAGE). (2010). *LGBT older adults and inhospitable health care environments.* Services & Advocacy for GLBT Elders (SAGE) and The Movement Advancement Project and SAGE & Center for American Progress. Retrieved from http://sageusa.org/resources/publications.cfm?ID=36#sthash.RHUrxMRG.dpuf.

Smith, D., & Matthews, W. (2007). Physician's attitudes toward homosexuality and HIV: Survey of a California medical society-revisited (PATHH-II). *Journal of Homosexuality, 53*(3–4), 1–9.

St. Pierre, M. (2012). Under what conditions do lesbians disclose their sexual orientation to healthcare providers? A review of the literature. *Journal of Lesbian Studies, 16*, 199–219.

Stein, G. L., & Bonuck, K. A. (2001). Physician—patient relationships among the lesbian and gay community. *Journal of the Gay and Lesbian Medical Association, 5*, 87–93.

Trompeter, S. E., Bettencourt, R., & Barrett-Connor, E. (2012). Sexual activity and satisfaction in health community-dwelling older women. *American Journal of Medicine, 125*, 37–43. doi:10.1016/j.amjmed.2011.07.036.

US Department of Health and Human Services (HHS). (n.d.). *A timeline of AIDS.* Retrieved from http://www.aids.gov/hiv-aids-basics/hiv-aids-101/aids-timeline/.

US Department of Health and Human Services, DHHS. (2010). *Healthy people 2020.* Retreived from http://healthypeople.gov/2020/topicsobjectives2020/overview.aspx?topicid=25#ten.

U.S. Department of Health and Human Services, Health Resources and Services Administration. (2011). *Women's health USA 2011.* Rockville, Maryland: U.S. Department of Health and Human Services.

Vann, M. (2014). Senior sex myths debunked. *Everyday Health.* Medically reviewed by Bass, P. F. Retrieved from http://www.everydayhealth.com/sexual-health/senior-sex-myths-debunked.aspx.

Wu, L. T., & Blazer, D. G. (2010). Illicit and nonmedical drug use among older adults: A review. *Journal of Aging and Health, 23*, 481–504.

LGBT Elders in Nursing Homes, Long-Term Care Facilities, and Residential Communities

21

John T. White and Tracey L. Gendron

Abstract

This article examines the opportunities and challenges faced by lesbian, gay, bisexual, and transgender elders who are aging in the long-term care continuum. From independent and community living, to adult day services, assisted living and nursing facilities, LGBT elders may face discrimination from administrators, direct care professionals, neighbors, and other residents/participants. Ironically, enduring a lifetime of fear and discrimination has many positive factors for LGBT elders' resiliency, self-esteem, and social networking. Further, LGBT individuals are now increasingly accepted into "mainstream" society. It is, however, important to understand that that the current cohort of LGBT elders may not only fear, but lack the funds to participate in, the long-term care continuum.

Keywords

LGBT · GLBT · Gay · Lesbian · Bisexual · Transgender · Elder · Older adult · Long-term care

Overview

In recent years, a good deal of scholarship has been amassed on the topic of sexual orientation, gender identify, and aging, and rightfully so. According to the National Resource Center on LGBT Aging (2010), there are approximately 1.5 million lesbian, gay, bisexual, and transgender elders currently residing in the USA. This number is expected to increase to approximately 3.5 million by 2030. To compound these statistics, social isolation affects a disproportionate numbers of LGBT elders as they continue to deal with stigma, discrimination, ageism, and even distancing within the LGBT umbrella.

National organizations, including the LGBT Aging Project, SAGE (Services and Advocacy for GLBT Elders), the National Resource Center on LGBT Aging, the American Society on Aging, and the Gerontological Society of

J.T. White (✉) · T.L. Gendron
Virginia Commonwealth University, Richmond, VA, USA
e-mail: whitejt2@vcu.edu

T.L. Gendron
e-mail: tlgendro@vcu.edu

© Springer International Publishing Switzerland 2016
D.A. Harley and P.B. Teaster (eds.), *Handbook of LGBT Elders*,
DOI 10.1007/978-3-319-03623-6_21

Terms for Discussion
Gay: Men who are attrached to other men
Lesbian: Women who are attracted to other women
Bisexual: Sexual attraction to both men and women
Transgender: Referencing gender identity and not sexual orientation. The gender identity often does not conform to assigned gender at birth.

Fig. 21.1 Terms for discussion gender identification

America, have published scholarly, evidence-based information on what it is to be an aging member of the gay, lesbian, bisexual, and transgender communities. This new wave of information is being presented after years of isolated studies that are still monumentally significant, but nonetheless lacking in statistical power. This is to be expected of studies of populations facing multitudinous stigmas of aging and sexual orientation or aging and gender identity, or any combination thereof.

The following chapter will focus on the barriers to inclusion for LGBT elders as they age into the long-term care continuum with the overarching message that current scholarship supports: getting older (and being gay, lesbian, bisexual, or transgender) has its distinct challenges though many LGBT elders are maintaining and even thriving. With support from a Gerontological Optimal Aging Framework, case studies, and emerging scholarship, the authors will help readers gain a better understanding of a strength-based approach to aging in the face of adversity.

Learning Objectives

1. Readers will have an increased understanding of the gerontological framework for optimal aging.
2. Readers will have an increased understanding of person-centered care philosophies and practice.
3. Readers will have an increased understanding of options for long-term care and the long-term care continuum.

4. Readers will have an increased understanding of barriers to inclusion for members of the aging LGBT aging population and the sociogenesis of these barriers.
5. Readers will have an increased understanding of case studies of LGBT individuals who have overcome barriers to optimal aging.
6. Readers will have an increased understanding of the difference between sexual orientation and gender identity (Fig. 21.1).

Introduction

This chapter uses a gerontological framework and person-centered care philosophy as lenses from which to evaluate the challenges LGBT elders face in the long-term care continuum, which includes a variety of settings from independent living to skilled nursing. This chapter also reviews and evaluates barriers to inclusion and opportunities for optimal aging that LGBT elders face as they age into the long-term care continuum. In order to comprehensively achieve this, issues related to person-centered care, cultural competence, and cultural humility throughout the care continuum will be identified and evaluated. A strength-based treatment is employed as the reader evaluates what it means to optimally age in a holistic manner: biologically, psychologically, sociologically, and spiritually.

We begin by exploring a brief history of the research and practice related to sexual orientation, gender identity, and the care continuum. We then identify and define options ranging from "aging in place" to long-term care, as well as the barriers and unique opportunities for successful aging in the long-term care continuum. We evaluate reasons why LGBT older adults may hide their sexual orientation or gender identity and spend time defining and treating the differences between sexual orientation and gender identity. We identify best practices for creating a supportive environment for LGBT elders and evaluate a case study on optimal aging.

This chapter presents a brief history of the research and reviews the current state of LGBT elders aging within the continuum of care. National organizations, movements, and policies that impact LGBT optimal aging will be identified, as well as state, local, and regional best practices for support and inclusion. In addition, examples of LGBT-inclusive housing developments throughout the nation, affordability of long-term care, and emerging options for aging in place are discussed. We conclude the chapter by evaluating academic and community stakeholders in service delivery to LGBT elders and the roles they can play in future optimal aging and engagement of LGBT elders.

Teaching Tool: http://lgbtagingcenter.org/training/buildingRespect.cfm
Complete the following one-hour presentation from the National Resource Center on LGBT Aging. Identify 5 key takeaway points from this presentation.

The Long-Term Care Continuum

The long-term care continuum consists of a variety of options that includes living at home completely independently to 24-h care provided in a long-term care facility. The long-term care continuum includes the following:

Aging in Place/Independent Living: Aging in the environment of an elder's choice.

In Home Care: Receiving assistance with activities of daily living through formal or informal care networks, while still living independently.

Adult Day/Senior Centers: Community-based organization where elders access programs, services, and resources ranging from socialization to nutrition to some basic care intended to support independent living/aging in place.

Assisted Living: Housing for elders or persons with disabilities that provides basic nursing care, housekeeping, and prepared meals as needed.

Skilled Nursing: A residential option that provides skilled or advanced care for elders, usually 24 h per day.

Hospice: Palliative care that focuses on the holistic needs of chronically or terminally ill patients.

Discussion: In what setting would you prefer to age and among the company of what individuals and groups? What personal resources and networks will you need to employ and maintain in order to you age in your preferred setting?

LGBT and Aging: A History of Research

Reviewing the research relating to the aging, LGBT population is a true learning experience in and of itself. It is not simply an exercise in uncovering scholarship, it is educational in the means of research methodology. The data collection methods are sobering.

As one might imagine, acquiring data and results with any statistical power from a marginalized population is a challenge. The LGBT population did not begin to "come out" until after the 1969 Stonewall Riot and the pioneering efforts of leaders such as Harvey Milk in the mid-1970s. Research from this time and throughout the 1980s and 1990s is, by and large, relegated to urban settings, bars, clubs and anecdotal, and qualitative studies (Johnson et al. 2005; Addis et al. 2009).

Until 1974, the American Psychological Association classified homosexuality as a deviant, pathological condition, and so it was not until after the mid-1970s that research on homosexuality shifted from a deviance model to that of a social-constructivist one (Johnson et al. 2005). The data for members of the transgender population have only recently been upgraded with the release of the DSM V, in 2013. In both cases, data derive from a younger cohort with a different view and values from their elder counterparts (Quam and Whitford 1992).

A quote by Berger and Kelly (1996) personifies just how stereotypes and antiquated data proliferate:

> The older lesbian...is purported to be a cruel witch. Cold, unemotional, and heartless, she despises men. Devoted solely to masculine interests and career pursuits, she has no friends and is repeatedly frustrated by the rejections of younger women. The older gay man is said to become increasingly isolated and effeminate as he ages. Lacking family and friends, he is portrayed as desperately lonely. He must settle for no sex life at all, or he must prey upon young boys to satisfy his lust. (Berger and Kelly 1996, p. 306)

Stereotypes such as these above originate within the lifetime of the current cohort of LGBT elders. They inform the conventional wisdom surrounding sexual orientation and one can only assume gender identity.

> Discuss the genesis of stereotyping. How can stereotyping impact optimal aging and person-centered care?

Major Issues of the Chapter Topic and Relevant Policies

Much of the existing literature has relatively few participants, and the data are skewed toward the environments in which they took place. The empirical data track heavily toward higher rates of smoking, alcohol use, and obesity (Hughes and Evans 2003). They tend to support older stereotypes of the LGBT population as immersed in a culture of alcoholism, depression, and poor health habits. Examples of real evidence-based qualitative and quantitative studies on LGBT elders begin to emerge in the 1990s and 2000s when data from national organizations (Human Rights Campaign, National Gay and Lesbian Task Force, SAGE) were mined. Although this represents an improvement, the data were collected from members of the LGBT population who are active, enfranchised, engaged, and more likely to participate in "out and proud" organizations. Much of the existing studies lack statistical power due to small sample size and high potential for participant bias. Therefore, it is unwise to unilaterally rely on research that is still emerging and calibrating. While there are indeed excellent, rich, statistically significant studies that have been completed, further research is needed that supports a person-centered model of care and inquiry.

Emerging scholarship tells us that elders who are isolated are at increased risk for premature death (Pantell et al. 2013). Compounding this, according to SAGE, LGBT elders are at increased risk for isolation. LGBT elders are over twice as likely to live alone with thinner support networks, three to four times less likely to have children, and twice as likely to be single as compared to the heterosexual population. LGBT elders have higher disability rates, struggle with economic insecurity, and have increased mental health concerns manifest from a lifetime of discrimination (SAGE 2010).

Visit www.gensilent.com and view the film trailer and review the following statistics in Fig. 21.2. What do you find most startling from this brief introduction to these cases? Why would any elder wait until near the end of life to reach out for assistance?

The Caring and Aging with Pride Study (2011) gives additional information on why the barriers to inclusion and "othering" of LGBT elders are so real and profound. The study found that 82 % reported having been victimized at least once, and 64 % reported experiencing victimization at least three times in their lives. The report notes: "The most common type of victimization is verbal insults (68 %), followed by threats of physical violence (43 %), and being hassled by the police (27 %). Nearly one in four (23 %) have had an object thrown at them, and one-fifth (20 %) have had their property damaged or destroyed. Nearly one in five (19 %) have been physically assaulted (i.e., punched, kicked, or beaten), 14 % threatened with a weapon, and 11 % have been sexually assaulted.

This discrimination continues into later life. According to a 2005 study of LGBT long-term care residents, LGBT elders fear discrimination from administration, direct care professionals, and other residents (Johnson et al. 2005). These responses varied widely with regard to the variables of age, income, gender, community size, and education level of the respondents but are concurrent with the notion that, even among healthcare professionals and, arguably, younger members of the LGBT community, that LGBT elders are "homogeneous, isolated, lonely, and without hope." (Johnson et al. 2005 p. 86).

- Older people without adequate social interaction are twice as likely to die prematurely
- This increased risk of mortality is comparable to smoking **15** cigarettes per day, **6** alcoholic beverages per day, and it is **twice** as dangerous as obesity.
- 43 % of elders experience social isolation
- 11.3 million elders live alone (8.1 million are women)
- Based on current demographic trends, 16 million elders will live alone by 2020
- Older adults without adequate social interaction are twice as likely to die prematurely

According to the National Gay and Lesbian Task Force, the fear of isolation is real among LGBT elders. For many elders who have experienced marginalization and disenfranchisement over the life span, with advancing age comes an increasing reliance on public programs and social services. There is less independence or ability to retreat from discrimination, reinforcing isolative behaviors, and leading to the negative health outcomes outlined above.

Further, housing discrimination based on sexual orientation and gender identity is prohibited in only 15 states and the District of Columbia: California, Colorado, Connecticut, the District of Columbia, Illinois, Iowa, Hawaii, Maine, Minnesota, New Jersey, Nevada, New Mexico, Oregon, Rhode Island, Vermont, and Washington. There are also six states that prohibit housing discrimination based on sexual orientation (but not gender identity): Delaware, Maryland, Massachusetts, New Hampshire, New York, and Wisconsin. In addition, many cities prohibit discrimination on

	LGBT Elders	General Elder Population
Live Alone	75%	33%
No Children	90%	20%
Single	80%	40%

Fig. 21.2 The film trailer and review the following statistics

Graphic: Barriers to Health Care Access

According to the US Department of Health and Human Services, LGBT Adults are:

+ Less likely to have health insurance coverage

+ More likely to delay or not seek medical care

+ Facing barriers to access as older adults due to isolation and a **lack of culturally competent providers. One study found 13% of older LGBT adults were denied or provided inferior health care.**

+ More likely to **delay** or not get needed **prescription medications**

+ More likely to receive health care services in **emergency rooms**

+ Fail to receive screenings, diagnoses and treatment for important medical problems. 22% of LGBT older adults do not reveal sexual orientation to physicians. In some states health care providers can decline to treat or provide certain necessary treatments to individuals based on their sexual orientation or gender identity.

+ Particularly distressed in nursing homes. One study indicates elderly LGBT adults face distress from potentially **hostile staff and fellow residents**, denial of visits from partners and family of choice, and refusal to allow same-sex partners to room together

Fig. 21.3 Graphic barriers to healthcare access

the basis of sexual orientation, including Atlanta, Chicago, Detroit, Miami, New York, Pittsburgh, and Seattle. While that status of the LGBT population is changing, anti-discrimination is by no means universal (Fig. 21.3).

> In terms of barriers to successful aging, why might the lesbian population be faced with different barriers than the gay male population? And what about the transgender population?

A Chilly Welcome?

Even given this newer trend toward LGBT positive aging, empirical data still indicate a fear among LGBT elders of aging into a long-term care environment. When one experiences decreasing voice and choice in the healthcare setting, concerns arise. And what about the relationship between direct care professionals and LGBT residents? According to the US Department of Labor and Human Services, direct care is a low-paying vocation. Personal Care Aides and Nursing Aides earn an average of $10.66/h or $21,320 annually based on a 2000 h year (Figs. 21.4, 21.5, 21.6, and 21.7).

According to the data, most direct care workers have limited education and lower household incomes. Women and immigrants are disproportionately represented among direct care workers, again according to the data. There is an increased prevalence of public assistance programs, and while we do not wish to engage in any stereotyping at all, we do need to evaluate external stressors and the ability to give good, person-centered care.

With these data, it is reasonable to assume increased stressors among direct care professionals. Lower income may mean that a second job is required. Less formal education may mean that lower levels of cultural competence may be expected. Research by Gendron et al. (2013) also underscores these findings. In a population of 158 direct care professionals, a majority represented a minority population, were female, and had a high school diploma or less.

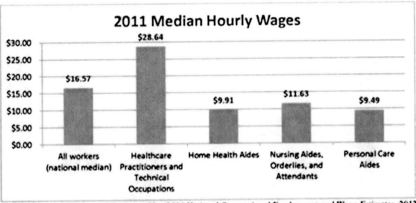

Fig. 21.4 Bureau of labor and statistics

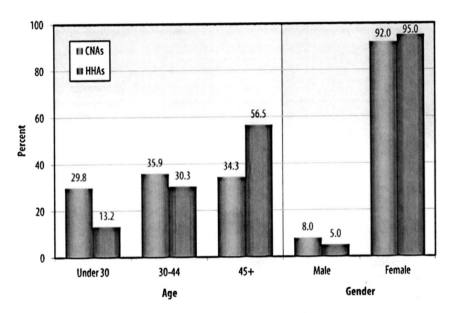

Fig. 21.5 Direct care workers have limited education and lower household incomes

The Unique Lens of Gender Identity, Gender Expression and Gender Classification

In addition to the social distance between direct care professionals and LGBT elders, there is the issue of the non-person-centered approach of integrating sexual orientation and gender identity. From the introduction of this chapter, we have defined sexual orientation and gender identity as two entirely different constructs. Lesbian, gay, and bisexual classification refers to sexual preference or attractions. A transgender classification entails gender identity, gender expression, or gender classification. Members of the transgender population are not necessarily gay or lesbian and, ironically, often face discrimination by members of the LGB population, in addition to the heterosexual population.

Transgender elders are both underserved and understudied in relation to their LGB

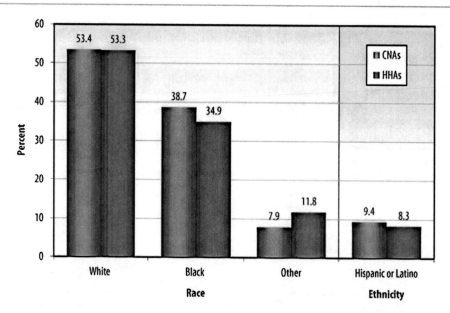

Fig. 21.6 Women and immigrants are disproportionately represented among direct care workers

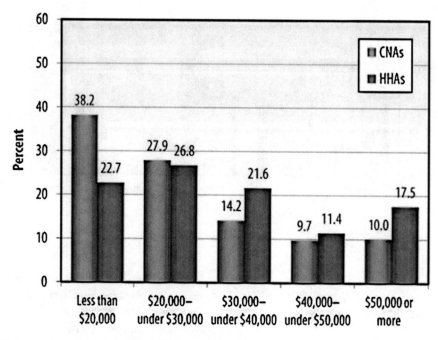

Fig. 21.7 Increased prevalence of public assistance programs

counterparts and most certainly in relation to heterosexual elders. According to Perrson (2009), the term transgender denotes a community of individuals whose biological sexual identity of birth is not always congruent with their manifested gender identity. Interestingly, though gender identity and sexual orientation are markedly different biological and psychological manifestations, aging may be seen as a unifier. Isolation, health issues, and personal finances are issues that universally challenge. The transgender population experiences these issues at heightened levels.

One of the most significant barriers to optimal aging that transgender elders face in the long-term care continuum is actual lack of knowledge by healthcare professionals. Transgender elders may present with characteristics of both their birth anatomy and transitional anatomy. They may have unique medication interactions. Unique healthcare screenings may be required based on an individual's biological sex, surgical status, declared gender, and hormonal therapies. There is significant anecdotal data from members of the transgender population of healthcare professionals refusing the treat "those people." This purposeful "othering" of transgender male and female elders further exacerbates social isolation and healthcare challenges associated with otherwise normal aging.

This "othering" of transgender individuals is also manifest in social supports. Like members of the LGB population, transgender individuals are often isolated from usual social support systems, such as parents, siblings, children, and spouses. Without identity with the homosexual or heterosexual community, many transgender elders face increased social isolation. While the increase in technological connectivity offers social supports via the World Wide Web, these supports are not adequate for direct care and socialization and may, ironically, perpetuate the physical isolation experienced by transgender elders.

Although great strides have been made over the last few years toward LGB rights, the transgender population continues to face institutional obstacles in employment, health care, and law enforcement.

Two West Virginia transgender women claim their recent DMV visits were especially harrowing as they attempted to update their names and change their driver's license photos. In separate incidents, both recount officials telling them their appearance looked too feminine for a driver's license issued to a male and that they would have to dress down for their photos. "(A manager) told me it was a DMV policy that people listed as male could not wear makeup," said Kristen Skinner. "The manager referred to me as "it" and told me to take off my makeup, wig and fake eyelashes." Skinner, whose hair and eyelashes were her own and not fake, eventually took the license photo after removing all facial makeup. The 45-year-old IT professional called the experience at the Charles Town office in Jefferson County on January 7 "humiliating." (**retrieved from** www.cnn.com)

According to the 2008 National Transgender Discrimination Survey, these heightened barriers to successful aging for transgender elders also translate into housing. Given the cost of aging into the long-term care continuum, incidences of homelessness persist among transgender elders. To combat this, in 2012, the US Department of Housing and Urban Development issued a proclamation making housing discrimination based on sexual orientation and gender identity illegal. The ruling also makes it possible for LGBT and T individuals and couples are included in HUD's definition of "family" and are, therefore, entitled to HUD's public housing and voucher programs.

Despite these advances, according to SAGE and the NCTE's 2012 report on improving policy and practice related to transgender elders, much more needs to be done. Long-term care administrators and public/private housing providers are not aware of the new protections for the transgender population; therefore, housing discrimination continues. As a result of amplified "othering" experienced by members of the transgender aging population, it is increasingly difficult to gather the personal, social, and financial resources necessary to combat housing discrimination across the long-term care continuum. This continues to be true even in the private sector, and even if adequate funding for long-term care is available.

Food for Thought: Discussion
Given the data, what are the implications for LGBT elders who age from community into a long-term care setting?

LGBT Older Adult Participants: Aging and Health Findings

▸ Nearly one-half have a disability and nearly one-third report depression.
▸ Most LGBT older adults (91%) engage in wellness activities.
▸ Almost two-thirds have been victimized three or more times.
▸ Thirteen percent have been denied healthcare or received inferior care.
▸ More than 20% do not disclose their sexual or gender identity to their physician.
▸ About one-third do not have a will or durable power of attorney for healthcare.
▸ Most needed services: senior housing, transportation, legal services, social events.

Fig. 21.8 Retrieved from www.caringandaging.org

New Trends in LGBT Aging

What is unique about the "Gen Silent" documentary is that it could have easily left the viewer with an image of the LGBT elder as defeated. Maggie Kuhn, founder of the Gray Panthers, referred to this as the "Detroit Syndrome" in the following passage:

> Only the newest model is desirable. The old are condemned to obsolescence; left to rot like wrinkled babies in glorified playpens – force to succumb to a trivial, purposeless waste of their years and their time. (Maggie Kuhn in Sheppard, 1982).

Instead, the viewer is left feeling inspired. Each story shows how, when faced with adversity, LGBT elders are able to recalibrate, refocus, and plot a new course for optimal aging. There are bittersweet moments, indeed. However, the viewer is left with the more contemporary vision of LGBT elders aging well, despite disparities. This is no way implies that the barriers to optimal aging for LGBT elders are not real. It simply showcases that in the face of adversity, LGBT elders can thrive.

According to the American Society on Aging (2014), LGBT elders display remarkable resilience, despite the many obstacles they face. Despite increased levels of poor general health, physical limitations, and mental distress as compared to heterosexuals, LGBT elders are remaining connected throughout the life span. The Caring and Aging with Pride study (2011) of 2,560 LGBT elders ages 50 to 95 finds an emerging cohort of positive aging. While the information is presented in a largely negative

manner, it supports the emerging notion. Read differently, the following graphic from the Caring and Aging with Pride study showcases that, two-thirds do not report depression, most engage in wellness activities, 90 % have received some form of healthcare, 80 % do disclose sexual orientation or gender identity to medical professionals, etc. This is not meant to undermine the absolute need for more culturally competent care for LGBT elders, rather it showcases an emerging trend toward positive aging. Continuing this path to improvement, especially in long-term care, is of paramount importance (Fig. 21.8).

How to Level the Playing Field?

According to a 2005 survey in the *Journal of Homosexuality*, diversity trainings for healthcare professionals, diversity trainings for long-term care residents, and the development of LGBT and LGBT-friendly retirement/care facilities would serve as the best remedies for discrimination. Ninety-three (93 %) of respondents believed that diversity/sensitivity trainings for staff would be of value, while 83 % felt that similar trainings would be of value for fellow residents. Nearly all (98 %) of respondents indicated that LGBT or LGBT-friendly facilities would be well-received.

In the last decade, we have seen a rise in the number of diversity and sensitivity training offered, as well as an increase in the number of LGBT-friendly communities. New communities that cater to the aging LGBT population have opened in California, New Mexico, Massachusetts, and the Blue Ridge Mountains of North Carolina. Federal Fair Housing law dictates that residential communities cannot exclude the heterosexual or non-transgender population but must be open and welcoming to all.

According to Gendron et al. (2013), in a mixed method study of 158 eldercare professionals who participated in an LGBT cultural competence training, 97 % expressed knowledge gain and positive feelings about participating in the training. Even with this professed knowledge gain and the growing resources for LGBT cultural competence training, the literature tells us that more needs to be done, particularly toward understanding the unique differences between sexual orientation and gender identity. Although the data absolutely support significant barriers to optimal aging throughout the care continuum, currents are changing, and LGBT elders are becoming increasingly engaged and self-advocating. Progress will continue with the assistance of social and policy advocates as issues of social isolation and support connectivity and engagement are addressed.,

Keys Facts in Social Isolation (adapted from SAGE)

> Social Isolation is a universal risk for all aging elders.
> Living alone is the predominant risk for social isolation and disproportionately affects LGBT elders.
> LGBT elders may face increased levels of social isolation due to disability, economic security, and mental health concerns.
> LGBT caregivers are also at risk for increased social isolation.
> Major life transitions, such as the death of a loved one or unemployment, may also impact social isolation disproportionately among the LGBT population.
> Aging in a rural environment, compounded with stigma and discrimination, may also impact social isolation.

Policy and Advocacy Solutions (adapted from *Improving the Lives of LGBT Older Adults, 2010*)

> Pass non-discrimination policies or ordinances at the state or local level. Increase awareness or enforcement of existing non-discrimination policies.
> Encourage service providers to adopt their own non-discrimination policies and actively promote them.
> Examine state laws on public health, nursing homes, assisted living facilities, and home care agencies for opportunities to support LGBT elders.
> Develop evidence-based, person-centered, and accessible cultural competency trainings to reach large number of healthcare professionals.
> Work with accrediting healthcare agencies, such as the National Board of Long-term Care Administrators, to develop standards for working with LGBT elders.
> Advocate for better training and support of states' long-term care ombudspeople.
> Seek to reinforce protections for LGBT elders under the federal Nursing Home Reform Act
> Work with US Department of Housing and Urban Development to create regulations that require nursing homes and assisted living facilities to allow same-gender couples and families of choice to share rooms.

Profile in LGBT in LGBT Leadership: Guy M. Kinman, Jr

Optimal aging for LGBT elders is easier said than done. It is important to evaluate case studies and anecdotal information for best practices for approaching optimal aging in the long-term care continuum for LGBT elders.

As of this writing, Guy M. Kinman, Jr., is 96 years old. He is currently a resident of Imperial Plaza, an assisted living facility in Richmond, Virginia's Bellevue community. After nearly thirty years of activity in Richmond's LGBT community, Guy is receiving a good deal of praise and attention for his early civil rights efforts. What is inspiring about Guy's message is that even though he recognizes that "and end" to life is real, this deadline has offered him the courage to be what he always wanted to be. He realizes that you often you cannot do everything, but you can focus on enough to find happiness. Guy is inspired by the Chinese philosophy that the definition of wisdom is knowing "what is enough."

Enough, however, continues to be a daily motivator for Guy. Enough is finding the things that "turn you on" and bring out the best in you, even given limited faculties, limited space, or limited time. Enough, today, for Guy is the election of the nation's first African-American president and even the opportunity to look beyond his approaching ninety-seventh birthday to offer praise and feedback for next year's Gay Pride Celebration in Richmond. Enough, for Guy Malcolm Kinman, Jr., is acquired through an outlook and ethic that has developed over a lifetime that matured and flourished over the last three decades, and continues to grow with each passing day. This wisdom will proliferate through Guy's informational and financial generosity with numerous charitable organizations as well as the Guy Kinman Research Award through the Virginia Historical Society and the Gay Community Center of Richmond. This legacy will allow subsequent generations the opportunity to learn from what has come before them to help construct their authentic self and, in doing so, to shine.

Guy was married for a number of years and did not come out as a gay man until his 60 s in the early 1980s. At this time of social conservatism where the Moral Majority and Christian Coalition were significant cultural players, Guy organized a billboard campaign in Richmond, Virginia.

By 1985, Guy had been retired for three years. He believed he had nothing to lose anymore by being "out." He felt his gay friends' fears and wish for them the freedom they deserved and the confidence he enjoyed. The mid-1980s were a time when the Moral Majority, headed by the Reverend Jerry Falwell, was at the high of its popularity. The LGBT community in Lynchburg and Roanoke were attempting to launch an educational campaign on billboards that read "Someone You Know Is Gay. Maybe Someone You Love." As president of the Richmond Virginia Gay and Lesbian Alliance, Guy spearheaded the fundraising efforts to erect 11 of these billboards throughout the Richmond region. The campaign launched in December of 1985 and provided Guy a vehicle to use his masterful sales and networking skills to raise the funds necessary to fund the project, as well as serve as spokesperson for the Richmond Virginia Gay and Lesbian Alliance on numerous occasions (Fig. 21.9).

Guy offers tribute to many of his colleagues in the development of The Billboard Program. In a

Fig. 21.9 Billboard from the 1985 Billboard Campaign in Richmond, Virginia

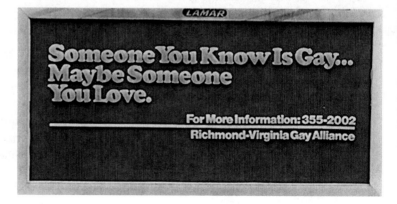

time when attitudes toward the LGBT community were predominantly negative and many members of the minority population were fleeing to larger cities, Guy worked with others to develop The Billboard Campaign to show not only the heterosexual community, but also the LGBT population in Richmond that there was hope for better treatment and a more positive attitude. The project offered a voice to those who felt like they were without one and helped Guy also develop his very loud, very clear, voice in order to shout, yet in a peaceful way. The Billboard Project was, for Guy, his golden opportunity to make his voice heard.

Guy was, and is, not bashful about speaking with the media and public with regard to The Billboard Project and on issues of LGBT civil rights in the years following. He and others orchestrated a meeting with the Richmond City Council to request that sexual orientation be added to the City's non-discrimination policy. Guy recalls that at the time, many of the people who attended this meeting at City Hall were afraid to have their faces shown on television. As a result, the media shot images of the feet of those in attendance to showcase the numbers as well as shooting the elected representative who was speaking the City Council from his back. Guy offers praise to those who were willing to even attend this meeting at a time when many felt like there would be a backlash if they were identified as LGBT.

In addition to television media, the Richmond print media would also offer a more narrow focus of the LGBT population. Guy took the initiative to contact a columnist with the Richmond Times-Dispatch who had written what Guy perceived as a very one-sided article. Guy met with the columnist and expressed his negative opinion with him. This act "impressed the hell" out of Guy's friends.

Another instance was when a representative of the American Legion made a derogatory remark about gays and lesbians. Guy took the initiative to contact the local NBC affiliate and orchestrated a debate between himself and the President of the American Legion. Though "terrified" at the prospect of the debate, Guy felt compelled to be interviewed and to have his voice heard on behalf of a community which had little voice at that time. While Guy credits himself with being a spokesperson for the LGBT movement in Richmond at that time, he also credits many other people who assisted in their own ways and within their own spheres of comfort and influence.

In addition to the media, Guy also felt compelled to reach out to the Richmond Police Department after the murder of two gay men. After returning from a visit to Washington, DC, Guy again sprang to action. Together with Tony Segura, one of Guy's heroes and founder of the Mattachine Society in New York, Guy made an appointment with a representative of the Police Department to express concerns that the investigation into the murders might be compromised because of the victims' sexuality. The media were present at the event in the meeting with the Richmond Sergeant, who offered equal protection of the law to members of the LGBT community in Richmond, a powerful message at a time when many did not feel that law enforcement was on their side.

Today, Guy continues to be an advocate for the LGBT movement in Richmond. As a resident of Imperial Plaza, guy is well-known as a gay activist. He has taken his former fear of discrimination and taken to the pulpit, pen, and public with his pro-gay message. He is a unique example of how LGBT elders are able to adapt to adversity and capitalize of innate strengths and environmental opportunities.

1. What unique characteristics does Guy Kinman have in order to adapt and succeed in what would have been a hostile and changing environment?
2. Are these characteristics and assets universal to members of the LGBT community?

Critical Resources and Philosophies

Two critical philosophies are emerging in contemporary research and scholarship of sexual orientation, gender identity, and aging. It is important for readers to note the emerging scholarship that supports positive aging and resilience, even in the face of adversity. It is equally important for readers to note the absolute difference between sexual orientation and gender identity and to approach the LGB and T lens with the steadfast philosophy that members of the transgender population are not necessarily gay, lesbian, or bisexual.

As students and scholars continue to research barriers to optimal aging for the LGB and T population, there are several resources that are critical to gathering evidence-based information. **Services and Advocacy for GLBT Elders (SAGE)** is the country's largest and oldest organization dedicated to improving the lives of lesbian, gay, bisexual, and transgender (LGBT) older adults. Our mission is to lead in addressing issues related to lesbian, gay, bisexual, and transgender (LGBT) aging. More information is located at www.sageusa.org.

In addition to these national organizations, several documentaries are useful teaching tools and sources for case studies and anecdotal data. As previously mentioned, the documentary **"Gen Silent"** (www.gensilent.org) follows stories of LGBT elders and their concerns about having to go back into the closet in order to survive the long-term care continuum. The VCU Department of Gerontology has developed, in conjunction with the director of "Gen Silent" and the LGBT Aging Project, a teaching tool titled **"A Caring Response: Giving Care to LGBT Elders."** Together, the documentary and curriculum are go-to resources for information on LGBT elders and the long-term care continuum.

Two additional documentaries serve as solid teaching and educational tools. **"Ten More Good Years"** and **"Beauty Before Age: Growing Older in Gay Culture"** offer a glimpse into the lives of LGBT aging and identity. The former resource offers viewers an idea of how socioeconomic status, sexual orientation, and gender identity impact the other. The latter gives viewers insight into the value that gay men often place on youth and attractiveness. It informs on how aging and isolation be of even greater concern.

The Service-Delivery Team

The long-term care continuum is a complex system that involves multiple disciplines of healthcare professionals, particularly as we look through the holistic gerontological lens. The VCU School of Allied Health Professions introduced a program some years back titled **"Grand Rounds"** that evaluated the care of an individual from this holistic perspective of Allied Health Professions. This model for interprofessional collaboration generated a truly holistic view of all disciplines that impact service delivery.

While gerontology looks at aging in its entirety, it is possible to focus on disciplines including rehabilitation counseling, occupational therapy, physical therapy, patient counseling, and social work to support LGB and T elders in their optimal aging. The challenge is creating a cohesive network of healthcare management for each LGB and T elder where treatments are comprehensively managed.

In addition to the allied health professions, it is important to look at a combination of Departments of Social Services, nonprofit organizations, and the faith-based community to support person-centered service delivery for LGB and T elders. According to the National Resource Center on LGBT and Aging, several states have initiated trainings to support positive aging for LGBT elders. In New York City, Jewish Home Life Care and Hebrew Home at Riverdale have engaged in trainings of their direct care professionals working with LGBT older adults. Wisconsin's Agency on Aging Resources and Aging and Disability Resource Center has also engaged in comparable cultural competence and awareness building trainings.

In Virginia, all assisted living and adult day centers are regulated by the Virginia Department of Social Services and are bound to specific regulations are care requirements. In addition to the Virginia Department of Social Services, we can look at the Virginia Department for Aging and Rehabilitative Services (DARS) and Area Agencies on Aging. Programs such as "No Wrong Door" support all elders regardless of sexual orientation or gender identity. Outside of the formal care continuum, we can look at non-profit organizations and the faith community for both formal and informal assistance and a more person-centered approach to care.

Summary and Opportunities for Future Research

In sum, we have reviewed barriers to, and opportunities for, successful aging in the LGB and T population. In many instances, the picture is not pretty. Discrimination is still rampant among lesbian, gay, bisexual, and transgender elders even in light of recent political and social progress. The plight for transgender elders is even more challenging, as we have identified increased barriers to inclusion and obstacles for this cohort. A long history of "othering" and stigmatization by the dominant hegemony has resulted in biological, psychological, sociological, and spiritual disenfranchisement. Othering, in short, creates "us versus them" relationship where a dominant group perceives and promoted another group as unequal or alien. Othering is antithetical to a gerontological and person-centered care model and is just one of many barriers experienced by LBG and T elders.

In addition to the social phenomenon of othering, equal access to formal and informal healthcare services and residential options for LGB and T elders is also evident. LGB and T elders are more likely to be single, less likely to have children, and more likely to be disconnected from family of origin. This phenomenon creates additional barriers to successful aging, especially in more structured and formal care environments, such as assisted living, skilled nursing, and hospice.

The message from emerging scholarship and personal accounts is equally clear. Many LGB and T elders are either "surviving and thriving" or "working at it" (VanWegenen et al. 2012, p. 1). They are delving into personal resources and networks to overcome and surpass barriers to successful aging, even in light of barriers.

So, where do we go from here? In keeping with the gerontological lens of optimal aging and person-centered care, it is important to understand that more studies are needed. Richer data are needed from more diverse portions of the LGB and T population. We need to engage isolated elders from rural areas. We need to engage elders who may not be involved in national organizations. And we need to understand that there are nearly 8,000,000 LGB and T elders right now who may one day be candidates for the long-term care continuum. We need to ask them about their preferences for care. We need to train direct care professionals in cultural competence and person-centered care. And we need to pay close attention to not creating a long-term care environment where "one size fits all."

Learning Exercise: Conducting an Equity Audit (adapted from Sklra et al. 2009 and *Gay and Gray: Welcoming LGBT Elders in Long-Term Care*)
If you are an administrator for a long-term care facility, how would you ensure a supportive environment for LGB and T elders? Consider using the following questions to inform your initial inquiry. Please circle 1 for No, 2 for Rarely, 3 for Not Sure, 4 for Often, and 5 for Always.

Am I aware of members of the LGBT population residing in my longterm care facility?

1 2 3 4 5

Is it possible to immediately identify a member of the LGBT population?

1 2 3 4 5

Does my facility honor residents' sexual orientation, gender identity, and racial, ethnic, and cultural heritage?

1 2 3 4 5

Do you have the ability to ask residents about their sexual orientation or gender identity in a safe and confidential manner?

1 2 3 4 5

Does your facility have special protocol or operating procedures for working with members of the LGBT population?

1 2 3 4 5

Is your facility's marketing material inclusive of sexual orientation and gender identity?

1 2 3 4 5

Does your facility offer special training for healthcare professionals for working with LGBT elders?

1 2 3 4 5

Score:
7–14: Indicates minimal LGBT equity consciousness
15–21: Indicates somewhat developed equity consciousness
22–29: Indicates well-developed equity consciousness
30–35: Indicates a highly developed equity consciousness

Call to Equitable Action: How will you engage in supporting LGBT equity throughout the long-term care continuum? Conduct a 3-min elevator speech to deliver to classmates and colleagues on barriers to inclusion for LBG and T elders and your specific action plan for addressing these issues in your community.

Learning Exercises for Knowledge Gain

1. Please identify 5 barriers for LGBT inclusion in the long-term care continuum.
   (Looking for fear of discrimination by direct care professionals, fear of discrimination by other elders, lack of a formal/family caregiver infrastructure to facilitate the transition from community to the long-term care continuum, and financial barriers.)
2. Please offer your definition of the difference between sexual orientation and gender identity.
   (Looking for sexual orientation being an individual's sexual attraction preference and gender identity being how an individual perceives his or her own gender, regardless of expression.)
3. Please identify 5 different care environments in the long-term care continuum.
   (Looking for independent living, adult day/senior centers, assisted living, skilled nursing facilities, and hospice).
4. What is ageism and how is it particularly prevalent among gay men?
   (Looking for ageism as discrimination or stereotyping based on age or perceived age. This is particularly prevalent among gay men in that youth and physical appearance are often revered and especially honored by gay men across the life span).

5. Despite the barriers to inclusion, please offer opportunities for members of the LGBT population to thrive in the long-term care continuum.
   (Looking for 80/20, socioemotional selectivity, and selective optimization with compensation. Also specific examples from the Guy Kinman case study.)

6. Why might direct care professionals benefit from training and education about minority or disenfranchised populations?
   (Looking for direct care professionals often having less of an educational background and being undercompensated with fewer incentives to provide person-centered, culturally competent care. They may have never been exposed to members of the LGBT population and be less aware of their unique care needs).

7. Please define gerontology and how the gerontological lens can be supportive of optimal aging for LGBT elders.
   (Looking for the definition of gerontology as the holistic (biological, psychological, sociological, and spiritual, study of aging. The gerontological lens allows more than just one view of the aging elder. It looks at mind, body, spirit, social connections, and more, to arrive at a more thorough diagnosis. It is also supports empowering elders rather than portraying them in a diminished capacity).

Multiple-Choice Questions

1. According to the National Gay and Lesbian Task Force there are currently __ LGBT elder Americans.
   (a) 1,500,000
   (b) 3,000,000
   (c) 250,000
   (d) 750,000
   (Answer: a)

2. The number of LGBT elder Americans is expected to increase to ____ by 2030.
   (a) 1,500,000
   (b) 750,000
   (c) 3,500,000
   (d) 6,000,000
   (Answer: c)

3. An holistic approach to optimal aging employs:
   (a) Biological, psychological, sociological, and spiritual aging
   (b) Only spiritual aging
   (c) Only psychological aging
   (d) Aging without dementia
   (Answer: a)

4. The elements of the long-term care continuum include:
   (a) Independent living and skilled nursing facilities
   (b) Independent living, skilled nursing facilities, and hospice
   (c) Independent living only
   (d) Independent living, adult day facilities, assisted living, skilled nursing facilities, and hospice
   (Answer: d)

5. A person-centered care philosophy is grounded in an individual's:
   (a) Dependence on others
   (b) Menu items of living choices
   (c) Choice, dignity, respect, self-determination, and purposeful living
   (d) None of the above
   (Answer: c)

6. Until ____, the American Psychological Association classified homosexuality as a deviant, pathological condition.
   (a) 1964
   (b) 1974
   (c) 1984
   (d) 1994
   (Answer: b)

7. The Caring and Aging with Pride Study (2011) states that ___ % of LGBT elders report being victimized.
   (a) 52 %
   (b) 62 %
   (c) 72 %

(d) 82 %

(Answer: d)

8. Elements of the direct care professional demographics include:
(a) Limited education
(b) More women and racial/ethnic minorities
(c) Higher use of public assistance programs
(d) All of the above

(Answer: d)

9. ___% of LGBT elders report engaging in a health and wellness activity
(a) 20 %
(b) 50 %
(c) 75 %
(d) 90 %

(Answer: d)

10. According to the literature, a universal risk for all elders, regardless of sexual orientation or gender identity is:
(a) Social isolation
(b) Financial concerns
(c) Premature death
(d) Elder abuse

(Answer: a)

Resources

AARP

American Association of Retired Persons is a nonprofit, nonpartisan organization, with a membership of more than 37 million, that helps people turn their goals and dreams into real possibilities, strengthens communities, and fights for the issues that matter most to families such as healthcare, employment security, and retirement planning. We advocate for consumers in the marketplace by selecting products and services of high quality and value to carry the AARP name as well as help our members obtain discounts on a wide range of products, travel, and services.

Web site: http://www.aarp.org/

Additional resources:

http://www.aarp.org/relationships/friends-family/aarp-pride.html?intcmp=AE-SEARCH-AARPSUGG-LGBT

http://www.aarp.org/politics-society/rights/info-06-2009/more_lgtb_resources_from_aarp.html

http://www.aarp.org/politics-society/rights/info-06-2009/lgbt_glossary.html

http://www.aarp.org/politics-society/rights/info-06-2009/wisdom_of_the_elders_aarp_and_sage.html

http://www.aarp.org/politics-society/rights/info-03-2010/marriage_and_gay_rights.html

http://www.aarp.org/relationships/love-sex/info-02-2008/aids_prevention_for_50plus_pushed.html

AIDS Community Research Initiative of America (ACRIA)

ACRIA is the first-ever activist, community-based approach to the study of new treatments for HIV. ACRIA studies the lives and needs of people with or at risk for HIV through its Behavioral Research Program; offers critical HIV healthcare education to HIV-positive people and their caregivers all around the world through its HIV Health Literacy Program; and provides a variety of consulting services (technical assistance, monitoring and evaluation, curriculum development, and Web-based learning among them) to strengthen AIDS and other service organizations across the country, enabling those groups to better serve their own clients. Additionally, through the ACRIA Center on HIV and Aging, the organization is recognized as an international authority on the emerging issue of older adults and HIV.

Web site: http://www.acria.org/

Additional resources: https://www.dropbox.com/s/eablp1lb1y6eyqh/Policy%20Recommendations%20Older%20Adults%20with%20HIV.pdf

American Society on Aging

The American Society on Aging is an association of diverse individuals bound by a common goal: to support the commitment and enhance the knowledge and skills of those who seek to improve the quality of life of older adults and their families. The membership of ASA is multidisciplinary and inclusive of professionals who are concerned with the physical, emotional, social, economic, and spiritual aspects of aging.

Web site: http://www.asaging.org/

Additional resources:

http://www.asaging.org/lain

http://www.asaging.org/national-resource-center-lgbt-aging-sage

FORGE Transgender Aging Network

The Transgender Aging Network (TAN) exists to improve the lives of current and future trans/SOFFA (significant others, friends, family, and allies) elders by the following: identifying, promoting communication among, and enhancing the work of researchers, service providers, educators, advocates, elders, and others who are interested in trans/SOFFA aging issues; promoting awareness of concerns, issues, and realities; advocating for policy changes in public and private institutions, services, organizations, programs, etc.; and providing communication channels through which trans/SOFFA elders can give and receive support and information.

Web site: http://forge-forward.org/aging/

Additional Resources:

http://www.lgbtagingcenter.org/

http://www.grayprideparade.com/

Gay Men's Health Crisis (GMHC)

GMHC is the world's first and leading provider of HIV/AIDS prevention, care, and advocacy. Building on decades of dedication and expertise, we understand the reality of HIV/AIDS and empower a healthy life for all. GMHC's mission is to fight to end the AIDS epidemic and uplift the lives of all affected.

Web site: http://www.gmhc.org/

Additional resources:

http://www.gmhc.org/about-us/links

http://www.gmhc.org/blog

The Graying of AIDS

The Graying of AIDS combines portraits and oral histories of both long-term survivors and older adults who contracted HIV later in life with HIV/AIDS information to increase awareness,

sensitivity, and collaboration among caregiving professionals.

Web site: http://www.grayingofaids.org/

Additional resources:

http://www.grayingofaids.org/modes-of-transmission/

http://www.grayingofaids.org/glossary/

http://www.grayingofaids.org/resource-links/

http://www.grayingofaids.org/training-materials/

Lambda Legal

Lambda Legal is the oldest and largest national legal organization whose mission is to achieve full recognition of the civil rights of **lesbians, gay men, bisexuals, transgender people,** and those with **HIV,** through impact litigation, education, and public policy work. As a nonprofit organization, we do not charge our clients for legal representation or advocacy, and we receive no government funding. We depend on contributions from supporters around the country.

Web site: http://www.lambdalegal.org/

Additional resources:

http://www.lambdalegal.org/know-your-rights

http://www.lambdalegal.org/states-regions

http://www.lambdalegal.org/help

http://www.lambdalegal.org/publications/all

http://www.lambdalegal.org/our-work

The LGBT Aging Project/Third Sector New England

A nonprofit organization dedicated to ensuring that lesbian, gay, bisexual, and transgender older adults have equal access to the life-prolonging benefits, protections, services, and institutions that their heterosexual neighbors take for granted.

Web site: http://www.lgbtagingproject.org/

Additional resources:

http://www.lgbtagingproject.org/resources-for-lgbt-seniors/

Medicare Rights Center

The Medicare Rights Center is a national, nonprofit consumer service organization that works to ensure access to affordable health care for older adults and people with disabilities through counseling and advocacy, educational programs, and public policy initiatives.

Web site: http://www.medicarerights.org/

Additional resources:

http://www.medicarerights.org/resources/additional-resources/

http://www.medicarerights.org/resources/consumer-fact-sheets/

http://www.medicarerights.org/resources/newsletters/medicare-watch/archive/6-26-14/

National Association of Area Agencies on Aging (N4A)

The **National Association of Area Agencies on Aging** (N4A) is the leading voice on aging issues for Area Agencies on Aging and a champion for Title VI Native American aging programs. Through advocacy, training, and technical assistance, we support the national network of 618 AAAs and 246 Title VI programs. We **advocate** on behalf of our member agencies for services and resources for older adults and persons with disabilities.

Web site: http://www.n4a.org/

Additional resources:

http://www.n4a.org/programs/resources-lgbt-elders/

http://www.n4a.org/files/programs/resources-lgbt-elders/InclusiveServicesGuide2012.pdf

http://www.n4a.org/pdf/ReadyToServe1.pdf

http://www.n4a.org/files/programs/resources-lgbt-elders/newTransClientFactSheet.pdf

National Caucus & Center on Black Aged

NCBA is a 501(c) (3) not-for-profit organization dedicated to preserving the dignity and enhancing the lives of low-income elderly African-Americans. As one of the largest minority focused organizations in the USA, NCBA addresses the needs of its constituency in the areas of health, affordable housing, and employment. NCBA works to facilitate the sharing of resources, information, and experience across a spectrum of policymakers, legislators, advocacy, and service organizations to address the issues that impact the quality of life for America's elderly minority population.

Web site: http://users.erols.com/ncba/

Additional resources:

http://www.ncba-aged.org/Resources.php

National Center for Transgender Equality

The National Center for Transgender Equality is a national social justice organization devoted to ending discrimination and violence against transgender people through education and advocacy on national issues of importance to transgender people. By empowering transgender people and our allies to educate and influence policymakers and others, NCTE facilitates a strong and clear voice for transgender equality in our nation's capital and around the country.

Web site: http://transequality.org/

Additional resources:

http://transequality.org/Resources/index.html

http://transequality.org/Resources/links.html

National Senior Citizens Law Center

This center espouses that poor seniors have a right quality health care, long-term services, and supports and that all seniors have a right to enough income to meet their basic needs. We advocate at the administrative and legislative levels to ensure that laws and regulations work for poor seniors. We train over 10,000 advocates and service providers on the rights of poor seniors every year. We litigate as necessary to ensure poor seniors have the benefits and services they need.

Web site: http://www.nsclc.org/

Additional resources:

http://www.nsclc.org/index.php/tag/lgbt/

The National Gay and Lesbian Task Force

The mission of the **National Gay and Lesbian Task Force** is to build the power of the lesbian, gay, bisexual, and transgender (LGBT) community from the ground up. We do this by training activists, organizing broad-based campaigns to defeat anti-LGBT referenda and advance pro-LGBT legislation, and building the organizational capacity of our movement. Our Policy Institute, the movement's premier think tank, provides research and policy analysis to support the struggle for complete equality and to counter right-wing lies. As part of a broader social justice movement, we work to create a nation that respects the diversity of human expression and identity and creates opportunity for all.

Web site: http://www.thetaskforce.org/

Additional resources:

http://www.thetaskforce.org/issues

http://www.thetaskforce.org/reports_and_research

References

Addis, S., Davies, M., Greene, G., MacBride-Stewart, S., & Shepherd, M. (2009). The health, social care and housing needs of lesbian, gay, bisexual and transgender older people. *Health and Social Care in the Community, 17*(6), 647–658.

Auldridge, A., Tamar-Mattis, A., Kennedy, S., Ames, E., & Tobin, H. (2012). *Improving the lives of transgender older adults.* Services and advocacy for glbt elders and the national center for transgender equality.

Alzheimer's Association of New York City. (2012). *Gay and gray: Welcoming LGBT elders in long term care.* May/June 2012.

Berger, R. M., & Kelly, J. J. (1996). Gay men and lesbians grown older. In R. P. Cabaj & T. S. Stein (Eds.), *Textbook of homosexuality and mental health* (pp. 305–316). Washington, DC: American Psychiatric Press.

Fredriksen-Goldsen, K. I., Kim, H.-J., Emlet, C. A., Muraco, A., Erosheva, E. A., Hoy-Ellis, C. P., et al. (2011). *The aging and health report: Disparities and resilience among lesbian, gay, bisexual, and transgender older adults.* Seattle: Institute for Multigenerational Health.

Gendron, T., Maddux, S., Krinsky, L., White, J., Lockeman, K., Metcalfe, Y., & Aggarwal, S. (2013). Cultural competence training for healthcare professionals working with LGBT older adults. *Educational Gerontology, 39*(6).

Grant, J., Mottet, L., Tanis, J., Harrison, J., Herman, J., & Keisling, M. (2011). *Injustice at every turn: A report of the national transgender discrimination survey.* Washington: National Center for Transgender Equality and National Gay and Lesbian Task Force.

Hughes, C., & Evans, A. (2003). Health needs of women who have sex with women. *BMJ, 327*(7421), 939–940.

Johnson, M., Jackson, N., Arnette, J., & Koffman, S. (2005). Gay and Lesbian perceptions of discrimination in retirement care facilities. *Journal of Homosexuality, 49*(2), 83–102.

McKenzie, K., & Skrla, L. (2011). *Using equity audits in the classroom to reach and teach all students.* Corwin: Thousand Oaks.

National Center for Transgender Equality. (March 2012). *Know your rights: Fair housing and transgender people.* Retrieved from www.transeqaulity.org.

National Resource Center on LGBT Aging. (2012). *A self-help guide for LGBT older adults and their caregivers and loved ones: Preventing, recognizing, and addressing elder abuse.* Retrieved from http://www.lgbtagingcenter.org/resources/pdfs/SELF-HELP_elderAbuse_Guide.pdf.

Pantell, M., Rehkopf, D., Jutte, D., Syme, S., Balmes, J., & Adler, N. (2013). Social isolation: A predictor of mortality comparable to traditional clinical risk factors. *American Journal of Public Health, 103*(11), 2056–2062.

Perrson, D. (2009). Unique challenges of transgender aging: Implications from the literature. *Journal of Gerontological Social Work, 52*, 633–646.

Quam, J. K., & Whitford, Gary S. (1992). Educational needs of nursing home social workers at the baccalaureate level. *Journal of Gerontological Social Work, 18*(3/4), 143–156.

The Equal Rights Center. (2014). *Opening doors: An investigation of barriers to senior housing for same-sex couples.* Retrieved from http://www.equalrightscenter.org/site/DocServer/Senior_Housing_Report.pdf?docID=2361.

VanWegenenn, A., Driskell, D., & Bradford, B. (2012). I'm still raring to go: Successful aging among lesbian, gay, bisexual, and transgender older adults. *Journal of Aging Studies, 27*, 1–14.

David Godfrey

Abstract

This chapter explores the end-of-life issues and what makes end-of-life issues different for LGBT adults. The laws and policies relating to end-of-life have many presumptions that favor family, specifically biological or adoptive family and family from marriage. These presumptions impact health care decision-making, visitation policies, health insurance, health benefits, retirement plans, taxation, and inheritance rules. The expansion of same-sex marriage is changing this picture, but a great deal of work remains to be done. Societal homophobia impacts access to care, relationship recognition, and even funeral planning. Ageism is common in some parts of the LGBT community, casting a shadow over many LGBT elders. Many of the current generation of LGBT elders survived the darkest days of AIDS and HIV, and this experience influences their views on aging and end-of-life.

Keywords

Ageism · Presumptions · Incapacity · Inheritance · Surrogate

Overview

This chapter will explore how personal relationships and family structure impact LGBT elders and end-of-life decisions. The chapter will examine how legal presumptions and bias in laws and standard protocol favoring marital and biological family impact LGBT elders. The chapter will review the basics of planning for incapacity health care decision-making and inheritance and how LGBT elders may need to plan ahead for the outcome they desire. Homophobia is still a factor in our society and is ageism can be especially virulent in the LGBT community. All of these factors influence later life and dying for LGBT elders.

D. Godfrey (✉)
American Bar Association, Chicago, IL, USA
e-mail: david.godfrey@americanbar.org

© Springer International Publishing Switzerland 2016
D.A. Harley and P.B. Teaster (eds.), *Handbook of LGBT Elders*,
DOI 10.1007/978-3-319-03623-6_22

Learning Objectives

1. Readers will develop an understanding of how family structure and possible estrangement from with biological family impact end-of-life for LGBT elders.
2. Understand how legal presumptions and bias in laws and standard protocols impact end-of-life issues for LGBT elders.
3. Articulate how the generation that survived the early years of HIV/AIDS is impacted by that experience.
4. Identify the basic tools for planning for incapacity and estate planning and why completing them is especially important for LGBT elders.
5. Identify ways that homophobia and ageism impact LGBT elders.
6. Understand the change that growing access to same-sex marriage will have on end-of-life for LGBT elders.

Introduction

The purpose of this chapter is to highlight the factors that make end-of-life issues different for LGBT adults. Many factors, including laws, social norms, and cultural values, impact how people live and the decisions they make near the end-of-life. Our personal beliefs and values, our interaction with loved ones and community, social and cultural expectations, and laws, all impact our ability to live and die as we choose. Everyone is going to die, and volumes are written every year about later life, dying, and death. The majority of the writing focuses on heterosexual families; however, this chapter will focus on what sets these issues apart for LGBT adults. LGBT elders are less likely to have children, more likely to be estranged from families of origin, less likely to have marital family (a spouse and in-laws), less likely to fully self-disclose to health care providers, likely to have experienced the death of a large number of contemporaries at a young age, and working in a legal system that favors via preemptions and assumptions martial and

biological family. Clearly, each of these situations can produce adverse outcomes for LGBT elders at the end-of-life.

Health Care

End-of-life health care issues for LGBT adults gained national attention in 2007 with the ordeal of Janice Langbehn and Lisa Pond. During the winter of 2007, Janice, Lisa, and their four children traveled from the state of Washington to Miami, Florida, to take a Caribbean cruise. Shortly before boarding, Lisa suffered a brain aneurysm and was rushed to a local hospital. Despite offering to fax a living will and durable power of attorney for health care, Janice was not allowed to make health care decisions or visit with Lisa for hours. Janice and the children were isolated from Lisa as her condition worsened and she was moved to intensive care. A hospital social worker told Janice that she was "in an anti-gay city and state." Janice and the children were not allowed to see Lisa until Lisa's sister arrived just minutes before Lisa died (McCorquodale 2013.) The saga made the national news when Lambda Legal sued the hospital. As part of a settlement, the hospital agreed to change policies and train staff to be more responsive to LGBT families (Legal 2008).

In April 2010, President Obama issued a memo directing the Department of Health and Human Services to take steps to assure health care decision-making and hospital visitation by LGBT families (The White House 2010, April 15). Fifteen months later, HHS released new regulations directing health care facilities that receive any federal funding (virtually all do by treating Medicare or Medicaid patients) to create new policies that include informing LGBT patients of their right to designate visitors and to not discriminate based on gender identity or sexual orientation (Legal 2008). As of 2013, only 26 states have addressed the issue of hospital visitation by statute, leaving this important issue up to individual facility policy in nearly half of the states (Human Rights Campaign 2013).

Hospital Visitation Laws [Fact sheet]. Retrieved from http://hrc-assets.s3-website-us-east1.amazo naws.com//files/assets/resources/hospital_visita-tion_laws_12-2013.pdf).

Discrimination and Bias

LGBT elders are at risk of bias and discrimination on multiple fronts. Despite great progress, we live in a society with a heterosexual bias. An opposite-gender spouse is the default assumption. Gender choices in application or information forms are limited to male and female, leaving intersex and trans persons with no appropriate choice. Homophobia is still common. A survey of LGBT elders found that the vast majority, if needing institutional long-term care, would choose to be closeted about their sexuality and, if ever receiving in home care, would fear mis-treatment by caregivers based on sexual orienta-tion or gender identity. LGBT (2010) older adults in long-term care facilities. A fear of discrimina-tion by health care service professionals is cited as a major fear among LGBT elders (Knauer 2010).

Ageism is widespread in society and in the LGBT community. Ageism especially impacts the gay male community with youth and sexual attractiveness being a significant focus of tradi-tional gay culture and society (Knauer 2009). Older gay men are rejected by their younger peers. For example, one man speculated that he could stand nude in the corner of gay bar and not be noticed. Another joked that a gay man is dead at 30 (Arana 2013, August 22). Much work is needed in legal, social, and policy areas for LGBT elders to age in dignity and without fear (Knauer 2010).

End-of-Life, Death, and Dying: What Makes LGBT Elders Different from Others?

Dying and death are a universal part of life. The difference for LGBT elders is in the likely mix-ture of family of origin, marital, and chosen family. Family of origin or biological family is the family a person is raised within, including birth or adoptive parents, siblings, and blood relatives. Marital family includes a spouse and in-laws. Chosen families are the "network of friends drawn together by affinity rather than consanguinity that provide a wide arrange of family support" (Knauer 2009.) For gay and lesbian adults, chosen family frequently takes the place of marital family. This is especially true in states that do not allow or recognize same-sex marriage. Some LGBT adults experience "estrangement and distance from families of origin" and form chosen families in the place or biological family (Knauer 2010.) The law, however, frequently views chosen families, as strangers and outsiders often leaving chosen family with little ability to make health care decisions without legal documents.

Adult children and grandchildren play a major role in end-of-life social interaction and health care. Adult children often provide a social net-work, act as caregivers, and participate in making end-of-life health care decisions. LGBT elders are less likely to have children, an estimated 37 % of LGBT adults have children (Gates 2013), and by comparison an estimated 74 % of all adults have children (Newport and Wilke 2013, September 25). Desire for children is still the norm in USA (Newport and Willke 2013). LGBT elders who do have children may be estranged from them. "Coming out" to children and the risk of rejection is a great fear of LGBT adults. The mixture of chosen, marital, and bio-logical family is a barrier, which complicate end-of-life issues for LGBT elders.

Society and the law create preferences or presumptions that favor families of origin and marital family. Heterosexuality is presumed in social interaction. When asking about a person's spouse, the societal norm is to ask about a spouse of the opposite gender. A female hospital or nursing home patient will, by default, be asked whether she has a husband. Statutes codify these presumptions and preferences in health care decision-making, visitation in a health care facilities, benefits eligibility, survivorship, funeral planning, taxes, and inheritance rights. Generally, preferences and presumptions in the law can be overcome with legal planning.

It Gets Complicated

When working with LGBT elders, it is easy to make generalizations and assumptions. As with any population, generalizations and assumptions can lead one astray. The first generalization is that LGBT adults are not married. Widespread same-sex marriage is a relatively recent development; estimates in early 2015 are that about 70 % of the US population lives in a place that allows or recognizes a same-sex marriage. Experts agree that there are over 1000 federal benefits for married couples. It is expected that same-sex marriage will become increasingly common in coming years. As of the production of this book, the US Supreme Court is hearing law suits against states that do not recognize same-sex marriage.

Discussion Box

1. Same-sex marriage is changing the face of LGBT life in the USA and much of western Europe. Experts agree that there are over 1000 federal benefits provided to legally married couples in the USA. Yet, there is significant religious opposition to same-sex marriage in the USA. Discuss separation of religious and governmental issues in same-sex marriage.
2. End-of-life is a time when families gather to provide care and say good-byes. Discuss how this is impacted when the person nearing the end-of-life is LGBT.
3. In a recent survey, the vast majority of LGBT adults responded that if they needed long-term care, in their home, in an inpatient setting, they would be reluctant to disclose their sexual orientation or gender identity to caregivers.

This fear forces committed couples in long-term relationships to act like close friends instead of spouses.

Discuss how this impacts quality of life and quality of care for LGBT elders.

During their lives, many lesbian and gay adults have entered into opposite-sex marriages. Marriage brings with it economic, legal, and social benefits and can be seen as a source of security. One article described gays and lesbians in opposite gender marriages as people who "hid (e) behind the pillars of convention" (LeDuff 1996, March 31). Some lesbian and gay adults enter into opposite-gender marriages hoping to blend in and live what prevailing society considers a normal adult life. Marriage can be the ultimate hiding place for sexual orientation or gender identity. A desire for children leads some lesbian or gay adults to enter into opposite gender marriages—sometimes with full knowledge by both partners—sometimes without.

For a bisexual adult, having an attraction to members of both genders is part of his or her core sexual orientation and gender identity. Many bisexual adults marry a person of the opposite gender, and some then act on their same-sex attraction, resulting in a complex mixture of marital and chosen family. It is not uncommon for a bisexual adult to be married to an opposite gender partner, with or without children, and at the same time to have a same gender partner. In many instances, the martial partner does not know about the same-sex partner, in other cases they do. This complex mixture of martial and chosen family is far outside the societal norm. In the event of a health crisis or end of life, this complex mixture may function as a family, or may exclude one of the partners from end of life and death.

Trans includes a spectrum of individuals whose primary sexual identity or gender expression is inconsistent with the gender assigned at birth. This can range from physical expression or dressing in a way not expected by society to persons seeking gender reassignment surgery.

A person, who self identifies as trans or gender non-conforming, or queer, may be heterosexual, bisexual, or gay/lesbian and may marry members of the same or opposite gender. Persons who have had gender reassignment surgery and legally changed the gender designation in official documents have overcome the barrier to opposite-sex marriage in many states. Disclosure of sexual orientation can be a choice: a person's appearance that is perceived as being inconsistent with societies gender expectations can be difficult or impossible to conceal.

Another generalization is that LGBT elders do not have children. Census data show that 37 % of LGBT adults have children (Gates 2013). A desire for children is a strong driver of human behavior. Most commonly LGBT adults have children from opposite-sex relationships, marital or non-martial. If the relationship breaks up after the children are born, sexual orientation or gender identity is sometimes, but not always, used to isolate the children from the LGBT parent. As children mature, some may reject or self-isolate from the LGBT parent. Increasingly, same-gender couples are having children. Same-sex couples can use surrogates, or artificial insemination. Some bypass the medical assistance to conceive children, sometimes resulting in child support and paternity issues (Narayan 2014). In many states, same gender couples can adopt, or one of the two can adopt. End of life issues are family issues, and any factor that isolates parents and children complicates end of life.

Case Study

Eddie's story

I was born in 1928 and grew up in Louisville, Kentucky. I knew I was different as a kid. I was drafted in World War II and spent three years in the Navy, and I fell in love. Fred was his name, and he was gorgeous. We served on the same ship, palled around ports in the south Pacific, and pledged our undying love to one another. We talked for hours about how we would spend our lives together. When the war ended, we were discharged on the west coast and went to Los Angeles. I worked as desk clerk in a hotel, and Fred and I shared a room and everything else for a few weeks. He went home to visit family in Iowa saying he would be back in a couple of weeks. Three weeks later I received a letter from him. He said what we did was not right, and he could not live like that and was going to marry the girl down the street and try hard to be normal. I was heartbroken. I only saw him once years later, and he denied that we ever loved one another.

After a few months, I went home to my mothers' house and started college. I was hanging out on the front porch talking with the girl next door. Over a couple of weeks, I told her everything, about Fred and love and broken promises. One day she said, "Why don't you marry me?" I explained that I really preferred guys. She reasoned that we both wanted children; she did not care about sex as long as I would do my part to have kids. She wanted a best friend for life. She said, "If I marry you, I will never be bored." We went across the river to Indiana one afternoon and got married by a justice of the peace. It was three weeks before I told my mother. Mom shook her head, saying it would never work. We have been married almost 50 years. We had three kids. We had a "don't ask don't tell policy." When she was away, I could go out with the boys. When I was out of town for work, anything goes, as long as I come home. Oh, the fun I have had over the years. If I had kept a diary, the book I could write. But, I never would have written anything down. In those days, people whispered behind their hands about someone being "different," in the end for me, it was always, but he is married with children. That saved my skin several times. We are best friends, we are good for one another, and we take care of one another. But, I have never stopped thinking about Fred, and love.

It is important to be careful about the generalization that LGBT adults will be estranged from marital and biological family. Many families are very accepting of LGBT family members, while others actively reject LGBT family members. An individual assessment of the nature of family relationships is essential to helping an LGBT elder with end-of-life issues. In any family, disagreement and strained relationships complicate end-of-life. The strain of illness and death can bring to the surface suppressed beliefs, feelings, and emotions. Families that have gotten along for decades, when faced with an end-of-life illness or death, may feel compelled to argue religious and societal views to urge an LGBT elder to change before death.

The last caution is that an LGBT individual can be "out" with one person and in the closet with the next person. Sexual orientation is generally invisible, and LGBT adults spend a lifetime deciding what to disclose to whom. When working with LGBT adults at the end-of-life, it is important to honor and respect the choices that they have made. Accidental disclosure can strain relationships and cause frustration and confusion at a time when the support of family and friends can be most important. Knowing what to say to whom is especially complicated if the LGBT elder near the end-of-life is unable to communicate their wishes regarding disclosure. If unsure of the level of disclosure, the best course of action can be to listen carefully for clues—while maintaining confidentiality.

End-of-Life Health Care Decision-Making

In an ideal world, every person would remain fully aware and able to make and communicate health care decisions until their last heartbeat and breath. In reality, most people experience at least a short period before death when they are unable to make or communicate decisions regarding the kind and extent of health care that they want or do not want to receive. Every adult has a fundamental right to make health care decisions.

Only when a person lacks the ability to make or communicate health care decisions does this right shift to someone else. Even when the transfer of health care decision-making is triggered, it is important that the individual be included in the decision-making process and that the known wishes of the patient be honored. Even if unable to make a decision, the individual may be able to express preferences or fears that can guide the decision-making process. The ultimate goal is for the decision that is made and to reflect the wishes, beliefs, goals, and values of the individual.

Default Decision Makers

Virtually, all states by statute or common law allow someone to make health care decisions for a person who is unable to do so (American Bar Association Commission on Law and Aging 2014). All of the default health care decision-making rules turn first to marital and biological family members. The most common provisions first ask the patient's spouse to make health care decisions. If there is no spouse, the person's adult children are generally second in line to make health care decisions (and the laws vary in how they treat disagreement among them.) If there are no adult children, the rules look to the person's parents. This process continues moving out through the family tree. Domestic partners are included on the statutory lists in five states, and best friends are included in 23 states—but only are called on to make health care decisions when there is no spouse or biological family higher up in the statutory list (ABA Commission on Law and Aging 2014). Default surrogate consent statutes). For an LGBT elder, a "close friend" or chosen family may be his or her preferred health care decision maker. The growth of same-sex marriage will change this picture, with more and more same-sex couples becoming spouses recognized by the law.

The spousal preference disproportionally impacts LGBT elders. Same-sex couples are less likely to be married than opposite-sex couples.

Until recently, few states allowed same-sex couples to marry. This is a rapidly changing area of the law. Time will tell if same-sex couples marry at the same rate as opposite-sex couples. Unmarried opposite-sex couples face the same issue as unmarried same-sex couples on this issue—with the major difference being that opposite-sex couples can marry in every state, and same-sex couples can only marry in some states. For same-sex couples who are married, the marital preferences apply.

The health care decision maker presumptions can be overcome by the naming of a health care surrogate. This is the same for all adults and requires specific legal steps.

Advance Care Planning

Advance care planning includes naming a health care surrogate and communicating health care goals, values, and beliefs to the health care surrogate and health care providers to guide decision-making when the elder is not able to make or communicate decisions. The process focuses on the needs, goals, preferences, cultural traditions, family situation, values, and the needs and preferences of surrounding family (Levine Feinberg 2013, May 1).

Successful planning involves a spectrum of people, including the patient, health care providers, marital, biological, and chosen family and the health care surrogate. Including the surrogate early in the process will help the surrogate gain insight into the choices and preferences of the person for whom they may someday need to make decisions (Tilly et al. 2007).

Naming and Empowering a Health Care Decision Maker

Everyone should name a health care surrogate; doing so is especially important for LGBT adults because of the potentially complex mixture of chosen, biological, and marital family. Naming a health care surrogate is a legal process involving designating someone in writing to make health care decisions in the event that the patient is unable to do so. A health care surrogate may be named in a durable power of attorney for health care, a declaration of a surrogate, or in a combination form that serves as a living will and appointment of a surrogate. The legal formalities of naming a health care surrogate vary from state to state, making it difficult to create a single form that works for everyone. There is multistate durable power of attorney for health care that works for most people in about 40 states (Giving someone a power of attorney for your health care) (Retrieved from ABA Commission on Law and Aging Web site: http://www.americanbar.org/content/dam/aba/administrative/law_aging/2011/2011_aging_hcdec_univhcpaform_4_2012_v2.authcheckdam.pdf). Many states have a standard form power of attorney for health care, or standard form living will directive. Frequently, state-specific forms can be found on the Web sites of the state attorney general, state department of health or aging services, or legal aid Web site.

The health care surrogate should be selected with great care. Being a health care surrogate can be very difficult. Surrogates are sometimes called upon to make life and death decisions. Health care surrogates, especially for LGBT elders, may find themselves at the middle of disputes between loved ones. Surrogates also need to be prepared to advocate with health care providers for the person-centered care in line with the goals, values, and beliefs of the person who appointed them. To be effective, a surrogate needs to understand the goals, values, and beliefs of the person, be willing and able to make decisions that reflect what the person would make, and have the strength to make decisions even if unpopular with others.

Empowering a surrogate is a human services process that starts with understanding the health care goals, beliefs, and values of the patient. For many adults, this starts with self-discovery, thinking about the kinds of care wanted or not wanted under various circumstances and who to include or exclude in a time of illness and dying. Tools such as "Five Wishes" (http://www.agingwithdignity.org/five-wishes.php.) and the

"Conversation Starter Kit" (www.theconversation project.org) can be very helpful both in helping the individual think about these issues and in starting conversations with others. Once the individual has a grasp on his or her health care goals, values, and beliefs, it is essential that this information be shared with the health care surrogate, family, and loved ones and health care providers. Without this conversation, the health care surrogate may lack critical information for making health care decisions. It is important to include health care providers in the advance planning conversations. Health care providers need to know who to turn to for health care decisions and to understand the health care goals and values of the patient. The potentially complex mixture of chosen, biological, and marital family increases the need for advance health care planning for LGBT elders. Without advance planning, health care providers will default to the standard assumptions and protocols with a heterosexual bias.

Human and aging services professionals must be careful not to give legal advice when assisting with standard forms. Providing a form is not the practice of law. Providing information is generally not the practice of law. The challenge is avoiding the tipping point between providing information and interpreting the law. When in doubt, ask an attorney what to do and where to stop. Alterations or changes in the standard forms should be done by an attorney. It is very easy when making changes to invalidate forms. Some states have specific language that must be included for an advance health care directive to be valid. Special care must be taken when creating clauses about specific treatment—to assess the impact on other treatment options. Most states have strict limitations on who can serve as a witness or notary when advance health care directives are signed. Missing any one of these can cause the planning to be ineffective.

Advance directives for trans elders need to include specific instructions. The forms should include provisions instructing health care providers on the preferred gender pronoun and name to use when communicating with or about the patient. The health care surrogate should be empowered to direct health care providers to address the elder by their preferred gender and name (The National Resource Center on LGBT Aging and Whitman-Walker Health 2014). Individuals who have had gender reassignment surgery have special medical needs; the surrogate needs to be empowered in a power of attorney for health care to advocate with health care providers and insurance companies for appropriate care.

Creating advance directives such as appointing a health care surrogate or completing a living will directive can be a do-it-yourself (DIY) project. However, there are risks in DIY planning. Many standard forms are poorly written, and few come with clear instructions on how to complete them. The witness or notary instructions are state-specific and must be followed precisely. Using a lawyer to complete advance directives costs money (though many legal aid programs provide this service free of charge for older Americans). The assistance of a trained professional can increase the likelihood of success. For LGBT elders, who fear a challenge to advance care planning by family members, working with an attorney on advance health care directives adds an additional layer of protection that the planning is done correctly, and at a time when the elder has capacity and is not subject to undue influence. Unmarried couples should avoid helping one another with advance health care directives, as this may be interpreted as undue influence and used to challenge the validity of the documents.

Advance care planning should not stop with the creation of documents. To be effective, advance care planning needs to include meaningful conversations with family, friends, and health care providers. The goal is for everyone to understand the goals, values, and beliefs of the individual regarding health care, especially end-of-life health care. Advance care planning carried out, without creation of legal documents, especially for LGBT elders who wish to appoint a surrogate different than the legal default, would be ineffective in that the preferred health care surrogate would lack the authority to do so. Creating legal documents without having meaningful conversations with loved ones and health care providers is equally doomed to failure—if no one knows what the plans are and what they mean—the plans are unlikely to be followed. Mentioned earlier, tools such as "Five Wishes" and "Your Conversation Starter Kit" are very helpful in planning and facilitating meaningful conversations about health care wishes.

Elder Law

Elder law is a growing area of practice, and planning for LGBT families is a popular topic for elder law attorneys. Elder law expands on traditional estate planning—work that focuses on who gets what after death—by focusing on issues likely to occur while the client is still alive. Elder law covers a broad spectrum of issues, including financial security, housing, living arrangements, caregiving, health care benefits, the possibility of incapacity, and the preservation and distribution of assets after death. Most adults stand to benefit from advice and assistance from an elder law attorney. Legal aid programs are able to help some low-income older adults. According to Legal Service Corporation, about 15 % of legal aid clients legal are age 60 and older (http://www.lsc.gov/about/lsc-numbers-2013#2013Ageand GenderofClients). Funding is provided under the Older Americans Act for legal assistance. Local senior centers, local area agencies on aging, or state offices on aging can direct low-income older adults to the attorneys funded under this program. There is a locator for free legal assistance for low-income older adults on the National Legal Resource Center Web site at http://nlrc.acl.gov/Services_Providers/Index.aspx.

Caregiving

Family, chosen, marital, and biological, are the most common caregivers of elders. There are an estimated 10 million Americans in need of long-term care services (Selected Long Term Care Statistics, Family Caregiver Alliance, viewed on 9/24/2014 at https://caregiver.org/selected-long-term-care-statistics.), and only about 1.4 million persons living in skilled long-term care facilities in the USA (CMS 2013) The vast majority of long -term care services are provided in the community by family and friends. For LGBT elders, home and community based care falls largely to chosen family.

If caregivers are paid, there should be a formal written caregiver agreement. Elder law attorneys craft these agreements to take into account the care needs, wishes of the parties, tax and employment laws, and Medicaid laws. No two individuals and no two families are the same, and the agreements should be written to specifically reflect the situation. This is especially important for caregivers of LGBT elders, as biological family may challenge the payments. Caregiver agreements spell out the caregivers' obligations and the terms of payment. The agreement and compliance with it can be a defense against accusations by family members or others that the caregiver was financially exploiting the elder.

Caregiver agreements are also essential if the elder ever applies for Medicaid. On average, 70 % of nursing home residents qualify for Medicaid. When an application is made for Medicaid benefits, the agency looks at gifts made within five years and may impose periods of ineligibility based on gifts. A caregiver agreement documents that payments to a caregiver were payments for services and not gifts.

Medicaid pays for health care for needy elderly and disabled adults when no other payment source is available. Medicaid is a needs-based program, meaning a beneficiary must establish a financial and medical need to be covered by the program. Medicare by contrast is available without regard to financial need. The financial need for Medicaid includes both limits on income and on assets. Congress created special provisions to protect a married couple from total impoverishment if one of them needs long-term care paid for by Medicaid. These are known as Medicaid spousal impoverishment protections. The protections exempt the average home, at least one motor vehicle, and allow the spouse not requiring Medicaid services to retain modest savings. The spousal impoverishment protections did not protect married same-sex couples, until the *Windsor* decision ruled parts of the Defense of Marriage Act unconstitutional (Windsor v. United States, 570 U.S.—(2013). Prior to this, the Department of Health and Human Services Centers for Medicare and Medicaid Services had issued policy letters saying that states could only protect same-sex couples by finding that not doing so was an undue hardship. This is still the only option in states that do not allow or recognize as valid same-sex marriage. The *Windsor* decision extends the spousal impoverishment provisions to hundreds of thousands of married same-sex couples. Same-sex couples should consult an experienced elder law attorney about the best options for paying for long-term care and Medicaid eligibility (possibly before they make a decision to marry.)

Estate Planning and Inheritance

An end-of-life concern for many people is who inherits what when they die. Inheritance issues for LGBT elders are complicated by defaults and presumptions in the law favoring martial and biological family. It is helpful to be familiar with the basic principles; the details of these issues fill a number of tomes.

When a person dies, laws or legal plans made by the person determine who inherits his estate. An estate includes personal property, money, investments, vehicles, furniture, household items, jewelry, the right to receive income, and real property. Without a will or estate plan, marital and biological families inherit the estate. To overcome the statutory presumptions, an adult needs a will, trust, or other estate-planning instrument. Estate planning is especially important for LGBT elders, as the statutory defaults do not include chosen family. LGBT adults nearing the end-of-life should review their estate plan with an attorney to assure that the outcome is what they want to have happen.

Social Security provides an essential income support for 93 % of all American elders. Social Security provides spousal, survivor, and widows and widowers benefits. Social Security spousal,

survivor, and widows benefits are becoming a bigger issue for LGBT elders as a result of the expansion of same-sex marriage and the Windsor decision. This is a rapidly evolving area of law and policy, and the Social Security Administration is expanding the availability of spousal, survivor, and widows benefits at a rapid pace. This is a complex area, married same-sex couples should be advised to check with an expert to see whether they are eligible for spousal benefits under Social Security.

Most private retirement plans or pensions are required by federal law to protect spouses by requiring a surviving spouse benefit as the default, unless waived by the non-employee spouse. Federal law imposes strict requirements on waiving the spousal benefit; these protections extend to married same-sex couples. For traditional defined benefit pensions, this means that when a married person retires, the retirement benefit is based on paying a benefit for the lifetime of both spouses, unless waived; if the wage earner dies before retiring, the surviving spouse is eligible for a survivor pension. For a defined contribution plan such as an IRA or 401 k, the default beneficiary for a married person is the spouse, unless waived. In addition, a surviving spouse is given preferential treatment in the federal tax law for an inherited tax deferred defined contribution plan (the typical IRA or 401 k plan). Post-Windsor, these provisions apply to married same-sex spouses, though it may take a few years for all of the account documents to be amended to reflect the changes in federal law. For LGBT elders with non-marital chosen family, it is essential that they name beneficiaries on all retirement plans.

When working with LGBT elders nearing the end-of-life, it is important to review beneficiary designations on pensions, retirement plans, life insurance, bank accounts, and investment accounts. For property that has a formal written form of ownership such as bank accounts, investment accounts, and motor vehicles, the ownership after death may be determined by form of ownership on the documents. There are two things to look for: is there more than one name on the ownership documents, or, is there a designation of a beneficiary, payable on death or transferable on death designation in the ownership paperwork?

Property owned in the name of more than one person is classified as joint property. Most bank accounts with more than one name on them are set up as "joint-with-right-of-survivorship." This means when one joint owner dies, the other joint owner(s) are presumed to own the account. It is also possible for jointly owned property to not be "joint-with-right-of-survivorship"—in which case the share of the deceased is an asset of their estate. Bank and investment accounts may also may list a beneficiary, frequently called a "payable on death" (POD) or "transferable on death" (TOD) designation. Accounts with POD or TOD designations pass automatically as an operation of law to the named beneficiary at the time of death. Life insurance pays to the named beneficiary, no document other than a form supplied by the insurance company, can change the beneficiary on a life insurance policy.

Housing and Home Ownership for LGBT Elders

A person can own a home in a wide array of legal forms. A critical issue for a person near the end-of-life is to assure that the person(s) they want to inherit or be able to continue living in the home have a legal right to do so. Evaluation of this requires looking at the ownership documents. This should be done by an attorney with expertise in real estate and inheritance laws of the state in which the home is located. It is common for the home occupied by an LGBT couple to be in the name of one person. This places the survivor at risk of not being able to remain in the home without advance legal planning.

For a lease, if both parties are not on the lease, the lease may terminate at the death of the named lessee, forcing the grieving member of the couple of negotiate with the landlord or move. In extreme cases, it can result in the person not on the lease being locked out of the home until probate court orders can be obtained granting

them access to the home. The right to remain in a leased home is especially valuable in areas with rent control.

A home is the largest single asset owned by the average American. The wording on the deed is essential to understanding joint ownership of real estate. If the deed to real property lists multiple owners, an expert in real property law in the state that the property is located should be called on to review who owns what interests. The two most common forms of joint ownership of real estate are tenants in common and joint tenancy. The death of an owner in a tenancy, in common, results in the estate of the deceased owning the deceased owners interest in the property. A joint tenancy is also known as "joint-with-right-of-survivorship". The death of a joint tenant results in the surviving joint owners inheriting the property automatically. There is a third less common form, called tenancy by the entireties, that is a super-strong form of joint-with-right-of-survivorship ownership only available to married couples. With the expansion of same-sex marriage, some couples may wish to change their form of ownership to tenancy by the entireties. The exact language that creates each of these varies from state to state. It is important to have an attorney familiar with the laws of the state the real estate is in review the deeds to verify that the outcome is as wished by the owners. LGBT elders need to be especially concerned with this, as homes purchased individually are not automatically inherited by chosen family and homes owned jointly, purchased before a same-sex marriage, may be in a tenancy in common and not create an automatic right to inherit.

End-of-life is a time that many adults engage in or review estate planning. Estate planning is especially important for LGBT elders because of the mixture of marital, biological, and chosen family. Without estate planning, all real and personal property not owned in a manner that transfers ownership at the time of death is inherited by marital or biological family—a process known as intestacy. The defaults under intestacy may not reflect wishes of LGBT elders. Estate planning varies from simple to very complex depending on the state the person lives or owns property in, the value of the estate, the complexity of the assets, and the goals of the individual. A consultation with an estate planning attorney, familiar with the complex issues faced by LGBT elders, is the best option to determine what is best for an individual.

Attitudes About End-of-Life

If this chapter were written in the 1980s or 1990s, HIV-Aids would be a major topic of consideration for end-of-life and LGBT adults. With advances in care, most persons who test positive for the HIV virus (HIV+) today are able to manage the infection as a long-term chronic illness. Over the past 20 years, the prognosis for an HIV+ adult has changed from a near certain death, to a near-normal life expectancy with diligent health care. Treatment for HIV+ infection is taxing; the drug regimens are complex and have side effects. Understanding the complex health care issues helps to understand the goals and needs of a person who is HIV+.

Many of today's LGBT elders lived through the darkest days of HIV, and some lost many friends and partners. There are many long-term survivors with HIV, and there are many who lived through the epidemic without being infected. HIV changed the way many LGBT elders view life and end-of-life issues. When a population sees large numbers of its contemporaries die young, many in the prime of life, it impacts the outlook on life and death. Just as soldiers who return from war after seeing fellow soldiers die are forever changed by the experience, LGBT elders who lived through the early years of HIV are similarly changed by the experience. Some feel guilty that they lived while others died. Some feel thankful to be alive. Yet, many others were overwhelmed by the sheer volume of illness and death that they experienced. Some want and need to talk about this experience, and others such as some old soldiers do not want to talk about the past. As an aging service professionals, the best we can do is politely open the door for

conversation and be a willing listener for those who wish to talk.

The end-of-life and death are a part of life. The unique factors for LGBT elders are based on the complex picture of marital, biological, and chosen family and the desire to disclose or not disclose sexual orientation and gender identity. There is a social media posting that makes the rounds from time to time that a real friend is the one you trust to go to your house when you die and delete the files on your computer, shred the pictures and DVDs, and dispose of the special box in the closet. For LGBT adults who have been protective of disclosing being LGBT in life, having someone they trust to "straighten up the house" after death can be a great relief. In working with LGBT adults on end-of-life issues, it can be very helpful to assure that they have someone they trust to sort through their personal artifacts after death.

Some LGBT adults are entirely open and transparent, but disclosure of sexual orientation and gender identity is a conscious choice for many LGBT adults. It is essential to understand the degree of comfort with disclosure of an individual, to be able to assist the individual in end-of-life issues. It is essential that aging services professionals develop a degree of trust with an LGBT elder, so that the LGBT elder will openly discuss what they want to disclosed, or not disclosed, and to whom. It is important that we help carry out those wishes. Do they want a rainbow flag at their memorial service? Do they need someone to clean out the closet? Do not assume anything. Worrying about disclosure can cause great stress for an LGBT elder. If you can help relieve this stress, you will ease the end-of-life transition.

Policy Boxes
To provide leadership and develop resources and expertise, the US Department of Health and Human Services funded the National Resource Center on

LGBT Aging in 2010. http://www.sageusa.org/programs/nrc.cfm.

Why is it important that this initiative and others continue?

End-of-life illnesses are very stressful for everyone involved. Families, who have been polite, accepting, and tolerant of LGBT chosen family, can be less polite and rejecting of chosen family in an end-of-life setting. It is not uncommon to hear families who welcomed the same-sex partner in the house for the past 25 holidays, demand that the partner be excluded from the hospital room or funeral. Stress brings out the worst in some people and the best in others. It is also common to see LGBT elders previously estranged from marital and biological family reach out to the family they have avoided for decades at the end-of-life. This can lead to a wide spectrum of experiences calling on all of the skills of human and aging services professionals.

The Last Act

Funeral and memorial arrangements are either an end-of-life concern for the dying or for the survivors. For many elders, planning a funeral is the last act. In virtually every state, the law defaults to marital and biological family to make arrangements for disposition of the bodily remains. For LGBT elders with a mixture of chosen, marital, and biological family, this can be a point of conflict. Some families have engaged in extended litigation over funeral plans and burial location. Pre-planning funeral arrangements make it clear what the elder wanted and is invaluable in the event of conflict. In some cases, pre-planning can be overridden by surviving family. The greatest likelihood of the last act being what the elder wants happens when the elder pre-plans and shares the plans with everyone.

Summary

LGBT elders live and die much the same as everyone else; the things that are different are the personal and family relationships, legal bias, and presumptions in favor of marital and biological family, the degree of disclosure of LGBT status, and cultural homophobia. Understanding these issues is the first step. The challenge for human and aging services professionals is to create a level of trust with LGBT elders, so that they share with you what their wishes are regarding end-of-life, so you can empower them to carry out those wishes. Extra care needs to be taken in planning for end-of-life health care, long-term care, financial management, and inheritance to assure that the wishes of LGBT elders are carried out.

Learning Exercise

Self-Check Questions

1. Explain five ways that expansion of same-sex marriage will change the end-of-life issues for same-sex couples.
2. Describe how homophobia, heterosexism, and ageism impact LGBT elders at the end-of-life.
3. Fred signed a living will directive form naming Tom his long-term partner as his health care surrogate at a community health fair and locked the documents away in his safe deposit box. What can he can he do to improve the effectiveness of his advance health care planning?
4. Barbie and Ken have long been hostile to their daughter Crystal being involved in relationships with other women. Crystal has terminal cancer. Crystal recently married Jane in part because she was afraid that her parents would try to exclude Jane from making health care decisions for her and interfere with Jane's inheritance from Crystal. How does the marriage change the picture? What does it not change?

5. Steve is gay and married Karen in 1965. They have raised two children. Steve has had a steady boyfriend, Paul for the past 25 years. Steve's kids refer to him as Uncle Paul; he has attended family gatherings and holidays with Karen and Steve for the past 20 years. Karen doesn't talk about her personal life. She and Steve are best friends. Discuss the ramifications on end-of-life issues for Steve. What can be done today to improve the odds that all are involved in end-of-life decisions and care?

6. James and Mark have been together for nearly 30 years and say they will get married when the state they live in recognizes same-sex marriage. Mark is quick to remark that they "have no dogs, no cats, no kids, nothing that makes noise and has to be cleaned up after." What are the implications as they age and face possible long-term care?

Experiential-Based Assignments

1. What programs and services are available in your community for older LGBT adults? Visit your local LGBT community center and ask about resources for older members of the community. Does your local senior center offer resources or programs for LGBT seniors?

2. LGBT adults tend to become invisible in long-term care settings. Visit local skilled nursing facilities or assisted living facilities and ask about programs to support the needs of LGBT residents and training for staff on meeting the needs of older LGBT adults.

3. Assemble a program on LGBT awareness and offer to present this program to staff at local aging services providers.

Multiple-Choice Questions

1. An important generalization to avoid when working with LGBT elders is:
   (a) They will only talk to you once they trust you

   (b) They tend to go back into the closet when in need of long-term care
   (c) They do not have children

2. Concealing one's sexual identity can be hardest for a person who is
   (a) Gay
   (b) Lesbian
   (c) Bisexual
   (d) Transgender

3. A person who identifies as transgender may be
   (a) Gay or Lesbian
   (b) Bisexual
   (c) Heterosexual
   (d) All the above

4. When a patient is unable to make or communicate health care decisions, the first place health care providers generally turn to is:
   (a) The patient's spouse
   (b) The patient's parents
   (c) The courts
   (d) Adult protective services

5. What is the most important step in person-centered advance care planning?
   (a) Having meaningful conversations with family and health care providers
   (b) Signing legal documents appointing a health care surrogate
   (c) Signing a living will
   (d) Omitting family of origin

6. What is the most important legal change that same-sex marriage causes?
   (a) Eliminates discrimination
   (b) Allows joint ownership of real property
   (c) Recognition under state and federal law as spouses
   (d) Encourages institutional collaboration

7. What is the most protective form of joint ownership of real estate?
   (a) Tenants in common
   (b) Tenancy by the entireties
   (c) Joint with right of survivorship
   (d) Inclusive specificity

8. What legal specialty focuses on issues before death
   (a) Estate planning
   (b) Advance care planning

   (c) Elder law

   (d) Preferential law

9. LGBT elders who lived through the early years of HIV/AIDS in the 1980s and 1990s may have an outlook on life similar to?

   (a) Cancer survivors

   (b) Soldiers returning from D-day

   (c) Person's with dementia

   (d) Persons with immigrant status

10. If you are unsure to whom an LGBT person has disclosed his or her sexual orientation or gender identity and if they are not able to communicate, your best course of action is to?

   (a) Tell everyone and let the chips fall where they may

   (b) Ask each person in the person's life if they knew

   (c) Listen for clues

   (d) Avoid the issue

Key

c

d

d

a

a

c

b

c

b

c

Resources

1. SAGE—Services and Advocacy for LGBT Elders—http://www.sageusa.org/

2. National Center for Lesbian Rights—http://www.nclrights.org/

3. Human Rights Campaign—http://www.hrc.org/

4. Leading Age—http://www.leadingage.org/LGBT.aspx

5. Caring and Aging with Pride—http://caringandaging.org/wordpress/

6. National Legal Resource Center—http://nlrc.acl.gov/Legal_Issues/LGBT_Aging/index.aspx

7. The Conversation Project—http://theconversationproject.org/

8. Aging with Dignity /Five Wishes https://www.agingwithdignity.org/index.php

9. ABA Commission on Law and Aging—http://www.americanbar.org/groups/law_aging.html

10. Lambda Legal—http://www.lambdalegal.org/

11. National Academy of Elder Law Attorneys—www.NAELA.org

References

American Bar Association Commission on Law and Aging, (2014, June). *Default surrogate consent statutes*. Retrieved from http://www.americanbar.org/content/dam/aba/administrative/law_aging/2014_default_surrogate_consent_statutes.authcheckdam.pdf.

Arana, G., (2013, August 22). *When I'm old and gay*. The American Prospect. Retrieved January 29, 2015 from http://prospect.org/article/when-im-old-and-gay.

CMS (2013). *Nursing home data compendium 2013*. Retrieved on September 24, 2014 from http://www.cms.gov/Medicare/Provider-Enrollment-and-Certification/CertificationandComplianc/downloads/nursinghomedatacompendium_508.pdf.

Gates, G. J., (The Williams Institute). (2013, February). *LGBT parenting in the United States*. Retrieved from http://williamsinstitute.law.ucla.edu/wp-content/uploads/LGBT-Parenting.pdf.

Human Rights Campaign (2013). *Hospital Visitation Laws [Fact sheet]*. Retrieved from http://hrc-assets.s3-website-us-east1.amazonaws.com/files/assets/resources/hospital_visitation_laws_12-2013.pdf.

Knauer, N. (2009). LGBT elder law: Toward equity in aging. *Harvard Journal of Law and Gender*, 1–58.

Knauer, N. (2010). *Gay and lesbian elders: Estate planning and end-of-life decision making*. Florida Coastal Law Review, pp. 163–215.

LeDuff, C. (1996, March 31). *Gay, getting old, getting by*. The New York Times. Retrieved from http://www.nytimes.com/1996/03/31/nyregion/gay-getting-old-getting-by.html.

Legal, L., (2008). Langbehn v. Jackson memorial hospital [Fact sheet]. Retrieved from http://www.lambdalegal.org/in-court/cases/langbehn-v-jackson-memorial.

Legal Service Corporation (2013). *LSC by the numbers*. Retrieved on January 24, 2015 from http://www.lsc.gov/about/lsc-numbers-2013#2013AgeandGenderofClients.

Levine, C., & Feinberg, L. (2013, May 1). *Transitions in care: are they person and family centered* [Blog post]. Retrieved from http://asaging.org/blog/transitions-care-are-they-person-and-family-centered.

LGBT older adults in long term care facilities (2010). Retrieved from Lambda Legal website: http://www.lambdalegal.org/sites/default/files/publications/downloads/ext_nsclc_stories-from-the_field.pdf.

McCorquodale, A., (2013, May 26). *Florida counties that don't recognize domestic partnerships*. The Huffington Post. Retrieved from http://www.huffingtonpost.com.

Narayan, C., (2014, January 24). *Kansas court says sperm donor must pay child support*. CNN. Retrieved from http://www.cnn.com/2014/01/23/justice/kansas-sperm-donation/.

Newport, F., & Wilke, J.. (2013, September 25). Desire for children still norm in U.S. *Gallop Organization*. Retrieved from http://www.gallup.com/poll/164618/desire-children-norm.aspx.

The National Resource Center on LGBT Aging & Whitman-Walker Health, (2014). *Creating end-of-life documents for trans individuals: An advocate's guide*. Retrieved from: http://www.lgbtagingcenter.org/resources/pdfs/End-of-Life%20PlanningArticle.pdf.

The White House. (2010, April 15). *Presidential memorandum—hospital visitation* [Press release]. Retrieved from http://www.whitehouse.gov/the-press-office/presidential-memorandum-hospital-visitation.

Tilly, J., et al., (2007). Dementia care practice recommendations for assisted living residences and nursing homes. *Alzheimer's Association Campaign for Quality Residential Care*. Retreived on January 24, 2015 from http://www.alz.org/national/documents/brochure_DCPRphases1n2.pdf.

Tracey L. Gendron, Terrie Pendleton and John T. White

Abstract

This chapter discusses the complexity of mental health among older lesbian, gay, bisexual, and transgender (LGBT) individuals. Mental health issues for LGBT older adults can potentially involve the long-term impact of stigma and discrimination, and the changing view of sexual orientation and gender identity as pathology to non-pathology. This chapter will address both the risk and protective factors that are relevant to mental health counseling of LGBT older individuals, will discuss the history of research and practice related to mental health, and will provide recommendations for creating culturally competent evidence-based training programs for mental health service providers working with LGBT older adults. As well, the chapter provides an overview of specific issues relevant to the LGBT community including depression and anxiety and body image concerns. Interdisciplinary perspectives to service delivery for LGBT older adults are highlighted.

Keywords

LGBT mental health · Mental health counseling · Minority stress theory · Depression and anxiety · Body image

Overview

This chapter provides an introduction to mental health counseling specifically addressing relevant issues for lesbian, gay, bisexual, and transgender (LGBT) older adults. The chapter begins with a broad discussion of mental health and then more specifically examines relevant history that impacts psychological services for LGBT clients.

T.L. Gendron (✉) · T. Pendleton · J.T. White
Virginia Commonwealth University, Richmond, USA
e-mail: tlgendro@vcu.edu

T. Pendleton
e-mail: terrie.pendleton@hms.com

J.T. White
e-mail: whitejt2@apps.vcu.edu

© Springer International Publishing Switzerland 2016
D.A. Harley and P.B. Teaster (eds.), *Handbook of LGBT Elders*,
DOI 10.1007/978-3-319-03623-6_23

Specific psychological issues are presented including depression and anxiety and body image and eating disorders. Potential barriers to accessing mental health services are described as well as how mental health counselors can become culturally competent service providers. This chapter addresses both the risk and protective factors that are relevant to mental health counseling of LGBT older individuals and specifically highlights issues that are unique for transgender older adults. Finally, recommendations for creating culturally competent evidence-based training programs for mental health service providers working with LGBT older adults are provided.

Learning Objectives

By the end of the chapter, the reader should be able to:

1. Understand the risk and protective factors that are important to the mental health of LGBT older adults.
2. Understand the difference between sexual orientation and gender identity in mental health risk factors and outcomes.
3. Understand the history of research and practice related to mental health of LGBT elders.
4. Understand culturally competent evidence-based mental health practice concepts for working with LGBT older adults.
5. Discuss the importance of understanding the developmental risk and protective factors of growing up as an LGBT individual to counselor competency and effective mental health service delivery.

Introduction

Mental health refers to the state of emotional and psychological well-being and is inextricably linked with physical health and quality of life. Mental health of older LGBT individuals is a complex issue involving the long-term impact of

stigma and discrimination, the changing view of sexual orientation and gender identity as pathology to non-pathology, and socioenvironmental stress that impacts individual psychosocial resources. Social stress theory and minority stress theory provide well-established frameworks emphasizing how stress can impact an individual's mental health and well-being from extended exposure to discrimination and stigma (Aneshensel 1992; Dohrenwend 2000; Meyer 1995, 2003). Minority stress is based on the premise that, due to stigma and marginalization, LGBT individuals may experience enduring psychological stress (Meyers 2003). Research has documented the negative impact of minority stress on the mental health of the overall LGBT population, including higher rates of mental disorders, substance abuse, and self-harm than heterosexual populations (Cochran and Mays 2000; King et al. 2007; Meyer 1995). However, research has also demonstrated that good mental health outcomes were indicated for those individuals that were "out" (i.e., people knowing about their sexual orientation or gender identity) who had a higher sense of social integration and lower internalized homophobia and transphobia (D'Augelli et al. 2001; Lombardi 2009). As with the heterosexual population, good mental health outcomes for older adults are related to self-acceptance, purpose in life, social support, and financial security. Some studies suggest that LGBT older adults may adjust to aging more successfully than their non-LGBT counterparts, due to increased resilience from dealing with prejudice, stigma, and loss (Gabbay and Wahler 2002; Orel 2004).

Although the term "LGBT" is utilized as an umbrella term, gender identity (transgender older adults) and sexual orientation (LGB older adults) are distinctive from each other with different mental health influences and outcomes. There are numerous reasons why mental health needs based on sexual orientation and gender identity differ, including the history of the categorization of homosexuality and gender identity as diagnosable conditions in the American Psychiatric Association's Diagnostic and Statistical Manual of Mental Disorders (*DSM*).

History of Research and Practice

The population of 65 and older LGBT individuals came of age during a time when they were considered mentally ill by mental health professionals and as often engaging in immoral and/or illegal by society's standards (Jacobson and Grossman 1996). Therefore, older LGBT individuals developed in a culture of being socially invisible in the twentieth century. This pervasive stigma was a major contributor to the decision for many to follow a "heteronormal lifestyle" or to conceal their sexual orientation/gender identity from family, friends, and employers (D'Augelli et al. 2001).

On the other hand, there was a growing culture shift during the 1960s and 1970s during which society began to embrace more diverse sexualities/identities and emphasized tolerance. Baby boomers—those born from 1946 to 1964—were the first generation to more openly dabble with "alternative lifestyles" (Rubin 2001), a variety of non-traditional family forms, including gay and lesbian relationships, open marriages, and multiple relationships.

History of Sexual Orientation. The development of mental health services for LGB people can be best understood in the context of the tumultuous history and society's ever-changing view of the morality of sexual orientation. Societal and religious objections to same-sex relationships and attraction have existed since at least the Middle Ages (Davenport-Hines 1990). In the 1950s–1980s, the characterization of homosexuality as a mental illness led to the oppression of sexual orientation and encouraged countless people to participate in psychoanalytic and psychiatric treatments to "cure" their homosexual tendencies (Smith et al. 2004). During the early to mid-twentieth century, psychoanalysis was the dominant perspective in psychiatry and argued that homosexuality was a "reparative" attempt to achieve sexual pleasure when a normal heterosexual outlet proved too threatening (Rado 1949). Homosexuality was identified in the *DSM* as an illness until 1973, and conditions pertaining to homosexuality were not entirely removed until 1987.

History of Gender Identity. Gender identity has faced a similar historical background of medical and psychological pathologization. Gender identity was characterized as a disorder until the emergence of the *DSM-V* in 2014, which replaced the term "gender identity disorder" with "gender dysphoria." Although transgenderism is still represented in the *DSM-V*, gender identity has been reclassified from a disorder with the new aim of therapy to assist people to live in the way that best suits their authentic gender.

There is tremendous variation and diversity among transgender individuals in terms of their mental health needs. Because mental health is intrinsically linked to physical, psychosocial, and spiritual health, successful mental health interventions with older transgender individuals require a holistic approach to health that includes both primary and psychosocial cares. Specific issues that impact mental health for transgender individuals include transphobia, the impact of gender issues on psychosocial and identity development, and psychological effects of hormones (Bockting et al. 2006). Refer to Discussion Box 1 for additional guidance on discussing transphobia.

> **Discussion Box 1**
> What is your definition of transphobia? Please provide an example, either real or hypothetical.

The LGBT older adult population may still remember a time when medical and mental health professions sexualized and pathologized their identity and behavior. Today, the mainstream view among mental health clinicians is that homosexuality is a normal human expression and is no more inherently associated with psychopathology than is heterosexuality (Herek and Garnets 2007). Although sexual orientation and gender identity are no longer considered disorders, lingering stigma and fear remain as barriers for older LGBT individuals to accessing mental health services.

Psychological Issues

Opinions and feelings about sexual orientation and gender identity are rampant, as are opinions and attitudes about aging. Surprisingly, there is not much empirical literature about aging among sexual minorities; therefore, there are comparatively few studies about the mental health needs of older LGBT people. However, there are a variety of known factors that can impact mental health among LGBT older adults. According to minority stress theory (Meyer 2003), LGBT individuals are at higher risk for psychological problems because they face chronic stressors as a result of their minority status. This can take the form of external, objectively stressful events, the expectation of external stressors, and the internalization of negative societal attitudes regarding their minority status (Meyer 2003). In addition, society is facing an uphill battle against ageism (fear of older people) and gerontophobia (fear of our own aging), as aging anxiety remains pervasive in the USA. Being LGBT and being older can result in "double jeopardy," whereby the older, sexual minority individual becomes even more vulnerable to psychological stressors. Therefore, older LGBT individuals may struggle with issues such as negative self-image and self-hatred, and self-imposed or societal isolation, and perhaps regret for not coming out earlier or at all (Makadon et al. 2008). Being older and LGBT increases obstacles to accessing adequate mental health services in a predominantly youth and heteronormative society (Orel 2004). Refer to the case study below as a guide to discuss what psychological issues can impact an LGBT older adult.

Case Study

Ms. Jones is an elder lesbian whose partner recently passed away. She lives in a rural, conservative community and has experienced increased incidences of anxiety and depression since her partner passed away. What are barriers to successful aging for Ms. Jones?

Depression and Anxiety

The National Alliance on Mental Illness (2014) reports that LGBT people are likely to be at higher risk for depression than their heterosexual counterparts. This statement is also as likely true of LGBT elders, as evidenced by The Aging and Health Report (2010) finding that 31 % of LGBT elders reported having depressive symptoms at a clinical level, with more than half having been told by a doctor that they had depression. In many areas of mental health, people of color and transgender people show higher rates of mental distress as well.

Exposure to stigma, discrimination, and resulting victimization based on sexual orientation and/or gender identity, coupled with ageism and victimization based on age, result in LGBT older adults being vulnerable to depression and anxiety. Evidence indicates that mental health outcomes are associated with the stress of having a stigmatized identity and living in a discriminatory environment (Meyer 2007). In addition, loss and grief can have an impact on mental health, especially if the loss is unacknowledged, which may often be the case with a grieving LGBT older adult (Glacken and Higgens 2008).

Anxiety disorders have received relatively little empirical attention among older adults compared to the research on mood disorders such as depression. However, generalized anxiety disorder (GAD) is thought to be the most common anxiety disorder among older adults (Hybles and Blazer 2003) and is associated with lower quality of life and increased risk of medical conditions (Mackenzie et al. 2011). The cause of depression and anxiety in the LGBT community, and specifically among LGBT elders, can be attributed to a variety of factors that include:

- Societal oppression as a part of a marginalized group;
- A societal norm that encourages the minimization of the LGBT experience;
- Stress specific to living in and navigating a homophobic culture;
- Societal pressures to fabricate an untrue self;

- Internalized oppression/internalized homophobia;
- Isolation;
- Grief/loss/loneliness;
- Denial of true self;
- Low self-esteem.

The diversity of the aging LGBT community requires an understanding of both the historical and social context of their lives. Some are of the "Greatest Generation," who came of age in the shadow of the Great Depression or in the McCarthy era (1950s). Others are of the baby boom generation, who came of age during the era of the civil rights movement (1960s) and the Stonewall riots (1969) (Fredriksen-Goldsen and Muraco 2010). Yet, others are from ethnic minority groups, which adds the influence of race as a historical and social context (see Chaps. 5, 6, 7, 8, 10). Many LGBT elders internalized the oppression, homophobia, and transphobia that have been ever present in our society. The internalization of the prevalent societal thinking regarding the LGBT community and the aging population in general makes it difficult to counter the negative messages with positive attributes. According to the National Alliance on Mental Illness (NAMI 2014), "LGBT people do not by definition have a mental illness, but they have to contend with societal stigma and negative experiences that likely contribute to an increased vulnerability to mental illness" (p. 2). Without family or community support, the hatred can manifest internally, impacting the LGBT older adult's belief about himself and others in his community. However, it is important to note that most LGBT individuals ultimately live happy and healthy lives (NAMI).

It is very likely that many LGBT elders did not have the experience of a positive family support system specific to their sexual orientation/gender identity during their formative years. Depending on the societal norms of the time, LGBT elders more often hid their sexual orientation/gender identity from family and friends, thus limiting important support systems. The lack of this support system and identity building block could have caused increased vulnerability for mental health disturbance, health-related deterioration,

and overall decrease in general life well-being. Isolation is another factor that can contribute to an increased risk of mental health disturbance (see Chap. 30 for further discussion on social isolation). Isolation can contribute to loneliness, low self-esteem, and sense of self-worth. Low self-esteem and/or self-worth can create a constant dissonance that can ultimately lead to a path of self-destruction (i.e., alcohol, drugs, risky behaviors, and violence to self and others), which in turn leads to depression and anxiety.

Although becoming a "whole" person can be a lifelong endeavor for most individuals, LGBT older adults who have engaged in this "denial of the true self" for a large percentage of their lives may have trouble attaining their "whole-person" potential during their lifetime. Treatment considerations with LGBT older adults, as with other minority groups, involve assisting the client in working toward self-acceptance. The acceptance of oneself is an important factor in decreasing depression and anxiety in the LGBT community. Use the following case study as a guide to discuss how to address the mental health concerns of an older LGBT individual.

Case Study

Ms. A. is an 82-year-old African-American woman who lives in her home in the community. Once a week, Ms. A. visits a hair stylist and talks about her life. During the course of one conversation, Ms. A. shared that she had never been married and had no children and that she had never felt a part of a "regular" group of people. The information shared led the stylist to believe that Ms. A might be a part of the LGBT community. The stylist, who was also a part of the LGBT community, continued to engage with Ms. A and talk with her about her life. Eventually, Ms. A confided that she was a lesbian. Ms. A also shared that she was no longer in contact with most of her lesbian friends and that she was felt isolated from the LGBT community. Ms. A also discussed feelings of sadness about her social isolation and lack of connection with people of her age in the LGBT community.

Questions for discussion: If you talking to Ms. A, how would you approach this situation? What would be your concerns about Ms A's mental health? How would you address these concerns?

Protective Factors against Depression and Anxiety. It is important to note that community epidemiological research has consistently demonstrated that the prevalence of major depression decreases with age and is especially low among those 65 and older (Beekman et al. 1999; Blazer and Hybels 2005; Jorm 2000). In addition, LGBT older adults may have protective factors that make them less likely to experience depression or anxiety as a result of stigma and discrimination. For example, Orel (2004) found that many older LGBT individuals demonstrated that the process of "coming out" helped develop psychological resilience that prepared them for psychological issues related to aging. The process of "coming out" may actually buffer LGBT people against later crises, a term called crisis competency (Kimmel 1978). Along with the likelihood of experiencing prejudice and stigma throughout their life, older LGBT people develop coping mechanisms that foster resilience. A sense of resilience brings strength to the aging process. In fact, research has demonstrated that older LGBT people report higher levels of life satisfaction and lower self-criticism (Barranti and Cohen 2000). For a more in-depth discussion of crisis competency, see Discussion Box 2.

Discussion Box 2
Given examples of what life experiences, in addition to coming out, those LGBT individuals may have experienced which support their "crisis competency."

Specific Issues in the older transgender population. Gender dysphoria and gender identity disorder are terms that have been used to describe the pathology associated with the anxiety and sadness that is experienced by those who feel that they are living as the wrong gender. Research has demonstrated that transgender individuals are at higher risk of poor mental health and attempted suicide (Clements-Noelle et al. 2001). Stigma, discrimination, and exposure to transphobia can have a profound impact on the development of mood and anxiety disorders. Transphobia can be described as a feeling of unease toward those who identify as transgender (Hill 2002). The scope and prevalence of discrimination and harassment is well documented in the literature. Studies have reported that it is common for transgender individuals to experience verbal harassment, employment discrimination, economic discrimination, housing discrimination, and physical abuse (Clements 1999; Lombardi 2001; Reback et al. 2001).

Body Image and Eating Disorders

Body image and eating disorders are important topics in relation to the older LGBT population in part because of the belief that these issues are restricted to white upper-class heterosexual girls. Body dissatisfaction has been found to be relatively stable over the life span, with the importance of body image just as salient for older adults as for younger and middle-aged adults (Webster and Tiggeman 2003). In addition, the ideal body image is continuing to become more rigid for both men and women in the LGBT community.

Body image is a multidimensional construct that emphasizes the degree to which individuals are satisfied with their appearance. Perception of one's shape and weight represents an important component of self-concept and self-esteem. Dissatisfaction with one's body can have a number of potential consequences, including disordered eating, depression, and anxiety (Forman and Davis 2005).

Body Image and Sexual Orientation. Recent research has suggested that sexual orientation in both men and women may play a significant role in body dissatisfaction and the development and onset of disordered eating, as there are a disproportionate number of men with eating disorders that are gay and/or bisexual (Feldman and Meyer 2007). Research has demonstrated that homosexual men are generally more dissatisfied with their weight and more likely to desire an underweight ideal and have more eating disturbances than heterosexual men (Frenchet et al. 1996; Herzog et al. 1991; Williamson and Hartley 1998). Gay and bisexual men are more likely than heterosexual men to view their bodies as sexual objects and therefore may be more vulnerable to experiencing body dissatisfaction (Siever 1994).

Sociocultural perspective is a theory that has been used to describe the presence of body dissatisfaction in the LGBT community. Sociocultural perspective postulates that the social and cultural values that inform the ideas of what constitutes an ideal body image are unobtainable by many (Yager 2000). According to the sociocultural perspective, gay and bisexual men are subject to similar demands and pressures as heterosexual women, which make them more likely to be affected by norms that guide ideal beauty. On the other hand, researchers have found that the application of sociocultural perspective to lesbian and bisexual women has the opposite effect; for example, lesbian and bisexual women may be less prone to eating disorders because they do not share the standards and ideals of feminine beauty embraced by heterosexual women (Feldman and Meyer 2007). However, it is a misnomer that a strong feminist perspective is protection against lesbian and bisexual women having body image concerns. Research on body image and eating disorders among lesbian and bisexual women has produced unclear results. For example, some studies demonstrate stronger associations between body esteem and self-esteem in homosexual women, with increased prevalence of disordered eating (Striegel-Moore et al. 1990; Wichstrom 2006), while others have shown fewer dysfunctional eating attitudes and behaviors in homosexual women (Lakkis et al. 1999; Strong et al. 2000). Clearly, there is more research needed regarding the relationship between body image and eating disorders among lesbian and bisexual women.

Body Image and Gender Identity. There is a dearth of research regarding the relationship between gender identity, body image, and eating disorders. However, eating disorders and body dissatisfaction are related to gender and gender roles (Murnen and Smolak 1997). It has been postulated that the constructs of masculinity and femininity may best explain the relationship between gender roles and disordered eating. In other words, those with more feminine characteristics, regardless of gender, are more likely to experience disordered eating or body dissatisfaction. However, research on gender role and eating pathology is contradictory and difficult to interpret. Although some studies suggest femininity associated with higher levels of eating disorders (Meyer et al. 2001), others reveal that higher masculinity was associated with abnormal eating behaviors (Pritchard 2008). Limited evidence exists supporting a possible relationship between being transgender and having an eating disorder. The limited research that does exist hypothesizes that male-to-female transgender individuals are at great risk of developing an eating disorder.

There is very little research on body image and eating disorders among older adults and almost nonexistent research about body image and eating disorders among LGBT older adults. However, LGBT older adults may be more at risk for issues related to body image and eating disorders than their heterosexual counterparts. With aging come biological changes that effect physical appearance: increased weight, slowed metabolism, graying of hair, and wrinkles. Although there is a developmental phenomenon that promotes a more adaptive body image with age, body image is relatively stable across the life span. Therefore, older adults often age alone with maladaptive body dissatisfaction and disordered eating. A lifelong pattern of a negative body image can be exacerbated by a fear of aging. Fear of aging includes increasing concern about physical appearance and attractiveness. Fear of aging is predominant in Western culture and equates physical beauty with youth. Fear of aging has also been associated with both body dissatisfactions and disinhibited eating (Lewis and Cachelin 2001). Given that men subscribe more importance to physical attractiveness than women, older gay men are at greater risk of being less satisfied with their bodies and more vulnerable to eating disorders in order to conform to the pressure of physical attractiveness. In a study of gay and lesbian perceptions of aging, Schope (2005) found that gay men feel that gay society views aging as something negative. Interestingly, gay men identified the age of 39 as "old" for a gay man. Therefore, gay men appear to experience increased difficulties sustaining positive self-images in the face of both societal homophobia and judgment from within their own community.

Research Box

Drummond, M. (2006). Ageing gay men's bodies. Gay and Lesbian Issues and Psychology Review, 2(2)60–66.
Title of the Research: Aging Gay Men's Bodies.
Objective: To examine emergent body-based issues for older gay men.
Method: In-depth interviews of three gay males. Results: Emergent themes identify that older gay males have concerns about their body image.
Conclusion: Older gay men experience challenges in regard to their body image, which subsequently impacts identity and self-esteem.
"Amidst a highly commodified consumer culture in which the body is central to youthfulness and vitality, arguably even more so in gay culture, aging gay men are increasingly confronted with such ageist notions."

Barriers to Service Utilization

The LGBT aging community is a growing and diverse population, and careful examination of the current systems and mechanisms of care is needed. As healthcare professionals work toward meeting the needs of all older adults, the aging services network will be challenged to provide competent, fair, and equitable services to the LGBT community. The lives of lesbian, gay, bisexual, and transgender older adults are often obstructed by the barriers they encounter in order to attain mental health services in addition to other services, including medical care, short- and long-term care services, nutritional and physical fitness programs, senior housing, assisted living, in-home health services, legal services, transportation, recreation, and support groups.

In fact, a study by McIntyre et al. (2011) found that the medical model of care contains particular access to barriers for LGBT people. Specifically, study results identified systems-level barriers which include barriers inherent within the medical model that diminish individuality, lack of availability of supportive services including insufficient financial support for LGBT mental health services, and lastly disincentives for trained and culturally competent LGBT providers. As well, fear of discrimination is a significant barrier to the solicitation of mental health services for many LGBT older adults. The stigma of being a target of homophobia, heterosexism, or transphobia is of great concern to LGBT elders. It is not uncommon for an older adult to remain closeted about his or her sexual orientation or gender identity out of fear of insensitivity or lack of understanding which can contribute to disparities in mental health services and treatment (Mays and Cochran 2001; McIntyre et al. 2011).

Another barrier to mental health services for LGBT older adults relates to the professionals' lack of knowledge of the LGBT community, their culture, and lifestyle preferences. Professionals, although well intentioned, may be undereducated, miseducated, or simply not educated concerning the mental health needs of the LGBT community. A negative experience with a health professional, limited availability of LGBT-friendly professionals, and lack of education and support can cause LGBT older adults to shy away from seeking mental health services.

The lack of knowledge of mental health professionals can be particularly salient for older transgender individuals. It is not uncommon for mental health professionals to lack the knowledge about gender identity that is necessary to provide effective person-centered care.

As a result, it often becomes necessary for the older adult to educate his or her own mental health provider or medical healthcare provider about issues related to the transgender experience.

As well, the LGBT community may be disproportionally affected by the ever-rising costs of healthcare services, creating another barrier to the acquisition of mental health services. This is illustrated by the SAMHSA report (2014) estimating that one in three LGBT Americans in the low- to middle-income base lack health insurance. In addition, SAMHSA (2014) reported that nationwide, about one in five gay and bisexual men and one in four lesbian and bisexual women are living in poverty and more than 25 % of transgender Americans report an annual household income of less than $20,000.

Creating a safe and welcoming clinical environment is essential to break down barriers that may prevent older LGBT clients from accessing mental health services. A welcoming environment creates an atmosphere where people feel safe and cared for as individuals. A safe and welcoming clinical environment would provide a nonjudgmental, safe space that includes messages of inclusiveness such as a non-discrimination policies, culturally competent intake forms, appropriate educational materials, and courteous and respectful staff. It would also require that providers and their staff be culturally competent and sensitive and willing to engage the individual "where they are at." Cultural sensitivity includes valuing and respecting diversity and being sensitive to cultural differences. Another feature of a safe and welcoming clinical environment includes the ability of the client to be able to engage in open and honest communication with their provider. This is essential to the development of an effective therapeutic relationship. Therefore, effective communication must be stressed on the part of both the provider and the client.

Confidentiality, quality of services, and ethical behavior are all important factors when seeking mental health care and treatment. Historically, many minority communities have been subject to an array of unethical and unprofessional behaviors as a result of the structure of the healthcare system. For the LGBT community, concerns regarding homophobia, transphobia, and discrimination may keep LGBT elders from seeking services as they often assume that they will not be welcomed. In a study by Browne et al. (2008), several departments within a hospital system were identified that would particularly benefit from increased LGBT sensitivity training including chronic disease (including cancer and diabetes) and long-term care, and mental health. Gaining understanding of the culture of institutions with a history of discrimination and insensitivity to minority populations is essential for the development of effective intervention strategies.

At present, there are only a few LGBT inclusive aging providers in the USA who provide specialized services to the LGBT community. These organizations acknowledge and understand the concern of LGBT elders and the requirement for sensitivity and respect. Services and Advocacy for Gay, Lesbian, Bisexual and Transgender Elders (SAGE) is one such organization. SAGE is dedicated to improving the lives of LGBT older adults by targeting services specifically to LGBT older adults.

Counselor Competency

Counselor competency specific to LGBT older adults requires understanding of the sexual minority experience, the aging experience, and the effect that those experiences have had on the life of an LGBT elder. The importance of training for therapists to improve culturally competent practice with LGBT clients is well noted in the literature (King and McKeown 2004; Mair 2003). Mental health therapists require an understanding of how the psychological development of growing up LGBT differs from mainstream heterosexual development. Core training on LGBT development and lifestyle is central to recognize and avoid heteronormative bias, to gain awareness of internalized bias in the LGBT client, to gain awareness of personal attitudes that could impact the therapeutic relationship, and to consider the advantages and disadvantages of self-disclosure of sexual orientation and identity (King et al. 2007). Conversion or reparative therapy describes a range of psychological treatments that aim to change sexual orientation from homosexual to heterosexual. As a culturally competent practitioner, it is essential to understand the impact of conversion therapy in terms of its anti-gay impact on the individual and on society. Research has demonstrated that attempts by mental health professionals to pathologize and treat or change sexual orientation are unwelcome and lead to dissatisfactions and lower perceived helpfulness of therapy (King et al. 2007).

Counselor competency is especially critical for LGBT older adults receiving mental health services from majority group members (i.e., heterosexual service providers). The long-term effect of living in a minority status leaves the LGBT elder with more vulnerability to experiencing low self-esteem and internalized homophobia. The counselor must acknowledge the synergy of the two minority statuses (age and LGBT) and assist the client in creating positive self-esteem that defies the negative messages from society.

Counselor competency in LGBT elder issues requires that the counselor be sensitive to the following:

- The social and historical context presented by the client

  The counselor must be cognizant of how LGBT elders have been affected by the physical and social setting of a society where the cultural normative was heterosexuality and where LGBT elders were identified as the "Other" (e.g., different and separated from the norm). The historical context (i.e., politics, culture, religion, economics, mood, and attitudes) of the time played a dominant role in the individual development of the LGBT elder both positively and negatively.

- The language utilized by the client specific to their historical context

  The counselor must be conscious of the language and the meanings conveyed by language associated with the societal and cultural environment. The language utilized by the LGBT elder should be seen as indicative of their perception of the larger society.

- Ageism, fear of aging, homophobia, and transphobia (i.e., attitudes and prejudices within the larger society and within the LGBT community)

  Counselor education regarding the effects of ageism, fear of aging, homophobia, and transphobia is essential to counselor competency. The counselor's ability to relate to, empathize with, and assist the LGBT elder in the navigation of systems that are negatively affecting the individual is an imperative.

- Empathy and compassion regarding the LGBT/minority experience

  The counselor's ability to comprehend and show compassion of the minority experience will have a profound effect on the professional relationship. What does the minority experience specific to sexual orientation and gender mean to the individual's self-identity? How does this particular minority experience influence the LGBT elder's relationship with others and with himself? What are the other minority experiences of the LGBT elder and how have they affected the individual's development?

- Understanding of the intersectionality between LGBT issues, race, ethnicity, and aging

  The counselor's ability to understand the intersectionality of LGBT issues, race, ethnicity, and aging is critical to a holistic perception of the LGBT elder. What have been the experiences of the LGBT elder because of their sexual orientation, gender, race, ethnicity, and aging? Have these factors intersected, collided, or both? All of the factors identified have presented the

LGBT elder with both positive and negative experiences.

- Provision of an inclusive environment
  Providing an inclusive environment is central to building trust within the counselor/client relationship. An inclusive and welcoming environment includes honesty, flexibility, recognizing and valuing differences, open dialogue, and respectful interactions.

The implications of empirical data on this topic suggest that the mental health system must do more than sensitize counselors to the issues that face LGBT older adults. It is critical to provide education and training to create culturally competent providers skilled at person-centered care. Counselor competency specific to LGBT older adults must incorporate an understanding of the stigma, discrimination, and long-term effects of the sexual minority experience coupled with the aging experience for LGBT people in a society where youth is valued and the aging process is often misunderstood.

Counselor competency with the LGBT community, and specifically LGBT older adults, requires ongoing training and translation. The goal of training is far greater than simply sensitizing counselors to issues that LGBT older adults face; training must include the voices of the LGBT community through face-to-face interaction in order to gain deeper insight and understanding of an LGBT individual. Counselor competency for LGBT elders and the larger LGBT community requires that the mental health system seeks out LGBT professionals with the intent to collaborate with, refer clients to, and dialogue about LGBT issues that benefit both clients and the larger community. It is imperative that counselors receive appropriate training regarding the LGBT culture and lifestyle and that there is honesty and empathy in their understanding of the long-term effects of living a minority status in mainstream society. Ultimately, competent counseling requires the provision of a safe and trusting environment. Therefore, a competent counselor will strive to provide a person-centered approach to care by creating a safe and nonjudgmental therapeutic environment that encourages honesty and self-acceptance.

Discussion Box 3
Is it important to know about the sexual orientation of an older adult client seeking mental health services? Why or why not?

In general, do you think LGBT individuals age well? Why or why not? What risk factors or protective factors do you think are important?

Discussion Box 4
In your own words, define counselor competency **specific to the needs** of LGBT older adults.

What does your definition of counselor competency include? Is your definition inclusive?

Profile
Ms. G and Ms. B are 70-year-old lesbians who have been in a loving committed relationship for 37 years. The couple was married in 2008 in California. Both Ms. G and Ms. B report that when they came out 40 years ago, neither of their parents was happy. Ms. G's parents made attempts to get Ms. G's ex-husband to secure sole custody of their children due to their homophobic attitudes and fear that their grandchildren would have emotional scars. However, he would not, and instead, they shared custody of their children. At age 70, Ms. G is a practicing mental health therapist and counsels LGBT clients. "During my training, we focused strongly on understanding the dynamics unique to the lives of minority clients including women, LGBTQ, and people of color." Question for discussion: What elements of Ms. G and Ms. B's lives support their optimal aging?

Critical Research to Mental Health Issues of LGBT Elders

Although very few empirical studies have been conducted on mental health of the aging LGBT population, studies that do exist have demonstrated high life satisfaction and positive attributes to aging as an LGBT individual (Berger 1992). A study conducted by D'Augelli et al. (2001) found that mental health in older adulthood was influenced by better physical health, better cognitive functioning, higher self-esteem, less loneliness, and a higher percentage of people knowing about the individual's sexual orientation. In addition, suicidal ideation was predicted by negative feelings about one's sexual orientation, loneliness, and few people knowing about the individuals' sexual orientation. D'Augelli et al. 2001 found that vast majority of LGBT older adults in their sample reported good-to-excellent mental health and unchanged or improved mental health over the past five years. Mental health was positively related to income, indicating better mental health for those with higher income, and was negatively correlated with victimization, indicating that people who reported more victimization had lower levels of mental health. D'Augelli and Grossman (2001) looked at how disclosure of sexual orientation and victimization related to mental health in a sample of LGBT older adults aged 60 and older. Study results indicated that almost three-quarters of participants reported some form of victimization (verbal and/or physical). Poor mental health, as indicated by lower self-esteem, more loneliness, and more suicide attempts were reported by those that had been physically attacked (D'Augelli and Grossman 2001).

Studies have demonstrated that the prevalence of mood and anxiety disorders, substance abuse, and suicide attempts is higher among LGBT individuals than among heterosexuals (Cochran et al. 2003; Lytle et al. 2014). A meta-analysis by King et al. (2007) found that sexual minority individuals have a 1.5 times higher risk for depression and anxiety disorders and are 2.5 times more likely to attempt suicide than

heterosexuals. Cochran et al. (2003) found that the prevalence of panic attacks was greater in gay or bisexual men than in heterosexual men and that lesbian or bisexual women had a significantly greater 12-month prevalence of GADs.

A study by Lombardi (2009) found that older transgender people reported more stress as a result of lifetime experiences of discrimination. Study results found that post-transition, older people reported more discrimination and stress, which continues as a constant experience for people even after they transition (Lombardi 2009).

Related Disciplines Influencing Service Delivery and Interdisciplinary Approaches

LGBT older adults will seek services from an interdisciplinary team of professionals as they age within their communities. This cadre of professionals will include gerontologists, social workers, psychologists, geropsychologists, administrators, and healthcare and allied healthcare professionals.

The National Association of Social Workers (NASW) states, as one of its dual missions, to "seek to enhance the effective functioning and well-being of individuals, families, and communities through its work and through its advocacy." Social workers assist individuals, families, and communities in their attempt to reach their full potential through a myriad of services. Working in a variety of fields, social workers provide services in schools, churches, hospitals, police departments, prisons, community mental health clinics, psychiatric hospitals, not-for-profit and for-profit organizations, retirement communities, nursing homes, substance abuse clinics, court systems, and in other arenas. In the provision of social work services to LGBT elders, social workers are integral in assisting LGBT elders to find their voice and advocate for themselves. Social workers can and do provide avenues for interdisciplinary service involvement through their participation in many different fields in the community. For example, a medical social worker providing case management services in the home of a client will have a better understanding regarding the struggles the older adult is having that is limiting his ability to take his medications. The social worker would be able to share with the medical team the client's issues, and an action plan would be put in place to decrease and/or eliminate concerns. Also, in the provision of services to LGBT elders, social workers offer support, advocacy, and a voice. Acting as a bridge and a support system, social workers engage other disciplines on behalf of the LGBT elder seeking services. The discipline of social work influences service delivery positively through the utilization of a holistic and strength perspective offering nonjudgmental interventions.

As a discipline, psychology studies the behavior of humans and how their minds work in order to improve human behavior. Psychologists and geropsychologists deliver mental health counseling, as well as administer psychological evaluations, testing, and diagnosis. A psychologist or geropsychologist can work with older adults to cognitive and mood assessments and individual and group counseling. The American Psychological Association (APA) has demonstrated a commitment to research and education to support LGBT mental health and has established a division (Div 44) for the psychological study of LGBT issues.

An interdisciplinary approach to service delivery for the LGBT aging community is essential to the provision of culturally competent care. Aside from mental health professionals, medical and allied health professionals will require education and training on specific issues relevant to aging as an LGBT individual. Medical and allied health professionals are often the first stop in the care continuum and are responsible for providing appropriate services and/or referrals to meet the needs of their clients. In order to break down the barriers to seeking mental health services, an interdisciplinary approach to service provision will be necessary to ensure quality mental health care for LGBT older adults.

Summary

Culturally competent practice is essential to address the mental health needs of the aging LGBT community. A culturally competent practitioner must have awareness of issues that specifically impact sexual minority clients along with topics that are relevant specifically to older adults. Practitioners must be aware of the diversity of cultures in which LGBT older adults developed in order to comprehensively address current mental health needs. In other words, both the potential risk factors and protective factors experienced over the course of the life span must be examined as a part of a holistic therapeutic plan for an LGBT older adult.

In addressing the mental health needs of LGBT older adults, it is essential to take a person-centered approach to care and service provision. Person-centeredness recognizes the uniqueness of each person and empowers the individual to be the driver of her own care. Becoming a culturally competent mental health provider requires taking a person-centered approach by recognizing that meeting one older person is meeting ONE older person. Culturally competent service providers and practitioners are aware of generalizations based on age, sexual orientation, and/or gender identity. Culturally competent service providers and practitioners take into account the unique history and life experiences of each individual and her life journey to provide holistic person-centered care.

Learning Exercises for Knowledge Gain

1. According to minority stress theory, LGBT individuals face disparities in health outcomes, which are explained by stressors induced by discrimination and victimization (Meyer 2003). How does minority stress theory specifically relate to an LGBT older adult? How does minority stress theory relate

to LGBT older adults seeking mental health services?

2. Identify 5 barriers for LGBT older adults that may prevent them from accessing mental health services.

3. Describe 5 essential components of culturally competent training for mental health providers working with older LGBT clients.

4. Why is body image and eating particularly prevalent among gay men? How does the view of aging within the LGBT community impact body image and eating disorders?

Multiple-Choice Questions

1. Which of the following is a cause of depression and anxiety in LGBT elders?
   (a) Low self-esteem
   (b) Isolation
   (c) Denial of true self
   (d) All of the above

2. George is a 75-year-old gay man who never came out with his family and friends. Which of the following would he likely be at an increased risk for?
   (a) GAD
   (b) Higher blood pressure
   (c) High cholesterol
   (d) A personality disorder

3. A welcoming environment would include all of the following except
   (a) An inclusive gender section (i.e., male, female, transgender)
   (b) A non-discriminatory policy
   (c) Male- and female-only restrooms
   (d) Courteous, respectful staff

4. Which of the following is a barrier to service utilization?
   (a) Open and honest communication
   (b) Fear of discrimination
   (c) Professional's knowledge of the LGBT community
   (d) Nonjudgmental, safe space that includes messages of inclusiveness

5. Which of the following is true regarding counselor competency?
   (a) It requires understanding of the sexual minority experience
   (b) Becoming a culturally competent mental health provider requires taking a psychoanalytic approach
   (c) Training and education on LGBT aging issues is important for promoting counselor competency
   (d) Both A & C

6. Counselor competency in LGBT elder issues requires that the counselor understands
   (a) Social and historical context presented by the client
   (b) Knowledge of the client's views on fashion
   (c) Understanding of the intersectionality between LGBT issues, race, ethnicity, and aging.
   (d) Both A & D

7. Transphobia is
   (a) A lack of understanding of the psychology of the transgender individual
   (b) A feeling of unease toward those who identify as transgender
   (c) A clinical terminology no longer used to describe men who dress as women
   (d) The fear of people who are bisexual

8. Transgender individuals often experience discrimination in the form of
   (a) Employment discrimination
   (b) Physical abuse
   (c) Verbal harassment
   (d) All of the above

9. What are the factors that can negatively impact the mental health of LGBT older adults?
   (a) Self-imposed or societal isolation
   (b) A pattern of out-of-control sexual behavior
   (c) Ageism
   (d) Both A & C

10. Research has demonstrated that good mental health outcomes were indicated for LGBT individuals
    (a) Who had lifetime partners
    (b) Had an active religious affiliation
    (c) Who were out about their sexual orientation or gender identify
    (d) Both A & C

Key

1. (D)
2. (A)
3. (C)
4. (B)
5. (D)
6. (D)
7. (B)
8. (D)
9. (D)
10. (C)

Field-Based Experiential Assignments

1. Interview a mental health practitioner that specializes in working with LGBT clients. What did you learn about addressing the psychological/mental health needs of LGBT elders? What advice were you given about how to be a culturally competent provider?

2. Attend training on a mental health topic for LGBT older adults. The training can be facilitated by a local LGBT organization or a national LGBT organization such as Services and Advocacy with Gay, Lesbian, Bisexual and Transgender Elders (SAGE) or another institute providing education and training to the community.

3. Volunteer with the local LGBT Community Center in your area to become more familiar with LGBT community needs and resources and specifically to investigate the community needs of the aging LGBT population.

Resources

1. National Alliance on Mental Illness. http://www.nami.org/Content/NavigationMenu/Find_Support/Multicultural_Support/Resources/GLBT_Resources.htm

2. LGBT Aging Resources Issues Clearinghouse (part of the American Society on Aging) http://asaging.org/lgbt_aging_resources_clearinghouse

3. National Resource Center on LGBT aging http://www.lgbtagingcenter.org/

4. The Pride Institute http://pride-institute.com/

5. National LGBT Health Education Center at the Fenway Institute www.lgbthealtheducation.org

6. Project HEALTH—A program of Lyon-Martin Health Services and the Transgender Law Center www.project-health.org

7. SAMHSA Top Health Issues for LGBT Populations Information and Resource Toolkit http://store.samhsa.gov/product/Top-Health-Issues-for-LGBT-Populations/SMA12-4684.

References

Aneshensel, C. S. (1992). Social stress: Theory and research. *Annual review of sociology, 18*(1), 15–38.

Barranti, C., & Cohen, H. (2000). Lesbian and gay elders: An invisible minority. In R. Schneider, N. Kropt, & A. Kisor (Eds.), *Gerontological social work: Knowledge, service setting, and special populations* (2nd ed., pp. 343–367). Belmont, CA: Wadsworth.

Beekman, A. T., Copeland, J. R., & Prince, M. J. (1999). Review of community prevalence of depression in later life. *British Journal of Psychiatry, 174*, 307–311.

Berger, R. M. (1992). Research on older gay men: What we know, what we need to know. In J. J. Woodman (Ed.), *Lesbian and gay lifestyles: A guide for counseling and education* (pp. 217–234). New York: Irvington.

Blazer, D. G., & Hybels, C. F. (2005). Origins of depression in later life. *Psychological Medicine, 35*, 1241–1252.

Bockting, W. O., Knudson, G., & Goldberg, J. M. (2006). Counseling and mental health care for transgender adults and loved ones. *International Journal of Transgenderism, 9*(3–4), 35–82.

Browne, D., Woltman, M., Tumarkin, L., Dyer, S., & Buchbinder, S. (2008). Improving lesbian, gay, bisexual and transgender access to healthcare at New York City health and hospitals corporation facilities.

Clements, K. (1999). *The transgender community health project: Descriptive results*. San Francisco: San Francisco Department of Public Health.

Clements-Noelle, K., Marx, R., Guzman, R., & Katz, M. (2001). HIV prevalence, risk behaviors, health care use, and mental health status of transgender persons: Implications for public health intervention. *American Journal of Public Health, 91*, 915.

Cochran, S. D., & Mays, V. M. (2000). Lifetime prevalence of suicide symptoms and affective disorders among men reporting same-sex sexual partners: Results from NHANES III. *American Journal of Public Health, 90*(4), 573.

Cochran, S. D., Sullivan, J. G., & Mays, V. M. (2003). Prevalence of mental disorders, psychological distress, and mental health services use among lesbian, gay, and bisexual adults in the United States. *Journal of Consulting and Clinical Psychology, 71*(1), 53.

D'Augelli, A. R., & Grossman, A. H. (2001). Disclosure of sexual orientation, victimization, and mental health among lesbian, gay, and bisexual older adults. *Journal of Interpersonal Violence, 16*(10), 1008–1027.

D'Augelli, A. R., Grossman, A. H., Hershberger, S. L., & O'Connell, T. S. (2001). Aspects of mental health among older lesbian, gay, and bisexual adults. *Aging and Mental Health, 5, 149.*

Davenport -Hines, R. (1990). *Sex, death and punishment: Attitudes to sex and sexuality in Britain since the Renaissance.* London: Collins.

Dohrenwend, B. P. (2000). The role of adversity and stress in psychopathology: Some evidence and its implications for theory and research. *Journal of health and social behavior,* 1–19.

Feldman, M. B., & Meyer, I. H. (2007). Eating disorders in diverse lesbian, gay, and bisexual populations. *International Journal of Eating Disorders, 40*(3), 218–226.

Fredriksen-Goldsen, K. I., & Muraco, A. (2010). Aging and sexual orientation: A 25-year review of the literature. *Research on Aging, 32*(3), 372–413.

French, S. A., Story, M., Remafedi, G., Resnick, M. D., & Blum, R. W. (1996). Sexual orientation and prevalence of body dissatisfaction and eating disordered behaviors: A population-based study of adolescents. *International Journal of Eating Disorders, 19,* 119–126.

Gabbay, S. G., & Wahler, J. J. (2002). Lesbian aging: Review of a growing literature. *Journal of Gay & Lesbian Social Services, 14*(3), 1–21.

Glacken, M., & Higgens, A. (2008). The grief experience of same sex couples within an Irish context: Tacit acknowledgement. *International Journal of Palliative Nursing, 14,* 297–302.

Herek, G. M., & Garnets, L. D. (2007). Sexual orientation and mental health. *Annual Review of Clinical Psychology, 3,* 353–375.

Herzog, D. B., Newman, K. L., & Warshaw, M. (1991). Body image dissatisfaction in homosexual and heterosexual males. *Journal of Nervous and Mental Disease, 179,* 356–359.

Hill, D. B. (2002). *Genderism, transphobia, and gender bashing: A framework for interpreting anti-transgender violence.* Thousand Oaks, CA: Sage.

Hybels, C. F., & Blazer, D. G. (2003). Epidemiology of late-life mental disorders. *Clinics in Geriatric Medicine, 19*(4), 663–696.

Jacobson, S., & Grossman, A. H. (1996). Older lesbians and gay men: Old myths, new images, and future directions. *The lives of lesbians, gays, and bisexuals: Children to adults,* pp. 345–373.

Jorm, A. F. (2000). Does old age reduce the risk of anxiety and depression? A review of epidemiological studies across the adult life span. *Psychological Medicine, 30,* 11–22.

Kimmel, D. (1978). Adult development and aging: A gay perspective. *Journal of Social Issues, 34,* 113–130.

King, M., McKeown, E. (2004). Gay and lesbian identities and mental health. In D. Kelleher & G. Leavey (Eds.), *Identity and Health.* London: Routledge.

King, M., Semlyen, J., Tai, S. S., Killaspy, H., Osborn, D., Popelyuk, D., & Nazareth, I. (2007). A systematic review of mental disorder, suicide, and deliberate self harm in lesbian, gay and bisexual people. *BMC Psychiatry, 8*(1), 70.

Lakkis, J., Ricciardelli, L. A., & Williams, R. J. (1999). The role of sexual orientation and gender related-traits in disordered eating. *Sex Roles, 41*(1–2), 1–16.

Lewis, D. M., & Cachelin, F. M. (2001). Body image, body dissatisfaction, and eating attitudes in midlife and elderly women. *Eating Disorders, 9,* 29–39.

Lombardi, E. (2001). Enhancing transgender health care. *American Journal of Public Health, 91*(6), 869–872.

Lombardi, E. (2009). Varieties of transgender/transsexual lives and their relationships with transphobia. *Journal of Homosexuality, 56,* 977–992.

Lytle, M. C., Luca, S. M., & Blosnich, J. R. (2014). The influence of intersecting identities on self-harm, suicidal behaviors, and depression among lesbian, gay, and bisexual individuals. *Suicide and Life-Threatening Behavior, 44,* 384.

Mackenzie, C. S., Reynolds, K., Chou, K. L., Pagura, J., & Sareen, J. (2011). Prevalence and correlates of generalized anxiety disorder in a national sample of older adults. *The American Journal of Geriatric Psychiatry, 19*(4), 305–315.

Mair, D. (2003). Gay men's experiences of therapy. *Counseling and Psychotherapy Research Journal, 3,* 33–41.

Makadon, H., Mayer, K., Potter, J., & Goldhammer, H. (2008). *The Fenway guide to gay, lesbian, bisexual and transgender health.*

Mays, V. M., & Cochran, S. D. (2001). Mental health correlates of perceived discrimination among lesbian, gay, and bisexual adults in the United States. *American Journal of Public Health, 91*(11), 1869–1876.

McIntyre, J., Daley, A., Rutherford, K., & Ross, L. E. (2011). Systems level barriers in accessing supportive mental health services for sexual and gender minorities: Insights from the provider's perspective. *Canadian Journal of Community Mental Health, 30*(2), 173–186.

Meyer, C., Blissett, J., & Oldfield, C. (2001). Sexual orientation and eating psychopathology: The role of masculinity and femininity. *International Journal of Eating Disorders, 29*(3), 314–318.

Meyer, I. H. (1995). Minority stress and mental health in gay men. *Journal of Health and Social Behavior, 36* (1), 38–56.

Meyer, I. H. (2003). Prejudice, social stress, and mental health in lesbian, gay, and bisexual populations: Conceptual issues and research evidence. *Psychological Bulletin, 129*(5), 674.

Meyer, I. H. (2007). Prejudice and discrimination as social stressors. In *The health of sexual minorities* (pp. 242–267). Springer US.

Murnen, S. K., & Smolak, L. (1997). Femininity, masculinity, and disordered eating: A meta-analytic review. *International Journal of Eating Disorders, 22,* 231–242.

National Alliance on Mental Illness. (n.d.). Retrieved August 18, 2014, from http://www.nami.org/Template.cfm?Section=Depression&Template=/ContentManagement/ContentDisplay.cfm&ContentID=144036.

National Institute on Mental Illness (2014). State Mental Health Legislation 2014: Trends, Themes & Effective Practices. NAMI.

Orel, N. A. (2004). Gay, lesbian, and bisexual elders: Expressed needs and concerns across focus groups. *Journal of Gerontological Social Work, 43*(2/3), 57–75.

Pritchard, M. (2008). Disordered eating in undergraduates: Does gender role orientation influence men and women the same way? *Sex Roles, 59*(3–4), 282–289.

Rado, S. (1949). A adaptational view of sexual behavior. In P. H. Hoch & J. Zubin (Eds.), *Psychosexual Development in Health and Disease.* New York: Grune & Statton.

Reback, C. J., Simon, P. A., Bemis, C. C., & Gatson, B. (2001). *The Los Angeles transgender health study: Community report.* Los Angeles: University of California at Los Angeles.

Rubin, R. H. (2001). Alternative lifestyles revisited, or whatever happened to swingers, group marriages, and communes? *Journal of Family Issues, 22*(6), 711–726.

Schope, R. D. (2005). Who's afraid of growing old? Gay and lesbian perceptions of aging. *Journal of Gerontological Social Work, 45*(4), 23–39.

Siever, M. D. (1994). Sexual orientation and gender as factors in socioculturally acquired vulnerability to body dissatisfaction and eating disorders. *Journal of Consulting and Clinical Psychology, 62*(2), 252.

Smith, G., Bartlett, A., & King, M. (2004). Treatments of homosexuality in Britain since the 1950s—an oral history: The experience of patients. *BMJ, 328*(7437), 427.

Striegel-Moore, R. H., Tucker, N., & Hsu, J. (1990). Body image dissatisfaction and disordered eating in lesbian college students. *International Journal of Eating Disorders, 9*(5), 493–500.

Strong, S. M., Williamson, D. A., Netemeyer, R. G., & Geer, J. H. (2000). Eating disorder symptoms and concerns about body differ as a function of gender and sexual orientation. *Journal of Social and Clinical Psychology, 19*(2), 240–255.

Substance Abuse and Mental Health Services Administration. (2014). Affordable care act enrollment assistance for LGBT communities, a resource for behavioral health providers. Rockville, MD, substance abuse and mental health services administration.

The Aging and Health Report Disparities and Resilience among Lesbian, Gay, Bisexual, and Transgender Older Adults. (2010). Retrieved August 18, 2014, from, http://caringandaging.org/wordpress/wp-content/uploads/2012/10/Full-report10-25-12.pdf.

Webster, J., & Tiggemann, M. (2003). The relationship between women's body satisfaction and self-image across the life span: The role of cognitive control. *The Journal of Genetic Psychology, 164*(2), 241–252.

Wichstrom, L. (2006). Sexual orientation as a risk factor for bulimic symptoms. *International Journal of Eating Disorders, 39*(6), 448–453.

Williamson, I., & Hartley, P. (1998). British research into the increased vulnerability of young gay men to eating disturbance and body dissatisfaction. *European Eating Disorders Review, 6,* 160–170.

Yager, J. (2000). Weighty perspectives: Contemporary challenges in obesity and eating disorders. *American Journal of Psychiatry, 157*(6), 851–853.

Substance Use Disorders Intervention with LGBT Elders

Debra A. Harley and Michael T. Hancock

Abstract

Substance use disorders (SUDs) and mental health problems frequently co-occur. SUDs are one of the most common psychiatric diagnoses in older adults. The purpose of this chapter is to discuss SUDs among LGBT elders. Information is presented on the scope of SUDs, prevalence and patterns of use, SUDs and aging comorbidity, assessment, diagnosis, and treatment of LGBT elders. This chapter provides the reader with a baseline for understanding issues that impact and influence LGBT elders' substance use. There is no suggestion that LGBT status is synonymous with addiction or mental illness disorders. Thus, the chapter explores the extent to which SUDs exist among LGBT elders.

Keywords

Substance use disorders · Addiction · Mental health · Alcohol · Drugs · Prescription medication

Overview

Substance use disorders (SUDs) are recognized as a public health issues in the United States and in many parts of the world. The reasons people use and/or abuse alcohol and other drugs are varied, ranging from use to cope with stress, pain, and to escape, to a means to relax and socialize, to being accepted by peers, and others.

Rarely do people say that they consume alcohol because they like the taste or use drugs because they are good for them. For many LGBT persons, the use of alcohol is an intrinsic part of the gay bar scene, which is a cultural norm of the gay community. For many LGBT elders who grew up during a time of secrecy about their sexual orientation and gender identity, the gay bar represented the only safe place for socialization. As many LGBT adults age, they become isolated, especially as a result of disability and chronic illness, and substances become a means to deal with isolation. In this chapter, we examine issues

D.A. Harley (✉) · M.T. Hancock
University of Kentucky, Lexington, USA
e-mail: dharl00@email.uky.edu

© Springer International Publishing Switzerland 2016
D.A. Harley and P.B. Teaster (eds.), *Handbook of LGBT Elders*,
DOI 10.1007/978-3-319-03623-6_24

473

related to substance used, including mental health concerns, for LGBT elders.

Learning Objectives

By the end of the chapter, the reader should be able to:

1. Identify issues of SUDs for LGBT elders.
2. Understand the co-occurrence of SUDs and mental health concerns for LGBT elders.
3. Identify issues related to assessment, diagnosis, and treatment of SUDs in LGBT elders.
4. Identify policy concerns for addressing SUDs among LGBT elders.

Introduction

Currently, almost half of men and slightly over half of women over the age of 60 consume alcoholic beverages (Barnes et al. 2010) and most do not abuse alcohol. The majority of older adults are considered social drinkers. In general, alcohol consumption decreases with increasing age (International Center for Alcohol Policies [ICAP] 2014). Alcohol and drug use in older adults can be late-onset or one that began in young adulthood. Nevertheless, SUDs, which include alcohol, drugs, prescription medication, nicotine, and caffeine (Diagnostic and Statistical Manual of Mental Disorders 2013), among older adults are major and growing problems (Substance Abuse and Mental Health Services Administration [SAMHSA] 2008). The extent of the problem may be greater than suspected because of a misconception that older adults do not abuse alcohol and other drugs (AODs); consequently, healthcare professionals do not need to worry about SUD in this population. As a result of these misperceptions, healthcare professionals typically are the first to identify SUDs in elderly persons and to screen infrequently for substance abuse in their older patients.

For LGBT elders, the issue of underdiagnosis and gross underestimation of SUDs may be even greater because they have fewer resources in the community and within healthcare systems for prevention, earlier diagnosis, assessment, and treatment, and they may not seek services or ask for assistance (Ellison 2012; Jessup and Dibble 2012). Thus, as the baby boom cohort reaches retirement age, it encounters a healthcare system ill-prepared to deal with older adults with SUDs (Doweiko 2015).

SUDs are the third most common psychiatric diagnosis in older adults (Luggen 2006). The presence of both substance abuse and mental illness within a person is known as co-occurring disorder (COD). Although the majority of LGBT elders are in good mental health, significant percentages have symptoms of depression, anxiety, and AOD abuse higher than the general population (King et al. 2008; SAMHSA 2012). Limited information on the actual rates of SUDs among LGBT elders suggests that substance use among this population is highly correlated with poor mental health (Conron et al. 2010) and is a response to stressors related to violence, discrimination, internalized homophobia, low self-esteem, loneliness, stigma, and experiences of victimization based on sexual orientation and gender identity or expression (Frederiksen-Goldsen and Muraco 2010). In comparison with the general population, LGBT persons are more likely to use alcohol and drugs, have higher rates of substance abuse, are less likely to abstain from use, and are more likely to continue heavy drinking into later life (SAMHSA 2012). Lesbians and gay men perceive themselves to be at increased risk of SUDs, have an increased need for treatment, and face barriers to treatment. Moreover, the rates of alcohol consumption among lesbians and gay men do not seem to decrease with age as quickly as they do among heterosexuals (Healthy People 2010 2010).

The purpose of this chapter is to identify SUDs issues pertinent to LGBT elders. Given that SUDs and mental health frequently co-occur, reference is made to both SUDs and mental illness throughout this chapter. Information is presented on the scope of SUDs; prevalence and patterns of use; alcohol, drugs, and aging comorbidity; detection, assessment, and diagnosis of SUDs; and treatment and intervention of LGBT elders. Finally, discussion of implications for policy is presented. The intent of this chapter is to provide the reader with baseline information for understanding issues that impact and influence LGBT elders' substance use behavior. Considerable individual variation exists regarding LGBT elders on the basis of age, gender, sexual orientation, and gender identity or expression. We stress that being LGBT is not synonymous with having an addiction (Beatty and Lewis 2003) or mental health disorders (see Chap. 23 for additional information on mental health).

The Scope of SUDs

Alcohol is the most commonly abused substance by elderly people; approximately 15 % of older drinkers have a concurrent drug abuse disorder (Ellison 2012). Prescription medication misuse (i.e., non-medical use) and abuse are growing public health problems among older adults in the United States. Most misused medications are obtained legally through prescriptions. Usually, problematic prescription medication use by older adults is unintentional and falls into the misuse category, though it can progress to abuse if they continue to use a medication for only the desirable effects it provides (Addiction Technology Transfer Center Network [ATTC] 2009). Regardless of age, individuals who seek a prescription with the aim to use the medication inappropriately and who may have already become addicted present with certain characteristics and behaviors (see Table 24.1).

Older adults are at high risk of medication misuse because of conditions associated with pain, sleep disorders and insomnia, and anxiety. Elders are more likely than their younger counterparts to receive prescriptions for psychoactive medications with misuse and abuse potential (e.g., opioid analgesics, benzodiazepines) (Administration on Aging 2012). According to Basca (2008), medication for persons age 65 and

older account for one-third of all medications prescribed, accounting for only 13 % of the population in the United States. Older women are at higher risk because they are more likely to use psychoactive medications, usually associated with divorce, widowhood, lower income, poorer health status, depression, and/or anxiety. Elderly women take an average of five prescription medications at a time for longer periods of time compared to older men (Basca). Prolonged use of psychoactive medications has been associated with confusion, falls, hip fractures, loss of motivation, memory problems, difficulties with activities of daily living, declines in personal grooming and hygiene, and withdrawal from normal social activities in older adults. The use of opioid analgesics can lead to excessive sedation, respiratory depression, and impairment in vision, attention, and coordination (Simoni-Wastila and Yang 2006). Moreover, adverse drug reactions are more common among the elderly.

Due to multiple chronic illnesses, an elderly person may be under the care of more than one doctor, none of whom may be fully informed about the complete range of medications the patient is taking. As drug regimens become more complex, there is increased probability of error by the patient as well as a greater potential for drug interactions. The chance of drug interactions is further complicated by an older adult's use of over-the-counter drugs. Many medications that once were available only by prescription are now available without one. Older adults take seven times more over-the-counter drugs than do persons of any other age-group (Kinney 2011). Unfortunately, physicians must rely on patient self-report about the type, dosage, and frequency of over-the-counter drugs being taken.

Many prescribed and over-the-counter drugs can interact with alcohol. Physiological changes that occur with aging that affect drug distribution and metabolism can contribute to the increased risk of drug–alcohol interactions. Certain medications commonly taken by older adults (e.g., aspirin, oral anticoagulants, antihistamines, oral medication for diabetes, pain medication) can present problems in the presence of alcohol. While the elderly exhibit alcohol and other drug

Table 24.1 Characteristics of prescription-seeking persons

Unusual behavior in the waiting room or extremes of either slovenliness or being over-dressed
Assertive personality, often demanding immediate attention
Having unusually detailed knowledge of controlled substances and/or giving their medical history with textbook symptoms, or, in contrast giving evasive or vague answers to questions regarding their medical history
Stating they have no regular doctor or health insurance, or they are reluctant or unwilling to provide that information
Making specific request for a particular controlled drug and unwillingness to consider a different drug that is suggested as an alternative
Not showing much interest in their diagnosis and not keeping an appointment for further test, or refusing to see another professional for consultation
Appearing to exaggerate medical problems
Exhibiting mood disturbances, suicidal thoughts, lack of impulse control, thought disorders, and/or sexual dysfunction, all of which may be an indication of the misuse of medications
State that they must be seen right away
Want an appointment toward the end of office hours
Call or come in after regular office hours
State that they are just traveling through town and visiting friends or relatives
Present with physical problems that can only be relieved with narcotic drugs
Present with anxiety, insomnia, fatigue, or depression that can be reduced with stimulants or depressants
State that non-narcotic pain relievers do not work or that they have an allergic reaction to them
Claim to be a client of another health professional who is not available
State that their prescription has been lost, spoiled, or stolen and needs replacing
Request refills more often than originally prescribed

Adapted from Department of Justice, Drug Enforcement Administration, Office of Diversion Control (1999)

(AOD) use, illicit drug use (e.g., marijuana, cocaine, heroin) is low (Kinney 2011). However, illicit drug use may be increasing in a small percentage of the elderly population, such as the baby boomers (SAMHSA 2006). Illicit drug use in elders is linked to long-term drug use. According to Simoni-Wastila and Yang (2006), "older addicts may simply represent younger addicts who have survived their drug-use disorder" (p. 383).

By 2020, it is estimated about 2.7 million older adults will present with a drug addiction (Colliver et al. 2006). Estimating the number of LGBT elders among those with SUDs is difficult for the following reasons: Many LGBT persons do not disclose their LGBT status, substance abuse programs do not conduct outreach specific or implement LGBT-inclusive services to this population, intake and application forms do not contain questions about sexual identity, and LGBT persons have difficulty fully accessing

substance abuse prevention and treatment services (Wilkinson 2008). Although much less is known about bisexual and transgender men and women, they may be at increased risk of substance abuse because in addition to being discriminated against by the heterosexual community, they are frequently further marginalized by the gay and lesbian community.

Prevalence and Patterns of Use

The patterns of substance use and associated problems vary among the older adults, as well as the reasons for abusing substances. For some of the elders, substance abuse is linked to the stresses of aging. In behavioral terms, the best predictor of future behavior is past behavior, especially true for how someone will handle growing old. For example, those who have demonstrated flexibility throughout their lives will adapt well to stresses associated with aging. In addition, individuals with strengths and resiliency will adjust more readily to age-related stresses (Kinney 2011). Stresses of aging include, but are not limited to the following: (a) social stresses in which aging is equated with obsolescence and worthlessness, the process of receiving medical care and paying medical bills, and inadequate insurance coverage, especially for preventive services; (b) psychological stresses, with the greatest one for the elderly being loss (e.g., illness and death of family and friends, geographical separation of family, earned income, losses accompanying retirement); (c) biological stresses including physical disability, depressive illness with a physiological basis such as changes in the levels of neurochemicals, and dementia; and (d) iatrogenic stresses (harm caused by efforts to heal), which are by-products of the healthcare system and its insensitivities to elders' unique physiological and psychological changes. Usually, iatrogenic stresses are the result of overprescribing medication, failing to take into account the way the elderly metabolize medications, and ignoring that alcohol is also a toxic drug (Kinney). Kinney points out that as people age, they become less similar to one another and more individualistic; therefore, service providers should pay more attention to individual differences among elders.

Attention to alcohol use among older adults is important even when it does not qualify as abuse because it may cause or aggravate a range of health problems (Doweiko 2015; Kinney 2011). As people age, they become more sensitive to the effects of alcohol and medication, requiring less of the substance to feel its effects. Also, older adults have more physical and mental health issues than do younger adults (Ruscavage et al. 2006). Medical comorbidity in the older adults requires adequate monitoring, especially because the addition of substance abuse (resulting in multimorbidity) can complicate accurate diagnoses, including the length of time in order to make one. Multimorbidity makes it difficult to find a treatment that takes into account contradictions,

side effects, and drug interactions between substances, and affects the evolution of disease and the patient's functional status and his or her survival (Incalzi et al. 1997; Valderas et al. 2009).

Addiction rates are high among LGBT populations because of higher rates of depression, a need to escape from the constant presence of social stigma and homo/transphobia, efforts to either numb or enhance sexual feelings, to ease shame and guilt related to LGBT identity, and for some LGBT persons, peer pressure (www.recovery.org/topics/find-the-best-gay-lesbian-bisexual-transgender-lgbt-addiction-recovery-centers/#). Most LGBT elders report societal factors (e.g., discrimination, hate crimes, historical legal prohibitions on sexual behavior) as the reason for an increased prevalence of SUDs. Other anti-LGBT discrimination in situations that are unique to or particularly difficult for older people includes discrimination in housing, medical treatment, and public accommodations. Many LGBT elders are open about their sexuality and gender identity, but others remain closeted because they feel vulnerable and fear discrimination, abuse, or social condemnation. In addition, closeted LGBT elders may experience a certain level of stress when they come out later in life. These feelings lead to stressors for which they might use AOD as a means of coping or to reduce stress. LGBT persons across the age spectrum experience stigma, minority stress, and anti-gay/anti-trans social prejudice (Stevens 2012).

Today's older LGBT persons came of age when there were very few places in which they could safely express their sexuality or identity. One such place was gay bars, which play a central role in the LGBT community. Gay bars offer a place where LGBT persons might go to socialize without fear of ridicule, to meet potential partners, to relax, or to learn about one's sexuality and its implications for daily life (Doweiko 2015). Gay bars serve multiple functions for LGBT persons and have been described as a combination of bar, country club, and community center (http://www.agingincanada.ca/lgbt_older_adults.htm). Substance abuse, especially alcohol, is a large part of life of some segments of the LGBT community (SAMHSA 2012).

Alcohol, Drugs, and Aging Comorbidity

The effects of AOD on older adults are quite different than on younger adults, the majority of which stem from physiological changes associated with the aging process. Adults over the age of 65 have at least one chronic illness, which can increase their vulnerability to the negative effects of alcohol and/or drug consumption. In addition, specific age-related changes affect the way an older person responds to alcohol: (a) decrease in body water and increase in fat content, (b) increased sensitivity and decreased tolerance to alcohol, and (c) decrease in the metabolism of alcohol in the gastrointestinal tract. Each of these physiological changes results in a greater concentration in the blood system and quicker intoxication for older adults (SAMHSA 2008). The effects of alcohol on reaction time in older adults may well be responsible for some of the accidents, falls, and injuries that are prevalent in this age-group (Doweiko 2015). The interaction of age-related physiological changes and the consumption of high levels of AODs can trigger or exacerbate other serious health issues among older adults (see Table 24.2). Conversely, small amounts of alcohol have been shown to provide health benefits in older adults who do not have

Table 24.2 AOD abuse and comorbidities in older adults

Malnutrition
Cognitive impairment
Decreased bone density
Gastrointestinal bleeding
Alcohol-related dementia
Sleep pattern disturbances
Cirrhosis and other liver diseases
Increased risk of hemorrhagic stroke
Mental health problems, including depression and anxiety
Impaired immune system and capacity to combat infection and cancer
Increased risk of hypertension, cardiac arrhythmia, myocardial infarction, and cardiomyopathy

Adapted from SAMHSA (2008)

certain medical conditions, taking certain medications, or a history of AOD abuse. For example, alcohol has been shown to be a protective factor against coronary heart disease, heart failure, and myocardial infarction, particularly in older men (Djousse and Gaziano 2007; Gronbaek 2006). For postmenopausal women, moderate drinking can contribute to an improvement in bone density and a reduction in the risk of osteoporosis (Rapuri et al. 2000). In both elderly women and men, light-to-moderate drinking is associated with a reduced incidence of type 2 diabetes mellitus (Djousse et al. 2007). Elders who consume moderate amounts of alcohol have demonstrated improved cognitive functioning compared to those who abstain or report heavy drinking (Deng et al. 2006; Stampfer et al. 2005; Xu et al. 2009), and delay in cognitive decline in older women (Stott et al. 2008). Other studies support psychological benefits of moderate alcohol consumption among the elders, including reduced stress and improved mood and sociability (Bond et al. 2005; McPhee et al. 2004).

Because of age-related physical changes, moderate alcohol consumption is defined as one standard drink (e.g., 1 ½ oz of liquor, 12 oz of beer, or 5 oz of wine) (National Institute on Alcohol Abuse and Alcoholism [NIH] 2005) in a 24-hour period, and hazardous alcohol use is defined as more than three drinks in one sitting or more than seven drinks in a 7-day period (Drew et al. 2010). It is important to note that, depending on factors such as the type of alcohol and the recipe, one mixed drink can contain from one to three or more standard drinks (NIH). Although moderate alcohol consumption has demonstrated some beneficial effects, elders should not increase their alcohol consumption for health reasons. Alcohol consumption among the older adults requires careful monitoring along with other lifestyle factors (ICAP 2014).

The age at which a person begins to use substances and eventually progresses to abuse has implications for effects in later life. Elderly persons with SUDs can be categorized as early-onset or late-onset abusers. For early-onset abusers, substance abuse develops before age 65. Early-onset abusers show higher incidences of psychiatric and physical problems than do late-onset abusers. For late-onset abusers, substance abuse behaviors are thought to develop subsequent to stressful life situations (e.g., death of a partner, retirement, social isolation). Late-onset abusers typically have fewer physical and mental health problems than early-onset abusers (Martin 2012). In both early- and late-onset abusers, the physical changes associated with aging can skew tolerance in elders. The more alcohol or drugs used by a person is an indication of an increase in tolerance. The signs of tolerance include more substance consumed, in large quantities, and over a longer period of time than initially intended. The case of Stanley (below) illustrates an elder gay man presenting risk factors and comorbidities of substance abuse.

Discussion Box 24.1: The Case of Stanley

Stanley is a 71-year-old white gay man. He was referred to the community alcohol treatment program after having numerous falls. Stanley grew up in a large city with a visible and vibrant LGBT community. He considered himself an active member of that community until about age 53. In fact, he met his partner there and they had been together until his death two years ago. Admittedly, Stanley was a moderate-to-heavy drinker during his 30s, 40s, and 50s. He had a period of abstinence for about 15 years. Upon the death of his partner, Stanley started to drink heavily. This was the first time that Stanley has lived alone in over 40 years. He displayed symptoms of insomnia, depression, and suicidal ideation. His doctor prescribed antidepressant medication, which Stanley has been on for the last 15 months.

Stanley attended the substance abuse treatment program for about two sessions before disengaging. Although he continued to attend session erratically, his rationale for doing so was that the sessions were not helpful and requited too much of his time, and he believed that drinking provided him

with more "balance" than did either the medication on counseling. Stanley was deemed to have the capacity to make his own decisions. Noticeably, his physical and mental health deteriorated, and he had multiple burses from frequent falls and talked often about how life was not worth living alone. Stanley refused any additional treatment. At such time, the treatment and psychiatric considered Stanley as a threat to himself. He was admitted to inpatient treatment and a psychiatric evaluation was done.

Questions

1. What is the recognizable association between major life events, psychiatric disorder, and alcohol abuse?
2. What are the implications of Stanley's long period of sobriety/abstinence and relapse?
3. What type of treatment plan would you consider for Stanley?
4. What resources and service professionals would you involve in the treatment for Stanley?

Comorbidities in LGBT elders with mental illness present unique challenges. These elders have quadruple stigma (e.g., sexual orientation/gender identity or expression, mental health disorder, SUD, age). The stigma faced may affect LGBT elders' psychological health, adding additional stress and anxiety and leading to increases in substance use and other high-risk behaviors. Research Box 24.1 contains a study of the prevalence of mood, anxiety, and SUDs for older adults. Keep in mind that the level of minority stress varies depending on the life content and experiences of the individual (Stevens 2012). Literature suggests that LGBT elders with comorbidities experience life circumstances and exhibit responses to circumstances that may exacerbate their internalized stereotypes, making them less likely to seek help for substance abuse or mental health issues.

Research Box 24.1

Gum, A. M., King-Kallimanis, B., & Kohn, R. (2009). Prevalence of mood, anxiety, and substance-abuse disorders for older Americans in the national comorbidity survey-replication. *American Journal of Geriatric Psychiatry, 17*(9), 769–781.

Objective: This study aimed to explore the prevalence of psychiatric disorders among older adults in the United States by age (18–44, 45–64, 65–74, and 75 years and older) and sex. Covariates of disorders for adults age 65 and over were explored.

Method: A cross-sectional epidemiologic study using data from the National Comorbidity Survey-Replication was used. The participants were representative of a national sample of community-dwelling adults in the USA. The World Health Organization Composite International Diagnostic Interview was used to assess Diagnostic and Statistical Manual of Mental Disorders (4th ed.) psychiatric disorders.

Results: Prevalence of 12-month and lifetime mood, anxiety, and substance use disorders was lower older adults (65 years and older) than younger age-groups: 2.6 % for mood disorder, 7.0 % for anxiety disorder, 0 for any substance use disorder, and 8.5 % for any of these disorders (for any disorder, 18–44 years = 27.6 %, 45–64 years = 22.4 %). Among older adults, the presence of 12-month anxiety disorder was associated with female sex, lower education, being unmarried, and three or more chronic conditions. The presence of a 12-month mood disorder was associated with disability. Similar patterns were noted for lifetime disorders (any disorder: 18–44 years = 46.4 %, 45–64 years = 43.7 %, and 65 years and older = 20.9 %).

Conclusion: This study documented the continued pattern of lower rates of formal diagnoses for elders. These rates likely underestimate the effects of late-life psychiatric disorders, given the potential for underdiagnosis, clinical significance of subthreshold symptoms, and lack of representation for high-risk older adults (e.g., mentally ill, long-term care residents).

Questions

1. If LGBT elders were included in this study, do you think that the results would have been the same, different, or similar?
2. In what ways could this be redesigned to explore prevalence of mood, anxiety, and SUDs for LGBT elders?
3. Do you think that criteria for SUDs in the DSM-5 would change the interpretation of these data?

Detection, Assessment, and Diagnosis

Detection of substance abuse in the older adults is difficult because the signs and symptoms of substance abuse and aging are similar. Older adults have more medical problems than do younger persons, which in the early stages of SUDs often mimic the symptoms of other health conditions. In addition, older adults who abuse substances tend to attribute the physical complications caused by their substance use to the aging process. Similarly, physicians and family members aid in this assumption because they do not inquire about possible substance abuse in elderly persons (Doweiko 2015; Drew et al. 2010). Some family members believe that the elders have reached an age in life in which they have earned the right to drink and to not have their behavior questioned (Kinney 2011). Another reason for difficulty with detection is that social isolation is often both a reason for and consequence of substance abuse (see Chaps. 22 and 31). However, for older adults who are socially active, their peers might encourage drinking well into their later adult years

(Brennen et al. 2010). Other ways in which detection of SUDs are difficult to detect are that they have non-specific presentations and rarely demonstrate the traditional warning signs of an addiction (e.g., legal problems, workplace behaviors) (Drew et al.). For elders still in the workforce who have SUDs, missing days from work because of substance abuse problems are explained away as age-related conditions or stress of taking care of a sick spouse or partner (Doweiko). After retirement, typically elders have more time on their hands and, for those who may have been functioning substance abusers while working and able to manage their addiction, may begin to manifest symptoms in retirement as their substance abuse progresses (Zak 2010).

Elders tend to hide inappropriate AOD usage, making detection more difficult. The SAMHSA Guidelines (i.e., Screening, Brief Intervention, Referral to Treat [SBIRT], http://www.samhsa. gov/prevention/sbirt/) recommends that the first step in a process of detection is a screening, using a test like the Short Michigan Alcohol Screening Instrument-Geriatric Version (SMART-G) (Blow et al. 1992), which is tailored to the needs of older adults. The SMART-G contains ten questions about the person's estimation about quantity of alcohol consumed, eating habits, physical response after drinking, memory, reasons for drinking, conversations with medical personnel about one's drinking, and the use of rules to manage one's drinking. If an elderly patient answers "yes" to two or more of the items on the SMART-G, it is indicative of an alcohol problem. Another commonly used screening instrument is the CAGE (Ewing 1984). The CAGE contains four "yes/no" question about drinking: (a) feeling one should "cut down" on drinking, (b) felt "annoyed" by others criticizing one's drinking, (c) felt "guilty" about one's drinking, and (d) needing a drink in the morning as an "eye opener." A "yes" response of two or more is considered clinically significant. The patient's responses are used to discuss the need to cut down on the amount of alcohol consumed. If the patient does not see a need for change, a referral should be made to a mental health practitioner or a geriatric psychiatrist

(Naegle 2012). Both the SMART and CAGE are psychological screening instruments. It is important to note that a screening is not a diagnosis, rather a means to identify at-risk AOD use.

If the screening process suggests the presence of a SUD, the next step in the process is to determine the severity of the SUD. This step is known as assessment. A comprehensive assessment involves collection of data about the quantity and frequency of use, and the social health consequences of drug use, including nicotine, prescription, over-the-counter, herbal and food supplements, recreational drugs, and alcohol (Naegle 2012). In addition, a comprehensive assessment should include a through physical examination along with laboratory analysis and psychiatric, neurological, and social evaluations (Martin 2012). Given that many elders take numerous medications, a basic assessment of their medications may require the shopping bag approach in which elders bring in all of their medications (i.e., a shopping bag filled with medication). The assessment of elderly substance abusers involves a biomedical, psychosocial approach in which it is determined whether the patient has a biological disease (e.g., depression that is producing the abuse) or whether the substance abuse has produced a biochemical brain disorder (e.g., dementia, delirium). Both the medical complications from the abuse and medical problems exacerbated by drug dependence must be examined. Psychological distress (e.g., anti-gay/anti-trans prejudices) can induce addictive behavior, requiring psychological interventions to address the problem. Elderly LGBT persons may have a complex combination of functional and social behaviors that exacerbate substance abuse and complicate treatment. Thus, the treatment team must elicit basic biomedical psychosocial information during the diagnostic phase and then use these data to construct an appropriate treatment approach (Geriatric Substance Abuse-Dementia Education & Training Program n.d.). Finally, assessment should consider the spiritual concerns and beliefs of LGBT elders (see Chap. 27). This understanding may aid in the recovery process and relapse prevention.

During assessment and diagnosis, the assessor must be cognizant of several issues to accurately diagnose SUDs in elderly adults. First, memory loss, particularly short-term, can sometimes cause an older person to forget to take his or her medication or to take too much unintentionally. Similarly, the elder person may have difficulty recalling information accurately to answer questions during an assessment interview. Second, the interplay of health issues makes diagnosing and treating SUDs in elders more complicated than for other age-groups (Ruscavage et al. 2006). Third, the diagnostic criteria in the *Diagnostic and Statistical Manual* were validated on young and middle-aged adults. Although tolerance of a substance is one diagnostic criterion for SUDs, it may not apply because of physiological changes related to aging, which may result in less alcohol intake with not apparent reduction in intoxication. Similarly, elders with late-onset substance abuse may not experience physiological withdrawal when the substance is suspended. Fourth, a criterion that describes the negative impact of substance abuse on work functions may be irrelevant for elders who live alone. The result is that abuse among the elderly may be miscalculated. In addition, the criterion of giving up activities may be of little use when assessing a retiree who has fewer regular activities and responsibilities to give up (Menninger 2002). Finally, assessment usually takes place over several days. Thus, the assessment process can be fatiguing for elderly patients. Other challenges when working with the elderly population include service providers' biases and belief about aging, substance abuse, and LGBT populations, and denial of substance use by the elderly (Martin 2012).

Treatment and Intervention

The majority of elders with SUDs or mental health problems, especially LGBT elders, do not receive the treatment they need (Martin 2012). LGBT persons who are in need of treatment for SUDs face several substantial dilemmas: (a) a lack of culturally relevant trained staff and specialists, (b) staff members and clients who will attempt to impose their own ideological beliefs on them, (c) programs that do not address issues related to sexual identity or gender expression, and (d) programs that do not address issues related to traumatic childhood experiences (Cochran et al. 2007). In a survey of substance abuse treatment providers' attitudes and knowledge about LGBT clients, ATTC (n.d.) found half had no education about lesbian, gay, and bisexual persons, and 80 % had no education regarding transgender persons. Although half of the counselors in the study had worked with lesbian, gay, or bisexual clients in the past and few had worked with transgendered persons, the majority reported that they lacked information about many important issues that affect LGBT clients. The counselors reported that they had little or no knowledge of LGBT persons regarding the following: legal issues (73 %), domestic partnership (69 %), family issues (54 %), internalized homophobia (48 %), and coping strategies (37 %). However, 25–50 % of substance abuse counselors had positive attitudes about LGBT clients. The counselors recognized that they needed training in these areas to be more effective with all clients, especially for relapse prevention and aftercare planning and to be aware of the potential stresses in the client's life related to their sexual orientation or gender identity.

Although the LGBT population is comprised of a unique group of individuals with a special set of commonalities, as a subpopulation, transgender persons require additional considerations in the treatment process. One vital consideration is the stage of transition in which the person is engaged. For example, a person who is in pre-surgery status and is living the role of the "to be assigned" gender might encounter a range of policies in an inpatient treatment setting. Such policies may range from non-acceptance to acceptance with conditions (e.g., separate living quarters and bathrooms or separate rooms with access to generic bathrooms) (Beatty and Lewis 2003).

For LGBT persons, certain questions come up in the treatment process. Some questions deal with sexual identity and others with trauma (see Table 24.3).

Treatment protocol and treatment success are influenced by several factors including severity of substance use, type(s) of substance used, and whether substances are used in combination with other substances. Therefore, the types of drugs abused, the location of abuse, and potential triggers for relapse present differently depending on the population (Singh and Lassiter 2012). Regardless of age or gender, polysubstance abusers present more challenges in the treatment process because substances used in combination increase risk factors (Rowan and Faul 2011). Emerging evidence-based research supports the efficacy of a variety of pharmacological and psychotherapeutic interventions for SUDs and major psychiatric disorders in elderly persons. In light of comorbidities being associated with increased healthcare utilization and significant healthcare expenditures among elders, targeted prevention and early intervention can offset substantial costs to patients, their families, healthcare organizations, and the government (Bartels et al. 2005). In fact, an integrated approach to treatment of comorbidities results in far better outcomes. Using a multidisciplinary team to treat comorbidities enhances cohesiveness of care and reduces conflicts between service providers. The argument is for both disorders to be treated as "primary" using a combination of different modalities such as outreach and case management, motivational techniques, psychotherapy, and psychopharmacology.

Motivational interviewing, cognitive-behavioral therapy, brief therapeutic interventions, and individual, group, and family counseling which are widely used in the treatment of SUDs have been implemented with elders (Martin 2012). Brief interventions, intervention (i.e., significant people in the person's life collectively confront the person with their firsthand experiences of his or her substance use), and motivational interviewing, the least intensive treatment options, are recommended first with elderly substance abusers as a pre-treatment strategy or as treatment itself (Cummings et al. 2009; Ruscavage et al. 2006). Least-restrictive treatment options have been found to be effective; older adults respond better to age-specific group treatment and cognitive-behavioral therapy-based programs (Brown et al. 2006; D'Agostino et al. 2006). Some elders may be in need of intensive treatment such as inpatient/outpatient, detoxification, recovery or group home housing, and specialized outpatient services. The treatment approach should be tailored to LGBT elders' individual circumstances and needs

Table 24.3 Service provider questions in SUDs treatment of LGBT persons

When does one raise the question of the client's sexual identity if it appears to be a clinical issue?
Trust is one of the major factors in the therapeutic relationship. If sexual identity is presented as a clinical issue, then it may be relevant for the therapist to raise the issue. First, start with non-threatening questions. If the client remains closed and the topic clearly is a clinical concern, use more direct questions

Should the therapist reveal his or her own sexual identity?
If the facility is identified as LGBT specific, this may not be an issue except for non-LGBT staff. Non-identified facilities may have several concerns: (a) safety for the staff person, (b) acceptance by administrators, (c) acceptance by facility peers, (d) the purpose of revealing, (e) social lifestyle of the staff person, (f) the size of the LGBT community, (g) the impact of this information being revealed

Are there issues/challenges a transsexual person encounters when in treatment?
The stage of transition (i.e., pre-reassignment vs. post-reassignment surgery) will determine whether specific issues must be addressed

How concerned should service providers be with HIV antibody testing and counseling of LGBT population?
Research supports sexual activity and substance use as strong HIV risk-related behaviors. The elderly is one of the fastest growing groups to be diagnosed with HIV. There is a misperception that risk is somehow diminished with age and the topic is not discussed by health providers (Funders for Lesbian and Gay Issues 2004)

Adapted from Beatty and Lewis (2003)

(e.g., self-esteem, perceptual, cognitive, sensory, literacy, and language needs). The *Treatment Improvement Protocol* (*TIP*) *26* (SAMHSA 2008) identified several key characteristics of treatment that contribute to positive outcomes for elders with SUDs. Given that the protocol is not specific to LGBT persons, as authors of this chapter we present the material to be LGBT inclusive (see Table 24.4). Equally as important in treatment is psychoeducation (i.e., teaching components of behavior change) in which elders receive information and gain knowledge about the risks of combining alcohol with medications and excessive alcohol use (Brown et al. 2006; D'Agostino et al. 2006; Doweiko 2015; Martin 2012). Often, LGBT elders with SUDs are in need of strategies for increasing social interactions and personal efficacy when refusing substances and/or peer pressure.

Being honest with oneself and others is a hallmark of efficacious treatment strategies. However, for LGBT persons, being open about their sexual identity presents several dilemmas in treatment: (a) If they come out, they face possible rejection and alienation; (b) if they do not come out, they are viewed as untruthful; (c) if they indicate their differences from heterosexual clients, they are seen as asking for special privileges

Table 24.4 Characteristics for LGBT elder treatment positive outcomes

Emphasis on age-specific rather than mixed-aged treatment
Emphasis on sexual identity-specific characteristics
Use of supportive, non-confrontational approaches that build self-esteem
Focus on cognitive-behavioral approaches to address negative emotional states
Development of skills for improving social interaction and support
Involve support systems, including friends and family of choice
Appropriate pace and content for LGBT elders
Capacity to provide referrals to medical, mental health, aging, and LGBT-specific services
Counselors and service delivery personnel trained to work with LGBT elders

Adapted from SAMHSA (2008)

or jeopardizing other clients' recovery; and (d) if they accept generic treatment, their own recovery is jeopardized (ATTC n.d.). In light of these perceptions, counselors and service providers should work with LGBT elders to determine whether, when, and how to come out or to reveal their sexual identity while in treatment. In addition, attention must be given to the type of counseling (e.g., individual, group) that is more appropriate. Thus, counselors and service providers are required to have cultural competence related to the LGBT population, aging, and ethnic minority groups. For counselors and service providers who are not culturally competent in working with LGBT populations, it is best to acknowledge it and refer the client to someone with such competency.

Because of negative experiences of LGBT elders have had due to their sexual orientation or gender identity and expression, it is important for treatment interventionists to ensure that their treatment facility, office, and organization in which they work send a clear message that the environment is safe for LGBT persons to disclose their concerns. For example, displaying LGBT-friendly literature in the waiting room and offices or a "Safe Zone" or rainbow sticker on the front door of the building or reception area are symbols universally recognized as safe places. It is important first to seriously assess the safety of the service delivery environment before deciding to display such a symbol (Singh and Lassiter 2012). Deciding to disclose one's sexual orientation or gender identity or gender expression must be given serious consideration because although federal and a number of state statutes protect recovering substance abusers from many forms of discrimination, LGBT persons are not afforded the same protections in many areas of the United States (SAMHSA 2012).

Programs that provide treatment to LGBT persons must be particularly vigilant about maintaining client's confidentiality because the consequences of an inappropriate disclosure can have devastating consequences and implications for safety, employment, housing, and social services (SAMHSA 2012). In addition, special support group meetings (e.g., Alcoholics Anonymous) oriented toward the specific needs of LGBT elders must give consideration to addressing both age and sexual orientation or gender identity issues that are relevant to recovery. Unfortunately, such 12-step meetings are usually only found in large cities (Doweiko 2015). Further, 12-step programs can be unwelcoming of LGBT persons because of traditional religious persecution of sexual minorities (Shelton 2011). See Chap. 29 for additional discussion on the role of religious leaders in addressing LGBT elders.

Treatment services for LGBT elders with SUDs require knowledgeable service providers who are skilled in the aspects of aging, with cultural competence in LGBT issues, able to understand the effects of comorbidities, and able to integrate biomedical, psychosocial, and physiological risk factors for addiction. Service planning and delivery should follow a logical and sequential progression to increase more positive outcomes. Inclusion of various service professionals from across disciplines on the treatment team for LGBT elders is one way to potentially improve the quality of service.

Policy on SUDs

Substance abuse services need to address deep-rooted age discrimination and heterosexist philosophies that continue to permeate mainstream services. Advocates in the United States assert that policies should allow LGBT elders to access the most appropriate clinical service on the basis of need and that age and sexual orientation or gender identity must not be exclusion criteria (SAMHSA 2012). Although, historically, SUDs were thought to be more prevalent in younger LGB populations, much of the research and many treatment programs and protocols continue to ignore LGBT elders. A critical need exists for LGBT-specific standards of care and treatment protocols that are generally acceptable or sanctioned by national accreditation organizations. Such standards could be used as the basis for certification of clinical staff or licensing

of treatment programs, and as the basis for staff training programs (Healthy People 2010 2010). In addition, AOD screening should be part of all elders' annual medical examination. The administering of the CAGE by nurses should be part of the series of questions asked during a doctor's visit by patients.

When assessing LGBT persons with SUDs, treatment programs should incorporate more inclusive language into their assessment instruments and retain staff. Assessments include relationships with family of origin, family of choice and friends, level of community or systems support, social interactions, level of self-esteem, understanding of self-identity, and work issues (SAMHSA 2012) (see *A Provider's Introduction to Substance Abuse Treatment for Lesbian, Gay, Bisexual, and Transgender Individuals*). For transgender persons, it is important to address them based on the gender with which they identity. Similarly, assessment instruments should be sensitive to the age of the individuals and the presence of coexisting conditions in order to accurately measure the extent of the problem.

Although some efforts have been put forward regarding practice on SUDs for LGBT elders, an impact policy is needed to prioritize and fund prevention and intervention as a healthcare concern. Screenings for mental health concerns, including substance abuse, should receive equal focus as an emphasis just as is physical disorders and diseases among the elderly (e.g., cancer, arthritis, cataract). Although Medicare covers treatment for mental health issues, copayments can be prohibitive for elders with lower incomes. The Positive Aging Act, an amendment to the Public Health Service Act, is a policy alternative that could address SUDs in elders. First, the act could demonstrate ways of integrating mental health services for elders into primary-care settings. Second, it could support the establishment and maintenance of interdisciplinary geriatric mental health outreach teams in community settings where older adults reside or receive social services (Gage and Melillo 2011). In addition, because doctor shopping is a common occurrence among the elders, a need exists for information sharing on prescription medication through as a state database.

Finally, it is important to establish an educational program on signs, symptoms, and risk factors of substance abuse, including LGBT-specific and age-related content as a part of a public health initiative. An educational program can serve the secondary purpose of helping LGBT elders understand the importance of medical evaluation and treatment for any health conditions, as well as promote their comfort with disclosing their sexual identity if it is clinically relevant. Too often, LGBT health issues are lumped together as if all LGBT elders are alike. Any educational program should address health and mental health issues contextually for lesbians, gay men, bisexual men and women, and transgender male-to-female and female-to-male. One avenue is to develop partnerships with LGBT-sensitive primary-care physicians and clinicians, therapists, and psychiatrists (SAMHSA 2012).

Summary

Research on SUDs in the aging population has increased; however, focus on LGBT elders remains somewhat limited. LGBT elders exhibit higher rates of SUDs than their heterosexual counterparts. Reasons for substance abuse range from discrimination and stigma to loneliness and a means of socialization. In general, elders have medical comorbidity and, the addition of SUDs and mental health disorders serves to further complicate diagnosis and treatment. In assessing and diagnosing LGBT elders for SUDs, it is critical to be aware of the vast differences within this population.

To be effective, service providers must understand the unique characteristics and challenges of LGBT elders with SUDs when assessing, diagnosing, and planning treatment. Whether LGBT elders have early or late onset of substance abuse, they will benefit from culturally specific strategies and comprehensive approaches.

Learning Exercises

Self-Check Exercises

1. What are some unique characteristics of LGBT elders who abuse substances?
2. What is the most commonly abused substance by elders?
3. Why is it difficult to estimate the number of LGBT elders with SUDs?
4. How difficult is it for LGBT elders to find AA groups that are specific to their needs?
5. What roles do gay bars play in the lives of LGBT persons?

Experiential Assignments

1. Interview an LGBT elder to determine what his or her specific needs would be in a support group (e.g., AA) designed specifically of LGBT elders.
2. Interview a substance abuse counselor, social worker, or medical professional/nurse to explore his or her knowledge about meeting the unique needs of a LGBT elder with SUDs and a mental health disorder.
3. Develop a manual on substance abuse and mental health resources in you local town or city region for LGBT elders.

Multiple-Choice Questions

1. Which type of treatment options is recommended first for elders with SUDs?
   (a) Least costly
   (b) Most comprehensive
   (c) Least intensive
   (d) Multilevel
2. Which type of medication is the elderly most likely to receive that has misuse and abuse potential?
   (a) Psychoactive
   (b) Diuretic
   (c) Inhalants
   (d) Anti-coagulant

(3) What is the purpose of a substance abuse screening is to do which of the following?
(a) Identify a treatment protocol
(b) Identify at-risk behavior
(c) Make a diagnosis
(d) Determine the existence of a family history of substance abuse

4. Which of the following is how comorbitity of substance abuse and mental illness be defined and treated?
(a) Both as secondary conditions
(b) One as a primary and the other as a secondary condition
(c) Both as primary conditions
(d) One as a primary condition and the other as a symptom

5. Which of the following usually result in iatrogenic stress?
(a) Overprescribing of medication
(b) Ignoring that alcohol is also a toxic drug
(c) Failing to take into account the way the elderly metabolize medications
(d) All of the above
(e) None of the above

6. How are LGBT persons viewed if they do not reveal their sexual orientation or gender identity while in treatment?
(a) Secretive
(b) Introverted
(c) Selfish
(d) Untruthful

7. Which of the following is ignored as a growing concern of LGBT elders in substance abuse treatment?
(a) HIV
(b) Dementia
(c) Illicit drugs
(d) Substance-specific syndrome

8. Why are LGBT elders with comorbidities less likely to seek treatment?
(a) More medical problems than younger people
(b) Internalized stereotypes
(c) Religious reasons
(d) Legally cannot be questioned about substance use

9. What is a unique challenge of residential substance abuse treatment that is specific to transgender adults?
(a) Age at which they come out
(b) Post-reassignment surgery status
(c) Pre-reassigned surgery status
(d) Unwillingness to provide information

10. How many "yes" responses to questions on the CAGE or SMAR-G are indicative of a substance abuse problem?
(a) One
(b) Two
(c) Three
(d) All

Key

1-C
2-A
3-B
4-C
5-D
6-D
7-A
8-B
9-C
10-B

Resources

CSAP Substance Abuse Resource Guide: Lesbian, Gay, Bisexual and Transgender Populations: http://www.health.org/referrals/resguides.asp?InvNum=MS489
LGBT Populations: A Dialogue on Advancing Opportunities for Recovery from Addictions and Mental Health Problems: www.samhsa.gov/recovery/doc/LGBTDialogue.pef
National Association of Lesbian & Gay Addiction Professionals (NALGAP): www.nalgap.org
Preventing Alcohol and Other Drug Problems in the Lesbian and Gay Community: www.prta.com

Royal College of Psychiatrists (London) College Report CR 165. (2011, June). Our invisible addicts—First report of the older persons' substance misuse working group of the Royal College of Psychiatrists: www.rcpstch.ac.uk/files.../cr165.pdf

SAMHSA: A Provider's Introduction to Substance Abuse Treatment for LGBT Individuals (2012): www.store.samhsa.gov

The Center: LGBT Community Center: http://gaycenter.org/recovery

References

Addiction Technology Transfer Center Network. (2009). Prescription medication abuse: Part 2—what you should know & look for. *Addiction messenger, 12* (2), 1–3.

Addiction Technology Transfer Center Network. (n.d.) *Center for excellence for lesbian, gay, bisexual and transgender persons substance abuse treatment provider survey results.* Retrieved September 21, 2014 from www.uiowa.edu/~/attc/ce-lgbt/ce-lgbt-survey.html.

Administration on Aging. (2012). *Older Americans behavioral health issue brief 5: Prescription medication misuse and abuse among older adults.* Available at www.aoa.gov/AoARoot/AoA_Programs/HPW/Behavioral/docs2/IssueBrief5PrescriptionMedMisuseAbuse.pdf.

Barnes, A. J., Moore, A. A., Xu, H., Ang, A., Tallen, L., Mirkin, M., ... Ettner, S. L. (2010). Prevalence and correlates of at-risk drinking among older adults. The project SHARE study. *Journal of General Internal Medicine.* doi:10.1007/s11606-010-1341-x.

Bartels, S. J., Blow, F. C., Brockmann, L. M., & Van Citters, A. D. (2005). *Substance abuse and mental health among older Americans: The state of the knowledge and future directions.* Rockville, MD: Substance Abuse and mental Health Services Administration.

Basca, B. (2008). *The elderly and prescription drug misuse and abuse.* Retrieved September 18, 2014 from www.cars-rp.org/publications/PreventionTatics/PT09.02.08.pdf.

Beatty, R. L., & Lewis, K. E. (2003). Substance use disorder and LGBT communities. *Resource Links, 2* (3), 1–7.

Blow, F. C., Bower, K. J., Schulenberg, J. E., Demo-Danaberg, L. M., Young, J. P., & Beresford, T. P. (1992). The Michigan alcoholism screening test-geriatric version (MAST-G): A new elderly specific screening instrument. *Alcoholism, Clinical and Experimental Research, 16*, 372.

Bond, G. E., Burr, R. L., McCurry, S. M., Rice, M. M., Borenstein, A. R., & Larson, E. B. (2005). Alcohol and cognitive performance: A longitudinal study of older Japanese Americans. *The Kame Project. International Psychogeniatrics, 17*, 653–668.

Brennen, P. L., Schutte, K. K., & Moos, R. H. (2010). Patterns and predictors of late-life drinking trajectories: A 10-year longitudinal study. *Psychology of Addictive Behaviors, 24*, 254–264.

Brown, S. A., Glasner-Edwards, S. V., Tate, S., McQuad, J. R., Chalekian, J., & Granholm, E. (2006). Integrated cognitive behavioral therapy versus twelve-step facilitation therapy for substance-dependent adults with depressive disorders. *Journal of Psychoactive Drugs, 38*, 449–460.

Cochran, B. N., Peavy, K. M., & Cauce, A. M. (2007). Substance abuse provider's explicit and implicit attitudes regarding sexual minorities. *Journal of Homosexuality, 53*(3), 181–207.

Colliver, J. D., Compton, W. M., et al. (2006). Projecting drug use among baby boomers in 2020. *Annals of Epidemiology, 16*, 257–265.

Conron, K. J., Mimiaga, M. J., & Landers, S. J. (2010). A population-based study of sexual orientation identity and gender differences in adult health. *American Journal of Public Health, 100*(10), 1953–1960.

Cummings, S. M., Cooper, R. L., & Cassie, K. M. (2009). Motivational interviewing to affect behavioral change in older adults. *Research on Social Work Practice, 19* (2), 195–204.

D'Agostino, C. S., Barry, K. L., Blow, F. C., & Podgorski, C. (2006). Community interventions for older adults with comorbid substance abuse: The geriatric addictions program. *Journal of Dual Diagnosis, 2*, 31–45.

Deng, J., Zhou, D. H., Li, J. C., Wang, Y. J., Gao, C. Y., & Chen, M. (2006). A 2-year follow-up study of alcohol consumption and risk of dementia. *Clinical Neurology and Neurosurgery, 108*, 378–383.

Department of Justice, DEA, Office of Diversion Control. (1999, December). Don't be scammed by a drug abuser, 1(1). Retrieved September 16, 2014 from www.deadiversion.usdoj.gov/pubs/brochures/pdfs/recognizing_drug_abuser_trifold.pdf.

Diagnostic and Statistical Manual of Mental Disorders. (2013). *Diagnostic and statistical manual of mental disorders—DSM-5.* Washington, DC: American Psychological Association.

Djousse, L., Biggs, M. L., Mukamal, K. J., & Siscovick, D. S. (2007). Alcohol consumption and type 2 diabetes among older adults: The cardiovascular health study. *Obesity, 15*, 1758–1765.

Djousse, L., & Gaziano, J. M. (2007). Alcohol consumption and risk of heart failure in the Physician Health Study. *Circulation, 115*, 34–39.

Doweiko, H. E. (2015). *Concepts of chemical dependency* (9th ed.). Stamford, CT: Cengage Learning.

Drew, S. M., Wilkins, K. M., & Trevisan, L. A. (2010). Managing medications and alcohol misuse by your older patients. *Current Psychiatry, 9*(2), 21–24, 27–28, 41.

Ellison, J. M. (2012, March 5–9). *Mental health and mental illness in our aging population with treatment implications.* Symposium conducted at Harvard Medical School Department of Continuing Education, Key Largo, FL.

Ewing, J. A. (1984). Detecting alcoholism: The CAGE questionnaire. *Journal of the American Medical Association, 252*, 1905–1907.

Frederiksen-Goldsen, K. I., & Muraco, A. (2010). Aging and sexual orientation: A 25- year review of the literature. *Research on Aging, 32*, 372–413.

Funders for Lesbian and Gay Issues. (2004). *Aging in equity: LGBT elders in America.* New York, NY: Author.

Gage, S., & Melillo, K. D. (2011). Substance abuse in older adults: Policy issues. *Journal of Gerontological Nursing, 37*(12), 7–11.

Geriatric Substance Abuse-Dementia Education & Training Program. (n.d.). *Geriatric substance abuse.* Retrieved September 27, 2014 from www.alzbrain.org/pdf/handouts/6000.GERIATRICSUBSTANCEABUSEINTHEELDERLY.pdf.

Gronbaek, M. (2006). Factors influencing the relationship between alcohol and cardiovascular disease. *Current Opinion in Lipiodology, 17*, 17–21.

Healthy People 2010. (2010). *Substance abuse.* Retrieved September 3, 2014 from http://www.nalgap.org/PDF/Resources/Substance_Abuse.pdf.

Incalzi, R. A., Capparella, O., Gemma, A., et al. (1997). The interaction between age and comorbidity contributes to predicting the mortality of geriatric patients in the acute-care hospital. *Journal of Internal medicine, 242*, 291–298.

International Center for Alcohol Policies. (2014). Module 23: Alcohol and the elderly. *The ICAP Blue Book: Practical guides for alcohol policy and prevention approaches.* Retrieved September 25, 2014 from http://icap.org/PolicyTools/ICAPBlueBook/BlueBookModules/23AlcholandtheElderly/tabid/181/Default.aspx.

Jessup, M. A., & Dibble, S. L. (2012). Unmet mental health and substance abuse treatment needs of sexual minority elders. *Journal of Homosexuality, 59*, 656–674.

King, M., Semlyen, J., Tai, S. S., Killaspy, H., Osborn, D., Popelyuk, D., & Nazareth, I. (2008). A systematic review of mental disorder, suicide, and deliberate self harm in lesbian, gay, and bisexual people. *BMC Psychiatry, 18*, 70.

Kinney, J. (2011). *Loosening the grip: A handbook of alcohol information.* Boston: McGraw Hill.

Luggen, A. S. (2006). Alcohol and the older adult. *Advice for Nurse Practitioners, 14*(1), 47–52.

Martin, L. (2012). Substance abuse in aging and elderly adults: new issues for psychiatrists. Psych Central. Retrieved September 26, 2014 from http://pro.psychcentral.com/substance-abuse-in-aging-and-elderly-adults-ne-issues-for-psychiatrists/001011.html.

McPhee, S. D., Johnson, T. R., & Dietrich, M. S. (2004). Comparing health status with healthy habits in elderly assisted-living residents. *Family and Community Health, 27*, 158–169.

Menninger, J. A. (2002). Assessment and treatment of alcoholism and substance related disorders in the elderly. *Bulletin of the Menninger Clinic, 66*, 166–183.

Naegle, M. A. (2012). Alcohol use screening and assessment for older adults. *Try this: Best Practices in Nursing Care to Older Adults, 17*, 1–2. Retrieved September 25, 2014 from www.consultgerirn.org/uploads/File/trythis/try_this_17.pdf.

National Institute on Alcohol Abuse and Alcoholism. (2005). What is a standard drink? *A pocket guide for alcohol screening and brief intervention.* Retrieved September 21, 2014 from http://pubs.niaaa.nih.gov/publications/Practitioner/PocketGuide/pocket_guide.htm.

Rapuri, P. B. V., Gallagher, J. C., Balhorn, K. E., & Ryschon, K. L. (2000). Alcohol intake and bone metabolism in elderly women. *American Journal of Clinical Nutrition, 72*, 1206–1213.

Rowan, N. L., & Faul, A. C. (2011). Gay, lesbian, bisexual, and transgendered people and chemical dependency: Exploring successful treatment. *Journal of Gay and Lesbian Social Services, 23*, 107–130.

Ruscavage, D., Hardison, C., & Tuohy, C. M. (2006). *A guide to developing a substance abuse awareness program for older adults.* Silver Springs, MD: Central East Addiction Technology Transfer Center.

Shelton, M. (2011). Treating gay men for substance abuse. *Counseling, 21*(1), 18–22.

Simoni-Wastila, L., & Yang, H. K. (2006). Psychoactive drug abuse in older adults. *American Journal of Geriatric Pharmacotherapy, 4*, 380–394.

Singh, A. A., & Lassiter, P. S. (2012). Lesbian, gay, bisexual, and transgender affirmative addictions treatment. In D. Capuzzi & M. D. Stauffer (Eds.), *Foundations of addictions counseling* (2nd ed., pp. 380–399). Boston: Pearson.

Stampfer, M. J., Kang, J. H., Chen, J., Cherry, R., & Grodstein, F. (2005). Effects of moderate alcohol consumption on cognitive function in women. *New England Journal of Medicine, 352*, 245–253.

Stevens, S. (2012). Meeting the substance abuse treatment needs of lesbian, bisexual and transgender women: Implications for research to practice. *Substance Abuse and Rehabilitation, 3*(1), 27–36.

Strott, D. J., Falconer, A., Kerr, G. D., Murray, H. M., Trompet, S., Westndorp, R. G., et al. (2008). Does low to moderate alcohol intake protect against cognitive decline in older people? *Journal of the American Geriatrics Society, 56*, 2217–2224.

Substance Abuse and Mental Health Services Administration. (2006). Results from the 2005 national survey on drug use and health: National findings (Office of Applied Studies, NSDUH Series H-30, DHHS Publication No. SMA 06-4194). Rockville, MD: Author.

Substance Abuse and Mental Health Services Administration. (2008). *Substance abuse among older adults:*

Treatment improvement protocol series 26. Washington, DC: Author.

Substance Abuse and Mental Health Services Administration. (2012). *A provider's introduction to substance abuse for treatment for lesbian, gay, bisexual, and transgender individuals.* Washington, DC: Author.

Valderas, J. M., Starfield, B., Sibbald, B., Salisbury, C., & Roland, M. (2009). Defining comorbidity: Implications for understanding health and health services. *Annals of Family Medicine, 7*(4), 357–363.

Wilkinson, W. (2008). *Strengthening linkages between substance abuse providers and LGBT community resources.* Retrieved September 18, 2014 from www.lgbt-tristar.com.

Xu, G. L., Liu, X. F., Yin, Q., Zhu, W. S., Zhang, R. L., & Fan, X. B. (2009). Alcohol consumption and transition of mild cognitive impairment to dementia. *Psychiatry and Clinical Neurosciences, 63,* 43–49.

Zak, P. D. (2010, July). *Substance misuse among elder gay men.* Retrieved September 18, 2014 from www.038212C.netsolhost.com/wp-content/uploads/2013/08/Substance-Misuse-Among-Elder-Gay-Men-2010_FINAL.pdf.

Part V

Family and Community

LBGT Elders in Rural Settings, Small Towns, and Frontier Regions

Debra A. Harley

Abstract

Rural areas have a higher percentage of older adults than the rest of the USA and are expected to experience the greatest increase in this age group, as many rural areas are becoming retirement communities. This chapter presents a trans-disciplinary examination of issues relevant to LGBT elders in rural settings (RS), small towns (ST), and frontier regions (FR). Information is presented on the characteristics of these areas, a profile of LGBT elders in these settings, issues of isolation and survival strategies, healthcare concerns and disclosure, and issues about integrated services and policy. For many LGBT elders, geographic location, in tandem with social, cultural, and economic issues, is a significant factor that influences how LGBT individuals experience aging.

Keywords

Rural · Small town · Frontier · Geographic location · Remote communities

Overview

Often, when people think of rural settings, their attention turns to agricultural landscapes, small towns (ST), isolation, and low population density. In fact, rural America is quite expansive and part of each state, with ten percentages of the US geography being urban and the remainder 90 % rural. Two-thirds of the 3142 counties in the USA are rural (Hartman and Weierbach 2013). Nearly three out of ten Americans live in a rural area or a very small city (US Census Bureau 2010a). At least 15 definitions exist for rural settings (RS), including eleven by the Department of Agriculture. In this chapter, the definition of a rural area is the same as that defined by the Health Resources and Services Administration of the US Department of Health and Human Services, which encompasses all population, housing, and territory not included within an urban area (www.hrsa.gov/rurhealth/policy/

D.A. Harley (✉)
University of Kentucky, Lexington, Kentucky, USA
e-mail: dharl00@email.uky.edu

© Springer International Publishing Switzerland 2016
D.A. Harley and P.B. Teaster (eds.), *Handbook of LGBT Elders*,
DOI 10.1007/978-3-319-03623-6_25

definition-of-rural.html). Characteristics of rural society are presented later in this chapter.

Learning Objectives

By the end of this chapter, the reader should be able to:

1. Identify characteristics of RS, ST, and frontier regions (FR).
2. Identify unique challenges of LGBT elders in rural, ST, and frontier settings.
3. Discuss resiliency among LGBT elders in rural areas.
4. Understand ways in which interdisciplinary collaboration is used to meet the needs of LGBT elders in RS.

Introduction

A higher percentage of older adults live in rural areas than in the rest of the USA (Institute of Medicine [IOM] 2006; US Census Bureau 2010b); these areas will likely experience the greatest increase in this age group (Cromartie and Nelson 2009). Many rural areas are becoming retirement communities, as people "age-in-place" and as changes in migration patterns where older people have moved in and younger ones have moved out (Clark and Leipert 2007; Colello 2007). Between 2010 and 2030, growth in the US population aged 65 and older will increase rapidly, precisely the time period during which baby boomers will age into this population (Glasgow and Brown 2012). For example, the state of Florida has the highest proportion of elderly people in the USA, many of whom live in rural areas (Gunderson et al. 2006). Although diversity is substantial in certain areas of rural America, many rural counties remain largely non-Hispanic white (Hartman and Weierbach 2013). The older adult population living there presents health-related, financial, social,

psychological, and spiritual challenges and transitions, many of which are exacerbated in rural areas, and are even greater for LGBT elders. LGTB elders in rural areas experience triple jeopardy because they must deal with issues related to aging, situations of living in RS, and challenges owing to their sexual orientation and gender identity. These challenges are accentuated by the fact that limited research has focused specifically on the experiences and situations of rural LGBT elders (Comerford et al. 2004; Rowan et al. 2013).

LGBT elders living in rural settings are diverse and represent various ethnicities, experiences, histories, affiliations, cultures, and family dynamics. Some grew up in rural areas, while others migrated there at some point in their lives. Although not all LGBT elders in rural areas face isolation and loneliness, a commonality of RS for LGBT elder residents is that they are at a distinct disadvantage in comparison with their urban counterparts with regard to health outcomes, availability of services and resources, proximity to urban areas and services (can range from a few miles to hundreds of miles), income and economic stability, access to an LGBT community, and socialization. According to Lee and Quam (2013), "geographic location is a significant variable that, due to social, cultural, and economic differences between rural and urban settings will influence how LGBT individuals experience aging" (p. 113).

The purpose of this chapter is to present a trans-disciplinary examination of issues relevant to LGBT elders in RS, ST, and FR. Although RS, ST, and FR each have different characteristics, throughout this chapter the term rural will be used as an umbrella term to refer to RS, ST, and FR. Characteristics are presented to define each of these terms. Additional information is presented on a profile of LGBT elders in rural areas, isolation, and survival strategies; unique concerns of healthcare delivery and disclosure; and integrated services and policy issues. Information is presented with general application to LGBT elders in rural areas, acknowledging that exceptions exist among this diverse population.

Characteristics of Rural Society, Small Town, and Frontier Regions

The focus of this chapter is on rural settings and ST because large rural towns may have more in common with metropolitan areas than they do with remote and isolated ST (Hart et al. 2005). Rural America today has moved predominantly to a post-agrarian society: large intergenerational families are a thing of the past, many rural residents no longer work at local jobs, and many commute long distances to work. Typically, residents of rural areas maintain strong religious beliefs and conservative ideals, stressing family values and moral behavior. In addition, older adults living in rural areas are more likely than their urban counterparts to have lower incomes, live in poverty, have less formal education, be in poorer health, own their own homes (more likely to be substandard dwellings), have less access to health and social services and transportation, and their health and long-term care needs are less likely to be met (Fowles and Greenberg 2012). On average, the population of rural areas includes more elderly people, higher unemployment and underemployment, lower population density with higher percentages of poor, uninsured and underinsured residents, higher costs associated with healthcare services, fewer healthcare providers, a greater emphasis on generalists, healthcare facilities with limited scopes of service, greater dependency on Medicare and Medicaid reimbursement, higher rates of chronic diseases, and different clinical practice behaviors (Hart et al. 2005; Lenardson et al. 2009; McBride 2009; Ziller and Coburn 2009). Rural Americans are generally regarded as hardworking individuals with a strong sense of family, community, and traditional religious beliefs (Kellogg Foundation 2002).

Despite their heritage, culture, or history, rural older adults nearly always have a set of rural core values (i.e., resiliency, diligence, autonomy, and spirituality) that infuse all areas of their daily life, including the challenges of aging in remote communities (Averill 2012). In a study of rural older adults, Averill concluded that older adults in rural communities display impressive strengths and assets alongside the problems they face. These strengths are summarized as "(a) individual peers, family members, and caregivers/providers, (b) community-wide advocacy groups and centers, and (c) an array of rural values that inform the older adults behavior, outlook, and belief systems" (p. 366). Moreover, "the strengths will play a key role in interventions aimed at reducing or eliminating inequities." (p. 366). Contrary to the notion that older adults are pervasive users of the healthcare system, participants in Averill's study defined health as avoiding the healthcare system, done in conjunction with the ability to get out of bed each morning and to remain active.

Frontier regions are characterized by geographic isolation and low population density. In 1998, Congress passed *Health Care in Rural Areas, Sect. 799A*, which defines a frontier as an area with less than seven persons per square mile (Frontier Education Center 1998). Almost all frontier counties are in the western states, covering Montana, down to Texas and including Alaska (Zelarney and Ciarlo n.d.). Contextually, the geographic isolation of frontier counties poses unique challenges relating to access to and delivery of healthcare and human services. Serving small populations dispersed over wide areas forces greater reliance on physicians who are generalists, the use of paraprofessional staff and informal family, and community support systems (Minugh et al. 2007). Because elderly people often require a healthcare workforce that is more skilled and trained in geriatric care, further stress is placed on the healthcare and human service delivery systems (Roger 2002). Rural Medicare patients receive health services primarily in physician offices (Gunderson et al. 2006). In a study of health system challenges, Nayar et al. (2013) found that both the elders and persons under age 18 have a greater need for primary care services, frontier counties have a higher proportion of the elderly above age 65 population, significantly lower median household income, lower unemployment rates, lower illiteracy rates, a higher proportion of Hispanic and

American Indian population, and a higher percentage of population who are not proficient in English. Residents of FR are described as having distinct cultural characteristics, including self-reliance, conservatism, a distrust of outsiders, religion, work orientation, family values, and individualism (Nayar et al. 2013).

Residents of frontier counties have low exposure rates to environmental hazards such as ozone and particulate matter. In addition, these residents have a significantly lower proportion of obese individuals, lower physical inactivity, and diabetes. However, more adverse behavioral risk factors include significantly lower access to healthy foods and recreational facilities, higher liquor store density, and significantly higher motor vehicle fatality rates than non-frontier counties (Nayar et al. 2013). In addition, frontier regions are described as having high rates of substance abuse and suicide (Minugh et al. 2007; Wagenfeld 2000).

Rural America is currently undergoing major demographic and social transitions. There is an outmigration of younger individuals and an increase in ethnic minority groups, especially from Mexico, South America, and Asia with the vast majority being Mexican or Hispanic (Glasgow and Brown 2012; Jensen 2006; Phillips and McLeroy 2004). However, non-Hispanic whites are still a majority group (about 79 %) (Johnson 2012). Compared to natives in rural areas, new immigrants are more likely to be aged 18–64 rather than children or elders. The majority of these immigrants are married, less well educated, but they are not necessarily unskilled. In addition, more new immigrants work in agriculture than do natives, are underemployed, more likely to be in poverty or near poverty than their urban counterparts, and are likely to report good health but may not have access to health insurance (Jensen 2006).

Similar to rural areas in the USA, rural poverty in the developing world (e.g., sub-Saharan Africa, Asia, India, the Pacific, Latin America, the Caribbean, the Middle East and North Africa) is very high, with a strong concentration of extreme poverty among landless farmers, indigenous peoples, women, and children. The developing world is still more rural than urban, with 55 % of the total population living in rural areas. In fact, several parts of the developing world have as their majority population elderly people in rural areas (Kumar et al. 2001). At least 70 % of the world's very poor people are rural; South Asia has the greatest number of poor rural people and sub-Saharan Africa the highest incidence of rural poverty. About 34 % of the total rural population of developing countries is classified as extremely poor. Across regions in the developing world, families live on less than US $1.5—US $2.00 a day (Rural Poverty Report 2011). The comparison of rural poverty in the USA and in developing countries is compositionally (i.e., the characteristics of the residents) and contextually similar (i.e., characteristics of rural areas).

In a study of the rural–urban divide in health services utilization among older Mexicans in Mexico, Salinas et al. (2010) found that older Mexicans living in most rural areas were significantly less likely to have been hospitalized in the previous year and visited the physician less often than their urban counterparts. One possible explanation for this outcome is having health coverage. However, certain health factors such as diabetes, previous heart attack, hypertension, depression, and functional limitations predicted frequency of physician visits and hospitalization, but they did not explain variations between rural and urban older Mexicans. In Mexico, the healthcare system is work-based (i.e., associated with the formal labor market of employment). Although the Mexican government provides free state-run health services for uninsured persons or those unable to pay, resources are limited. Another possible explanation for the low number of doctor visits by rural older Mexican residents is that the elderly people tend to remain in their traditional locations (e.g., ST, villages). Given the elevated levels of poverty and lack of services in rural areas, older Mexicans are at greater risk for experiencing negative health consequences associated with material disadvantage.

Lack of access to quality care is the primary modifiable risk factor for mortality disparities in rural Mexico (Salinas et al. 2010).

Research suggests that in the USA (Centers for Disease Control 2013) and in developing countries, longevity is associated with healthcare access over the entire life course (Gu et al. 2009). In general, older adults report high levels of quality of life; however, rural older adults age 65 and over have lower social functioning than their urban counterparts. Moreover, older African Americans and Hispanics have lower levels of quality of life across several dimensions (Baernholdt et al. 2012), including socialization, fellowship, mobility, and self-care. Clearly, the world's elderly population living in these areas is more vulnerable to greater socioeconomic and health marginalization (Kumar et al. 2001).

Profile of LGBT Elders in Rural Society

Rural elderly LGBT persons present unique characteristics. The literature suggests several details are known about LGBT elders in rural communities. First, LGBT persons are shunned from rural society and experience heightened stigma because of its traditional values, fundamentalist religious beliefs, and strong conservative ideals found within these communities. In tandem with these characteristics and a sense of cultural heterosexism in rural communities, LGBT elders remain "closeted' because of fear of harassment of violence (Harley et al. 2014). Second, the anonymity often found in large cities is nonexistent in rural areas. The closeness and interdependence in rural areas and ST often blur boundaries of privacy; the behavior of residents is easily known and information is shared through local venues throughout the community. In a secondary analysis of data from the MetLife Mature Market Institute (2010a) "*Still Out, Still Aging*" survey, which compares supports for LGBT persons (i.e., baby boomers) aging in rural versus urban areas, Lee and Quam (2013) found that rural individuals reported lower levels of outness, guardedness with people including siblings and close friends, and lower levels of

household income. In a similar study among midlife and older lesbians and gay men in the desert of California, Gardner et al. (2014) found that almost one-third maintain some fear of openly disclosing their sexual orientation. Third, LGBT persons face potential isolation due to the lack of a visible gay community and fewer opportunities for social connection (Bostwick 2007; Hastings and Hoover-Thompson 2011). Fourth, rural elderly lesbians are among the poorest of the poor, with those with disabilities experiencing the most severe poverty (Brault 2012; Fowles and Greenberg 2011) (see Chap. 32).

Fifth, psychosocial and economic stressors are exacerbated in rural areas due to lower levels of education, limited opportunities, lack of availability of services, lack of transportation, and isolation (Fowles and Greenberg 2011). One area in which these factors are evident is the higher rate of mental health issues as compared to urban counterparts (Ziller et al. 2010). Many LGBT elders living in RS and who experience mental illnesses do not seek care. Research indicates a number of barriers to finding LGBT-friendly mental health providers and programs in rural areas (Willging et al. 2006a). For example, fears of harassment or violence prevent LGBT providers from working with LGBT persons to create networks and resources (Willging et al. 2006b). Moreover, most information about LGBT persons' mental health is related to counseling or psychotherapy and limited information about those with serious mental illness or those who require service other than therapy (Bostwick 2007). However, given the disparities in both mental health research and services of the LGBT population in general and certain LGBT populations, including rural populations, an appropriate inference is that LGBT elders in rural areas are underdiagnosed. Sixth, many LGBT persons have limited access to health care, are uninsured, underinsured, and lack financial resources for essential and preventive health care (Baker and Krehely 2012; Hunter 2005). Finally, LGBT persons living in rural areas face the same issues (e.g., poverty, lower quality of housing, scarce health and mental health resources, need of assistance with activities of daily living, and transportation) that heterosexual residents face resulting from political and economic inequities (e.g., relevance of rural areas, vulnerabilities, strengthening alliances, constituency size, and concentration) between rural and urban areas that perpetuate inequities in the system (Comerford et al. 2004; Hartman and Weierbach 2013).

Many LGBT elders in rural areas may be reluctant to define themselves openly as lesbian, gay, bisexual, or transgender because of the overt discrimination; physical, emotional, and psychological intimidation and abuse; involuntary outing; and generalized societal oppression of sexual minorities (Comerford et al. 2004). The degree to which LGBT elders experience stigma around their sexual identity greatly influences how they engage with supportive healthcare and social or human services (Masini and Barrett 2008). Older gay men and lesbians maintain some discomfort in their use of adult social services; the majority report some comfort accessing LGBT-friendly identified services and programs. In addition, lesbians report greater fear and discomfort than do gay men; older gay men and lesbians report less comfort in accessing LGBT-friendly services and programs than younger lesbians and gay men (Gardner et al. 2014). Because of discomfort in using health and social services in tandem with lack of family support, which is common for LGBT elders, it is necessary to make a greater effort to develop other sources of support, intensified in rural areas (Comerford et al. 2004). The case of Amanda and Susan below illustrates some of the problems faced by LGBT elders in rural areas as they age in place.

Discussion Box 25.1

Amanda, 73, is a retired nurse and a lesbian. She spent her entire professional career working a rural area and continues to live in the same area. She has been working as an advocate for LGBT healthcare equity for over 40 years. A year ago Amanda began to care for a friend, Susan, whose partner died three years ago. Susan

is in failing health and faces eviction from her home. Amanda and other friends in the community have taken steps to intervene on behalf of Susan with various social service agencies and healthcare providers. The social worker has requested that Susan be placed in a nursing home facility. Agency personnel, the caseworker, and healthcare providers will not communicate with anyone other than Susan.

This situation illustrates that caregiving extends beyond kinship ties. Mainstream care and service agencies do not understand that it takes a community to support LGBT elders who grow old in place. In addition, service providers have not given consideration to the potential homophobia and isolation that Susan may experience in a nursing facility.

Questions

1. What legal issues may be barriers to Amanda and other friends in advocating on behalf of Susan?
2. What characteristics of rural culture present barriers?
3. What are the policy implications for LGBT elders and their allies in rural areas?
4. What are the implications of aging-in-place for LGBT elders in rural areas?

Some research suggests that a gender difference exists in residential preference. For example, lesbians may elect to live in rural areas because it is conducive to the role of the butch lesbian and easily acceptable by rural dwellers who may see lesbians as hard-working women (Comerford et al. 2004). Others may elect to live in rural settings because of an affinity to the land and nature. Conversely, gay men tend to prefer urban settings because of increased opportunity for socialization. Rural areas demand independence and self-reliance, and often lesbians learn to do a wide range of cross-gendered, life-supporting activities on their own. Comerford et al. (2004), in a studied of fifteen elderly lesbians (average age of 60) in rural Vermont and found social isolation, took on an added dimension as a function of the fear of being rejected because of sexual orientation and fewer lesbians available for support within the population as a whole. In this study, social isolation was mediated by wellness and mobility factors, as the participants were able to leave their communities to socialize and gain support of lesbians in other areas. Although the participants were able to enlist heterosexual neighbors to help with living-related tasks, they did not rely on them for emotional support.

Comerford et al. (2004) also found that the majority of the women felt comfortable with their sexual identity as long as it remained private but became less so when their identity became public due to fear of potential consequence. In addition, these women promoted intentional construction of informal support networks as a central aspect of living as a lesbian because lesbians of their generation frequently lacked family support. Comerford hypothesized that as lesbians in rural areas age, they may need additional help to access transportation services, existing networks, and to develop new sources of social support. The use of technology (e.g., Internet, Web-based programs, tele-technology) to provide connection and social support is recognized as helpful; however, Internet access does not always exist for various rural and urban areas (Lewis and Marshall 2012). Many adults over age 65 are vulnerable to digital exclusion. Also, not all elderly people are computer literate (Clark and Leipert 2007). For frontier regions, availability and access to technology remain remote. Similar outcomes are found among elders in Europe (Burholt and Dobbs 2012).

In the rural culture, volunteerism is a strong component and can enhance social support (Clark and Leipert 2007). Volunteers are a vital force in rural communities and an investment in the people of the community. Rural culture enacts gender differences in how social supports are maintained and accessed, with women being primarily responsible for providing voluntary care. However, gender subscription is less prevalent in volunteering among LGBT populations. For example, lesbians in RS pride themselves on being independent and able to do whatever type of work to take care of themselves. Thus, in doing carpentry, older lesbians may be seen as doing "man's work." Even if others in rural communities do not label them as lesbians, they will view them as not being lady-like. Given the overwhelming traditional and conservative values in RS, older lesbians are seen often as hardy women.

Isolation and Survival Strategies

Elderly LGBT persons living in rural areas may become more isolated from their families of origin than others. Because elderly lesbians and gay men are more likely than their non-lesbian and non-gay counterparts to be single, childless, and estranged from family members, they must often rely on friends and "informal families of choice" (Baker and Krehely 2012, p. 19). As they age, LGBT elders may lose their visibility within the lesbian community (having little to no voice in the political agenda of the LGBT community), which can exacerbate their endemic loneliness in rural communities. They may be excluded or marginalized by the younger LGBT community to form community discussions and issues pertinent to them and absent from the mainstream LGBT political agenda. The experience of ageism in the LGBT community may compound psychological, victimization, and despair issues. Many experience the loss of a long-term partner and may have to hide the grieving process from others so as to hide the relationship (Hunter 2005). Thus, as LGBT elders in rural communities become more isolated, they eventually transform into the "truly invisible" (Comerford et al. 2004, p. 420).

For LGBT elders who manage to thrive in rural communities, a number of specific strategies are used, including finding a network to help cope with adversity and to gain access to certain resources, traveling to keep in touch and engaged because older adults sometimes prefer to meet face-to-face rather than by virtual means (e.g., Internet), managing disclosure or coming out because it may not always be safe to come out or coming out may negatively influence opportunities and access to services or further marginalization, and gaining access to sufficient resources to function better in one's environment (Rowan et al. 2013, see Research Box 25.1). Ironically, withholding disclosure about one's sexual identity, refraining from seeking assistance for health needs, and avoiding association with LGBT communities are employed as survival strategies by LGBT elders in anticipation of facing discrimination from service providers (Lee and Quam 2013). Downplaying or hiding one's sexual orientation and identity in rural, more conservative settings where the negative climate is believed, in some ways, to restrict self-acceptance and development of LGBT community cohesion and support is considered necessary for survival. Yet, out of necessity, the sparse population in RS almost force LGBT persons in rural areas to forge more close-knit connections and sense of family, especially in times of need, compared to their urban counterparts (Oswald and Culton 2003).

Research Box 25.1
Rowan, N. L., Giunta, N., Grudowski, E. S., & Anderson, K. A. (2013). Aging well and gay in rural America: A case study. *Journal of Gerontological Social Work, 56* (3), 185–200.

Objective: To explore the experience of one older gay man who lives in a rural community where he has lived throughout his life.

Method: A qualitative case study approach was used. The case was purposively as the participant appeared to be unique in his circumstances, primarily in the fact that he did not appear to have experienced the caustic elements thought to be present in rural communities for gay men. The case

---

was selected based upon existing contact with the participant in social interactions. The participant is an 80-year-old gay man. Person-environment fit theory was selected to help guide this study through in-depth interviews and thematic analysis.

Results: An overarching theme of life satisfaction clearly emerged, along with themes regarding supportive social networks and disclosure management of his sexual orientation.

Conclusion: The findings suggest that although it is important to understand the challenges faced by the LGBT community in rural environments, it is equally important to shed light on the ways in which older adults age well within these communities.

Questions

1. Do the experiences of LGBT elders who lived in rural areas for their entire life differ than those who moved there as adults?
2. What are the positive psychosocial issues LGBT elders in rural areas exhibit?
3. What factors contribute to healthy aging of LGBT elders in rural communities?

LGBT persons are considered to have unique strengths. Due to the oppression and stigma associated with sexual minority status (see Chap. 2), LGBT persons often adapt to many life situations, including discrimination, violence, and exclusion of legal recognition for couples/marriage. This trait of adaptability has led to LGBT persons being described as resilient and having strengths that will aid in successful aging (Crisp et al. 2008). LGBT elders regard that benefits of being a sexual minority help them prepare for aging by enhancing personal/interpersonal strengths and overcoming adversity. More specifically, they identify key strengths as (a) being more accepting of others, (b) not taking anything for granted, (c) being more resilient or having a stronger inner strength, (d) having greater self-reliance, (e) being more careful in legal and financial matters, and (f) having a chosen family (MetLife 2010b). Earlier studies on the advantages of being an aging sexual minority reveal that these individuals are not reliant on family, not limited to male or female roles, have more awareness of planning for the future, and have mature psychological and spiritual dimensions of life (Kimmel 1978; Lucco 1987). In fact, Kimmel described how early family stressors, especially around the coming out process, may provide LGBT elders with "crisis competency" or resilience that insulates the person again in later crises (p. 117). Research suggests that LGBT elders who had managed not to internalize stigmatizing messages, homophobia, and heterosexism were better able to face the challenges that come with later life. In addition, these individuals reported higher self-esteem, were more self-accepting, were better connected with family members, were actively engaged in social supports and community and social causes, and could assess their lives as having been worthwhile and purposeful (Smith and Gray 2009).

Conversely, Subhrajit (2014) suggests that due to institutionalized heterosexism, social isolation, and ageism within the LGBT community itself, many LGBT elders may retreat into the closet, thus reinforcing isolation. Some cope by passing for being heterosexual. Research suggests that disclosure decreases with increasing age (Gates 2010; Rawls 2004). Moreover, as LGBT persons grow older, they enter a world of services that may be unfamiliar. Any discussion of isolation related to LGBT elders must be understood in context. Elder and Retrum (2012) remind us, "it is useful to consider that each person has a different history and subsequent propensity for isolation depending on his or her behaviors and choices throughout life" (p. 17). Isolation may be voluntary or involuntary. The way in which a person becomes isolated is variable and multifaceted (see Chap. 29).

Unique Needs of Rural LGBT Elders and Concerns About HealthCare Service Delivery and Disclosure

One of the greatest challenges of the twenty-first century is ensuring the quality of life of an unprecedented large and growing elderly population (Kumar et al. 2001). Older adults in the general population and among LGBT groups tend to be the most frequent users of healthcare services in the USA. In the case of access and utilization, limited attention has been given to health care among elderly LGBT persons. However, LGBT people of all ages are much more likely than heterosexual adults to delay or not seek medical care (de Vries et al. 2011). Lesbians experience many life circumstances differently than do their heterosexual counterparts, including seeking, accessing, and using human services (Hash and Netting 2009; Maccio and Doueck 2002). For older LGBT adults, health concomitants of aging may be exacerbated by factors associated with gender and sexual orientation (de Vries et al. 2011). Specific challenges exist for older bisexual persons, including being unwelcome in the gay and lesbian community, being ignored or oppressed by gays and lesbians, and feeling like they need to present themselves as gay or lesbian in order to be accepted by gays and lesbians (Crisp et al. 2008). For bisexual persons, added discrimination is another barrier. Life within a context marked by fear and secrecy can have long-lasting, multiple, and frequently significant impact on many LGBT elders (Comerford et al. 2004).

According to the behavioral model, access to health care is determined by system factors (availability and supply of healthcare providers) and by consumers' predisposing (biological and social characteristics thought to affect an individual's propensity to use health services), enabling (though to affect an individual's ability to obtain health services), and need (thought to have the biggest impact on whether an individual seeks health care) characteristics (Xu and Borders 2003). Xu and Borders contend that one phenomenon that has the potential to further undermine the accessibility of health services in rural areas is migration or "outshopping" (seeking physician services outside of their local market area) for health services. For LGBT elders in rural areas, migration may be seen as a better choice to ensure confidentiality and to reduce discrimination. Despite being more likely to have usual source of care (USC), which is one of the factors that increases the use of preventive care services and decreases risk of having unmet health needs (Newacheck et al. 2000), rural adults are somewhat less likely to receive certain preventive care services than are urban adults (Ziller and Lenardson 2009). In addition, rural residents have more travel time and distance to a healthcare provider, which can adversely affect their ability to access a provider, especially among those needing specialty care (Chan et al. 2006).

In interviews with late middle-aged and older lesbians in a rural area, Butler and Hope (1999) found that their fears included panic when they thought about ever having to go to a nursing home because of heterosexual assumptions of the whole institution, being punished for being a lesbian, being old and fearful of having to deal with extremely hostile prejudice of the radical political right, and denying themselves the health care they needed because of lack of affordability. In fact, older lesbians may feel that revealing their identity is not important if it means receiving inferior healthcare services (Hunter 2005). In a study of lesbians deciding who to see for health and mental health care, Saulnier (2002) found that lesbians encountered a continuum of provider reactions that shaped their decisions: (a) homophobia, (b) heterosexism, (c) tolerance, (d) lesbian sensitivity, and (e) lesbian affirmation. See Table 25.1 for a list of fears of discrimination.

Based on the limited available studies on LGBT persons with serious mental illness, research findings suggest that they are subjected to poor treatment, particularly in the public mental health system (Bostwick 2007). LGBT persons feel compelled to hide their sexual orientation or gender identity in an effort to protect themselves from ridicule, abuse, or maltreatment from service providers and peers. In addition,

Table 25.1 Fears of discrimination from healthcare providers

Hostility
Rejection
Invisibility
Deny care
Reduced care
Stigmatization
Anti-gay violence/safety
Inadequate/substandard health care
Refrain from touching a patient who is lesbian
Careless management of private information and identity disclosure
Inappropriate verbal and/or nonverbal responses from providers and office staff
Refusal of service providers and healthcare systems to recognize extended families within the gay community

Adapted from Saulnier (2002)

concealing a fundamental part of themselves (e.g., identity) can often interfere with successful treatment because they are not able to bring the entirety of who they are into treatment (Lucksted 2004).

In a study of interactions between community-based aging service providers and LGBT older adults, Hughes et al. (2011) found very few services specific to the needs of older LGBT adults and very little outreach to this community. Knochel et al. (2012) surveyed leaders of Area Agencies on Aging, in which half of the existing agencies in the USA participated, in order to understand their services, training, and beliefs about serving LGBT older adults. Results showed that few agencies provided LGBT outreach services, one-third had trained staff around LGBT, and four-fifths were willing to offer training. Moreover, those agencies that provided, or were willing to provide training, were typically urban-based.

Sexual minorities encounter two unique obstacles: homophobia and heterosexism. Navigating healthcare, social, and human services can be further complicated by the degree to which lesbians self-disclose to others (Maccio and Doueck 2002). Providers along the healthcare continuum of caregivers ranging from doctors to pharmacists to hospitals and nursing home staff, may be hostile toward LGBT elders, untrained to work with them, unaware that older LGBT adults even exist, may lack knowledge about health disparities affecting LGBT people, and may lack skills of appropriate behavior dealing with closeted LGBT individuals (Public Advocate for the City of New York 2008). Of great concern is the number of LGBT elders who report experiencing victimization, physical assault, sexual assault, stalking, property damage, and financial exploitation motivated by homophobia (Gugliucci et al. 2013) (see Research Box 25.2). In addition, many LGBT older adults are not able to advocate for themselves—their families and facility staff are unaware of federal protections under the *Nursing Home Reform Act of 1987.*

Research Box 25.2

Gugliucci, M. R., Weaver, S. A., Kimmel, D. C., Littlefield, M., Hollander, L., & Hennessy, J. (2013). *Gay, lesbian, bisexual and transgender (GLBT) aging in Maine: Community needs assessment.* AARP.

Objective: To initiate the establishment of a Services and Advocacy for Gay, Lesbian, Bisexual and Transgender Elders (SAGE) Affiliate Chapter in Maine. The secondary purpose is to advance awareness of LGBT aging in Maine, and to improve services and support systems for Maine's older LGBT community.

Method: An online (survey Monkey) and paper survey was used with a convenience sample of 468 and three focus groups with a snowball sample of 36 participants. Survey questions were grouped under four categories: (1) health care, (2) personal safety, (3) social services, and (4) social well-being. Focus group discussions included four issues: (1) experience, understanding, and navigating the healthcare system; (2) awareness, opinions, and concerns about special healthcare services; (3) knowledge of legal documents necessary for protection; and

(4) accessing mental health services/maintaining one's mental health. Data were analyzed using descriptive statistics and theme classification.

Results: The results were varied. Most participants had adequate financial resources, access to LGBT-sensitive healthcare providers, and have taken steps to plan for aging through legal arrangements. Long-term care facilities and life planning were the issues for many respondents. More than half the respondents feel safe in their community, live openly as LGBT, and do not feel isolated. There is a sense of belonging in a faith community. Of concerns was the number of respondents reporting having experienced victimization, assault, stalking, financial exploitation, and property damage motivated by homophobia. In addition, the respondents expressed concerns about discrimination by healthcare providers, mental health practitioners, and social workers.

Conclusion: Regardless of financial status or community connections, LGBT elders are at risk of isolation and discrimination based on their minority status and vulnerability.

Questions

1. What are the limitations of sample selection?
2. What are the advantages and disadvantages of using research mix-methodology?
3. What other data analysis could have been used?

Improving the Lives of LGBT Older Adults (Sage and MAP 2010) identified key challenges facing LGBT elders: social sigma and prejudice, reliance on informal families of choice, and unequal treatment under laws, programs, and services. The three challenges impede LGBT elders' successful aging by reducing financial security, health/health care, and community support. The lifetime of discrimination faced by older LGBT elders and the resulting effects on financial security is compounded by major laws and safety net programs (e.g., Social Security, Medicaid, tax-qualified retirement plans, retiree health insurance benefits, veterans' benefits, inheritance laws) that fail to protect and support them equally with their heterosexual peers (Baker and Krehely 2012).

Persons who require multiple services from different service providers tend to receive appropriate services when the services are well coordinated and integrated. For LGBT elders in rural areas, the need for services to be integrated is increasingly important because of such factors as limited availability or proximity to services, costs of services, and transportation, which are often the result of policies established regarding eligibility for services, which are discussed below.

Integrated Services and Policy Issues

Several factors affect service provision for LGBT elders in rural areas. First, the ability of rural elders to access necessary care in the community they consider home is important. Second, elders benefit from the best possible care when congruency exists between standards of practice and licensure (Hartman and Weierbach 2013). Finally, as elders require care beyond the role of the healthcare provider, it is essential that the provider collaborate with professionals who are qualified through professional standards of practice and credentials to meet the needs of elders (Robert Wood Johnson Foundation 2011; IOM 2011). When elders seek services, the expectation is that the service provider will meet their needs, and moreover, they trust that the service provider has the knowledge, skills, and abilities to meet their needs (Hartman and Weierbach). This expectation is the same among LGBT elders, and the service provider should reciprocate in meeting this expectation. Fredriksen-Goldsen et al. (2011) found that only

28 % of the participants in their study currently use programs or services available in their community. When LGBT elders were asked what services and programs they believe are most needed, they identified senior housing, transportation, legal services, social events, and support groups, with all groups (i.e., lesbians, bisexual women, gay men, bisexual men, and transgender) endorsing the first four being the most needed. In rural settings, LGBT elders face barriers in accessing each of these services. Participants in Averill's study (2012) identified areas in which work is needed to counteract a "patchwork service network" because of a lack of organized, coordinated efforts (see Table 25.2).

Healthcare reform is anticipated to improve access to health care and health outcomes for LGBT populations in rural areas. "The *Affordable Care Act* is the most significant and far-reaching reform of America's health system since the creation of Medicare and Medicaid in the 1960s" (Baker and Krehely 2012, p. 21). The *Affordable Care Act* (ACA) introduces new protections and options for consumers in the private health insurance market, expands access to more comprehensive benefits and services, focuses on improving the nation's health, emphasizes lowering healthcare cost, and removes barriers for preexisting health conditions. The ACA is viewed as a historic

Table 25.2 Needed organized and coordinated efforts for service delivery

Accurately document which agencies offer what services
Various eligibility requirements
Funding sources that support programs
Kind of strategic planning to sustain programs in the future
Plans for linking to other services and programs in the region
How specific information about health and social services is disseminated, communicated, assessed for adequacy, evaluated for effectiveness, and revised in response to analysis and critique
How necessary personnel levels can be maintained or expanded

Adapted from Averill (2012)

opportunity to change the way people conceptualize how the healthcare industry provides care and promotes wellness, and is seen as the strongest foundation for closing LGBT disparities (Baker and Krehely 2012; National Coalition for LGBT Health 2012). For all LGBT groups, the ACA also undergirds efforts to (a) expand cultural competency in the healthcare workforce to include LGBT issues, (b) improve data collection to better identify and address health disparities, and (c) recognize the increasing diversity of America's families. Despite these improvements, ACA is not without challenges to healthcare services in rural areas. Approximately an additional 8.1 million rural residents are projected to be insured through Medicaid or state health exchanges due to implementation of ACA (UnitedHealth Center for Health Reform & Modernization 2011). The challenges of implementing ACA in rural areas may include, but not limited to: (a) the increase in the number of persons entering the insurance rolls may amplify existing pressures on an already overextended rural healthcare workforce, (b) the health professional shortage in certain specializations may further hinder timeliness of service, and (c) hospitals will be challenged to find new avenues to improve care and reduce cost in the health reform era (Choi 2012). See Chap. 19 for further discussion of the impact of ACA for LGBT elders.

The delivery of healthcare services to LGBT elders should involve understanding the "person-in-environment" or "person-in-situation" (Wheeler 2003). Healthcare providers must understand that LGBT elders cannot be understood apart from multifaceted contexts (e.g., familiar, social, political, spiritual, economic, and physical). With a person-in-environment framework, healthcare providers must be uniquely equipped to assess both the medical and psychological aspects of elders and intervene in a culturally competent manner, especially critically given the complex psychosocial issues underlying unmet healthcare needs, life style-related medical conditions and treatment non-adherence challenges that pose significant barriers in LGBT elders receiving optimal health care. To facilitate an understanding of the needs of LGBT elders,

especially in rural areas, interdisciplinary, multidisciplinary, transdisciplinary, and integrated approaches to training service providers are needed to reduce the discrepancy between pedagogy of training and the execution of producing competent professionals across the disciplines (Harley et al. 2014).

The way in which services are delivered to LGBT elders in rural areas in the USA, Canada, the United Kingdom, and other parts of the world is interchangeable to a certain extent. However, it is important for relevance and utility that context-specific knowledge be identified and applied to advance the quality of life of rural LGBT elders within the rural setting and service delivery system that is specific to their country (Clark and Leipert 2007). This is not to say that cross-cultural exchanges are not valuable. Building a strong coalition of allies with expertise to address the complexities of LGBT elders, both nationally and internationally, is warranted. SAGE and MAP (2010) assert that allies can bring resources, expertise, policy know-how, political connections and influence, and the ear of the mainstream aging community to the LGBT aging agenda. Moreover, collaboration between LGBT aging and mainstream aging entities is a natural partnership because many heterosexual elders are also affected by the same issues and barriers as LGBT elders. Policy to potentially achieve a process to improve the health of all residents in rural communities is offered in the strategic planning section of *Rural Health People 2020* (Bolin and Bellamy 2012, see Policy Box 25.1).

Policy Box 25.1

Strategic Planning for Rural Healthy People (RHP) 2020

Convene RHP 2020 Advisory Board to include representatives from funding partners, rural health providers, state rural health agencies, and national rural health agencies (including LGBT-specific services and programs).

Assess the extent to which the previous RHP 2010 achieved its objectives.

Through national engagement of stake-holders, initiate a Delphi process to iden-tify the highest priority rural-based HP 2020 focus areas and, within those, objec-tives to be achieved by RHP 2020.

Continuously work with rural stakeholder and advocacy groups for continued national focus on and support of RHPM2020.

Update and expand invitations for sub-mission of RHP 2020 Models for Practice to be published on an ongoing basis.

Work with CDC-PRC's Community Guide for Preventive Services leadership to develop and disseminate relevant entries (to serve as a resource to local, state, and national program directors in developing programs and policies in their communi-ties) to the Community Guide through collaboration with PRC's leadership.

Engage rural health researchers to update and refine rural health research and literature reviews by RHP 2020 priority focus areas.

Develop priority area toolkits for rural communities to employ in preparing local and state-specific proposals.

Use existing Web-based dissemination mechanisms and develop additional dis-semination mechanisms.

Adapted from Bolin and Bellamy (2012).

Any effort undertaken to improve current policy should take a multi-pronged approach. First, real and personal stories should be used to educate the public about how inequities affect LGBT elders. Putting a human face on discrim-ination and neglect illustrates the harmful effects of current policies. Second, debunking myths about LGTB populations can serve to sensitize others to the realities and challenges facing LGBT elders. Third, policy and practice should be informed by evidence-based research. Often, barriers for LGBT elders in accessing and receiving quality care are a function of a lack of adequate training and supervised clinical practice with this population. Appropriate training requires an understanding of effective interven-tion practices in RS. Fourth, funding for research that focuses on the experiences of LGBT elders living in rural areas is needed. Both rural elders and the community can benefit when partnerships are created to promote programs based on the research (NRHA 2011). Fifth, rural areas in gen-eral and specific population in RS in particular often need an advocacy infrastructure. Ideally, a national infrastructure is also needed (SAGE and MAP 2010); however, a grass-roots approach may produce a more immediate impact for LGBT elders living in rural areas. Activism among rural LGBT persons is marked by geographic distinc-tion in how they view differences between rural and urban LGBT persons. That is, rural LGBT persons tie activism to an urban phenomenon (Kazyak 2011). Too often rural areas lack the capacity to engage in advocacy to advance social, political, economic, and quality of life concerns. Finally, policy makers and service providers need to understand nuanced needs of rural residents. The assumption that a "one-size-fits-all" approach is sufficient is a disservice to LGBT elders in RS.e to LGBT elders in RS.

Summary

LGBT elders in rural areas have diverse social, physical, and economic characteristics. Collec-tively, they share characteristics of other residents in rural areas, and individually and as minority groups, they present unique challenges and con-cerns regarding service needs. LGBT elders in rural areas are both visible (i.e., seen with each other) and invisible (i.e., interconnected nature of rural life). Collectively, rural LGBT elders are poorer, have more health disparities, and have less social support than their heterosexual counter-parts. These factors may present additional con-cerns when aggregated by race.

Although some rural LGBT elders are healthy, well adjusted, and socially active, many others are not. Underutilization of services is more than a function of limited availability and access; it is also a manifestation of founded fears concerning receiving poor quality of service because of their sexual orientation and sexual identity. Overall, LGBT elders in rural settings are known to be at risk across numerous categories and to experience challenges that are compounded to a greater extent than their urban counterparts. Given the vulnerabilities of this population, recent changes in health reform, and the repeal of the Defense of Marriage Act (DOMA), the impact on the quality of life of LGBT elders in rural areas remains to be seen.

Learning Exercises

Self-Check Questions

1. RS in the USA make up a substantial portion of the country. Do the majority of people live in rural or urban areas?
2. FR are characterized by geographic isolation and low population density. As a result of being dispersed over wide areas, upon what type of physician do residents rely the most?
3. Some LGBT elders in rural areas are open about their sexual orientation and identity; however, many are not. What are the major reasons for them concealing their identity?
4. What challenges does the Affordable Care Act have for rural communities?
5. Why is it considered difficult to maintain privacy in rural communities?

Field-Based Experiential Assignments

1. Visit a local gathering spot or community center in a rural setting and one in an urban area and compare and contrast them. What did you observe about participants' interactions? How diverse were the participants? Did you observe an inclusive or welcoming environment for LGBT elders?
2. Volunteer to assist an LGBT elder in a rural area with transportation, chores, escort to a social event, and so forth.
3. Help to establish an advocacy network for LGBT elders in a rural community.

Multiple Choice Questions

1. The elderly in rural areas are more likely than urban elders to have which of the following?
   a. High income
   b. Live poverty
   c. Own their own car
   d. Graduate from college
2. Which type of healthcare workforce does the elderly require?
   a. General practitioner
   b. Skilled in tele-care
   c. Trained in geriatric care
   d. Understand aging of in-migration in rural areas
3. Which of the following influences how LGBT elders in rural areas engage with supportive healthcare or social services?
   a. Stigma around their sexual identity
   b. Age of the service provider
   c. Guidance received from social networks
   d. The number of older persons receiving services
4. What are LGBT elders in rural areas doing when they withhold disclosure about one's sexual identity, refrain from seeking assistance for health needs, and avoid association with LGBT communities?
   a. Exhibiting denial
   b. Relinquishing avoidance behavior
   c. Exercising cohort identity
   d. Employing survival strategies
5. Why can "outshopping" for health services be of benefit LGBT elders in RS?
   a. Reduce out-migration of older persons
   b. Increase confidentiality and reduce discrimination

c. Decrease admission to long-term care facilities

d. Increase priorities for funding of rural health care

6. Why is geographic location a significant variable for LGBT elders in RS?
   a. Rural locations provide more specialized health care
   b. Location influences how persons experience aging
   c. Urban locations provide better proximity to attractive amenities for retirement
   d. Location determines amount of internalized oppression persons experience

7. What types of coping strategies do LGBT elders employ most often to thrive in rural areas?
   a. Use of the Internet
   b. Church attendance
   c. Finding a network
   d. Internalizing stigmatizing messages

8. What is a barrier to establishing activism among rural LGBT persons?
   a. Activism is seen as an urban phenomenon
   b. Capacity to engage in advocacy
   c. Both of the above
   d. None of the above

9. Which of the following may provide LGBT elders with resilience in dealing with stressors?
   a. Crisis competency
   b. Cultural competency
   c. Futuristic planning
   d. Psychoanalysis

10. What is a recommended approach of understanding the needs of LGBT elders in RS?
    a. Person-in-globalization
    b. Medical model
    c. Psychological model
    d. Person-in-environment

Key

1-B
2-C
3-A
4-D
5-B
6-B
7-C
8-C
9-A
10-D

Resources and Websites

Elder Care Locator: www.eldercare.gov/Eldercare.NET/Public/Index.aspx

National Research Center on LGBT Aging: www.lgbtagingcenter.org

National Rural Health Association: www.ruralhealthweb.org

Rural Assistance Center: www.raconline.org

"USDA Rural Development—Rural Repair and Rehabilitation Loans and Grants for Seniors" Program: www.programsforelderly.com/housing-usda-rural-repair-and-rehab-loans-grants-senior-homeowners.pdf

References

Averill, J. B. (2012). Priorities for action in a rural older adults study. *Family Community Health, 35*(4), 358–372.

Baernholdt, M., Yan, G., Hinton, I., Rose, K., & Mattos, M. (2012). Quality of life in rural and urban adults 65 years and older: Findings from the National Health and Nutrition Examination Survey. *The Journal of Rural Health, 28,* 339–347.

Baker, K., & Krehely, J. (2012). How health care reform will help LGBT elders. *Public Policy and Aging Report, 21*(3), 19–23.

Bolin, J. N., & Bellamy, G. (2012). Rural healthy people 2020. Retrieved September 3, 2014, from http://www.sph.tamsc.edu/srhrc/docs/rhp2020.pdf.

Bostwick, W. B. (2007). *Disparities in mental health treatment among GLBT populations.* Arlington, VA: National Alliance on Mental Illness.

Brault, M. W. (2012). Americans with disabilities: 2010. *Household economic studies.* Retrieved January 12, 2013, from www.census.gov/prod/2012pubs/p70-131pdf.

Burholt, V., & Dobbs, C. (2012). Research on rural ageing: Where have we got to and where are we going in Europe? *Journal of Rural Studies, 28,* 432–446.

Butler, S. S., & Hope, B. (1999). Health and well-being for late middle-aged and old lesbians in a rural area. *Journal of Gay and Lesbian Social Services, 9*(4), 27–46.

Centers for Disease Control. (2013). *The state of aging and health in America 2013*. Atlanta, GA: Centers for Disease Control, U.S. Department of Health and Human Services.

Chan, L., Hart, L., & Goodman, D. (2006). Geographic access to health care for rural medicine beneficiaries. *Journal of Rural Health, 22*, 140–146.

Choi, J. Y. (2012). A portrait of rural health in America. *Journal of Rural Sciences, 27*(3), 1–16.

Clark, K. J., & Leipert, B. D. (2007). Strengthening and sustaining social supports for rural elders. *Online Journal of Rural Nursing and Health Care, 7*(1), 13–26.

Colello, K. J. (2007). Supportive services programs to naturally occurring retirement communities. Retrieved August 14, 2014, from http://aging.senate.gov/crs/aging15.pdf.

Comerford, S. A., Henson-Stroud, M. M., Sionainn, C., & Wheeler, E. (2004). Crone songs: Voices of lesbian elders on aging in a rural environment. *Affilia, 19*(4), 418–436.

Crisp, C., Wayland, M. S., & Gordon, T. (2008). Older gay, lesbian, and bisexual adults: Tools for age-competent and gay affirmative practice. *Journal of Gay and Lesbian Social Services, 20*(1/2), 5–29.

Cromartie, J., & Nelson, P. (2009). Baby boom migration and its impact on rural America. United States Department of Agriculture. Economic Research Service. Economic Research Report 79. Retrieved August 14, 2014, from http://www.ers.usda.gov/Publications/ERR79/ERR79.pdf.

de Vries, B., et al. (2011). *The health of lesbian, gay, bisexual, and transgender people: Building a foundation for better understandin*. Washington, DC: The National Academic Press.

Elder, K., & Retrum, J. (2012, May 30). *Framework for isolation in adults over 50*. Washington, D.C.: AARP.

Fowles, D. G., & Greenberg, S. (2011). A profile of older Americans: 2011. Washington, DC: Administration on Aging, U.S. Department of Health and Human Services.

Fowles, D. G., & Greenberg, S. (2012). *A profile of older Americans: 2012*. Washington, DC: Administration on Aging, Department of Health and Human Services.

Fredriksen-Goldsen, K. I., Kim, H. J., Emlet, C. A., Muraco, A., Erosheva, E. A., Hoy-Ellis, C. P., Goldsen, J., & Petry, H. (2011). *The aging and health report: Disparities and resilience among lesbian, gay, bisexual, and transgender older adults*. Seattle, WA: Institute for Multigenerational Health.

Frontier Education Center. (1998). *The final report of the Consensus Development Project, Frontier: A new definition*. National Clearinghouse for Frontier Communities. Retrieved August 14, 2014, from http://www.frontierus.org/documents/consensus'paper.htm.

Gardner, A. T., de Vries, B., & Mockus, D. S. (2014). Aging out in the desert: Disclosure, acceptance, and service use among midlife and older lesbians and gay men. *Journal of Homosexuality, 61*, 129–144.

Gates, G. J. (2010). *Sexual minorities in the 2008 general social survey: Coming out and demographic characteristics*. Los Angeles, CA: Williams Institute.

Glasgow, N., & Brown, D. L. (2012). Rural ageing in the United States: Trends and context. *Journal of Rural Studies, 28*, 422–431.

Gu, D., Zhanf, Z., & Zeng, Y. (2009). Access to healthcare services makes a difference in healthy longevity among older Chinese adults. *Social Science Medicine, 68*(2), 210–219.

Gugliucci, M. R., Weaver, S. A., Kimmel, D. C., Littlefield, M., Hollander, L., & Hennessy, J. (2013). *Gay, lesbian, bisexual and transgender (GLBT) aging in Maine: Community needs assessment*. Washington, D.C.: AARP.

Gunderson, A., Menanchemi, N., Brummel-Smith, K., & Brooks, R. (2006). Physicians who treat the elderly in rural Florida: Trends indicating concerns regarding access to care. *The Journal of Rural Health, 22*(3), 224–228.

Harley, D. A., Stansbury, K. L., Nelson, M., & Espinosa, C. T. (2014). A profile of rural African American lesbian elders: Meeting their needs. In H. F. O. Vakalahi, G. M. Simpson, & N. Giunta (Eds.), *The collective spirit of aging across cultures* (pp. 133–155). New York: Springer.

Hart, L. G., Larson, E. H., & Lishner, D. M. (2005). Rural definitions for health policy and research. *American Journal of Public Health, 95*(7), 1149–1155.

Hartman, R. M., & Weierbach, F. M. (2013). *February)*. Rural Health Congress: Elder health in rural America.

Hash, K. M., & Netting, F. E. (2009). It takes a community: Older lesbians meeting social and care needs. *Journal of Gay and Lesbian Social Services, 21*(4), 326–342.

Hastings, S. L., & Hoover-Thompson, A. (2011). Effective support for lesbians in rural communities: The role of psychotherapy. *Journal of Lesbian Studies, 15*(2), 197–204.

Hughes, A. K., Harold, R. D., & Boyer, J. M. (2011). Awareness of LGBT aging issues among aging services network providers. *Journal of Geronotological Social Work, 54*(7), 659–677.

Hunter, S. (2005). *Midlife and older LGBT adults: Knowledge and affirmative practice for the social services*. New York: Haworth Press.

Institute of Medicine. (2006). *Rebuilding the unity of health and the environment in rural America*. Washington, DC: The National Academies Press.

Institute of Medicine. (2011). *The future of nursing: Leading change, advancing health*. Washington, DC: The National Academics Press.

Jensen, L. (2006). New immigrant settlements in rural America: Problems, prospects, and policies. *Reports on Rural America, 1*(3), 1–34.

Johnson, K. M. (2012). Rural demographic change in the new century: Slower growth, increased diversity. *Issue Brief No. 44*. Durham, NH: Carsey Institute. Retrieved September 4, 2014, from http://www.carseyinstitute.

unh.edu/publications/IB-Johnson-Rural-Demographic-Trends.pdf.

Kazyak, E. (2011). Disrupting cultural selves: Constructing gay and lesbian identities in rural locales. *Qual Sociology, 34*, 561–581.

Kellogg Foundation. (2002, December). Perceptions of rural America. Available at http://www.wkkf.org/resource-directory/resource/2002/12/perceptions-of-rural-america

Kimmel, D. (1978). Adult development and aging: A gay perspective. *Journal of Social Issues, 34*(3), 113–130.

Knochel, K. A., Croghan, C. F., Moone, R. P., & Quam, J. K. (2012). Training, geography, and provisions of aging services to lesbian, gay, bisexual, and transgender older adults. *Journal of Gerontological Social Work, 55*(5), 426–443.

Kumar, V., Acanfora, M., Hennessy, C. H., & Kalache, A. (2001). Health status of rural elderly. *The Journal of Rural Health, 17*(4), 328–331.

Lee, M. G., & Quam, J. K. (2013). Comparing supports for LGBT aging in rural versus urban areas. *Journal of Gerontological Social Work, 56*(2), 112–126.

Lenardson, J., Ziller, E., Coburn, A., & Anderson, N. (2009, July). Health insurance profile indicates need to expand coverage in rural areas. In *Challenge for improving health care access in rural America: A compendium of research and policy analysis studies of rural health research and policy analysis centers* (pp. 11–12). Retrieved August 14, 2014, from www.raconline.org/pdf/research_compendium.pdf.

Lewis, M. K., & Marshall, I. (2012). *LGBT psychology: Research perspectives and people of African descent.* New York: Springer.

Lucco, A. (1987). Planned housing preferences of older homosexuals. *Journal of Homosexuality, 14*, 35–36.

Lucksted, A. (2004). Lesbian, gay, bisexual and transgender people receiving services in the public mental health system: Raising issues. *Journal of Gay and Lesbian Psychotherapy, 8*(3/4), 25–42.

Maccio, E. M., & Doueck, H. J. (2002). Meeting the needs of the gay and lesbian community: Outcomes in the human services. *Journal of Gay & Lesbian Social Services: Issues in Practice, Policy & Research, 14*(4), 55–73.

Masini, B. E., & Barrett, H. A. (2008). Social support as a predictor of psychological and physical well-being and lifestyle in lesbian, gay, and bisexual adults aged 50 and over. *Journal of Gay and Lesbian Social Services, 20*, 91–110.

McBride, T. (2009, June). A rural-urban comparison of a building blocks approach to covering the uninsured. In *Challenges for improving health care access in rural America: A compendium of research and policy analysis studies of rural health research and policy analysis centers* (pp. 15–22). Retrieved August 14, 2014, from www.raconline.org/pdf/research_compendium.pdf.

MetLife Mature Market Institute. (2010a). *Still out, still aging: The MetLife study of lesbian, gay bisexual, and transgender baby boomers.* Retrieved August 21, 2014, from http://www.metlife.com/assets/cao/mmi/publications/studies/2010/mmi-still-out-still-aging.pdf.

MetLife Mature Market Institute. (2010b). Out and aging: The Metlife study of lesbian and gay baby boomers. *Journal of GLBT Family Studies, 6*, 40–57.

Minugh, P., Janke, S., Lomuto, N., & Galloway, D. (2007). Adolescent substance abuse treatment resource allocation in rural and frontier conditions: The impact of including organizational readiness to change. *The Journal of Rural Health, 23*(1), 84–88.

National Coalition for LGBT Health. (2012). *The Affordable Care Act.* Retrieved March 15, 2013, from http://lgbthealth.webolutionary.com/affordable-care act.

National Rural Health Association. (2011). Elder health in rural America. Available at http://www.ruralhealthweb.org

Nayar, P., Yu, F., & Apenteng, B. A. (2013). Frontier America's health system challenges and population health outcomes. *The Journal of Rural Health, 29*, 258–265.

Newacheck, P. W., Hughes, D. C., Hung, Y.-Y., Wong, S., & Stoddard, J. J. (2000). The unmet health needs of America's children. *Pediatrics, 105*, 989–997.

Oswald, R. F., & Culton, L. S. (2003). Under the rainbow: Rural gay life and its relevance for family providers. *Family Relations, 52*, 72–81.

Phillips, C. D., & McLeroy, K. R. (2004). Health in rural America: Remembering the importance of place. *American Journal of Public Health, 94*(10), 1661–1663.

Public Advocate for the City of New York. (2008, December). *Improving lesbian, gay, bisexual, and transgender access to healthcare at New York City health and hospitals coorporation facilities.* Available at http://transgenderlegal.org/media/uploads/doc_84.pdf

Rawls, T. (2004). Disclosure and depression among older gay and homosexual men: Findings from the Urban Men's Health Study. In G. Herdt & B. de Vries (Eds.), *Gay and lesbian aging: Research and future directions* (pp. 117–142). New York, NY: Springer.

Robert Wood Johnson Foundation. (2011, November). Implementing the future of nursing-Part II: the potential of interprofessional collaborative care to improve safety and quality. *Charting Nursing's future, reports on policies that can transform patient care,* 1–8. Available at www.rwjf.org/goto.cnf.

Roger, C. C. (2002). The older population in 21st century rural America. *Rural America, 17*(3), 2–10.

Rowan, N. L., Giunta, N., Grudowski, E. S., & Anderson, K. A. (2013). Aging well and gay in rural America: A case study. *Journal of Gerontological Social Work, 56*(3), 185–200.

Rural Poverty Report. (2011). Rural poverty in the developing world. *Facts and figures: Rural poverty report 2011.* Retrieved August 14, 2014, from www.ifad.org/rpr2011/media/kit/factsheet_e.pdf.

Sage and MAP. (2010, March). *Improving the Lives of LGBT Older Adults.* Available at www.lgbtmap.org and www.sageusa.org.

Salinas, J. J., Snih, S. A., Markides, K., Ray, L., & Angel, R. J. (2010). The rural-urban divide: Health services utilization among older Mexicans in Mexico. *The Journal of Rural Health, 26,* 333–341.

Saulnier, C. F. (2002). Deciding who to see: Lesbians discuss their preferences in health and mental health care providers. *Social Work, 47*(4), 355–365.

Smith, M. S., & Gray, S. W. (2009). The courage to challenge: A new measure of resilience in LGBT adults. *Journal of Gay and Lesbian Social Services, 21,* 73–89.

Subhrajit, C. (2014). Problems faced by LGBT people in the mainstream society: Some recommendations. *International Journal of Interdisciplinary and Multidisciplinary Studies, 1*(5), 317–331.

UnitedHealth Center for Health Reform & Modernization. (2011). *Modernizing rural health care: Coverage, quality, and innovation* (Working Paper 6). Minnetonka, MN: UnitedHealth Group. Retrieved September 4, 2014, from http://www.unitedhealthgroup.com/hrm/UNH_WorkingPaper6.pdf.

U.S. Census Bureau. (2010a). Retrieved March 13, 2014, from www.census.gov/geo.reterence/urban-rural-2010.html.

U.S. Census Bureau. (2010b). *American community survey, 2005–2009.* Washington, DC: Department of Commerce.

Wagenfeld, M. (2000). Delivering mental health services to the persistently and seriously mentally ill in frontier areas. *Journal of Rural Health, 16*(1), 91–96.

Wheeler, D. P. (2003). Methodological issues in conducting community-based health and social services research among Urban Black and African American LGBT populations. In W. Meezan & J. I. Martin (Eds.), *Research methods with gay, lesbian, bisexual, and transgender populations* (pp. 65–78). New York: Haworth Press.

Willging, C. E., Salvador, M., & Kano, M. (2006a). Pragmatic help seeking: How sexual and gender minority groups access mental health care in a rural state. *Psychiatric Services, 57,* 871–874.

Willging, C. E., Salvador, M., & Kano, M. (2006b). Unequal treatment: mental health care for sexual and gender minority groups in a rural state. *Psychiatric Services, 57,* 867–870.

Xu, K. T., & Borders, T. F. (2003). Characteristics of rural elderly people who bypass local pharmacies. *The Journal of Rural Health, 19*(2), 156–164.

Zelarney, P. T., & Ciarlo, J. A. (n.d.). Defining and describing frontier areas in the United States: An update. Frontier Mental Health Services Resource Network. Letter to the Field No. 22. Retrieved August 14, 2014, from http://www.wiche.edu/MentalHealth/Frontier/letter22.asp.

Ziller, E., Anderson, N. J., & Coburn, A. F. (2010). Access to rural mental health services: Service use and out-of-pocket costs. *Journal of Rural Health, 26*(3), 214–224.

Ziller, E., & Coburn, A. (2009, April). Private health insurance in rural areas: Challenges and opportunities. In *Challenges for improving health care access in rural America: A compendium of research and policy analysis studies of rural health research and policy analysis centers* (pp. 13–14). Retrieved August 14, 2014, from www.raconline.org/pdf/research_compendium.pdf.

Ziller, E., & lenardson, J. (2009, June). Rural-urban differences in health care access vary across measures. In Challenges for improving care access in rural America (pp. 33–35). Retrieved August 14, 2014, from www.raconline.org/pdf/research_compendium.pdf.

Law Enforcement and Public Safety of LGBT Elders

26

Randy Thomas

Abstract

This chapter discusses the issues associated with law enforcement and the LBGT community. It describes the structure of law enforcement in the USA, the role that law enforcement plays in the criminal justice system and the current relationship between law enforcement and the LBGT community. This chapter also focuses on the victimization of LBGT elders, the criminal justice response, and the need for better outcomes. Information is presented on the legal structure that impacts law enforcement response and the need to understand the interaction between LBGT elders and the criminal justice system. This chapter will also look at law enforcement training and possible prescriptive actions needed to improve to elder LBGT victimization.

Keywords

Law enforcement · Criminal code · LBGT community · Law enforcement policies · Law enforcement training

Utah Police Officer on Leave for Refusing Gay Pride Parade Assignment

A Salt Lake City police officer has been put on leave due to allegations that he refused to work this weekend's Utah Pride Parade. "If you refuse to do an assignment, that's going to be a problem inside the police department," police spokeswoman Lara Jones said Friday of the officer's need to follow orders. Internal affairs are investigating the officer's refusal, while he is on paid leave Jones confirmed. She would not discuss the officer's reason for refusing the assignment, but said "the vast majority of

R. Thomas (✉)
Exodus International, Orlando, USA
e-mail: Cdr251@gmail.com

© Springer International Publishing Switzerland 2016
D.A. Harley and P.B. Teaster (eds.), *Handbook of LGBT Elders*,
DOI 10.1007/978-3-319-03623-6_26

officers, when they come to work, they understand that they leave their personal opinions at home and serve the community."

The Salt Lake Tribune, June 9, 2014

Overview

The purpose of this chapter is to discuss the issues associated with law enforcement and the LGBT community. It will explore the structure of law enforcement in the USA, the role that law enforcement plays in the criminal justice system, and the current relationship between law enforcement and the LGBT community. It will also focus on the victimization of LGBT elders, the criminal justice response, and the need for better outcomes. Additional discussion will be presented addressing the legal structure that impacts law enforcement response and the need to understand the interaction between LGBT elders and the criminal justice system. The chapter will also examine law enforcement training and possible prescriptive actions needed to reduce elder LGBT victimization.

Learning Objectives

By the end of the chapter, the reader will be able to:

1. Identify relevant issues of policing that impact the LGBT community.
2. Discuss the history of police/LGBT community relations.
3. Identify the critical issues associated with LGBT elder victimization.

4. Describe service models and intervention strategies that are effective in addressing police/LGBT victimization.

Introduction

Historically, a challenge of law enforcement has been "policing" a diverse population. Confronted with daily contact that can often be viewed from the complex perspectives of both the officer and any individual, the risk of misunderstanding can be great. This is particularly true of the officer's interactions with what is often characterized as the "minority" community. This could focus on such elements as race, gender, and sexual orientation. This chapter will specifically address LGBT issues and the complex interactions with law enforcement. The challenge will be in not only addressing the concerns of the LGBT community as a whole but also the elders who identify as LGBT.

The primary function of all law enforcement agencies is to protect the public and ensure that laws are obeyed. Law enforcement officers are charged with the duty to enforce laws created by legislative bodies and are most often the gatekeepers to the broader criminal justice system. The system is comprised of law enforcement, prosecutors, courts, and corrections. As a rule, the focus of law enforcement is on investigating crimes. All elements of the criminal justice system share a common ethical principle of equitably enforcing the law and protecting the public. Generally, applying this principle means that the system owes a duty to the community and to the public at large, rather than to an individual victim. Any criminal conduct is viewed as an act against the entire community and not just a private wrong. It is critical that any issue involving law enforcement includes a comprehensive understanding of the structure and function of law enforcement at every level (Brandl et al. 2007).

The complexity and diversity of the law enforcement function in the USA is not often understood. Media and television entertainment frequently present a false picture of the nature of policing at every level. Popular shows such as *Law and Order: SVU* and *Cops* (one a creative product, the other a reality show) never truly present the complexity of the average officer's day. The dramatic depictions never address the fact that there are over 17,000 law enforcement agencies in the USA at the local level (United States Department of Justice 2011). Television most often creates the impression that every agency is similar to those in New York or Los Angles and has vast resources and expertise to apply to every case. In fact, over half of the law enforcement agencies in the USA have less than 10 personnel (United States Department of Justice 2011). We are a nation that prides itself on the ability to provide law enforcement services, even at the lowest level of government.

This fragmentation of policing makes it difficult to draw wide inferences about police–community interaction. This situation is further complicated by the fact that there is no national standard addressing the delivery of police services in an individual community. The very definition of what constitutes a criminal act is determined by each state. Therefore, the statutory construct that establishes the legal environment for law enforcement is state-specific and can vary to a large degree from state to state. Differences in state and local perceptions and experience affect how officers approach the LGBT community. Recent legal issues such as defining sexual behavior, marriage equality, and discrimination directed toward LGBT individuals have demonstrated and highlighted cultural differences in every state. The relationship between sexual orientation and the code of laws of individual states only compounds the difficulty in discussing police behavior and the LGBT community.

Unfortunately, and all too often, the legal structure has defined the LGBT community in terms of behavior that has been codified as criminal. Although the courts have overturned many of these criminal statutes, they can often create an environment for law enforcement in which LGBT individuals are viewed as "criminals" rather than victims. Specifically, this is found in an aggressive enforcement or moral's offenses such as solicitation and indecent exposure. Often this is done in the context of community policing.

Defining "To Protect and Serve"

Before addressing specific issues of the LGBT community and law enforcement, it is important to clarify the concept of "protect and serve" and the reality of providing police services. While the entire concept of protect and serve makes an ideal short statement to put on the side of police vehicles, it does not explain who gets "protected" or "served." The words do not provide sufficient guidance or detail as to the complex nature of responding to community calls for service.

Though the primary focus of law enforcement is to respond to reports of suspected criminal activity, in many communities law enforcement is the only public service agency with a 24-hour, 7-day a week response capability. Other public agencies that have this ability are often limited in their mandate to respond (e.g., emergency medical services, fire departments). It is often the case that the public contacts law enforcement to respond to incidents that are clearly not related to any criminal offense, an example being civil disputes. This type of response represents the "serve" function.

Since the 1980s, with the rise of community policing, the "protect" part of the law enforcement function has changed significantly. Community policing was based on the recognition that law enforcement had become "removed" from the environment that they were serving. These efforts were an acknowledgment that law enforcement had a larger role to play in creating safe communities that addressed the concerns of all members of a community. It was not simply responding to calls from the public.

The actual outcomes of this approach have not always been effective; however, they do show that law enforcement has made an effort to promote a more inclusive service approach. This approach has not always reduced the tension between certain segments of society and the police. A recent Executive Session on Policing conducted by the Harvard Kennedy School and the National Institute of Justice focused on the concept of "rightful policing," an approach that challenges concept of simply enforcing the laws but on the importance of the perception citizens have of their contact with the police. Simply put, it is critical that this contact be respectful and legitimate, an important concept when addressing the concerns of the LGBT community (Meares 2015). Critical to all this discussion is an understanding of whom law enforcement is protecting and serving with respect to the LGBT population. In a research brief prepared by the National Center on Elder Abuse (National Center on Elder Abuse 2013), it has been estimated that 9 million Americans identify as LGBT, and of those, 1.5 million may be over 65. These data provide a clearer picture of who may be in need of both service and protection. It is probably safe to assume that these numbers may underestimate the size of LGBT persons because of reluctance to disclose their sexuality. While valid victimization rates for this group are difficult to ascertain, LGBT elders have responded to studies indicating that they have been victimized due to sexual orientation and gender identity. The National Center on Elder Abuse emphasizes that such incidents take place in both community and facility settings and that the LGBT population has been largely ignored in research (Walsh et al. 2011). This situation is further compounded by barriers to reporting abuse, such as homophobia, fear of authorities, and legal issues (Cook-Daniels 1997).

LGBT elders have been subjected to various forms of abuse (see Chap. 17). The most prevalent is verbal abuse based upon their sexual orientation and gender identity. Financial exploitation of gay elder men is also an issue (Meyer 2011). However, this situation is clearly seen in the one form of victimization that almost always creates a law enforcement response—

domestic violence. Many states have domestic violence statutes that do not recognize same-sex relationships in the statute (Network for Public Health, n.d.). Law enforcement then must rely on general criminal statutes pertaining to assault. The ability to provide victim services such as orders of protection is not available because of this deficit in the law. The lack of legal recognition of relationships can hamper law enforcement attempts to craft a solution that holds an offender accountable and protects the victim. LGBT domestic violence is a significant problem and one that most often confronts law enforcement. The ramifications of reporting domestic violence by a victim can be extremely negative. Doing so can result in family rejection, isolation, and a lack of concern by the community at large. Coupled with a lack of services and a legal structure that supports the victim, it is fair to assume that reporting will be very low.

Of special concern is the treatment of transgender persons. The most frequently occurring issue is the profiling of transgender persons as "sex workers." Other issues may be targeting these individuals by asking for identification and "policing" of public bathrooms designated as male or female. Sometimes, this law enforcement behavior may be coupled with racial profiling that treats these individuals as potential "suspects." A difficult issue for law enforcement is how to handle transgender persons if they are arrested. The most common practice is to place them in cells based upon genitally determined sex rather than their gender identity. While this places them at great risk of abuse by fellow detainees, it should be understood that this creates a practical challenge for jail/corrections administrators (Amnesty International 2005). The Atlanta (GA) Police Department adopted a policy outlining how to interact with transgender, intersex, or gender nonconforming individuals (APD.SOP.6180). It requires that officers treat these persons in a manner appropriate to their gender identity even though it may be different than that assigned at birth. It also addresses concerns with how this will be recorded on written documents and does so in way that meets the requirements of the agency and the individual (Atlanta Police Department 2014).

In 2014, the United States Department of Justice began a program addressing the issue of law enforcement and transgender persons, particularly women (The Crime Report 2014). It will be a program that will provide transgender cultural training to local agencies across the country. The core dilemma for law enforcement is developing policies that address such issues as how to address transgender persons, and how are they recorded on a report and the housing in detention. All require not only sensitivity by the officer but administrative procedures that acknowledge the issue but still meet the legal and data collection requirements of the criminal justice system (Police 2013).

Of significant importance is the lack of victimization data for elders. That fact, coupled with the hidden issue of LGBT elder abuse, makes any discussion of law enforcement response difficult. It must be understood that law enforcement can be "data driven." Any evaluation of police services often relies upon crime statistics. The primary vehicle for this discussion is the reporting mechanism used nationally by most law enforcement agencies, the National Incident Based Reporting System (NIBRS). It utilizes standardized definitions of criminal behavior and captures data with respect to the level of crime by type, victim, and offender characteristics and the relationship between them. This issue becomes critical when attempting to evaluate the impact of crime on the LGBT community. It is almost impossible to determine victimization levels given the manner in which the data are captured. Consequently, it is difficult for law enforcement to make a data-driven case that there exists a problem of crime directed toward the LGBT community and almost impossible to focus on elders. This is most important when law enforcement is developing problem-based enforcement services. Much more needs to be done in this area.

The History of Police and the LGBT Community

The relationship between the police and the LGBT community has historically been an adversarial one. The criminalization of same-sex behavior has put law enforcement in the position of enforcing laws that specifically target the LGBT community. This creates a climate in which LGBT persons are not protected from criminal behavior of others (Amnesty International 2005). Also, this creates conflict whereby same-sex conduct can result in an individual being treated as either a criminal or a victim, depending on the circumstances and the law enforcement response to a specific incident. Police interaction with individuals is often determined by the officer's biases and the department's organizational attitude toward a particular group. This is reflected in the quoted newspaper article at the beginning of this chapter. The Amnesty International Report (2005) discusses police targeting of LGBT individuals and selective enforcement of moral offenses such as lewd conduct and solicitation. For example, a common occurrence is a transgender person walking down the street being stopped and questioned about solicitation. This targeting creates a large barrier to addressing positive change and reflects current practice and policy of many law enforcement agencies.

This targeting of moral offenses also reflects a concept in Community-Oriented Policing that targets "quality of life" issues. This approach is designed to create a safer community by aggressively enforcing laws against minor offenses such as public drunkenness, loitering, vandalism, or public urination. The prime example of this style of policing is found in the New York Police Department. Although many contend that this has led to a significant reduction in overall crime in New York, it has also led to accusations of targeting minority populations (Amnesty International 2005). Therefore, it is also an accurate observation that these quality of life offenses can also be used to target the LGBT community.

A survey by Lambda Legal of LGBT individuals as well as those with HIV found that 73 % of respondents (1682 of 2376) reported negative face-to-face contact with the police. These interactions are divided between those that address misconduct and those that demonstrate an unsatisfactory response. Overall, the results demonstrate not only a pattern of hostile attitudes but also an inadequate response to reports of victimization (Lambda Legal 2012).

Little has been done to determine whether LGBT elders are treated differently than their heterosexual counterparts. When the issue of sexual orientation or gender identity is factored into a situation of mistreatment of elders, reliable inferences are difficult to make about treatment of LGBT elders. Most of the literature addressing law enforcement and the LGBT community does not account for age differences.

Creation of a positive relationship. While there are certainly many more studies of negative police conduct toward the LGBT community than positive conduct, there has been a national trend toward law enforcement agencies developing policies that emphasize the creation of a more positive relationship with this community. One strategy is to create an LGBT unit or one nested in another community-based function. However, as mentioned above, the majority of law enforcement agencies within the USA had less than 10 officers, and so the creation of a specialized unit or function is not possible.

Policy Box 26.1: A model structure for a LGBT function within a department

The mission of the LGBT Liaison Unit/Person includes:

- Fostering positive relations between the LGBT community and the department by providing a liaison for community members who may be crime victims and have information or issues of concern to the police department.
- Working with the various units in areas with a large, visible LGBT community

within them, to address concerns of that area.
- Assists in productive dialogue with investigative units concerning LGBT-related crimes.
- Works in partnership with other city agencies, other law enforcement entities, and community-based organizations, education, and involvement in other LGBT-related issues.
- Maintaining an interactive role in recruit-based and in-service police trainings regarding the LGBT community.
- Assisting the department in assessing and adjusting current policies and procedures and their impact on the LGBT community.

Legal structure and crimes perpetrated against LGBT persons. Another significant issue is the legal structure as it relates to crimes against LGBT individuals. The criminal code in most states is gender-neutral. This becomes a problem with those codes that address interpersonal violence (e.g., domestic violence statutes). As stated earlier, many states do not recognize same-sex relationships, which affect how law enforcement reacts to an incident. The recent United States Supreme Court decision regarding marriage equality (*King v. Burwell*) will significantly impact domestic violence statutes and law enforcement enforcement response.

Of significance is the problem of hate crimes. Only five states do not have a hate crime law (i.e., Arkansas, Georgia, Indiana, South Carolina, and Wyoming); however, considerable variations exist in who is covered by these laws. Fifteen states recognize neither sexual orientation nor gender identity, 15 states only recognize sexual orientation, and 15 states recognize both sexual orientation and gender identity (Human Rights 2013). These disparities create a confusing and state-specific issue when it comes to designing a law enforcement response that fits all agencies in the USA. In 2009, Congress passed the Matthew Shepard and James Byrd, Jr. Hate Crimes Act (NOLO 2015). The key provisions of the act that impact local law enforcement are focused on providing technical, forensic, and prosecutorial support to agencies when they investigate a violent crime that may be motivated by sexual orientation, gender identity, or a violation of local hate crime laws. It also provides for financial support for expenses associated with the investigation. On the surface, this is a very positive step in furthering a better system for responding to crimes against LGBT persons. However, it does require a local law enforcement agency to apply for the assistance. It also may be difficult to build a prosecutable case if the state statutes do not address hate crimes or the hate crime definition does not include LGBT persons.

Creating an Effective Police Response

The law enforcement community has long been recognized the need to address the issue of diversity. Mentioned earlier, many agencies have created specialized units to create a better response. Training standards have been adjusted to include policing diverse communities, and many communities have developed policies and procedures that recognize concerns of minorities. With the majority of law enforcement agencies having so few officers (US Department of Justice 2008), specialized units are located only in large, resource-rich agencies. What then, are the ideal responses to improve services to the LGBT community and in particular the elderly population?

Tailoring the response. The initial challenge is to design a police response that pertains to most agencies, regardless of size. First, there has to be a problem statement or description that will provide the framework for change. The central issues will be training and accountability. All significant changes in law enforcement have

resulted in changing the content of training. The other issue will be the need to provide for accountability in police interactions with the community. Both areas are critical to creating and sustaining an effective change in law enforcement.

In the USA, police officers receive their training through a system that contains initial entry, in-service, and advanced courses. While there are no national standards for law enforcement training, each state or local government establishes a system of police officer standards and training designed to meet their needs. The length and content of training varies widely, with a requirement to receive in-service training after entering the force not always applied.

Law enforcement training academies are varied in how they are structured. In some states, they are operated by the state and train all law enforcement candidates, and in others, they are operated by individual agencies or regional academies meeting the needs of several jurisdictions. In others, they are part of a technical school system and students fund their own training and there is no agency sponsorship. Although every state sets the training requirements for law enforcement certification and curriculum content, it is often very fragmented system in terms of quality. The average length of initial entry training is 761 hour (about 19 weeks), and the longest training time is about 965 hours, with some as short as 604 hours. Many academies require an additional field training experience ranging from a high of 1678 hours to a low of 225 hours. The majority of training time is spent in two areas–firearms and self-defense. Both of these areas are considered low-frequency events with high risk (driving is often considered in this area as well) (United States Department of Justice 2009).

Special topics. Important to any discussion of LGBT issues training will often fall under community policing or special topics. In most academies, the average number of hours for cultural diversity topics is eleven and content devoted to hate/bias crimes is four (United States

Department of Justice 2006). Training experts support the contention that the most effective way to train law enforcement is through discussion and application through practical problems (Amnesty International 2005). A key issue is also the content of bias/diversity training. Unless it is sensitive to the needs of the officers and content has been developed with community input, such training may lack validity. Any training program directed toward changing behavior (in this case, toward the LGBT community) must have the strong support of agency administration and must emphasize institutionalized and long-term effects. While there have successful efforts in training and policy and procedures for addressing persons with disabilities or mental health needs, the same effort has not been done for the LGBT community. This could serve as a model.

Accountability. Accountability is another key component of a more effective response and relies on standards set by the agency and its leadership. Its foundation is a set of policies that present a commitment to diversity and fair and equitable responses to community needs that include mechanisms to handle complaints. Most law enforcement agencies have some sort of internal affairs' process to handle citizen complaints. A central issue is whether a citizen feels comfortable filing a complaint and that is there a perception that the process is fair and open. There are many different ways to approach this problem; all rely on the public's perception of fairness and transparency. A critical issue for LGBT individuals is the perception of fair and respectful treatment. The model for meeting this need is often the creation of a special function within the agency to address LGBT issues.

Discussion Box 26.1: Improving the Police Response to LGBT Victims

Officers from the Thomasville Police Department have responded to a domestic violence call. Upon arriving, they discovered that the person who called, John Roberts, had been assaulted by Pete Sanger. After separating the parties, the officers conducted an initial investigation that

---

included interviewing both individuals, observing injuries to John, and documenting indications of a struggle in the living room. Thomasville is in a state that has a mandatory arrest domestic violence statute.

Discussion Questions:

1. What steps can the officers take to protect the victim and hold the offender accountable?
2. What victim services might be available to the victim?
3. What training should the department do to address the issue of victimization in the LGBT community?
4. How would the officer's personal bias impact the response?
5. What policies should the department have to address this issue?

An Effective Response Model. Many law enforcement agencies have created an organizational function that recognizes diverse groups. Often, this is a reaction to a crisis or a series of negative actions. These agencies represent a diverse range of communities with respect to size and resources available to law enforcement. In Fort Worth, Dallas, New York, Washington, D. C., Chicago, and Salem, Massachusetts have created LGBT liaison units (Stiffler 2010). What they all have in common is best reflected in the mission statement of the New York Police Department's Community Affairs LGBT Liaison Unit, which includes fostering positive relations, providing a liaison for community members who may be victims of a crime, and maintaining an interactive role in recruit-based and in-service training. These activities are critical in addressing the need to better serve the needs of the LGBT community (NYPD-Lesbian, Gay, Bisexual, Transgender Liaison Unit, n.d.).

Discussion Box 26.2: Developing Effective Policies and Procedures to Improve Police Response to LGBT Victims

Your department has seen an increase in crime directed at LGBT elderly individuals. A concern has been expressed by advocacy groups that your department has not responded appropriately in many cases and that there is a feeling that your officers are not adequately sensitive to their needs. You have been asked by the city administrator to develop and a plan to improve the department's response to this issue.

Discussion Questions:

1. What steps need to be taken to assess the scope of the problem?
2. What are the key elements in developing a policy in this area?
3. How will you address officer concerns?
4. What training should the department do to address the issue of victimization in the LGBT community?
5. How will you evaluate the effectiveness of any change in policy or procedure?
6. Who should be included in the development of the policy?

International approaches. The international community has a less than stellar record respecting the rights of LGBT persons. This is reflected in the global media attention to violent acts directed at LGBT individuals and includes state-sponsored legislation negatively impacting the rights of those individuals. The United Nations (UN) is slowly recognizing this problem and its rightful place in the larger issue of human rights. In 2011, the UN Office for the High Commissioner for Human Rights (OHCHR) issued a brochure calling attention to criminalizing homosexuality. It specifically addresses such topics as the death penalty for consensual sex acts, age of consent for homosexual and heterosexual acts, and enabling LGBT persons fleeing prosecution to avoid returning to their home countries. How this impacts the law enforcement function in the various nations remains to be seen.

Often policing borrows effective techniques and procedures from the larger international system of law enforcement. However, it is virtually impossible to conduct a reasonable discussion of this issue with respect to the international law enforcement community. The model for law enforcement in the USA has its genesis in the British system. That system is found in most of the former Commonwealth countries such as Canada or Australia. We can often share a common approach to policing; however, these countries have a more centralized form of policing and are not as fragmented as in the USA. The best example of a positive response is to look at a Canadian law enforcement example. While we share many similarities with our northern neighbor, law enforcement in Canada is a more centralized system with local, provincial, and federal agencies. The major cities have control over their local law enforcement, and there are other more regional structures such as Quebec and Ontario. The law enforcement function in the rural areas and those local governments that lack resources is the Royal Canadian Mounted Police (RCMP). The RCMP provides law enforcement support to all levels of government. During the period 2012–2013, the Ontario Association of Chiefs of Police (OACP) developed a resource document for the LGBT community (Ontario Association of Chiefs of Police 2013). It addresses concerns across the entire spectrum of issues in police/LGBT interactions and could serve as a model for police response in the USA.

Summary

Challenges facing law enforcement and the public safety of LGBT elders are complex. A "one size fits all" approach will not address the diversity of the law enforcement function in the USA. A severe lack of sufficient research on the victimization of elders, particularly among members of the LGBT community, makes it difficult to explore in-depth the law enforcement response to these individuals. Admittedly, the law enforcement response to the LGBT community has historically focused on the enforcement of offenses that target their sexual orientation rather than crime perpetrated against them. While many of these offenses have either been overturned by the courts or are no longer enforced, this legal approach clearly puts these individuals in the category of offenders and ignores the fact that they are often victims of crime. This problem is exacerbated by a lack of understanding by law enforcement officers of the complex lives these people may live.

Finally, there is a lack of understanding on the part of many citizens of the fragmented system of policing in the USA, a problem further complicated by the fact that the criminal code varies from state to state and that enforcement of these laws is part of a system response that includes prosecutors and the courts. Over 17,000 law enforcement agencies make it difficult to craft a response addressing the needs of every agency. The response to the challenge of providing public safety to the LGBT elder community lies in the need to recognize that a growing problem exists to craft a solution that fits an individual community and then to implement it in such a way that institutionalizes that solution.

Learning Exercises

Self-check Questions

1. What types of challenges do law enforcement agencies face when responding to the concerns of LGBT elders?
2. What makes the victimization of LGBT elders difficult?
3. What statutory constraints impact responding to the victimization of LGBT elders?
4. What does research tell us about the concerns of LGBT individuals when dealing with law enforcement?
5. How does the criminal code make it difficult for law enforcement to adequately protect LGBT elder victims?

6. How effective are hate crime statutes in providing protection to LGBT individuals?

Experiential Exercises

1. Identify a law enforcement agency that has a specialized unit addressing LGBT persons and interview the officers assigned to this unit.
2. Develop a training program for law enforcement that focuses on LGBT issues.
3. Develop a model policy for law enforcement response to LGBT concerns.
4. Identify a LGBT victim and conduct an interview that details their experience with law enforcement.

Multiple-choice Questions

1. The primary function of law enforcement is to provide_____?
   (a) Service
   (b) Protection
   (c) Enforce the laws
   (d) Enforce private actions
2. Law enforcement owes a duty to_____?
   (a) An individual
   (b) The criminal justice system
   (c) The courts
   (d) The community
3. One of the major issues confronting any study of law enforcement is_____?
   (a) Fragmentation
   (b) Policy
   (c) Training
   (d) Community studies
4. Enforcement of criminal statutes is based upon_____?
   (a) State statutes
   (b) Federal guidelines
   (c) Individual officer decisions
   (d) Community pressure
5. There are over _____ local law enforcement agencies?
   (a) 14,000
   (b) 15,000

(c) 16,000

(d) 17,000

6. The majority of local law enforcement agencies have less than_____officers?

   (a) 9

   (b) 10

   (c) 11

   (d) 20

7. The standards for the delivery of police services are set by_____?

   (a) The state

   (b) The local government

   (c) The federal government

   (d) Not anyone

8. Community-Oriented Policing targets what type of activity?

   (a) Quality of life

   (b) Crime

   (c) Service

   (d) Victimization

9. The creation of specialized units addressing LGBT issues is complicated by what fact?

   (a) Community standards

   (b) Size of the department

   (c) Laws

   (d) Training standards

10. Law enforcement training standards are set at what level?

   (a) The state

   (b) The federal government

   (c) The local government

   (d) The individual agency

Key

1. c

2. d

3. a

4. a

5. d

6. b

7. b

8. a

9. b

10. a

Resources

American Civil Liberties Union: www.aclu.org/lgbt-rights

International Gay and Lesbian Human Rights Commission: www.iglhrc.org

References

Alberty, E. (2014, June 6). Utah police officer on leave for refusing gay pride parade assignment. *The Salt Lake Tribune*. Retrieved June 9, 2014, from http://www.sltrib.com.

Amnesty International. (2005). *Stonewalled: Police abuse and misconduct against lesbian, gay, bisexual and transgendered people in the U.S.* Retrieved January 14, 2015, from http://www.amnesty.org/en/library/info/AMR51/122/2005.

Atlanta Police Department. (2014). *Transgender interaction policy* Retrieved February 25, 2015, from http://www.atlantapd.org/pdf/news-releases/175C2728-D143-4E88-BB16-43E1923D1F3A.pdf.

Brandl, B., Dyer, C., Heisler, C., Otto, J., Stiegel, L., & Thomas, R. (2007). *Elder abuse detection and intervention: A collaborative approach*. New York: Springer.

Cook-Daniels, L. (1997). Lesbian, gay male, bisexual and transgendered elders: elder abuse and neglect issues. *Journal of Elder Abuse and Neglect, 9*(2), 35–49.

Human Rights Campaign. (2013). *State hate crime laws*. Retrieved January 15, 2015, from http://www.hrc.org/statelaws.

Lambda Legal. (2012). *Protected and served?* Retrieved January 15, 2015, from http://www.lambdalegal.org/protected-and-served-police.

Meares, T. L. (2015). Rightful policing. *New perspectives in policing bulletin*. Washington, D.C.: U.S. Department of Justice, National Institute of Justice, NCJ 248411.

Meyer, H. (2011). *The LGBT senior population's risk of elder abuse*. Retrieved January 16, 2015, from http://www.ecarediary.com/viewblog.aspx?BlogID=530.

National Center on Elder Abuse. (2013). *Mistreatment of lesbian, gay, bisexual, and transgender (LGBT) elders*. Retrieved January 14, 2015, from http://www.ncea.aoa.gov/Resources/Publication/docs/NCEA_LGBT_ResearchBrief_2013.pdf.

New York Police Department-Lesbian Gay Bisexual Transgender Liaison Unit. (n.d.). Retrieved January 16, 2015, from http://www.nyc.gov/html/nypd/html/community_affairs/lgbt.shtml.

NOLO: Law for All. (2015). *Hate crimes act (Mathew Shepard Act)*. Retrieved February 25, 2015, from http://www.nolo.com/legal-encyclopedia/content/hate-crime-act.html.

Ontario Association of Chiefs of Police. (2013). *Best practices in policing and lgbtq communities in Ontario*. Retrieved February 25, 2015, from http://www.oacp.on.ca/Userfiles/Files/NewAndEvents/OACP%20LGBTQ%20final%20Nov2013.pdf.

Police. (2013). *Dealing with transgender subjects*. Retrieved February 25, 2015, from http://www.policemag.com/blog/training/story/2013/01/dealing-with-transgender-subjects.aspx.

Stiffler, S. (2010). *Police LGBT liaison units: how effective are they?* Retrieved January 16, 2015, from http://www.edgeboston.com/news/national///102392/police_lgbt_liaison_units:_how_effective_are_they?.

The Crime Report. (2014). *How cops can learn how to protect trans gender women*. Retrieved February 25, 2015, from http://www.thecrimereport.org/news/inside-criminal-justice/2014-05-can-cops-learn-how-to-protect-trans-women.

The Network for Public Health Law. *Domestic violence and same-sex relationships fact sheet*. (n.d.). Retrieved January 20, 2015, from https://www.networkforphl.org/_asset/lmb0yo/Master-List-of-SameSex-Domestic-Violence-Protections-Updated-1262012.pdf.

United States Department of Justice, Office of Justice Programs. (2011). *Census of state and local law enforcement agencies, 2008*. Retrieved June 10, 2014, from http://www.bjs.gov/index.cfm?ty=pbdetail&iid=2216.

United States Department of Justice, Office of Justice Programs. (2009). *State and local law enforcement training academies, 2006*, (Revised 4/1/09). Retrieved January 16, 2015, from http://www.bjs.gov/index.cfm?ty=pbdetail&iid=1207.

Walsh, C., Olson, J., Ploeg, J., Lohfeld, L., & MacMillan, J. (2011). Elder abuse and oppression: Voices of marginalized elders. *Journal of Elder Abuse and Neglect, 23*(1), 17–42.

The Role of Religious and Faith Communities in Addressing the Needs of LGBT Elders

Debra A. Harley

Abstract

Religious and faith communities occupy unique and specific roles and functions in society. Although information is presented on specific views about LGBT persons of certain religious affiliations, it is not the intent of this chapter to present a philosophical discussion of the concepts of religion and spirituality, nor to promote the views of any particular faith or denomination. The purpose of this chapter is to present information on the impact, role, and perceptions of faith communities in the lives of LGBT elders. Specifically, information is presented on the attitudes and perceptions of the "church" toward LGBT persons, the value placed on religion and spirituality by LGBT persons, and the ways in which religious leaders can provide care and support to LGBT elders. A discussion of implications of the role of religious leaders in policy development that affect LGBT persons is also presented.

Keywords

Religion · Spirituality · Faith communities · Religious leaders · Politics

Overview

Religion, spirituality, and faith are often discussed in unison and as interchangeable concepts, when, in essence, they are different and have individualized meaning for each person. The information presented in this chapter is intended to explore the role of religion, spirituality, and faith in the lives of LGBT elders. In addition, attention is given to attitudes and perceptions of faith communities toward LGBT persons. Although it is beyond the scope and intent of this chapter to present information about all faith communities and religious denominations, reference is made to specific beliefs and practices of various denominations to illustrate a point. The reader is encouraged to consider the information in this chapter not as endorsement or as criticism of a specific religion or religious beliefs, values, or practices.

D.A. Harley (✉)
University of Kentucky, Lexington, USA
e-mail: dharl00@email.uky.edu

© Springer International Publishing Switzerland 2016
D.A. Harley and P.B. Teaster (eds.), *Handbook of LGBT Elders*,
DOI 10.1007/978-3-319-03623-6_27

525

Learning Objectives

By the end of the chapter, the reader should be able to:

1. Understand how LGBT persons might define and connect to religion, spirituality, and faith communities.
2. Understand similarities and differences of various religious denominations' beliefs and attitudes about sexual orientation and gender identity.
3. Understand the cultural implications of religious beliefs about sexual orientation and gender identity or expression.
4. Identify how religion and politics are intertwined in regard to sexual orientation and gender identity and expression.

Introduction

Religious and faith communities occupy important, unique, and specific roles and functions in society. Although spirituality is different than religion/religiosity, it is often subsumed under religion and frequently used interchangeably. Rose (2012) suggests that in modern life, the two terms have an "uneasy relationship," and for many people, the two terms have become conflated, with spirituality as the default term used when referring to religion or religious practices. For some, the two terms are unrelated—religion often represents a dogmatic set of demands for behavior and beliefs seemingly incompatible with a diverse modern world. Others view *spirituality* as a cafeteria approach indicative of narcissism and lack of commitment (Rose). In a study of the meanings and manifestations of religion and spirituality among LGBT adults, Halkitis et al. (2009) found that LGBT persons defined spirituality largely in relational terms (e.g., in terms of one's relationship with God and with self) and religion largely in terms of communal worship and in terms of its negative

influences in their lives and communities. In this chapter, religion and spirituality are recognized and discussed separately, but supportive of each other. Religiosity is defined as a set of beliefs about the cause, nature, and purpose of the universe, especially of a superhuman agency, usually involving devotional and ritual observances, and often containing a moral code governing the conduct of human affairs (www.dictionary. reference.com/browse/religion). Spirituality is that which lies at the center of each person's being (e.g., God), an essential dimension, which brings meaning to life. Others may find relationships with other people as providing central or core meaning in their lives (MacKinlay 2006).

It is not the intent of this chapter to present a philosophical discussion of the various concepts of religion and spirituality. Moreover, this chapter does not promote the views of any particular faith or denomination. However, information is presented related to specific views about LGBT persons in relation to certain religious affiliations, acknowledging the existence of conservative and liberal theologies and beliefs about sexual minorities and fixed propositions and theological plurality. The term faith community is used to refer to both religion and spirituality and is considered as more inclusive of the two. Religion is salient in the lives of many people across different cultures and consists of various denominations and religious practices that are observed and practiced in different ways. Religious coping has been shown to reduce levels of depression and anxiety in connection with stressful situations and events, and social support within religious communities has been demonstrated as a vital factor in better health outcomes in older adults (Banerjee et al. 2014; Musick et al. 2004). Spirituality has been shown to protect older adults from negative attitudes and declines in physical health (Lowry and Conco 2002).

Many LGBT elders came of age during a time when homosexuality was seen as a psychiatric disorder, the goal of which was to "cure" them. In religious practices, the cure was one of conversion therapy (i.e., ex-gay ministry) or exorcism. The stressors of aging faced by many LGBT elders are compounded by the trauma inflicted by religion and society around their sexual orientation and gender identities (Mahru 2014).

The purpose of this chapter is to present information on the impact, role, and perceptions of religion, spirituality, and faith communities in the lives of LGBT elders. First, information is presented on the historical and contemporary functions of religion, spirituality, and faith communities. The attitudes and perceptions of the church toward LGBT persons and behaviors are examined. Next, the value placed on religion and spirituality by LGBT persons and how they express or practice those values and their experiences are discussed. In addition, the chapter includes ways in which religious leaders can provide care of and support to LGBT elders. Finally, political implications of the role of religions and religious leaders are discussed. Wherever possible, information is included from a cross-cultural perspective. Throughout this chapter, the term homosexual/homosexuality is used in the context of biblical reference, a term that is antiquated in contemporary times.

The Functions of Religions, Spirituality, and Faith Communities

Until the fifth century, the only persons who were punished for same-sex behavior were "passive men". Subsequently, Emperor Justinian interpreted same-sex intimacy as "against nature," and, therefore, a religious misdemeanor punishable by God that resulted in double punishment from God and law. In essence, the law became the weapon of the church (Dreyer 2008a, p. 749). Mainstream religions of Christianity, Judaism, and Islam have been described as being at best negative and at worst destructive toward LGBT persons (Lynch 1996). Religion has been used to legitimize the ostracism of LGBT persons. Sacred religious texts have been referenced consistently as authoritative means of verifying that LGBT patterns of attraction and intimacy are

sinful, to make claims that inevitably LGBT persons will receive divine punishment and damnation, and to monitor and control the behaviors and identities of LGBT persons (Halkitis et al. 2009).

This section examines the general function of religions, acknowledging that the purposes of religion are extensive and grounded in philosophical constructs, cultural contexts, and sociological assumptions. Beliefs about the function of religion have evolved over time. For example, Karl Marx and Frederick Engels asserted that the function of religion was to disguise the realities of the underlying economic system and reduce or cover up the suffering of the laboring masses. The structural–functional approach to religion has its roots in Emile Durkheim's work on religion, *Elementary Forms of the Religious Life* (1917). Durkheim believed that religion is the celebration of, and to a certain extent, self-worship of human society. According to Durkheim, religion provides three major functions in society: (a) social cohesion to help maintain social solidarity through shared rituals and beliefs, (b) social control to enforce religious-based morals and norms to help maintain conformity and control in society, and (c) meaning and purpose to answer existential questions (Carls 2012). Critics of the structural–functional approach to religion argue that it overlooks religion's dysfunctions (e.g., to incite violence, war, terrorism, hate crimes).

Lenkeit and Lenkeit (1997) expanded on the work of Durkheim and classified the value of religions to society into eight categories (see Table 27.1). The disciplinary function of religion is in many ways disproportionately applied to LGBT persons. As a disciplinary function, religion provides a paradigm for moral behavior and the promise of both natural and supernatural punishments for perceived breaches of conduct. Further efforts to explain the functions of religions are offered by Goldberg's (2010) list of functions: (a) transmission—to impart to each generation a sense of identity through shared customs, rituals, stories, and historical continuity; (b) translation—to help individuals interpret life

Table 27.1 Function of religion to society

Cohesive—helps to organize society, promote a unified group identity, and delineate between insiders and outsiders
Explanatory—helps to explain things that would otherwise remain inexplicable, both unexplained material phenomenon and deeper questions
Education—a role in instruction, especially moral instruction, and helps to pass down cultural values that might otherwise be lost
Euphoric—religious rituals provide feelings of awe, excitement, relief, enlightenment, and so forth. These experiences are often transformative, leading to changes in personality or motivation, and tend to cement cultural and moral values in the minds of participants, while motivating further action
Revitalize—rituals reinforce and reinvigorate the structures and values of society, and its subsets, such as family bonds. Most public holidays are good examples of this function in action
Ecological—mediates the contact between human groups and their environment, by adding critical moral value to decisions that are otherwise decided through self-interest
Disciplinary—provides a paradigm for moral behavior and promises both natural and supernatural punishments for perceived breaches of conduct
Supportive—being agents of redistribution, taking in contributions of money and resources, and redistributing on the basis of need. Also, providing individual support such as counseling, spiritual guidance, and material assistance in times of trouble

Adapted from Lenkeit and Lenkeit (1997)

events, acquire a sense of meaning and purpose, and understand their relationship to a larger whole, socially and cosmically; (c) transaction—to create and sustain health communities and provide guidelines for moral behavior and ethnical relationships; (d) transformation—to foster maturation and ongoing growth, helping people to become more fulfilled and more complete; and (e) transcendence—to satisfy the longing to expand the perceived boundaries of the self, become more aware of the sacred aspect of life, and experience union with the ultimate ground of being. These viewpoints on the functions of religion may or may not be representative of past or current functions or representative of different cultural aspects. Religiosity and scriptural liberalism (the degree to which one interprets the scriptural literally), associated with traditionalism, also influence faith communities' views of LGBT persons and behaviors.

Turner and Stayton (2014) contend that religious leaders face a wide variety of sexual needs and concerns, sexual expressions, and sexuality issues within their faith communities. Sexuality issues range from reproductive technologies to sexual abuse to sexual orientation and gender identity and expression. "Not only are faith communities filled with people experiencing difficult and complex situations involving sexuality, they are turning to their clergy and religious leaders for guidance and help in the belief that these same leaders are trained in, and capable of, dealing with this vast range of concerns" (p. 485). Given the sexual issues and the growing conflicts, awareness, and acknowledgement around them and across the spectrum of religious denominations, religious leaders remain ill prepared to deal with them (Turner and Stayton). When people in their congregations bring questions, concerns, or dilemmas, many religious leaders realize that they have inadequate information, understanding, or training to be good counselors or to address the interwoven spiritual nature of congregants' concerns. Turner and Stayton contend that "religious leaders are in a unique position to transform, inform, and influence society's understanding of sexuality and religion—through the pulpit, pastoral care of individuals and families, and involvement in local communities, the media, and policies" (p. 485). Unfortunately, sexuality and sex education are not a part of seminary education and religious training. See the case of Alex, an example of an older gay man coming to his religious leader for guidance on a situation around his sexuality.

The Case of Alex

Alex is a 71-year-old gay man. He has just returned to his hometown after an absence of 50 years. After the death of his partner, Alex decided to move back home to be close to his family, especially since acquiring some health issues. During attendance at church, one of the church members approached Alex and invited him to dinner, indicating that she wanted him to meet her mother who is recently widowed. The woman, oblivious to the possibility that Alex is gay, is trying to fix him up with her mother. Alex has declined several invitations. He likes being back home and participating in the church in which he grew up, however, is not comfortable with telling any of the church members that he is gay. He decided to go back "in the closet" and is experiencing some stress because he cannot be open about his sexual orientation. Alex decided to talk with his minister.

Questions

1. What are some possible reactions from the minister for which should Alex be prepared?
2. What type of knowledge and skill should the minister have to assist Alex?
3. How would you counsel Alex?

In understanding the functions of religion, spirituality, and faith communities in the lives of LGBT persons, one can argue that in each, there is diversity and inclusion, not division and exclusion. Sexuality and spirituality are integral parts of everyday life in multiple faith traditions around the world in which both sexual wholeness and spiritual wholeness are intricately connected (Turner and Stayton 2014). Religious leaders are often the first point of contact for concerns of their faith community members.

Religious Attitudes and Perceptions Toward LGBT Populations—Cultural and Denominational Differences

Faith communities are broadly categorized as Buddhism, Christianity, Islam, Hinduism, Humanism, and Judaism. Within each, subcategories exist concerning the way in which congregations interpret and practice their doctrines. Faith communities may range from traditional/conservative to contemporary/progressive. According to Gold (2010), the views of differing denominations range from punishment by Fundamentalist Christianity to full acceptance by Quakers or Unitarian Universalists, with other churches encompassing both ends of the spectrum by advocating love for the sinner (the person), but hate of the sin (gay behavior). A strong relationship exists between the messages religious leaders promote regarding LGBT acceptance and support and the attitudes held by their congregations (Dutwin 2012). In fact, Hoffman et al. (2006) suggest that "developing a religious identity allows a person to develop a sense of identity and worth in relation to God and his or her place in the universe", thus, "religion may affect a person's LGB identity development" (p. 11). The geographic location of faith communities also influences religious beliefs. For example, in the "Bible Belt" (i.e., states in the West South Central, East South Central, and South Atlantic), much of which adheres to Christian fundamentalist dogma about homosexuality (e.g., homosexuals are bad, diseased, sinful), Christianity permeates other social institutions such as schools, homes, and entertainment venues (Barton 2010). For faith positions of various faith communities, the reader is referred to the Human Rights Campaign (http://www.hrc.org/resources/entry/faith-positions). Barton asserts that the majority of research on

homosexuality has explored heterosexual attitudes toward homosexuals with a focus on the
relationship between prejudice, right-wing,
authoritarianism, and dimensions of religiosity.
Much of religion has been used to create and
cultivate hostility against LGBT persons.

Stances of faiths on LGBT issues in Islam are
difficult to summarize because of its enormous
geographic, linguistic, and cultural diversity. To a
large extent, attitudes depend on how individual
Muslims and Islamic sects interpret the Holy
Quran and other theological sources. Nevertheless, a majority of Muslims express very negative
attitudes toward LGBT persons. However, only a
few passages in the Quran and several hadiths
(sayings attributed to the prophet Muhammad)
refer to sex between two males. Specifically, the
story of Lut (or Lot as he is known in Jewish and
Christian Bibles) is mentioned, but the Quran does
not call for a specific punishment for this behavior.
While most Islamic institutions have not explicitly
addressed transgender issues, they do make reference to cross-dressing, those transgressing traditional gender roles, and sex-reassignment
surgery (Human Rights Campaign, n.d.).

The beliefs about and responses to LGBT
issues in Judaism vary across Orthodox and
Reform Judaism. The Torah clearly states that
the act of homosexuality is prohibited. The Torah
refers to homosexuality as *Toaviva*-abomination
(i.e., abhorrent to God) (Amsel, n.d.). The Tal-
mud says that in the act of homosexuality, the
person is "straying" from one of the primary
goals in life—to procreate and populate the earth.
It is in the straying that homosexuality is prohibited. That is, it is not the "unholiness" of the
homosexual relationship, but rather, the violation
of one's purpose on earth (Amsel). For Jews, the
law of the Torah is the all-encompassing and
governs every single part of living, general,
societal, and personal (Shaffer, n.d.). Conversely,
Reform Judaism has a long history of working
for the full inclusion of LGBT persons in Jewish
life (Appell, n.d.). According to Appell, Reform
Jews "are guided by the very basic belief that all
human beings are created *b'tselem Elohim* (in the
Divine image)" (p. 1). The Reform Movement

believes that, "regardless of context, discrimination against any person arising from apathy,
insensitivity, ignorance, fear, or hatred is inconsistent" with the fundamental belief of *b'tselem
Elohim*, "for the stamp of the Divine is present in
each and every one of us" (Rabbi David Saper-
stein cited in Appell).

Homosexuality is discussed seven times in the
Christian Bible: Genesis 19, Judges 19, Leviticus
18, Leviticus 20, Romans 1, Corinthians 6, and 1
Timothy 1 (Dwyer 2007). These passages serve
as the foundation for most of the abuse projected
on LGBT persons in some churches (Atchison
2013). In response to these biblical references,
adherents claim that God condemns homosexuality or homosexuals. In response, Dwyer wrote
the book, *Those 7 References: A Study of 7
References to Homosexuality in the Bible*.
Dwyer's rationale was to allow LGBT persons
who have been abused by the "misuse" of
scripture to have a voice about a different interpretation of God's voice to be heard in these
passages in ways that had been silenced for many
for a long period of time. In her reflections about
the seven references, Atchison (2010) asserts that
often the Bible is used (and misused) in two
extreme interpretations to oppress and harm
members of sexual minority groups. The Bible is
used either blindly as "The Word" and the use of
certain texts as a self-flagellation (referring to self
and others of their community as "sin"), or with
complete dismissal of the whole book and
Christianity itself, allowing Christian fundamen-
talists to unanimously dictate what is righteous
and what is good.

Atchison (2013) suggests that for people who
teach and preach about the seven references, it is
necessary to understand that, the Bible, although
relevant for today, was written in a particular
historical context, making it often difficult to
apply something written for a particular ancient
audience to a contemporary lived experience.
This view is consistent with that of Dreyer
(2006a) who espouses that theologians and exe-
getes cannot ignore the changes that have
occurred in social life from biblical times,
through the ages, to our modern and postmodern

worlds. A postmodern view is that sexuality is not a homogeneous entity, rather the result of an infinite variety of ever changing factors. LGBT persons feel that they are "being" a sexual minority and God made them this way.

Different religions and denominations have varying attitudes toward sexual orientation and sexual identity; experience may vary greatly depending on the nature of the religious community. The experiences of LGBT persons in faith communities are as diverse as the type of practices and ceremonies in which they engage. "Religion has been a source of both solace and suffering for many LGBT Americans" (Human Rights Campaign 2014). For some LGBT persons, neither their sexual orientation, their religion, nor the intersection of the two is a problem, while others struggle with the attitudes of those around them, religious leaders, or their own internalized attitudes toward sexual orientation or sexual identity (Pace 2013). Many LGBT persons have been raised in an organized religion but have been forced to leave those communities because of condemnation. However, in recent years, there has been a shift in a growing number of organized religious groups in the United States to issue statements officially welcoming LGBT persons as members. As an example, some religious organizations have taken supportive stands on issues that affect LGBT persons (e.g., freedom from discrimination, right to marry, ordination of openly gay clergy) (Human Rights Campaign 2014).

Religion-based bigotry, "the attitudes of prejudice hostility or discrimination toward gay people that are falsely justified by religious teachings or belief," causes enormous harm to LGBT persons (Faith in America 2010). Negative social attitudes about sexual orientation and gender identity can cause harmful consequences in the lives of LGBT persons, creating the "fear of going to hell" depression, low self-esteem, feelings of worthlessness, self-doubt, and internalized homo/bi/transphobia (Barton 2010; Mahru 2014). In a study of LGBT persons in Ireland, Reygan and Moane (2014) found that while participants lived in an increasingly pluralistic Irish society, the negative dividend of religious homophobia created intrapsychic

tension for participants and led some to abandon religion altogether. The authors also found that a changing Irish society is characterized by increased diversity, openness, and respect for minority rights including LGBT rights. Some denominations welcome the inclusion of all persons, including those who are LGBT (e.g., Episcopalian, United Methodist, Unitarian Universalist), at the same time that others overtly condemn them (e.g., Christian fundamentalist, Baptist). The current policy (as of 2012) of the United Methodist Church' states, "We implore families and churches not to reject or condemn lesbian or gay members and friends. We commit ourselves to be in ministry for and with all persons". Although the United Methodist Church bans discrimination at the congregational level and recognizes the "scared worth" of all persons, church doctrine also states that homosexuality is incompatible with Christian teachings and bans financial support of all LGBT-based groups. More progressive factions among clergy and laity have defied church doctrines in an effort to reclaim the Bible's call for social justice as it applies to marriage and ordination (Human Rights Campaign 2014).

In Canada, The United Church has developed policies about sexual orientation and transgender and gender identity, affirming all human being regardless of sexual orientation. The timeline of policy decisions on sexual orientation of The United Church of Canada includes the following: (a) in 1984, affirmed acceptance of all human beings as made in the image of God, regardless of sexual orientation, acknowledged that the church has condoned the rejection of lesbians and gays, and called the church to repent; (b) in 1988, declared that "all persons, regardless of sexual orientation, who profess faith in Jesus Christ and obedience to him, are welcome to be or become full members of the church;" (c) in 1992, began creating resources for same-sex covenants; and (d) in 2003, called on the Government of Canada to recognize same-sex marriage in marriage legislation (http://affirmunited.ause.ca). More recently, The United Church of Canada passed policies on gender identity and the participation and ministry of transgender people, instructing staff to develop resources to encourage the participation and ministry of transgender persons in the life of the church and to prepare individuals and churches to receive such participation and ministry.

Another international perspective of challenging prejudice toward LGB persons is recommendations from Scotland and England. In Scotland, the proportion of people who have religious faith and those who do not is significant, including LGB persons (Donnelley 2008). Attitudes of Scottish people of faith toward LGBT persons vary greatly, with 21 % believing that same-sex couples should not be allowed to marry (15 % for people who have no religion or seldom attend religious meetings and 43 % for people who attend religious meeting at least once a week), and 32 % of those who attend religious meetings at least once a week agreed same-sex couples should be allowed to marry (Scottish Government Social Research 2007). Across Britain, 71 % of people with a religious belief state that they would be comfortable if their local religious representative was gay (Guasp and Dick 2012). These attitudes of many people of faith do not necessarily correspond to the positions taken by faith leaders, nor is the majority view of people within a faith widely reported as representative of that faith (Donnelley).

Within the Christian tradition, LGBT persons can experience the rejection of the Church community and even further oppression when they negotiate their gendered identities in relation to their church community's construction of sexuality (Sharma 2008). Although LGBT persons may be welcomed in the faith community and regarded as devoted Christians, church officials are still allowed to exclude LGBT persons who are honest about their gay lifestyle. Taylor (1989) refers to this as the "ethics of inarticulacy." Although sexuality as a social construct is forever changing, the challenge for institutional religion is that these institutions cannot easily accept these changes (Dreyer 2008a, b). The impact of negative messages from the Christian faith community about LGBT persons in regard to who they are, how they may or may not love, and what their value is in the eyes of God is

summarized by Martin (1996) as resulting in a denial of self-identity (see Discussion Box 27.1).

Discussion Box 27.1

Any interpretation of scripture that hurts people, oppresses people, or destroys people cannot be the right interpretation, no matter how traditional, historical, or exegetically respectable. There can be no debate about how the fact that the church's stand on homosexuality has caused oppression, loneliness, self-hatred, violence, sickness, and suicide for millions of people. If the church wishes to continue with its traditional interpretation, it must demonstrate, not just claim, that it is more loving to condemn homosexuality than to affirm homosexuals ... Is it really better for lesbians and gay teenagers to despise themselves and endlessly pray that their very personalities be reconstructed so that they may experience romance like their straight friends? It is really more loving for the church to continue its worship of "heterosexual fulfillment" ... while consigning thousands of its members to a life of either celibacy or endless psychological manipulations that masquerade as "healing"?

Questions

1. What are the main points being made by Martin?
2. What is the difference between condemning homosexuality and affirming heterosexuality?
3. Both LGBT persons and heterosexuals express sexuality. In what ways do LGBT persons experience a tension between their faith and reality as sexual beings as compared to heterosexuals.

Martin (1996).

In a Pew (2013) survey of LGBT Americans' ($n = 1197$) attitudes, experiences, and values in changing times, the overwhelming majority

(92 %) said that society has become more accepting of them in the past decade. The participants attribute this change to various factors ranging from people knowing and interacting with someone who is LGBT to advocacy on behalf of high-profile public figures to LGBT adults raising families. However, LGBT persons report that many religions are not accepting of them. They describe the Muslim religion (84 %), the Mormon Church (83 %), the Catholic Church (79 %), and evangelical churches (73 %) as unfriendly. Fewer than half of LGBT participants indicated that the Jewish religion and mainline Protestant churches were unfriendly, and one-in-ten described them as friendly, with the remainder indicating that they were neutral.

Overwhelmingly, research on religion and sexual minorities has focused on lesbians and gays. There is limited to no attention given either to bisexuality or transgenderism and religion and/or spirituality. Donnelley (2008) states that while many of the religious issues identified for LGBT persons apply to transgender persons, the pattern of attitudes toward transgender persons is significantly different than toward LGB persons. For instance, issues for transgender persons of faith can be different: there are fewer trans-persons than LGB persons, and the law covers trans and LGB persons differently. All of these factors suggest that differences in approach may be needed for trans and LGB issues (Donnelley).

Research on LGBT Elders' Religious and Spiritual Beliefs and Practices and Experiences

Both the religious beliefs and the way in which individuals worship is a matter of choice, personal preference, and familial teaching. For many LGBT persons, participation in organized religion may be detrimental to their mental health because of negative messages about their sexual orientation and gender identity that are communicated through religious teachings, institutionally imposed sanctions against openly LGBT members, and the prohibition against gay religious leaders (Lease et al. 2005). The conflict

between one's sexual orientation or gender identity and one's religious identity may lead to dissonance because full acceptance of one aspect of the self implies full rejection of another (Gold 2010). Ways that religiosity may shape sexual identity and ways in which LGBT persons' engage in worship practices are altered by their experience within hostile or affirming religious communities. Some LGBT persons elect to eschew organized religion entirely, while others self-define as atheists. Yet others may reject public religious life but may express their religious and spiritual commitment by engaging in private acts of devotion, meditation, and prayer. LGBT persons who remain committed to participating in organized religious life may choose to ignore or minimize the relevance of anti-gay doctrines and sentiments within their faith community (Halkitis et al. 2009).

A study by Halkitis et al. (2009) included 498 participants ranging in age from 18 to 75. Of these participants, only 24.5 % ($n = 122$) reported that they held a membership in a religious institution such as a church, synagogue, or mosque, and those who indicated membership tended to be older than non-members. The majority of participants were raised in religious households. Although it is unclear whether the findings that older LGBT persons tended to hold membership in organized religion is a reflection of a developmental effect, they may suggest that as LGBT persons age, they will have a need for organized communities in which they can express their religious and spiritual beliefs. Moreover, these individuals will have a particular need for welcoming and affirming religious communities, ones that can help them negotiate the challenges associated with aging (Halkitis et al.).

As people get older, their support networks often shrink. Rose (2012) found that spiritual and religious experiences were an important source of support and strength for many LGBT elders. Conversely, it was also a source of pain, due to religiously linked experiences of stigma, usually in childhood or young adulthood. For all of the participants in Rose's study, sexual orientation or gender identity set them apart in some way from the heterosexual mainstream of their generation and required them to define themselves spiritually. Those participants had a variety of individual experiences, but most were in the mainstream of American traditions (e.g., church, synagogue, other religious institutions). According to Rose, the individuals grew up during a time when the majority of American society held religious and social conservative views about homosexuality, bisexuality, and gender non-conformity. Moreover, "to acknowledge one's identity, was, for the majority of study participants, to find oneself in a world where religious leaders, social arbiters and, often, one's own family, would almost universally condemn you" (p. 12).

For many of the LGBT elders in Rose's (2012) study, the spiritual community provided a place to perform service to others. The majority of participants indicated substantial involvement with their spiritual or religious community. LGBT elders played various roles and performed important functions in their faith community including the role of deacons, celebrants, taking care of the place of worship or fellow congregants, and mentor of younger members. In addition, LGBT elders provided spiritual and personal support and advice to others struggling with issues of identity or with personal crises. These LGBT elders highly valued their spiritual community and regarded it as a place for them to fulfill the tasks of adulthood that they might not have had the opportunity to do if they were disconnected from it. All of the LGBT elders in the study stated that in one way or another, having a religious or spiritual practice, community, or perspective helped them cope with life stressors, coming out, health issues, and changes in life circumstances.

Similarly, Espinoza (2014) found that 40 % of LGBT elders say that their support networks have become smaller over time, as compared to 27 % of non-LGBT older people. Among LGBT elders who consider the church or faith community as part of their support networks, 26 % are African American, 8 % are White, and 8 % are Hispanic/Latino. (See Chaps. 6, 7, 8, 9, and 10 for discussion of the role of religion in the lives of ethnic populations). Research shows that involvement in religious and spiritual practice corresponds to better health-related outcomes regardless of age (Beery et al. 2002; Brennan 2004; Newlin et al. 2008), and may provide social support and a sense of well-being, which promotes better overall mood (Mitchell and Weatherly 2000).

A Gallup Poll on LGBT populations and religious affiliation in the USA found that LGBT persons are significantly less likely than non-LGBT persons to be highly religious and significantly more likely to be classified as non-religious. Religiosity among national adults found that 24 % of LGBT identify as highly religious, 29 % as moderately so, and 47 % as not religious compare with non-LGBT at 41, 29, and 30 %, respectively. A comparison by gender reveals that male gay, bisexual, and transgender persons compared with non-gay, bisexual, and transgender were classified 25 % versus 36 % as highly religious, 26 % versus 28 % as moderately, and 49 % versus 35 % as not religious (Newport 2014). Some LGBT persons find that no specific religion's teachings are fully in accordance with their personal identity and worldview, but take comfort from the idea of a spiritual presence in the world. Others find that spirituality fits more easily into their identities than religion, although many do also maintain a strong belief in the teachings of particular faiths (Pace 2013). A national survey of American congregations from 2000 to 2010 (conducted in 2000, 2005, 2008, and 2010) identified substantial changes including a net overall result of fewer persons in the pews and decreasing spiritual vitality (Roozen 2011) (see Table 27.2).

Similarly, a Pew study (Taylor 2013) found that LGBT adults are less religious than the general public. Approximately 48 % reported no religious affiliation compared to 20 % of the public at large. Of those LGBT adults with religious affiliation, one-third said there is conflict between their religious beliefs and their sexual orientation or gender identity, and 29 % said they have been made to feel unwelcome in a place of worship.

The results from each of the studies discussed above reveal that while societal views about

Table 27.2 American congregations 2000–2010

Continued increase in innovative, adaptive worship
Rapid adoption of electronic technologies
Increase in racial/ethnic congregations, many for immigrant groups
Increase in the breadth of both member-oriented and mission-oriented programs
Increase in connection across faith traditions
Change in the historical pattern of religious involvement in support of the electoral process
Significant decrease in financial health
Continuing high levels of conflict
Aging membership
Fewer persons in the pews
Decreasing spiritual vitality

Adapted from Roozen (2011)

LGBT persons have shifted relatively dramatic over the past decade, highly religious people remain more likely than others to believe that sexual behavior and identity of LGB persons should not be accepted by society. This view serves to marginalize, stigmatize, and perpetuate stereotypical views and attitudes at a time that many LGBT persons of all ages are coming out and speaking out.

In response to the two extremes of how the Bible is used and misused that were discussed earlier in this chapter, Atchison views these two extremes as black and white (absolute and opposite) and as inhabiting a gray area in between. See Discussion Box 27.2 for Atchison's interpretation of existing in a gray area.

Discussion Box 27.2

Gabrie'l J. Atchison is a feminist, an African American, and a member of the LGBT community. She has a doctorate in Women's Studies and a master's of religion with a concentration in Women, Gender and Sexuality Studies. Dr. Atchison has created "healing spaces" for women, including Angel's Refuge whose vision is to create peaceful spaces for those who are experiencing grief and loss or have experienced trauma (http://angelsrefuge.wordpress.com/about/).

Inhabiting a Gray Area:

"I believe that God loves me as I am"... "He made me the way that I am"... "He also made me the way that I am for a purpose" ... "In my uniqueness, I am here to serve a specific Devine purpose" ... "I trust God" ... "My challenges are about self-acceptance, deepening my faith and learning to love His people" ... "My challenge is not about trying to repress, hide or deny part of myself" ... "I know that God loves me, and nothing I read will change my mind."

Questions

1. What is Gabrie'l's view of her relationship with God and faith?
2. What are Gabrie'l's challenges?
3. If you were to have a conversation with Gabrie'l, how would you respond to her inhabiting a gray area?

Adapted from http://angelsrefuge.wordpress.com/2010/06/08/homosexuality-and-the-bible-part-1-of-7/

Hoffman et al. (2006) align LGB faith development with the stages of LGB identity development in an attempt to explain LGB religious experience. The authors indicate that with many models, conflict along with resolution is at the core of transition from one stage to the next. For LGB persons, a conflict may exist between growing acceptance of their own sexual identity and religious beliefs and attempts to relieve this conflict often leads initial attempts to deconstruct religious beliefs deemed unquestionable.

Wood and Conley (2014) reviewed the need for counselors and researchers to address the effects of LGBT person's loss of religious and spiritual (R/S) identity and to examine the concepts of R/S abuse and R/S struggle. R/S abuse refers to physical, sexual, or psychological abuse perpetrated by those in power within R/S communities (Gubi and Jacobs 2009). S/R struggles are "efforts to conserve or transform a spirituality that has been threatened or harmed" (Pargament et al. 2005, p. 247). Wood and Conley concluded that as LGBT persons experience R/S abuse, they might experience R/S struggle, which may then lead to loss of R/S identity. See Research Box 27.1.

Research Box 27.1: Religious/Spiritual Identities

Wood and Conley (2014). Loss of religious or spiritual identities among the LGBT population. Counseling and Values, 59, 95–111

Objective: The purpose of this article is to underscore the need for counselors and researchers to address the effects of LGBT persons' loss of R/S identity and to examine the concepts of R/S abuse and R/S struggle.

Method: This is a conceptual article. The authors include institutional and denominational components of religion in the definition of R/S abuse. To understand the impact of R/S abuse on LGBT persons, the authors explore S/R abuse using Ward's (2011) types of R/S abuse, integrate microaggressions as defined by Sue et al. (2007), and expand microaggressions to include sexual microaggressions (Shelton and Delgado-Romero 2011). A case study of an individual who suffers from loss of R/S identity is presented to explore the implications for counselors and researchers.

Results: The concepts that are discussed in this article, although important, do not have empirical bases. Counselors should use these concepts with caution because individual differences exist in experiences of R/S abuse, R/S struggle, and loss of R/S identity. Further qualitative research (e.g., grounded theory) and quantitative (e.g., predictors of loss) research are necessary to assess the validity of the negative effects of

lass of R/S identity as well as generalizability to different individuals.

Conclusion: As LGBT persons experience R/S abuse, they may experience R/S struggle, which may then lead to loss of R/S identity. Because of the non-finite nature of loss of R/S identity, LGBT persons can experience negative mental health effects. Multiple facets of LGBT persons' identities can be affected and require attention, thus counselors can help them experience loss in the most functional way possible.

Questions

1. What type of qualitative research study would you design?
2. What variables would you use in a quantitative research design
3. What type of LGBT characteristics would you consider in designing either a qualitative or quantitative study?

Religious Leaders' Pastoral Care Provided to LGBT Elders

Dreyer (2008b) suggests that the ambiguity in pastoral care with gay people in many institutional Christian communities exacerbates the "unhealed wound" of gay persons. The unhealed wound refers to the ambiguity in ecclesial approaches to pastoral care with LGBT persons. That is, the ministries of churches that reach out to educate or counsel LGBT persons sound positive; however, LGBT persons to whom they want to reach out are labeled as deviant and stigmatized. Even in many faith communities that have moved toward greater tolerance toward LGBT persons, this more tolerant approach is conditional—gays should confess that same-sex behavior is sinful and should either be "healed" and "become heterosexual" or remain celibate for the duration of their lives (Dreyer 2008b).

If indeed "one of the main tasks of the church is to help heal people's wounds, this should include those wounds caused by outdated social codes that express prejudice against sexual orientation and behaviors that differ from heteronormative conventions" (Dreyer 2008b, p. 1237).

Many LGBT elders have encountered negative experiences and have been hurt deeply by religion. Thus, they may have strong initial suspicions of religious leader and their motives. In interactions with LGBT elders, it is the responsibility of religious leaders to convey a non-judgmental presence during visits or in counseling and to affirm them as they are and assure them that they are safe (Mahru 2014). Pastoral engagement with sexual minorities is affected by religious leaders' disposition, which is related to their religious views. Thus, self-reflection on and awareness of religious leaders' own personal disposition, theological views, and values will prepare them for engaging openly and respectfully with those whose belief system may differ from theirs (Dreyer 2008b). According to Dreyer (2005, 2006b), the mental, physical, and spiritual well-being of all people of faith is the concern of pastoral caregivers. Thus, Dreyer (2008b) advocates for practical theologians to expose all harmful attitudes toward others, including LGBT persons. Whereas therapists and counselors have an ethical obligation to refrain from imposing their views on clients and to be non-judgmental about clients' belief systems, many religious leaders may find it difficult to do so. The issue of maintaining a value-free approach may be even more difficult for religious leaders from "a tradition where religious propositions are presented as undeniable truths, and especially when dealing with sexual minorities where social and religious morality and values are significant issues" (Dreyer 2008b, p. 1244).

Anonymous pastoral care (APC) is one option for assistance in concerns pertaining to sexuality (Van Drie et al. 2014). APC eliminates the risk of rejection or judgment by their religious leaders. APC is especially positioned to counsel LGBT persons because of socially contested sexual issues such as lesbianism, gayness, bisexuality, and transgenderism. Van Drie et al. (2014) assert that the World Wide Web offers ease and anonymity with which persons can obtain advice and reassurance. Although LGBT adults are heavy users of social media (80 %) as compared to the general public (58 %), older LGBT persons are less like to do so (Taylor 2013).

The Need for LGBT-Affirmative Congregations. Generally, LGB persons have three options when dealing with religious and spiritual issues: (a) reparative or conversion therapy—attempts to help the person change their sexual orientation, (b) the use of therapy to help the person live a celibate life, and (c) abandonment of their religious beliefs and work through the issues related to the anticipated loss of meaning and support in their lives (Hoffman et al. 2006). Despite being proven as ineffective and outdated, conversion therapy is highly regarded among religious leaders as a way to change a person's sexual orientation. Hoffman et al. offer another option an affirming or welcoming model for those who do not believe that their sexual orientation is sinful or wrong and wish to maintain their religious beliefs. LGBT-affirmative congregations and spiritual communities may be more in line with the biblical teachings of both justice and love. In this vein, Dreyer (2008b) suggests several LGBT-affirmative considerations for religious leaders. First, religious leaders who adopt such a theology and philosophy will be more advantageous when engaging LGBT persons, and an open view of the scripture will be conducive to finding a way that the Bible does not damage, reject, or condemn individuals. Second, openness to the voices of the marginalized is conductive to a pastoral and therapeutic responsibility to listen to and understand the experience of the other from the inside. Finally, the willingness of religious leaders to struggle with the Bible and with other voices rather than adhere to a set of prescribed answers is helpful when dealing with the complex personal, social, and religious sectors of LGBT persons.

In 2006, the Social Issues and Resources Panel of the Presbyterian Church in Ireland put forward General Assembly Resolution (GAR) guidelines (http://www.presbyterian ireland.org/getmedia/c89505dc-f8a9-4640-ad20-

ab20-ab9f6bed106/Pastoral-Guideline), which advocated for "the need for the church to be the church," meaning that "the church has a crucial responsibility to create an environment of love, understanding, acceptance, patience, forgiveness, openness, and grace." In addition, the GAR guidelines stipulated that the role of pastoral care is not to force gay and lesbian persons into counseling, let alone suggest demonic activity. The guidelines asserted the danger of suggesting that sexual minorities are sick and need to be healed, and clarifying that all people, in various ways, are in need of the healing graces.

In a survey of members of the congregation of Dignity, Lutherans Concerned, and Integrity churches, institutions that seek to affirm LGB sexual orientation among their congregants, Lease et al. (2005) found less internalized homonegativity and higher spiritual scores among members. The authors concluded that overt behaviors and attitudes that convey acceptance are important in offsetting the negative messages from mainstream religious denominations. Moreover, Gold (2010) believes that in light of the current situation, "empathy for the spiritual plight of LGB persons must serve as the basis for grieving what may have to be sacrificed and for

rejoicing in what must be discovered in order to integrate and live out one's spiritual and sexual orientation" (p. 210).

Strategies for making gay and lesbian persons and their families feel welcome in one's faith community were adapted by Fortunate Families and Concerned Catholics for lesbian and Gay Inclusion (2014, www.kcprovince.org/kcprovince/wp-content/uploads/2014/01/Pastors-resource.pdf). These strategies ranged from ensuring general hospitality for all to homily development inclusive of references to LGBT persons to being patient/sensitive to the possibility that LGBT persons may be present. Contemporary theological reactions to sexual minorities offer a more inclusive approach for LGBT persons while challenging religious leaders to reexamine their judgmental stance (see Table 27.3).

Political Implications

Over the years, much of the opposition to equality for LGBT persons in America has come from organized religion, especially from conservative religious leaders and faith-based groups.

Table 27.3 Contemporary theological reactions on sexual minorities

John McNeill

Through the lenses of scriptural interpretation and psychological insight, McNeill argues that, in justice, the Church needs to abandon its traditional opposition to committed, sexually active lesbian or gay relationships. He proposes, "The same moral norms should be applied in judging the sexual behavior of a true homosexual as we ordinarily apply to heterosexual activity." Additionally, he argues "there is the possibility of morally good homosexual relationships and that love which unites the partners in such a relationship, rather than alienating them from God, can be judged as uniting them more closely"

Sister Margaret Farley

She observes that the church's teaching on sexuality is based in an act-centered morality (i.e., what is judged god or bad or bad is an activity). She proposes that the church adopt a relationship-centered morality (i.e., what is judged good or bad is the quality of the relationship between people). Principles such as free consent of the partners, equality between partners, a sense of commitment, and permanency, she argues, provide a better basis for evaluating the good in a partnership that the Church's current teaching with its heavy biological emphasis

Bishop Geogrey Robinson

He asks two critical questions: (1) Why are sexual sins considered offenses against God and not against people? (2) Why does the Church's sexual morality have such little Biblical, and specifically New testament, support? He proposes that the Church could develop a new sexual ethnic from the Gospels by looking at the principles that Jesus taught about how people should treat one another

www.kcprovince.org/Kcprovince/wp-content/uploads/2014/01/Pastors-Resource.pdf

Beyond preaching and teaching that sexual minorities represent a violation of God's will, many religious leaders and groups have worked in the political arena to oppose legislation and policies that provide human rights and equality for LGBT persons (Thistlethwaite and Cook 2011). Thistlethwaite and Cook argue that while it is important to support the First Amendment rights of faith communities to voice their beliefs, it is equally important "to oppose their effects to impose their theology on a pluralistic democracy and deny justice and equality to millions of LGBT Americans" (p. 1). The quest is to expand and reframe the debate that will allow for moral equality to be as important as legal and social equality.

One area of considerable debate surrounds the separation of church and state. In the United States, on one side of the political debate (the Religious Right) are organizations that identify themselves as family focused and for traditional values, and believe that their religious views should be that of all Americans. On the other side (the Left) are organizations that support separation of church and state and oppose the imposition of religious views about homosexuality and gay marriage as espoused by the Religious Right. Although religious groups have the right to hire whomever they want and to restrict to whom they will offer services, many view that they should not have a right to accept government funding to operate programs and then refuse to offer services to certain classes of people such as LGBT persons. For faith-based organizations to do so is tantamount to government-sponsored discrimination on the grounds of sexual orientation and gender identity.

Prominent religious leaders of the Christian Right openly influence public policy that restricts and denies LGBT rights (White 2006). In July of 2014, over 100 religious clergy, theologians, and faith leaders sent a letter to President Obama urging him not to include religious exemptions in an executive order prohibiting federal contractors from using hiring policies that discriminate against LGBT persons. Those religious leaders stressed that it is unjust for any person or corporation to use their religious beliefs to trample the rights and beliefs of others and stipulated that such actions run contrary to the "Golden Rule" articulated in every world religion.

Grzymala-Busse (2012) argues that religion has had clear and significant impacts in several domains of politics. These include voting and political behavior; as institutional players, lobbyists, and coalition partners; in the origins of institutions and the long-term outcomes through specific ideas and norms regarding appropriate institutional solutions; on attitudes toward and polices of social welfare; and through the influence of regime type and durability by legitimizing and lending support to secular regimes, or conversely, withdrawing that support and opposing particular secular incumbents and governing structures. These domains demonstrate that "organized religion and the secular state are in constant interaction, if not conflict" (Grzymala-Busse, p. 433). Religious loyalties continue to structure political thought and action because, as suggested by Grzymala-Busse, once religion is introduced into politics, it becomes very difficult to disinvite it. In 1991, Demerath described the presence and impact of religion in politics and policy development and this perception is as relevant today. According to Demerath, "Not only do its absolutist criteria clash with the politics of compromise, but religion tends to be emotionally 'hot and accompanied by it own experts who are frequently difficult to control ... very few state officials relish publicly opposing religious considerations once they have been activated" (p. 30). The comingling of religion and politics regarding polices on LGBT persons has proven to be a battle between individual freedom and personal choice and imposition of mandated doctrines and narrow interpretations of the Bible for everyone (Americans United for Separation of Church and State, n.d.).

Summary

Religion and spirituality are related but distinct entities. A person can be spiritual without being religious. Many LGBT persons identify as spiritual, defining it as their connection to the world and their place in it. LGBT elders are involved with religion and spirituality in different ways and at various levels. There seems to be reciprocity between the way in which religion influences sexual identity and the way in which LGBT persons engage in worship practices.

Some religions have used scripture and religious writings to justify the marginalization and oppression of LGBT persons. Conservative religious leaders continue to pronounce sexual minorities and sinners and immoral persons and to oppose LGBT rights across social, economic, employment, and religious spectrums. They hold this stance even in light of more accepting attitudes of the general public toward LGBT persons. Opponents of anti-LGBT views of some religious leaders and faith communities is that these leaders and communities are holding to scripture of the Old Testament and not to gospel, which is more applicable to modern times. Moreover, opponents believe that religious documents were written at a time when those who penned the scripture could not envision the world of modern times.

In summary, many faith communities have taken increasingly favorable and supportive stances on the issues that affect LGBT persons. In addition, many faith communities exhibit clearly supportive and welcoming environments for LGBT persons. It is difficult to say if and when the anti-LGBT sentiment of many religious leaders and faith communities will be resolved. However, it is feasible to suggest that the religious leaders take the stance espoused by Dreyer (2008b): making the church whole by "bringing together in on created humanity the people that the church has so often separated and polarized … heterosexuals form sexual minorities, glorifying the one pole and demonizing or demeaning the other" (p. 1251).

Learning Exercises

Self-check Questions

1. What is the difference between religion and spirituality?
2. What was the response of faith communities to LGBT elders during the era in which they grew up?
3. How prepared are religious leaders to address concerns of LGBT members in their congregations?
4. What are the characteristics of Christian Fundamentalist dogma?
5. How many times is homosexuality discussed in the Christian Bible?

Field-based Experiential Assignments

1. Develop a presentation in which you defend the rights of LGBT persons to be equally recognized and supported in faith communities.
2. Interview religious leaders on their knowledge of LGBT issues and how qualified they believe they are to provide pastoral care to LGBT elders.
3. Select a denomination and volunteer to review and modify/update their policies on LGBT members in the church and/or develop a resource directory of available service.

Multiple-choice Questions

1. Which historical figure determined that same-sex intimacy was against nature and a crime?

    (a) Moses
    (b) Jesus
    (c) King Solomon
    (d) Emperor Justinian

2. Which of the following books of the Bible does not mention homosexuality?

(a) Mark

(b) Romans

(c) Genesis

(d) Leviticus

3. Which of the following is a postmodern view of sexuality?

(a) Homogeneous

(b) Bi-modal

(c) Heterogeneous

(d) Moralistic

4. Which of the following context was sexual diversity not considered by writers of the Bible?

(a) Behavioral

(b) Ceremonial

(c) Cultural

(d) Marriage

5. Negative religious attitudes about sexual minorities can lead to which of the following in LGBT persons?

(a) Depression

(b) Low self-esteem

(c) Feelings of worthlessness

(d) All of the above

(e) None of the above

6. In Rose's study, how do LGBT elders rate their faith community?

(a) Tolerant and guarded

(b) Source of strength and supportive

(c) Intolerant and dismissive

(d) Supportive and judgmental

7. Which of the following is true of LGBT persons' religious identity?

(a) Less religious than non-LGBT persons

(b) More likely to identify as non-religious

(c) Equally religious as non-LGBT persons

(d) Both a and b

(e) None of the above

8. Which of the following is an ethical requirement for therapist, but religious leaders may find more difficult when working with LGBT persons?

(a) Non-judgmental and not impose beliefs

(b) Impose beliefs and suggest conversion treatment

(c) Non-judgmental and promote the views of the faith community

(d) Assist LGBT persons to understand how their behavior is sinful

9. Which of the following should be given consideration when looking at religious issues for LGBT persons?

(a) Issues are consistently the same for LGBT persons

(b) Transgender issues may be different and require different approaches

(c) Gay men are discriminated against more in faith communities

(d) Lesbians are readily accepted in faith communities

10. Which of the following do LGBT elders report about their social support network?

(a) Gets larger as they age

(b) Remains unchanged

(c) Includes more younger people looking mentors

(d) Gets smaller as they age

Key

1-d

2-a

3-c

4-c

5-d

6-b

7-d

8-a

9-b

10-d

Resources

A Wider Path: Spiritual Experiences of LGBT Seniors (film): http://youtu.be/ESQzndjLre0

Gay Buddhist Sangha: www.gaybuddhistsangha.org

Gay Christian Network: www.gaychristian.net

Gay Church: www.gaychurch.org/

Imaan (Muslim): www.imaan.org.ku

Jewish Gay and Lesbian Group: www.jglg.org.uk

LGBT Ministries Books & Videos for Education and Discussion: www.lgbtq/discussion/index.shtml

North Como Presbyterian Church. (2005). *Ordination Standards: Biblical, Theological, and Scientific Perspectives*. Roseville, MN: iUniverse, Inc.

Outreach & Public Witness for LGBTQ Rights: www.lgbt/witness/index.shtml

Sarbat (Sikhs): www.sarbat.net

Stringfellow, Roland Rev. (2011). Amber Hollibaugh—The Role of Congregations in Supporting LGBT Seniors (film): vimeo.com/27884144

Unitarian Universalist LGBT History and Facts: www.lgbtq/history/index.shtml

Welcoming and Inclusive Congregations: www.lgbtq/welcoming/index.shtml

References

Americans United for Separation of Church and State. (n. d.). *Church, state and tour freedom at risk! The religious right's war on LGBT Americans*. Washington DC. Retrieved November 10, 2014 from http://www.au.org/resources/publications/the-religious-rights-war-on-lgbt-americans.

Amsel, N. (nd). Homosexuality in Orthodox Judaism. Retrieved November 9, 2014 from www.lookstein.org/resources/homosexuality_amsel.pdf.

Appell, V. (nd). What does Reform Judaism say about homosexuality? Retrieved November 9, 2014 from http://www.reformjudaism.org/practice/ask-rabbi/what-does-reform-judaism-say-about-homosexuality.

Atchison, G. J. (2010, July 8). *Homosexuality and the Bible (part 1 of 3) Genesis 19*. Retrieved November 6, 2014 from http://angelsrefuge.wordpress.com/2010/06/08/homosexuality-and-the-bible-part-1-of-7/.

Atchison, G. J. (2013, June 2). *Homosexuality and the Bible: The New Testament (part 3 of 3)*. Retrieved November 6, 2014 from http://anglesrefuge.wordpress.com/2013/06/02/homosexuality-and-the-bible-part-3-of-7/.

Banerjee, A. T., Strachan, P. H., Boyle, M. H., Anand, S. S., & Oremus, M. (2014). Attending religious services and its relationship with coronary heart disease and related risk factors in older adults: A qualitative study of church pastors and parishioners' perspectives. Journal of Religion and Health, 53, 1770–1785.

Barton, B. (2010). "Abomination"—Life as a Bible belt gay. *Journal of Homosexuality, 57*, 465–484.

Beery, T. A., Baas, L. S., Fowler, C., & Allen, G. (2002). Spirituality in persons with heart failure. *Journal of Holistic Nursing, 20*(1), 5–25.

Brennan, M. (2004). Spirituality and religiousness predict adaptation to vision loss among middle-age and older adults. *International Journal of Psychology and Religion, 14*(3), 193–214.

Carls, P. (2012). Emile Durkheim. Internet encyclopedia of philosophy. Retrieved October 27, 2014 from www.iep.tum.edu/durkheim/.

Demerath, N. J. (1991). Religious capital and capital religions: Cross-cultural and non-legal factors in the separation of church and state. *Daedalus, 120*(3), 21–40.

Donnelley, R. R. (2008, February). Challenging prejudice: Changing attitudes toward lesbian, gay, bisexual and transgender people in Scotland. Edinburgh: Scottish Government.

Dreyer, Y. (2005). Sexuality and shifting paradigms—setting the scene. *Hervormde Teologiese Studies, 61*(3), 729–751.

Dreyer, Y. (2006a). Heteronomatiwiteit, homofobie en homoseksualiteit – 'n roetekaart vir 'n inklusiewe kerk. *Hervormde Teologiese, 62*(2), 445–471.

Dreyer, Y. (2006b). Prejudice, homophobia and the Christian faith community. *Verbum et Ecclesia, 27*(1), 155–173.

Dreyer, Y. (2008a). Pastoral care and gays against the background of same-sex relationships in the *Umwelt* of the New Testament. *Hervormde Teologiese Studies, 64*(2), 739–765.

Dreyer, Y. (2008b). A pastoral response to the unhealed wound of gays exacerbated by indecision and inarticulacy. *Hervormde Teologiese Studies, 64*(3), 1235–1254.

Dutwin, D. (2012). LGBT acceptance and support: The Hispanic perspective. Social Science Research Solutions. Retrieved October 28, 2014 from www.ncir.org/images/uploads/publicagions/LGBTAS_HispanicPerspective.pdf.

Dwyer, J. F. (2007). *Those 7 references: A study of 7 references to homosexuality in the bible*. Charleston, SC: BookSurge Publishing.

Espinoza, R. (2014). *Out and visible: The experiences ad attitudes of lesbian, gay, bisexual, and transgender older adults, ages 45–75*. New York, NY: Services and Advocacy for LGBT Elders.

Faith in America. (2010). *Addressing religious arguments to achieve LGBT equality*. Retrieved November 9, 2014 from www.faithinamerica.org/2010-2/2p-content/uploads/2010/11/FIA_ConfrontingReligiousArguments.pdf.

Gold, J. M. (2010). *Counseling and spirituality: Integrating spiritual and clinical orientations*. Upper Saddle River, NJ: Merrill.

Goldberg, P. (2010, June 21). Toward a broader understanding of religion's functions. Retrieved October 31, 2015 from www.huffingtonpost.com/phillip-goldberg/toward-broader-understa_b_545314.html.

Grzymala-Busse, A. (2012). Why comparative politics should take religion (more) seriously. *Annual Review of Political Science, 15*, 421–442.

Guasp, A., & Dick, S. (2012, January). *Living together— British attitudes to lesbian and gay people in 2012*. Retrieved November 13, 2014 from www.socialwelfare.bl.uk/subject-areas/services-client-groups/minoritygroups/stonewall/160499living_together_2012.pdf.

Gubi, P. M., & Jacobs, R. (2009). Exploring the impact on counselors of working with spiritually abused clients. *Mental Health, Religion and Culture, 12*, 191–204.

Halkitis, P. N., Mattis, J. S., Sahadath, J. J., Massie, D., Ladyzhenskaya, L., Pitrelli, K., et al. (2009). The meanings and manifestations of religion and spirituality among lesbian, gay, bisexual, and transgender adults. *Journal of Adult Development, 16*, 250–262.

Hoffman, L., Knight, S. K., Boscoe-Huffman, S., & Stewart, S. (2006). *Religious experience, gender, and sexual orientation*. Retrieved November 11, 2014 from www.saybrook.edu.newexistentialists/files/media/ReligiousExperienceGenderandSexualOrientation.pdf.

Human Rights Campaign. (nd). Stances of faith on LGBT issues: Islam. Retrieved November 9, 2014 from http://www.hrc.org/resources/entry/stances-of-faith-on-lgbt-issues-islam.

Human Rights Campaign. (2014). Faith positions. Retrieved October 26, 2014 from http://www.hrc.org/resources/entry/faith-positions.

Lease, S. H., Horne, S. G., & Noffsinger-Frazier, F. (2005). Affirming faith experiences and psychological health for Caucasian lesbian, gay, and bisexual individuals. *Journal of Counseling Psychology, 52*, 378–388.

Lenkeit, D., & Lenkeit, R. (1997). *Introducing cultural anthropology*. Mountain View, CA: Mayfield Publishing Company.

Lowry, L. W., & Conco, D. (2002). Exploring the meaning of spirituality with aging adults in Appalachia. *Journal of Holistic Nursing, 20*(4), 388–402.

Lynch, B. (1996). Religious and spirituality conflicts. In D. Davies & C. Neal (Eds.), *Pink therapy: A guide for counselors and therapists working with gay, lesbian, and bisexual clients* (pp. 199–207). Buckingham, England: Open University Press.

Mackinlay, E. (2006). Spiritual care: Recognizing spiritual needs of older adults. *Journal of Religion, Spirituality and Aging, 18*(1–2), 59–71.

Mahru, J. (2014). *Pastoral care and LGBT seniors*. Berkeley, CA: Center for gay and lesbian studies in religion and ministry. Retrieved October 26, 2014 from www.clgs.org/files-clgs/CLGS_LGBTSeniorsFinal.pdf.

Martin, D. B. (1996). Arsenokoites and malakos: Meaning and consequences. In R. L. Brawley (Ed.), *Biblical ethics and homosexuality: Listening to scripture* (pp. 117–136). Louisville, KY: Westminster.

Mitchell, J., & Weatherly, D. (2000). Beyond church attendance: religiosity and mental health among rural older adults. *Journal of Cross Cultural Gerontology, 15*(1), 37–54.

Musick, M. A., House, J. S., & Williams, D. R. (2004). Attendance at religious services and morality in a national sample. *Journal of Health and Social Behavior, 45*, 198–213.

Newlin, K., Melkus, G. D., Tappen, R., Chyun, D., & Koenig, H. G. (2008). Relationships of religion and spirituality to glycemic control in Black women with type 2 diabetes. *Nurse Res, 57*(5), 331–339.

Newport, F. (2014, August 11). LGBT population in the U.S. significantly less religious. Retrieved October 26, 2014 from http://www.gallup.com/pool/174788/lgbt-population-significantly-less-religious.

Pace. (2013). *Religion and LGBT issues*. London, England. Retrieved October 26, 2014 from www.pacehealth.org.uk/files/2013/6551/5626/Religion_and_LGBT_issues.pdf.

Pargament, K. I., Murry-Swank, N., Magyar, G. M., & Ano, G. G. (2005). Spiritual struggle: A phenomenon of interest to psychology and religion. In W. R. Miller & H. D. Delaney (Eds.), *Judeo-Christian perspectives on psychology: Human nature, motivation, and change* (pp. 245–268). Washington, DC: American Psychological Association. Doi:10.1037/10859-013.

Reygan, F., & Moane, G. (2014). Religious homophobia: The experiences of a sample of lesbian, gay, bisexual and transgender (LGBT) people in Ireland. *Culture and religion: An Interdisciplinary Journal, 15*(3), 298–312.

Roozen, D. A. (2011). *A decade of change in American congregations 2000–2010*. Hartford, CT: Hartford Institute for Religious Research. Retrieved October 26, 2014 from www.FaithCommunityToday.org/sites/faithcommunitiestoday.org/files/DecadesofChangeFinal_0.pdf.

Rose, E. (2012). *A wider path: Spiritual experiences of LGBT seniors-An exploratory manual to accompany the film*. Retrieved October 28, 2014 from www.nyam.

org/social-work-leadership-institute-V2/geriatic-social-work/hppae/for-students/LGBT-Spirituality-Capstone-Project.pdf.

Scottish Government Social Research. (2007). *Attitudes to discrimination in Scotland: 2006.* Edinburgh: Scottish Government.

Shaffer, B. (nd). Do homosexuals fit into the Jewish community? Retrieved November 9, 2014 from http://www.chabad.org/library/article_cdo/aid/663504/jewish/Do-Homosexuality-fit-into-the-Jewish-Community.htm.

Sharma, S. (2008). Young women, sexuality and protestant church community. *European Journal of Women's Studies, 15,* 345–359.

Sheldon, K., & Delgado-Romero, E. (2011). Sexual orientation microaggressions: The experience of lesbian, gay, bisexual, and queer clients in psychotherapy. *Journal of Counseling Psychology, 58,* 210–221.

Sue, D. W., Capodilupo, C. M., Torino, G. C., Bucceri, J. M., Holder, A. M. B., Nadal, K. L., & Esquilin, M. (2007). Racial microaggressions in everyday life: Implications for clinical practice. *American Psychologist, 62,* 271–286.

Taylor, C. (1989). *The sources of the self: The making of the modern identity.* Cambridge, MA: Harvard University Press.

Taylor, P. (2013, June 13). *A survey of LGBT Americans: Attitudes, experiences, and values in changing times.* Retrieved November 9, 2014 from http://www.pewsocialtrends.org/2013/06/13/a-survey-of-lgbt-americans/7/.

Thistlethwaite, S. B., & Cook, M. (2011, January). *Keeping the faith: Faith organizing for lesbian, gay, bisexual, and transgender moral and civil rights in southern states.* Washington DC: Center for American Progress.

Turner, Y., & Stayton, W. (2014). The twenty-first century challenges to sexuality and religion. *Journal of Religion and Health, 53*(2), 483–497.

Van Drie, A., Ganzevoort, R. R., & Spiering, M. (2014). Anonymous pastoral care for problems pertaining to sexuality. *Journal of Religion and Health, 53,* 1634–1652.

Ward, D. J. (2011). The lived experience of spiritual abuse. *Mental Health, Religion & Culture, 14,* 899–915.

Wood, A. W., & Conley, A. H. (2014). Loss of religious or spiritual identities among the LGBT population. *Counseling and Values, 59,* 95–111.

White, M. (2006). *Religion gone bad: The hidden dangers of the Christian right.* New York: Penguin Group.

Brian McNaught

Abstract

To understand and address the unique challenges faced by lesbian, gay, bisexual, and gender diverse seniors requires an awareness of what drives workplace diversity initiatives, and cultural competence on the multiple differences represented by the limiting acronym, LGBT.

Keywords

LGBT elders · Workplace · Public policy · Law

This brief chapter on the issues facing lesbian, gay, bisexual, and transgender (LGBT)[1] seniors in the workplace is a reflection based upon my 40-year career working as an educator on LGBT concerns. I'm not an academician, and so this chapter is somewhat different from other chapters in this book.

When approaching this topic, you work with the assumption that there is a war for talent in the workplace that somewhat evens the playing field. In theory, companies cannot afford to lose the best and brightest workers because their workplace is unwelcoming. To attract and retain highly qualified people and to maintain a competitive edge, most companies seek to create conditions in which the diversity of their workforce is celebrated and fully tapped. That should mean that older lesbian, gay, bisexual, and transgender people are seen as having the potential to be among the company's best and brightest employees, thus increasing the odds of profitability.

That said, the working conditions for LGBT employees of all ages can vary in the same company, depending upon the mentality of middle management. When the middle manager, influenced by any number of variables such as religious beliefs, familiarity with gay and transgender people, race, and gender, among other factors, does not ascribe to his or her company's

---

[1] While I will occasionally use the acronym LGBT in writing and speaking, I believe it is preferable to write and say the words lesbian, gay, bisexual, and transgender. These four words represent four distinct communities, each with its own concerns. The LGBT acronym enables people not to say the words, diminishes the difference in issues, and is often confusing to the reader or listener. "Is it a sandwich?".

B. McNaught (✉)
Brian McNaught & Associates, Ft. Lauderdale, Florida, US
e-mail: brian@brian-mcnaught.com

© Springer International Publishing Switzerland 2016
D.A. Harley and P.B. Teaster (eds.), *Handbook of LGBT Elders*,
DOI 10.1007/978-3-319-03623-6_28

values, the lesbian, gay, bisexual, and transgender worker is vulnerable to increased risk of harassment.

When considering harassment, or other hostile working conditions, the reader needs to allow for the possibility of the worst behavior in the workplace, such as physical and emotional abuse, but he or she is encouraged to focus more on problems created by unconscious incompetence. Excluding examples of termination, hiring discrimination, and overt hostility, the majority of LGBT people in the workplace complain about feeling isolated because of their sexual orientation or gender identity or expression. Fear of isolation is what keeps many LGBT people in the closet. The isolation is created by the lack of social interactions with colleagues, especially conversations having to do with personal life.

One of the challenges in creating a clear picture of workplace issues for lesbian, gay, bisexual, and transgender seniors is that the culture is changing so quickly that the picture will never be complete or reliable. For instance, marriage equality is now the law of the land, some politicians insist they will continue to resist it. Though progress is being made in state-by-state passage of non-discrimination ordinances, there are now efforts to pass statewide legislation that grants religious liberty to employees to discriminate on the basis of their personal beliefs. Eventually, the Federal Employment Non-Discrimination Act (ENDA) will be passed, but probably not for many years. The current fear of gender diversity on the part of many members of Congress keeps the legislation locked up. That will change, or the legislation will change, and it will be passed, but it will still not cover housing and public accommodation, which might have an impact on a discussion of LGBT workplace issues. If a gay senior faces discrimination in housing, is it possible for him or her to live near the workplace?

We are aware of the quickly changing culture, which in the Western world is becoming more comfortable with the full range of sexual orientation and gender expression, and we are aware of the increase in protective legislation. But, understanding the challenges faced by senior

lesbian, gay, bisexual, and transgender workers means being aware of the rapidly paced changes in language and attitudes in LGBT communities. When I first began working on this issue, the focus was on gay people. It then became about lesbian and gay people. Bisexuality was soon added to the topic. Then, transgender issues became part of the discussion. Not long ago, the organization that was originally called the National Gay Task Force changed its name to include letters in the acronym to accommodate the issues of people who identify as queer, questioning, intersex, and asexual. Further, the new preferred term for transgender people is gender diverse, and the new preferred term for transitioning (the process of physically becoming one's true self) is realignment. Although I have been familiar with these issues for decades, I need to constantly update my educational resources on the topic because of these changes in language and attitudes.

What began as a workplace concern in the United States, with me introducing the topic as a business issue in 1985, is now being discussed throughout the world because of the multi-national identity of most major corporations. Creating an office culture that is welcoming to LGBTQQIA people is not just important in New York, but also in Mumbai. Wall Street banks brought me to India, Japan, Hong Kong, and Singapore to train their employees on gay and transgender issues. That work has rapidly expanded throughout those countries and many others. Understanding LGBT senior workplace issues requires familiarity with the cultures of those individual countries, especially as they relate to age, sexual orientation, and gender expression diversity.

Gay and transgender discrimination has become an issue of importance to the United Nations. The Roman Catholic Church is said to be softening its approach because of the statement by Pope Francis, "Who am I to judge?" Gay issues are now part of the discussion on where the Olympics will be held. Economic sanctions are being imposed on countries that discriminate against gay people. The words "lesbian, gay, bisexual, and transgender" were all used by President Obama in his State of the Union address in 2015.

Another component of the discussion is the very important shift in approaching the transgender topic. The number of people in a society who identify as transsexual or as transgender is very small, but the number of people who are discriminated against because of the diversity of their gender expression is huge. Heterosexual men who are considered effeminate and heterosexual women who are considered masculine can experience more discrimination on the job than a masculine gay man or a feminine lesbian. What is considered acceptable behavior or expression for males and females varies widely from culture to culture. Hand holding by heterosexual men is common in India but not in Great Britain.

One more consideration when analyzing workplace concerns for lesbian, gay, bisexual, and transgender people is the differences between the individuals. Some LGBT people are highly qualified and are likely to be accommodated easily. People who bring in money are highly valued despite their age. If the senior gay person in question is black, Latino, female, foreign, Muslim, economically challenged, or has a disability, he or she will generally fair less well than a gay white Christian male, at least in the United States. If the transgender person in question is transsexual, and passes easily because he or she fits neatly in the male or female box and is physically attractive, he or she will fare much better than the person, who after realignment, does not look attractive or is easily identifiable as a man or woman. Cross-dressing men have a much more difficult time than cross-dressing women, partly because of sexism, and partly because they sometimes do not pass easily as a female. If the person's appearance is considered by others as "peculiar," it is more likely that he or she will suffer discrimination in the workplace.

Realtors tell us that the primary factor in selling a house is location, location, location. My message to companies is that the only reliable way to create a workplace that feels safe to lesbian, gay, bisexual, and transgender people of all ages is education, education, education. Most people want to be supportive but do not know how.

They do not start conversations with gay or transgender people because they fear making a mistake, and so they keep quiet. The silence is interpreted as hostility or at least disapproval. Education through diversity training creates more competent and confident allies and lowers the chances of unwelcoming behaviors. In addition to continuing education, a company that wants to diminish the chances of discriminating against LGBT seniors needs to nurture an LGBT employee resource group that will help the company stay ahead of the game, in properly adjusting to the changes in the culture, the rules, and the issues.

The following essay is an updated newspaper column/Internet blog that I wrote, which was reprinted by groups working with lesbian, bisexual, and transgender seniors.

Essay on LGBT Seniors—No Money, No Work, and You're Old

The dream is recurring. I'm in a panic because I don't have a job, and I question if I've ever worked. I'm sure that I'm too old to find meaningful employment, but I need money. I eventually become conscious that I'm dreaming, and I remind myself that I've had a personally rewarding career and that I don't need to work.

Perhaps the dream is prompted by my struggle with the idea of retirement, or having been fired for being gay at age 26, or almost always working for myself, or maybe it is because it took many years before my father and mother accepted that educating others on lesbian, gay, bisexual, and transgender (LGBT) issues was a real job. It is a bad dream that takes me a while to shake.

Yet, for many people my age and younger, there is no waking from the bad dream, and there is no shaking off the emotional toll it takes. Being unemployed and needing money are the most pressing issues of their lives. They fear running out of money before they die and ending up being dependent on others to survive.

The people who live these nightmares most often are older workers who, regardless of their sexual orientation or gender identity, have watched the depletion of their savings and the diminished value of their skills. They have either lost, or fear they soon will lose, their jobs because of profit loss, automation, or their inability to keep pace with information technology.

If these unemployed older people are lesbian, gay, bisexual, or transgender, their situation may feel more precarious. In addition to feeling less needed, they may also feel less wanted. If they are closeted, they may be seen as lacking the fortitude to face the challenges of the ever-changing workplace. Closeted LGBT people, I suspect, are rarely unknown and often disparaged as unable to lead. If they are out of the closet, they may fear that being out will be a factor in their not being kept or re-hired. Despite how many corporate promises are made about not discriminating on the basis of sexual orientation or gender identity, many people feel that the promise only counts in the war for talent when the gay or transgender employee is seen as exceptional in what he or she does. Additionally, most states allow for such workplace discrimination.

Until the ENDA passes Congress and is signed into law by the President, LGBT people can be discriminated against in employment in several states. Even if ENDA passes, gay and gender diverse-people can be denied housing and public accommodation. Attempts to pass laws that guarantee religious liberty make employment rights for LGBT people even more tenuous.

Discrimination against gay, lesbian, bisexual, and gender diverse people in the workplace ranges from physical violence to silence. Depending upon the location of the workplace, and the age, race, gender, religious affiliation, and education of fellow employees and managers, the workplace harassment can be unrelenting and unchecked, or more a matter of subtle social isolation because of cultural incompetence. Without protective legislation, LGBT people, including seniors, suffer higher rates of unemployment and income inequality.

Transgender people are particularly affected by a lack of protections. Ninety percent of this group reports discrimination in the workplace. These individuals are twice as likely as the general population to be unemployed and four times as likely to live at the poverty level.

According to the State of Georgia Department of Labor (2012), 4.7 % of the workforce is 65 years of age or older. Pew Research (Drake 2013) speculates that by 2022, 31.9 % of people 65–74 will still be working. In the private sector, 6.48 per cent of those people will be LGBT seniors, according to the Williams Institute on Sexual Orientation Law and Public Policy (2011) of 65 in order to make ends meet. A significant percentage of those people are LGBT. Questions that need to be asked are, will these LGBT seniors have legal protections against discrimination on the job, and what unique challenges do they face because of their sexual orientation or gender diversity?

Many older people would like to retire, but what if their nest egg has been depleted because the value of their house has depreciated, they have had unexpected health care costs, or their pension was cut—they have no alternative but to find work. But what work? How does the 55-year-old gay man find work after his money-making "companion" dies and leaves the bulk of his assets to his children and grandchildren? The single lesbian near retirement is not seen as being as needy of steady income as the man who has dependents. If she is let go in downsizing, how does she find work to make up the lost income? And, what happens to an older person who is transsexual? Where does the average, senior, transgender person find work unless he or she is extraordinary at what he or she does?

The old career development resource book, *What Color is Your Parachute* (Bolles 2015), and every similar book published since, tells us that our best chance of finding a job is knowing someone who can help. Job hunters are encouraged to make lists of the people they know who might be able and willing to pull strings or make introductions. What good connections do older LGBT people have? What if they have pulled back from straight family and friends because they wanted to be out and proud? Are their gay or straight friends comfortable putting their reputations on the line by making a call or giving them a letter of recommendation? Will the names of younger lesbian, gay, bisexual, and transgender employees be on the list of possible connections? Do younger LGBT employees relate to, or even like, their older counterparts? Are corporate LGBT Employee Resource Groups (ERGs), headed by younger workers, aware of the struggles of Baby Boom gay and transgender employees, and do they see such issues as worthy of their attention, and of inclusion in their limited budget?

In the corporate world, finding allies who understand and support the specific issues of older LGBT persons is critical to having their needs championed. While older workers, in general, can feel alienated by the attitudes of younger workers, it can be particularly disenfranchising for a senior gay worker. To hear gay worker to hear the offensive word "queer" used as a proud self-description by younger LGBT employees, and to see that there is no awareness on the part of youth of the many sacrifices that have been made to create such a welcoming work environment for them, can prompt senior workers to pull away from ERGs. Younger workers can be seen as ungrateful upstarts who are competing for the jobs needed to secure the older worker's sustainability. Older employees can be seen as stubborn and out of touch with cultural advances and as obstacles to promotions.

If older LGBT workers hope to secure the support of younger LGBT workers, attention must be given to changing attitudes. Older transgender workers are sometimes seen by many younger transgender job seekers, not as pioneers, but as sad vestiges of the time when people felt forced to pick one gender over the other. Today's youth are far more fluid in their queer identity and feel less the need for full transition surgery. Closeted older, lesbian, gay, and bisexual workers can be seen by some younger LGB employees as roadblocks to the success of equal treatment in the workplace, especially in regional offices and foreign countries. Focusing attention on the issues facing LGBT seniors requires corporate ERGs to ask seniors questions about the challenges they face and about how best to be allies.

Outside the workplace, unemployed gay and transgender seniors, like their heterosexual peers, can find support in their search for work from AARP, the American Association of Retired People. AARP has a 17 % success rate in finding work for its members. But unemployed older LGBT people can also get training and guidance from SAGE, Services and Advocacy for LGBT Elders, a national organization with regional affiliates. They have a 25 % success rate in helping senior clients find employment.

That still leaves 75 % of the LGBT seniors who have sought help from SAGE, and the many more who have not heard of, or tried to get such help, living daily in the nightmare that only occasionally visits me in my dreams. If young lesbian, gay, bisexual, and transgender activists are looking for the next cause to take on after marriage equality, the bread and butter issues of LGBT seniors is an issue needing immediate attention.

Learning Exercises

1. What factors go into helping LGBT seniors remain in the workforce? Who is likely to do so and why?
2. What factors prevent LGBT seniors from entering the workforce? How can these be surmounted?
3. What factors do you take in consideration in addressing the needs of the older LGBT employee or those seeking employment?

Experiential Exercises

1. Describe your experience working with an older lesbian, gay, bisexual, transgender employee. Was there a particular situation that occurred within the workplace setting that you remember? If yes, why?
2. If you know a senior who is working and LGBT, ask him or her to describe a situation

in his or her work where he or she was treated well and where he or she was treated poorly.

References

Bolles, R. N. (2015). *What color is your parachute? A practical manual for job-hunters and career-changers.* New York: Random House LLC.

Drake, B. (2013). Number of older Americans in the workforce is on the rise. Facttank: Pew Research Center. Retrieved 20 February 2015 at http://www.pewresearch.org/fact-tank/2014/01/07/number-of-older-americans-in-the-workforce-is-on-the-rise/.

Georgia Department of Labor. (2012). Workforce statistics. Retrieved on 25 February 2015 at www.dol.state.ga.us/.

LGBT Intersection of Age and Sexual Identity in the Workplace

29

Debra A. Harley and Pamela B. Teaster

Abstract

LGBT older workers represent a diverse and growing segment of the workforce. Often, older LGBT workers must contend with unfair laws and discriminatory policies in the labor force. They must overcome the typical barriers to employment such as lack of modern skills, stereotypes, and disincentives of fringe benefits. Federal, state, and local governments and private business must examine their policies that adversely affect LGBT workers and aging workers. Collectively, LGBT workers are subjected to legalized discrimination, which can result in job loss or demotion. LBGT workers endue an unfair burden because of their sexual orientation and gender identity or expression. America is at a policy crossroads and is being tested for its response to legally sanction discrimination and violation of the civil right of LGBT workers. The future of the American work force may well be determined by its response to LGBT workers.

Keywords

LGBT elders · Workplace · Public policy · Legislation · Discrimination

Overview

Older workers have always faced barriers to employment. Although older workers are less likely to be unemployed compared to their younger counterparts, those who do become unemployed tend to have significantly longer periods of job seeking (Government Accountability Office 2012). Research suggests that trends in labor market outcomes of older workers are dependent upon characteristics such as race, educational attainment, geographic location, and sexual orientation and gender identity. Higher rates of unemployment exist among ethnic minorities, residents of rural areas, those with lower educational attainment, and among LGBT

D.A. Harley (✉)
University of Kentucky, Lexington, USA
e-mail: dharl00@email.uky.edu

P.B. Teaster
Virginia Tech, Blacksburg, VA, USA

© Springer International Publishing Switzerland 2016
D.A. Harley and P.B. Teaster (eds.), *Handbook of LGBT Elders*,
DOI 10.1007/978-3-319-03623-6_29

persons, especially those who are transgender (MAP, Human Rights Campaign, & Center for American Progress 2013). According to Make (2013), the loss of a job or income can be financially devastating for LGBT older adults, who have a higher-than-average risk of poverty. In addition, certain exemptions in the Federal Employment Non-Discrimination Act (ENDA) allow discrimination against LGBT persons in the workplace. According to Wolff (2014, p. 1), "the religious exemption in the current version of ENDA would enshrine the idea that LGBT equality is incompatible with the free exercise of religion." Discrimination in the workplace is becoming even more relevant to LGBT elders because many of them must stay in the workforce longer out of economic necessity.

The purpose of this chapter was to discuss workplace challenges faced by LGBT elders. Information is presented on the status of older job seekers, workplace issues for LGBT workers, and changing workplace culture for LGBT elders. The reader is encouraged to put himself or herself in the place of LGBT older workers and examine workplace issues through the lens and weight of oppression and discrimination, challenges that LGBT elders often experience.

Learning Objectives

By the end of this chapter, the reader should be able to:

1. Identify workplace issues that affect LGBT workers in general and LGBT elders in particular.
2. Understand ways that legislation includes discriminatory exemptions against LGBT workers.
3. Understand ways in which sexual orientation, gender identity or expression, and age intersect in the workplace.
4. Identify ways in which workplace culture can be hanged to be more LGBT-supportive.

Introduction

Many, if not most, progressive thinkers agree that discrimination in the workplace is wrong and have recognized the importance of LGBT-inclusive workplace protections as a solution to this problem (Center for American Progress 2013). According to Badgett et al. (2013b), employment discrimination based on sexual orientation and gender identity undermines workplace performance and prevents highly qualified workers from achieving the success that should be earned through hardwork. Badgett et al. contend that because of the lower cost and/or higher revenues that diversity in the workplace creates, employers have considered the economic benefits of adding LGBT-supportive policies, including sexual orientation and gender identity nondiscrimination polices and domestic partner benefits polices. In a review of thirty-six studies evaluating the impact of LGBT-supportive employment policies and workplace climates on business outcomes, Badgett et al. found a strong positive relationship between LGBT-supportive policies or workplace climates and business-related outcomes, while few or none showed a negative relationship or no relationship (see Research Box 29.1).

Research Box 29.1 Badgett, M. V. L., Durso, L. E., Kastanis, A., & Mallory, C. (2013b, May). *The Business impact of LGBT-supportive workplace policies*. Los Angeles, CA. The Williams Institute. **Objective:** To evaluate all published research evaluating the impact of LGBT-supportive employment policies and workplace climates on business outcomes in order to answer two questions: (1) Does research show that LGBT-supportive policies bring about the specific benefits mentioned by private companies that enact them, or are they associated with other similar economic benefits that may have an impact on the bottom line? and (2) If LGBT-supportive policies bring about certain benefits, does research show that these benefits actually have an impact on the bottom line, and if so, is it possible to estimate that effects in quantitative terms?

Method: First, relevant materials that were cited in previous Williams Institute reports and internal memos on this topic were collected. Second, all of the scholarship cited in those materials was gathered. Third, computerized searches using Google Scholar and Library article searches function were gathered from databases. Systematic combinations of words were used in the search. Fourth, relevant scholarship cited in the materials in the databases was gathered. Finally, systematic combinations of terms were used to search the Internet. In addition, a set of study characteristics that helped to determine the overall methodological strength of each paper was used.

Results: Most studies found a positive relationship between LGBT-supportive policies or workplace climates and business-related outcomes, while few or none found a negative or no relationship.

Conclusion: Researchers and business officials should collaborate to fully utilize data collected by employers and to make findings available to policymakers, the public, and other businesses.

Questions

1. What other research questions would you investigate from the literature on LGBT-supportive workplace policies?
2. What do you anticipate would be the outcome when looking at the interaction of age and sexual orientation and gender expression?
3. How would you design a study to evaluate the impact of LGT-supportive workplace policies based on the size of the business (e.g., small vs. medium vs. large)?

Although attitudes and perceptions concerning LGBT persons are gradually changing in the workplace landscape, discrimination remains a major challenge. On the one hand, for Fortune 500 companies, 62 % offer domestic partner health insurance benefits, 87 % have nondiscrimination policies based on sexual orientation and 94 % of Fortune 100 companies have nondiscrimination policies that include sexual orientation (Human Rights Campaign 2011a), and 46 % have nondiscrimination policies that include gender identity or gender expression, compared to 69 % of Fortune 100 companies (2011b). On the other hand, in a survey of employment discrimination and how it impacts LGBT employees, The Williams Institute (2011) found that 27.1 % of all LGBT employees experienced discrimination, as compared to 37.7 % of LGB employees who were out, and 27.1 % of LGB employees experienced harassment, compared to 38.2 % of those who were out. For transgender employees, 97 % experienced harassment or mistreatment in their workplace, and 47 % were fired, not advanced, or not hired due to their gender identity (National Center for Transgender Equality and the National Gay and Lesbian Task Force 2009). Fifty-eight percent of LGBT workers reported that a coworker makes a joke or derogatory comment about LGBT people at least once in a while and 67 % of LGBT employees do not report anti-LGBT remarks to human resources or management (Human Rights Campaign 2009).

Most LGBT elders have had to deal with the effects of a lifetime of discrimination on the basis of sexual orientation and gender identity or expression. According to Cray (2013), "the effects of employment discrimination against older LGBT workers are not static or confined to the workday" (p. 1). Often, LGBT older adults are denied pension plan options that provide financial protection for a surviving partner, even though LGBT employees earn their pension in the same ways as their heterosexual counterparts (MAP, SAGE, & Center for American Progress 2010). For many LGBT elders, the lines between work life and daily living are both marred by acts of discrimination, heterosexism, and homogeneity.

Status of Older Job Seekers and Older LGBT Workers

The economic downturn beginning in 2007 has led to an increase in labor force participation for may older workers. For those ages 55–64, the upward trend was driven almost exclusively by the increased labor force participation of women; the male participation rate was flat to declining. However, among older adults ages 65 or over, the rate increased for both females and males during 2007–2008 (Copelan 2014). As a growing segment of the population, older workers face challenges in finding and maintaining employment. In part, this is due to competing with younger, more technologically savory workers as well as having to stay in the labor force for longer periods of time for a variety of reasons (e.g., unexpected expenses, death of a spouse or partner, supplementing retirement accounts, financing health care). On positive note, older workers continue to work because of the removal of barriers that traditionally prevented them from working in their later years (e.g., increased life expectancy, better health outcomes, employment opportunities that require less physical labor) (Johnson 2004). Increasingly, various segments of the labor market are recognizing the value of and demanding that they employ older workers (Society for Human management, 2010).

The unemployment rate among older workers is lower than the national average for all workers (Heidkamp et al. 2012). Older workers are generally less likely to lose their jobs than younger workers because their tenure on the job provides them with some protection. Munnell et al. (2006) found that the lower probability of job loss for older workers was based on the correlation between age and tenure, but controlling for tenure, age does not protect workers from displacement. In fact, Munnell et al. found that the probability of displacement actually increases with age. Research also suggests that older workers who lose a job have a more difficulty than their younger counterparts in reconnecting

to the labor market (Johnson and Park 2011; Maestas and Li 2006; Li 2010). The reemployment rate for older displaced workers ages 55–64 was only 39 %; for those 65 and over, the rate was 22 % (Bureau of Labor statistics 2010). For older job seekers, long periods of unemployment are cause for serious concern because of the effects on mental health as well as job readiness (Heidkamp et al.). The problem of job opportunity also has a geographic component, because unemployment is associated with declining local and regional economies (Report of the Taskforce on the Aging of the American Workforce, 2008). In addition, for older workers who are not successful in finding new jobs, many are forced to accept steep cuts in pay (Johnson and Mommaerts 2011).

Older job seekers encounter obstacles due to employers' reluctance to hire them. They harbor the following negative perceptions, believing that older workers are (a) more expensive, including wages, health insurance, and the cost to train them; (b) less productive than younger workers and deliver lower quality work; and (c) less flexible in adapting to change in the workplace (Walker 2007). On the supply-side challenges (i.e., woeker characteristics), older job seekers encounter skill limitations combined with limited access to training programs, limited job searching skills, and health- and disability-related challenges that often accompany aging (Heidkamp et al. 2012). Overall, older job seekers face a plethora of real and perceived challenges that may contribute to poor outcomes: a weak demand from employers, possible age discrimination, and outdated skills in a technological job market.

Older LGBT workers experience high rates of discrimination in the workplace, and unfortunately, state and federal laws often fail to protect them. Over the past seventy years, Presidential executive orders requiring workplace protections from discrimination, including federal contractors, have not been overturned by courts, Congress, or subsequent Presidents. Under current federal law, it is entirely legal to fire someone based on sexual orientation or gender identity. Furthermore, LGBT workers lack adequate legal protection from employment discrimination (Badgett, Burns, Hunter et al. 2013a).

The LGBT Workforce. MAP, SAGE, and the Center for American Progress (2013) reported that the US workforce includes an estimated 5.4 million LGBT workers. The LGBT workforce is diverse but has common characteristics. The first characteristic is that LGBT workers are geographically dispersed: 93 % of same-sex couples live in all US counties. As many as 4.3 million LGBT persons live in states without state laws providing employment protection based on sexual orientation or gender identity or expression. Second, LGBT workers are racially and ethically diverse, 33 % of whom are persons of color, compared to 27 % of non-LGBT individuals. Third, a significant number of LGBT workers are raising children, thus heightening the importance of making family benefits available. In addition, if the norm of non-LGBT grandparents who are raising children holds true for LGBT grandparents, it is reasonable to assume that a substantial number of older LGBT workers are raising grandchildren (i.e., grandparents raising grandchildren). A fourth characteristic is that varying levels of education exist among LGBT workers. Data are mixed—some suggest that individuals with lower educational levels are more likely to identify as LGBT, while other data indicate a higher probability that persons in same-sex couples have at least a bachelor's degree than their opposite-sex counterparts. Similarly, transgender persons had much higher educational attainment than the population as a whole (National Transgender Discrimination Survey 2011). Fifth, the literature consistently suggests that LGBT workers experience unemployment at an equal or higher rate than do other workers, with transgender persons' unemployment rates twice that of the US populations as a whole. Rates for transgender persons of color are as high as four times the national unemployment rate (MAP, Human Rights Campaign, & Center for American Progress). Finally, LGBT workers in the USA are at higher risk of poverty than are other workers.

Workplace Issues for LGBT Workers

LGBT persons, their advocates, and their allies agree that some progress has been made for LGBT persons in the workplace. Most of the progress made has been through diversity programs. However, general acceptance of LGBT persons in the workplace may lead to complacency about the need for continued progress. A challenge is continuing harassment or discrimination based on sexual orientation and gender identity. Surprisingly, persons' blatantly offensive comments based on sexual orientation or gender identity are tolerated in workplaces that would never tolerate such comments based on religion or race (Madell 2012a). Another challenge is the inability to address family needs in the same ways that non-LGBT couples can. For example, the majority of companies does not offer domestic partner benefits (Madell 2012a).

Although organizations highlight polices and benefits for LGBT employees from corporate headquarters, a lack of education and information exists beyond that which is provided in offices located outside main branches (Madell 2012b). This limited scope of education beyond the corporate office has implications for LGBT persons in companies with global offices. Given that attitudes and practices toward LGBT persons are cultural, countries have practices that range from total acceptance and integration of LGBT persons to placing them in prison to putting them to death (Madell 2012b). Many workers in organizations do not know how to behave toward LGBT persons, and so they just ignore them (Madell 2012b). For example, non-LGBT workers may not invite LGBT coworkers out after work. Given that networking and decision-making often take place in social settings, LGBT workers are completely left out of this process.

Another persistent problem in companies is the lack of accountability processes to ensure that managers and supervisors create the right culture of acceptance of LGBT workers (Madell 2012b). Consequently, some managers or supervisors fail to pass along the right message or model LGBT-supportive behavior to their employees.

Yet another challenge for LGBT persons is deciding whether or not to come out in the workplace. Due to discrimination and concern for safety, many LGBT persons remain closeted. Finally, the overarching challenge to LGBT persons in the workplace remains the continued lack of legal protection (Wyatt 2015). Understanding these challenges from the perspective of LGBT persons is paramount if workplace culture is to change in any meaningful way.

Changing Workplace Culture for LGBT Elders

Workplace inequality and discrimination are harmful to all LGBT employees. Mentioned earlier, the impact on LGBT elders is intensified by economic reasons that have lead to them remain in the workforce longer or re-enter the job market upon retirement. Even with federal laws such as the Age Discrimination in Employment Act, age-based workplace discrimination persists. Compared to younger persons, older job applicants are more likely to be passed over for interviews and more likely to be paid less. For older LGBT workers, the effects of age-based discrimination may be compounded by discrimination on the basis of sexual orientation, gender identity, or gender expression (Cray 2013). Discrimination in employment has long-term implications for LGBT elders. Over the course of their work history, many LGBT elders have experienced years of job instability and unequal pay, which can contribute to financial insecurity well after retirement and for the rest of an elder's life (Grant et al. 2010). In addition, underemployment, extended unemployment, and lower wages can contribute to elevated poverty rates among LGBT elders (Badgett et al. 2013c).

At the core of the American work ethic is that if people work hard and meet their responsibilities, they should be able to get ahead. This "basic bargain is embedded in laws that promote equal access to jobs and that protect workers from unfair practices" (MAP, Human Rights Campaign, & Center for American Progress 2013, p. 1).

For LGBT persons, however, this bargain remains broken, resulting in bias, fewer workplace benefits, and higher taxes, despite the passage of federal and state laws aimed expressly at prohibiting discrimination against LGBT workers.

Increasingly, it is important to examine the role of unions in advocating for the rights of LGBT workers. In 2012, the American Federation of State, County, and Municipal Employers (AFSCME) set forth a resolution calling for equality for LGBT workers (http://www.afscme.org/members/conventions/resolutions-and-amendments/2012/resolutions/lesbian-gay-bisexual-and-transgender-workers). The global counterpart to AFSCME is Population Services International (PSI), a global union federation of health care, municipal, community, and government workers that champions human rights, advocates for social justice, and promotes universal access to pubic services in over 150 countries. PSI asserts that LGBT workers' rights are actually trade union rights, and trade union rights are human rights. Thus, "trade unions are committed to fight against discrimination and for an inclusive non-violent society" (http://www.world-psi.org/en/issue/lgbt). Understanding the connection between workplace rights, safe work environments, and economic development and work productivity is becoming increasingly important in understanding how to meet challenges faced by LGBT persons in the workplace. Supportive-LGBT workplace policies and workplace climates are linked to positive outcomes for LGBT workers ranging from greater job commitment to greater openness about being LGBT (see Table 29.1).

MAP, Human Rights Campaign, & Center for American Progress (2013) identified barriers to equal and fair treatment of LGBT and other workers concerning a lack of legal protection, which makes it harder to find and keep a good job, and fewer benefits and more taxes that put LGBT workers and their families at risk (see Table 29.2). In 2013, 278 businesses and employers submitted a brief to the US Supreme Court in which they argued that unequal treatment of LGBT workers and their families under federal law harms business by the following:

Table 29.1 Positive outcome of LGBT-supportive workplace policies

Greater job commitment
Improved workplace relationships
Increase job satisfaction
Improved health outcomes
Less discrimination against LGBT employees
More openness about being LGBT
Increase productivity for LGBT employees

Adapted from Badgett et al. (2013b)

Table 29.2 Barriers to legal protection in workplace discrimination

Bias and discrimination in recruitment and hiring
On-the-job inequity and unfairness
Wage gaps and penalties
Lack of legal protection
Unequal access to health insurance benefits
Denial of family and medical leave
Denial of spousal retirement benefits
Unequal family protections when a worker dies or is disabled
Higher tax burden for LGBT families
Inability to sponsor families for immigration

Adapted from MAP et al. (2013)

1. Creating complex and difficult compliance burdens by requiring businesses to treat married LGBT employees as single for federal taxes, payroll taxes, and certain workplace benefits but as married for all other purposes in states that recognize same-sex couples.
2. Requiring employers to implement and enforce discriminatory treatment of employers in their own companies, even when doing so goes against core corporate values and basic business sense.
3. Creating an environment that makes it harder for LGBT workers to perform at their best.
4. Negatively impacting the employer's ability to compete for and hire top talent (MAP, Human Rights Campaign, & Center for American Progress 2013).

Contained in the report, businesses and companies state clearly that, if discrimination on the basis of sexual orientation in the laws of the states blocks them from recruiting, hiring, and retaining the very best employees, they will be unable to achieve the success that each is capable of achieving with a workforce constituting the best and brightest employees.

The conundrum is how to move forward to ensure an LGBT-inclusive workplace. Recommendations were made by MAP, Human Rights Campaign, & Center for American Progress (2013) to address barriers to legal protection and to fewer benefits and more taxes. The first set of recommendations pertains to reducing discrimination and increasing responsiveness to inclusiveness and to timeliness to data gathering and processing: (a) pass nondiscrimination laws and policies, (b) increase wage discrimination protections, (c) ensure effective and swift discrimination claims processing, (d) foster diverse and inclusive workplaces, (e) ensure transgender workers can update the gender marker on their identity documents, and (f) increase data collection on LGBT workers. The second set of recommendations addresses equal access to individual and family benefits: (a) recognize the families of LGBT workers, (b) advance equal access to individual and family health insurance benefits, (c) provide equal access to individual and family medical leave, (d) provide equal access to spousal retirement benefits, (e) provide equitable economic protections when a worker dies or is disabled, (f) revise the IRS tax code to provide equitable treatment for LGBT workers, and (g) provide pathways to immigration and citizenship for binational LGBT families. The key to moving toward a more equitable workplace is for all levels of government and businesses to adopt policies for the fair treatment for LGBT workers. The issue of fairness is critical for LGBT workers, because employer benefits and disparities have economic implications for them over their lifespan.

In a report, *Time for a Change: The Case for LGBT-Inclusive Workplace, Leave Laws &*

Table 29.3 Federal Job Anti-Discrimination Laws

Age Discrimination in Employment Act (ADEA)—prohibits discrimination against persons 40 years of age or older

Americans With Disabilities Act of 1990 (Title I andTitle V), as amended ADA)—prohibits employment discrimination against qualified individuals with disabilities in the private sector, and in state and local government

Civil Rights Act of 1964 (Title VII)—prohibits employment discrimination based on race, color, religion, sex, or national origin

Civil Rights Act of 1991—made changes in the federal laws against employment discrimination enforced by EEOC; reverse Supreme Court decisions that limited the rights of persons protected by these laws; authorizes compensatory and punitive damages in cases of intentional discrimination

Equal Pay Act of 1963 (EPA)—protects men and women who perform substantially equal work in the same establishment from sex-based wage discrimination

Genetic Information Nondiscrimination Act of 2008 (GINA)—prohibits employment discrimination based on genetic information about an applicant, employee, or former employee

Rehabilitation Act of 1973 (Sections 501 and 505)—prohibit discrimination against qualified individuals with disabilities who work in the federal government

Older Workers Benefit Protection Act of 1990 (OWBP)—forbids discrimination by employers based on age when providing employee benefits

Adapted from EEOC (www.eeoc.gov/facts/qanda.html)

Nondiscrimination Protections, Make (2013) opined that "given health disparities and high rates of family poverty in the LGBT community, LGBT workers have a critical need for LGBT-inclusive laws and polices that strengthen job security and provide time off for personal health and family caregiving needs" (p. 2). To better support the health and family needs of LGBT workers, Make offered needed policy and legal changes. First, expand marriage equality. The ruling of the Supreme to strike Section 3 of the Defense of Marriage Act was a victory for LGBT equality. Although the federal government now recognizes same-sex marriages, many LGBT persons live in states without marriage equity. The second recommendation is to broaden the definition of spouse under the Family Medical Leave Act (FMLA). For private sector workers, the FMLA defines spouse according to the marriage laws of the state in which a worker resides, which often excludes many same-sex couples. A third recommendation is in response to the ineligibility of many LGBT workers for FMLA leave because of the size of their employer, the number of hours worked, or length of time a worker has been employed. In addition, the FMLA's definition of family is narrow. The federal government and states should pass legislation to expand access to

FMLA and pass LGBT-inclusive family and medical leave laws (Make). Fourth, pass LGBT-inclusive and job-protected paid leave laws at all levels of government, especially important to LGBT workers who are unable to afford unpaid time off work. Fifth, government at all level should serve as a model employer by instituting strong nondiscrimination protections and LGBT-inclusive workplace leave policies for government employers. Sixth, federal, state, and local governments should pass employment nondiscrimination laws that prohibit discrimination on the basis of sexual orientation and gender identity or expression. These laws can provide LGBT workers with recourse against harassment and discrimination and protection to those who otherwise fear disclosing their family relationships and caregiving responsibilities (Make). The last two recommendations involve building and strengthening collaborations between the LGBT community and workplace leave coalitions, so that they work with businesses to identify model employers and to develop spokespersons for LGBT-inclusive leave laws and police (Mark).

Identification of options for helping older LGBT workers either find or maintain employment requires discussion among and input from various government and business entities. Many LGBT older workers may need assistance with job searches; require flexible work arrangements; or need training, education, or flexible job opportunities. The majority of older workers are healthy and do not require any accommodations. Beyond limitations that may be associated with aging, many older workers are hindered by negative perceptions by employers and coworkers. For service providers working with LGBT persons, advocates working on behalf of LGBT persons, and LGBT persons themselves, the key to advancing equity and nondiscrimination in the workplace is obtaining legal protections in all states. Table 29.3 contains select federal laws that prohibit job discrimination. The Equal Employment Opportunity Commission (EEOC) enforces these laws and provides oversight and coordination of all federal equal employment opportunity regulations, practices, and policies.

Summary

LGBT older workers represent a diverse and growing segment of the workforce. Often, older LGBT workers must contend with unfair laws and discriminatory polices in the labor force. They must overcome the typical barriers to employment such as lack of modern skills, stereotypes, and disincentives of fringe benefits. Federal, state, and local governments and private business must examine their policies that adversely affect LGBT workers and aging workers. Collectively, LGBT workers are subjected to legalized discrimination, which can result in job loss or demotion. LBGT workers endue an unfair burden because of their sexual orientation and gender identity or expression. America is at a policy crossroads and is being tested for its response to legally sanction discrimination and violation of the civil right of LGBT workers. The future of the American work force may well be determined by its response to LGBT workers.

Learning Exercises

1. What factors go into helping LGBT elders remain in the workforce? Who is likely to do so and why?
2. What factors prevent LGBT elders from entering the workforce? How can these be surmounted?
3. What factors do you take in consideration in addressing the needs in addressing the older LGBT employee or those seeking employment?
4. In what ways does ENDA discriminate against LGBT workers?
5. What type of LGBT-supportive workplace policies have businesses put in place?

Experiential Exercises

1. Describe your experience working with an older lesbian, gay, bisexual, transgender employee. Was there a particular situation that occurred within the workplace setting that you remember? If yes, why?
2. If you know an elder who is working and LGBT, ask him or her to describe a situation in his or her work where he or she was treated well and where he or she was treated poorly.
3. Imagine that you have been invited to testify before Congress to provide arguments in support of LGBT-supportive workplace legislation. What evidence would you present?

Multiple-Choice Questions

1. Which of the following is a reason that loss of a job can be devastating for LGBT workers?
   (a) Many LGBT persons live in poverty
   (b) Many LGBT persons cannot afford to live near their jobs

(c) Most LGBT workers have large families

(d) Most LGBT workers are past their prime

2. Which of the following types of businesses have implemented LGBT-inclusive policies?
   (a) Small businesses
   (b) Government agencies
   (c) Fortune 500
   (d) Universities

3. FMLA defines spouse by which of the following?
   (a) Federal government
   (b) The state
   (c) DOMA
   (d) Business model

4. The federal Nondiscrimination Employment Act includes which of the following exemptions for businesses?
   (a) Companion
   (b) Public accommodation
   (c) Religious
   (d) Transgender

5. Which of the following is a rationale of why businesses have added LGBT-inclusive policies?
   (a) Low cost
   (b) Higher revenue
   (c) Economic benefit
   (d) All of the above
   (e) None of the above

6. Which of the following prohibits discrimination in employment?
   (a) American Association of Retired People
   (b) Age in Discrimination in Employment Act
   (c) Age and Wage Fairness Act
   (d) Older Persons Fair Employment Act

7. LGBT workers who work hard and meet their responsibilities and are denied fairness in hiring and promotion are aside to be victims of which of the following?
   (a) A broken bargain
   (b) An unofficial promise
   (c) A misunderstanding
   (d) An unintentional act

8. Why is it important to address instability in employment and job discrimination for LGBT workers?
   (a) To avoid workplace violence
   (b) Implications for financial insecurity well after retirement
   (c) To reduce the high cost of treatment for HIV/AIDS
   (d) Implications for family planning

9. Which of the following groups report the highest rate of discrimination and harassment in the workplace?
   (a) Lesbians
   (b) Gay men
   (c) Bisexuals
   (d) Transgender persons

10. People who may want to be supportive of LGBT persons in the workplace, but do not know how, may remain silent. The silence may be taken for which of the following?
    (a) Hostility
    (b) Approval
    (c) Avoidance
    (d) Mining one own business

Key

1-A
2-C
3-B
4-C
5-D
6-B
7-A
8-B
9-D
10-A

Resources

A Better Balance: www.abetterbalance.org.

American Association of Retired People (AARP): www.aarp.org.

American Federation of State, County, and Municipal Employers: www.afscme.org.

Equal Employment Opportunity Commission (EEOC): www.eeoc.gov.

Human Rights Campaign: www.hrc.org/resources/entry/lgbt-employee-resources.

Human Rights Campaign—Corporate Equality Index 2015: Rating American Workplaces on Lesbian, Gay, Bisexual and Transgender Equality: www.hrc.org/campaigns/corporate-equality-index.

Lambda Legal: www.lambdalegal.org.

LGBT Equality in the Workplace: A TUC Guide for Union Negotiators on LGBT Issues (UK): www.rmt.org.uk/news/publications/lgbt-equality-in-the-workplace.pdf.

PFLAG: www.pflag.org.

Population Services International (PSI): www.world-psi.org.

References

Badgett, M. V. L., Burns, C., Hunter, N. D., Krehely, J., Mallory, C., & Sears, B. (2013a, February 13). *An executive order to prevent discrimination against LGBT workers*. Retrieved March 2, 2015 from http://www.americanprogress.org/issues/lgbt/report/2013/02/19/53931/an-executive-order-to-prevent-discrimination-agsinst-lgbt-workers/.

Badgett, M. V. L., Durso, L. E., Kastanis, A., & Mallory, C. (2013b, May). *The business impact of LGBT-supportive workplace policies*. Los Angles, CA: The Williams Institute. Retrieved February 28, 2015 from http://www.WilliamsInstitute.law.ucla.edu/wp-content/uploads.Business-Impact-of-lgbt-supportive-workplace-policies.pdf.

Badgett, M. V. L., Durso, L. E., & Schneebaum, A. (2013c, June). New patterns of poverty in the lesbian, gay, and bisexual community. Los Angles, CA: The Williams Institute.

Bureau of Labor Statics. (2010). *Long-term displaced workers by age and employment status in January 2010*. Washington, DC: Author.

Center for American Progress. (2013, August 7). *Older LGBT workers protected by ENDA*. Retrieved February 28, 2015 from http://www.lgbtsr.org.2013/08/07/older-lgbt-workers-protected-by-enda/.

Cray, A. (2013). *Advancing employment equity for LGBT older adults*. Retrieved February 27, 2015 from http://www.lgbtagingcenter.org/resources/resource.cfm?r=621.

Copelan, C. (2014). Labor-force participation rates of the population ages 55 and older, 2013. *Employee Benefit Research Institute Notes, 35*(4), 2–4. Washington, DC: Employee Benefit Research Institute.

Government Accountability Office, (2012, April). *Unemployed older workers: Many experience challenges regaining employment and face reduced retirement security*. Washington, DC: Author. Retrieved February 28, 2015 from www.gao.gov/assets/600/590408.pdf.

Grant, J. M., Koskovich, G., Frazer, M. S., Bjerk, S. & SAGE. (2010). *Outing age 2010: Public policy issues affecting lesbian, gay, bisexual, and transgender elders*. Washington, DC: National Gay and Lesbian Task Force Policy Institute. Retrieved February 27, 2015 from http://www.Williamsinstitute.law.ucla.edu/up-content/uploads/LGB-Poverty-Update-Jun-2013.pdf.

Heidkamp, M., Mabe, W., & Degraaf, B. (2012, March). *The public workforce system: Serving older job seekers and the disability implications of an aging workforce*. New Brunswick, NJ: NTAR Leadership Center.

Human Rights Campaign. (2009). *Degrees of equality: A national study examining workplace climate for LGBT employees*. Retrieved February 28, 2015 from http://www.hrc.org/resources/entry/degrees-of-equality.

Human Rights Campaign. (2011a). *LGBT equality at Fortune 500*. Retrieved February 28, 2015 from http://www.hcr.org/resources/entry/lgbt-equality-at-fortune-500.

Human Rights Campaign. (2011b). *Workplace discrimination: Policies, laws, and legislation*. Retrieved February 28, 2015 from http://www.hrc.org/resources/entry/Workplace-Discrimiation-Policy-Laws-and-Legislation.

Johnson, R. (2004, July). Trends in job demand among older workers, 1992–2002. *Monthly Labor Review*, 48–56.

Johnson, R. W., & Mommaerts, C. (2011). *Age difference in job loss, job search, and reemployment*. Washington, DC: The Urban Institute.

Johnson, R. W., & Park, J. S. (2011). *Can unemployed older workers find work?*. Washington, DC: The Urban Institute.

Li, X. (2010). *Extending work lives of older workers: The impact of Social security policies and the labor market*. [Abstract] (Dissertation). The Pardee Rand Graduate School.

Madell, R. (2012a). *LGBT: Progress and problems in the workplace, Part 1*. Retrieved March 3, 2015 from http://www.theglasshammer.com/news/2012/06/25/lgbt-progress-and-problems-in-the-workplace=part-1/.

Madell, R. (2012b). *LGBT: Progress and problems in the workplace, Part 2*. Retrieved March 3, 2015 from http://www.theglasshammer.com/news/2012/06/28/lgbt-progress-and-problems-in-the-workplace-part-2/.

Make, J. (2013, November). *Time for a change: The case for LGBT-inclusive workplace leaves laws and non-discrimination protections*. New York, NY: A Better Balance. Retrieved February 27, 2015 from www.

abetterbalance.org/web/images/stroies/Document/general/reports/TimeforaChangeFinalReport.pdf.

MAP, Human Rights Campaign, & Center for American Progress. (2013, June). *A broken bargain: Discrimination, fewer benefits and more taxes for LGBT workers.* Retrieved February 28, 2015 from http://www.lgbtmap.org/file/a-broken-bargain-full-report.pdf.

MAP, SAGE, & Center for American Progress. (2010, September). *LGBT older adults and pensions.* Retrieved March 2, 2015 from http://cdn.americanprogress.org/wp-content/uploads/issues/2010/09/pdf/lgbt_pensions.pdf.

Masetas, N., & Li, X. (2006). *Discourage workers? Job search outcomes of older workers* [Abstract]. University of Michigan, Michigan Retirement Research Grant.

Munnell, A., Sass, S., Soto, M., & Zhivan, N. (2006). *Has the displacement of older workers increased?* Boston: Center for Retirement Research at Boston College. Retrieved March 2, 2015 from http://www.nber.org/programs/ag/rrc/6.1.pdf.

National Center for Transgender Equality and the National Gay and Lesbian task Force. (2009, November). *National Transgender Discrimination Survey.* Retrieved February 28, 2015 from http://www.transeqaulity.org/issues/national-transgender-discrimination-survey.

Report of the Taskforce on the Aging of the American Workforce. (2008). Retrieved March 2, 2015 from www.doleta.gov/reports/FINAL_Taskforce_Report_2-11-08.pdf.

National Transgender Discrimination Survey. (2011). Retrieved March 2, 2015 from http://www.endtransgenderdiscrimination.org/report/html.

Society for Human Resource management. (2010, November 17). *Statement of Cornelia Gamlem on behalf of the Society for human Resource Management, present to the U.S. Equal Employment Opportunity Commission.* Retrieved March 2, 2015 from http://www.shrm.org/Advocacy/PublicPolicyStatusReports/Courts-Regulations/Documents/SHRM%20testimony%20before%20EECO%20discussing%20effective%20practices%20for%20older%20workers.11172010.pdf.

The Williams Institute. (2011, July). *Documented evidence of employment discrimination and its effects on LGBT people.* Retrieved February 28, 2015 from http://www.freedomtowork.org?page_id=533.

Walker, D. M. (2007). *Older workers: Some best practices and strategies for engaging and retaining older workers.* Washington, DC: U.S. Government Accountability Office. Retrieved from http://www.gao.gov/new.item.d07433t.pdf.

Wolff, T. B. (2014, June 20). *How ENDA still allows discrimination against LGBT workers.* The Nation. Retrieved February 28, 2015 from http://www.thenation.com/aerticle/180358/how-enda-still-allows-discrimination-discrimination-against-lgbt-workers.pdff.

Wyatt, C. (2015). *5 workplace issues LGBT candidates still encounter.* Retrieved March 3, 2015 from http://www.ttidiversity.com/.

Isolation, Socialization, Recreation, and Inclusion of LGBT Elders

30

Debra A. Harley, Linda Gassaway and Lisa Dunkley

Abstract

As people age, social support systems are essential, especially for LGBT persons who might be at greater risk of social isolation. Each person has a different experience and subsequent propensity for isolation. For many LGBT elders, social inclusion continues to be aspirational, with limited authentic and sustained progress having been made in this area. In this chapter, the influencing issues of socialization and inclusion/exclusion of LGBT elders are examined. The unique circumstances across the life span for LGBT elders that may either help or hinder opportunities for socialization and inclusion are discussed. Social inclusion to successful aging of LGBT elders is reviewed to gain insight into some of the explanations of their withdrawal from social and recreational functions. The significance of family involvement is explored. Finally, policy on social inclusion of elders is presented.

Keywords

Socialization · Inclusion · Isolation · Exclusion · Recreation · Senior citizen centers

Overview

Social inclusion is a term used to describe how government, policy makers, community, business, professional service entities, and individuals collaborate to ensure that all people have the best opportunities to enjoy life and do well in society, making sure that no one is left out or forgotten in our community (Rimmerman 2013). However, social inclusion has not been defined in its own right, but rather as a desired goal or with respect to challenges and deficits (Repper and Perkins 2003). In essence, social inclusion is the opposite of social exclusion. Cobigo et al. (2012) suggest that the main challenges in understanding social inclusion are that social inclusion is (a) at risk of being an ideology and

D.A. Harley (✉) · L. Gassaway · L. Dunkley
University of Kentucky, Lexington, USA
e-mail: dharl00@email.uky.edu

© Springer International Publishing Switzerland 2016
D.A. Harley and P.B. Teaster (eds.), *Handbook of LGBT Elders*,
DOI 10.1007/978-3-319-03623-6_30

may lead to ineffective and potentially harmful strategies; (b) still mainly defined as the acceptance and achievement of the dominant societal values and lifestyle, which may lead to moralistic judgments; (c) often narrowly defined and measured; and (d) often limited to the measure of one's participation in community-based activities. For many LGTB elders, social inclusion continues to be aspirational, with limited authentic and sustained progress having been made in this area. It is not being a sexual minority or being an elderly person that is the main cause of social exclusion of LGBT elders; instead, it is the way in which society responds discriminately to them. The purpose of this chapter is to discuss influencing issues of socialization and inclusion/exclusion of LGBT elders. First, information is presented on a framework of isolation affecting elderly adults, which highlights the unique circumstances across the life span for LGBT elders who may either help with or limit opportunities for socialization and inclusion. Second, the role of socialization, recreation, and inclusion in the lives of LGBT elders is presented to identify the extent to which LGBT elders are able to remain active and have a sense of contributing to causes and points of interest. Third, unique social inclusion challenges to successful aging of LGBT elders are reviewed to gain insight into some of the explanations of their withdrawal from social and recreational functions. Fourth, the significance of family involvement is explored. As individuals age, their roles in the family take on a different meaning; thus, understanding family involvement with LGBT elders is important. Finally, a review of the impact of policy on social inclusion of LGBT elders is presented.

Learning Objectives

By the end of the chapter, the reader should be able to:

1. Understand the concepts of social inclusion/exclusion.

2. Identify contributing factors to social isolation of LGBT elders.
3. Understand social inclusion challenges to successful aging of LGBT elders.
4. Identify the extent to which LGBT elders are able to remain active and contribute to causes and points of interest.
5. Understand the role of family involvement in socialization of LGBT elders.
6. Identify areas in which policy is needed to promote inclusivity of LGBT elders in various mainstream settings and services.

Introduction

As a movement, social inclusion has origins in three paradigms. The first of which is in 1970s' French ideas of social solidarity conceived by Lenoir (1974) (Burchardt et al. 2002), which referred to people who have slipped through the net of the social insurance system and are subsequently administratively excluded by the state (Boardman 2010). The second paradigm is the specialization paradigm that is dominant in the USA and UK and that is frequently associated with discrimination. In the USA, the American counterpart to the social model, Minority Group Model, emerged in the late 1970s and was influenced by the Civil Rights Movement. The third is the monopoly paradigm, which is commonly used in Western Europe to strengthen group monopoly (Rimmerman 2013) to include marginalized groups. Other manifestations of the social exclusion concept include a link to poverty, financial well-being, consumption, and income adequacy (Buckmaster and Thomas 2009); a lack of recognition of fundamental human and civil rights; and the existence of an underclass (Rafaelic 2012). From a sociological perspective, "social inclusion and exclusion function as apparati that problematize people on the margins, and by extension, contribute to their governance and control" (Allman 2013, p. 2).

Isolation of elders occurs when conditions necessary for maintaining a functional social network break down (Walker and Herbitter 2005).

Individual and societal factors contribute to the degree to which elderly people become isolated. Individual factors include living arrangements, mobility, ethnicity, socioeconomic status, gender, and sexual orientation and gender expression along with a host of subjective factors such as attitudes and expectations. Societal factors include prejudices, discrimination, homo/bi/transphobia, community characteristics, and American society's emphasis on individual self-sufficiency and remaining independent at all costs. In addition, the degree to which elders receive social support from family and friends, participate in activities, and have access to information influences the degree to which they experience isolation (Walker and Herbitter 2005). The lack of social support is a contributing factor to abuse of older adults by Acierno et al. (2010). See Chaps. 16 and 17 for further discussion on elder mistreatment and victimization.

As people age, social support systems are essential especially for LGBT persons who might be at greater risk of social isolation and offer elders social interaction and connectedness, reduce social isolation and loneliness, and can assist with daily tasks of living (Espinoza 2014).

However, such support may be lacking for LGBT elders (Espinoza 2013). In comparison with their heterosexual peers, LGBT elders are significantly more likely to be isolated, twice as likely to live alone, half as likely to be partnered, half as likely to have close relatives to call for help, and more than four times more likely to be childless (Movement Advancement Project and SAGE 2010). Moreover, the relationship between diminished social and caregiving supports with a range of health problems that can have serious consequences for older adults can result in premature institutionalization, which contributes to even greater social isolation for LGBT elders. Once institutionalized, LGBT elders may experience isolation not only from external connections, but also within the facility, especially if homophobia and heterosexism and a lack of awareness of the needs of LGBT residents among staff and peers exist. Depending on his or her behaviors and choices throughout life, each person has a different experience and subsequent propensity for isolation (Elder and Retrum 2012). To facilitate an understanding of terminology used throughout this chapter, a glossary of terms is presented in Table 30.1.

Table 30.1 Glossary of terms

Loneliness—is actually a state of mind with an emotional response to lack of human interaction and companionship (Cacioppo and Patrick 2008)

Objective isolation—is a quantifiable status that can be determined outside of an individual's perception (Elder and Retrum 2012)

Social disconnectedness—is characterized by a lack of contact with others and is indicated by situational factors (e.g., small social network, infrequent social interaction, lack of participation) (Cornwell and Waite 2009)

Social engagement—is the level to which a person is involved in social activity (James et al. 2012)

Social integration—occurs when a person is involved in a range of social relationships and when a person feels a strong sense of identity with his or her role (Brissette et al. 2000)

Social isolation—refers to objective physical separation from other people or perceived isolation even if others are present: the distancing of an individual, psychologically or physical, or both, from his or her network of desired or need relationships with other people (Biordo et al. 2009)

Social networks—are interconnected webs of relationships in which people are naturally embedded (Biordo et al. 2009)

Social supports—are psychological and material resources that help people adapt to change and cope with stress (Elder and Retrum 2012)

Subjective isolation—refers to how an individual perceives his or her experience and if he or she feels isolated (Elder and Retrum 2012)

Framework for Isolation in LGBT Elders

Isolation in later life occurs within certain contextual psychosocial and social factors (see Table 30.2). Biordo and Nicholson (2009) distinguished between voluntary and involuntary isolation and developed a typology that identifies individuals' isolation along a continuum. Individuals are either (a) integrated (i.e., not isolated), (b) become isolated slowly over time, (c) recently isolated due to an acute event, or (d) lifelong isolates. Thus, social isolation is a loss of place within one's group(s). It should be noted that a solitary lifestyle is not an accurate indicator of isolation (Elder and Retrum 2012). A solitary lifestyle is one in which an individual enjoys spending a significant amount of time alone and enjoy pursuing activities independently. Oldham and Morris (1995) describe the solitary personality type as being alone, remaining independent, maintaining autonomy, being self-contained, and being uninfluenced by praise or criticism among others. In a study of quality of life (QoL) in rural and urban adults aged 65 and older, Baernholdt et al. (2012) examined associations between three dimensions of QoL: social functioning, emotional well-being, and needs and health behaviors. The results suggest that while older adults reported high levels of QoL, they had lower social functioning with older African Americans and Hispanics scoring lower than Whites on two QoL dimensions. Many of the participants expressed a need for educational, cultural, and recreational programs, as well as

Table 30.2 Contextual factors for isolation in later life

Income
Mobility
Societal factors
Social networks
Social supports
Individual history
Physical environment
Social engagement and integration

Adapted from Elder and Retrum (2012), British Columbia Ministry of Health (2004)

spiritual and religious programs that would respect their sexual and gender identities. The researchers concluded that rural older adults may be socially isolated and may need interventions to maintain physical and mental health, strengthen social relationships and support, and to increase their participation in the community to promote QoL. See Chap. 25 for further discussion on elders in rural areas.

When asked to describe their living arrangements and support systems over time, LGBT adults aged 45–75 overwhelmingly indicated that they are more likely than their non-LGBT peers to live alone, have smaller support networks over time (40 % compared to 27 % for non-LGBT elders), and are less satisfied with the information that they receive related to support systems. For ethnic minority groups, African American LGBT elders are more likely than their peers to report that people from their faith communities are part of their support networks. In comparison with 21 % of their non-LGBT peers, approximately 34 % of LGBT elders live alone and 48 % of LGBT elders live with spouses or partners compared to 70 % of their non-LGBT peers. Older lesbian and bisexual women (59 %) are far more likely than their gay male counterparts (43 %) to live with a partner or spouse and less likely to live alone (25 and 38 %, respectively) (Espinoza 2014). These national data are similar to earlier data of LGBT elders in San Diego in which 41 % were either married, in a domestic partnership, or had a significant other (Zians 2011).

One area of concern is the ability of LGBT elders to access adequate social care as they age. Social care is defined as the broad-based system of informal social network resources (i.e., family, friends, church) and the network of community-based formal services (e.g., home health care, senior citizen centers) (Cantor and Brennan 2000). To age independently and maintain quality of life, the social care network is considered an important component (Brennan-Ing et al. 2014, see Research Box 30.1). In Cantor and Mayer's (1978) text on *Hierarchical Compensatory Theory*, when older adults need assistance, they turn first to immediate family. However, many LGBT elders are estranged from their biological families (Espinoza 2013; MAP and SAGE, 2010). If family are unavailable, older adults will turn to more distant relatives, than friends and neighbors, and finally to formal supports. Older LGBT adults usually do not have informal social resources as robust as their heterosexual counterparts, with less than half of LGBT elders having a partner or spouse and even less having at least one child (Espinoza 2014; Fredriksen-Goldsen et al. 2011). The alternative for LGBT elders is reliance on the family of choice, which comprises close friends and neighbors (de Vries and Hoctel 2007; Brennan-Ing et al. 2014). Zians (2011) found that most LGBT elders (73 %) report having younger friends; however, only 30 % believe that they could count on these younger friends to assist them while growing older. Of this group studied, 495 indicated that they were uncertain whether they could count on these younger friends for assistance and 32 % believed that they definitely could not count on them as they grow older.

Research Box 30.1

Brennan-Ing et al. (2014).

Objective: To explore the social care networks of older LGBT adults, with a focus on the viability of the social support network, formal service utilization, and unmet needs for assistance.

Method: Data were obtained in 2010 and 2011 from a convenience sample of older LGBT adults recruited through the Center on Halsted (COH) in Chicago. COH offers diverse public programs and social services, including mental health counseling, HIV testing and prevention, and community cultural programs and older adult program among others. Participants were also recruited at various AIDS service organizations, health fairs, and community events in Chicago. To qualify, participants had to identify as LGBT and be at least 50 years of age and sufficiently fluent in English. Two hundred thirty-three

participants were recruited, resulting in 210 usable surveys. The average age was 60, 71 % were men, 24 % were women, and 5 % were transgender or intersex. One-third was Black, and 62 % were Caucasian. Data were analyzed using a mixed-methods approach with the quantitative portion using a correlational design and the qualitative portion using a grounded-theory approach.

Results: Quantitative assessments found high levels of morbidity and friend-centered support networks. Need for and use of services was frequently reported. Content analysis revealed unmet needs for basic supports, including housing, economic supports, and help with entitlements. Limited opportunities for socialization were strongly express, particularly among older lesbians.

Conclusion: Implications suggest that for those who are isolated due to illness, stigma, or an absence of friends and family members, the risk is that these LGBT elders will fall through the cracks if we are unable to better address their social care needs.

Questions

1. Do you think that results would be different across aging categories (old, old-old, and oldest-old)?
2. What is the purpose of using a mixed-methods approach?
3. How do these results generalized to the general older LGBT population?

Several barriers are present with the use of informal networks for support. For example, non-family members may not be empowered to make decisions regarding health care. In addition, negative interactions can result between biological family members and informal support members when decisions need to be made regarding LGBT elders' health care, long-term, last wishes, or financial security. Finally, the lack of legal recognition of same-sex partners in most jurisdictions excludes informal networks and partners from making caregiving decisions (Breenan-Ing et al. 2014), despite recent developments with the repeal of Defense of Marriage Act (DOMA). Regardless of these challenges, the early assertion of Dorfman et al. (1995) holds true that in some situations, "support from friends is actually more desirable because it is given freely and without obligation," as opposed to help and support from relatives, which can be considered more stressful "due to increased expectations and demands" (p. 40). In regard to individuals living away from urban and suburban areas, the ability to access social networks is even more challenging for LGBT elders because of the nature of their rural geographical settings (see Chap. 25).

One of the underlying factors determining the prevalence of those considered as isolated is their living status (i.e., live alone) (Elder and Retrum 2012). In a study of living arrangement and loneliness among LGB elders, Kim and Fredriksen-Goldsen (2014) found that compared with LGB older adults living with a partner or spouse, both those living alone and those living with others reported higher degrees of loneliness (see Research Box 30.2). It is estimated that 17 % of Americans over 65 years of age are isolated because they live alone. For LGBT elders, 53 % feel isolated from others (Fredriksen-Goldsen et al. 2011). Moreover, these individuals face one or more barriers related to geographical location (e.g., rural), language, physical or mental disability, economic instability, losing a partner and/or close friends, losing an important role such as employment, having a small social network, and having poor-quality social relationships. Community-level risk factors for isolation include feeling safe to leave one's home, access to transportation, availability of local events conducive to meaningful activities as defined by the older person, and lacking or having limited opportunities for social interaction and access to resources. Societal-level risk factors consist of ageism, racism, sexism, or homophobia, and discrimination

(Cornwell and Waite 2009; Ortiz 2011; Rosenbloom 2009). For ethnic minority LGBT elders, social isolation might be heightened because they might be isolated from their racial and ethnic communities as LGBT older adults as well as from the mainstream LGBT community as people of color (Fredriksen-Goldsen et al. 2011).

Research Box 30.2

Kim and Fredriksen-Goldsen (2014).

Objective: To examine the relationship between living arrangement and loneliness among LGB older adults using the loneliness model. The potential correlated including social resources and personal constraints were taken into consideration.

Method: The data from a national survey of LGB adults aged 50 and older ($N = 2444$) were used. Types of living arrangement include living with a partner or spouse, living alone, and living with someone other than a partner or spouse.

Results: Compared with LGB older adults living with a partner or spouse, both those living alone and those living with others reported higher degrees of loneliness, even after controlling for other correlates. The results of a multivariate regression analysis reveal that social support, social network size, and internalized stigma partially account for the relationship between living arrangement and loneliness.

Conclusion: Living arrangement was found to be an independent correlate of loneliness among LGB elders. Targeted interventions are needed to reduce loneliness in part by enhancing social resources and reducing risks of internalized stigma. Eliminating discriminatory policies against same-sex partnerships and partnered living arrangements is recommended.

Questions

1. Do you think that the results would be different when examining the same variables for transgender elders?

2. How can this study be redesigned to examine living arrangements and loneliness for urban versus rural?
3. What other variables do you recommend be examined as part of this study?

A strong correlation exists between isolation and morbidity; isolation is considered a risk factor in the development of illness and impairments in the presence of illness. Evidence suggests that loneliness is a predictor of depression, isolation is predictive of cognitive impairment in older women, and isolation rates are associated with higher rates of rehospitalization (Cacioppo et al. 2010; Crooks et al. 2008; Curtis et al. 2006; Tomaka et al. 2006). Loneliness, which commonly coexists as a precursor to isolation, has a wide range of negative effects on a person's physical and mental health, including weight gain or loss, poor nutrition generally, and lack of adherence to medication regimen. In addition, loneliness can be attributed to low self-esteem and is strongly linked to genetics. Kuyper and Fokkema (2010) examined factors that contributed to loneliness in LGB elders who are in a "more adverse position in general" (e.g., being less socially embedded, having more health problems, differing in living conditions and socioeconomic status) (p. 1171) and that might also be impacted by LGB-specific factors which, when experienced, can "be stressful and lead to adverse mental health outcomes" (Meyer 1995, 2003). Similar results were found between social embeddedness and loneliness among LGB adults in the Netherlands (Fokkema and Kuyper 2009). Compared with their heterosexual counterparts, older LGB adults were more likely to have experienced divorce, to be childless, or to have less intensive contact with their children. Furthermore, they had less intensive contact with other members of their families and were less frequent churchgoers.

Minority Stress. Meyer (1995, 2003) identified and described five "processes of minority stress" which include (1) external objective stressful events (e.g., discrimination, negative attitudes, victimization), (2) expectation of negative events and therefore having to be "on guard," (3) internalized homophobia, (4) concealment of identity, and (5) an ameliorating factor that can actually counteract the effects of the first four factors. Kuyper and Fokkema (2010) found that although the general factors were found to contribute to loneliness, a significant portion of the variance in loneliness remained unexplained. Kuyper and Fokkema suggest that minority stressors contribute to higher levels of loneliness among older LGB persons. Moreover, they found that minority stress processes added overwhelmingly to explain the variance of models that predicted loneliness in which "social embeddedness and non-social variables were already incorporated" (p. 1177). Table 30.3 provides a list of health risks associated with loneliness.

Table 30.3 Health risks of loneliness

Suicide
Anxiety
Dementia
Depression
Substance abuse
Antisocial behavior
Cognitive impairment
Altered brain function
Poor decision-making
Increased stress levels
Decreased memory and learning
Cardiovascular disease and stroke
The progression of Alzheimer's disease
Adapted from Cacioppo and Patrick (2008)

Role of Socialization, Recreation, and Inclusion in the Lives of LGBT Elders

Human beings are considered as social creatures that thrive from interaction with others. People assign value to being included in activities, both at work and in social settings. As individuals age, socialization may become curtailed for a number of reasons at a time in their lives when many people find themselves able to engage in social or recreational activities. Brennan-Ing et al. (2014, p. 41) surveyed LGBT elders to learn about their social care needs and reported that respondents expressed an "interest in a wide range of educational and recreational services, including computer and technology classes, and culinary programs." The use of the Internet is on the rise by seniors in general, as many Baby Boomers enjoy relative ease of access and use of technology. However, for many LGBT elders, access and use of technology is not easily accomplished. One respondent expressed concern over financial barriers getting in the way of accessing culture and arts programs. Others wanted spiritual programs but stressed that such programs must not discriminate based on differences inherent in LGBT elders. Recreational sports and programs such as yoga, exercise classes, and card games were requested as well. Although many cities and communities allow LGBT elders to participate in their programs, the same fears experienced with regard to housing and assisted living, for example, tend to hold true in this arena. Many LGBT elders fear being discriminated against, made fun of, or alienated by the staff or their heterosexual peers in the chosen activities. If LGBT older adults do in fact underutilize service and avoid participation in activities, the result is a sort of self-imposed exclusion and isolation in addition to that which imposed upon them by society.

Participants in the Brennan-Ing et al.'s (2014) study also expressed their desire for alternative venues for meeting people. One man stated, "I don't know where to go to meet other gay men my own age in a healthy setting, rather than the bar" (p. 42). An older lesbian commented that there are limited social environments for those who are aged 50 and older. The "bar scene" is for younger women, and fund-raisers that combine socialization are too expensive for participants. Older gay men and older lesbians both seem to face similar challenges with socializing and meeting potential romantic partners, citing ageism as a significant barrier. In a needs assessment of LGBT seniors in San Diego, Zians (2011)

found that 47 % of all respondents experienced difficulty in finding opportunities for friendship or social connection. Of these respondents, 31 % reported moderate difficulty, 12 % serious, and 4 % severe. There was no difference in response based on gender or ethnicity.

Overall, LGBT elders have positive feelings of belonging to the LGBT community; however, distinct differences also exist. Specifically, lesbians are more likely to feel more positive about belonging to the LGBT community than do bisexual women. Older gay and bisexual men tend to have similar feelings of belonging, while transgender elders are less likely to have such positive feelings (Fredriksen-Goldsen et al. 2011). The extent to which LGBT elders perceive acceptance and inclusion both in the community at large and in the LGBT community may be a function of social selection, which is the tendency for individuals sharing certain characteristics and specific cultural backgrounds to live in similar neighborhoods and participate in similar activities (Bread and Petitot 2010).

In an examination of urban space from a non-heterosexist perspective, Nusser (2010) explored how LGBT persons experience everyday space in the city, particularly the places in which they feel the most (i.e., spaces preferred) and least comfortable (i.e., spaces avoided) being a sexual minority. The study explored two research questions: (a) How do relationships between the design, management, and spatial characteristics of spaces communicate values about sexual orientation and gender identity? and (b) How could planners and designers create more inclusive spaces? Nusser contends that while urban design and service planning has always interacted with issues of sexuality, "the failure of the literature to address these practices explicitly has led to the silencing of minority sexualities in planning discourse and the severe marginalization of many queer people in cities" (p. 1). Although reference is not made specifically to LGBT elders, presumably the confluences of the urban planning process produce similar marginalization. Not all heteronormative space is anti-LGBT; however, most spaces in the USA are heteronormative. LGBT persons in

Cambridge and in two US cities were interviewed to ascertain their observations about LGBT and anti-LGBT spaces. Nusser found that LGBT spaces were perceived as highly enclosed and had rigid boundaries imposed discrete entrance (informal entrance in the USA), attached parking lot, near public transportation, and near LGBT-tested places. Anti-LGBT spaces had activity concentrated in the interior, which were enclosed, and exposed entrances were at the lowest elevation of the space.

Socialization and inclusion promote positive feelings about belonging to communities in general and to the LGBT community for older LGBT adults. Although self-disclosure about ones' sexual orientation and gender identity can lead to rejection and victimization, "it can also provide opportunities for community and social support that can be crucial to older adults' wellbeing" (Fredriksen-Goldsen et al. 2011, p. 16). The willingness to be "out" and participating in the community can provide LGBT elders with access to resources and support systems about which they may have been unaware. For many LGBT elders, the key is to find ways to deal with the "social and legal convention" in society to "discriminate against, ridicule, and abuse" them "within the foundational institutions" of the family, workplace, health care, social service programs, and recreational settings (Grant et al. 2011, p. 6). A persistent challenge for LGBT elders is to find support systems that are nonjudgmental.

Social Inclusion Challenges to the Successful Aging of LGBT Elders

Although many LGBT elders live alone, living alone does not mean that they are living in isolation, are facing stresses, or are lonely. In this day and time, communication technologies are more widely used than ever and may expand opportunities for elders to communication, therefore decreasing social isolation and loneliness (British Columbia Ministry of Health 2004). Furthermore, not all LGBT elders lack social support. However, when older adults living alone

lack social support or support systems, they are at much greater risk for a host of psychosocial adjustment issues. MAP and SAGE (2010) identify four major obstacles to social support and community engagement for LGBT elders: (1) lack of support from and feeling unwelcome in mainstream aging programs, (2) lack of support from and feeling unwelcome in the broader LGBT community, (3) lack of sufficient opportunities to contribute and volunteer, and (4) housing discrimination adds to the challenge LGBT elders face in connecting to their communities. In response to these obstacles, MAP and SAGE offer a series of recommendations to overcome these barriers (see Table 30.4). Each barrier adds to an LGBT elders' sense of rejection.

Unwelcoming mainstream aging programs. Senior citizen centers and other aging programs (e.g., civic groups) and churches often do not consider the possibility that participants may be LGBT. Some of these settings discriminate based on omission of inclusive services, while others do so intentionally through denial of services and harassment. Many LGBT elders distrust service providers and avoid local agencies, consequently, missing out on services and sense of community of their peers. Only a small number of agencies that provide services for the aging citizens engage in outreach programs designed to welcome LGBT elders (e.g., see New York City Department for the Aging, www.nyc.gov/html/dfta/html/services/lgbt.shtml). Often, these agencies also are not "prepared to address incidents of discrimination toward LGBT elders by other older people" (MAP and SAGE 2010, p. 48). MAP and SAGE reported that barriers encountered by LGBT elders at mainstream centers include (1) denial of services, (2) harassment from providers and heterosexual elders, and (3) having specific needs ignored. It is because of these types of barriers that many LGBT elders conceal their sexual identity when participating in activities offered by mainstream aging programs.

Unwelcoming LGBT community. Even though the LGBT community is diverse, ageism abounds, especially among gay males. LGBT

Table 30.4 Recommendations to inclusion barriers of LGBT elders

Solutions for making LGBT elders more welcome in general aging programs
• Address cultural competency and discrimination issues among mainstream aging service providers and programs
• Partner with aging service providers to welcome LGBT elders and increase on-site LGBT elder programs and services at mainstream facilities
Solutions for making LGBT elders more welcome in LGBT programs
• Make LGBT elders more welcome in the LGBT community at large
Solutions to increase LGBT elder opportunities to contribute and volunteer
• Improve overall opportunities for all elders to engage in volunteerism and civic engagement
• Involve LGBT elders in general LGBT and LGBT elder advocacy
Solutions to help LGBT elders secure needed housing
• Add sexual orientation to the non-discrimination provisions of the federal Fair Housing Act (FHA) and parallel state policies to render existing housing LGBT-friendly
• Consider supporting LGBT elder housing projects

Adapted from MAP and SAGE (2010)

elders feel unwelcome by younger generations of LGBT persons, ignored because of their age, marginalized as they grow older, and experienced diminished social support. Gender differences in socialization exist between LGBT elders. For example, older gay men report a greater sense of rejection from their younger counterparts than do lesbians, owing in part to a "loss of social valuation as physical and sexual changes affect what has been a source of self-esteem" (MAP and SAGE 2010, p. 490). Research suggests that older lesbians tend to retain a higher level of socialization through political involvement and mentoring of younger lesbians. Younger gay men tend to be more dismissive of older gay men, in part because of their emphasis on physical attributes (MAP and SAGE). In addition, many gay men feel that very little is done by the LGBT movement to engage LGBT elders in social events. Elder lesbians, on the other hand, report that their social networks were more resilient and "showed less fluctuation in response to changes with aging" (p. 49). Bisexual elders face the challenge of general distrust toward them by some segments of society, which may include heterosexual, gay, and lesbian individuals, who believe that bisexual persons simply choose to be open to both male and female partners out of convenience and that these individuals may simply choose an opposite-sex partner to avoid being labeled gay or lesbian. Such stigma and distrust most certainly can contribute to bisexual elders' concern about aging, identity, and social isolation (Hillman 2012). Hillman suggests that some transgender elders align themselves with the LGBT community, whereas others do not because of discrimination from among the gay community itself. Moreover, with the availability of options for support groups via the Internet, it is unclear what proportion of transgender elders use or even have access to this informational system (Hillman). On a positive note, the movers and shakers in the LGBT movement are allotting more time and effort toward issues related to their elder constituents, especially as the Baby Boomers advance into old age (Diverse Elders Coalition 2012).

Lack of sufficient opportunities to contribute. LGBT elders are often overlooked as potential volunteers and providers of support to others. Given their vast experiences, LGBT elders have the potential to make enormous contributions as advocates. Doing so can provide them with a sense of purpose while decreasing social isolation. The reasons elders volunteer include altruism, filling leisure time, enhancing social contacts, a need for affiliation, a sense of duty, to feel competent, or to contribute to the functioning of their communities. Unlike younger age groups, elders rarely volunteer to gain work experience or employment-related contacts (British Columbia Ministry of Health 2004). Adults who have opportunities for continued work and/or volunteer activities have better mental and physical health, vitality, quality of life, and, indirectly, physical activity (Cullinan 2006; King and King 2010).

Three large volunteer programs exist (i.e., RSVP, Foster Grandparent Program, Senior Companion Program) under the Senior Corps umbrella, which is administered by the federal government. Participation tends to be hampered by "income eligibility, service scope, and time requirements" (MAP and SAGE 2010, p. 50). MAP and SAGE recommend that national volunteer programs should reach out to elder LGBT citizens. Another avenue for contribution is self-advocacy. "Sage and other organizations working with LGBT older adults have long recognized that the greatest resource available to LGBT older adults is often themselves" (2010, p. 50). Considering that many of today's LGBT elders have participated in civic action in support of LGBT people at some time in their lives, they can bring to the table a great deal of knowledge, experiences, and problem-solving skills, to mention a few. SAGE (2010) cites that the following LGBT aging organizations were started by older adults: Gay and Gray in the West (Denver, CO), the Silver Haired Legislature (Missouri), Old Lesbians Organizing for Change (OLOC), and the Leadership Academy of Lavender Seniors of the East Bay (San Leandro, CA).

Housing discrimination. Discrimination in housing is a growing concern for sexual minorities of all ages; however, for LGBT elders, the problem is often magnified because of economic reasons. In addition to being denied housing, including residency in mainstream retirement communities, LGBT elders might find themselves facing homelessness due to economic reasons. Homelessness among older adults in general and LGBT elders in particular is increasing because many are finding themselves either outliving their retirement income and having not saved enough for retirement, or their social security income not keeping pace with the rate of inflation and cost of living. Limited lifetime earnings place LGBT elders at high risk for poverty in old age. Older Americans who lack affordable housing must spend a large portion of their budget on housing, leaving less money for essential needs (Funders for Lesbian and Gay Issues 2004). LGBT elders rank housing as their number one priority (Plumb and Associates 2003–2004).

LGBT elders face special challenges in the area of housing. For example, health issues and disabilities often decrease their ability to continue living independently and to age in place. For many LGBT elders who are not partnered, who do not have children, or who are estranged from or closeted to members of their family, supports are absent. Furthermore, LGBT elders are hesitant to access home health care or other assisted living services because of the fear of inviting judgmental or hostile care providers into their homes, and "having a stranger come into their home—maybe the only place that the elder was truly able to be out and express their sexual identity—can be as terrifying as living communally with people who will presume that they are straight" (Plumb and Associates 2003–2004, p. 18). Although they need them, studies reveal that LGBT elders access essential services (e.g., senior citizen centers, food stamps, meal plans, visiting nurses) much less frequently than the general population (MAP and SAGE 2010).

A discussion of housing as a challenge for LGBT elder is incomplete without discussion of the major demographic transition toward urbanization, which has influences on the health and quality of life of older persons. The type of neighborhood in which LGBT elders live suggests that communities more conducive to "active aging" and "aging in place" can influence health (e.g., accessible and affordable health and healthcare services, opportunities to stay active), participation (e.g., accessible public transportation, information services, recreational programs, social connections, volunteer opportunities, places to worship, a sense of being valued and respected), and security (e.g., home and community safety, transportation safety, affordable housing) (Beard and Petitot 2010). This ecological perspective of aging (Lawton and Nahemow 1973) assumes an interface between a person's functional capacity, adaptation, and his or her physical and social environment. These components link to related concepts of urban design and service planning for disability and aging (e.g., universal design, accessibility, walkable communities) (Alley et al. 2007).

Family Involvement

The definition of family has changed to varying degrees to be more inclusive of different compositions. Over the course of a century, a movement toward modified family structures based on individual choice and circumstance has occurred. Clearly, LGBT elders have a family of origin (biological). In addition, they may have an established family (partnership/marriage). Frequently, LGBT elders have a chosen or created family comprised of people selected for inclusion, such as close friends, other LGBT persons, and trusted neighbors. Rarely does the chosen family include blood relatives. Many LGBT elders found it necessary to create an alternative family for reasons such as being closeted, being rejected by the family of origin, or because of logistics that made contact with and support from blood relative difficult. Thus, LGBT elders often exist in a familial structure that is chosen, whose research overwhelmingly focuses on as a social support system (Fredriksen-Goldsen et al. 2011; Muraco et al. 2008; Orel 2004).

Given the limited family supports of many LGBT elders, Espinoza (2013) examined the role of friendship for LGBT people as they age through an interview with two longtime leaders in LGBT aging (Jesus Ramirez-Valles and Gina D'Antonio). The two leaders suggested the following: (a) Social spaces in which LGBT persons live should be welcoming as they age, (b) LGBT culture prefers young people, and (c) the likelihood of losing social connections and friendships happens at moments when they are often most needed, such as facing chronic illness. One aspect that has changed for aging

LGBT persons is that friendships in the workplace have increased because LGBT persons are more open about their identity.

In a study of the intersection of family, community, and disclosure in the lives of gay and lesbian elders, LGBT elders regarded traditional family members such as siblings, children, parents, aunts, and cousins as part of their familial makeup. When questioned about support networks, all participants expanded their definitions of family beyond biological ties to include friends, community members, and ex-partners. These digressions from the family of origin revealed the creation of a "chosen family." All participants indicated their sexual identity as influential on their familial experiences (Irizarry 2011).

Several demographic trends may exacerbate social isolation and loneliness of LGBT elders. According to the British Columbia Ministry of Health (2004), the family structure of the Baby Boom generation differs dramatically from the current generation of elders. For example, heterosexual Baby Boomers have married later, had fewer children, have a higher divorce rate, and increased longevity than did previous generations. Lesbian and gay couples who have biological children or who have adopted children have fewer offspring than did previous generations. The result may be that more childless elderly people are living alone. Further, the trend toward smaller family size in the family of origin for Baby Boomers may reduce the capacity of kin networks to provide formal support to LGBT elders. Also, the Baby Boom generation is highly mobile, which may mean that few family members live in close proximity.

The impact of how family is defined in the general population and among LGBT populations has yet to be determined. However, it is likely that the conceptualization of family has changed in both meaning and scope among different cultures, across generations, and within LGBT and non-LGBT groups. Therefore, as a result, the development of policy on social inclusion may be influenced by more non-traditional interpretations and expectations of what people envision as important to their inclusion and social well-being.

Impact of Policy on Social Inclusion

LGBT elders are often excluded from, or at least not represented in, national survey databases that are used to make evidence-based policy. Recently, the US Department of Health and Humans Services (2011) has taken steps to rectify this problem by requiring the inclusion of sexual orientation and gender identity questions on national surveys. Brennan-Ing et al. (2014) identify two areas in which policy can have positive outcomes for LGBT elders: One is in housing, and the other is in reauthorization of the *Older Americans Act* (see Chap. 17). Declaring LGBT elders a population of "greatest social need" would earmark federal funding supporting state and local area agencies on aging to meet the health, housing, economic, and social service needs of this population (Brennan-Ing et al.).

In a study to identify the role of our society in producing senior isolation and to determine what can society do to combat it, Walker and Herbitter (2005) identified both individual and societal factors (described earlier in this chapter) and stressed that isolation of elders can be found in even the most densely populated areas. The authors suggested that settlement houses, community centers, and other locally based service organizations are ideally suited to identify and assist isolated seniors because of their intimate knowledge of their communities, networks, and web of contacts. In addition to providing increased support to existing programs, Walker and Herbitter recommended the following steps for local government along with nonprofit and private sectors: (a) a citywide assessment of elderly needs to better gauge the severity of the problem, (b) development of voluntary check-in registry to track the well-being of elders, (c) implement a citywide public education and anti-discrimination campaign, along with a clearly written, widely publicized protocol for individuals to follow when they become concerned about the welfare of an elder in their neighborhood, (d) conduct extensive outreach to ensure that seniors are aware of available services, (e) tailor services to the elder population's unique and changing needs, (f) organizations should reevaluate their approach to service delivery and consider new, more inclusive methods of outreach and service delivery, and (g) strategic planning should be developed to engage elders in the social service system as early as possible, before a crisis situation occurs or isolation develops. Although these recommendations are for elders in general, their policy implications for LGBT elders are discussed below to offer an opportunity to be more inclusive of varying sexual orientation and sexual identity and to address isolation issues specific to them.

A defining characteristic of an inclusive society is participation in social and community life. The Australian government stresses that to achieve social inclusion means delivering policies and programs that support people to learn and strengthen their ability to participate in their communities. To that end, we borrow the following approaches to social inclusion principles from the Australian government (www.meetingpoint. org.au/assets/mp_s12_sipfa.pdf) for application to LGBT elders. The first is to make the most of LGBT elders' strengths such as families, communities, and culture. Assuming, promoting, and supporting a positive view of LGBT identity and culture are particularly important ways to reduce social exclusion and discrimination while working parallel with specific initiatives to improve their health, housing, family relationships, and support networks. Working in parallel with other initiatives is the second approach, which is paramount in building partnerships with key stakeholders. Strong relationships between government, community, private, and other stakeholders are key to strengthening service provision and social innovations over time. It is suggested that the sharing of expertise to produce innovative solutions is required for sustainable outcomes (Australian Government n.d.).

The development of tailored services to meet each person's different needs is a third approach (Austrian Government n.d.). For LGBT elders who are at risk of significant exclusion, mainstream services may not be sufficient or appropriate to counter against exclusion. On the one hand, it is not to necessarily create new programming, but rather to expand existing services and link them for greater inclusivity. On the other hand, it is necessary to develop program interventions for socially isolated and lonely LGBT elders because the one-size-fits-all approach to policy and program design is contra-indicated (Children's, Women's and Seniors Health Branch, British Columbia Ministry of Health 2004). For LGBT elders at high risk for social exclusion, reduction in the fragmentation of services systems is particularly important in relation to transitions from adulthood to old age or to retirement. Moreover, tailoring services for LGBT elders can be concentrated to specific locations (e.g., rural, urban, ethnic community). This approach lends itself to increasing buy-in from LGBT elder participants. A fourth approach is giving high priority to early intervention and prevention. The strategy is to head off isolation and exclusion by understanding root causes (e.g., poverty, disability, transportation) (Austrian Government, n. d.). Identifying root causes of isolation for LGBT elders and the connection between different types of disadvantage allows interventions to be designed to either prevent the occurrence of exclusion or provide more effective support to LGBT elders who are vulnerable before exclusion and isolation become entrenched.

A fifth strategy is to use evidence and integrated data to inform policy. "Progress toward social inclusion must be accompanied by better information, faster learning and better use of knowledge to improve outcomes" (Australian Government n.d., p. 4). We are living in an era in which programming and policy are influenced by evidence-based practices. Interventions should draw on the practical experience of service and support networks, existing research and the evidence-based practices, monitoring and evaluating strategies as they develop, and focus on outcomes (summative), as well as documentation of progress. The monitoring and evaluating of interventions should be designed in a way which builds on this evidence-base. The use of clear indicators and reporting from the perspective of

the LGBT elder, the family, the support networks, and the community should identify the essence of the problem and have a clear and accepted interpretation (Austrian Government n.d.).

The final approach is to plan for sustainability. Strategies that will help LGBT elders and communities deal more effectively with problems, barriers, and challenges in the future, as well as solving current problems, are essential to ensure that LGBT elders build capacity and develop protective factors to enable them to self-manage through life-course events (Austrian Government n.d.). A planning process for sustainability must include establishing benchmarks, adopting formal qualified targets that are attainable, measurable, and time specific, focusing on long-term policy goals, and integrating long-term social inclusion objectives in broader reform efforts (e.g., budgetary reform) (Austrian Government n.d.).

Many social inclusion principles for older adults, especially LGBT elders, are aspirational. In the USA, Canada, Austria, and European Union, programs or services such as visiting senior programs (i.e., to provide friendship to elders who are homebound or living alone) are managed through an existing service agency as part of an outreach component (Adelman et al. 2006; British Columbia Ministry of Health 2004). The Children's, Women's, and Seniors Health Branch British Columbia Ministry of Health (2004) acknowledges the potential harmful effects of social isolation for elders and suggests that policy implications can be separated into two categories: areas for further research and developing future interventions (see Policy Box 30.1). Clearly, future research is needed across multiple areas of exclusion and social isolation for LGBT elders including disability and ethnicities. In addition, transgender elders are probably the most neglected segment of LGBT persons in research and service provision. Consideration needs to be given to contextualize these implications for all LGBT elders.

Policy Box 30.1 Policy Implications
Future work is about social isolation and loneliness of LGBT elders.

Future Research:

Explore and document the experiences of different ethnicities with social isolation and loneliness.

Explore and document the interaction of social isolation and loneliness with poverty.

Explore and document the experiences of individuals whose spouses/partners have a disability or physical or cognitive decline.

Explore and identify the direct links between social isolation and loneliness and service usage.

Identify the specific health-enhancing elements of social support.

Develop a discourse on best practices for addressing the adverse effects of social isolation and loneliness among elders.

Increase the qualitative element in studies on social isolation and loneliness.

Program Development:

Support transportation initiatives for elders.

Use communication technologies to reduce isolation.

Increase community awareness of services specific for LGBT elders.

Support informal caregiving.

Increase the service delivery capacity of small community agencies.

Support the development of volunteer-based outreach programs.

Adapted from Children's, Women's and Seniors Health Branch, British Columbia Ministry of Health (2004).

Summary

Social isolation and loneliness contribute to negative effects on the health, premature functional decline, and mortality of LGBT older adults. Other factors such as income level, educational attainment, geographical location, and relationship with family members are associated with elevated levels of loneliness and isolation. Isolation can be exaggerated when LGBT elders do not know who can be relied upon or trusted for professional services and personal support. Many LGBT elder may be unaware of the availability of certain social services in the community or may become aware of them very late. Efforts are acutely needed to identify which groups among LGBT elders are underutilizing services and targeting those seniors and their support networks.

Other efforts are needed in curriculum design of health and human and social service educational and training programs. In addition, partnerships between government, community, and nonprofit service agencies are important to support needs of LGBT elders. The capacity to provide services to LGBT elders is expanded through collaboration. For programs and services offered to LGBT elders, it is critical that policy makers move toward policies and budgetary appropriations that are inclusive and responsive to all segments of this population. In the final analysis, society must assist LGBT elders to move from what Walker and Herbitter (2005) refer to as "aging in the shadows."

Learning Exercises

Self-check Questions

1. What are the ways in which older lesbians and older gay men differ in how they are perceived by younger lesbians and gay males?
2. What are some of the societal factors that contribute to the degree in which the elderly become isolated?
3. In comparison with heterosexual elders, how do LGBT elders differ in their social support systems?
4. What are some contextual factors for isolation in later life?
5. How does social isolation differ from a solitary lifestyle?

Field-Based Experiential Assignments

1. Conduct a survey of staff at a senior citizen center to determine their attitudes toward inclusion of LGBT elders.
2. Work with a senior citizen center, a church, or a senior living community to develop inclusive programming and activities for LGBT elders.
3. Develop a documentary on "A Day in the Life of an LGBT Elder."

Multiple-Choice Questions

1. Which of the following LGBT elders are more likely to report that people from their faith communities are part of their support networks?
   (a) African Americans
   (b) Asian Americans
   (c) Hispanic Americans
   (d) White Americans
2. Which of the following is considered an important component to age independently and maintain quality of life?
   (a) Recreation
   (b) Faith community
   (c) Social care network
   (d) Culturally competent service providers
3. Which of the following is a primary underlying factor determining the prevalence of those considered as isolated?
   (a) Age of spouse/partner
   (b) Living status
   (c) Low self-esteem
   (d) Genetics
4. Feeling safe to leave one's home, access to transportation, and availability of local events describe which of the following risk factors for isolation?
   (a) Societal-level risk factors
   (b) Personal-level risk factors
   (c) Geographical-level risk factors
   (d) Community-level risk factors
5. Which of the following group of LGBT elders report a greater sense of rejection because of physical and sexual changes?
   (a) Lesbians
   (b) Gay men
   (c) Bisexual women
   (d) Bisexual men
6. Which of the following contributes to higher levels of loneliness among older LGBT persons?
   (a) Minority stress
   (b) External subjective events
   (c) Internalized homophobia
   (d) All of the above
   (e) None of the above
7. Denial of services, harassment from providers and heterosexual elders, and having specific needs ignored at mainstream centers and programs lead to which of the following behaviors in LGBT elders?
   (a) Concealing their sexual identity
   (b) Advocating for inclusion
   (c) Accepting marginalization
   (d) Dismissing heterosexism
8. Which of the following demographic trends may exacerbate social isolation and loneliness in the future of LGBT Baby Boomers?
   (a) Decreased longevity than previous generations
   (b) Larger number of children than previous generations
   (c) Smaller family size in the family of origin
   (d) Less mobility
9. The types of neighborhood in which LGBT elders live suggest that communities are more conducive to which of the following?
   (a) Accessing services
   (b) Aging in place
   (c) Civic engagement
   (d) Employment contacts
10. In which areas can isolation of elders be found?
   (a) Rural
   (b) Densely populated

(c) Urban

(d) Only a

(e) All of the above

Key

1-a

2-c

3-b

4-d

5-b

6-d

7-a

8-c

9-a

10-e

Resources

Diverse Elders Coalition: www.diverseelders.org

FORGE Transgender Aging Network: www. forge-forward.org

Human Rights Campaign: www.hrc.org/index.htm

LGBT Eder Initiative: www.lgbtei.org

National Resource Center on LGBT Aging: www.lgbtagingcenter.org

Old Lesbians Organizing for Change: www. oloc.org

Osage, P., & McCall, M. (2012). *Connecting with socially isolated seniors: A service provider's guide.* Baltimore, MD: Health Professions Press.

References

Acierno, R., Hernandez, M. A., Amstadter, A. B., Resnick, H. S., Steve, K., Muzzy, W., & Kilpatrick, D. G. (2010). Prevalence and correlates of emotional, physical, sexual, and financial abuse and potential neglect in the United States. The National Elder Mistreatment Study. *American Journal of Public Health, 100,* 292–297. doi:10.2105/ajph.2009.163089.

Adelman, M., Gurevitch, J., de Vries, B., & Blando, J. A. (2006). Openhouse: Community building and research in the LGBT aging population. In D. Kimmel, T. Rose, & S. David (Eds.), *Lesbian, gay, bisexual, and transgender aging: Research and clinical perspectives* (pp. 247–264). New York, NY: Columbia University Press.

Alley, D., Liebig, P., Pynoos, J., Banerjee, T., & Choi, I. H. (2007). Creating elder-friendly communities: preparations for an aging society. *Journal of Gerontological Social Work, 49,* 1–18.

Allman, D. (2013). *The sociology of social inclusion.* Retrieved March 14, 2014 from http://sgo.sagepub.com/content/3/1/2158244012471957.full.print.

Austrian Government. (n.d.). *Social inclusion principles for Austria.* Retrieved January 2, 2015 from www.meetingpoint.org.au/assets/mp_s12_sipfa.pdf.

Baernholdt, M., Yan, G., Hinton, I., Rose, K., & Mattos, M. (2012). Quality of life in rural and urban adults 65 years and older: Findings from the National Health and Nutrition Examination Survey. *The Journal of Rural Health, 28,* 339–347.

Beard, J. R., & Petitot, C. (2010). Ageing and urbanization: Can cities be designed to foster active aging? *Public Health Review, 32*(2), 427–450.

Biordo, D. L., Nicholson, & Social isolation, N. R. (2009). *Chronic illness: Impact and interventions* (7th ed.). Sudbury, MA: Jones and Bartlett Publishers.

Boardman, J. (2010). Concepts of social exclusion. In J. Boardman, A. Currie, H. Killaspy & G. Mezey (Eds.), *Social inclusion and mental health* (pp. 10–12). RC Psych Publications.

Brennan-Ing, M., Seidel, L., Larson, B., & Kariak, S. E. (2014). Social care networks and older LGBT adults: Challenges for the future. *Journal of Homosexuality, 61*(1), 21–52.

Brissette, I., Cohen, S., & Seeman, T. E. (2000). Measuring social integration and social networks. In S. Cohen, L. Underwood, & B. Gottlieb (Eds.), *Social support measurement and intervention: A guide for health and social scientists* (pp. 53–85). New York, NY: Oxford Press.

British Columbia Ministry of Health. (2004). *Social isolation among seniors: An emerging issue.* British Columbia, ON: Author.

Buckmaster, L., & Thomas, M. (2009). *Social inclusion and social citizenship—Towards a truly inclusive society. Research paper no. 08 2009–10.* Australia: Department of Parliamentary Services, Parliamentary Library.

Burchardt, T., Le Grand, J., & Piachaud, D. (2002). Introduction. In J. Hills, L. Le Grand, & D. Piachaud (Eds.), *Understanding social exclusion* (pp. 1–2). Oxford: Oxford University Press.

Cacioppo, J. T., Hawkley, L. C., & Thisted, R. A. (2010). Perceived social isolation makes me sad: 5-year cross-lagged analyses of loneliness and depressive symptomatology in the Chicago Health, Aging, and Social Relations Study. *Psychology and Aging, 25*(2), 453–463.

Cacioppo, J., & Patrick, W. (2008). *Loneliness: Human nature and the need for social connection*. New York: W. W. Norton & Company.

Cantor, M. H., & Mayer, M. (1978). Factors in differential utilization of services by urban elderly. *Journal of Gerontological Social Work, 1*(1), 47–61.

Cantor, M. H., & Brennan, M. (2000). *Social care of the elderly: The effects of ethnicity, class, and culture*. New York: Springer.

Children's, Women's and Seniors Health Branch, British Columbia Ministry of Health. (2004). *Social isolation among seniors: An emerging issue*. Retrieved January 2, 2015 from http://www.health.gov.bc.ca/library/publications/year/2004/Social_Isolation_Among_Seniors.pdf.

Cobigo, V., Ouellete-Kuntz, H., Lysaght, R., & Martin, L. (2012). Shifting our conceptualization of social inclusion. *Stigma Research and Action, 2*(2), 75–84.

Cornwell, E. Y., & Waite, L. J. (2009). Social disconnectedness, perceived isolation, and health among older adults. *Journal of Health and Social Behavior, 50*(1), 31–48.

Crooks, V. C., Lubben, J., Petitti, D. B., Little, D., & Chiu, V. (2008). Social network, cognitive function, and dementia incidence among elderly women. *American Journal of Public Health, 98*(7), 1221–1227.

Cullinan, P. (2006). November-December). Late-life civic engagement enhances health for individuals and communities. *The Journal on Active Aging, 5*(6), 66–73.

Curtis, S., Copelan, A., Fagg, J., Congdon, P., Almong, M., & Fitzpatrick, J. (2006). The ecological relationship between deprivation, social isolation and rates of hospital admission for acute psychiatric care: A comparison of London and New York City. *Health and Place, 12*(1), 19–37.

De Vries, R., & Hoctel, P. (2007). The family, friends of older gay men and lesbians. In N. Teunis & G. Herdt (Eds.), *Sexual inequalities and social justice* (pp. 213–232). Berkeley, CA: University of California Press.

Diverse Elders Coalition. (2012). *Securing our future: Advancing economic security for diverse elders*. Retrieved December 27, 2014 from www.globalaging.org/health/us/2012/SecuringourFutureAdvancingEconomicSecurityforDiverseElders.pdf.

Dorfman, R. A., Lubben, J. E., Mayer-Oakes, A., Atchison, K., Schweitzer, S. O., DeJong, F. S., et al. (1995). Screening for depression among a well elderly population. *Social Work, 40*, 295–304.

Elder, K., and Retrum, J. (2012, May 30). *Framework for isolation in adults over 50*. Retrieved December 19, 2014 from www.aarp.org/content/dur/aarp/aarp_foundation/2012_PDFs/AARP-Foundation-Isolation-Report-Framework-Highlights.pdf.

Espinoza, R. (2013). Friendship a pillar of survival for LGBT elders. *Aging Today, 34*(3), 1–3.

Espinoza, R. (2014). *Out & visible: The experiences and attitudes of lesbian, gay, bisexual and transgender older adults, Ages 45–75*. New York, NY: SAGE.

Fokkema, C. M., & Kuyper, L. (2009). The relationship between social embeddedness and loneliness among older lesbian, gay, and bisexual adults in the Netherlands. *Archives of Sexual Behavior, 38*, 264–275.

Fredriksen-Goldsen, K. I., Kim, H. J., E, Let, C. A., Muraco, A., Erosheva, E. A., Hoy-Ellis, C. P. et al. (2011). *The aging and health report: Disparities and resilience among lesbian, gay, bisexual, and transgender older adults*. Seattle: Institute for Multigenerational Health.

Funders for Lesbian and Gay Issues. (2004). *Aging in equity: LGBT elders in America*. Author.

Grant, J. M., Mottet, L. A., Tanus, J., Harrison, J., Herman, J. L., & Keisling, M. (2011). *Injustice at every turn: A report of the National Transgender Discrimination Survey*. Washington, DC: National Center for Transgender Equality and National Gay and Lesbian Task Force.

Hillman, J. (2012). *Sexuality and aging with LGBT populations. Sexuality and aging: Clinical perspectives*. New York, NY: Springer Science Business Media.

Irizarry, N. (2011, April 25). *All in the family: Looking at the intersection of family, community and disclosure in the lives of gay and lesbian elders*. Undergraduate Library Research Award. Paper 3. Digital Commons at Loyola Marymount University and Loyola Law School Retrieved August 26, 2014 from http://digitalcommons.lmu.edu/ulra/awards/2011/3.

James, J. B., Besen, m E, Matz-Costa, C., & Pitt-Catsouphes, M. (2012). *Engaged as we age*. Boston: Boston College, The Sloan Center on Aging and Work.

Kim, H. J., & Fredriksen-Goldsen, K. I. (2014). Living arrangement and loneliness among lesbian, gay, and bisexual older adults. *The Gerontologist*.

King, A. C., & King, D. K. (2010). Physical activity for an aging population. *Public Health Reviews, 32*(2), 401–426.

Kuyper, L., & Fokkema, T. (2010). Loneliness among older lesbian, gay, and bisexual adults: The role of minority stress. *Archives of Sexual Behavior, 39*, 1171–1180.

Lawton, M. P., & Nahemow, L. (1973). Ecology and the aging process. In C. Eisdorfer & L. Nashemow (Eds.), *The psychology of adult development and aging* (pp. 464–488). Washington, DC: American Psychology Association.

Lenoir, R. (1974). *Les Exclus: Un Francais sur Dix*. Edition du Seuil.

Meyer, I. H. (1995). Minority stress and mental health in gay men. *Journal of Health and Social Behavior, 36*, 38–56.

Meyer, I. H. (2003). Prejudice, social stress, and mental health in lesbian, gay, and bisexual populations: Conceptual issues and research evidence. *Psychological Bulletin, 129*, 674–697.

Movement Advancement Project and SAGE. (2010). *Improving the lives of LGBT older adults*. New York: Author.

Muraco, A., LeBlanc, A. J., & Russell, S. T. (2008). Conceptualizations of family by older gay men. *Growing Older: The millennial LGBTs, 20,* 69–90.

Nusser, S. P. (2010). *What would a non-heterosexist city look like? A theory on queer spaces and the role of planners in creating the inclusive city.* Thesis, Massachusetts Institute of Technology, Cambridge, MA: Department of Urban Studies and Planning. Available at http://dspace.mit.edu/handle/1721.1/59581.

Oldham, J. M., & Morris, L. B. (1995). *The new personality self-portrait: Why you think, work, love, and act the way you do.* New York, NY: Bantam.

Orel, N. (2004). Gay, lesbian and bisexual elders: Expressed needs across focus groups. *Journal of Gerontological Social Work, 43,* 57–77.

Ortiz, H. (2011). *Crossing new frontiers: Benefits access among isolated seniors.* National Center for Benefits Outreach and Enrollment (NCBOE). National Council on Aging. Retrieved August 26, 2014 from www.CenterforBenefits.org.

Plumb, M., & Associates. (2003–2004). *SAGE national needs assessment: A report prepared for senior action in a gay environment.* Retrieved November 6, 2014 from www.marjplumb.com/pdfs/SAGENationalNeedsAssessment.pdf.

Rafaelic, A. C. (2012). The importance of social inclusion in personalized care. *Dialogue in Praxis: A Social Work International Journal, 1*(14), 141–149.

Repper, J., & Perkins, R. (2003). *Social inclusion and recovery: A model for mental health practice.* London: Elsevier Health Sciences.

Rimmerman, A. (2013). *Social inclusion of people with disabilities: National and international perspectives.* Cambridge: Cambridge University Press.

Rosenbloom, S. (2009). Meeting transportation needs in an aging-friendly community. *Generations, 33*(2), 33–43.

Tomaka, J., Thompson, S., & Palacio, R. (2006). The relation of social isolation, loneliness, and social support to disease outcomes among the elderly. *Journal of Aging and Health, 18*(3), 359–384.

U.S. Department of Health and Human Services. (2011). *Affordable Care Act to improve data collection, reduce health disparities.* Washington, DC: Author.

Walker, J., & Herbitter, C. (2005). *Aging in the shadows: Social isolation among seniors in New York City.* New York, NY: United Neighborhood Houses of New York.

Zians, J. (2011). LGBT San Diego's trailblazing generation: Housing & related needs of LGBT seniors. Retrieved October 2, 2014 from www.thecentersd.org/pdf/programs/senior-needs-report.pdf.

Part VI

Counseling and Human Services Delivery

Steven D. Johnson and Anthony Fluty Jr.

Abstract

Although little empirical information exists on what constitutes effective psychotherapy specifically for LGBT elders, gay affirmative treatment approaches are increasing among practicing clinicians. LGBT elders as a specific population have certain unique issues that should be considered by clinicians when providing psychotherapy and counseling. While not all issues pertain to every individual, concerns about coming out, internalized oppression, sexual minority stress, and stereotyping are issues that should be considered by clinicians when counseling LGBT elders. Having an understanding of these issues promotes culturally competent practice. Using a gay affirmative approach in counseling allows the clinician to utilize different theoretical psychotherapeutic approaches when working with LGBT elders. Cognitive-behavioral therapy, person-centered therapy, and existential therapy lend themselves to effective counseling strategies when combined with a gay affirmative approach. Other theoretical approaches may also be equally effective with LGBT elders. Besides individual counseling, LGBT elders may benefit from group therapy, couples counseling, or pastoral counseling if indicated.

Keywords

LGBT seniors · Gay affirmative therapy · Cultural competence · Gay psychotherapy

Overview

The purpose of this chapter is to explore issues that are unique to LGBT elders and how certain psychotherapies and counseling techniques might prove to be beneficial for LGBT elders.

S.D. Johnson (✉) · A. Fluty Jr.
University of Kentucky, Lexington, USA
e-mail: sjohn5@email.uky.edu

© Springer International Publishing Switzerland 2016
D.A. Harley and P.B. Teaster (eds.), *Handbook of LGBT Elders*,
DOI 10.1007/978-3-319-03623-6_31

While there are unique issues for this population, one should keep in mind that not all issues pertain to every individual. As with all counseling, understanding the client's unique journey is paramount in developing an effective treatment strategy. This chapter will outline issues specific to LGBT elders, describe individual theories for counseling these issues, and discuss other treatment modalities to help students and clinicians become culturally competent when counseling LGBT elders.

Learning Objectives

By the end of the chapter, the reader should be able to:

1. Identify and understand unique issues for LGBT elders for clinical practice.
2. Understand specific counseling theories of cognitive-behavioral therapy and their application with LGBT elders.
3. Understand specific counseling theories of person-centered therapy and their application to LGBT elders.
4. Understand specific counseling theories of existential therapy and their application to LGBT elders.
5. Understand how to implement effective counseling strategies with LGBT elders based upon the above theories.

Introduction

To date, limited empirically validated information exists on what constitutes effective psychotherapy for LGBT elders. The life-span psychological and mental health issues of LGBT individuals as a whole have continued to be practically absent from the mainstream psychological literature, with even less being written about LGBT elders specifically (Bieschke et al. 2007; David and Cernin 2007; Mabey 2011; Quam and Whitford 1992; Ritter and Terndrup 2002). However,

psychotherapy with LGBT individuals has evolved significantly in the last few decades. Until the 1970s, psychotherapy with this population had focused on treating a mental disturbance. It was not until 1973 that homosexuality was removed from the *diagnostic and statistical manual of mental disorders* (DSM) as a psychological disorder (Krajeski 1996). Even with this significant change, anti-gay sentiment continued for many mental health clinicians, with treatment still focused on reparative and conversion-type therapies (Lebolt 1999). While professional organizations such as the American Psychiatric Association, the American Psychological Association, and the National Association of Social Workers have clearly mandated these conversion therapies to be counter-therapeutic and likely harmful, they unfortunately still exist and are regarded by some as an option for therapeutic treatment (Bieschke et al. 2007).

While this is a small proportion of the type of therapy conducted today with the LGBT community, there still is a significant gap between historic ideas of "curing" the gay client and current beliefs about what types of psychotherapies are most efficacious for LGBT individuals. Likewise, most graduate training programs in behavioral health still lack a comprehensive inclusion of LGBT issues across their curricula (Biaggio et al. 2003). Yet, many psychotherapists and counselors work with LGBT individuals who present for psychotherapy to deal with a variety of issues, including those specifically related to being a sexual minority.

Cultural Competence with LGBT Elders

What is Cultural Competence? In 2007, NASW saw the need to formally identify the important role that diversity plays in client service. With the profession embracing this understanding, NASW published *Indicators for Cultural Competence in Social Work Practice*. In it, cultural competence is defined as "the process by which individuals and systems respond respectfully and effectively to people of all cultures, languages, classes, races, ethnic backgrounds, religions, and other diversity factors in a manner that recognizes, affirms and values the worth of individuals, families, and communities and protects and preserves the dignity of each" (NASW 2007, p. 12). Keeping this definition in mind, let us explore how it might be applied to counseling LGBT elders.

Senior adults in general face many challenges as they grow older, including health, finances, and decreasing support, as well as possible ageism and discrimination (Gratwick et al. 2014). In counseling elders, it is important to keep these concerns in mind as well as possible other concerns unique to older adult LGBT individuals. Coming out, internalized oppression, sexual minority stress, and stereotyping are unique issues counselors may encounter when working with senior sexual minorities.

Issues Specific to LGBT Elders

Coming Out

Coming out is a unique developmental milestone for LGBT individuals. It involves disclosing one's minority sexual orientation to others. Far from being a singular event, coming out may often be filled with both significant highs and lows. Self-acceptance of one's LGBT sexual orientation is usually a significant part of the coming out process. Often seen as a process that may take many years to complete, coming out can be a time of doubt, distress, and discomfort for many LGBT individuals (Beckstead and Israel 2007). Fortunately, for some, however, it can be a time of growth, connection, and self-acceptance (Riggle and Rostosky 2012).

Psychotherapists working with LGBT clients should bear in mind that most of these clients will have a coming out narrative to share (Johnson 2012). Clients may be in different stages of coming out from denial or unawareness about their sexual orientation to feeling like they are completely out to family and friends. No

matter what stage of coming out a client might be experiencing, this process is still something developmentally unique to the LGBT community (Smith 1997). While coming out issues may or may not be the focus of psychotherapy, clinicians should consider this unique phenomenon during their initial assessment with LGBT clients, just as one would likely assess for Post-Traumatic Stress Disorder in returning combat veterans.

There have been several developmental theories that describe the coming out process in the context of identity formation. Typically, these developmental models refer mostly to lesbians and gay men (Ritter and Terndrup 2002). It would be beneficial for clinicians to be familiar with these theories when working with LGBT elders or other clients who are coming out. Grace (1992), a social worker, proposed a five-stage model of gay and lesbian identity formation that included acknowledging and understanding the unique challenges faced by lesbians and gays in a homophobic society. Grace noted that environmental barriers of a homophobic society create oppressive effects reflected in the development of lesbians and gays (Grace 1992).

Grace's (1992) first level of identity development in his coming out model is emergence. In this stage, individuals sense that they are different, yet realize they must conform to heterosexist norms. They work at passing for being heterosexual, although they may begin to experience same-sex attraction. Next, Grace identifies stage 2 as acknowledgment. In this stage, feelings of fear and shame may increase prior to accepting one's sexual orientation. This stage typically occurs during adolescence, but may occur later in life for some. "Fear of acknowledging their same-sex feelings leads many to deny, rationalize, or bargain in order to limit conscious awareness of their emerging sexual identities" (Grace 1992, p. 42).

Stages 3 and 4 may be different for lesbians and gay men. For lesbians, Grace identifies the third stage as first relationships, followed by the fourth stage of finding a community. For gay men, this is typically reversed. Gay men, according to Grace, will first explore the gay community before finding their first relationship. The final stage is self-definition and reintegration. He describes this as on open-ended, ongoing, and lifelong process with each new situation and relationship. As LGBT individuals meet new people, they are faced with whether or not to disclose their sexual orientation.

For elders, coming out is still a lifelong process. For example, as individuals transition from independent living to an assisted living or skilled nursing facility, they may be faced with having to come out again or return to the closet for safety reasons. Counseling sessions may involve dealing with these coming out issues. As the climate is now safer and more socially acceptable, some individuals may be facing coming out for the first time in their lives. For example, it may be that some LGBT seniors who may have felt pressured to be in a traditional marriage may now be more open to the idea of coming out and exploring a different life arrangement.

Case Vignette 32.1

Mr. Tucholski is a 79-year-old Polish immigrant who recently moved into an assisted living facility outside of Trenton, NJ. Prior to moving into the facility, Mr. Tucholski led an openly gay life with his partner of 37 years. When his partner died a year ago, Mr. Tucholski sold his home that was too much to take care of on his own and moved into the assisted living facility. At his first counseling session, Mr. Tucholski relates significant concern about sharing with his neighbors the fact that he is gay. He tells you that he wants to live authentically but is afraid that his neighbors might not accept his sexuality. He also relates that the activity director at his facility has invited him to religious services that appear to be of a conservative nature. He is concerned that there might be repercussions if this individual and other staff members know that he is gay. In his counseling sessions, it becomes apparent that coming out issues are once again a significant stress for this LGBT elder.

Internalized Oppression

Internalized oppression can be defined as the LGBT individual's manifestation of society's anti-LGBT attitudes (Nadal and Mendoza 2014). This internalization of negative attitudes is theorized to lead to conflicts within the individual, lowered self-regard, and self-deprecating attitudes (Meyer and Dean 1998). Several researchers have applied the idea of internalized oppression in LGBT individuals to the internal stress of minority stress as noted below. According to certain theorists (e.g., Gonsiorek 1988; Meyer 1995; Nadal and Mendoza 2014), the effects of internalized oppression will likely be most intensely felt early in the coming out process. However, due to the long-lasting effects of early socialization experiences and the persistent experience of minority stress, internalized oppression will continue to influence the LGBT individual throughout his/her lifetime (Newcomb and Mustanski 2011). Viewed through this conceptualization of internalized oppression as a component of minority stress, it follows that internalized oppression would likely be related to a variety of different psychological and physical health outcomes (Igartua et al. 2003; Newcomb and Mustanski 2011).

For some LGBT elders, self-acceptance and working through internalized oppression may still be a significant obstacle prevalent in psychotherapy. Having lived through years of oppression and societal discrimination, many individuals may internalize their sexual identity as negative. This lack of self-acceptance may impact an individual's self-confidence and interpersonal relationships. Counseling and psychotherapy may be helpful in identifying and ameliorating negative self-beliefs.

Historically, individuals' negative self-concepts may have been reinforced not only by society but also by religious beliefs or doctrine (Haldeman 2004). See Chap. 27 for further discussion on religious and faith communities' responses to LGBT persons. Unfortunately, it is not uncommon for LGBT elders to have faced negative messages from religious institutions and society as a whole. Helping LGBT elders replace negative schemas and develop new beliefs about their sexual identify may foster a healthier self-identify.

Sexual Minority Stress

Besides dealing with ageism and other stressors, many senior LGBT individuals also may have to cope with sexual minority stress. Sexual minority stress theory posits that in addition to general stress experienced by all people, LGBT individuals experience unique, chronic stressors (both internally and externally) and are continually forced to adapt and cope with societal stigmatization (Meyer 2003). Internal stressors include perception of stigma associated with being LGBT, internalized heterosexism, self-concealment, and emotional inhibition. External stressors include such things as experiences of harassment, discrimination, bullying (see Chap. 18), and anti-LGBT violence (Szymanski et al. 2008). Minority stress theorists have asserted that these stressors can lead to mental health problems for LGBT individuals (Meyer 2003; Szymanski 2005).

Minority stressors can include visible issues that are well-documented in the news media. These stressors can also take on more subtle forms that do not gain public attention. For example, Szymanski et al. (2008) point out that bisexuals experience unique minority stressors in that they are often stereotyped as being promiscuous and untrustworthy or they are viewed as being gay or lesbian persons who refuse to embrace their real sexuality. Persons who identify as bisexual may also be seen as unwilling to give up their heterosexual privilege and, therefore are subject to discrimination from the gay and lesbian community as well as the heterosexual community (Israel and Mohr 2004).

Many LGBT elders have lived through years of oppressive climates (Mabey 2011). Discrimination against LGBT individuals was the norm with strong messages from local, state, and national legislative policies that condoned discrimination against sexual minorities. Thus, for some LGBT elders, sexual minority stress may have become a chronic condition that may have affected their mental health and well-being (Meyer and Frost 2013). When working with LGBT elders, clinicians should keep in mind the cumulative effects of sexual minority stress and assess for this phenomenon in individual and group therapy.

Stereotyping

Stereotypes are generally considered to be "beliefs about the characteristics, attributes, and behaviors of members of certain groups" (Hilton and von Hippel 1996, p. 240). Hilton and von Hippel (1996) note the connection between stereotypes and prejudice and how this affects perception of certain social groups. The LGBT community is a social group that has been the target of many stereotypes (Clausell and Fiske 2005). LGBT elders grew up in an era where gay stereotypes were often prevalent. Many elders may have been victims of negative stereotyping themselves. For some individuals, these stereotypes may have included bullying and teasing, negatively affecting the individual's self-concept. Negative stereotypes can lead to self-doubt and negative thoughts about self. Believing negative stereotypes can lead to internalized oppression and even self-loathing (Smith and Gray 2009). Assessing and processing for how negative stereotypes may have affected an individual may be essential in successful counseling and psychotherapy. Particularly with LGBT Elders, loss of independence that results in having to depend on professional caregivers may elicit fear of discrimination and stereotyping. Counselors should assess for these concerns, particularly if there has been a new life transition such as moving to new community to be closer to family or perhaps a skilled care facility that might involve the stress of coming out again.

In summary, there are unique issues that might arise when working with LGBT elders. Having an understanding of these unique issues will better help clinicians to plan appropriate interventions for their clients. However, clinicians should always be cautious in assuming what will be significant in working with each individual LGBT elder. In other words, clinical judgment should always supersede assumptions of what issues might be significant to the LGBT older adult presenting for counseling. Clinicians should always remember that each individual case is unique and not stereotype based on population characteristics.

Individual Counseling

As mentioned previously, little empirical research exists in the psychotherapy literature on what counseling techniques are most helpful for LGBT individuals in general. Even less exists that is specific for LGBT elders (Bieschke et al. 2007; Ritter and Terndrup 2002). This is due, in part, to the fact that until the early and mid-1980s, most of the psychotherapy literature still focused on curing clients of homosexuality (Stein and Cabaj 1996). Empirical outcome studies for the effectiveness of psychotherapy in general is improving for some psychotherapy modalities, but overall, nothing specific exists for this particular population. However, there has been an increase of scholarly publications on gay affirmative therapy.

Gay Affirmative Therapy

What exactly is gay affirmative therapy? And how has it come to be viewed by many professionals as the appropriate therapeutic modality for working with LGBT individuals? To understand how the counseling and psychotherapy community have arrived at this point, a quick overview of the historical path will be useful.

When homosexuality was removed as a disorder from the DSM, thoughts of homosexuality began shifting from pathology to a naturally occurring lifestyle. Psychotherapy treatment for

LGBT individuals also shifted from conversion-type therapies, still common in the 1980s and 1990s, to acceptance-model therapies. In 2000, the American Psychological Association adopted 16 positive and affirming guidelines for psychotherapy with LGBT individuals (American Psychological Association 2000). This perspective has helped shift the focus of treatment toward a gay affirmative approach that seeks to understand the effects of discrimination, rejection, concealment of identity, and internalized oppression that many LGBT individuals experience (Meyer 2003).

In an attempt to define what was being called gay affirmative therapy, one researcher conducted a literature review asking the following questions: "(1) Does gay affirmative therapy exist? (2) Can gay affirmative therapy be defined? (3) Are there any distinguishing features implicit in gay affirmative therapy? and (4) What issues emerge which have wider implications for counseling clients who are gay?" (Harrison 2000). To explore these questions, he reviewed 33 journal articles and summaries of conference papers dated between 1982 and 1995. He concluded from his thematic analysis that gay affirmative therapy included a non-pathological view of homosexuality and knowledge by the therapist that is appropriate for working with gay clients (Harrison 2000). He noted that some articles expanded the definition to include the role of the therapist as challenging oppression in self and others, identifying societal discrimination, and advocating for social change.

Langdridge (2007), writing from the United Kingdom, also noted that this "more developed" or "strong" affirmative therapy is different from what is usually considered gay affirmative therapy, or in his words "ethically affirmative therapy." Langdridge argued that ethically affirmative therapy is nothing more than ethically appropriate therapy involving LGBT clients. Thus, true LGBT affirmative therapy to Langdridge must include not only the understanding and acceptance but also the "positive affirmation to directly ameliorate the effects of heterosexism." (Langdridge 2007, p. 30). Langdridge also pointed out that while many refer to their therapeutic work as gay affirmative therapy, no one specifically identified significant theoretical or technical modifications to clearly define unique characteristics of gay affirmative therapy. This reinforces Harrison's (2000) conclusions that what exists in the literature is actually a gay affirmative approach to therapy rather than a gay affirmative therapy.

Even though no conclusive research exists on what constitutes effective psychotherapy with LGBT clients, many in the mental health field have identified the importance of psychotherapists using gay affirmative therapy or a gay affirmative approach with their clients. In the *Handbook of Counseling and Psychotherapy with Lesbian, Gay, Bisexual, and Transgender Clients*, Ruperto Perez, one of the book's editors, defines gay affirmative therapy as "the integration of knowledge and awareness by the therapist of the unique development and cultural aspect of LGBT individuals, the therapist's own self-knowledge, and the translation of this knowledge and awareness into effective and helpful therapy skills at all stages of the therapeutic process" (Bieschke et al. 2007, p. 408). Although this definition lacks a unique theoretical framework, it clearly aligns with most counseling philosophies. In the following sections, we explore how to apply gay affirmative therapy or a gay affirmative approach to several common therapeutic modalities that lend themselves to treating LGBT elders.

Cognitive Behavior Therapy

Cognitive-behavioral therapy (CBT) is a form of psychotherapy that focuses on examining the relationships between thoughts, feelings, and behaviors. It has its roots in Rational Emotive Therapy (Ellis 1962) and later work on cognitive therapy by Aaron Beck. The basic proposition of CBT is that cognitions or beliefs strongly determine our feelings and actions. In other words, how an individual's situation is perceived is a defining feature of how an individual feels and behaves (Beck et al. 1979). This is significant, as

individuals continually process information from their external and internal environments. For example, ending a romantic relationship could elicit many feelings associated with the event. These feelings and subsequent behaviors will be determined by what the individual believes about the situation.

Essentially, in the therapy session, clinicians help clients explore patterns of thinking that can lead to negative feelings and actions. Individuals learn to modify their patterns of thinking to improve coping (Beck 1995). CBT is a type of psychotherapy that is different from traditional psychodynamic psychotherapy in that the therapist and the patient will actively work together as a team to help the patient recover from agreed upon problems. CBT deals with the here and now and is a practical therapy that often makes use of in-session teaching as well as homework assignments. CBT is a short-term psychotherapy that typically completed in 8–12 sessions.

In CBT, clinicians help patients address negative life views or schemas. For LGBT elders, these might include negative thoughts about being gay or transgendered (internalized oppression). These long-term negative beliefs may inhibit the individual from fully enjoying life and experiencing healthy relationships. The CBT model would have the patient to identify specific situations causing distress. The therapist would then help the patient identify any negative or irrational thoughts about sexuality or gender identity pertaining to the specific situation. By examining these thoughts, the therapist and client determine which beliefs are rational or irrational and may be contributing to negative emotions. By continuing this process, the therapist helps the client identify patterns in thinking that create negative schemas. By substituting counter thoughts for irrational thinking, the client is able to adopt new ideas that lead to corrected schemas and improved mood. This is one example of negative or automatic thoughts that a therapist might encounter when working with LGBT elders. Others might include distorted thoughts about self-worth, physical appearance, relationships, family, and acceptance in the heteronormative community.

When working with LGBT elders who may have held negative beliefs about themselves for years, clinicians may find challenging such beliefs to be especially difficult. However, because CBT is done in the context of a collaborative relationship, building a therapeutic alliance with the client may aid positive therapeutic success. Homework task is an essential element of CBT. These might include reading assignments, thought monitoring and challenging, or behavioral tasks. Ultimately, the goal of CBT is for clients to become their own therapist and be able to apply CBT techniques on their own (Beck 1995).

Person-Centered Therapy

Person-centered therapy is primarily based upon the relationship between the therapist and the client. According to Carl Rogers, the founder of person-centered therapy, all individuals have the ability to resolve their problems and actualize their full potential (Rogers 1951). Person-centered therapy is a non-directive psychotherapy meaning the client, not the therapist, sets the agenda for the therapy sessions. The therapist is responsible for creating an empathetic, caring, and genuine environment in the therapy sessions. To this end, the therapist must demonstrate the core therapeutic values of congruence, unconditional positive regard, and empathy creating a foundation of trust in the therapeutic relationship (Rogers 1957).

Person-centered therapy gained popularity during the 1960s and 1970s (Knopf 1992). According to Knopf (1992), Rogers was open-minded and accepting of the gay lifestyle. He was known to have lesbian, gay, and bisexual colleagues working with him prior to the declassification of homosexuality from the DSM. There are close parallels with current gay affirmative therapy and the strong tenets of acceptance contained in person-centered therapy.

Therapists wishing to use person-centered therapy with LGBT elders should begin with mastering the three tenets of empathy,

unconditional positive regard, and congruence. Empathy is a consistent appreciation of the subjective experience of the client. Beyond reflective listening or mirroring, empathy is carried out in a personal, nonjudgmental way to truly understand the client's internal frame of reference. Beyond the therapist's empathetic understanding is the importance in appreciating the complete world of the client. This creates a way in which the therapist gets closer and closer to the true meaning and feelings of the client, thus fostering a deeper therapeutic relationship based upon respect for and understanding of the other person (Corsini and Wedding 2005).

Unconditional positive regard is another fundamental aspect of person-centered therapy. Therapists must demonstrate total acceptance of the client's right to his or her feelings. Sometimes described as prizing the client in a total rather than conditional way, Rogers felt unconditional positive regard was necessary for an authentic therapeutic relationship and for the self-actualizing tendency to the full development of one's potential (Rogers 1986). This may be particularly important for LGBT elders who may not have experienced unconditional acceptance.

Congruence involves a genuineness of the therapist to express feelings being experienced with the client. Rather than assume a professional distance, the therapist attends to any persistent feelings created in the therapeutic relationship and expresses them authentically to the client. By being transparent or genuine, the therapist increases the likelihood that the client will change and grow in a constructive manner (Rogers 1957).

Case Vignette 32.2

Ryan has set up an initial appointment to see you in an outpatient-counseling center. During your initial assessment with Ryan, you learn that he is a female-to-male transgendered client. Ryan is 61 years old and works as a marketing consultant for a local Fortune 500 company. He is feeling depressed because of a recent breakup with his partner. He is seeking counseling to deal with this significant transition. Besides relationship issues, Ryan continues to deal with some internalized oppression, work stress, and family acceptance. At this first session, Ryan tells you

"I just dread getting up every morning. Everything seems like such a chore. I'm just tired of putting forth so much effort only to be faced with failure. I am not suicidal, but I just sometimes wish I could take a break. I just feel so worthless at times and full of guilt and hate for myself. I thought things would be better when I transitioned, but some days it just seems really hard. Now that I am getting older, I wonder if I will ever find anyone with whom I can share my life."

1. The therapeutic relationship is the core of person-centered therapy. Knowing what you do about Ryan, how would it be for you to develop a relationship with him? Is there anything that might get in your way with him? Do you really feel you could listen in a non-judgmental way?
2. What do you mainly hear Ryan saying?
3. After establishing a therapeutic relationship with Ryan, what do you feel are the first issues that should be addressed in the counseling session?

Existential Therapy

Existential therapy is as much a philosophical approach as it is psychotherapy. It grew out of philosophical questions of Kierkegaard and Nietzsche who addressed questions of the meanings of life. It emphasizes choice, freedom, responsibility, and self-determination. In short, we are the authors of our life story. Existential therapy places primary focus on understanding the client's current experience and not so much in using specific therapeutic techniques.

Yalom (1980) identified six key features of existential therapy: (1) We have the capacity for self-awareness. (2) Because we are basically free beings, we must accept the responsibility that accompanies our freedom. (3) We have a concern to preserve our uniqueness and identity; we come to know ourselves in relation to knowing and interacting with others. (4) The significance of our existence and the meaning of our life are never fixed once and for all; instead, we recreate ourselves through our projects. (5) Anxiety is part of the human condition. (6) Death is also a basic human condition, and awareness of it gives significance to living. Using these tenets, existential therapy usually focuses on four broad themes or concerns of the human condition: freedom, isolation, meaninglessness, and death (Yalom 1980).

Yalom (1980) identified freedom as a source of anxiety as individuals are the authors of their lives and therefore responsible for their actions and destiny. This can be particularly significant for LGBT elders in that it forces the realization that individuals are responsible for creating their own life story. Oftentimes, individuals feel victimized by circumstances. Existential therapy challenges the clients to use the concept of freedom in creating positive meaning for their life (Frankl 1967).

Next is the idea of existential isolation. Individuals come into existence alone, create their life through choices and decisions, and ultimately leave existence in isolation. Being unable to fully accept this idea can lead individuals into unhealthy relationships, in which they look toward others for meaning and significance. By acknowledging this fact, Yalom (1980) believed that individuals gained the capacity to relate to others on a deeper level. In working with LGBT elders, clinicians may find that clients may be dealing with this concept of existential isolation. Helping them work through the anxiety of being alone may offer an opportunity for more self-understanding and actualization. Fear of existential isolation can create a great deal of interpersonal psychopathology. Helping clients sort through this anxiety can resolve both conscious and unconscious conflicts.

Human beings have a strong desire to create meaning. Conversely, the lack of meaning can be one of great existential concern. In existential therapy, clients are faced with finding unique meaning for their lives in a world where meaning is self-defined. Discovering a sense of meaning is essential in creating a hierarchy of values. Values provide a blueprint for life conduct. Our life values tell us not only why we live, but also how to live. Helping LGBT elders establish meaning may be an essential part of the therapeutic process. The last stages of identify development involve an integrated sense of self, finding meaning in being part of the gay community, and also finding meaning in other areas of life.

Yalom's fourth existential theme is death. Awareness that death is inevitable contrasted with a strong desired to live can create inner conflict. Each human being must face his or her own mortality. Likewise, each human being creates defenses against facing death. People tend to busy themselves with daily distractions so that they do not have to think about what ultimately awaits them. In a sense, they are in denial about death. In existential therapy, clients strive to find a balance between the ultimate reality of death and total denial of its existence. If the individual cannot create balance, internal psychopathology may occur. Clinicians working with LGBT elders will encounter individuals struggling with this existential crisis. Being able to talk openly with clients about how they have created meaning and their thoughts about death

allow them to experience a healthy level of anxiety versus neurotic anxiety. For LGBT elders, these issues may be something that they have avoided thinking about due to other life stress(es). Being able to process thoughts and feelings about death with LGBT elders offers a productive time of reflection. Existential therapy offers LGBT elders a way to address the large questions of their existence.

Cognitive-behavioral therapy, person-centered therapy, and existential therapy are broad in scope and work well when combined with a gay affirmative approach for a variety of issues. Below is a chart containing suggestions on what approach might work well for certain issues (Table 31.1).

It should be noted that cognitive behavior therapy, person-centered therapy, and existential therapy were discussed in this chapter as approaches the authors thought would fit well with issues LGBT elders might face along with compatibility with a gay affirmative approach. There is no research to support that these specific therapeutic approaches might work better than other therapeutic modalities. Other psychotherapeutic approaches such as psychodynamic therapy, gestalt therapy, interpersonal therapy, and behavioral therapy may also be effective when combined with a gay affirmative approach when working with LGBT elders. Clinicians should always use their clinical judgment when selecting a treatment modality and planning psychotherapeutic interventions.

Tables 31.1 Suggested therapeutic approaches for specific issues

Cognitive behavior therapy	Person-centered therapy	Existential therapy
Anger	Self-esteem issues	Anxiety
Depression	Guilt	Guilt and shame
Anxiety	Grief and loss issues	Loss and suffering
Life transitions	Relationship issues	Value clarification
Social anxiety	Growth work	Meaning
Caregiver distress	Insecurity	Mortality
Addictions	Aging	Life choices
Relationship issues	Coming out issues	Life transitions
Aging		
Stress		
Coming out issues		

LGBT Dating for Older Adults

It would not be uncommon for LGBT elders to discuss issues of dating in their counseling sessions. Consider the following unique situations that a clinician might face when working with an LGBT Elder:

- A lesbian presents for counseling after losing her wife of 31 years. Having resolved her grieving, the patient now inquires about how to meet someone new.
- A 65-year-old gay man who had been married to a woman has recently "come out" and is wanting to begin dating men. He is seeking advice on the best way to meet other single gay men.
- A bisexual woman has just ended her relationship with a man. She expresses a desire to start dating women. She does not want to go to bars or to religious-sponsored events and is perplexed about how best to find other bisexual women or lesbians.
- A 58-year-old male to female (MTF) transgendered client has recently completed sexual reassignment surgery. She is seeking to begin dating for the first time as a female. She is concerned about whether to disclose being transgender with new dating partners.

How would you deal with each of the above situations in a counseling session? Remember, your role as a therapist is not to offer advice but to support the client in resolving their issues.

Other Counseling Modalities

While individual psychotherapy may be beneficial for many LGBT elders, other treatment modalities may also be effective for certain issues.

The next section discusses how group counseling, couple's counseling, and pastoral counseling may be helpful to certain LGBT elders.

Group Counseling

Group counseling is another form of psychotherapy that can be advantageous for LGBT elders (Ross et al. 2007). Group counseling offers different opportunities for individuals that are not available in individual counseling sessions. Some unique features of this modality are a therapy environment that replicates real-world situations, an opportunity to practice interpersonal skills, real-time feedback from peers, and social support (Yalom and Leszcz 2005). In the group setting, individuals are able to have their issues normalized by meeting with others who share similar issues or problems. This commonality allows them to not only work on their own specific issues, but to help others with their problems as well.

Frost (1997) notes that group psychotherapy can be advantageous for senior gay males, primarily because the format itself forces them to address a number of significant issues. Because typically in groups, there is an agreement to "stay until the work is done" (p. 275), members are forced to stay and deal with their interpersonal anxiety rather than leaving a stressful situation. He also notes that group psychotherapy may provide a way for gay men to increase their sense of self-worth by practicing new ways to relate positively to other men. For many group members who struggle with intimacy and vulnerability, the group dynamic provides a way to build a healthy sense of trust and connection with other group members (Ritter and Terndrup 2002).

Couples Counseling

Same-sex couples seek counseling for issues similar to those affecting all couples. Communication problems, infidelity and affairs, substance abuse, and decision-making about staying together or separating are issues faced by all clients (Cabaj and Klinger 1996). Besides these common issues, however, LGBT couples have unique issues that impact their relationships. According to Green (2004), most same-sex couples face similar issues, including (1) coping with societal homophobia and heterosexism; (2) defining a relationship despite the lack of a societal or legal model for same-sex relationships; (3) creating social networks that provide emotional support and establishing families of choice; and (4) maintaining flexible gender roles (thus avoiding over-dependency in female couples or emotional disengagement and competition in male couples).

Additional issues that may face same-sex couples are coming out issues. Stages of coming out may differ for each person in the relationship thus creating tension for the couple as to how "out" they are to other people. In other words, if one member is out to family and friends and the other is not, this may create tension in the relationship. Additionally, family dynamics may cause problems for same-sex couples. If the families of origin are not supportive, same-sex couples may have to negotiate discrimination not only from society, but also from their families. Being in a relationship that is not validated by one's family can add to sexual minority stress (Connolly 2004).

With the legalization of same-sex marriage, some same-sex couples may be facing adjustment issues surrounding their newly defined relationships. While in the past they may have had to downplay or disguise their relationship, they are now able to openly share their relationship publicly. This may cause some issues of adjustment for the couple. Couples counseling may include ways to adjust to this new dynamic (Segal and Novack 2008).

Pastoral Counseling

Many older LGBT people may have felt oppressed by and now subsequently feel alienated from the religious traditions into which they were born (i.e., their spiritual traditions of origin). This may be especially true of those whose religious traditions are highly rigid or fundamentalist (Blando 2009). However, for some LGBT elders, organized religion and spirituality have been and continue to be a source of comfort and support (Halkitis et al. 2009; Rostosky et al. 2012) especially if the religious organization to which they belong is seen as gay-affirming (Sowe et al. 2014). If a client presents in counseling with issues surrounding religion and spirituality, it would be germane for the clinician to address those issues as thoroughly as possible within the scope of their training. At times, it may be best to refer the client for pastoral counseling if the issues fall beyond what the clinicians feel they are able to provide. Pastoral counseling may be provided by individuals specifically trained in religious counseling techniques. While each counseling situation is unique, pastoral counseling might be indicated for LGBT elders with strongly self-identified religious backgrounds, individuals having a type of religious crisis, or those contemplating existential or end-of-life issues (Halkitis et al. 2009). Clinicians should be sure to discuss pastoral counseling with the client before making a referral to be sure they both agree that it is therapeutically appropriate.

Summary

Although little empirical information exists on what constitutes effective psychotherapy for LGBT elders, positive strides have been made in moving from treatment focused on reparative or conversion-type therapies to gay affirmative treatment. LGBT elders as a specific population have certain unique issues that should be considered by clinicians when providing psychotherapy and counseling. While not all issues pertain to every individual, concerns about coming out, internalized oppression, sexual minority stress, and stereotyping are issues that should be considered by clinicians when counseling LGBT elders. Having an understanding of these issues promotes culturally competent practice.

Using a gay affirmative approach in counseling allows the clinician to combine different theoretical psychotherapeutic approaches when working with LGBT elders. Cognitive-behavioral therapy, person-centered therapy, and existential therapy lend themselves to effective counseling strategies when combined with a gay affirmative approach. Other theoretical approaches may also be equally effective with LGBT elders. Besides individual counseling, LGBT elders may benefit from group therapy, couples counseling, or pastoral counseling if indicated.

Learning Exercises

Explore the Services and Advocacy for Gay, Lesbian, Bisexual, and Transgender Elders (SAGE) Web site at http://sageusa.org/. Read one article or select a topic from the Web site that you feel would help your understanding of counseling LGBT seniors.

Self-check Questions

1. Define cultural competence and how it relates to LGBT elders.
2. According to the authors, what are the unique issues faced when counseling LGBT elders? Can you think of other issues that you may encounter when working with this population?
3. Why is it important to understand the different stages of coming out? Are these stages different for LGBT seniors than younger adults?
4. Discuss the differences between being culturally competent and stereotyping clients when working with LGBT elders.
5. Do you feel that sexual minority stress is less for LGBT elders than younger adults? Why or why not?
6. Some might argue that using a gay affirmative approach is appropriate for use with all clients. What do you think this means?

7. How might a therapist use existential therapy when working with a client dealing with internalized oppression?

Multiple-Choice Questions

1. Cultural competence can be defined as:
   A. Responding respectfully to people of all cultures, languages, classes, and races
   B. Affirming the values and the worth of individuals, families, and communities
   C. Protecting and preserving the dignity of diversity factors
   D. All of the above
2. A unique developmental milestone for LGBT individuals involving disclosing one's minority sexual orientation to others is known as:
   A. Internalized oppression
   B. Self-actualization
   C. Coming out
   D. Reverse stereotyping
3. A gay man meets with a counselor because he still feels shameful and guilty about his sexuality. These negative feelings toward himself can best be described as:
   A. Internalized oppression
   B. Obsessive-compulsive thoughts
   C. Gay stereotyping
   D. Narcissistic injury
4. The first stage of coming out involves coming out to:
   A. Family
   B. Close friends
   C. Intimate partners
   D. Self
5. A gay affirmative approach in psychotherapy can be used with:
   A. Cognitive-behavioral therapy
   B. Person-centered therapy
   C. Existential therapy
   D. All of the above
6. In cognitive-behavioral therapy, the main focus of the therapeutic process involves:
   A. Processing childhood events
   B. Changing negative beliefs
   C. Analyzing dreams and wishes
   D. Answering questions about life's meaning

7. Focusing on empathy, congruence, and unconditional positive regard are therapeutic characteristics of:
   A. Person-centered therapy
   B. Psychodynamic therapy
   C. Cognitive-behavioral therapy
   D. Existential therapy

8. Existential therapy is an approach used to address:
   A. Irrational beliefs
   B. Homonegativity
   C. Purpose and life meaning
   D. Risky behaviors

9. Unique counseling issues to LGBT seniors include all of the following EXCEPT:
   A. Coming out
   B. Internalized oppression
   C. Sexual dysfunction
   D. Sexual minority stress

10. Having to deal with ongoing stress, both internally and externally, connected to being LGBT can be defined as:
    A. Sexual minority stress
    B. Psychosocial stress
    C. Post-traumatic stress
    D. Stereotypical stress

Key

1. D
2. C
3. A
4. D
5. D
6. B
7. A
8. C
9. C
10. A

Resources

1. National Association of Social Workers (NASW)—Indicators for the achievement of NASW standards for cultural competence in social work practice: http://www.social workers.org/practice/standards/NASWCulturalStandardsIndicators2006.pdf

2. American Psychological Association (APA)—Guidelines for psychotherapy with lesbian, gay, and bisexual clients: http://www.apa.org/practice/guidelines/glbt.pdf

3. National Association of Social Workers (NASW)—Press understanding and working with lesbian, gay, bisexual, and transgender persons: https://www.naswpress.org/publications/diversity/inside/affirmative-chap.html

4. American Association of Retired Persons (AARP)—information and resources for LGBT seniors: http://www.aarp.org/relationships/friends-family/aarp-pride/

5. National Resource Center on LGBT Aging: http://lgbtagingcenter.org/

6. Services and Advocacy for Gay, Lesbian, Bisexual, and Transgender Elders (SAGE): http://sageusa.org/

References

American Psychological Association. (2000). Guidelines for psychotherapy with lesbian, gay, and bisexual clients. *American Psychologist, 55*(12), 1440–1451.

Beck, A. T., Rush, A. J., Shaw, B. F., & Emery, G. (1979). *Cognitive therapy of depression.* New York: Guilford Press.

Beck, J. S. (1995). *Cognitive therapy: Basics and beyond.* New York: Guilford Press.

Beckstead, L., & Israel, T. (2007). Affirmative counseling and psychotherapy focused on issues related to sexual orientation conflicts. In K. J. Bieschke, R. M. Perez, & K. A. DeBord (Eds.), *Handbook of counseling and psychotherapy with lesbian, gay, bisexual, and transgender clients* (pp. 221–245). Washington, DC: American Psychological Association.

Blando, J. A. (2009). Buddhist psychotherapy with older GLBT clients. *Journal of GLBT Family Studies, 5*(1–2), 62–81.

Biaggio, M., Orchard, S., Larson, J., Petrino, K., & Mihara, R. (2003). Guidelines for gay/lesbian/bisexual/-affirmative educational practices in graduate psychology programs. *Professional Psychology: Research and Practice, 34*(5), 548–554.

Bieschke, K. J., Perez, R. M., & DeBord, K. A. (2007). *Handbook of counseling and psychotherapy with lesbian, gay, bisexual, and transgender clients.* Washington, DC: American Psychological Association.

Cabaj, R. P., & Klinger, R. L. (1996). Psychotherapeutic interventions with lesbian and gay couples. In R. P. Cabaj & T. S. Stein (Eds.), *Textbook of homosexuality and mental health* (pp. 485–501). Arlington: American Psychiatric Association.

Clausell, E., & Fiske, S. T. (2005). When do subgroup parts add up to the stereotypic whole? Mixed stereotype content for gay male subgroups explain overall ratings. *Social Cognition, 23*, 161–181.

Connolly, C. M. (2004). Clinical issues with same-sex couples: A review of the literature. In J. J. Bigner & J. L. Wetchler (Eds.), *Relationship therapy with same-sex couples* (pp. 3–12). New York, NY, US: Haworth Press.

Corsini, R. J., & Wedding, D. (2005). Current psychotherapies (7th ed., instr. ed.). Belmont, CA, US: Thomson Brooks/Cole Publishing Co.

David, S., & Cernin, P. A. (2007). Psychotherapy with lesbian, gay, bisexual, and transgender older adults. *Journal of Gay & Lesbian Social Services: Issues In Practice, Policy & Research, 20*(1–2), 31–49.

Ellis, A. (1962). *Reason and emotion in psychotherapy.* Oxford, England: Lyle Stuart.

Frankl, V. (1967). *Psychotherapy and Existentialism: Selected Papers on Logotherapy.* Harmondsworth: Penguin.

Frost, J. C. (1997). Group psychotherapy with the aging gay male: Treatment of choice. *Group, 21*(3), 267–285.

Gonsiorek, J. (1988). Mental health issues of gay and lesbian adolescents. *Journal of Adolescent Health Care, 9*, 114–122.

Grace, J. (1992). Affirming gay and lesbian adulthood. In N. J. Woodman (Ed.), *Lesbian and gay-lifestyles: A guide for counseling education* (pp. 33–47). New York: Irvington.

Gratwick, S., Jihanian, L. J., Holloway, I. W., Sanchez, M., & Sullivan, K. (2014). Social work practice with LGBT elders. *Journal Of Gerontological Social Work, 57*(8), 889–907.

Green, R. J. (2004) Foreword. In J. Bigner & J. Wetchler (Eds.), Relationship therapy with same-sex couples (p. xiv). New York: Haworth Press.

Haldeman, D. C. (2004). When sexual and religious orientation collide: Considerations in working with conflicted same-sex attracted male clients. *The Counseling Psychologist, 32*(5), 691–715.

Halkitis, P. N., Mattis, J. S., Sahadath, J. K., Massie, D., Ladyzhenskaya, L., Pitrelli, K., et al. (2009). The meanings and manifestations of religion and spirituality among lesbian, gay, bisexual, and transgender adults. *Journal of Adult Development, 16*(4), 250–262.

Harrison, N. (2000). Gay affirmative therapy: a critical analysis of the literature. *British Journal of Guidance & Counseling, 28*(1), 37–53.

Hilton, J. L., & von Hippel, W. (1996). Stereotypes. *Annual Review of Psychology, 47*, 237–271.

Igartua, K. J., Gill, K., & Montoro, R. (2003). Internalized homophobia: A factor in depression, anxiety, and suicide in the gay and lesbian population. *Canadian Journal Of Community Mental Health, 22*(2), 15–30.

Israel, T., & Mohr, J. J. (2004). Attitudes toward bisexual women and men: Current research, future directions. *Journal of Bisexuality, 4*, 117–134.

Johnson, S. D. (2012). Gay affirmative psychotherapy with lesbian, gay, and bisexual individuals: Implications for contemporary psychotherapy research. *American Journal of Orthopsychiatry, 82*(4), 516–522.

Kertzner, Barber, & Schwartz, (2011). Mental health Issues in LGBT elders. *Journal of Gay & Lesbian Mental Health, 15*(4), 335–338.

Knopf, N. (1992). On gay couples. *The Person-Centered Journal, 1*(1), 52–62.

Krajeski, J. (1996). Homosexuality and the mental health professions: A contemporary history. In R. P. Cabaj & T. S. Stein (Eds.), *Textbook of homosexuality and mental health* (pp. 17–32). Washington, DC: American Psychiatric Press.

Langdridge, D. (2007). Gay affirmative therapy: A theoretical framework and defence. *Journal of Gay and Lesbian Psychotherapy, 11*(1/2), 27–43.

Lebolt, J. (1999). Gay affirmative psychotherapy: A phenomenological study. *Clinical Social Work Journal, 27*(4), 355–370.

Mabey, J. (2011). Counseling older adults in LGBT communities. *The Professional Counselor: Research and Practice, 1*(1), 57–62.

Meyer, I. H. (1995). Minority stress and mental health in gay men. *Journal of Health and Social Behavior, 36,* 38–56.

Meyer, I. H. (2003). Prejudice, social stress and mental health in lesbian, gay, and bisexual populations: Conceptual issues and research evidence. *Psychological Bulletin, 129,* 674–697.

Meyer, I. H., & Dean, L. (1998). Internalized homophobia, intimacy and sexual behavior among gay and bisexual men. In G. Herek (Ed.), *Stigma and sexual orientation* (pp. 160–186). Thousand Oaks, CA: Sage Publications.

Meyer, I. H., & Frost, D. M. (2013). Minority stress and the health of sexual minorities. In C. J. Patterson & A. R. D'Augelli (Eds.), *Handbook of psychology and sexual orientation* (pp. 252–266). New York, NY, US: Oxford University Press.

Nadal, K. L., & Mendoza, R. J. (2014). Internalized oppression and the lesbian, gay, bisexual, and transgender community. In E. R. David (Ed.), *Internalized oppression: The psychology of marginalized groups* (pp. 227–252). New York, NY, US: Springer Publishing Co.

National Association of Social Workers. (2007). *Indicators for the achievement of NASW standards for cultural competence in social work practice.* Washington, DC: National Association of Social Workers.

Newcomb, M. E., & Mustanski, B. (2011). Moderators of the relationship between internalized homophobia and risky sexual behavior in men who have sex with men: A meta-analysis. *Archives of Sexual Behavior, 40*(1), 189–199.

Quam, J. K., & Whitford, G. S. (1992). Adaptation and age-related expectations of older gay and lesbian adults. *The Gerontologist, 32*(3), 367–374.

Riggle, E., & Rostosky, S. (2012). *A positive view of LGBTQ Embracing identity and cultivating well being*. Lanham, Maryland: Rowman & Littlefield Publishing Group.

Ritter, K. Y., & Terndrup, A. I. (2002). *Handbook of affirmative psychotherapy with lesbians and gay men*. New York: The Guilford Press.

Rogers, C. R. (1951). *Client-centered therapy*. Boston: Houghton Mifflin.

Rogers, C. R. (1957). The necessary and sufficient conditions of therapeutic personality change. *Journal of Consulting Psychology, 21*, 95–103.

Rogers, C. R. (1986). Client-centered therapy. In I. L. Kutash & A. Wolf (Eds.), *Psychotherapist's casebook: Therapy and technique in practice* (pp. 197–208). San Francisco: Jossey-Bass.

Ross, L. E., Doctor, F., Dimito, A., Kuehl, D., & Armstrong, M. S. (2007). Can talking about oppression reduce depression? Modified CBT group treatment for LGBT people with depression. *Journal Of Gay & Lesbian Social Services: Issues In Practice, Policy & Research, 19*(1), 1–15.

Rostosky, S. S., Johnson, S. D., & Riggle, E. (2012). Spirituality and religion in same-sex couples' therapy. In J. J. Bigner & J. L. Wetchler (Eds.), *Handbook of LGBT-affirmative couple and family therapy* (pp. 313–326). New York: Routledge Taylor and Francis Group.

Segal, C. A., & Novack, S. L. (2008). Members of the wedding: The psychological impact of the legalization of same-sex marriage in Massachusetts. *Studies in Gender And Sexuality, 9*(2), 208–213.

Smith, A. (1997). Cultural diversity and the coming-out process: Implications for clinical practice. In B. Greene (Ed.), *Ethnic and cultural diversity among lesbians and gay men* (pp. 279–300). Thousand Oaks, CA, US: Sage Publications Inc.

Smith, M. S., & Gray, S. W. (2009). The courage to challenge: A new measure of hardiness in LGBT adults. *Journal of Gay & Lesbian Social Services: Issues In Practice, Policy & Research, 21*(1), 73–89.

Sowe, B. J., Brown, J., & Taylor, A. J. (2014). Sex and the sinner: Comparing religious and nonreligious same-sex attracted adults on internalized homonegativity and distress. *American Journal of Orthopsychiatry, 84*(5), 530–544.

Stein, T. S., & Cabaj, R. P. (1996). Psychotherapy with gay men. In R. P. Cabaj & T. S. Stein (Eds.), *Textbook of homosexuality and mental health* (pp. 413–432). Arlington, VA, US: American Psychiatric Association.

Szymanski, D. M. (2005). A feminist approach to working with internalized heterosexism in lesbians. *Journal of College Counseling, 8*, 74–85.

Szymanski, D., Kashubeck-West, S., & Meyer, J. (2008). Internalized heterosexism. *The Counseling Psychologist, 36*, 510–524.

Yalom, I. D. (1980). *Existential Psychotherapy*. New York: Basic Books.

Yalom, I. D., & Leszcz, M. (2005). *The theory and practice of group psychotherapy* (5th ed.). New York, NY, US: Basic Books.

Advocacy and Community Needs Assessment

32

Robert Espinoza

Abstract

This chapter provides an overview of the current public policy dilemmas faced by lesbian, gay, bisexual, and transgender (LGBT) older people in areas such as economic security and employment, health equity and healthcare access, housing, HIV and aging, data collection and research, and major federal legislation meant to protect older people in this country. It summarizes the current research and literature on LGBT aging and offers an assessment of the national advocacy capacity of national, state, and local nonprofit organizations working to support LGBT elders. The chapter closes with future considerations for strengthening policy supports for a growing, vulnerable, and neglected demographic of LGBT older adults.

Keywords

Policy · Aging · Advocacy · Legislation · LGBT

Overview

The purpose of this chapter is to provide an overview of the most pressing public policy issues currently faced by LGBT older people. Attention is given to the historical context behind these issues, key research and policy recommendations, recent policy advancements, an assessment of the infrastructure of LGBT aging organizations and programs, and future consid- erations for strengthening the policy apparatus that can spur political change for LGBT older people. The intent is to spur the reader to understand advocacy, as well as identify ways in which he or she might be able to become an advocate on behalf of LGBT elders.

Learning Objectives

By the end of this chapter, the reader should be able to:

1. Understand recent, current, and pressing policy issues faced by LGBT older persons.

R. Espinoza (✉)
SAGE, New York, USA
e-mail: respinoza@sageusa.org

© Springer International Publishing Switzerland 2016
D.A. Harley and P.B. Teaster (eds.), *Handbook of LGBT Elders*,
DOI 10.1007/978-3-319-03623-6_32

2. Identify relevant policy that affects LGBT older persons.

3. Understand the multidisciplinary infrastructure of national, state, and local organizations working to advance policy change for LGBT elders.

Introduction

In the last decade, the visibility of lesbian, gay, bisexual, and transgender (LGBT) older adults has grown considerably, gaining significant traction in federal public policy discussions on aging, long-term care, and LGBT rights. The broader societal awareness about aging and long-term care can be partially attributed to a demographic shift that has rapidly changed the age composition of the US population; estimates forecast that the percentage of people aged 65 and older will grow from 13.7 % of the US population in 2012 (or 43.1 million people) to 21 % in 2040 (or nearly 80 million people) (Administration on Aging, Administration for Community Living 2013). This aging shift has captured the attention of policy government officials, nonprofit leaders, health and aging professionals, and mainstream media. Additionally, the increased visibility and acceptance of LGBT people have enabled a concurrent growth in organizations and programs focused on LGBT older people, many of which produce landmark policy analysis and spearhead advocacy to remove the policy barriers faced by LGBT people as they age. Conservative estimates suggest that there are at least 1.5 million LGBT people aged 65 and older in this country and that this number will double in the next two decades (Movement Advancement Project and SAGE 2010). Yet despite the policy progress made over the last five years in regard to LGBT elders (Espinoza 2013b), policy leaders often omit LGBT elders from major discussions and proposals focused on improving the health and wellness of US seniors. Concurrently, the LGBT aging sector that is positioned to steer a policy

agenda for LGBT elders remains marginal, especially when compared to the magnitude of the population and its large-scale concerns, or when contrasted with the much larger national aging and long-term care field.

This chapter begins by reviewing the policy research and literature on LGBT older people, notably the research that was produced from 2010 to the present. The chapter then examines various policy issues in depth, including the Older Americans Act; economic security, employment, and poverty; affordable housing and safe, long-term care; health equity and healthcare access; HIV and aging; and data collection and research. The chapter proceeds to describe the multidisciplinary infrastructure of national, state, and local organizations working to advance policy change for LGBT elders and proposes a variety of issues that should be resolved through future scholarship, such as developing best practices for integrating LGBT issues into national surveys and clinical settings so that LGBT elder advocates can draw from data for future policies and programmatic interventions.

Policy Research and Literature on LGBT Older People

The policy research and literature on lesbian, gay, bisexual, and transgender (LGBT) aging dates back to 2000, though most policy reports on this subject were produced from 2010 to the present. In *Outing Age: Public Policy Issues Affecting Gay, Lesbian, Bisexual, and Transgender Elders*, the first in-depth policy report on LGBT elders, Cahill et al. (2000) outline a variety of political, social, and cultural challenges faced by LGBT older people, including the lack of LGBT-friendly social services, unequal treatment in safety net programs such as Medicaid and Medicare (among others), ongoing discrimination in housing and nursing homes, and a general lack of policies that protect LGBT people. They note that ageism in the LGBT community coupled with heterosexism in the aging field has colluded to exclude the realities of LGBT older people from policy conversations on aging, long-term care, health, and LGBT rights.

> This landmark policy report both lays the groundwork and anticipates the policy advocacy movement that will emerge on LGBT elders in the ensuing two decades: Today we stand at the edge of two tidal waves: a growing wave of GLBT people aging and entering the social service and community institutions which care for and advocate for the elderly; and a tidal wave of reaction against government, and against government funding for social service needs. How will GLBT people fare as these waves wash over our communities? To date, aging service providers are not ready for the new wave of GLBT elders, policy makers are running away from it, and until very recently, frankly, the GLBT community has not faced this wave either (p. iv).

In 2010, the Movement Advancement Project and SAGE (Services and Advocacy for GLBT Elders) revive this LGBT aging policy agenda by positing that LGBT older adults deal with three overarching challenges: the long-term consequences of stigma and discrimination; the over-reliance of LGBT older people on "families of choice" that are not legally protected and are often rendered secondary to spouses and biological next of kin in public policies, legal protections, and within most mainstream aging service provision; and the general unequal treatment of LGBT people in aging services and under the law. The authors surmise that these challenges compound to impair LGBT elders' financial security, proper health and healthcare access, and their level of social support.In response, the authors enumerate more than 50 policy recommendations in areas such as Social Security, Medicaid, Veteran's Benefits, visitation and medical-decision-making, housing and more (pp. 65–68). The report also elicits the support of a few national aging organizations, including AARP (formerly the American Association of Retired Persons), the American Society on Aging, and the National Senior Citizens Law Center, which forecasts how mainstream national aging organizations will become more supportive of an LGBT elder policy agenda in the years that follow.

Subsequent policy reports focus on discrete policy areas or subpopulations of LGBT older people who face additional barriers and considerations. SAGE (2011b) describes the opportunities offered by the Older Americans Act to support LGBT elders, citing recommendations for this signature legislation to amend its definitions to specify LGBT older adults; require data collection and reporting on the extent to which local services and programs serve LGBT older people; broaden definitions of "family" to include families of choice; and support LGBT cultural competence training nationwide. The National Senior Citizens Law Center (2011) profiles the stories of more than 700 LGBT older people and their loved ones in long-term care settings, describing harrowing incidents throughout the country of verbal and physical harassment from staff and other residents, as well as stories of staff members refusing to use a resident's preferred (gendered) name or to provide basic care or services, among other stories of hardship. In its recommendations, the report calls for additional research on the experiences of LGBT elders in long-term care facilities and more LGBT cultural competence training for nursing home and other aging professionals, as two notable examples. The National Academy on an Aging Society (2011) examines a variety of current policy topics related to LGBT elders, including the policy barriers faced by older adults with HIV, the role of public policy in creating culturally competent aging services for LGBT elders, and how the Affordable Care Act explicitly supports both older people and LGBT people, among other issue areas. This report represents the first multi-issue policy report on LGBT aging published by a national organization focused on aging: the Gerontological Society of America. SAGE and the National Center for Transgender Equality (2012) offer more than 60 recommendations for policy and practice in regard to supporting transgender older people, including recommendations related to privacy and documentation, violence, aging service and healthcare barriers, employment and housing discrimination, and more. The reader is referred to Chap. 14 in this book for further discussion on transgender elders. SAGE (2013a) identifies 10 policy areas that can promote health equity among LGBT older people of color, including data collection, strengthening Social Security, increasing funding for culturally and linguistically competent aging supports, and more. The author notes that though LGBT elders of color represent an important segment of the demographic shift that is rapidly diversifying and aging the US population, "the available research shows that they often face heightened health disparities and are largely rendered invisible in public policy discussions on aging" (p. 1). The reader is referred to Chaps. 6–8 in this book for further discussion on LGBT elders of color. The National Hispanic Council on Aging (2014) focuses on the importance of funding and delivering LGBT-friendly culturally and linguistically appropriate services to LGBT Latino older people. The needs assessment finds that LGBT Latino people deal with multiple barriers to accessing supportive communities when they age, including the biases of more conservative people of faith, the lack of environments that embrace LGBT Latino elders as people with multiple identities, and the compounding challenges of having survived discrimination rooted in one's sexual and gender identity, as well as one's racial and ethnic realities. The Equal Rights Center (2014) argues for stronger LGBT-friendly non-discrimination protections in housing based on a 10-city investigation among older same-sex couples. The investigation finds that in 48 percent of the tests, older same-sex couples experienced at least one form of differential treatment when seeking housing in senior-living facilities, such as being provided less information about additional units, or being required to pay additional fees or costs, and undergo a more extensive application process, among other hurdles. The Diverse Elders Coalition (2014) argues for policy improvements in eight areas related to HIV and aging, including funding HIV prevention programs aimed at older people, increasing Medicaid expansion across states, developing and propagating clinical care guidelines for treating older people with HIV, and more. The report also calls for the inclusion and funding of HIV and aging as a significant need in the upcoming 2015 White House

Conference on Aging, the existing Ryan White Care Program, and the current reauthorization of the Older Americans Act.

Policy Issues Faced by LGBT Older Adults

LGBT older people face an array of policy barriers in areas related to the Older Americans Act, economic security and employment, health equity, HIV and aging, affordable housing and long-term care, and data collection and research. LGBT elders are not explicitly accounted for in most public policies that are meant to support older people, and many LGBT elders face unequal treatment under the law as LGBT people and as same-sex couples. LGBT elders concurrently experience differential treatment in accessing aging and health services, housing, and long-term care—with marginal legal protections or policy-funded interventions. The data and research on LGBT older people remain thin and underfunded. Nevertheless, policy advocates have advanced a variety of protections in recent years, widening opportunities to protect LGBT elders in safety net programs, aging services, and federal and state public policy.

Older Americans Act

The Older Americans Act (OAA) serves as the country's largest vehicle for funding and delivering services to older people in the USA; estimates suggest that its funding scope is more than $2.3 billion annually (National Health Policy Forum 2012). The OAA also emphasizes reaching older people with the "greatest social need," which includes economically vulnerable people and racial and ethnic minorities. However, the OAA does not include LGBT-specific provisions that would increase funding for programs, services, and research related to LGBT older people. Without these provisions, the national array of service providers and local and state government agencies that comprise the country's "aging network" are not compelled, encouraged, or mandated to consider LGBT people as a population worthy of targeted supports (SAGE, n.d.b).

The reauthorization of the OAA, which takes place every five years, provides an opportunity to amend this legislation in ways that address these concerns. In response, national LGBT and aging advocates have proposed that the OAA be amended to specify LGBT older adults as a population of "greatest social need." Additionally, advocates propose that OAA require that state and area agencies on aging report the extent to which they serve LGBT older people; that OAA increase funding for both research and programs focused on LGBT elders; and that the National Resource Center on LGBT Aging, a technical assistance and training center seeded by the US Department of Health and Human Services (HHS) in 2010 and led by SAGE, be permanently established in the OAA (SAGE, n.d.b).

These recommendations have garnered widespread support from leading national nonprofits in the aging field such as the Leadership Council of Aging Organizations, as well as from members of Congress and federal agencies (SAGE 2011a). A proposed 2012 Senate bill and a proposed 2014 House bill on OAA reauthorization included these LGBT-friendly recommendations (Tax 2014). In July 2012, the Administration for Community Living (ACL) at HHS issued guidance recommending that LGBT older people be considered by ACL's grantees as a population of greatest social need in local planning efforts (SAGE 2014a). In addition to the legislative remedies outlined above, federal agencies can exercise their authorities to issue regulatory and administrative changes that move forward many aspects of these recommendations.

Economic Security, Employment, and Poverty

A lifetime of discrimination in the workforce and in public benefit programs has diminished retirement savings, exacerbated economic security, and spurred higher poverty rates for many LGBT older people, notably LGBT people of color who deal with the added burdens of multiple forms of discrimination (MAP and SAGE 2010). These economic conditions are worsened by the current recession, the general increase in healthcare costs over the years, the pervasiveness of age-related bias (as early as age 40), and LGBT-specific discrimination in the employment process and the workplace (Cray 2013). The federal government does not prohibit workplace discrimination based on sexual orientation and gender identity, while 29 states lack protections for both sexual orientation and gender identity in the workplace (Human Rights Campaign 2014a, b). Additionally, many LGBT older people and their families do not have other assurances such as adequate paid leave protections that would allow them or their primary caregivers to take time off from work to care of their loved ones when they are ill; paid leave protections nationwide are sparse; and typically "families of choice" who are friends and caregivers of many single LGBT older people, are not protected by leave protections (Make 2013a). The reader is referred to Chap. 29 in this book for further discussion on LGBT issues in the workplace.

Finally, unequal treatment for same-sex couples in federal programs such as Medicaid and Social Security has left many LGBT older couples without the financial resources they need to live financially secure in old age (MAP and SAGE 2010). The June 2013 Supreme Court decision that effectively struck down the federal Defense of Marriage Act has spurred numerous improvements for same-sex couples in accessing important federal benefits, though the breadth of these benefits continues to evolve as the federal administration implements this decision across programs (Tax 2014). Two notable policy tensions are whether federal benefits should be available to all legally married same-sex couples regardless of whether they reside in a state that does not sanction same-sex marriage and whether these benefits should extend beyond marriage and support couples or dyads in civil unions, domestic partnerships, and/or mutually dependent caregiver relationships (Freedom to Marry 2013; Movement Advancement Project and SAGE 2010). The reader is referred to Chap. 36 in this book for further discussion on the implications of the Supreme Court ruling on same-sex marriage.

To improve the economic security of LGBT older people, policy leaders propose an array of policy remedies. Congress could pass the Employment Non-Discrimination Act, which would provide critical workplace protections related to sexual orientation and gender identity to millions of LGBT workers (Cray 2013). Additionally, the President could issue an executive order that prohibits federal contractors from discriminating on the basis of sexual orientation and gender identity (Ford 2014). Federal, state, and city governments could enact paid leave laws that expand legal recognition to same-sex couples and broader "families of choice," allowing LGBT older workers and their caregivers to support one another in times of illness (Make 2013b). The federal government could ensure that LGBT people, same-sex couples, and their families of choice in all states have access to federal benefits across areas such as Medicare, Social Security, Veteran's Benefits, the Family and Medical Leave Act, and more (Lambda Legal 2013). The Social Security Administration could exercise its authority to ensure that same-sex couples in marriages, civil unions, and domestic partnerships have equal access to Social Security spousal, survival, and death benefits, regardless of the state in which they reside (Novak 2014).

The federal administration has made significant progress following the June 2013 Supreme Court decision that invalidated the Defense of Marriage Act. In June 2013, the Social Security Administration (SSA) announced that transgender people could update their Social Security records to reflect their proper gender identities, and in April 2014, SSA issued updated guidance that a gender transition does not affect the validity of transgender people and their spouses (with additional review required in some states) (National Center for Transgender Equality 2013; 2014a).

In April 2014, the US Department of Health and Human Services released guidance that legally married same-sex couples are eligible for Medicare benefits, regardless of where the couple lives (2014). In May 2014, the Administration for Community Living issued guidance to its grantees that they could include same-sex married couples in their definitions of "spouse," "family," and "relative" and that grantees should follow the "place of celebration" rule, meaning that same-sex marriages will be affirmed for ACL programs, regardless of the state in which they reside (SAGE 2014a). Finally, a bill has been introduced in the US Senate—the Social Security and Marriage Equality (SAME) Act of 2014—that would extend spousal, survival, and death benefits under Social Security to married same-sex couples in all states (Goodwin and Knox 2014).

Affordable Housing and Safe Long-Term Care

Many LGBT older people struggle with securing safe and affordable housing. Research shows that LGBT older people encounter various forms of differential treatment when attempting to buy or rent homes and apartments, as well as access senior housing (Movement Advancement Project and SAGE 2010; Equal Rights Center 2014). Additionally, many LGBT elders encounter bias and discrimination from staff members and fellow residents in independent living and assisted-living facilities, nursing homes, and home care (National Senior Citizens Law Center 2011). Espinoza (2014) notes that while a crop of affordable LGBT senior housing complexes have been developed around the country, generating significant media attention and widespread interest from LGBT older people and their advocates, the availability of these complexes and the limited stock of units cannot meet the demand of millions of LGBT older people who might want to reside in these residences; advocates posit that housing solutions for LGBT elders must be more innovative and expansive.

The author also argues that a lifetime of discrimination has hampered the economic security and limited the housing options of many LGBT older people, notably people of color, transgender people, and women. The broader housing crisis, recession, and foreclosure crisis has only worsened these housing realities for LGBT elders.

Policy advocates argue for the importance of federal and state-level non-discrimination protections that include sexual orientation and gender identity and which cover public accommodations to account for nursing homes and other long-term settings (Human Rights Campaign 2014a). To support LGBT senior housing complexes as well as a range of housing supports geared at LGBT older adults (i.e., LGBT sensitivity training for housing providers, know-your-rights resources for LGBT elders who are seeking housing, and more), federal and state governments could increase funding for these types of housing developments and supports (U. S. Department of Housing and Urban Development, n.d.). The Older Americans Act, the US Department of Housing and Urban Development, and the Centers for Disease Control and Prevention could play critical roles in funding and promoting senior housing communities that offer more skilled long-term services to LGBT older people, as well as promote independent living communities that allow for aging in place. Finally, increased funding for LGBT cultural competence training that reaches long-term care staff and housing providers around the country could help ensure that LGBT elders live in homes and long-term care facilities that feel more welcoming and safe (SAGE 2013b).

A February 2014 report on housing discrimination among same-sex older adults garnered widespread media attention and visibility on LGBT elders and housing (Equal Rights Center 2014). Around the country, housing developers and community advocates have increasingly spearheaded the creation of LGBT senior housing complexes, including Los Angeles, Minneapolis, Philadelphia, and more (SAGE 2013a). The National Resource Center on LGBT Aging continues to train hundreds of aging providers nationwide on the issues faced by LGBT elders, increasing knowledge and supportiveness for LGBT elders among aging professionals (National Resource Center on LGBT Aging 2014). State advocates have also led LGBT sensitivity trainings for housing providers to reduce bias and discrimination aimed at LGBT older people (Wayland 2014).

Health Equity and Healthcare Access

Fredriksen-Goldsen et al. (2011) conducted a national study of LGBT older adults that found significant disparities in areas related to physical and mental health, including obesity, high blood pressure, cholesterol, arthritis, cataracts, asthma, cardiovascular disease, diabetes, and other areas. In regard to mental health, the authors found that more than half of the study's respondents had been told by a doctor that they had depression and 39 % had seriously thought about suicide. And in many of the health areas examined in the study, LGBT older people of color and transgender people faced higher health disparities. The research shows that many LGBT older people report avoiding or delaying care for fear of discrimination; as one example, older people with HIV are often more likely to be dually diagnosed with HIV and AIDS than their younger counterparts, a medical designation that suggests that older people are not seeking proper care to detect HIV, older people are not speaking candidly about their sexual health with their providers, and/or older people are not being screened properly by medical professionals, many of whom might mistakenly assume that sexual activity diminishes or goes away in old age (National Resource Center on LGBT Aging 2011). One systematic barrier to LGBT-friendly patient-centered health care is that questions about sexual orientation and gender identity, which would identify LGBT patients to doctors, nurses, and other medical professionals, are rarely asked in the patient intake process. Conversely, evidence suggests that these questions improve candor and can lead to important interventions related to common LGBT health concerns (The Fenway Institute and The Center for American Progress, 2013).

To address national health disparities, the Affordable Care Act (ACA) put into place a number of enhancements for LGBT people and seniors, including new provisions that prevent health insurers from denying coverage based on preexisting conditions such as a person's sexual orientation, gender identity or HIV status, and various supports for people aged 65 and older, including assistance with prescription drug costs and increased access to more prevention services (SAGE 2013d). The extent to which ACA has improved healthcare access for LGBT older people remains unknown, though the need for improved health coverage is more substantiated. The Center for American Progress (2013a) has found that 34 % of LGBT people were uninsured at the beginning of the open enrollment period (October 2013) for the ACA's marketplaces. Twenty-eight percent of LGBT people aged 50–64 were uninsured in this research (K. Baker, personal communication, May 28, 2014). Additionally, 82 % of uninsured LGBT people reported discrimination when trying to access their partners' plans; 67 % had been without health insurance for more than two years, and 60 % reported delaying medical care for the past 12 months because they could not afford the costs of health care (Center for American Progress 2013b). The reader is referred to Chap. 19 in this book for further discussion on the impact of health reform on LGBT elders. Finally, transgender older people in particular struggle with accessing health care; lifelong discrimination has limited their job security, their incomes, and their access to private employer insurance. In turn, many transgender older people rely largely on federal programs such as Medicare and Medicaid, which have historically contained arbitrary exclusions for transition-related health care, placing the financial burden for these procedures entirely on the transgender patient (SAGE and NCTE 2012, pp. 15–16).

A 2013 report on health equity (SAGE) outlined various policy proposals to improve the health of LGBT older people, in particular people of color who face multiple health and aging-related challenges. The report recommends passage of two legislative bills related to the Older Americans Act, which would facilitate support programs geared at LGBT older people, as well as culturally and linguistically appropriate supports for people of color and limited-English-proficient people, a percentage of whom are LGBT. The US Department of Health and Human Services (HHS) and its relevant agencies could exercise their authorities to fund programs that target LGBT older people, while encouraging other grantees and community-based partners to work closely with LGBT nonprofits when implementing their health initiatives. Because the federal and state marketplaces did not collect data on the sexual orientations and gender identities of new enrollees, it remains unclear how many LGBT people are included in the roughly 8 million people who enrolled in the ACA marketplace (K. Baker, personal communication, May 28, 2014). Thus, SAGE (2013b) recommends that the federal regulations on state exchanges explicitly account for LGBT older people, which could include LGBT data collection on enrollees. Additionally, in May 2014, HHS declared that Medicare could no longer arbitrarily exclude transition-related surgery, regardless of a person's medical condition. This decision means that transgender people can obtain this surgery if it is approved by a medical provider that accepts Medicare and if they are able to cover the remaining medical costs such as deductibles and co-pays (National Center for Transgender Equality 2014b).

HIV and Aging

Since its onset in the early 1980s, the HIV/AIDS epidemic has disproportionately affected LGBT people, notably men who have sex with men, transgender people, and people of color. As HIV treatment drastically improved in the mid-1990s, HIV/AIDS became less of a death sentence and more of a chronic and manageable illness, profoundly altering the age composition of the epidemic into the present (SAGE, n.d.a). By 2015, one in two people with HIV in the USA will be aged 50 and older—and by 2020, this proportion will increase to nearly three in four people (or 70 %). Research also shows that new infections are on the rise among older people, many of whom report not being screened or tested by healthcare providers who mistakenly assume that sexual activity ends in older age. Additionally, older people are often dually diagnosed with both HIV and AIDS, a clinical designation that means the virus has worsened to a state of medical and financial crisis (Cahil et al. 2010). A growing body of medical research indicates that people with HIV in their early 50s exhibit the same number of comorbidities as people without HIV in their early 70s; the virus, the anti-retroviral treatment, and a range of socioeconomic factors compound to spur aging and disability faster and sooner among people with HIV (American Academy of HIV, Medicine, American Geriatrics Society and AIDS Community Research Initiative of America 2011). More broadly, few organizations, government agencies, or health and aging service providers account for the existence or the growing needs of older adults with HIV, many of whom are LGBT and/or people of color (Diverse Elders Coalition 2014).

Advocates propose a range of policy interventions to support this demographic, as recently described in a policy report authored by the Diverse Elders Coalition (2014). The Ryan White Care Program, which provides essential services to people with HIV throughout the country, must be sufficiently funded to support the growing population of older people with HIV. The Centers for Disease Control and Prevention (CDC) could dedicate funding for HIV prevention campaigns aimed at older people, as well as better promote its testing guidelines to reach older populations. HHS could implement and promote guidelines for the clinical care of older people with HIV, given the number of earlier age-related comorbidities; these guidelines were recently created by a national team of HIV experts from different fields and disciplines (American Academy of HIV, Medicine, American Geriatrics Society and AIDS Community Research Initiative of America 2011). The reauthorization of the Older Americans Act and the 2015 White House Conference on Aging provide critical opportunities to integrate policy changes and recommendations for older people with HIV. Finally, if every state opted to expand Medicaid coverage through the Affordable Care Act (ACA), and every person with HIV was in care, this change would provide coverage to more than 200,000 people with HIV who otherwise might not receive appropriate health care.

The visibility of HIV and aging has grown in the last few years. In fall 2013, a Congressional hearing and briefing examined the policy barriers faced by older adults with HIV, gathering experts from around the country (ACRIA 2013). In 2013, the CDC issued a landmark surveillance report tracking HIV among people aged 50 and older in five-year increments; this report allows researchers to better track the course of the epidemic as older people age (Centers for Disease Control and Prevention 2013). In May 2014, national advocates representing older people, people with HIV, LGBT people, and communities of color held a historic national teleconference and released an updated policy report on HIV and aging, calling for action on eight policy recommendations that would dramatically improve the health and wellness of older adults with HIV (Diverse Elders Coalition 2014).

Data Collection and Research

Espinoza (2013a) describes the various challenges faced by the systematic data collection and research on LGBT older adults. The large-scale quantitative data and research on LGBT older people remain thin and sparse, which prevents the knowledge that would substantiate and inform properly designed programs, policies, and interventions that target LGBT elders.

Questions that capture a person's sexual orientation and transgender status are not included in most federal surveys, from the US Census to the broad array of federal surveys on health, retirement, long-term care, and other matters relevant to LGBT elders. This means that statistics on the total number of LGBT older people in this country are conservative estimates at best. Further, where questions are asked, the related sample sizes for people aged 50 and older are often too small to form representative findings; few, if any, questions related to sexual orientation and gender identity are assessed for their clarity and accuracy among older populations, many of whom might have generational traits that shape their understanding of these research questions as well as their willingness to respond. Moreover, the challenges with securing older adult samples in representative surveys intensify when researching LGBT elder subgroups. For example, researchers struggle with reaching low-income, racially, and ethnically diverse transgender older people; most studies on transgender people have older adult samples that are more likely to be white and have higher income than their younger counterparts (SAGE and NCTE 2012, p. 4).

Along the same lines, questions on sexual orientation and gender identity are rarely captured in the patient intake process by most public and private health and aging entities, despite evidence that these questions can improve patient candor and patient care; further, when properly aggregated and reported, the responses to these questions could help illuminate health disparities (The Fenway Institute and The Center for American Progress 2013). Finally, state and area agencies on aging are not encouraged or required to measure the extent to which they outreach and serve LGBT older people in their areas, which limits the public understanding on the types of services and supports that LGBT elders receive in different parts of the country (SAGE, n.d.b). Research shows that too few state and area agencies on aging provide outreach to LGBT communities or LGBT-friendly services through their agencies (Knochel et al. 2011).

To broaden the data and knowledge on LGBT older adults, advocates and researchers propose various policy solutions (SAGE 2013b). The US Department of Health and Human Services (HHS) and agencies within HHS such as the Administration for Community Living (ACL) and the Centers for Disease Control and Prevention could develop, include, and test elder-sensitive questions on sexual orientation and gender identity in their national survey instruments. The Office of the National Coordinator for Health Information Technology could include data collection on sexual orientation and gender identity within its meaningful use standards for electronic health records. State health departments could integrate questions on sexual orientation and gender identity into their patient intake processes for people entering the Medicaid-funded system, similar to recent efforts in New York State (Espinoza 2013a, b). HHS could track data on discrimination and mistreatment of LGBT older people through the National Ombudsman Reporting System, and ACL could require that state and area units on aging to collect data that measure the extent to which LGBT older people are being served by the national aging network, especially in more conservative, less LGBT-friendly areas (SAGE 2013b).

In 2013, the CDC began testing a question on sexual orientation in its National Health Interview Survey and encouraged states to use questions on both sexual orientation and gender identity in the CDC's Behavioral Risk Factor Surveillance System (U.S. Department for Health and Human Service 2013). In 2013, the New York State Department of Health integrated questions on sexual orientation and gender identity into its statewide patient intake process for specific Medicaid-funded facilities, and the New York State Office for the Aging also revised its intake forms to include these questions (Espinoza 2013a, b). Both developments signal opportunities for other federal and state agencies to modify their surveys and patient intake processes to include LGBT-specific questions, ideally with elder-appropriate methodologies that collect robust samples of LGBT older people.

To protect LGBT elder clients and patients, these questions should be accompanied with protocols for collecting data, LGBT cultural competence training for professionals, and resources that educate LGBT patients on their legal rights in aging and long-term care settings (National Resource Center on LGBT Aging 2013). The reader is referred to Chaps. 22 and 34 in this book for further discussion on healthcare practices with LGBT elders, and the ethical standards and practices in human services and health care.

Related Disciplines

To better understand the political progress that has been achieved for LGBT elders, as well as what can be accomplished in the future, it is important to map the sector of organizations, programs, and coalitions working on federal, state, and local advocacy for LGBT older people. These organizations work across disciplines and sectors, yet their policy endeavors are generally focused on policy analysis and joint advocacy activities such as holding briefings for lawmakers, offering legal guidance to federal and state agencies, and building public awareness and support for LGBT elder policy concerns. While extremely successful in the last 10 years, advocates argue that the LGBT aging sector must significantly expand in order to continue achieving large-scale change for future generations of LGBT older adults.

LGBT Aging Organizations, Programs, and Coalitions

While the visibility of LGBT aging has increased dramatically since 2007, as well as the number of nonprofit actors working to address the lives of LGBT older people, this sector continues to be comparatively small when compared to the broader aging and LGBT rights fields and to the national nonprofit sector. Only a few national organizations and less than 50 state and local organizations are primarily focused on LGBT aging in their missions and programs, a percentage of which are leading policy analysis and advocacy. As evidence of the national underfunding and marginalization of LGBT aging, Funders for LGBTQ Issues has reported that US foundation giving to organizations and programs serving LGBT older people grew marginally from $1.9 million to $3.5 million between 2007 and 2012 (Funders for LGBTQ Issues 2009; Funders for LGBTQ Issues 2013). More broadly, US foundations awarded more than $49 billion to nonprofits in 2012 (Foundation Center 2013), meaning that foundation giving to LGBT aging is a minute fraction of total foundation giving in the USA. A sufficiently funded LGBT aging sector of national and state organizations— working in coalition with their partner organizations in the aging and long-term care field— will be vital to support the growing millions of LGBT older people over the next few decades.

National Organizations

While the sector of organizations working to support LGBT older people has expanded in the last decade, it remains a small field led by a few national organizations and a few dozen organizations working largely at the local level. SAGE (Services and Advocacy for GLBT Elders), which was founded in 1978, remains the largest and oldest national organization focused primarily on LGBT older people, coordinating direct services for LGBT elders, providing training to aging providers on LGBT cultural competence (through its National Resource Center on LGBT Aging, seeded in 2010 by the US Department of Health and Human Services), spearheading federal and state policy improvements with national and state partner organizations, and producing online consumer resources for LGBT elders related to health, legal, and financial planning, caregiving, and more (SAGE, n.d.f). Old Lesbians Organizing for Change (OLOC) is a national network for lesbians aged 60 and older; its signature programming includes regional and national gatherings, as well as trainings and resources focused on the manifestations of ageism, a system of attitudes, behaviors, and institutional practices that devalue older people based on faulty or overstated presumptions about old age (Old Lesbians Organizing for Change, n.d.). Additionally, a small group of national organizations have focused programs and initiatives on LGBT older people over the last five years, including among others, the Center for American Progress, the Equal Rights Center, FORGE, the Human Rights Campaign, the National Center for Lesbian Rights, and the National Gay and Lesbian Task Force (SAGE, n.d.d). Notably, the American Society on Aging coordinates a national network focused on LGBT aging issues that convenes key experts and produces research, news, analysis, and scholarship on matters relevant to LGBT older adults (American Society on Aging, n.d.).

State Organizations

SAGE affiliates exist in 26 cities and towns around the country (across 19 states and Washington, DC) providing aging services to LGBT elders and engaging in local and state advocacy (SAGE, n.d.e). These affiliates tend to be small in budget size and programmatic scope, and they exist as programs within broader-themes nonprofits or as autonomous organizations (S. Worthington, personal communication, 2014). Additionally, local organizations focused on LGBT elders exist in other parts of the country; notable examples include GLBT Generations (Minneapolis, MN); the LA Gay and Lesbian Center of LA (Los Angeles); Lavender Seniors of the East Bay (Oakland, CA); Openhouse (San Francisco); SunServe (Wilton Manors, FL); and Training to Serve (St. Paul, MN). Three organizations focus on LGBT older people of color: the Azteca Project (Chula Vista, CA); the Detroit Elder Project at KICK (Detroit, MI); and GRIOT Circle (Brooklyn, NY) (SAGE, n.d.d).

Partnerships and Coalitions

To address the policy barriers faced by LGBT older people, nonprofits have formed partnerships and coalitions on a range of issues. SAGE has partnered with the Movement Advancement Project and the National Center for Transgender Equality to author policy reports on LGBT aging and transgender elders, respectively, and it has partnered with groups such as the Equal Rights Center and the National Hispanic Council on Aging to support the research methodologies and report releases of policy studies on housing discrimination and LGBT Latino older people, respectively (Equal Rights Center 2014; Movement Advancement Project and SAGE 2010; National Hispanic Council on Aging 2014; SAGE and National Center for Transgender Equality 2012). In 2010, seven organizations formed the Diverse Elders Coalition, a coalition focused on federal policy improvements for elder of color and LGBT elders; since 2010, the coalition has increased policy awareness and led advances in areas such as the Older Americans Act, the Affordable Care Act, and HIV and aging, among others. This coalition has highlighted how organizations with different marginalized populations can find common areas of interest and leverage their institutional power to affect large-scale change (Espinoza 2011, pp. 8–12). The National Gay and Lesbian Task Force coordinates a "New Beginning Initiative" focused on administrative and regulatory policy opportunities for LGBT people, including a working group of 10–12 national organizations focused on LGBT aging (National Gay and Lesbian Task Force, n.d.). Organizations such as ACRIA (AIDS Community Research Initiative of America), the Gay Men's Health Crisis, and SAGE have coled national policy research and advocacy related to HIV and aging (SAGE, n.d.). Around the country, nonprofits and individual advocates have formed coalitions and task forces to support policy change for LGBT elders. Three noteworthy examples are the LGBT Aging

Policy Task Force in San Francisco; the LGBT Older Adult Coalition in Detroit, MI; and the LGBT Elder Initiative in Philadelphia, PA. These networks have overseen LGBT elder needs assessments, brought together advocates to produce policy reports and recommendations, and organized meetings and educational seminars on issues affecting LGBT older adults in their communities (Bajko 2013; LGBT Elder Initiative, n.d.; The LGBT Older Adult Coalition, n. d.).

How did this LGBT aging sector come to be, and what can it accomplish in the future, as the needs of LGBT elders grow larger? Adams (2011) describes the historical context, possibilities, and limitations behind the relative growth of the LGBT aging sector since 2005, when the White House Conference on Aging first included LGBT delegates in its decennial gathering. Between 2007 and 2011, Adams notes that SAGE, the largest organization in this field, grew from a $1.5 million annual budget to nearly $7 million, and its local affiliates grew from six to 21. Adams argues that early leaders in the LGBT aging field succeeded in developing necessary local services for LGBT older people in different parts of the country, as well as in identifying the various policy barriers affecting LGBT elders, but they struggled with developing the type of institutional capacity (e.g., organizations, networks, coalitions) that could move political and cultural change at the federal and national levels and that could connect the dots among local groups to form a national grassroots movement. The author acknowledges that the election of an LGBT-friendly Presidential administration in 2008, the increased awareness of elders brought on by the aging of the Baby Boom generation, and the pivotal support of a handful of private foundations all contributed to a climate in which organizations such as SAGE could build its infrastructure and policy apparatus. It also created a climate where more organizations could prioritize LGBT older people, at least through discrete programs and initiatives. Nevertheless, the author emphasizes the urgency of policy change that can open up many more government funding streams to LGBT elder programs and

warns that the underfunded LGBT aging field is limited in its ability to focus on large-scale legislative reforms and culture change.

> Adams (2011) writes: At the same time, the experience of LGBT aging advocates also highlights some of the likely limits to progress during difficult times, as forward movement is shaped and restricted by who has the capacity to engage in the advocacy process, what issues stronger and larger institutions are effective at advancing, and in a still underdeveloped space like the LGBT aging field, what remains beyond the reach of even the field's strongest leaders (p. 18).

Issues to Be Resolved Through Research and Other Scholarship

A 2011 report on LGBT health from the Institute of Medicine calls for additional research on various issues related to later adulthood, including broader demographic and descriptive research (i.e., the number and percentage of elders who are LGBT, across their full diversity); family and interpersonal relations, including the role of families of choice; experiences with health services, including barriers to access and quality of care; physical and mental health; and sexual and reproductive health, including HIV and aging. The report also calls for more research on transgender and bisexual elders (Institute of Medicine 2011, pp. 283–284). More research in these areas could inform the types of programmatic interventions needed to support the full breadth of LGBT older adults. Additionally, the research could yield insight into the specific policy barriers faced by LGBT older people across the spectrum; for example, further research on bisexual older people would identify a host of policy opportunities to support aging among this population.

Further research should also assess the proper implementation of various policy proposals, including how to properly ask elder-appropriate questions related to sexual orientation and gender identity in both surveys and clinical settings—in ways that preserve confidentiality, yield accurate information, and shield LGBT respondents from prejudice, stereotypes, and discrimination from health providers and social service staff collecting these data (Espinoza 2013a, b). Elder-friendly questions in surveys and clinical questions should be routinely tested and validated, and best practices on these questions should be widely shared across sectors that interact with LGBT older people. Policy proposals also request that agencies within the national aging network, such as state and area units on aging, report the extent to which they conduct outreach to LGBT communities, as well as track the number of LGBT older people they serve (SAGE, n.d.b). Recognizing the possible biases of staff members within the aging network, and the limited resources afforded to aging services in many areas of the country, further research should understand the feasibility of revising local intake forms to better capture these data, as well as how to provide data on LGBT people in cost-effective ways. Around the country, aging providers and LGBT community organizations are developing and implementing programs and services that are meant to support the health, community, and financial security of LGBT older people (Barrios-Paoli and Thurston 2011). Research should assess the impact and effectiveness of these programs, with advice on which programs could yield the best outcomes with the most efficient resources and which programs can be properly replicated throughout the country. The LGBT aging field could benefit from a slate of evidence-based practices that address the various subpopulations that comprise LGBT elders, as well as the range of later adulthood issues outlined in the 2011 IOM report on LGBT health.

Summary

LGBT older people are at the center of a demographic shift that is rapidly changing the US population. As the Baby Boom generation continues turning age 65, millions of LGBT people will become more visible in the aging and long-term care field. This increase in elder

numbers and LGBT visibility has sparked the imagination of policy advocates who have produced a vast literature documenting the many policy barriers faced by LGBT older people. In general, LGBT elders lack the community support, economic security, and proper health and healthcare access to age successfully. They face an array of concerns, from health and economic security, to data collection and housing, to reforming major legislation such as the Older American Act and much more. Recent advances in regard to marriage equality for same-sex couples have shifted the economic supports for legally married LGBT older adult couples, but these federal benefits related to marriage constitute only a small fraction of the inequalities and hardships faced by the broader LGBT older adult population, in particular transgender people, poor and low-income people, and people of color.

Is the current LGBT aging sector sufficiently resourced to meet this demand? Many advocates fear that it is not. The LGBT aging sector needs to grow in its scope and strength, and the broader aging and long-term care must become increasingly responsive to LGBT issues in order to address the profound aging of America. Recently, progress has been made as mainstream aging organizations have begun to lend their support and resources to partnerships and coalitions that are focused on repairing the policy inequities of LGBT older people.

Yet any forward movement in public progress also raises more questions. If the LGBT aging field is able to convince the aging network to track the extent to which they serve LGBT older people, what's the best and most inexpensive way to accomplish this goal, given that we live in an economic era of restrained financial resources? If health and aging providers become increasingly aware about the existence of LGBT people in their clientele, how should we equip these thousands of practitioners with the tools and training to work with this growing demographic? Policy implementation and enforcement is as important as policy advancement, especially when dealing with vulnerable populations.

The LGBT aging field has made significant strides in moving the aging field to the point where it can ask these more difficult questions—now it needs the large-scale private and public support to move the national dial in support of LGBT elders nationwide.

Learning Activities

Self-check Questions

1. What role do LGBT elders play in self-advocacy?
2. What are the barriers to inclusion of LGBT elders in discussion on aging policy?
3. What are the challenges faced by systemic data collection of LGBT elders in research?

Experiential Exercises

1. Conceptualize ways in which you can advocate on behalf of LGBT elders.
2. Develop an interdisciplinary approach in which LGBT elder can plan and implement self-advocacy strategies.
3. Start a letter writing campaign to state legislators and policy makers to promote fairness and equity for LGBT elders.

Multiple-Choice Questions

1. Which of the following contributed to a climate in which organizations such as SAGE could build it infrastructure and policy apparatus?
   (a) Election of an LGBT-friendly Presidential administration in 2008
   (b) Increased awareness of elders brought on by the aging Baby Boom generation
   (c) Support of a handful of private foundations

(d) All of the above
(e) None of the above

2. Which of the following is the largest organization in the LGBT aging sector?
   (a) PFLAG
   (b) SAGE
   (c) AARP
   (d) EEOC

3. Which of the following is a barrier to accessing supportive communities for LGBT Latino people as they age?
   (a) Biases of more conservative people of faith
   (b) Lack of environments that embrace LGBT elders as people with multiple identities
   (c) Compounding challenges of having survived discrimination rooted in their sexual and gender identity
   (d) All of the above
   (e) None of the above

4. Which of the following legislation contains an array of barriers in affordable housing, HIV and aging, economic security, and employment?
   (a) Older Americans Act
   (b) Senior Citizen Protection Act
   (c) Elders Anti-Victimization Act
   (d) LGBT Aging Act

5. When seeking housing in senior-living facilities, LGBT people often experience which of the following treatment?
   (a) Subsidized funding
   (b) More information about additional units
   (c) Required to pay additional fees or cost
   (d) Undergo an abridged application process

6. Which of the following usually impair LGBT elders' financial security, healthcare access, and level of social support?
   (a) Broad definition of family
   (b) Affordable Care Act requirement of routine medical tests
   (c) Reliance of families of choice that are not legally protected

(d) Extensive reporting protocols

7. Which of the following is considered a landmark policy report for laying the groundwork and anticipates the policy advocacy movement on LGBT elders?
    (a) The Aging and Health Report
    (b) Outing Age
    (c) Expanded and Improved Medicare for All Act
    (d) Older Workers; Employment Preferences

8. Which of the following legislation put into place a number of enhancements for LGBT people and seniors to prevent health insurers from denying coverage based on preexisting conditions such as a person's gender identity or HIV status?
    (a) Affordable Care Act
    (b) Anti-Transgender Discrimination Act
    (c) Senior Health Care Equity Law
    (d) Medicare

9. Which of the following is a systematic barrier to LGBT-friendly patient-centered health care?
    (a) Questions about sexual orientation and gender identity are stated negatively
    (b) Questions about sexual orientation and gender identity are too intrusive
    (c) Questions about sexual orientation and gender identity are rarely asked
    (d) Questions about sexual orientation and gender identity are only intervention-focused

10. Which of the following is the primary reason for LGBT older people avoiding or delaying services?
    (a) Fear of diagnosis
    (b) Fear of not being screened properly by medical professionals
    (c) Fear of being identified by the wrong gender pronoun
    (d) Fear of discrimination

Key

1-d
2-b
3-d
4-a
5-c
6-c
7-b
8-a
9-c
10-d

References

ACRIA (AIDS Community Research Initiative of America). (2013, September 18). *ACRIA testifies at congressional hearing on HIV and aging* (Press release). Retrieved from http://www.acria.org/news/acria-testifies-at-congressional-hearing-on-hiv-and-aging.html.

Adams, M. (2011). Reflections on advancing an LGBT aging agenda. *Public Policy & Aging Report: Integrating Lesbian, Gay, Bisexual, and Transgender Older Adults into Aging Policy and Practice, 21*(3), 14–18.

Administration on Aging, Administration for Community Living. (2013). *A profile of older Americans: 2013.* Washington, DC: U.S. Department of Health and Human Services.

American Academy of HIV Medicine, American Geriatrics Society and AIDS Community Research Initiative of America. (2011). *The HIV and aging consensus project: Recommended treatment strategies for clinicians managing older patients with HIV.* Retrieved from http://hiv-age.org/clinical-recommendations/.

American Society on Aging. (n.d.). *LGBT aging issues network.* Retrieved from http://www.asaging.org/lain.

Bajko, M. (2013, February 7). Report details SF LGBT senior issues. *The Bay Area reporter.* Retrieved from http://www.ebar.com/news/article.php?sec=news&article=68486.

Barrios-Paoli, L., & Thurston, C. (2011). Bridging the service gap: LGBT older adults, public–private partnerships and program innovation. *Public Policy & Aging Report: Integrating Lesbian, Gay, Bisexual, and Transgender Older Adults into Aging Policy and Practice, 21*(3), 28–29.

Cahill, S., Darnell, B., Guidry, J., Krivo-Kaufman, A., Schaefer, N., Urbano, L., et al. (2010). *Growing older with the epidemic: HIV and aging.* New York, NY: Gay Men's Health Crisis.

Cahill, S., South, K., & Spade, J. (2000). *Outing age: Public policy issues affecting gay, lesbian, bisexual and transgender elders.* New York, NY: The Policy Institute of the National Gay and Lesbian Task Force.

Center for American Progress. (2013a). *LGBT Communities and the Affordable Care Act: Findings from a national survey.* Washington, DC: CAP.

Center for American Progress. (2013b). *Uninsured LGBT People and the Affordable Care Act: Research on* outreach and communication strategies from the Center for American Progress. Washington, DC: CAP.

Centers for Disease Control and Prevention. (2013). Diagnoses of HIV infection among adults aged 50 years and older in the United States and dependent areas, 2007–2010. HIV Surveillance Supplemental Report 2013. Retrieved from http://www.cdc.gov/hiv/topics/surveillance/resources/reports/#supplemental.

Cray, A. (2013, August 6). ENDA provides protections for older LGBT Americans. Retrieved from http://www.americanprogress.org/issues/lgbt/news/2013/08/06/71553/enda-provides-protections-for-older-lgbt-americans/.

Diverse Elders Coalition. (2014). 8 policy recommendations for improving the health and wellness of older adults with HIV. New York, NY: DEC.

Equal Rights Center. (2014). Opening doors: An investigation of barriers to senior housing for same-sex couples. Washington, DC: ERC.

Espinoza, R. (2011). The diverse elders coalition and LGBT aging: Connecting communities, issues, and resources in a historic moment. Public Policy & Aging Report: Integrating Lesbian, Gay, Bisexual, and Transgender Older Adults into Aging Policy and Practice, 21(3), 8–12.

Espinoza, R. (2013a, November 2013). The unmeasured LGBT life. The Huffington Post. Retrieved from http://www.huffingtonpost.com/robert-espinoza/the-unmeasured-lgbt-life_b_4261203.html.

Espinoza, R. (2013b, July 31). Five years of political progress for LGBT older people—but more remains. (Blog post). Retrieved from http://blog.sageusa.org/blog/2013/07/five-years-of-political-progress-for-lgbt-older-peoplebut-more-remains-1.html#sthash.I6fG0hGz.dpuf.

Espinoza, R. (2014, February 28). LGBT people: Our longing for home, our right to housing. The Huffington Post. Retrieved from http://www.huffingtonpost.com/robert-espinoza/lgbt-people-our-longing-f_b_4858491.html.

Ford, Z. (2014) Why an LGBT nondiscrimination executive order would not be 'redundant.' Think Progress. Retrieved from http://thinkprogress.org/lgbt/2014/04/04/3422936/why-an-lgbt-nondiscrimination-executive-order-would-not-be-redundant/.

Foundation Center. (2013). Key facts on U.S. Foundations. New York, NY. Foundation Center.

Freedom to Marry. (2013, July 3). After DOMA: What it means for you. Retrieved from http://www.freedomtomarry.org/resources/entry/after-doma-what-it-means-for-you.

Fredriksen-Goldsen, K. I., Kim, H.-J., Emlet, C. A., Muraco, A., Erosheva, E. A., Hoy-Ellis, C. P., et al. (2011). The aging and health report: Disparities and resilience among lesbian, gay, bisexual, and transgender older adults. Seattle, WA: Institute for Multigenerational Health.

Funders for LGBTQ Issues. (2009). Lesbian, gay, bisexual, transgender and queer grantmaking by U.S. Foundations (2007). New York, NY: Funders for LGBTQ Issues.

Funders for LGBTQ Issues. (2013). 2012 tracking report: Lesbian, gay, bisexual, transgender and queer grantmaking by U.S. Foundations. New York, NY: Funders for LGBTQ Issues.

Goodwin, L., & Knox, O. (2014). Murray bill would force Social Security to pay same-sex spouses survivor benefits. Yahoo News. Retrieved from http://news.yahoo.com/murray-bill-would-force-social-security-to-pay-same-sex-spouses-survivor-benefits-220923730.html.

Human Rights Campaign. (2014a). Housing for LGBT people: What you need to know about property ownership and discrimination. Retrieved from http://www.hrc.org/resources/entry/housing-for-lgbt-people-what-you-need-to-know-about-property-ownership-and.

Human Rights Campaign. (2014b, May 15). Employment Non-Discrimination Act. Retrieved from http://www.hrc.org/laws-and-legislation/federal-legislation/employment-non-discrimination-act.

Institute of Medicine. (2011). The health of lesbian, gay, bisexual, and transgender people: Building a foundation for better understanding. Washington, DC: The National Academies Press.

Knochel, K., Croghan, C., Moone, R., & Quam, J. (2011). Ready to serve? The aging network and LGBT and T older adults. Minneapolis, MN: University of Minnesota College of Education and Human Development.

Lambda Legal. (2013). The Supreme Court ruling on the defense of Marriage Act: What it means. After DOMA. Retrieved from http://www.lambdalegal.org/publications/after-doma.

LGBT Elder Initiative. (n.d.). About us. Retrieved from http://www.lgbtei.org/p/about-us.html.

Make, J. (2013a). Time for a change: The case for LGBT-inclusive workplace leave laws & nondiscrimination protections. New York, NY: A Better Balance.

Make, J. (2013b, June 7). Why paid leave is an LGBT aging issue (Blog post). Retrieved from http://blog.sageusa.org/blog/2013/06/why-paid-leave-is-an-lgbt-aging-issue.html.

Movement Advancement Project and SAGE (Services and Advocacy for GLBT Elders). (2010). Improving the lives of LGBT older adults. Denver, CO: MAP.

National Academy on an Aging Society. (2011). Public policy & aging report: Integrating lesbian, gay, bisexual, and transgender older adults into aging policy and practice. Boston, MA: The Gerontological Society of America.

National Center for Transgender Equality. (2013). Transgender people and the Social Security administration. Washington, DC: NCTE.

National Center for Transgender Equality. (2014a, April 1). Victory: Social Security admin clarifies benefits applications for trans people and their spouses (Blog post). Retrieved from http://transgenderequality.wordpress.com/2014/04/01/victory-social-security-admin-clarifies-benefits-applications-for-trans-people-and-their-spouses/.

National Center for Transgender Equality. (2014b). *Fact sheet on medicare coverage of transition-related care.* Washington, DC: NCTE.

National Gay and Lesbian Task Force. (n.d.) *New beginning initiative.* http://www.thetaskforce.org/newadmin/newbeginning_intro.html.

National Health Policy Forum. (2012). *Older Americans Act of 1965: Programs and funding.* Washington, DC: George Washington University.

National Hispanic Council on Aging. (2014). *In their own words: A needs assessment of hispanic LGBT older adults.* Washington, DC: NHCOA.

National Resource Center on LGBT Aging. (2011). *HIV/AIDS and older adults: Fact versus fiction.* Retrieved from http://www.lgbtagingcenter.org/resources/resource.cfm?r=322.

National Resource Center on LGBT Aging. (2013). *Inclusive questions for older adults: A practical guide to collecting data on sexual orientation and gender identity.* New York, NY: SAGE.

National Resource Center on LGBT Aging. (2014). Our trainings. Retrieved from http://www.lgbtagingcenter.org/training/index.cfm.

National Senior Citizens Law Center. (2011). *Stories from the field: LGBT older adults in long-term care facilities.* Washington, DC: NSCLC.

Novak, S. (2014, January 6). Expand Social Security benefits to same-sex couples, no matter what the state. *Huffington Post.* Retrieved from http://www.huffingtonpost.com/scott-novak/same-sex-couples-social-security-benefits_b_4538692.html.

Old Lesbians Organizing for Change. (n.d.). About OLOC. Retrieved from http://www.oloc.org/about/index.php.

SAGE (Services and Advocacy for GLBT Elders). (2011a). Leadership Council of Aging Organizations issues official document on older Americans act-supporting LGBT elders in reauthorization (Press release). Retrieved from http://sageusa.org/newsevents/release.cfm?ID=35.

SAGE (Services and Advocacy for GLBT Elders). (2011b). *LGBT older adults and reauthorization of the older Americans Act.* New York, NY: SAGE.

SAGE (Services and Advocacy for GLBT Elders). (2013a). Affordable housing for LGBT older adults. National Resource Center on LGBT Aging. Retrieved from http://www.lgbtagingcenter.org/resources/resource.cfm?r=654.

SAGE (Services and Advocacy for GLBT Elders). (2013b). *Health equity and LGBT elders of color:* *Recommendations for policy and practice.* New York, NY: SAGE.

SAGE (Services and Advocacy for GLBT Elders). (2013d). *Why new health coverage options matter to me.* New York, NY: SAGE.

SAGE (Services and Advocacy for GLBT Elders). (2014a, May 8). SAGE applauds new guidance by ACL that extends benefits to same-sex married couples (Blog post). Retrieved from http://blog.sageusa.org/blog/2014/05/sage-applauds-new-guidance-by-acl-that-extends-benefits-to-same-sex-married-couples.html.

SAGE (Services and Advocacy for GLBT Elders). (n.d.a). *The issues: HIV and aging.* Retrieved from http://sageusa.org/issues/hiv.cfm.

SAGE (Services and Advocacy for GLBT Elders). (n.d.b). *The issues: Older Americans Act.* Retrieved from http://sageusa.org/issues/oaa.cfm.

SAGE (Services and Advocacy for GLBT Elders). (n.d.c). National LGBT aging roundtable. Retrieved from http://sageusa.org/programs/roundtable.cfm.

SAGE (Services and Advocacy for GLBT Elders). (n.d.d). *Our partners.* Retrieved from http://sageusa.org/about/partners.cfm.

SAGE (Services and Advocacy for GLBT Elders). (n.d.e). SAGENet. Retrieved from http://sageusa.org/advocacy/sagenet.cfm.

SAGE (Services and Advocacy for GLBT Elders). (n.d.f). What we do. Retrieved from http://sageusa.org/about/what.cfm.

SAGE (Services and Advocacy for GLBT Elders) and National Center for Transgender Equality. (2012). *Improving the lives of transgender older adults: Recommendations for policy and practice.* New York, NY: SAGE.

Tax, A. (2014). The latest news from D.C. *SAGE Matters,* 6.

The Fenway Institute and The Center for American Progress. (2013). *Asking patients questions about sexual orientation and gender identity in clinical settings: A study in four health centers.* Boston, MA: The Fenway Institute.

The LGBT Older Adult Coalition. (n.d.). About the coalition. Retrieved from http://lgbtolderadults.com/about/.

U.S. Department for Health and Human Service. (2013). Healthy People 2020. Washington, DC. Available at http://www.healthypeople.gov/2020/default.aspx.

Wayland, S. (2014). Year in review: A national resource makes an impact. Available at http://www.lgbtagingcenter.org/about/NRC/_YearInReview.pdf.

Disabilities and Chronic Illness Among LGBT Elders: Responses of Medicine, Public Health, Rehabilitation, and Social Work

33

Debra A. Harley

Abstract

Aging is frequently marked by chronic conditions and disability involving physical, psychological, and sensory disorders. Individuals with adult or later onset of chronic illness or acquired disability (CIAD) tend to experience more adjustment difficulties than those with early onset. Although most elderly adults remain healthy throughout the aging process, many LGBT elders do have chronic conditions and disabilities that affect their health and successful aging. This chapter reviews disabilities and chronic conditions that affect LGBT elders, challenges they face in dealing with disabilities and chronic illness, and implications of health care and health policy.

Keywords

Disability · Chronic illness · Late onset · Acquired disability

Overview

Aging is frequently marked by chronic conditions and disability involving physical, psychological, and sensory disorders. Normal age-related changes occur within various body systems, affecting physiological, pharmacological, behavioral, and cognitive responses. The rate of disability is higher in the elderly population in comparison with the general population and disproportionately higher in LGBT elders than non-LGBT elders, with the highest rates among ethnic minorities (Espinoza 2011). A disability may be due to a developmental stage of the aging process, the result of an accident, environmental factors, lifestyle, or congenital factors. Although the prevalence of various disabilities gradually increases with advancing age, it starts to accelerate after age 70 and causes a growing need for assistance, especially after age 80 (Heikkinen 2003). However, most elderly persons report good health in the presence of chronic illness, in part because they may expect illness as a natural consequence of aging and therefore alter their definition of health (Fredriksen-Goldsen 2011).

D.A. Harley (✉)
University of Kentucky, Lexington, USA
e-mail: dharl00@email.uky.edu

© Springer International Publishing Switzerland 2016
D.A. Harley and P.B. Teaster (eds.), *Handbook of LGBT Elders*,
DOI 10.1007/978-3-319-03623-6_33

The purpose of this chapter is to discuss disabilities and chronic conditions that affect LGBT older adults. Information is presented on the definitions of disability and chronic illness; the status of aging, health, and disability; characteristics and challenges of chronic illness and disability among LGBT elders; targets for intervention; and health care and policy issues.

Learning Objective

By the end of this chapter, the reader should be able to:

1. Understand the concept of disability.
2. Understand co-occurring disabilities and chronic conditions in the elderly.
3. Understand how LGBT elders are impacted by disabilities and chronic conditions.
4. Understand health disparities, interventions, and healthcare policies for LGBT elders.

Introduction

Individuals with adult or later onset of chronic illness or acquired disability (CIAD) tend to experience more adjustment difficulties than do those with early onset. It is hypothesized that those with early onset and longer duration have had more time to adjust to a disability. Individuals with CIAD are faced with significant changes in their social and familial relationships, vocational functions, and life roles while dealing concurrently with psychosocial distress, physical pain, loss of role identity and status, prolonged medical treatment, and gradually decreasing performance of self-care and daily activities (Bishop 2012; Falvo 2014). In addition, mental health plays an important role in physical health; poor mental health can increase risk of developing chronic health conditions or aggravate

existing conditions (Fredriksen-Goldsen et al. 2011).

The prevalence of disability among LGBT elderly is approximately 50 % (Fredriksen-Goldsen et al. 2011; Fredriksen-Goldsen et al. 2013). Wallace et al. (2011) found that LGB adults aged 50–70 had higher rates of physical disability compared to their heterosexual counterparts. Further inspection of these results based on the gender reveals that about 31 % of lesbians and 24 % of gay men report a disability as defined as a condition that substantially limits one or more basic instrumental activities of daily living (IADL). Heikkinen (2003) asserts that on the one hand disability in old age has identified non-modifiable risk factors such as age, gender, and genetics. On the other hand, disability in old age has modifiable risk factors such as age-related diseases, impairments, functional limitations, poor coping strategies, sedentary lifestyles and other unhealthy behaviors, as well as social and environmental obstacles, many of which stem from earlier phases of life and the prevalent socioeconomic conditions. Moreover, diseases, particularly multiple chronic illnesses, are the main causes of old-age disability. LGBT elders with disabilities must also contend with ableism; like homophobia and transphobia, it is pervasive in society.

The information in this chapter is not intended to stereotype elders as sick, depressed, cognitively or physically impaired, or fragile. Nevertheless, because most elderly adults remain healthy throughout the aging process and reside in their homes (Zians 2011), many other older adults, especially LGBT elders, develop chronic conditions and disabilities that affect their health and successful aging. Successful aging is identified with three important components: (a) avoiding disease, (b) staying engaged in life, and (c) maintaining high cognitive and physical functioning (Zians 2011). Nevertheless, the literature is consistent in the acknowledgment that with increasing age comes increased likelihood of disability.

Definition of Disability and Chronic Illness

The term "successful aging," which emphases that not all aging is negative, may inadvertently stigmatize older adults who have a disability (Chappell and Cooke 2010). Thus, Chappell and Cooke advance the notion of Kennedy and Minkler (1998), who argue that aging consists of both able bodies and disabled bodies and the notion of Zola (1993) that for individuals, disability "is not whether but when, not so much which one, but how many and in what combination" (p. 10). Disability is defined from various aspects including medical, vocational, and perceptual, and is interpreted from conceptual, legal, and cultural perspectives. In the broadest sense, disability refers to the functional limitations of activity that result from impairment (Falvo 2014). Conceptually, disability is not a condition that is inherent in the individual, but rather the result of the interaction between the person and the environment that imposes limitations on the person. The concept of disability has historical, social, legal, and philosophical influences on its interpretation (Disability World 2012). In some contexts, disability is considered a social phenomenon; however, the ability to carry out one's roles in life is also a medical entity (Fried et al. 2004). Culturally, a person may not consider him or herself as having a disability because he or she is still able to perform many activities of self-care and maintain a certain level of social interaction.

In the USA, legally, disability is defined in Section 504 of the Rehabilitation Act of 1973 and the Americans with Disabilities Act of 1990 as (a) "a physical or mental impairment that substantially limits one or more of the major life activities of such individuals, (b) a record of such an impairment, or (c) being regarded as having such an impairment" (Colker 2005, p. 101). The World Health Organization (WHO) (2011) defines disability as an umbrella term, which covers impairments (i.e., a problem in body function or structure), activity limitations (i.e., a difficulty encountered in executing a task or action), and participation restrictions (i.e., a problem experienced in involvement in life situations). Although there is no universal international legal definition of disability (Degener 2006), increasingly, the global community is utilizing the International Classification of Impairments, Disabilities and Handicaps (ICIDH) definition of disability, which describes three dimensions: impairment, disability, and handicap in the context of health experience (see Table 33.1). A new version of ICIDH is currently being drafted and may be published simultaneously with the release of this book. The new ICIDH will allow for more specific recognition of the third dimension of disability, with renaming it "participation" and recognition of the critical role played by the environment or contextual factors in restricting fill participation of persons with disabilities (Disability World 2012).

Table 33.1 ICIDH dimensions of disability

Impairment—Any loss or abnormality of psychological, physiological, or anatomical structure or function. Impairment is considered to occur at the level of organ or system function
Disability—Any restriction or lack (resulting from an impairment) of ability to perform an activity in the manner or within the range considered normal for a human being. Disability is concerned with how functional performance affects the whole person
Handicap—A disadvantage for a given individual, resulting from impairment or a disability, that limits or prevents the fulfillment of a role that is normal (depending on age, sex, and social and cultural factors) for that individual
The third dimension—Handicap focuses on the person as a social being and reflects the interaction with and adaptation to the person's surroundings. The classification system for handicap is not hierarchical, but is constructed of a group of dimensions, with each dimension having an associated scaling factor to indicate impact on the individual's life

Adapted from WHO (2011)

Across the life span, disability is typically defined in terms of difficulties in one or more physical activities of daily living (PADLS) (e.g., bathing, dressing, feeding, and toileting) or in one or more IADLs (e.g., walking, housekeeping, shopping, using the phone, taking medication, climbing stairs, reaching, and lifting or carrying large objects) (Heikkinen 2003; Wallace et al. 2011). Loss of the ability to care for oneself appropriately results in further loss of independence and can lead to the need for care in an institutional setting (Centers for Disease Control and Prevention [CDC] 2013). Moreover, Heikkinen contends that the general pattern of an increase in disability with advancing age is fairly consistent across industrialized countries, even though there may be significant differences in the prevalence of particular disabilities and underlying factors.

Just as development is not static or finite, neither is disability. The effects of chronic illness and disability may differ depending on individual attributes and on different stages of development, impeding the development of certain skills associated with a particular stage of life. For example, for older adults, illness or disability can present physical or cognitive limitations in addition to those commonly associated with the aging process. An individual grows old gradually and does not suddenly become old when he or she turns age 60, 65, or 70 (Chappell and Cooke 2010). Disability is a process of continuous adaptation to changes across the life span (Sheets 2010). Eventually, disability limits autonomy, introduces dependence, reduces quality of life, and increases risk of assisted living or custodial care and premature death (Fried et al. 2004; Heikkinen 2003).

One of the essential functions to an individual's everyday life is mobility. In fact, mobility is considered central to an understanding of health and well-being among older populations. Limited or lack of mobility significantly narrows an older person's world and ability to do things that bring enjoyment and meaning to life (Centers for Disease Control and Prevention 2013).

The physical environment offers the potential to assist an individual to intrinsic disability (i.e., ability to perform an activity regardless of context) through the removal or modification of environmental barriers. Thus, for persons with disabilities the goal is to enhance an individual's actual ability (i.e., ability to perform an activity when supported by the physical or social environment) (Chappell and Cooke 2010; Verbrugge and Jette 1994). The challenge for many older adults with disabilities and chronic illness is that aging-in-place (remaining at home) may be compromised by environmental hazards and barriers, common in the homes of older adults (Chappell and Cooke). Table 33.2 identifies modifications often needed for older adults to remain at home as they age. In addition, fear of discrimination and stigma drives many LGBT elders to avoid services that might enable them to stay in their homes and avoid premature institutionalization (Funders for Lesbian and Gay Issues 2004).

Without traditional support systems that allow them to age-in-place, many LGBT elders end up relying on nursing homes or other facilities to provide long-term care (MAP and SAGE 2010).

Table 33.2 Modifications necessary for elders to age-in-place

Automatic door openers or door handles instead of doorknobs
Flashing lights connect to doorbell for those hard-of-hearing
Frequently used items in a lower location/easier to reach
Handrails in showers, bathtubs, and around toilet area
Wider doorways, hallways, and circulation paths
No carpet and fewer transitions in flooring
Lower counters, tables, and cabinets
Step-free entry into shower
Enhanced ringer on phone
Handrails on walls
Large print dials
Brighter lighting
Exterior ramps

Status of Aging, Health, and Disability

Throughout the world, people are living longer, and their quality of life, to a large extent, is determined by their health status. Over the past century, a major shift occurred in the leading cause of death for all age groups, from infectious diseases and acute illnesses to chronic diseases and degenerative illnesses. Global estimates for disability are increasing due to population aging and the rapid spread of chronic diseases, as well as improvements in the methodologies used to measure disability (WHO 2011). Moreover, WHO (2011) suggests that disability is part of the human condition in which everyone will be temporarily or permanently impaired at some point in life. Persons who reach old age will experience increasing difficulties in functioning. Two out of every three older Americans have multiple chronic conditions and accounts for 66 % of the country's healthcare budget (Centers for Diseases Control and Prevention 2013; National Institute on Aging [NIA], National Institutes of Health [NIH] 2011). The National Report on Healthy Aging reports on 15 indicators of older adult health, which are grouped into four areas: health status, health behaviors, preventive care and screening, and injuries. Eight of the 15 indicators are contained in *Healthy People 2020*. To date, the USA has met six of the *Healthy People 2020* targets (i.e., leisure time physical activity, obesity, smoking, taking medications for high blood pressure, mammograms, and colorectal cancer screenings), with most states ahead of schedule on four health indicators for older adults (i.e., obesity, medications for high blood pressure, mammography, smoking), and with significant work to do on other indicators for older adults (i.e., flu vaccine, pneumonia) (Centers for Disease Control and Prevention). The Centers for Disease Control and Prevention identifies the areas where services are most needed for LGBT elders: housing, transportation, legal services, and chronic disease prevention.

Heart disease and cancer pose the greatest risks as people age, and for older adults, other chronic diseases and conditions including Alzheimer's disease, diabetes, chronic lower respiratory, stroke, influenza, and pneumonia represent the major contributors to deaths (Centers for Disease Control and Prevention 2013; WHO 2011). Typically, older adults have multiple illnesses; the varied nature of these conditions requires intervention from multiple healthcare specialists, various treatment regimens, and prescription medications that may not be compatible. Because of these multiple conditions, older adults are at an increased risk for having conflicting medical advice, adverse drug effects, unnecessary and duplicative tests, and avoidable hospitalizations (Centers for Disease Control and Prevention).

Although disability correlates with disadvantage, not all persons with disabilities are equally disadvantaged. Women, the elderly, the poorest, and those with more severe impairments experience greater discrimination and barriers (WHO 2009, 2011). LGBT elders are represented consistently across these groups. The documentation of widespread evidence of barriers that are identified by WHO (2011) (see Table 33.3) for persons with disabilities parallels the barriers experienced by LGBT elders.

The status of aging, health, and disability discussed in this section is relevant to LGBT elders. In addition, LGBT older adults have complex outcomes for chronic illness and disabilities. The following section examines the occurrence of health and disability-related conditions that are specific to LGBT elders.

Chronic Illness and Disability Among LGBT Elders

Physical disability occurs frequently in older adults and is "an outcome of diseases and physiological alterations with aging, with the impact of these underlying causes modified by social, economic, and behavioral factors as well as access to medical care" (Fried et al. 2004, p. 256). With the diversity of life span, health

Table 33.3 Barriers for persons with disabilities

Inadequate policies and standards—policy design does not always take into account the needs of persons with disabilities, or existing policies and standards are not enforced
Negative attitudes—beliefs and prejudices constitute barriers to education, employment, health care, and social participation
Lack of provision of services—persons with disabilities are particularly vulnerable to deficiencies in services such as health care, rehabilitation, and support and assistance
Problems with service delivery—poor coordination of services, inadequate staffing, and weak staff competencies can affect the quality, accessibility, and adequacy of services for persons with disabilities
Inadequate funding—resources allocated to implementing policies and plans are often inadequate
Lack of accessibility—many built environments, transportation systems, and information are not accessible to all. Lack of access is a frequent reason for persons with disabilities being discouraged from seeking employment, inclusion, or accessing health care
Lack of consultation and involvement—many persons with disabilities are excluded from decision making in matters directly affecting their lives
Lack of data and evidence—a lack of rigorous and comparable data on persons with disabilities and their circumstances and evidence on programs that work can impede understanding and action

Adapted from WHO (2011)

outcomes, and other individual variations among older persons, elders are frequently identified as vulnerable because of comorbidity (multiple chronic conditions), frailty, and disability. Fried et al. assert that these clinical entities are distinct but causally related in that both frailty and comorbidity predict disability, disability exacerbates frailty and comorbidity, and comorbid diseases may contribute, at least additively, to the development of frailty. No distinction is made between the older population and older LGBT adults for these clinical entities. Over two decades ago, Fine and Asch (1988) asserted that almost all research on adults with disabilities seemed to assume the irrelevance of sexual orientation and presume that having a disability eclipses social experience. To date the majority of research on aging and disability and chronic illness continues to ignore LGBT elders. For LGBT persons with disabilities, a disability is likened to living in the "second closet" (Benedetti 2011). Thus, only estimates of the full extent of LGBT health disparities are possible due to a consistent lack of data collection. The main areas of disparity are access to health care, HIV/AIDS, mental health, and chronic physical conditions (MAP and SAGE 2010).

Understanding chronic conditions and disability among LGBT elders is increasingly important for several reasons: (a) advances in medicine, public health, rehabilitation, and technology have increased life expectancy for persons with disabilities; (b) LGBT elders have limited access to culturally sensitive and LGBT-affirmative service; (c) older adults are remaining in the workforce longer; (d) LGBT elders are among the poorest of the poor, especially women; (e) LGBT elders have higher rates of health disparities; and (f) quality of life is compounded by the intersection of age, sexual orientation or gender identity, and disability (Harley 2015). Increasing numbers of older adults living to reach old age (including LGBT elders) have changed the demographics of disability (Sheets 2010). The case of Gloria below is an illustration of a lesbian who acquired a disability earlier in life and additional chronic illnesses as she aged.

Case Study of Gloria Gloria is a 67-year-old African American lesbian. She was diagnosed with multiple sclerosis at age 36. Gloria worked as a college professor until her disability forced her to retire at age 57. Subsequently, she was diagnosed with arthritis in her hands and knees at age 48 and recently with macular degeneration of the eye. Gloria does not go to the doctor on a regular basis. She waits until the symptoms of her illnesses become, as she describes them, intolerable.

Gloria was married and divorced at age 23. She has two grown children who live in other states. Gloria served in the army for eight years. Gloria has ongoing contact with her children.

Gloria is still able to drive, but has reduced the distance that she will drive because of muscle weakness, severe headaches, and vision problems. She is not active in the LGBT community, but she does have several lesbian and gay friends with whom she socializes. Gloria regards herself as an advocate for lesbians and women's rights.

Questions

What are the functional implications related to Gloria's disabilities?
What type medical specialists will Gloria have to see?
What are the cultural considerations in working with Gloria?
What do you need to know about Gloria's family dynamics and support system?
What issues must be addressed with regard to the intersection of age, disability, and ethnicity?

LGBT older adults are at an elevated risk of disability and mental distress, with 31 % reporting depression and more than 53 % of transgender older adults at risk of both disability and depression. The rates of disability among LGBT elders are also distinguishable by gender, with sexual minority women's health being significantly lower than men and heterosexual women. Older gay and bisexual men are more likely to experience poor physical health compared to heterosexual men. Bisexual men have significantly higher rates of cardiovascular disease than gay men. Transgender older adults are more likely than non-transgender older adults to have obesity, cardiovascular disease, asthma, and diabetes. Lesbians and bisexual women have similar rates of vision, hearing, and dental impairments; bisexual men have more vision impairments than gay men, and transgender older adults have more sensory and dental impairments than their non-transgender counterparts. Older lesbians are significantly more likely to engage in heavy drinking as compared to older bisexual women (Fredriksen-Goldsen 2011; Fredriksen-Goldsen et al. 2011).

In a study of disparities and resilience among LGBT older adults, Fredriksen-Goldsen et al. found that 41 % of the participants in the project had limitations in their physical activities as a result of physical, mental, or emotional problems. Of this percentage, 21 % were using adaptive equipment. An examination of the combination of LGBT older adults with limits in physical activities and the use of adaptive equipment reveals that 47 % have a disability, including 53 % of lesbians, 51 % of bisexual women, 41 % of gay men, 54 % of bisexual men, and 62 % of transgender older adults. Collectively, LGBT elders have diagnoses of high pretension (45 %), high cholesterol (43 %), arthritis (35 %), cataracts (22 %), asthma (16 %), diabetes (15 %), hepatitis (11 %), and osteoporosis (10 %). It is unknown if the rate of Alzheimer's disease among LGBT elders is different than the general elderly population.

The American Community Survey (ACS) is a general household survey conducted by the US Census Bureau and is designed to provide communities with reliable and timely demographic, economic, and housing information. An examination of ACS (Population Association of America 2014) data, from the 2009–2011, reveals that the prevalence of disability among older adults in same-sex relationships varies by gender and relationship type, and by type of disability. Overall, 17.5 % of older men in same-sex relationships were living with a disability compared to 20.8 % of married men and 21.5 % of unmarried men in opposite-sex relationships. Men in same-sex relationships were less likely to report difficulty in cognitive, ambulatory, self-care, and sensory functions compared to married and unmarried men in opposite-sex relationships. However, men in same-sex relationships were slightly more likely to report difficulties with independent living. On the other hand, women in same-sex relationships reported higher levels of almost all disability types compared to their married and unmarried counterparts in opposite-sex relationships, including any disability and difficulty in ambulatory, self-care, sensory, and independent living functions. The prevalence of cognitive difficulty for women in same-sex relationships was less than that of women in unmarried opposite-sex relationships, but more than that of women in married opposite-sex relationships. In summary, these data provide evidence of national disparities in disability between older adults in same-sex relationships compared to older adults in opposite-sex relationships. And, this relationship is especially strong and consistent for women (Populations Association of America).

Overall, mental health of LGBT elders is good (70.8 on a scale of 0 = very poor to 100 = excellent). In rating satisfaction with their life, lesbians report (71.8), bisexual women (65.6), gay men (71.7), bisexual men (65.6), and transgender older adults (62.7). Thirty-one percent of LGBT elders report some type of depressive symptoms, with 53 % having been told by a doctor that they have depression. Transgender older adults have the highest rate of depression (48 %), and lesbians (27 %) and gay men (29 %) have the lowest, and 24 % of LGBT older adults have been told they have anxiety (Fredriksen-Goldsen et al. 2011). Two of the most alarming mental health issues for LGBT elder are loneliness and social isolation (see Chap. 30). Both of these issues can lead to negative health consequences or be the result of chronic illness and disability. Older bisexual women and men exhibit higher rates of loneness than lesbians and gay men. The rates of neglect experienced by LGBT elders are similar to the general elderly population, and their rates of mistreatment tend to be higher (see Chaps. 16, 17, and 21 in this text). Across the categories of physical and mental health, transgender older adults fair worst than other LGB elders. The prevalence of physical and mental health problems is elevated among LGBT elders even taking into account differences in age distribution, income, and education; however, those LGBT elders with lower incomes and lower education are at more heightened risk (Fredriksen-Goldsen et al.).

Much of the sparse research that has been done on LGBT elders with disabilities has looked at either physical or mental disabilities. There is a clear lack of focus on LGBT older adults with developmental disabilities. This is especially disconcerting for two reasons. First, many persons with developmental disabilities have the same life expectancy as the general population. Second, while most people begin to experience the effects of aging in their 40s, some persons with a developmental disability may require a greater level of support at a younger age than the general population. The later reason requires more attention be given to factors associated with aging such as changes in social roles, activity levels, behavior patterns, and response to occurrences in the environment and health conditions (Connect Ability 2010). Some characteristics of aging may mask symptoms of a developmental disability and vice versa. For example, an older adult with Alzheimer's may exhibit a lack of insight or an inability to articulate what he or she is experiencing, both of which are characteristic of cognitive impairment associated with a developmental disability and Alzheimer's disease.

LGBT elders with disabilities and chronic conditions may find themselves facing issues of coming out or coming out again as needs for social services increase (Sue and Sue 2013). It is important for them to understand and be prepared for the potential negative responses they may receive as they complete the application process for services. For example, the answers that they provide on an application may inadvertently expose them to discrimination. Thus, LGBT elders' application for services because of a disability may be overshadowed by a service provider's preoccupation and bias with their sexual orientation or gender identity. Discussion Box 33.1 provides some examples of implications for practice.

Discussion Box 33.1

Implications for practice with LGBT older adults

Avoid use of heterosexist language.

Be aware if the person has competency issues.

Do not use labeling language (e.g., disabled person).

Be aware of a change in name of a transgender person.

Ask the person by what name he or she want to be addressed.

To the extent possible, give the person as much autonomy as possible.

Be aware that LGBT clients have specific concerns about confidentiality.

Recognize the historical affects of stigma related to sexual identity and age.

Be knowledgeable of the person's support system or the need to establish one.

Understand the functional limitations of disabilities/chronic conditions for the individual.

Do not assume that the presenting problem is the result of sexual orientation, or gender identity.

Assist the person in identifying concerns that have to be addressed in the short-term and long-term (e.g., housing, end-of-life issues).

Recognize that mental health issues may be the result of stress related to homophobia/transphobia, internalized homophobia, the coming out process, or lack of support systems.

Questions

1. What are the ways that you can prepare to address these issues?
2. Do you know the resources that can assist you in supporting your efforts to work with LGBT elders with disabilities?
3. How can the intersection of disability, age, and sexual identity impact service delivery?

Service Needs and Intervention

Disability is complex, and the interventions to overcome the challenges associated with disability are multiple and systemic, varying with the context (WHO 2011). An area of critical concern for elders is affordable housing as they age-in-place. LGBT elders identify housing as the number one priority for action in a needs assessment conducted by Senior Action in a Gay Environment (SAGE) (Funders for Lesbian and Gay Issue 2004). Moreover, housing discrimination is of primary concern, including "trepidation" about mainstream senior housing options (Knauer 2009; National Gay and Lesbian Task Force 2006). Implicit in affordability is accessible housing that will allow elders to maintain independence, quality of life, and safety in terms of both the condition of the dwelling and residential location. The ability to obtain adequate and safe housing affects all aspects of life (e.g., employment, proximity to friends and family, access to services), and the relationship between housing and other aspects of everyday life is particularly important for older persons who may be more restricted because of their mobility, income, and support systems (Equal Rights Center 2014).

The Equal Rights Center (2014) conducted an investigation to determine the extent of adverse, differential treatment experienced by a senior seeking housing for oneself and a same-sex spouse. The study used matched pair testing (i.e., one LGB senior tester and one heterosexual senior tester) in 200 tests across 10 states. In 96 (48 %) of the 200 tests conducted, the LGB tester experienced at least one type of adverse, differential treatment as compared to the heterosexual tester with an opposite-sex spouse. The differential treatment was not as blatant as refusal or rejection by a housing provider. Instead, barriers to equal housing opportunity ranged from differences in availability, pricing, fees and costs, incentives to rent, amenities available, and application requirements. Sometimes, housing providers refused to recognize the same-sex couples, encouraging them to apply separately or restricting them from living together. More blatant cases of differential treatment include housing providers making degrading remarks, being less than inviting, or being hostile. Although this study did not include transgender persons, discrimination is also a widespread problem against them, regardless of their sexual orientation, which typically results in being denied a home or apartment, being evicted because of being transgender or gender non-conforming, and homelessness (Grant et al. 2011). Other studies found that gay or lesbian home seekers were subject to unfavorable treatment 27 % of the time (Michigan Fair Housing Centers 2007), and when emailing the same housing provider to inquire about housing availability, opposite-sex couples were more likely to receive a response than same-sex couples (Davis et al. 2013). See Chap. 21 for additional discussion on housing concerns of LGBT elders.

Many older adults with disabilities rely on assistive animals (e.g., service animals, support animals, assistance animals, therapy animals) to perform tasks or provide support that alleviates at least one of the functional limitations or effects of a disability. Persons with an assistive animal who are refused rental housing or required to pay an additional fee or deposit essentially deny persons with disabilities access to housing. Despite legal protection, persons who use assistive animals are frequently denied required accommodations (Equal Rights Center 2012). The Equal Rights Center found that housing providers or leasing agents either do not know the reasonable accommodation policies in place for their properties, or do not obtain and provide this information for a potential tenant with a disability on request.

Healthcare and Other Services. Often, providing healthcare services, counseling, and other social services to LGBT elders is challenging because of stigma and discrimination from service providers. According to the American Medical Association (2009), the failure of physicians to recognize patient's sexual orientation and gender identity and patients non-disclosure can result in serious medical problems, inferior health care, or denial of appropriate services. The distribution of discrimination by service providers against LGBT elders is even more so against transgender elders. In a survey of 320 area agencies and state units on aging, Knochel et al. (2011) found that more than one in four reported that transgender older adults would either not be welcomed by local service providers or the agency was unsure of how welcome they would be. The Institute of Medicine (2011) verifies that major research gaps in transgender aging, elder abuse, substance abuse, risk and best practices for long-term hormone therapy, sexual health, and cancers as areas in which more transgender researches are needed. Often, both fear and reality of discrimination lead to underutilization of services (Tobin 2011). Table 33.4 contains examples of discrimination and victimization experienced by LGBT elders and that create obstacles to accessing and utilizing necessary health and social support services. In addition, racism affects the health and healthcare experiences of ethnic minority LGBT elders differently than their non-minority counterparts (see Chaps. 5–8, and 10 in this text). The combination of ageism and homophobia or transphobia serves to demean, devalue, and denigrate older LGBT adults and pathologize their lives. Furthermore,

Table 33.4 Obstacles to LGBT elders accessing health and social support services

Ageism
Hostility
Harassment
Homophobia
Tansphobia
Lack of affordability
Threats of being "outed"
Denial or provision inferior services
Threats of physical violence
Violation of confidential information
Panic over dealing with heterosexual assumptions
Verbal insults and inappropriate nonverbal responses from service providers and staff
Refusal of healthcare systems to recognize extended families within the GBT Community

the discriminatory behavior of practitioners may result in inaccurately assessing LGBT elders presenting problems, refraining from providing appropriate services and referrals, increasing LGBT elders dependency on caregivers and service providers, and offering inappropriate treatments (Crisp et al. 2008).

Another area of critical concern for LGBT elders with disabilities is the need of support systems, both informal (e.g., family and friends) and formal (e.g., institutional care). Overreliance on informal support system often results in emotional stress, physical fatigue, and financial burden for those individuals. Reliance on institutional supports can result in increased dependency for LGBT elders. An overlapping and critical concern for LGBT elders with disabilities and chronic conditions is decision making about end-of-life issues (see Chap. 22). In the absence of a living will or healthcare directive, older LGBT adults may rely on members in their informal network to make decisions. These members may be denied access to an elder at the end of the life due to provisions in the Health Insurance Portability and Accountability Act (1996), one intention of which was to provide greater safeguards concerning medical records.

Most importantly, LGBT elders with disabilities and chronic conditions need to achieve recognition as a distinct minority group with needs unique from their heterosexual counterparts. The assumption of heterosexuality by service providers serves to not only relegate LGBT elders to secondary status because of age, disability, sexual orientation, and gender identity, but also to dismiss the reality that they exist. This belief informs the delivery of health care, social services, and social programs (Kimmel 2014). In fact Kimmel et al. (2015) use very explicit adjectives to describe the perceptual impact on LGBT elders by implicit heterosexual assumptions in various service arenas. These descriptions include how assumptions "limit" the language used in intake forms and communication, "prevent" discussion, "interfere" with, "preclude," "marginalize," and "alienate" LGBT seniors. In an effort to counteract these negative and aversive assumptions, the guidelines developed by The Joint Commission (2011) for hospitals and medical settings can be implemented by various human and social service entities (see Table 33.5).

The intent of identifying health disparities and other service needs of LGBT elders is to illuminate and define them in a way that advances the formulation of public policy and legislation (Gamble and Stone 2006). Too often, policies have discriminated against LGBT persons, failed to recognize them as deserving of equal protection under the law, and erected barriers to seeking and securing needed services for health and mental health. The overall objective of policy should be to decrease, eventually eliminate discriminatory practices, and level the playing field. The following section discusses policy implications for LGBT elders with disabilities.

Policy Issues

The disparities in disability between LGBT elders and their heterosexual counterparts in tandem with their status as an already vulnerable population should raise concern for practitioners and policymakers alike (Population Association of America 2014). As the overall population ages, the numbers of the most vulnerable (e.g., persons with disability, the elderly, women living alone, minorities) will grow as well. Clearly, an older population with health, disability, and mobility issues will drive the demand for home modifications, housing options that facilitate delivery of services and help prevent premature entry into assisted living facilities and nursing homes, flexible housing zoning polices, and aggressive enforcement of the requirements of the Fair Housing Act and the ADA to help LGBT elders age-in-place (Lipman et al. 2012). Of course, a critical concern is how to pay for the services to help LGBT elders with disabilities and chronic conditions age-in-place.

Developing policy that is responsive to the needs of LGBT elders with disabilities and chronic conditions does not always require the reinvention of services. Rather, modifications can be made in existing policy used to respond to

Table 33.5 Guidelines for provision of care

Create a welcoming environment that includes LGBT clients
Prominently post the program's non-discrimination policy
Ensure that waiting rooms and other common areas reflect and include LGBT clients and families (e.g., rainbow flag, LGBT-friendly periodicals)
Create or designate unisex or single-stall restrooms
Ensure that visitation policies are implemented in a fair, non-discriminatory manner
Foster an environment that supports and nurtures all clients and families
Avoid assumptions about a person's sexual orientation or gender identity based on the appearance
Be aware of misconceptions, biases, stereotypes, and other communication barriers
Promote disclosure of sexual orientation and gender identity while remaining aware that disclosure or "coming out" is an individual process
Make sure that all forms contain inclusive, gender-neutral language that allows for self-identification
Use neutral and inclusive language in interviews and when talking to all clients. Ask the client what pronoun is preferred
Listen to and reflect the client's choice of language when describing his or her own sexual orientation and how the client refers to his or her relationship or partner
Provide information and guidance for the specific health concerns of LGBT persons
Become familiar with online and local resources available for LGBT persons
Seek information and stay up-to-date on LGBT health topics
Be prepared with appropriate information and referrals

Adapted from The Joint Commission (2011)

barriers imposed on persons with disabilities and disadvantaged groups (e.g., WHO 2011). For example, emphasis should be placed on early intervention with the provision of services as close as possible to individuals' residence or community. For established services, the focus should be on improving efficiency and effectiveness by including LGBT-sensitive programming and improving quality and affordability. In less-resourced settings, the focus should be on accelerating the supply of LGBT-appropriate services, complemented by referrals to secondary services. Integrating LGBT services specific to elders with disabilities into primary and secondary healthcare settings can improve availability if these settings have practitioners who are sensitive to and competent in working with this population. In addition, referral systems between different modes of service delivery (e.g., inpatient, outpatient, home-based care), levels of health service provision (e.g., primary, secondary, and tertiary care facilities), and types of human and social service assistance (e.g., food

stamps, housing, and protection and advocacy) can improve access. For persons with disabilities, community-based services are a critical part of the continuum of care (WHO 2011).

An area in which policy issues and social concerns are lagging behind is in addressing older adults with HIV. Over time, AIDS has shifted from being dubbed the "gay" disease to equally affecting heterosexuals and disproportionately affecting women and people of color. People are living an almost typical life span if diagnosed and treated early. A growing number of older adults are getting HIV because they do not believe that they are at risk. In fact, older adults are more vulnerable to HIV infection than younger people due to biological changes associated with aging (e.g., thinner mucosal membranes in the anus and vagina) (Tietz and Schaefer 2011). In terms of policy, Tietz and Schaefer assert that the problem is that virtually no comprehensive, federal HIV prevention initiatives have been funded to target older adults in light of HIV being one of many treatable chronic conditions affecting this population. Therefore, several recommendations are presented for the Centers for Disease Control regarding HIV and older adults. First, the CDC needs to extend its age cap (ages 16–64) for recommended annual HIV testing to include adults over age 64, especially since many are sexually active. Second, develop HIV prevention models aimed specifically at older adults and should include a social messaging component to end the HIV and anti-gay stigma often seen in nursing homes, senior centers, and other senior programs. As part of its reauthorization, the Older Americans Act (OAA) can make legislation more responsive to older adults living with and at risk for HIV. Defining older adults with HIV as a population of greatest social need within the OAA will allow the Administration on Aging to dedicate critical resources for community planning and social services, research and development projects, and personnel training in the field of aging (Tietz and Schaefer).

Although there are existing aging services, public policy, and research initiatives intended to support older adults in times of need, most are inaccessible to LGBT elders and their loved ones. In addition, available services and programs are geared toward the general population and do not take into consideration the unique circumstances facing LGBT elders with disabilities and chronic conditions (Fredriksen-Goldsen et al. 2013). Moreover, policy and legislation for persons with disabilities do not include specific reference to LGBT persons with disabilities.

Summary

Almost half of the LGBT elders over age 50 have a disability. LGBT elders are at an elevated risk of disability, chronic conditions, and mental distress. Some of the disabilities and chronic health conditions of LGBT elders are a result of the aging process and others are related to stressor experienced as a result of a lifetime of stigma and discrimination. Similar to other groups, LGBT elders possess both strengths and

resilience and challenges and barriers that impact their health outcomes. Not all aging is negative. They must address the pervasiveness of ableism, homophobia, and transphobia. Certain health behaviors are more prevalent among older LGBT adults as compared to their heterosexual counterparts.

As a group, LGBT elders are one of the least understood in terms of their chronic health conditions and aging-related needs. The types of chronic conditions among LGBT elders vary according to gender. The severity of disability also affects the person's level of independence, mobility, their ability to age-in-place, and social inclusion.

Overwhelmingly, research on adults with disabilities has not focused on LGBT elders. Understanding LGBT elders within the context of disability has implications for the development of services and programs and policy. LGBT elders with disabilities have different attributes and characteristics that interact with age than their differently able peers, and deserve no less than having their differing and unique needs understood and served.

Research Box 33.1

Objective: To comprehensively examine disability among LGB adults through the use of population-based data.

Method: Estimated prevalence of disability and its covariates and compared by sexual orientation by using data from the Washington State Behavioral Risk Factor Surveillance System collected in 2003, 2005, 2007, and 2009. Multivariate logistic regression was used to analyze the relationship between disability and sexual orientation after controlling for covariates of disability.

Results: The prevalence of disability is higher among LGB adults compared with their heterosexual counterparts; LGB adults with disabilities are significantly younger than heterosexual adults with disabilities. Higher disability prevalence among lesbians and among bisexual women and men remained significant after we controlled for covariates of disability.

Conclusion: Higher rates of disability among LGB adults are of major concern. Efforts are needed to prevent, delay, and reduce disabilities as well as to improve the quality of life for lesbian, gay, and bisexual adults with disabilities. Future prevention and intervention efforts need to address the unique concerns of these groups.

Questions

1. What type of methodology might have been more appropriate for this study?
2. What is the importance of this study to public healthcare cost associated with disability in LGB adults as they age?
3. What implication does this study have for planning for intrinsic ability and actual ability of LGB adults as they age and want to age-in-place?
4. What are the limitations to this study?

Learning Exercises

Self-Check Questions

1. Do individuals with later onset of chronic illness or acquired disability (CIAD) or with early onset disability experience more adjustment difficulties?
2. At what age does disabilities start to accelerate?
3. What identifiable non-modifiable risk factors are associated with disability in old age?
4. What are the main causes of old-age disability?
5. What are the three important components of successful aging?

Field-Based Experiential Assignments

1. Interview an older lesbian, gay man, bisexual person, or transgender person with a disability. Based on the interview, help the person set up a resource guide.
2. Participate in advocacy services or activities for persons with disabilities through (a) attending public hearings, (b) doing background research for a protection and advocacy agency, or (c) attending a public demonstration for persons with disabilities.
3. Examine your own views of minority sexuality and aging. Next, examine how your views impact your ability and willingness to work with LGBT elders with disabilities. What are the ethical implications of your beliefs? Finally, consider that you or a family member are an LGBT elder with a disability or chronic condition and examine how you will feel.

Multiple-Choice Questions

1. A person with a disability who does not consider him or her self as having a disability because he or she can perform many activities of self-care and is able to maintain a certain level of social interaction, is exhibiting which of the following?
   (a) A condition inherent in the individual
   (b) Cultural perception of disability
   (c) A philosophical perception of disability
   (d) Denial
2. The definition of disability that states a disability is a physical or mental impairment that limits one or more of the major life activities, a record of impairment, or a person being regarded as having impairment, is the definition of which of the follow?
   (a) World Health Organization
   (b) Classification of Impairments, Disabilities, and Handicaps

(c) Americans with Disabilities Act

(d) Rehabilitation Act of 1973

3. Activities such as walking, dressing, feeding, and toileting are known as which of the following?

   (a) Physical activities of daily living

   (b) Instructional activities of daily living

   (c) Instrumental activities of daily living

   (d) Disability continuum of daily living

4. Which of the following groups among LGBT elders have the highest overall rate of disability?

   (a) Lesbians

   (b) Gay men

   (c) Bisexual men

   (d) Bisexual women

5. What are the two most alarming mental health issues for LGBT elders?

   (a) Bipolar disorder and loneliness

   (b) Loneliness and social isolation

   (c) Social isolation and depression

   (d) Depression and anxiety

6. At what age does the Centers for Disease Control cap it recommendation for annual HIV testing?

   (a) 55

   (b) 64

   (c) 67

   (d) 70

7. What is the rate of Alzheimer's disease among LGBT elders as compared to the general elderly population?

   (a) Lower

   (b) Higher

   (c) Unknown

   (d) About the same

8. Which of the following do LGBT elders identify as the number one priority for action?

   (a) Social support systems

   (b) Food stamps

   (c) Transportation

   (d) Housing

9. Which of the following presents more adjustment difficulties to disability or chronic illness?

   (a) Early onset

   (b) Midlife onset

   (c) Later onset

   (d) None of the above

10. Which of the following refers to older adults remaining in their home?

   (a) Aging-in-place

   (b) Assistive living

   (c) Structural support

   (d) Group home

Key

1-b

2-d

3-c

4-a

5-b

6-b

7-c

8-d

9-c

10-a

Resources and Websites

Center for Disability and Aging: www.acl.gov/Programs/CDAP/OIP/ADRC/index.aspx

National Coalition for LGBT Health (Being LGBT with a Disability): www.lgbthealth.webolutionary.com/content/being-lgbt-disability

National Council on Independent Living: www.ncil.org

National Organization on Disability: www.nod.org

Services and Advocacy for Gay, Lesbian, Bisexual and Transgender Elders (Disability: www.sageusa.org/issues/disability.cfm

US General Services Administration: www. gas.gov

US Government Disability Resources: www. Disability.gov

References

American Medical Association. (2009). *AMA policy regarding sexual orientation: H-65.973 health care disparities in same-sex partner households.* Houston, TX: Author. Retrieved July 19, 2014 from http://www.ama-assn.org/ama/pub/about-ama/our-people/member-groups-sections/glbt-advisory-committee/ama-policy-regarding-sexual-orientation.page.

Benedetti, M. (2011). *The second closet: LGBTs with disabilities.* Retrieved September 12, 2014 from http://www.myhandicap.com/gay-lesbian-disability.html.

Bishop, M. (2012). Quality of life and psychosocial adaptation to chronic illness and acquired disability: A conceptual and theoretical synthesis. In I. Marini & M. A. Stebnicki (Eds.), *The psychological and social impact of illness and disability* (pp. 179–191). New York: Springer.

Centers for Disease Control and Prevention. (2013). *The state of aging and health in America 2013.* Atlanta, GA: Centers for Disease Control and Prevention, US Department of Health and Human Services.

Chappell, N. L., & Cooke, H. A. (2010). Age related disabilities—Aging and quality of life. In J. H. Stone & M. Blouin (Eds.), *International encyclopedia of rehabilitation.* Available at http://cirrie.buffalo.edu/encyclopedia/en/article/189/.

Colker, R. (2005). *The disability pendulum.* New York: New York University Press.

Crisp, C., Wayland, S., & Gordon, T. (2008). Older gay, lesbian, and bisexual adults: Tools forage-competent and gay affirmative practice. *Journal of Gay & Lesbian Social Services, 20*(1/2), 5–29.

Davis, M. & Company. (2013). *An estimate of housing discrimination against same sex couples.* Retrieved September 9, 2014 from http://www.huduser.org/portal/Publications/prf/Hsg_Disc_against_SameSexCpls_v3.pdf.

Degener, T. (2006). The definition of disability in German and foreign discrimination law. *Disability Studies Quarterly, 26*(2). Available at http://www.dsq-sds.org/article/view/696/873.

Disability World. (2012, June 28). *Definitions of disability.* Retrieved July 18, 2014 from http://www.disabled-world.com/definitions/disability-definitions.php.

Equal Rights Center. (2012). *Misguided: Housing discrimination against individuals using guide dogs.* Washington, DC: Author.

Equal Rights Center. (2014). *Opening doors: An investigation of barriers to senior housing for same sex couples.* Washington, DC: Author.

Espinoza, R. (2011). The diverse elders coalition and LGBT aging: Connecting communities, issues, and resources in a historic moment. In R. B. Hudson (Ed.), *Public policy & aging report: Integrating lesbian, gay, bisexual, and transgender older adults into aging and practice* (pp. 8–13). Washington, DC: National Academy on an Aging Society.

Falvo, D. (2014). *Medical and psychosocial aspects of chronic illness and disability* (5th ed.). Sudbury, MA: Jones & Bartlett.

Fine, M., & Asch, A. (1988). *Women with disabilities: Essays in psychology, culture, and politics.* Philadelphia: Temple University Press.

Fredriksen-Goldsen, K. I. (2011). Resilience and disparities among lesbian, gay, bisexual, and transgender older adults. In R. B. Hudson (Ed.), *Public policy & aging report: Integrating lesbian, gay, bisexual, and transgender older adults into aging policy and practice* (pp. 3–7). Washington, DC: National Academy on an Aging Society.

Fredriksen-Goldsen, K. I., Kim, H. J., Barkan, E. E., Muraco, A., & Hoy-Ellis, C. P. (2013). Health disparities among lesbian, gay, and bisexual older adults: Results from population-based study. *American Journal of Public Health, 103*(10), 1802–1809.

Fredriksen-Goldsen, K. I., Kim, H. J., Emlet, C. A., Muraco, A., Erosheva, E. A., Hoy-Ellis, C. P., et al. (2011). *The aging and health report: Disparities and resilience among lesbian, gay, bisexual, and transgender older adults.* Seattle: Institute for Multigenerational Health.

Fried, L. P., Ferrucci, L., Darer, J., Williamson, J. D., & Anderson, G. (2004). Untangling the concepts of disability, frailty, and comorbidity: Implications for improved targeting and care. *Journal of Gerontology: Medical Sciences, 59*(3), 255–263.

Funders for Lesbian and Gay Issues. (2004). *Aging in equity: LGBT elders in America.* New York, NY: Author.

Gamble, V. N., & Stone, D. (2006). US policy on health inequities: The interplay of politics and research. *Journal of Health Politics, Policy and Law, 31*(1), 93–126.

Grant, J. M., Mottet, L. A., Tanis, J., Harrison, J., Herman, J. L., & Keisling, M. (2011). *Injustice at every turn: A report of the national transgender discrimination survey.* Washington, DC: National Center for Transgender Equality and National Gay and Lesbian Task Force.

Harley, D. A. (2015). Disabilities among LGBT elders. In A. E. Goldberg (Ed.), *The SAGE encyclopedia of LGBT studies.* Thousand Oaks, CA: Sage.

Heikkinen, E. (2003). What are the main risk factors for disability in old age and how can disability be prevented? Copenhagen WHO Regional Office for Europe (Health Evidence Network report). Available at http://www.euro.who.int/document/E82970.pef.

Institute of Medicine. (2011). *The health of lesbian, gay, bisexual and transgender people: Building a foundation for better understanding.* Washington, DC: The National Academic Press.

Kennedy, J., & Minkler, M. (1998). Disability theory and public policy: Implications for critical gerontology. *International Journal of Health Services, 28*(4), 757–776.

Kimmel, D. (2014). Lesbian, gay, bisexual, and transgender aging concerns. *Clinical Gerontologist, 37,* 49–63.

Kimmel, D. C., Hinrichs, K. L., & Fisher, L. D. (2015). Understanding lesbian, gay, bisexual, and transgender elders. In P. A. Lichtenberg & B. T. Mast (Eds.), *APA Handbook of clinical geropsychology.* Washington, DC: American Psychological Association.

Knauer, N. J. (2009). LGBT elder law: Toward equity in aging. *Harvard Journal of Law & Gender, 32,* 1–58. Retrieved 9, 2014 from http://worlks.bepress.com.

Knochel, K. A., Croghan, C. F., Moone, R. P., & Quam, J. K. (2011). *Ready to serve? The aging network and LGB and T adults.* Washington, DC: National Association for Area Agencies on Aging.

Lipman, B., Lubell, J., & Salomon, E. (2012). *Housing an aging population: Are we prepared?.* Washington, DC: Center for Housing Policy.

MAP & SAGE. (2010). *Improving the lives of LGBT older adults.* New York: Author.

Michigan Fair Housing Centers. (2007). *Sexual orientation and housing discrimination in Michigan: A report of Michigan's Fair Housing Centers.* Retrieved September 9, 2014 from www.fhcmichigan.org.

National Gay & Lesbian Task Force. (2006). *Make room for all: Diversity, cultural competency & discrimination in an aging America.* Retrieved November 7, 2014 from www.thetaskforce.org/static_html/downloads/reports/reports/MakeRoomForAll.pdf.

National Institute on Aging, National Institutes of Health. (2011). *Global health and aging.* Retrieved July 23, 2014 from www.nia.nih.gov/sites/default/files/global_health_and_aging.pdf.

Population Association of America. (2014). *Disability among older adults in same-sex relationships: Working Paper.* Population Association of America Annual Meeting. Boston, MA: Author. Retrieved September 10, 2014 from www.paa.2014.princeton.edu/papers/141954.

Sheets, D. (2010). Aging with physical disability. In J. H. Stone, & M. Blouin (Eds.), *International encyclopedia of rehabilitation.* Available at http://cirrie.buffalo.edu/encyclopedia/en/article/288/.

Sue, D. W., & Sue, D. (2013). *Counseling the culturally diverse: Theory and practice* (6th ed.). Hoboken, NJ: Wiley.

The Joint Commission. (2011). *Advancing effective communication, cultural competence, and patient-and family-centered care for the lesbian, gay, bisexual, and transgender (LGBT) community: A field guide.* Oakbrook Terrace, IL: Author. Available at www.jointcommission.org/assets/1/18/LGBTFieldGuide.pdf.

Tietz, D., & Schaefer, N. (2011). The policy issues and social concerns facing older adults with HIV. *Public Policy & Aging Report, 21*(3), 30–33.

Tobin, H. J. (2011). Improving the lives of transgender older adults. In R. B. Hudson (Ed.), *Public policy & aging report: Integrating lesbian, gay, bisexual, and transgender older adults into aging policy and practice* (pp. 12–13). Washington, DC: National Academy on an Aging Society.

Verbrugge, L. M., & Jette, A. M. (1994). The disablement process. *Social Science and Medicine, 38*(1), 1–14.

Wallace, S. P., Cochran, S. D., Durazo, E. M., & Ford, C. L. (2011). *The health of aging lesbian, gay, and bisexual adults in California.* Los Angles, CA: UCLA Center for Health Policy Research.

World Health Organization. (2009). *World health survey, World Health Organization, 2002–2004.* Retrieved September 11, 2014 from http://www.ho.int/health-info/survey/en.

World Health Organization. (2011). *World report on disability: Disability and rehabilitation.* Retrieved September 11, 2014 from www.who.int/disabilities/world_report/2011/report/en.

Zians, J. (2011). *LGBT San Diego's trailblazing generation: Housing & related needs of LGBT seniors.* Retrieved July 23, 2014 from www.thecentersd.org/pdf/programs/senior-needs-report.pdf.

Zola, I. (1993). Disability statistics, what we count and what it tells us: A personal and political analysis. *JDPS, 4*(2), 10–39.

Part VII
Conclusion

Ethical Standards and Practices in Human Services and Health Care for LGBT Elders

34

Pamela B. Teaster and Amanda E. Sokan

Abstract

Understanding and working with a population as diverse as LGBT elders is not possible without a grounding in ethics and its application to real-world problems faced by the older adults and their families. Principles of autonomy, beneficence, nonmaleficence, justice, fidelity, and veracity are critical for professionals to understand when confronting dilemmas that LGBT elders face. In this chapter, the authors use a case study to illustrate a real-world example of ethical and moral action. The purpose of this chapter is to provide a grounding in ethical principles and frameworks, as well as discuss pertinent codes of ethics, in order to make the case that an understanding of ethics is essential when dealing with the complex dilemmas that LGBT elders face.

Keywords

Autonomy · Beneficence · Nonmaleficence · Justice · Fidelity · Veracity · Codes of ethics

Overview

Understanding and working with a population as diverse as LGBT elders is not possible without a grounding in ethics and its application to real-world problems faced by the older adults and their families. Principles of autonomy, beneficence, nonmaleficence, justice, fidelity, and veracity are far more easily understood in theory than in application when professionals are confronted with dilemmas that LGBT elders face. Because of their status as a sexual minority, their historic ostracization, their fears related to outing, and vulnerabilities acquired by some as they age, it is imperative to understand and adhere to ethical principles and frameworks embedded in disciplinary codes of ethics. In this chapter, the authors use a case study to illustrate a real-world example of ethical and moral action.

P.B. Teaster (✉)
Virginia Tech, Blacksburg, VA, USA
e-mail: pteaster@vt.edu

A.E. Sokan
University of Kentucky, Lexington, Kentucky, USA

© Springer International Publishing Switzerland 2016
D.A. Harley and P.B. Teaster (eds.), *Handbook of LGBT Elders*,
DOI 10.1007/978-3-319-03623-6_34

639

The purpose of this chapter is to provide the reader with a grounding in ethics and ethical principles and frameworks in order to make the case that an understanding of ethics is essential when dealing with LGBT elders.

Learning Objectives

By the end of the chapter, the reader should be able to:

1. Understand basic principles of ethics.
2. Understand how ethics are applied to health and healthcare situations.
3. Understand ethical codes for law, social work, and medicine as they apply to human services and health care for LGBT elders.
4. Identify future areas for the intersection of ethics, human services, and health care for LGBT elders.

Introduction

In order to introduce and frame this section, we will start with an illustrative case, one that actually occurred (with names changed to protect confidentiality). We will refer to it and expand on it throughout the chapter.

> It was an unremarkable day at the office for Ann Fields, researcher, the only notable difference being that her hair had been cut and colored (she liked to say "clipped and dipped"). Having her hair cut always made her feel better, but likely that had more to do with the strong bond that she had forged with her hairdresser, Bill, of over 10 years. The two discussed everything, including her research work on elder abuse. Over the years, she had come to realize, as depicted in the stage play and movie, Steel Magnolias, how much intimate interaction occurred between a hairdresser and a long-time client. She had even mentioned to Bill that the next effort that she would make on raising the visibility of the issue of elder abuse would be to contact the hairstyling association in their state to see what they might be able to add on their website about the topic.
>
> On that typical day at work, Bill telephoned her using her office phone (not typical). When he

asked for her, he was far less jovial than he was usually. Dr. Fields, this is Bill Smock. I have a gentleman here who wants to speak with you—about possible elder abuse. Can you talk with him? He is sitting here in my chair getting his hair trimmed. Bill had her attention. And of course she had time and of course she would take the call.

The man explained that he thought that his mother was being exploited by his nephew, a young man who had just never been able to hold a job. The man explained that his mother would become really agitated when the nephew's name was mentioned, particularly if asked about the increasingly frequent loans that she had made to him. The man confessed that he did not want to put his nephew in jail, but that talking directly with him (and his mother) had only emboldened the nephew. And he mentioned that his mother was more than a little confused, confined to her home, and more and more relied on her wheelchair rather than her walker. And there was one more thing to add about his mother—she had come out ten years ago to the family. Really and all along, she was a lesbian.

Ann Fields sighed. The information seemed like a case study that she might write for her students someday, but the wrinkle was that she was not a direct services provider and that her dear friend Bill was intervening immediately and on his client's behalf. At the end of the conversation, she recommended that the man call Adult Protective Services (APS), and she provided the number for him. Then, she called an APS worker who was also a friend, and told him to be on the lookout for the report. She hoped that she had done the right things, and she also hoped that the right things would be done, whatever they turned out to be. Contextual factors would make this a more complicated case than some. And, Ann also knew that, due to confidentiality, she would not know anything more about the report.

The case above is emblematic of the very real and urgent importance of ethical and moral action. A number of these issues are at work in the case illustration above. The son's ethical and legal duty was to report the suspicion (his state was an "any person" state), and his ethical responsibility was to protect his mother from being harmed. At the point he made the call to Ann Fields, it was her moral responsibility to assist a fellow human being seeking help, and her relationship to Bill had often been one she characterized as being one of a brother and sister. At the point the son reported the suspicion to APS (if he in fact did), other ethical codes also would come into play—those most typically of the professions of social work, law, and medicine, all of which will be discussed below. The purpose of this chapter is to provide the reader with a grounding in ethics and ethical principles and framework in order to make the case that an understanding of ethics is essential when dealing with LGBT elders. We first anchor this chapter on ethics by providing the reader with a basic understanding of ethics and its importance. Then, we discuss how human services codes of ethics and those of law and medicine both complement and confound helping LGBT elders.

What Is Ethics?

What ought to be in a given circumstance (s).

The Oxford English Dictionary (1996) provides a simple definition of ethics as a system of moral principles or values that govern or provide rules of conduct. Ethics is the sphere within the discipline of philosophy that explores morals, values, and virtues of human conduct, not as they are but as they ought to be (Pozgar 2012). Ethics are universal principles that provide a basis to guide, regulate, prescribe, or understand behavior on both micro- (individual) and macro- (group, culture) levels. However, ethics is not law, and so does not carry legal force, and is not binding. (Darr 2011). These principles aid in making distinctions between good versus bad, right versus wrong, and in determining what may be considered acceptable or unacceptable, or what ought to be in a given circumstance. Ethics is more than feelings, or what is legal, moral, religious, socially normative, or acceptable by society. Ethics often find representation in theories and principles, some of which are presented in brief below.

Ethical Theories. There are a variety of theories that provide a range of ethical perspectives. Often they detail parameters for actions that are considered ethical and provide a premise for doing so. For instance, normative ethics focuses on moral standards of human behavior—that which is good and right (Summers 2009), communicative ethics focuses on the importance of negotiation and communication in ethical conflict resolution (Moody 1992), utilitarian theories emphasize the greater good for all, consequential theories, on the other hand, focus on outcomes and context (situational ethics), while ethical relativism considers the impact of different cultures on notions of what is morally right or wrong (Pozgar 2012).

Ethical principles. Ethics can also be looked at in terms of principles distilled from various theories to help inform and guide ethical conduct and behavior. Principlism, as an ethical framework, provides a universal set of principles or rules of conduct most commonly recognized in general discourses of ethics, namely beneficence, nonmaleficence, justice, and autonomy (Beauchamp and Childress 2012). Simply put, *beneficence* exhorts us to do good to others, *nonmaleficence* urges against doing harm to others, and while *justice* reminds us of the importance of fairness in distributive justice, *respect for autonomy* focuses on self-determination and requires us to recognize and acknowledge the right of individuals (and groups) to make their own choices and decisions (Pozgar 2012; Beauchamp and Childress 2012) (see Table 34.1).

These principles have been applied to the field of aging, although some have voiced reservations about issues of interpretation and application (Moody 1992; Polivka and Moody 2001). Holstein and Mitzen (2001) and Holstein et al. (2011) argue that principlism fails to consider the heterogeneity of older adults, while others have argued that strict or rigid applications of these principles may result in undesirable results. For example, an overemphasis on nonmaleficence may lead to paternalism, thereby limiting freedom of action for competent older adults, and upholding autonomy may detract from recognizing the importance and responsibilities of membership in social and collective networks (Polivka and Moody 2001; Holstein and Mitzen 2001; Holstein et al. 2011). Thus, these perceived limitations of using principlism, including the emphasis on individuals to the detriment of community, neglect or nonconsideration of factors such as context, circumstance, and agents to which it is applied, and its

Table 34.1 Ethical theories, proponents, and premises

Theory/approach	Proponent(s)	Premise	Focus
Utilitarianism	Jeremy Bentham, John Stuart Mill	Ethical actions provide the greatest balance of good than evil	Utility and consequences
Rights approach	Immanuel Kant	Ethical actions protect individual dignity and freedom of choice	Self-determination; individual rights
Deontology	Kant, Descartes, Calvinists	Ethical actions comply with divine command	Duty and right by God's law
Fairness and justice approach	Aristotle	Ethical actions are fair and equal for all	Consistency; equal distribution of benefits and burdens
Common good approach	Plato, Aristotle, Cicero, John Rawls	Ethical actions serve the common good	Interconnectedness of individual and communal good
Virtue ethics	Aristotle, Thomas Aquinas	Ethical actions are virtuous	Virtuousness (e.g., prudence, compassion, integrity, honesty, courage)

tendency to view relationships as adversarial because of its origins in law and philosophy, have led to the exploration and development of alternative frameworks more suited to addressing aging (Hofland 2001). These frameworks are presented below; what they share in common is the focus placed on the perspectives of agents, subjects, and context in the consideration of ethics (see Table 34.2).

In addition to the creation of alternative frameworks, other avenues have been explored for a more meaningful interpretation and application of ethics in aging. For instance, other principles, such as honesty, integrity, compassion, caring, and privacy, are of particular resonance when dealing with older adults and can be used as tools to guide ethical action and decision-making. Finally, principlism still has relevance, in as much as the principles of beneficence, nonmaleficence, justice, and autonomy are evaluated, interpreted, and applied with due consideration for how well they can be manipulated or adapted to address aging issues meaningfully. For instance, a consideration of what constitutes ethical standards and practices relating to LGBT elders must consider their personal and group history and experience as it relates to sexual orientation and/or gender identity, and the implications for the provision of care and other services.

Table 34.2 Ethical frameworks

Framework	Premise	Focus
Phenomenology	Ethics should consider shared experience, understanding, and meaning	Perspectives of participants themselves
Hermeneutics	Ethics should respect diversity of experiences and relativity of ethical situations	Meaning and validation
Narrative ethics	Ethics should consider more facts of the case	Experience, dimensions of meaning as well as facts
Virtue ethics	Virtuous character leads to ethical acts	Moral character, not actions performed
Ethics of care	Caring for others as human activity, based on action and practice, not rules	Care that is attentive, responsible, competent, and responsiveness

Sources Hofland (2001), Tronto (1993)

Why Ethics Is Important for Working with LGBT Elders

Understanding ethics as applied to elders, particularly the LGBT elder population, is important for a number of reasons (i.e., decision-making, habilitation, resource allocation, dementia, end of life), which are discussed below. Older LGBT adults represent a special population highly deserving of ethical considerations and treatment. The aging population, of which LGBT elders are a part, presents unique and confounding ethical challenges for healthcare and human services professionals. The complexities of an aging society include ethical considerations heretofore historically unheard of as recently as the 1900s when the average US life expectancy was age 47, to today, when it is 76 (World Health Organization 2014). Several domains pertinent to aging LGBT individuals warrant ethical attention.

Decision-Making. Competent elders are often capable of making decisions for themselves, even until the end of their lives. However, their ability to make decisions for themselves can become compromised due to such reasons as medication interactions, chronic illness, dementia, general weakness, or all of the previous reasons in combination. Also, because of vulnerabilities that some elders experience at the end of their lives, they may be the focus of unhealthy dependencies by their care providers (formal or informal) and so may become the unwitting victims of undue influence (Nerenberg 2000) when making decisions.

For elders who are competent and who wish to authorize another individual to make decisions for their health care, finances, or both, a power of attorney (POA) document must be executed, while the older adult still has the capacity to make decisions (see Chap. 22). Such a document executed under undue influence or when an older adult no longer possesses the capacity to make decisions is not a legally executed or binding document. In addition, should an older adult fail to appoint a surrogate or become incompetent without executing a POA, many states have a statutorily established order of surrogacy, which

usually begins with the spouse of the elder, followed by a son or daughter and continuing to next of kin. This designation can be particularly problematic for older LGBT persons, since the law in many states does not recognize the marital status of a same-sex partner. Due to divided acceptance of an elder coming out, some family members are estranged and so may be very poor surrogates for the incapacitated elder. Also, the isolation that some older LGBT persons experience may make surrogate decision-making even more challenging, because his or her wishes for health care and service acceptance may not be discernable or followed. This situation would be particularly difficult should an LGBT elder require that a guardianship be initiated due to his or her incapacity (Teaster et al. 2010).

The emphasis on autonomy to the exclusion of other ethical principles (Holstein and Mitzen 2001; Holstein et al. 2011) is one not as deeply held in other countries (and actually, not by all older adults) as it is in the USA. Some countries have far different approaches toward treating persons who are dying or persons who are suffering from a terminal illness. For example, Moody (2001) describes the conundrum faced when a US-based and indoctrinated medical team faces the wishes of an Asian family concerning the issue of veracity. The US team wants to tell the old Asian mother that she has terminal cancer, but the family members, acting within the value system of their culture, want to withhold this information.

Habilitation. Unlike the majority of their younger counterparts, older adults live in both community and facility settings, and many will live in both at some point in their lives (Congressional Budget Office 2013). The meaning of place and where an elder identifies his or her home reflects important ethical concepts of belonging, respect for persons, autonomy, and justice (Beauchamp and Childress 2012; Holstein and Mitzen 2001). For many adults, the home in which they intended to live for the remainder of their days may become inappropriate for them: Upkeep or house payments may become too expensive, the neighborhood is no longer safe, the elder is no longer able to traverse stairs, and little accommodation is possible, or the elder experiences dementia and cannot attend to activities of daily living or instrumental activities of daily living. Making decisions concerning one's habilitation is life-altering and may be irreversible, a situation different from when they were a younger adult.

One of the most wrenching decisions that many families face is whether or not to have an elder leave his or her home and move to either an assisted-living facility (if resources allow it) or a nursing home (synonymous with death for some elders) (Kane and Caplan 1990; Powers 2003). Bed availability and quality of care are ongoing concerns for care provision in nursing homes (see, generally, Web sites for the Centers for Medicare and Medicaid Services and National Consumer Voice for Quality Long-Term Care). For LGBT elders, there is an added concern, which is that of being outed in a care environment that may be inhospitable to him or her. Some facilities have staff members who are vicious and abusive, and some such facilities, which may provide excellent and loving care, may be the only one available within a huge radius, as is often the case in rural areas. Here, ethical dilemmas revolve around limiting freedoms to protect and preserve safety. This aspiration may not be realized if the care environment does not welcome LGBT elders (see Chaps. 16, 17, 25, and 28).

Resource Allocation. Resource allocation is yet another arena in which ethics informs how healthcare providers and service professionals treat the needs of LGBT elders. Even though approximately 20 % of the population will be composed of older adults, policy tends to lag both scholarship and demographic realities. In addition, uncomfortable questions arise as to deservingness. Whose interests have primacy? Young children? Adolescents? Young or old LGBT persons? Gay or straight? The allocation of resources is usually not so blatantly black or white. More often than not, simmering below the surface are issues of who gets what, when, and where. When resources are scarce, these issues become even more heated. Guns or butter, or in another interpretation, guns or canes, is a frequently debated issue, particularly at the national level. Ethical issues of justice (Callahan 1995; Moody 1992; Rawls 2009) come to bear when resources are allocated. As an example, a goal of the 2010 Affordable Care Act has been to widen healthcare coverage for persons who have heretofore been unable to access it. Questions concerning the fairness of compelling persons to purchase health care, despite hardship, strike at the bedrock principle of autonomy, one fiercely guarded in the USA.

In addition to this, the allocation of healthcare resources is the developing conundrum concerning access to technology (Lesnoff-Caravaglia 1999). Perhaps nowhere in the USA is the digital divide more keenly felt than that which divides generations coupled with those who are well off and those who are not. As an illustration, LGBT elders with the ability to teleconnect via some form of computer (e.g., laptop, mobile phone, iPad) with others are thus able to reduce isolation and its effect on health and well-being. Elders who are able to live in homes that are becoming increasingly "smart" may be able to reduce injuries at rates far higher than their poorer and older counterparts. Also, elders with means are able to afford better assistive devices such as canes, walkers, mobile scooters, and the like far more easily than elders who have limited means to acquire them.

Dementia. Also, unlike their younger counterparts, older adults, who are disproportionately affected by the problem, may develop a type of dementia (Binstock et al. 1992; Post 2000; Purlita and ten Have 2004). About 4–5 million people in the USA have some degree of dementia at any given time, a number expected to increase over the next few decades due to the aging of the population. Dementia affects about 1 % of people aged 60–64 years and 30–50 % of people older than 85 years. Dementia is the leading reason for placing elderly people in institutions such as nursing homes. Dementia is a serious condition that results in significant financial and human costs (Alzheimer's Association 2014). Dementias are not all alike. In the USA, 50,000–60,000 new cases of Parkinson's disease (PD) are diagnosed each year, adding to the one million people who currently have PD (National Parkinson Foundation, n.d.), while an estimated 5.2 million Americans of all ages had Alzheimer's disease in 2014, including an estimated 5 million people aged 65 and older and approximately 200,000 individuals under the age of 65 (Alzheimer's Association 2014).

Regardless of type, cures do not yet exist, and the march of such chronic diseases is relentless. When persons become deeply forgetful (Post 2000), it is all the more important to provide respectful care to such afflicted individuals who may be unable to remember that they are lesbian or for that matter, their very name. It is in these particular positions of vulnerability that afflicted LGBT elders must be treated with dignity and respect for personhood, though many former vestiges may become unrecognizable.

End of Life. Finally, considerations of what is ethical come to bear at the terminus of a long life. This is not to say that end-of-life issues do not affect younger populations, but living to an old age involves the certainty that older adults are nearing the end of their lives, a time when the complexities that append to living a long life intersect (Ellingston and Fuller 2001; Gaventa and Coulter 2005). End of life can involve addressing real pain encountered through chronic illness and that encountered as a consequence of living. Personal pain can be acute when families and friends fail to accept the needs and wishes of an LGBT elder. Ideally, end-of-life circumstances allow for the resolution of a life that is coming to an end, one that requires special attention and care if the dying elder is LGBT. It may be very important to the elder that, despite years of friction, family conflict is confronted and resolved. Issues of religiosity and spirituality are also highly important at this time in life (see Chap. 29).

The ethical issues presented above that are germane to an aging LGBT population are not exhaustive of those that may arise. They are, however, illustrative of why an understanding of ethics is critical when healthcare and service professionals confront conundrums of aging LGBT persons. The following section explores the application of ethical principles and approaches to specific issues that such professionals encounter as well as offers suggestions for ways to approach ethical dilemmas.

Application of Ethics

Ethics can be applied in a variety of ways. Ethics can be used as rules of conduct "moral code" for individual behavior, as well as for groups such as those adopted as professional codes of ethics, as a means to determine rights, duties, and responsibilities to others as well as to inform decision-making (Pozgar 2012). Applying ethics to LGBT elders requires considering not only what rights accrue to LGBT older adults, but also what duties and responsibilities are incumbent on health and social services providers in order to effectively care and serve this population. It is also important to consider what ethical considerations need to inform optimal decision-making and how current ethical principles can be interpreted to reflect LGBT elders' reality.

Interpreting ethical principles through the LGBT perspective can help develop an ethical framework or "moral map" for caring for LGBT elders and the unique ethical dilemmas that may arise. Such applications must at the very least affirm LGBT elders, address prejudice, recognize inequalities and vulnerability, and be flexible.

One alternate framework, whose precepts provide a good starting point for application of ethics to LGBT elders, is Joan Tronto's *Ethic of Care* (1993). Care is defined as "activity that includes everything that we do to maintain, continue, and repair our 'world' so that we can live in it as well as possible. That world includes our bodies, our selves, and our environment, all of which seek to interweave in a complex, life-sustaining web" (Fisher and Tronto 1990, p. 40, as cited in Tronto 1993, p. 61). According to Tronto, how we "care" for others is a human activity, and because it is an action and practice, rather than a set of rules, which is based upon a flexible standard, what constitutes good and thus ethical care reflects "the way of life, the set of values and conditions, of the people engaged in the caring practice" (Tronto 1993, p. 61). Also, four phases of care and the correlating ethical principle have been recognized:

Phase 1: Caring about—*Attentiveness* as the ethical quality (dimension) of being able to perceive the needs of others and one self.

Phase 2: Caring for—assuming the *Responsibility* for responding to the identified need for care.

Phase 3: Caregiving—ethical requirement of *Competence* in performing the functions of care.

Phase 4: Care receiving—relates to the *Responsiveness* of recipients of care, to care received, and the ability of care to meet/address identified needs.

Applying the ethics of care to LGBT elders requires health and social services providers to become knowledgeable about the unique needs and challenges these elders face, as a necessary foundation in order to properly discern the needs to be addressed, as well as to determine the scope of responsibility. It requires competence not only with regard to the nature of work performed, but also cultural competence in issues affecting sexual orientation, gender identity, and how these may interact with aging to determine unique needs and inform appropriate interventions. Additionally, by considering the response of LGBT elders, the application of the ethics of care places the LGBT elder in the epicenter of decision-making and action, ensuring a voice in the issues that affect them, such as the efficacy of services received.

Another way to promote the application of ethical standards and practices with LGBT elders is to embed appropriate ethical principles and values in the professional codes of conduct for the different disciplines that work with LGBT elders. These codes are important because they prescribe agreed-upon standards and expectations of conduct, as well as consequences for breach, if that occurs (Pozgar 2012; Resnik 2011). Professional codes of ethics protect both

providers and LGBT elders by promoting responsibility, accountability, and professionalism in service delivery. They can provide a method, lens, or perspective to guide decision-making, problem identification, and solution, as well as promote the social and moral values that they consider important (Resnik 2011). It is critical, therefore, that these codes clearly include ethical principles germane to working with LGBT elders.

Codes of Ethics

In order to provide guidance for elevating members' behavior and to instill confidence (both within and outside the organization), various disciplines as well as government and professional organizations have developed and subsequently adopted codes of ethics that guide the conduct of professional behavior (Plant 2001). Most codes of ethics, also called codes of conduct, explicate an organization's values, mission, and vision. Additionally and typically grounded in the ethical principles and frameworks delineated earlier in this chapter, an organization's code of ethics provides direction to its members on appropriate standards of conduct, including how to adhere to them (Adams et al. 2001). Most mature professions have developed codes of ethics or conduct (e.g., social work, law, medicine, gerontology). Such guidance is critical for the complex situations that can arise when working with older members of a sexual minority. Below, we return to our case study earlier and discuss codes of ethics for social work, law, medicine, and gerontology, highlighting how they might guide members' treatment of LGBT elders.

The man who sat in the chair of the beauty salon did, in fact, make a report to Adult Protective Services. The report was logged in the state system, and an APS worker was assigned to investigate the case. The APS worker had a Master's of Social Work and belonged to the National Association for Social Work.

Code of Ethics for Social Work. According to the preamble of the Code of Ethics for Social

Work, promulgated by the National Association of Social Work (NASW) (2008),

The primary mission of the social work profession is to enhance human well-being and help meet the basic human needs of all people, with particular attention to the needs and empowerment of people who are vulnerable, oppressed, and living in poverty. A historic and defining feature of social work is the profession's focus on individual well-being in a social context and the well-being of society. Fundamental to social work is attention to the environmental forces that create, contribute to, and address problems in living.

The preamble of the code stresses that the profession should promote social justice and social change with and on behalf of clients whom they serve. The code stipulates that the term "clients" is used inclusively and refers to "individuals, families, groups, organizations, and communities" and that "social workers are sensitive to cultural and ethnic diversity and strive to end discrimination, oppression, poverty, and other forms of social injustice." Core values of the NASW include service, social justice, dignity and worth of persons, importance of human relationships, integrity, and competence.

Most pertinent to clients who are LGBT is Section 1 of the code, "Social Workers' Ethical Responsibilities to Clients." Subsections within Section 1 include social workers' commitment to clients, respect for clients' self-determination, informed consent, professional competence, cultural competence and social diversity, conflict of interests, privacy and confidentiality, access to records, sexual relationships, physical contact, sexual harassment, derogatory language, payment for services, clients who lack decision-making capacity, and interruption and termination of services. Particularly salient for social workers who are addressing the needs of older LGBT clients is the guidance that the code provides on self-determination and cultural competency, which defer to the ethical principles of autonomy, nonmaleficence, and justice. According to the Section 1.02 on self-determination,

Social workers respect and promote the right of clients to self-determination and assist clients in their efforts to identify and clarify their goals. Social workers may limit clients' right to self-determination when, in the social workers' professional judgment, clients' actions or potential actions pose a serious, foreseeable, and imminent risk to themselves or others.

Goals for LGBT elders may be to remain in the home as long as possible, to direct their own health care, or to discontinue life support in the event that medical treatment is deemed futile. An elderly LGBT person's self-determination may have to be limited, for example, if the older adult were determined to be self-neglecting (see Chap. 16).

Also highly important for working with older LGBT clients is Section 1.05, i.e., Cultural Competence and Social Diversity. The section directs social workers to "understand culture and its function in human behavior and society, recognizing the strengths that exist in all cultures." Further, "social workers should obtain education about and seek to understand the nature of social diversity and oppression with respect to race, ethnicity, national origin, color, sex, sexual orientation, gender identity or expression, age, marital status, political belief, religion, immigration status, and mental or physical disability."

Section 1.05 includes the strongest admonition of the code to respect and understand the particular needs and situations of older LGBT clients, tenets that reflect the ethical principles of beneficence and nonmaleficence, as well as the ethics of care discussed earlier. It is notable that the code was revised in 2008 to specifically mention sex, sexual orientation, gender identify, and expression (NASW).

Upon investigation of the report to APS, the social worker assigned to the case substantiated it for physical abuse and financial exploitation by the nephew. It had not taken the older woman long to admit that her nephew had been threatening to out her in the intimate assisted living facility in which she was currently living. The woman was adamant that she wanted the exploitation to end (she never quite admitted that the bruises on her arms were the result of his striking her) but that she did not want her nephew to go to jail. But the social worker knew that exploiting an elder was a crime as was physical abuse. She referred the case to the local commonwealth's attorney.

Code of Ethics for Law. The American Bar Association's (ABA) rules of professional conduct for members of the legal profession are codified in Model Rules of Professional Conduct, adopted by the ABA House of Delegates in 1983. Commonly known as Model Rules, this code has nationwide application and has been modified and adopted by most states as the format for state-level disciplinary codes or rules of professional conduct, with the exception of the state of California (ABA 1983). The nature and extent of a lawyer's professional responsibility are delineated in the preamble and scope of the Model Rules of Professional Conduct. The preamble emphasizes that the Model Rules provide a framework to guide practitioners in the ethical practice of the law and a basis for disciplinary action against those who fail to comply with the prohibitions and obligations imposed.

According to Sections 1 and 2 of the preamble, a lawyer has multiple responsibilities—"as a member of the legal profession, is a representative of clients, an officer of the legal system and a public citizen having special responsibility for the quality of justice." It also spells out clearly, the various capacities in and through which the lawyer acts a representative of his/her client(s):

> [2] As a representative of clients, a lawyer performs various functions. As advisor, a lawyer provides a client with an informed understanding of the client's legal rights and obligations and explains their practical implications. As advocate, a lawyer zealously asserts the client's position under the rules of the adversary system. As negotiator, a lawyer seeks a result advantageous to the client but consistent with requirements of honest dealings with others. As an evaluator, a lawyer acts by examining a client's legal affairs and reporting about them to the client or to others.

Thus, a lawyer's functions and roles include advising, advocacy, negotiation, evaluation, and reporting as clients' needs and circumstances dictate. In addition, the preamble indicates that a lawyer may serve as "third-party neutral" in dispute resolutions without a representational role to parties involved. Section 4 requires that

lawyers perform these functions with competence, promptness, and diligence. These roles and performance requirements are pertinent and useful considerations when dealing with allegations or reports of elder mistreatment (see earlier discussions in Chap. 16).

ABA core values for professional conduct address client–lawyer relationships, the roles of lawyers as counselor/advisor and advocate, as well as transactions with nonclients. For instance, Rules 1.1, 1.3, and 1.6 and Rule address values of competence, diligence, and confidentiality, respectively, in client–lawyer relationships:

> Rule 1.1 Competence: A lawyer shall provide competent representation to a client. Competent representation requires the legal knowledge, skill, thoroughness and preparation reasonably necessary for the representation.

> Rule 1.3 Diligence: A lawyer shall act with reasonable diligence and promptness in representing a client.

As stated earlier, these values are pertinent when dealing with LGBT elder clients. Competence requires that a lawyer be culturally competent in LGBT issues, including knowledge and awareness of the history of prejudice and stigma, attitudes of clients themselves as well as others to issues of sexual orientation or gender identity, and how these impact the experience of clients or issues at stake. Also, the potential to reduce or ameliorate harm suffered by LGBT elder clients through prompt and timely action is anchored on the capacity to act with diligence and recognition of the need and benefits from doing so.

Because of the history of prejudice and stigma that LGBT people endure as a result of sexual orientation and/or gender identity, the value placed on confidentiality of information in client–lawyer relationships is critical. Subject to exceptions in subsection (b), such as the protection from harm or death, and commission of crimes or fraud, Rule 1.6 (a) provides that,

> A lawyer shall not reveal information relating to the representation of a client unless the client gives informed consent, the disclosure is impliedly authorized in order to carry out the representation or the disclosure is permitted by paragraph (b).

Further, subsection (c), which requires that

> A lawyer shall make reasonable efforts to prevent the inadvertent or unauthorized disclosure of, or unauthorized access to, information relating to the representation of a client.

is also germane to protecting LGBT privacy interests, especially in light of the fears of persecution, discrimination, backlash, and other undesirable consequences following disclosure of sexual orientation or gender identity often harbored by LGBT elders. For instance, research indicating that such fears are significant contributors to nondisclosure of LGBT status in health care encounters (Durso and Meyer 2012; Fredriksen-Goldsen et al. 2011).

The value of communication also addressed in Model Rules is important because it works in tandem with confidentiality and informed consent, both of which are tied to the ethical principle of *autonomy*. Appropriate, timely, honest, open, and clear communication is necessary in order to serve LGBT elder clients because it facilitates decision-making and enhances trust and understanding in the client–lawyer relationship.

Model Rules also provide guidance for dealing with clients with diminished capacity, which may be relevant in some cases involving LGBT elders with increased levels of vulnerability due for instance to cognition, or other circumstance. Rule 1.14 states,

> (a) When a client's capacity to make adequately considered decisions in connection with a representation is diminished, whether because of minority, mental impairment or for some other reason, the lawyer shall, as far as reasonably possible, maintain a normal client-lawyer relationship with the client.
>
> (b) When the lawyer reasonably believes that the client has diminished capacity, is at risk of substantial physical, financial or other harm unless action is taken and cannot adequately act in the client's own interest, the lawyer may take reasonably necessary protective action, including consulting with individuals or entities that have the ability to take action to protect the client and, in appropriate cases, seeking the appointment of a guardian ad litem, conservator or guardian.

The goal of protection can be linked to the ethical principle of *nonmaleficence* (i.e., do no harm). This section also provides that a lawyer may disclose or reveal information about the client whether it is necessary to protect the client's interests. This is potentially a useful safeguard that may be necessary in effecting communication with and informed action by other stakeholders or professionals such as social workers, healthcare providers, and/or criminal justice system on behalf of the client.

Model Rules also provide guidance in terms of the roles that a lawyer might play in relation to an LGBT elder client and how to execute these ethically. These roles help shape goals of behavior when working with LGBT elders on issues, such as elder mistreatment. As advisor, in Rule 2.1, lawyers are required to "exercise independent professional judgment and render candid advice" and to consider beyond the law, "other considerations such as moral, economic, social and political factors that may be relevant to the client's situation." Again, this is pertinent when dealing with LGBT elders because their sexual identity and/or gender identity reflect and impact moral, social, and political realities of the day with implications for both these LGBT elders and society in general. Counselor and advocate are two other roles addressed in Model Rules. The conduct of either role can bear on the ethical principle of *autonomy and respect for persons*, because they require considerations of the rights to self-determination of LGBT elders, to make choices and decisions. They also reflect the duty of truth-telling and fidelity to clients (Darr 2011). As counselor, emphasis is placed on the ethical responsibility to obtain informed consent and to protect client's interests (Rule 2.3/4). In the role of advocate (Rule 3), lawyers are required to exhibit the values of candor, fairness, and truthfulness and to act in good faith in the interests of the client. In order to do so effectively, again the importance of LGBT cultural competence (sensitivity, knowledge, and awareness) cannot be overstated.

Finally, the Model Rules also recognize a duty of lawyers for public service, such as through provision of *pro bono* services to those of limited means. This reflects the ethical principle of beneficence (do good) as well as *justice* (fairness). According to Rule 6, lawyers should provide services—at free or reduced rates "to persons of limited means" (6.2); or "to individuals, groups or organizations seeking to secure or protect civil rights, civil liberties or public rights... where the payment of standard legal fees would significantly deplete the organization's economic resources or would be otherwise inappropriate" (6.1). Because the life experiences of LGBT elders often reflect a curtailment of their rights and result in socioeconomic disparities in later life, the provisions of Rule 6 are of particular salience to this population, by assuring extending access to legal representation, regardless of financial wherewithal to do so.

Although the Model Rules of Professional Conduct do not specifically mention issues of sexual orientation or gender identity, the espoused core values lend themselves to the ethical treatment of LGBT elders by detailing acceptable behaviors in client–lawyer relationships, as well as expectations and responsibilities to act as advisor/counselor and advocate in service to all clients. Appropriate service in these roles requires at the very least a willingness to understand the challenges facing LGBT elders, LGBT cultural competence, and collaboration with other caregivers, stakeholders, or professions as necessary to assure the interests of LGBT elder clients.

> The local commonwealth's attorney reviewed the report in front of him, as well as the notes he had made during his conversation with the social worker. Cognizant of his ethical role as counsellor and advocate, he wanted to be sure that he left no stone unturned in dealing with the matter. However, from past experience and anecdotal conversations with other colleagues, he knew that he would need more information before he could determine how to proceed, for example what extra issues did the question of sexual orientation create, which should be considered, and how to establish evidence of the physical abuse alleged. He recalled a recent article written by a physician about the forensics of physical abuse and mental health concerns in vulnerable adults. He wondered if there was any benefit to speaking to a health care provider as he prepared to work on this case.

Code of Ethics for Medicine. The American Medical Association's (AMA) Code of Medical Ethics provides nine ethical statements that constitute the professional code of ethics for physicians. The first professional code of ethics for physicians was adopted at the inception of the AMA in 1847 (Darr 2011). Since then, it has undergone a number of revisions as recently as 2001 (AMA 2015). According to its preamble, this code that sets the standards of honorable conduct or behavior for physicians was designed primarily for the protection of patients and requires that

> As a member of this profession, a physician must recognize responsibility to patients first and foremost, as well as to society, to other health professionals, and to self.

A review of the nine ethical statements that make up the Code of Medical Ethics (the Code) reveals the following core values—competence, compassion, respect for human dignity and rights, honesty, confidentiality, respect for the law, professionalism, and duty to patients and wider community. Of particular relevance here, Principle I requires that—

> A physician shall be dedicated to providing competent medical care, with compassion and respect for human dignity and rights.

The requirement of competence and compassion in providing care touches on the ethical principal of respect for persons and autonomy. Competence also requires that the physician seeks knowledge and resources necessary to support the provision of compassionate and appropriate care to LGBT elders. In addition, Principle IV emphasizes the importance of respect for patient rights, thus ensuring the protection of privacy and confidentiality—important considerations when dealing with LGBT elders as stated earlier. The ethical responsibility to seek LGBT cultural competence finds support in Principle V, which states that—

> A physician shall continue to study, apply, and advance scientific knowledge, maintain a commitment to medical education, make relevant information available to patients, colleagues, and

the public, obtain consultation, and use the talents of other health professionals when indicated.

As stated earlier (see Chap. 20), provider awareness and sensitivity improves disclosure in health encounters and enhances outcomes (Lambda Legal 2010; Durso and Meyer 2012; The Joint Commission 2011). Compliance with Principle V also encourages collaboration with other service and care providers, or working in multidisciplinary teams, which augur well for care. The code recognizes the physician responsibility to improve community and public health (Principle VII). This responsibility to "do good" in a broader level can serve as the impetus for encouraging more rigorous participation of physicians in efforts to identify and address elder mistreatment generally and within the LGBT community.

Finally, Principles VIII and IX contain the following provisions:

VIII. A physician shall, while caring for a patient, regard responsibility to the patient as paramount.
IX. A physician shall support access to medical care for all people.

Taken together, these principles have ramifications for physician behavior in the care of LGBT elders. It requires that the well-being of LGBT elder patients be the key consideration in healthcare encounters. To ensure this, the needs and challenges faced by LGBT elders and barriers to quality care, including access to care, must be addressed. It requires recognition of the moral or ethical context of care, for instance the need to balance autonomy with protection, or beneficence with nonmaleficence; the understanding that care requires a holistic approach that combines medical and social factors and thus, the value in seeking out those outside the medical community who are in positions to provide insight and assistance.

The doctor to whom the case was referred was helping a gerontologist at the university in town (Dr. Ann Fields, a Fellow of the Gerontological Society of America) conduct a National Institute of Justice funded study on testing theories and outcomes of elder abuse. He had agreed to put out some flyers describing the study in his office and to mention it to patients for whom he thought and

understood that the study was appropriate. He passed the information on to his recovering patient. He always liked helping with the research endeavor though his clinical practice took nearly all the time and focus he had.

Code of Ethics for the Gerontological Society of America. A Code of Ethics for members of the Gerontological Society of America (GSA) was developed by members of the Research, Education, and Practice Committee and approved by GSA Council 2002. Its stated purpose is to guide "professional behavior for the members of the Gerontological Society of America," who are directed to conduct themselves in a manner consistent with the statements set out in the Code (GSA 2002). The intention of the Code is to "promote discussion and provide general guidelines for ethically responsible decisions" (GSA 2002). The statement applies, but is not limited, to members' relationships with "research subjects, colleagues, students, employees and society at large as we carry out our aging related work" (GSA). Pertinent to the research alluded to above is the following set of statements.

To those we study we owe disclosure of our research goals, methods, and sponsorship. The participation of people in our research activities shall only be on a voluntary basis and only on research projects approved by an appropriate institutional review board. We shall provide a means through our research activities and in subsequent publications and reports to maintain the confidentiality of those we study. The people we study and their proxies must be made aware of the likely limits of confidentiality and must not be promised a greater degree of confidentiality than can be realistically expected under current legal circumstances in our respective nations. We shall, within the limits of our knowledge, disclose any significant risks or limits of possible benefits to those we study.

Other statements from GSA's code direct members to respect the dignity, integrity, and worth of individuals, families, and communities touched by members' activities, which would include LGBT elders involved in the research endeavor and concepts addressing the ethical principles of autonomy, beneficence, and fidelity. Additional topics addressed under the code are appropriate treatment of colleagues and factual reporting of research findings (reflects the principle of veracity), nondiscriminatory access to education, accurate and timely reporting of qualifications, and adherence to the responsibility of communicating and advancing and communicating an understanding of human aging to the society at large (GSA 2002).

Included in the codes for the professions described above, although not explicitly stated but certainly implied, is how professionals should treat LGBT elders. Such treatment can involve juggling the values of many professions, which can even be conflicting at times. Another persistent conflict mentioned above arises about the professions' primacy placed on autonomy, one that can be at loggerheads with the directive to do no harm or to simply do good. A thorough understanding of ethical frameworks and principles is essential to resolve such challenging dilemmas.

Summary

Any understanding of a group as diverse as are LGBT elders is bereft without a thorough understanding of ethics and its application to real-world problems. Values of autonomy, beneficence, nonmaleficence, justice, fidelity, and veracity are far more easily understood in principle than in application when confronted with the complex dilemmas faced when trying to assist LGBT elders. Due to their status as a sexual minority, their historic ostracization, their fears related to outing, and vulnerabilities acquired by some as they age, it is imperative that professionals of all stripes have a grounding in ethics and adhere to the code of ethics promulgated by their profession.

Policy Box

You have been selected to serve on the Mayoral Council for Sustainability (Sustainability Council) in your city. This is part of a broader mandate to create a sustainable and livable community for all persons. As a member of the subcommittee on health, you recently attended a health conference organized by the local Rainbow Alliance for aging LGBT. You have been working as an advocate and would like to see a more open and inclusive policy in the local health department, to help promote the delivery of quality services to all persons in the community. As a result of what you learned at the conference, you would like the policy to specifically include the growing population of LGBT elders in your community. You have decided that a good starting point would be to create a code of ethics for the local health department.

Questions

(a) How would you go about this project?
(b) What factors should you consider and what ethical principles might be relevant?
(c) Who should be involved?
(d) Create a draft policy for consideration by the subcommittee on health and leadership of the local health department.

Learning Activities (Both)

Self-Check Questions

1. What are ethical issues particular to older adults? How does being an LGBT elder increase the complexity of the issues?
2. Explain the ethical principles of autonomy, beneficence, nonmaleficence, and justice. Provide an example of when one principle contradicts another.
3. What is Tronto's ethic of care?
4. What are components of the ethical codes described above that are similar in each? Different?
5. Why is understanding ethics important for healthcare and social services professionals?

Experiential Exercises

1. Identify a social worker and discuss with him or her an experience in which he or she worked with an LGBT elder and how the social work code of ethics helped or hindered the work.
2. Explore the ethical principle that you think most important and why.
3. What is your profession's code of ethics? Explore its implications for how you will conduct your work.

Multiple-Choice Questions

1. Which of the following is not considered a universal ethical principle under principlism?
   (a) Autonomy
   (b) Beneficence
   (c) Confidentiality
   (d) Nonmaleficence
   (e) Justice
2. Which of the following statements about professional codes of ethics is *not* true?
   (a) Most professions have a code of ethics
   (b) Codes of ethics set accepted standards for behavior and practice
   (c) Codes of ethics reflect the core values of the profession
   (d) Codes of ethics have legal force/force of law
   (e) Codes of ethics provide an ethical framework for self-regulation
3. Ethics can be defined as _____
   (a) Feel good factors people should consider
   (b) System of moral principles or values that provide rules of conduct
   (c) System of legal principles or values that provide rules of conduct
   (d) Universal principles that help regulate and understand individual or group behavior
   (e) Both b and d

4. The ethical theory that focuses on moral standards of behavior and what is good and right is _____
   (a) Communicative ethics
   (b) Normative ethics
   (c) Utilitarian ethics
   (d) Consequential ethics
   (e) Ethical relativism
5. The ethical theory that focuses on the importance of negotiation in ethical conflict resolution is _____
   (a) Communicative ethics
   (b) Normative ethics
   (c) Utilitarian ethics
   (d) Consequential ethics
   (e) Ethical relativism
6. _____ is the ethical theory that emphasizes a balance of good than evil and the greater good for all.
   (a) Communicative ethics
   (b) Normative ethics
   (c) Utilitarian ethics
   (d) Consequential ethics
   (e) Ethical relativism
7. According to _____, ethics should consider the impact of different cultures or notions of what is morally right or wrong.
   (a) Communicative ethics
   (b) Normative ethics
   (c) Utilitarian ethics
   (d) Consequential ethics
   (e) Ethical relativism
8. Tronto's "Ethics of care" is an alternative ethical framework which is based on the premise that _____
   (a) Caring for others is a human activity based on action and practice and not rules
   (b) Virtuous character leads to ethical acts
   (c) Ethics should consider experience and dimensions of meaning in addition to facts
   (d) Ethics should respect diversity of experience and the relativity of ethical situations

(e) Ethics should consider shared meaning from the perspectives of participants themselves

9. Which of the following is *not* a true statement about the limitations of applying principlism to the field of aging?
   (a) It emphasizes individuals to the detriment of community
   (b) It considers the heterogeneity of older adults
   (c) It neglects such factors as context, circumstance, and agents to whom it is applied
   (d) It has a tendency to view relationships as adversarial
   (e) Strict application may result in undesirable results

10. In working with LGBT elders, health and social services professionals can apply ethics to _____
    (a) Decision-making
    (b) Habilitation
    (c) Resource allocation
    (d) All of the above
    (e) a and b only

Key

1. c
2. d
3. e
4. b
5. a
6. c
7. e
8. a
9. b
10. d

Resources

American Bar Association. Model of Model Rules of Professional Conduct. http://www.americanbar.org.

American Medical Association (AMA). Code of Medical Ethics—American Medical Association. http://www.ama-assn.org/go/codeofmedicalethics.

Centers for Medicare and Medicaid Services. http://www.cms.gov/.

National Association of Social Workers. Code of Ethics. http://www.socialworkers.org/pubs/code/code.asp.

National Adult Protective Services Association. Code of Ethics. http://www.napsa-now.org/about-napsa/code-of-ethics/.

National Consumer Voice for Quality Long-Term Care. http://theconsumervoice.org/.

Gerontological Society of America. Code of Ethics. http://www.geron.org/code-of-ethics.

References

Adams, J. S., Tashchian, A., & Shore, T. H. (2001). Codes of ethics as signals for ethical behavior. *Journal of Business Ethics, 29*(3), 199–211.

Alzheimer's Association. (2014). *What we know today about Alzheimer's disease and dementia*. Retrieved March 03, 2015 at http://www.alz.org/research/science/alzheimers_research.asp.

American Bar Association (ABA). (1983). *Model rules of professional conduct*. The Center for Professional Responsibility. Available at www.americanbar.org.

American Medical Association (AMA). (2015). *Code of medical ethics—American Medical Association*. Available at http://www.ama-assn.org/go/codeofmedicalethics.

Beauchamp, T. L., & Childress, J. F. (2012). *Principles of biomedical ethics.*(7th ed.). Oxford: Oxford University Press.

Binstock, R. H., Post, S. G., & Whitehouse, P. J. (Eds.). (1992). *Dementia and aging: Ethics, values, and policy choices*. Baltimore, MD: The Johns Hopkins University Press.

Callahan, D. (1995). *Setting limits: Medical goals in an aging society*. Washington, DC: Georgetown University Press.

Congressional Budget Office. (2013). *Rising demand for long-term services and supports for elderly people*. Retrieved online March 05, 2015 at http://www.cbo.gov/sites/default/files/44363-LTC.pdf.

Darr, K. (2011). *Ethics in health services management* (5th ed.). Baltimore: Health Professions Press.

Durso, L. E., & Meyer, I. H. (2012). Patterns and predictors of disclosure of sexual orientation to healthcare providers among lesbians, gay men, and bisexuals. *Sexuality Research and Social Policy, 1.* UCLA: The Williams Institute. Retrieved from: http://escholarship.org/uc/item/08b546b6.

Ellingston, S., & Fuller, J. D. (2001). A Good Death? In M. Holstien & P. Mitzen (Eds.), *Ethics in community-based elder care* (pp. 200–207). New York: Springer Publishing Company.

Fredriksen-Goldsen, K. I., Kim, H.-J., Emlet, C. A., Muraco, A., Erosheva, E. A., Hoy-Ellis, C. P., Goldsen, J., Petry, H. (2011). *The aging and health report: Disparities and resilience among lesbian, gay, bisexual, and transgender older adults—Key findings fact sheet*. Seattle: Institute for Multigenerational Health. Retrieved from http://depts.washington.edu/agepride/wordpress/wp-content/uploads/2012/10/factsheet-keyfindings10-25-12.pdf.

Gaventa, W. C., & Coulter, D. L. (2005). *End-of-life care: Bridging disability and aging with person-centered care*. Binghamton, NY: The Haworth Pastoral Press.

Gerontological Society of America. (2002). Code of ethics. Retrieved March 03, 2015 at http://www.geron.org/code-of-ethics.

Hofland, B. F. (2001). Ethics and aging: A historical perspective. In M. B. Holstein & P. B. Mitzen (Eds.), *Ethics in community-based elder care*. New York: Springer.

Holstein, M. B., & Mitzen, P. (Eds.). (2001). *Ethics in community-based elder care*. NewYork: Springer Publishing.

Holstein, M. B., Parks, J. A., & Waymack, M. H. (2011). *Ethics, aging, and society: The critical turn*. New York: Springer Publishing.

Johnson, T. F. (Ed.). (1999). *Handbook on ethical issues in aging*. Westport, CT: Greenwood Press.

Kane, R. A., & Caplan, A. L. (Eds.). (1990). *Everyday ethics: Resolving dilemmas in nursing home life*. New York: Springer Publishing Company.

Legal, Lamda. (2010). *When health care isn't caring: Lamda legal's survey of discrimination against LGBT people and people with HIV*. New York: Lamda Legal.

Lesnoff-Caravaglia, G. (1999). Ethical issues in a high-tech society. In T. F. Johnson (Ed.), *Handbook on ethical issues in aging* (pp. 271–288). Westport, CT: Greenwood Press.

Moody, H. R. (1992). *Ethics in an aging society*. Baltimore, MD: The Johns Hopkins University Press.

Moody, H. R. (2001). Cross-cultural geriatric ethics. In M. Holstein & P. Mitzen (Eds.), *Ethics in community-based elder care* (pp. 249–260). New York: Springer Publishing Company.

National Association of Social Workers. (2008). *Code of ethics*. Retrieved on March 02, 2015 at http://www.socialworkers.org/pubs/code/code.asp.

National Parkinson Foundation. (n.d.). *Parkinson's disease overview*. Retrieved March 03, 2015 at http://www.parkinson.org/parkinson-s-disease.aspx.

Nerenberg, L. (2000). Developing a service response to elder abuse. *Generations, 24*(2), 86.

Plant, J. F. (2001). Codes of ethics. In T. Cooper (Ed.), *Handbook of administrative ethics* (pp. 309–333). New York: Marcel Dekker.

Polivka, L., & Moody, H. R. (2001). A debate on the ethics of aging: Does the concept of autonomy provide a sufficient framework for aging policy? *Journal of Aging and Identity, 6*(4), 223–237.

Post, S. G. (2000). *The moral challenge of Alzheimer disease: Ethical issues from diagnosis to dying* (2nd ed.). Baltimore, MD: The Johns Hopkins University Press.

Powers, B. A. (2003). *Nursing home ethics: Everyday issues affecting residents with dementia*. New York: Springer Publishing Company.

Pozgar, G. D. (2012). Healthcare ethics. *Legal aspects of health care administration* (11th ed., pp. 367–398). Jones and Bartlett Learning: Sudbury, MA.

Purlita, R. B., & ten Have, H. A. M. J. (Eds.). (2004). *Ethical foundations of palliative care for Alzheimer disease*. Baltimore: Johns Hopkins University Press.

Rawls, J. (2009). *A theory of justice*. Boston: Harvard University Press.

Resnik, D. B. (2011). *What is ethics in research and why is it important?* Retrieved February 27, 2015 from http://www.niehs.nih.gov/research/resources/bioethics/whatis/index.cfm, NIEHS website: http://www.niehs.nih.gov/.

Summers, J. (2009). Theory of healthcare ethics. In E. E. Morrison (Ed.), *Health care ethics: Critical issues for the 21st century* (pp. 3–40). Jones and Bartlett: Sudbury, MA.

Teaster, P. B., Wood, E., Schmidt, W., Lawrence, S. A., Mendiondo, M. (2010). *Public guardianship after 25 years: In the best interest of incapacitated people?* New York: Praeger Publishing Company.

The Joint Commission (2011). *Advancing effective communication, cultural competence, and patient- and family-centered care for the lesbian, gay, bisexual, and transgender (LGBT) community: A field guide*, Oak Brook, IL.

Tronto, J. C. (1993). *Moral boundaries: A political argument for an ethic of care*. New York: Routledge.

World Health Organization. (2014). *World Health Statistics 2014*. Retrieved March 03, 2015 at http://www.who.int/mediacentre/news/releases/2014/world-health-statistics-2014/en/.

Trends, Implications, and Future Directions for Policy, Practice, and Research on LGBT Elders

Pamela B. Teaster and Debra A. Harley

Abstract

LGBT elders remain nearly invisible to advocates, researchers, educators, practitioners, administrators, and policy makers. The topics of sexual orientation and gender identity are rarely addressed in health and human service delivery or educational degree programs, and their relevance to LGBT elders is further marginalized or omitted from these venues. In this chapter, we identify trends and anticipate future directions and implications for policy practice and research on LGBT elders. This chapter serves simultaneously as a capstone of the previous 34 chapters and as a roadmap for advancing a research and service delivery agenda to address the challenges of LGBT elders.

Keywords

Research · Future trends · Policy · Practice · LGBT elders

Overview

LGBT elders struggle with the same issues about aging as the broader community and with unique concerns that are not represented by mainstream institutions and laws (Abercrombie and Johnson 2007). This chapter is both a capstone of the previous chapters in this book and a roadmap for discussion of trends and future directions of policy, practice, and research on LGBT elders. The intent is to focus on gaps that remain to be addressed. Legal standing for same-sex couples is a hotly debated issue. Over the past two decades, American voters have voted numerous times on the rights of LGBT persons, and more often than not, the outcomes have not been favorable (Russell 2012). Integration of sexual orientation and gender identity into current legislation pertaining to aging and older persons remains tenuous at best. Comprehensive healthcare and social policies and practices that are inclusive and sensitive to the unique needs of LGBT elders remain elusive. In addition, variation in state and local policy regarding LGBT persons adds another dimension for consideration. Although policy, practice, and research on

P.B. Teaster (✉)
Virginia Tech, Blacksburg, VA, USA
e-mail: pteaster@vt.edu

D.A. Harley
University of Kentucky, Lexington, Kentucky, USA
e-mail: dharl00@email.uky.edu

© Springer International Publishing Switzerland 2016
D.A. Harley and P.B. Teaster (eds.), *Handbook of LGBT Elders*,
DOI 10.1007/978-3-319-03623-6_35

LGBT elders are limited in comparison with their non-LGBT counterparts, transgender persons are the most marginalized, excluded, and discriminated against of all sexual minorities or gender-variant persons. However, there appear to be hopeful signs that the tide of public opinion is changing with such initiatives as the repeal of DOMA and the election of an openly gay bishop by one of the mainline churches.

Learning Objectives

By the end of the chapter, the reader should be able to:

1. Identify future trends in policy, practice, and research that will impact LGBT elders.
2. Identify the core competencies for practice with LGBT elders.
3. Discuss existing gaps in policy, practice, and research on LGBT elders.

Introduction

It is difficult to imagine that any sector of the aging population as a whole has been ignored or under-investigated, particularly given the plethora of scholarly and practice gerontological literature that has been produced over the past fifty years. Robert Hudson, highly recognized scholar of aging policy for over 30 years, observes, "… LGBT older adults have remained nearly invisible to the community of advocates, researchers, practitioners, administrators, and politicians who associate themselves with the modern aging enterprise" (Hudson 2011, p. 1). Though topics of sexual orientation and gender identity among middle-age and older adults are rarely addressed in health and human service delivery training or in educational degree programs (Fredriksen-Goldsen et al. 2014), more clinicians, counselors, social workers, and human service providers are finding themselves working with LGBT elders. In order to help LGBT persons at any age, it is important to understand LGBT issues and stigma, as well as to become aware of available resources, or the lack thereof (Hillman 2012). According to Fredriksen-Goldsen et al. (2014), "health and human service providers must comprehend the intersectionalities of history, social structures, and cultural factors and how they have shaped the life experiences of LGBT elders. In addition, practitioners must identify the typical and the highly unique, yet normative experiences of LGBT people as they age, recognizing distinct transitions over the life course, such as identity management (e.g., coming out or not), and how they influence service use" (p. 86).

Although older, baby boom, and younger LGBT persons share common themes such as concerns about coming out, difficulties with prohibitive religious beliefs, anxiety about HIV and AIDS, disparities in health care and job opportunities, fear of discrimination, concerns about support networks, and legal issues related to same-sex marriage and partnerships, important differences exist between these age cohorts (Hillman 2012). Many LGBT elders came of age when the prevailing social norm was to ignore or subvert homosexual tendencies and to ascribe to traditional family values and relationships. Consequently, they (a) are less likely to receive vital information about HIV education, treatment, and prevention (Makadon and Cahill 2012; National Institute on Aging 2009), (b) have fewer family members available to tend to basic and instrumental needs, (c) are more likely to have endured persecution by the community at large, (d) encounter difficulties forming informal social support groups or romantic relationships because they are less likely to easily identify one another due to concern about revealing LGBT identity, and (e) were raised in a generation in which one was not forthcoming about one's sexual preferences (Hillman 2012; MetLife Mature Market Institute 2010). Each of these issues influences policy development, service delivery, and research foci for LGBT elders.

Disparities in Outcomes for LGBT Elders and Older Heterosexual Populations

Substantial differences with their heterosexual counterparts persist for LGBT elders in important domains such as health care, housing, socioeconomic status, social isolation, equal treatment under the law, and targeted programming. At both younger and older ages, LGBT persons remain "invisible" in healthcare settings (Makadon and Cahill 2012). Clinicians, most of whom receive little or no training regarding sexual orientation and gender identify, rarely if ever inquire about their patient's sexual history, sexual orientation, and gender identity (Makadon and Cahill).

As with practice settings, a growing body of research literature suggests that LGBT elders are discriminated against by health and social service providers: many have received substandard care because of their LGBT identities (Gratwick et al. 2014). Even when providers of aging services indicate a willingness to become more responsive to the needs of LGBT elders (e.g., relevant staff training), evidence suggests that they rarely follow through (Knochel et al. 2012). According to Gehlert et al. (2010, p. 408), "because the determinants of disparities occur at multiple levels, from the molecular to societal and interact with one another in ways not yet fully understood, they represent a challenge to researchers attempting to capture their complexity."

The San Francisco LGBT Aging Policy Task Force (2014) identified key areas of concern and associated solutions to address: data collection, cultural competency, health and social services, housing, and legal services (see Table 35.1). In (2012), a summit hosted by Healing Detroit (an African American LGBT initiative) and the LGBT Older Adult Coalition was held to explore the needs and experiences expressed by LGBT elders on their experiences and concerns about aging in the Detroit area. The Coalition attracted a mainly Caucasian audience from the suburbs, while Healing Detroit attracted primarily an inner city African American audience. In exploring

Table 35.1 Concerns and solutions for LGBT elders

Concern 1: Lack of data on gender identity and sexual orientation among city agencies prevents understanding of service needs and utilization in the LGBT population

• *Solution*: Collect data on gender identity and sexual orientation whenever other voluntary demographic data are collected

Concern 2: Senior service providers do not have adequate cultural competence to appropriately serve LGBT seniors

• *Solution*: Require training to improve cultural competency of service providers in working effectively with LGBT elders

Concern 3: LGBT elders lack information and enrollment support for social services, financial support, benefits counseling, legal advocacy, and health insurance access

• *Solution*: Develop and implement an information, referral, enrollment assistance, and case management referral program that provides a single place for LGBT elders to receive information, referral, and enrollment assistance for a wide range of available social services and health care

Concern 4: Availability of limited supportive services to aid in the provision, coordination, and planning of care to address unique challenges facing LGBT elders

• *Solution*: Develop and implement an LGBT elder case management and peer specialist program

Concern 5: Availability of limited support services to address the emotional, behavioral health, and social isolation challenges of LGBT elders

• *Solution*: Develop and implement an LGBT elder peer counseling program and an LGBT peer support volunteer program

Concern 6: LGBT elders have unique barriers to accessing information about and services for Alzheimer's and dementia care

• *Solution*: Create an LGBT-targeted education and awareness campaign and increase availability of related support groups

Concern 7: LGBT elders struggle with low income and poor financial literacy

• *Solution*: Develop and implement financial literacy training services targeting LGBT elders

Concern 8: LGBT elders are especially vulnerable to losing their residential housing as a result of eviction and physical barriers to aging in place, and the consequences of losing housing late in life are severe for most LGBT elders

• *Solution*: Improve eviction prevention protections for LGBT elders through rental and homeowner assistance,

(continued)

Table 35.1 (continued)

legal services, and increased restriction on evictions and increase resources for LGBT elder homeowners

Concern 9: LGBT elders need more access to affordable housing

• *Solution*: Increase availability of and access to affordable housing by including LGBT elders in planning processes, prioritizing developments that target them, and providing LGBT-focused housing counseling and rental assistance

Concern 10: Conditions in apartments and single room occupancy (SRO) where many LGBT elders live are often unacceptable

• *Solution*: Improve conditions in apartments and SROs through improved Department of Building Inspections (DBI) policies and enhance work on habitability

Concern 11: Many LGBT elders feel unsafe and unwelcome in city shelters

• *Solution*: The city should address unsafe and unwelcoming treatment of LGBT elders in city shelters by providing targeted shelter services and implementing training at existing shelters

Concern 12: LGBT elders in long-term care facilities face systemic discrimination and abuse

• *Solution*: Improve legal protections and resources for LGBT elders in long-term care facilities

Concern 13: LGBT elders face obstacles to and lack resources for drafting appropriate life-planning documents

• *Solution*: Promote LGBT life-planning legal clinics, referral protocols, and sample documents, and develop resources to aid LGBT elders who wish to complete the planning process

Adapted from San Francisco LGBT Aging Policy Task Force (2014)

similarities and differences faced by each of these groups, Lipscomb and LaTosch (2012) reported that (a) mature LGBTQ persons are isolated by their community, and their peers are self-afflicted; (b) if they relocated to a senior living facility, mature LGBTQ persons are most likely sent back into the closet; (c) the LGBTQ community is youth-oriented to the point that women and men aged 55 and over cannot relate to the present social network; (d) financially and career successful women and men aged 55 and over are becoming increasingly isolated by their education, career climbing, and inadequately developed partnerships and community network

building; (e) current LGBTQ women and men aged 55+ have lived an isolated lifestyle that has not condoned discussion of issues such as physical illness, financial troubles, and personal relationships; and (f) the younger cohort of baby boomers includes women and men aged 55+ who are not as economically able for their final years as their same-gender counterparts. Older and retired LGBT persons have concerns (e.g., healthcare affordability, competent care) different from their younger counterparts (e.g., housing, independence).

The most common concern for both inner city African American LGBT elders and their suburban Caucasian counterparts was social isolation created by feeling unwelcome at social activities in an LGBT community geared for younger persons, fear of social ostracism within the mainstream senior social community, and unwelcome senior living communities. The most significant difference between them was African American LGBT elders' challenges of living in the city (e.g., unemployment, poverty, systemic racial inequity issues) and Caucasian suburban LGBT elders' challenges for acquiring culturally competent healthcare and appropriate housing options (Lipscomb and LaTosch 2012). Findings by Lipscomb and LaTosch are consistent with results from other studies (e.g., Espinoza 2013, 2014; Fredriksen-Goldsen et al. 2011; Kim and Fredriksen-Goldsen 2014) and other sources reported in this book.

In addition to health disparities, research findings point to other legal, political, and social issues that significantly impact the health and well-being of LGBT persons (Ard and Makadon 2012). One important and highly visible issue is the heated debate over the legality of same-sex marriage, along with it associated benefits. According to Badgett (2011), the right to marry is associated with greater feelings of social inclusion among LGBT persons, whether married or not. Another issue is that, across the lifespan, LGBT elders may experience **violence and mistreatment** at higher rates than do heterosexual elders and are at high risk for elder abuse, neglect, and exploitation (MAP et al. 2010). Although his work on elder mistreatment did not address LBGT elders, the national prevalence study by Acierno et al. (2010) identifies that elders most at risk are those who have a lack of social support and who were previously exposed to a traumatic event, situations that are very common for LGBT elders. A third issue is that gay men and lesbians tend to place high value on self-sufficiency and thus may **hesitate to accept assistance** in old age (SAGE and MAP 2010). Such hesitation may well increase the vulnerabilities to mistreatment cited previously. Finally, in addition to hereditary factors, general socioeconomic, cultural, and environmental conditions; living and working conditions; social and community influences; and individual lifestyle factors constitute **social determinants** influencing disparities between and among LGBT elders (Makadon and Cahill 2012).

Interdisciplinary Perspective to the Study of Aging and Sexual Minorities

Three major approaches to collaboration are multidisciplinary, interdisciplinary, and transdisciplinary. *Multidisciplinarity* involves experts, researchers, or service providers from a variety of disciplines working together, but with each approaching the issue at hand through his or her own disciplinary lens. *Interdisciplinarity* has the goal of transferring knowledge from one discipline to another and allowing experts, researchers, or service providers to inform one another's work and discuss and compare their individual findings. *Transdisciplinarity* is collaboration in which experts, researchers, or service providers operate outside their disciplines or specialties (Gehlert et al. 2010). Each represents an improvement over a monodisciplinary approach in that it can capture the multifaceted and complex nature of the causes and consequences of group differences, "with disciplinary scholars operating in concert at more than one level throughout the entire research process" (Gehlert et al. 2010, p. 410). Similarly, service providers gain a better understanding of the multiple needs

of LGBT elders and of how to provide services in a more integrated and comprehensive way. Although the approach used to collaborate may be determined by one's discipline, specialty, or setting, the acknowledgment of different perspectives to service delivery will advance access and quality of service to LGBT elders.

Human and social service, medical, nursing, and health sciences disciplines represent many of the professions that knowingly or unknowingly work with LGBT elders. A major challenge across disciplines is the lack of understanding concerning how to educate people to engage in an interdisciplinary approach for examining the impact of contextual factors on the lives of LGBT elders. Disciplines typically teach and train service providers in isolation, resulting in disciplinary myopia—a lack of awareness and understanding of competencies and expectations of practitioners with whom they will work in delivering services to LGBT elders. Effective communication across disciplines is crucial in order to implement the latest educational approaches and evidence-based strategies to address challenges facing LGBT elders.

Bridging the Gap Between Policy and Practice

Chance (2013) argued that while the Affordable Care Act (ACA) will likely help remedy some of the discrimination that results in the LGBT community's disparate access to health care, it is ineffective in combating broader LGBT healthcare discrimination. Its reformatory focus is on increasing access to care; however, it fails to address the specific needs of the LGBT community and the stigma that results from lower quality care. Chance believes that the social stigma associated with a patient's LGBT status is the driver of gaps in access to quality healthcare services, the result of which causes him or her to delay seeking health care when needed or to avoid it altogether. Thus, there is a need to shift the policy and regulatory focus toward improving the quality of health care for LGBT persons, to remedy the LGBT community's disparate healthcare status, and to require cultural competency training for healthcare providers. Also, Chance proposes that as a national legislative and regulatory effort should be launched amending the ACA to focus on provisions aimed at the discrimination that causes substandard provision of care to LGBT persons as well as cultural competency training to students in medical schools and existing practitioners. The justification to amend the ACA to include provisions requiring applicable agencies to issue rules aimed at increasing implementation and utilization of LGBT-specific cultural competence training is predicated upon the older adults' participation in Medicare and Medicaid programs and the agencies' recipients of federal research dollars.

LGBT persons, especially transgendered persons, are subject to arbitrary and discriminatory practices in private insurance coverage, which limit access to safe and competent care. Private health insurance plans often exclude coverage for medically necessary care related to gender transition, which can range from psychotherapy to medication, gender-specific examinations, and surgical care (Auldridge and Espinoza 2013; Feldman and Goldberg 2007). Auldridge and Espinoza concluded that these practices are more devastating for LGBT elders of color who are concentrated in low- and fixed-income statuses. The result is a wide disparity in health care for rich and poor and for Caucasian and ethnic and sexual minority elders.

Innovative Approaches to Improve Services for LGBT Elders

Cultural differences of LGBT elders are poles apart from other older adults and should be taken into consideration during assessment and in service provision in order to reduce health, housing, and economic disparities (Pugh 2005). An example of a program taking this approach is the *Los Angeles Gay & Lesbian Center's Seniors Services Department* (hereafter referred to as the Center). The Center responds to the needs of LGBT elders with a three-pronged service approach that includes opportunities for socialization, supportive case management services, and training to help other service providers develop affirmative, supportive practices with helping these populations. The Center is the largest LGBT community center in the world and includes a comprehensive health clinic, mental health clinic, legal services, senior services, youth shelter and services, substance abuse programs, and community cultural arts (Gratwick et al. 2014). The Center's continuum of services is akin to the interdisciplinary approach mentioned earlier in this chapter. The Center is integrated in that it provides services to LGBT persons and to their heterosexual counterparts aged 50 and older.

In an exploration of how to work toward an interdisciplinary approach to assisting the LGBT aging community, Abercrombie and Johnson (2007) reported the major themes of a *Town Hall meeting on aging in the LGBT community convened in Decatur, Georgia*. The goal of the meeting was to answer two questions: (1) What are the LGBT community's most significant concerns about its aging community members? and (2) What are the approaches and actions that can best improve the quality of life of the growing number of aging LGBT community members? The most significant concerns identified included a fear of aging; concerns about the availability of money, housing, and services; and retaining the ability to maintain as much control over their lives as possible. The most important approaches and actions to mollify these concerns were as follows: (1) mobilization of the LGBT community, (2) creation of alternative housing and healthcare opportunities, (3) increase education and research, (4) increase planning and advocacy, (5) foster greater collaboration, and (6) more effective communication through new technologies. Attention to such efforts, conducted on multiple levels and through a truly interdisciplinary effort, would allow the reduction of socioeconomic disparities for LGBT elders.

Services and Advocacy for Gay, Lesbian, Bisexual and Transgender Elders (SAGE) and Movement Advancement Project (MAP) (2010) offered broad-based recommendations for building change and improving the lives of LGBT elders. The first recommendation was to provide immediate relief for LGBT elders through increasing funding for and provision of LGBT elder programs, affording immediate access to volunteer-based care, and providing education tools and legal services to LGBT elders. The second recommendation was to create an effective LGBT aging infrastructure through the creation and support of a much-needed advocacy infrastructure by building a strong coalition of allies. The third recommendation was to expand an understanding of LGBT aging issues through advocating for more research on LGBT older adults and generating a national public discussion about LGBT aging issues.

Electronic Medical Records. In addition, the agendas outlined above are the issue of electronic record keeping and the data fields it captures. Documenting patients and clients' progress is frequently linked to data. Given this situation, it is only logical to gather data on sexual orientation and gender identity (a) to increase providers' ability to screen, detect, and prevent conditions more common in LGBT persons; (b) to create a better understanding of LGBT persons' lives; (c) to allow comparison of patient/client outcomes with national survey samples of LGBT persons (Makadon and Cahill 2012); and (d) to enhance the patient–provider interaction and regular use of health care (Healthy People 2020). Supporting the institution of these practices, in 2003, the Institute of Medicine recommended collecting data on sexual orientation and gender identity in electronic health records (EHR) (see Table 35.2 for the core functions of EHR) and

Table 35.2 Core functions of electronic health records

Health information and data
Result management
Order management
Decision support
Electronic communication and connectivity
Patient support
Administrative processes and reporting
Reporting and population health

Adapted from Institute of Medicine (2003)

recommended the creation of structured data elements to allow for comparing and pooling data to analyze the unique needs of LGBT persons. However, in a study of the use of EHRs in US hospitals, Jha et al. (2009) found that, contrary to a consensus that the use of information technology should lead to more efficient, safer, and higher quality care, no reliable estimates of the prevalence of adoption of EHR existed (see Research Box 35.1).

Research Box 35.1

Jha, A.K., Des Roches, C.M., Campbell, E. G., Donelan, K.D., Rao, S.R., Ferris, T.G., Shields, A., Rosenbaum, S., & Blumenthal, D. (2009). Use of electronic health records in US hospitals. *New England Journal of Medicine, 360*, 1628–1638.

Objective: This study aimed to determine the extent to which large hospitals, teaching hospitals, non-teaching hospitals, and private hospitals adopt electronic health records.

Method: All acute hospitals that are members of the American Hospital Association were surveyed for the presence of specific electronic record functionalities. Using a definition of EHR based on expert consensus, the proportion of hospitals that had such systems in their clinical areas was determined. In addition, the relationship of adoption of EHR with specific hospital characteristics and factors that were reported to be barriers to or facilitators of adoption were examined.

Results: Based on responses from 63.1 % of hospitals surveyed, only 1.5 % of US hospitals have a comprehensive EHR system in all clinical units and an additional 7.6 % have a basic system in at least one clinical unit. Computerized provider order entry for medications has been implemented in only 17 % of hospitals. Larger hospitals in urban areas and teaching hospitals were more likely to have EHR. Capital requirements and high maintenance costs were cited as the primary barriers to implementation, although hospitals with systems were less likely to cite these barriers than hospitals without such systems.

Conclusion: The very low levels of adoption of EHR in US hospitals suggest that policy makers face substantial obstacles to the achievement of healthcare performance goals that depend on health information technology. A policy strategy focused on financial support, interoperability, and training of technical support staff may be necessary to help with adoption of such systems in US hospitals.

Questions

1. How can this study be redesigned to do a comparative study of US hospitals and international hospitals in developed countries?
2. What were the independent and dependent variables?
3. If VHA hospitals were excluded from this study, how differently would the results be?

In Canada, many consider EHR systems to be critical for achieving another goal of interdisciplinary collaboration: improved continuity of care, reduced duplication, and decreased incidents of adverse events. However, a number of potential barriers continue to exist (e.g., creating safe, accessible computer-generated records, the ability of health professionals to generate, add to and share documents) (Deber and Baumann 2005). To surmount these barriers, Deber and Baumann recommend attention to three aspects to promote the initiative they support: How health care is financed, how health care is funded, and how it is delivered. Upon resolution of these conundrums, they contend that attention must be paid to the barriers created by interpretations by provincial governments of legal definitions inherent in the Canadian Constitution and the Canadian Health Act.

Future Directions and Implications for Policy, Practice, and Research on LGBT Elders

The National Academy on an Aging Society published *Public Policy & Aging Report* (2011) in which they explore several topics related to LGBT elders, including the absence of research and public policies devoted to LGBT populations, the failure of existing general aging policies to incorporate LGBT needs and interests, the need of cultural competency training among service personnel, partnerships between organizations working with LGBT elders and elders of color to advance common policy goals, and the implications of a demographic estimate showing that one in two Americans living with HIV will be aged 50 and older by 2015 (Hudson 2011). Adults over the age of 50 who receive a diagnosis of HIV are more likely to receive a concurrent AIDS diagnosis (51 %) compared to their younger peers (33 %) (Centers for Disease Control 2013). Moreover, the stigma of HIV may be perceived to be greater in the elderly population, leading them to hide their diagnosis or avoid testing. HIV prevention campaigns that exist do not typically target elders (Pratt et al. 2010). It is critical that the spheres of research and practice come together to reliably and appropriately inform each other so that desirable policies affecting the very real issues that LGBT persons face be created, developed, and implemented wisely and well.

Policy. For decades, the lives of LGBT persons have been restricted and dictated by public opinion and exploited by the homophobia and heterosexism that pervades the cultural and political landscape of many institutions (Russell 2012). Public opinion has often been the arbiter of public policy, which, in the main has not been sympathetic to the plight of many LGBT persons, including upholding and expanding their rights under the law. According to Russell, when the political and the personal collide, LGBT persons are often vulnerable political targets. On a more positive note, the passage of the ACA provides new health coverage options that should benefit LGBT elders. Prior to the ACA, one in three lower income LGBT adults in the USA had no health insurance. To remedy that situation, Section 1557 of the ACA prohibits discrimination against individuals based on sex, sex stereotyping, and gender identity. Even in light of the potential benefits of the ACA for many LGBT elders, Heinz and Choi (2014) contend that the sweeping policy is only effective if people are aware of it and if outreach, education, and communication are instituted to ensure that LGBT persons have access to quality, affordable health care, and freedom from discrimination. Until these efforts are realized, LGBT elders will be marginalized and oppressed, victims of a variety of disparities, health care being paramount among them.

Practice. Culturally competent practice with LGBT elders in health and human services is an area of critical need. Various disciplines and professional organizations (e.g., American Psychological Association, America Counseling Association, Commission on Certified Rehabilitation Counselors, Council on Social Work Education) "prioritize multicultural competency as an essential factor in both educational training and practice, with the inclusion of sexual and gender minority groups in definitions of multiculturalism" (Fredriksen-Goldsen et al. 2014, p. 82). The implementation of standards and policy statements by professional organizations in their respective Codes of Ethics has propelled LGBT persons into the forefront as populations that traverse a variety of practice settings and are worthy of appropriate and quality treatment. Fredriksen-Goldsen et al. outline 10 core competencies to improve professional practice and service development to promote the health and well-being of LGBT elders (see Table 35.3) in an effort to provide a blueprint for addressing the increasing needs of this population, their families, and their communities. Those competencies were developed from existing LGBT health and aging literature and, although the focus is on social work competencies, they are applicable to other disciplines. Until these competencies are addressed in part or in whole, the lives of LGBT

Table 35.3 Core competencies for practice with LGBT elders

Critically analyze personal and professional attitudes toward sexual orientation, gender identity, and age, and understand how culture, religion, media, and health and human service systems influence attitudes and ethical decision-making

Understand and articulate the ways that larger social and cultural contexts may have negatively impacted older adults as a historically disadvantaged population

Distinguish similarities and differences within the subgroups of LGBT elders, as well as their intersecting identities (i.e., age, gender, race, health status) to develop tailored and responsive health strategies

Apply theories of aging and social and health perspectives and the most up-to-date knowledge available to engage in culturally competent practice with LGBT elders

When conducting a comprehensive biopsychosocial assessment, attend to the ways that the larger social context and structural and environmental risks and resources may impact LGBT elder

When using empathy and sensitive interviewing skills during assessment and intervention, ensure the use of language is appropriate for working with LGBT elders to establish and build rapport

Understand and articulate the ways in which agency, program, and service policies do or do not marginalize and discriminate against LGBT elders

Understand and articulate the ways that the local, state, and federal laws negatively and positively impact LGBT elders, to advocate on their behalf

Provide sensitive and appropriate outreach to LGBT elders, their families, caregiver and other supports to identify and address service gaps, fragmentation, and barriers that impact LGBT elders

Enhance the capacity of LGBT elders and their families, caregivers, and other supports to navigate aging, social, and health services

Adapted from Fredriksen-Goldsen et al. (2014)

elders will continue to be compromised by their relegation to less than full citizenship status.

Research. Although more research on LGBT elders is available than in previous years, there remains a general lack of empirical research (Hillman 2012) to inform future research as well as the practice community. In part, two major factors appear to contribute to limited research on LGBT elders: non-self-disclosure of sexual minority status and lack of data collection on sexual minority status by investigators and service providers (Gratwick et al. 2014). Discussed earlier, the Town Hall meeting on aging in the LGBT community, preparing for the future meeting in Decatur, Georgia, identified specific recommendations in the areas of education and research: to educate the LGBT community about aging issues and to educate both the general public and the organizations that should serve the needs of LGBT elders (Abercrombie and Johnson 2007).

HIV/AIDS and its implications for LGBT elders is another arena where research is needed. Although HIV/AIDS has evolved into a chronic, manageable disease due to the success of anti-retroviral therapy, many persons aging with HIV are living with considerable consequences of the disease as a result of early onset (i.e., often in their 50 s) and of multiple comorbid health conditions, elevated mental health issues, substance abuse, stigma driven social isolation, and concomitant loneliness. Many LGBT elders who are living with HIV face the disease without the social support networks that they need to age successfully, despite the fact that they have exhibited significant levels of resilience as long-term survivors. Consequently, there continues to be an increased need for research focused on the medical management of HIV in the older population, including sexual minorities. In addition, medical providers must become better educated in the care of older patients with HIV and risk assessment for HIV (Brennan-Ing and Karplak 2011). And, as a part of an older patients' health assessment, questions about exposure to HIV should become normative rather than atypical.

Summary

One of the most important issues that must be addressed is the present gap between policy and practice for LGBT elders. Does the gap exist because of a lack of evidence-based practices to inform policy, or because of a lack of policy to chart a course for interventions to be developed? Several common themes are explicit in policy issues, practice, and research pertaining to LGBT persons and aging: (1) discriminatory practices are a health risk; (2) stigma is associated with aging, sexual orientation, and gender identity; (3) service providers are in need of education and training about aging and LGBT issues; and (4) research is needed to understand health and health outcomes for LBGT elders. Without attention to these themes, improvements in the health and well-being of LGBT elders will be sporadic—another in the list of disparities that this growing and deserving population of elders faces.

Resources

Center for Population Research in LGBT Health: www.lgbtpopulationcenter.org

LGBT Aging Project: www.lgbtagingproject.org

Movement Advancement Project (MAP): www.lgbtmap.org

Public Policy & Aging Report: www.aging-society.org

Services & Advocacy for Gay, Lesbian, Bisexual & Transgender Elders (SAGE): www.sageusa.org

The Fenway Institute: www.thefenway-institute.org

The National Gay and Lesbian Task Force: http://thetaskforce.or13

Learning Exercises

Self-Check Questions

1. What are some of the commonalities and difference across age cohorts of LGBT persons?
2. What is one of the major challenges across disciplines to an interdisciplinary approach to addressing issues relevant to LGBT elders?
3. How can the Affordable Care Act be improved to address broader LGBT healthcare discrimination?

4. What are the major contributing factors to limited research on LGBT elders?
5. What concerns have LGBT elders identified as the most important?

Experiential Exercises

1. Imagine that you have the ability to develop or influence policy pertaining to LGBT elders. Select a specific area (e.g., health care, housing, employment) and outline issues that need to be addressed, specify potential policy/solutions, and how you would implement them.
2. Research an LGBT elder who has influenced policy on older LGBT adults. How has he or she been able to establish or change current policies?

Multiple-Choice Questions

1. Which type of approach to collaboration occurs when experts or practitioners operate outside their disciplines or specialty?
   (a) Interdisciplinary
   (b) Transdisciplinary
   (c) Multidisciplinary
   (d) Intradisciplinary
2. The Affordable Care Act has been criticized for failure to do which of the following for LGBT persons?
   (a) Ensure access to health care
   (b) Promote life care planning
   (c) Ensure quality of care
   (d) Promote a full spectrum of services
3. In addition to health disparities, which of the following may be a reason for disparities between LGBT and non-LGBT elders?
   (a) LGBT elders place high value on self-sufficiency
   (b) Non-LGBT elders are able to better handle criticism from family members
   (c) LGBT elders are able to use their domestic partners' health insurance
   (d) Unmarried non-LGBT elders are able to use their domestic partners' health insurance

4. Which of the following legislation prohibits discrimination bases on sex, sex stereotyping, and gender identity?
   (a) Americans with Disabilities Act
   (b) Civil Rights Act
   (c) Affordable Care Act
   (d) Medicare
5. Which of the following is a logical reason to gather data on sexual orientation and sexual identity?
   (a) Increases ability to screen, detect, and prevent conditions more common in LGBT persons
   (b) Helps develop a better understanding of patients' lives
   (c) Allows comparison of patient outcomes with national survey samples of LGBT person
   (d) All of the above
   (e) None of the above
6. Which of the following is the intended purpose of electronic health records?
   (a) Reduce duplication
   (b) Allow clinician to share information
   (c) Improve quality of care
   (d) All of the above
   (e) None of the above

Key

1-b
2-c
3-a
4-c
5-d
6-d

References

Acierno, R., Hernandez, M. A., Amstadter, A. B., Resnick, H. S., Steve, K., Muzzy, W., & Kilpatrick, D. G. (2010). Prevalence and correlates of emotional, physical, sexual, and financial abuse and potential neglect in the United States: The National Elder Mistreatment Study. *American Journal of Public Health, 100,* 292–297. doi: 10.2105/ajph.2009.163089.

Abercrombie, J., & Johnson, S. (2007, June 17). *Aging in the LGBT community: Preparing for the future—*

Report on the 2nd *Town Hall meeting.* Retrieved February 24, 2015 from www.Sageatl.org/doc/ TownHallreport-AgingLGBTCommunity.pdf.

Ard, K. L., & Makadon, H. J. (2012). *Improving the health care of lesbian, gay, bisexual and transgender (LGBT) people: Understanding and eliminating health disparities.* Boston, MA: The Fenway Institute. Retrieved January 3, 2015 from www. lgbthealtheducation.org/wp-content/uploads/12-054_ LGBTHealtharticle_v3_07-09-12.pdf.

Auldridge, A., & Espinoza, R. (2013). *Health equity and LGBT elders of color: Recommendations for policy and practice.* New York, NY: SAGE.

Badgett, M. V. L. (2011). Social inclusion and the value of marriage equality in Massachusetts and the Netherlands. *Journal of Social Issues, 67*(2), 316–334.

Brennan-Ing, M., & Karpalk, S. (2011, September). HIV & aging research: A roadmap for the future. Retrieved January 5, 2015 from http://www.lgbtagingcenter.org/ resources/print.cfm?=324.

Centers for Disease Control. (2013, November). HIV among older Americans. Retrieved February 25, 2015 from www.cdc.gov/hiv/pdf/library_factsheet_HIV_ AmongOlderAmericans.pdf.

Chance, T. F. (2013). "Going to pieces" over LGBT health disparities: How an amended Affordable Care Act could cure the discrimination that ails the LGBT community. *Journal of Health Care Law and Policy, 16*(2), 375–402.

Deber, R., & Baumann, A. (2005). *Barriers and facilitators to enhancing interdisciplinary collaboration in primary health care.* Ottawa, ON: EICP. Retrieved February 25, 2015 from www.eicp.ca/en/resources/ pdf/Barriers-and-Facilitators-to-Enhancing-Interdisciplinary-Collaboration-in-Primary-Health-Care.pdf.

Espinoza, R. (2013). Friendship a pillar of survival for LGBT elders. *Aging Today, 34*(3), 1–3.

Espinoza, R. (2014). *Out & visible: The experiences and attitudes of lesbian, gay, bisexual and transgender older adults, ages* (pp. 45–75). New York, NY: SAGE.

Feldman, J. L., & Goldberg, J. M. (2007). Transgender primary medical care. *International Journal of Transgenderism, 9*(3–4), 3–34.

Fredriksen-Goldsen, K. I., Hoy-Ellis, C. P., Goldsen, J., Emlet, C. A., & Hooyman, N. R. (2014). Creating a vision for the future: Key competencies and strategies for culturally competent practice with lesbian, gay, bisexual, and transgender (LGBT) older adults in the health and human services. *Journal of Gerontological Social Work, 57*, 80–107.

Fredriksen-Goldsen, K. I., Kim, H. J., Let, C. A., Muraco, A., Erosheva, E. A., Hoy-Ellis, C. P., et al. (2011). *The aging and health report: Disparities and resilience among lesbian, gay, bisexual, and transgender older adults.* Seattle: Institute for Multigenerational Health.

Gehlert, S., Murray, A., Sohmer, D., McClinton, M., Conzen, S., & Olopade, O. (2010). The importance of transdisciplinary collaborations for understanding and resolving health disparities. *Social Work in Public Health, 25*, 408–422.

Gratwick, S., Jihanian, L. J., Holloway, I. W., Sanchez, M., & Sullivan, K. (2014). Social work practice with LGBT seniors. *Journal of Gerontological Social Work, 57*, 889–907.

Heinz, M., & Choi, J. K. (2014, April 15). *Enhancing health care protections for LGBT individuals.* Retrieved January 5, 2015 from http://www.hhs.gov/ healthcare/facts/blog/2014/04/health-care-protections-for-lgbt-individuals.html.

Hillman, J. (2012). Sexuality and aging with LGBT populations. In *Sexuality and aging: Clinical perspectives.* New York, NY: Springer.

Hudson, R. (2011). *Study highlights gaps in policy and research on LGBT older adults.* The Gerontological Society of America. Retrieved January 7, 2015 from http://www.news-medical.net/news/20111117/Study-highlights-gaps-in-policy-and-research-on-LGBT-older0adults.aspx.

Institute of Medicine. (2003). *Key capabilities of an electronic health record system.* Washington, DC: Author. Retrieved February 25, 2015 from www.nap. edu/catalog/10781/key-capabilities-of-an-electronic-health-record-system-letter-report.

Jha, A. K., DesRoches, C. M., Campbell, E. G., Donelan, K., Rao, S. R., Ferris, T. G., et al. (2009). Use of electronic records in US hospitals. *New England Journal of Medicine, 360*, 1628–1638.

Kim, H. J., & Fredriksen-Goldsen, K. I. (2014). Living arrangement and loneliness among lesbian, gay, and bisexual older adults. *The Gerontologist*, doi:10.1093/ geront/gnu083.

Knochel, K. A., Croghan, C. F., Moone, R. P., & Quam, J. K. (2012). Training, geography, and provision of aging services to lesbian, gay, bisexual, and transgender older adults. *Journal of Gerontological Social Work, 55*, 426–443.

Lipscomb, C., & LaTosch, K. (2012, July). *Exploring the needs of lesbian, gay, bisexual, and transgender elder in metro Detroit.* Retrieved February 22, 2015 from http://e-kick.org/exploring-the-needs-of-lesbian-gay-bisexual-and-transgender-elders-in-metro-detroit/.

Makadon, H. J., & Cahill, S. (2012, April 30). *Aging in LGBT communities: Improving servicesand eliminating barriers to care.* Health Care and Aging National Primary Care Conference on Aging. Boston, MA: The Fenway Institute. Retrieved February 25, 2015 from www.healthandtheaging.org/wp-content/uploads/ 2012/05/Aging-Conference-FINAL-JW-3-13.pdf.

MAP, SAGE, & CAP. (2010). *LGBT older adults: Facts s a glance.* Retrieved February 25, 2015 from www. lgbtagingcenter.org/resourdes/resource.cfm?r=22.

MetLife Mature Market Institute & The Lesbian and Gay Aging Issues Network of the American Society of Aging. (2010). Out and aging: The MetLife study of lesbian and gay baby boomers. *Journal of GLBT Family Studies, 6*, 40–57.

National Institute on Aging. (2009, March). *Age page: HIV, AIDS, and older people.* Retrieved February 25,

2015 from www.nia.nih.gov/sites/default/files/hiv_aids_and_older_people_0.pdf.

Pratt, G., Gascoyne, K., Cunningham, K., & Turnbridge, A. (2010). Human immunodeficiency virus (HIV) in older people. *Age and Ageing, 39*(3), 289–294.

Pugh, S. (2005). Assessing the cultural needs of older lesbians and gay men: Implications for practice. *Practice: Social Work in Action, 17*, 207–218.

Russell, G. M. (2012). When the political and the personal collide: Lesbian, gay, bisexual, and transgender people as political targets. In S. H. Dworkin & M. Pope (Eds.), *Casebook for counseling lesbian, gay, bisexual, and transgender persons and their families* (pp. 329–339). Alexandria, VA: American Counseling Association.

SAGE & MAP. (2010, March). *Improving the lives of LGBT older persons*. New York, NY: Author.

San Francisco LGBT Aging Policy Task Force. (2014, March). *LGBT aging at the golden gate: San Francisco policy issues & recommendations*. Retrieved February 23, 2015 from www.sf-hrc.org/sites/sf-hrc.org/files/LGBTAPTF_FinalReport_FINALWMAFINAL.pdf.

Implications of DOMA and the Supreme Court Ruling on Same-Sex Marriage for Spousal Benefits

36

Debra A. Harley and Pamela B. Teaster

Abstract

The purpose of this chapter is to examine the implications of the Defense of Marriage Act (DOMA) and the Supreme Court ruling on same-sex marriage pertaining to spousal benefits. The focus is on same-sex marriage, not necessarily civil unions or registered domestic partnerships. Given this ruling; first, this chapter will identify issues of concern emanating from both sides of the debate on gay marriage that were presented to the Supreme Court. Second, implications after DOMA in regard to Medicaid and Medicare spousal protections; Supplemental Security Income (SSI) for the elderly, blind, and persons with disabilities; military and spousal benefits; immigration; and private employment issues and benefits are discussed. Implications for inheritance, power of attorney, and families of choice in hospital visitations and medical decision-making are dispersed throughout the discussion. The information presented in this chapter is intended to present information to help guide thinking and actions of service professionals.

Keywords

The Defense of Marriage Act · DOMA · Same-sex marriage · Gay marriage

Overview

LGBT persons in the USA have long been viewed as undeserving of equal rights and recognition in same-sex marriages. The Defense of Marriage Act (DOMA), a federal law that allows states to refuse to recognize same-sex marriage granted under laws of other states, was enacted in 1996. In 2013, Section 3 of DOMA was declared unconstitutional, in conjunction with other statutes that had barred same-sex couples from being legally recognized as spouses for purposes of federal laws, effectively barring lesbians and gay persons from receiving federal marriage benefits. The affirmation of the Supreme Court that DOMA is discriminatory was hailed as a major victory for LGBT persons. The US Supreme Court ruled in favor of same-sex marriage on June 24, 2015.

D.A. Harley (✉)
University of Kentucky, Lexington, USA
e-mail: dharl00@email.uky.edu

P.B. Teaster
Virginia Tech, Blacksburg, VA, USA
e-mail: pteaster@vt.edu

© Springer International Publishing Switzerland 2016
D.A. Harley and P.B. Teaster (eds.), *Handbook of LGBT Elders*,
DOI 10.1007/978-3-319-03623-6_36

Many supporters view same-sex marriage as the most pressing civil rights issue of this era.

The purpose of this chapter is to examine the implications of DOMA and the Supreme Court ruling on same-sex marriage pertaining to spousal benefits. The focus is on same-sex marriage, not necessarily civil unions or registered domestic partnerships. First, we will identify issues of concern emanating from both sides of the debate on gay marriage were presented to the Supreme Court. Second, implications after DOMA in regard to Medicaid and Medicare spousal protections; Supplemental Security Income (SSI) for the elderly, blind, and persons with disabilities; military and spousal benefits; immigration; and private employment issues and benefits are discussed. Implications for inheritance, power of attorney, and families of choice in hospital visitations and medical decision-making are dispersed throughout the discussion. The information presented in this chapter is not intended to serve as legal advice or as guidance in decision-making about spousal benefits, but rather, we present information to help guide thinking and actions of service professionals. The terms same-sex marriage and gay marriage are used interchangeably throughout the chapter.

Objectives

By the end of this chapter, the reader should be able to:

1. Identify the general arguments in support of and against same-sex marriage.
2. Identify the intent of DOMA, legal challenges, and implications of the Supreme Court's ruling.
3. Understand the implications of DOMA for federal, healthcare, and employment benefits as well as immigration concerns
4. Understand policy for LGBT persons in order to make decisions about whom they consider family and their role in medical decision-making.

Introduction

Historically, lesbians and gay persons have been deemed as different from other groups of people and contextualized only by their sexual orientation. LGBT persons have been stereotyped based on their relationships, type of work, athleticism, appearance, and a host of other characteristics. Thus, LGBT persons, especially older lesbians and gay men, have lived a substantial part of their lives being denied equal protection under the law in the areas of a non-discriminatory workplace, health and social services, housing, social activities, stalking, financial security, and dating violence and marriage. The consequences of exposure to lifetime experiences of de facto legally sanctioned discrimination and victimization have thwarted the quality of life and contributed to chronic stressors and psychological distress for many LGBT persons.

After the court ruled that Section 3 of DOMA was unconstitutional, courts across the nation, with the exception of the Cincinnati Appeals Court, have struck down a series of state prohibitions on same-sex marriage, many of them passed by voters in referendums. In fact, many of those court decisions compared the prohibitions to the ones on interracial marriage that the Supreme Court struck down in 1967 in *Loving v. Virginia* (Barnes 2015). To date, 37 states and the District of Columbia have legalized gay marriage or are poised to do so. Meanwhile, 13 states have constitutional amendments banning gay marriage (Pew Research Center 2015). In the DOMA case, *USA v. Windsor*, the majority decision written by Justice Anthony Kennedy stated, "the federal government could not refuse to recognize or provide benefits to people in same-sex marriages that were conducted in states where they were legal." In his opinion, from a federalist perspective, Kennedy wrote that withholding federal recognition of same-sex married couples "places them in an unstable position of being in second-tier marriages" and "demeans the couple, whose moral and sexual choices the Constitution protects … and whose relationship the state has sought to dignify." Moreover,

Kennedy wrote that allowed same-sex marriages "conferred upon them a dignity and status of immense import." Further, Kennedy asserted that DOMA was written to convey moral disapproval of homosexuality and "a stigma upon all who enter into same-sex marriages made lawful by the unquestioned authority of the states" (Gay & Lesbian Advocates & Defenders [GLAAD] 2015) (see Table 36.1 for a list of consenting and dissenting justices). Essentially, the repeal of Section 3 of DOMA expanded protections for legally married same-sex couples, granting them the same benefits received by opposite-sex married couples. Dozens of lower court judges interpreted Kennedy's opinion to mean that states' bans violate constitutional rights as well (GLAAD 2015).

A fact sheer series produced by the Human Rights Campaign (n.d.) produced the fact sheets series, *After DOMA: What it Means for You*, and begins with the following response:

> The Supreme Court victory in USA v. *Windsor* striking down the discriminatory federal Defense of marriage Act (DOMA) affirms that all loving and committed couples who are married deserve equal legal respect and treatment from the federal government. The demise of DOMA marks a turning point in how the US government treats the relationships of married same-sex couples for federal programs that are linked to being married. At the same time, a turning point is part of a longer journey, not the end of the road. There is much work ahead before same-sex couples living across the nation can enjoy all the same protections as their different-sex counterparts (http://www.hrc.org/resources/entry/doma-get-the-facts).

Ilona Turner, legal director of the Transgender Law Center in San Francisco, indicated that marriage equality is an issue that affects many transgender persons in the USA. Turner added,

"transgender people who are in marriages that may be legally considered same-sex can now be confident that their marriages will receive the full respect and recognition they are entitled to from the federal government" (http://www.transgenderlawcwnter.org/archieves/8493). For transgender persons, recognition of their marriage as valid depends on what state they live in, what medical procedures they have undergone, and whether or not an employer or insurer challenges their marriage's validity (http://www.transgenderlawcenter.org/archieves/8493). Additional information about transgender persons and marriage law is available at www.lambdalegal.org/know-your-rights/transgender/trans-marriage-law-faq (see Chap. 14 in this text for further discussion on transgender persons).

Supreme Court Ruling on Same-Sex Marriage: To Be Determined

The process that determines the fate of the legal recognition of same-sex marriage is set in motion. The High Court heard oral arguments in April and rendered a decision on June 26, 2015. The Supreme Court decided that freedom to marry a person of one's choice is a constitutional right. Prior to this ruling, both proponents and opponents of same-sex marriage agree that the Supreme Court has set the stage for a potentially historic ruling. According to Sherman (2015):

> Proponents of same-sex marriage said they expect the high court to settle the matter once and for all with a decision that invalidates state provisions that define marriage as between a man and a woman. On the other side of the issue, advocates for traditional marriage want the court to let the political process play out, rather than have judges order states to allow same-sex couples to marry. (p. 1)

The ruling on the constitutionality of same-sex marriage marks the fourth time in 27 years that the court will be weighed in on major gay rights issues. Its first ruling occurred in 1986 when the court upheld Georgia's anti-sodomy law. The most recent decision was

Table 36.1 Consenting and dissenting justice on DOMA

Consenting	Dissenting
Ruth Bader Ginsburg	John G. Roberts, Jr.
Stephen G. Breyer	Antonin Scalia
Sonia Sotomayor	Clarence Thomas
Elena Kagan	Samuel A. Alito, Jr.

Table 36.2 Hospitals' written policies and procedures on patients' visitation rights

Inform each patient of his or her right to receive visitors whom he or she designates, including domestic partner
Do not restrict or limit visitation rights based on sexual orientation and gender identity, among other factors
Ensure that all visitors have full and equal visitation rights, consistent with a patient's wishes

Adapted from http://www.hrc.org/resources/entry/hospital-visitation-guide-for-lgbt-families

in 2013 when it struck down part of DOMA in a decision that has paved the way for lower court rulings across the country in favor of same-sex marriage rights (Sherman).

The Supreme Court accepted cases from Michigan, Ohio, Kentucky, and Tennessee, in which restrictions about same-sex marriage were upheld by a Cincinnati, Ohio, Appeals Court on November of 2014. The parties on each side of the debate addressed two questions: (1) whether the Constitution requires states to issue marriage licenses to same-sex couples, and (2) whether states must recognize same-sex marriages performed in other states in which they are legal (Barnes 2015).

Defense of Marriage Act (DOMA)

In 1996, President Clinton signed DOMA into law. Two significant parts of DOMA are of interest to our discussion in this chapter. The first is Section 3 of DOMA, which prevented the federal government from recognizing any marriages between gay or lesbian couples for the purpose of federal laws or programs, even if those couples were considered legally married by their home state. The second is that individual states do not have to recognize the relationships of gay and lesbian couples who were legally married in another state. Although the Supreme Court stuck down Section 3, it did not challenge Section 2 of DOMA, which declares that all states and territories have the right to deny recognition of any marriage of same-sex couples that originated in states where they are legally recognized (GLAAD 2015). The Supreme Court's ruling in *Windsor* applies only to the federal government. See Policy Box 36.1.

Policy Box. 36.1: The Reach of DOMA
Prior to a June 2013 ruling by the US Supreme Court, the Defense of Marriage Act (DOMA) singled out lawfully married same-sex couples for unequal treatment under federal law. The law discriminated in two important ways: (1) Section 2 of DOMA allowed states to refuse to recognize valid civil marriages of same-sex couples; and (2) Section 3 of the law carved all same-sex couples, regardless of their marital status, out of all federal statutes, regulations, and rulings applicable to all other married people, with the effect of denying them over 1100 federal benefits and protections.

In June 2013, the US Supreme Court held that Section 3 of DOMA was unconstitutional (Windsor v. USA). However, steps must still be taken to fully repeal this discriminatory law. First, Section 2 of DOMA was not part of the *Windsor* case and remains the law of the land. Second, there is no uniform standard across the federal government for determining whether a couple's marriage is valid for federal purposes. To the extent possible, the administration has advanced a broad implementation of the *Windsor* decision, ensuring that lawfully married same-sex couples are fully recognized wherever they may live in areas such as immigration, federal employee, and service member spousal benefits and federal taxation. However, there are a few areas, such as Social Security and veterans benefits, in which this issue remains unsettled, and a resolution may require action by Congress.

Excerpted from http://www.hrc.org/resources/entry/respect-for-marriage-act (March 2015)

Discussion Questions:

1. How have some states dealt with the *Winsor* ruling?
2. What question is now before the Supreme Court and what effect could a decision either way have for same-sex couples?
3. What are early indicators (search the Internet for DOMA February 2015) concerning how the court might rule?

Similar to the ongoing debate around same-sex marriage in the USA, Canada legalized same-sex marriage nationwide in 2005, making it the fourth county in the world and the first outside Europe to do so. In *Halpern v. Canada*, the Ontario Court of Appeal concluded that the traditional definition of marriage unconstitutionally violated persons' *Charter* right to equality. The Civil Marriage Act provided a gender-neutral definition. The legal definition of marriage under the Act is, "Marriage, for civil purposes, is the lawful union of two persons to the exclusion of all others." In addition, the Act extended full legal benefits and obligations of marriage to same-sex couples as received by married different-sex couples under Canada's business corporation and cooperative laws, and with regard to veterans' benefits, divorce, and income taxes (http://www.mapleleafweb.com/features/same-sex-marriage-canda#civil). Most legal benefits commonly associated with marriage had been extended to cohabitating same-sex couples since 1999 (http://www.nytimes.com/2005/06/29/world/americas/29iht-web.0629canada.html?_r=0).

The repeal of DOMA has substantial implications for families concerning a number of different federal rights that provide necessary marital benefits. Several marital benefits now granted to same-sex couples in legal marriages include social security benefits, multiple tax categories, military family benefits, healthcare benefits, political contribution laws, rights to creative and intellectual property, and hospital visitation and decision-making rights. GLAAD (2015) noted that couples married in a state where marriage equality is legal, but who are living in a state where it is not may have a more difficult time receiving benefits. In addition, the federal government's recognition of benefits under DOMA will allow binational couples to sponsor foreign-born spouses for US residency. For example, individuals who are legally married have begun to receive green cards following the High Court decision on DOMA (GLAAD).

Marital Benefits After DOMA

In the USA, marriage confers 1138 rights, protections, and benefits in federal law that both are legal and practical (Human Rights Campaign n. d.). Generally, society considers that the spouse is the most privileged party, an important factor in making medical decisions or receiving benefits on behalf of a spouse, or executing rights that would otherwise require a power of attorney or similar legal document. Marriage also gives the right to sue on behalf of a spouse (http://www.myfamilylaw.com/library/legal-rights-and-benefits-of-marriage/?more=yes). Regardless of age, those rights are conferred upon different-sex married couples in the USA. With the repeal of DOMA, federal benefits emanating from federal law are extended to same-sex couples. Below, we discuss several key marital benefits now extended to same-sex couples. We stress that this information is not intended to be legal advice or legal opinion, nor is it inclusive of all aspects. Most of the information below is either summarized or verbatim from the Human Rights Campaign (n.d.) fact sheet series, *After DOMA: What it Means for You*.

Federal Taxes. The federal government has a growing list of Code provisions tied to marital status and the impact of marriage on personal taxes. It is important to understand that every couple's situation is unique and may change from year to year. With the invalidation of DOMA, the following are a few tax issues that may affect married same-sex couples. For filing status (i.e., single, head of household, married filing jointly, married filing separately), only married couples can file as married, whether jointly or separately. Filing status is determined on the last day of the year. For example, persons who are married on the last day of the year are considered married for the entire year. It is believed that the Internal Revenue Service (IRS) will instruct married same-sex couples to file income taxes as married, whether jointly or separately. If the individual is considered married in his or her state of permanent residence, that practice seems to suggest that only people in states that license or recognize marriages of same-sex couples and in the D.C. can expect to be treated as married by the IRS. However, the IRS does not always follow this practice; for example, the IRS recognizes "common law" marriages for federal tax purposes no matter where a couple resides as long as their marriage was valid where entered (http://hrc-assets.s3-website-us-east-1.amazonaws.com/files/assets/resources/Post-DOMA_FSS_Federal-Taxes_v3.pdf).

Social Security. Although the Social Security Administration (SSA) has yet to issue specific guidance on eligibility for benefits for same-sex couples nationwide, including eligibility depending on whether persons live in a state that bars marriages, a state with some alternative status such as civil unions, domestic partnerships, or designated beneficiaries, or living in a marriage state, SSA should still accept an application for benefits, while these determinations are being made. Nevertheless, in 2013, the SSA announced that it was processing some retirement spousal claims for same-sex couples (http:///hrc-assets.s3-website-us-east-1.amizonaws.com/files/assets/resources/Post-DOMA_FSS_Federal_Social-Security_v3.pdf). Additional information from SSA about benefits for same-sex couples and family members is available at http://ssa.gov/doma/.

Supplemental Security Income (SSI). The SSI programs pay cash benefits to people who are at least age 65 and meet financial limits or have severe disabilities and very limited income and resources (www.ssa.gov/pgm/ssi.htm). It is more difficult for a married couple living together to qualify for SSI than when not living together. A married couple (both age 65 years or older) living together who meets the Social Security Act disability standard must apply for SSI as a couple. For married couples living together, with only one spouse meeting the age of disability standard, the qualifying spouse must apply as an individual. However, the income and resources of the ineligible spouse will be considered (i.e., deemed) to constitute the income and resource of the spouse applying for SSI as stipulated by a formula set forth in SSI regulations. Marital status is based under the statute on "appropriate state law," and regulations further specify that the law of the state where the couple principally lives (i.e., domicile) at the time of application should apply. Under additional statutory provisions, even if the marriage is not recognized by the state where the couple lives, the couple will nevertheless be considered married for SSI purposes if a spouse can inherit personal property from the other without a will under the state's law as would a spouse (http://hrc-assets.s3-website-us-east-1.amazonaws.com/files/assets/resources/Post-DOMA_SSI_v2.pdf).

A married same-sex couple living in a state that respects the marriage will be regarded as married for SSI purposes, and the income and resources of both spouses will be taken into account to determine SSI eligibility and benefits. It is uncertain what this means for married same-sex couples who live in a state that does not recognize their marriage. The couple would not be regarded as married under the law of their state of domicile. However, it is possible that the couple could be construed as "holding themselves out" as married to the community and hence subject to the rules for married couples for federal SSI purposes. A section of the Social Security Act provides that, even if there is no recognized marital relationship, if two individuals hold themselves out as "husband and wife" to the community in which they reside, they will be regarded as a married couple for SSI eligibility purposes. Efforts may be made in non-recognition states to apply this "holding out" provision to same-sex partners in evaluating eligibility for SSI (http://hrc-assets.s3-website-us-east-1.amazonaws.com/files/assets/resources/Post-DOMA_ssI_v2.pdf).

Medicaid. Medicaid is a federal-state health insurance program targeted for very low-income people who meet certain guidelines. Medicaid also provides insurance coverage for long-term care for persons who qualify. Each state has it own Medicaid program that is partially funded by the federal government. Although there are some federal requirements that states must follow, each state has different rules about who qualifies for Medicaid and what is covered. The Affordable Care Act (ACA) made Medicaid available to all very low-income people regardless of whether they have a child, a disability, or are elderly; however, under the recent Supreme Court ruling about ACA, not every state has to expand Medicaid under the law. In states that choose not to expand Medicaid, the old eligibility rules will still apply. Many states that have marriage equality did not treat same-sex married couples as married for many Medicaid programs. Given that the Medicaid program is limited to very low-income people, who is considered to be a family member for the purposes of determining family income and assets impact eligibility for Medicaid (http://hrc-assets.s3-website-us-east-1.amazonaws.com/files/assets/resources/Post-DOMA_MEDICAID_v3.pdf). Additional information is available at www.helthcare.gov or www.medicaid.gov.

Medicare Spousal Protections. Medicare is a federal health insurance program for adults aged 65 and older, as well as for certain younger people with disabilities. Medicare has four parts: (a) Part A, hospital insurance; (b) Part B, medical insurance; (c) Part C, Medicare Advantage Plans, which are private health plans that contract with Medicare to provide both Part A and Part B benefits; and (d) Part D, prescription drug coverage. For most people, becoming eligible for

Medicare is as simple as turning 65 years old, but other aspects of the program, such as requirements and amounts of premiums, eligibility for certain types of plans, and timing of enrollment, may depend on work history, access to other health care, health status, and income. In several situations, having a spouse may alter the way benefits are accessed. Additional information is available at www.medicare.gov or www.ssa.gov/pgm/medicare.htm.

Medicare defines the same definitions as Social Security. According to the Medicare guidelines, a person is a spouse if (a) he or she has a valid marriage under the law of the state where he or she lives at the time of filing for benefits, or (b) he or she has the same rights as a husband or wife for purposes of the distribution of intestate personal property under the laws of the state where he or she lives at the time of filing for benefits. This definition also applies to married same-sex couples who live in a state that recognizes their marriage. For married same-sex couples living in states that discriminate against their marriages, federal law likely prevents them from accessing spousal benefits. If a partner applied for benefits while living in a state that recognized the marriage or allowed the spouse to inherit without a will as a spouse and only moved after the commencement of receiving benefits, he or she should continue receiving Medicare benefits in the new home state, regardless of the relationship recognition laws in that state because benefits are determined by the marital status in the state in which application was made for benefits (http://hrc-assets.s3-website-us-east-1.amazonaws.com/files/assets/resources/Post-DOMA_Medicare_v3.pdf).

Military Spousal Benefits. For members who are in the active military, reserves, and National Guards, by statute a spouse is a husband or wife as the case may be. In 2013, the Secretary of Defense wrote in a memo that:

> In the event that the Defense of marriage Act is no longer applicable to the Department of Defense, it will be the policy of the Department to construe the words "spouse" and "marriage" without regard to sexual orientation, and married couples, irrespective of sexual orientation, and their

dependents, will be granted full military benefits (http://www.defense.gov/news/Same-SexBenefitsMwemo.pdff).

With the High Court striking down DOMA, the DOD construes the statutory definition of spouse as inclusive. Generally, the military considers marriage valid if it was valid in the state where the marriage took place. A state-issued marriage certificate is normally all the evidence necessary to demonstrate that the marriage was considered valid by the state. Generally, marriages entered into foreign countries to foreign nationals must be approved by the military service beforehand. The military determines a marriage to be valid based on the law of the state where the marriage took place; thus, it should not matter in what state the couple lived when they married, what state they moved to after the marriage, or where a spouse was stationed around the world. Once a spouse is recognized by the military as a spouse, the laws of the state in which the couple lives no longer play a role in whether either spouse is eligible for spousal benefits from the military (http://hrc-assets.s3-website-us-east-1.amazonaws.com/files/assets/resources/POST-DOMA_MilitarySpousalBenefits_v3.pdf).

Veteran's Spousal Benefits. Two categories of veterans receive benefits from the Department of Veterans Affairs (DOA): qualified non-retired (those who meet eligibility requirements for specific benefits usually related to time-in-service and discharge characterization) and retirees (those who served at least 20 years in the military and who formally retired from military service). A veteran spouse or surviving spouse is defined as a person of the opposite sex who is a wife or husband. However, the repeal of DOMA appears to make these definitions constitutionally invalid and no longer enforceable. On the other hand, the statutes that govern veteran's benefits contain problematic provisions for determining when a marriage is valid. Because determination of marriage validity derives from federal statues, action will likely be required by the courts or Congress. A better standard would be a "place of

celebration" rule, so that spousal status is assessed according to the law of the state where one married or secured a spousal status. This is the standard DOD and the military use, where there is no statute specifying a place of residence rule. Unless a "place of celebration" rule is established for the VA, if a veteran and his or her spouse traveled from a state that would not recognize the marriage in order to marry in a state that recognizes the marriage of same-sex couples and lived in a non-recognition state when their veteran's benefits took effect, they will likely not be considered married for purposes of the VA (http://hrc-assets.s3-website-us-east-1.amizonaws.com/files/assets/resources/Post-DOMA_FSS_Veteran_Spousal_Benefits_v3.pdf.

Immigration (binational). Immigration is a complicated area of law, with many factors specific to each individual. Before the repeal of DOMA, LG persons were advised not to marry their partner, because for the most common type of non-immigrant visas (e.g., tourist, student), the foreign national entering the USA must demonstrate to US immigration officials that he or she does not have the intent to remain in the USA. Now, however, it is anticipated that for those seeking permanent resident status in the USA based on marital relationship, in many cases it will make sense to marry and file for permanent benefits. Furthermore, in many cases, an LG person can marry his or her partner and sponsor him or her for a green card. Options for families will vary from case to case, based upon a number of factors including whether the partners are living together or in different countries; whether the partners are living together in the USA or abroad; whether the partners have married; whether the partners can marry; and for families together in the USA, whether the non-US citizen partner arrived here after having been inspected by an immigration officer or whether the partner entered without inspection. Same-sex couples will also have to meet the general criteria for marriage-based immigration. Other considerations are specific for immigrants who are in lawful immigration status versus those who are out of status (http://hrc-assets.s3-website-us-east-1.amazonaws.com/files/assets/resources/Post-DOMA_FSS_Immigration_v3.pdf). For additional information about the procedure to apply for marriage-based immigration petitions on behalf of foreign spouses who are inside the U.S., see Immigration Equality's adjustment of status (www.immigrationequality.org/issues/transgender/adjustment-of-status-procedural-steps/). For foreign spouses who are outside the USA, see Immigration Equality's consular processing (www.immigrationequality.org/issues/transgender/consular-processing-procedural-steps/) (see Chapter 13 in this text for further discussion on LGBT immigrants).

Private Employment Issues and Benefits. Although discrimination against married same-sex couples under the DOMA did not bar private employers from offering most spousal employment benefits to employees' same-sex spouses, it subjected them to discriminatory tax treatment and other forms of unequal treatment. If a spouse is covered under an employer's health plan and is considered validly married by the federal government, both partners should be eligible for the following additional federal protections: (a) The value of the spouse's health insurance will not be treated as taxable income to the employee or to the spouse; (b) the spouse and children have the right to remain covered by the employed spouse's health plan regardless of loss of job or reduction of hours, or if divorced or separated (COBRA coverage or COBRA continuation coverage); and (c) while most health plans only allow enrollment at specific times, marriage or divorce are "qualifying events" that will permit enrollment or un-enrollment outside specific time periods. In addition to these protections, the partners may have other rights under state law. If the couple lives in a state that recognizes the marriage, for benefit purposes, the federal government will consider the marriage valid, and thus, the partners have a right to all the protections offered to spouses under federal law. In states that do not recognize same-sex marriage, there may be some initial uncertainty because the IRS ordinarily follows the law of the state of primary residence in determining whether to recognize a marriage. Because the IRS and Department of Labor regulate some programs, it may take some time to obtain guidance as to which marriages will be treated as valid by the federal government (http://hrc-assets.s3-website-us-east-1.amazonaws.com/files/assets/resources/Post-Doma_Private_FEDERAL_TAXES.pdf). For more information about federal regulation of employee benefits, see www.dol.gov/cbsa/faqs/faq_compliance_pension.html and www.aging.senate.gov/crs/pension7.pdf.

For persons in same-sex marriages, recognition of the marriage by the federal government carries different implications than those of the state, especially in states that do not respect or recognize same-sex marriage. Among LGBT advocates and supporters, the general tone is that the repeal of DOMA is a major victory in equity to spousal benefits for LGBT persons. Most LGBT persons regard recognition of same-sex marriage in all states as the ultimate victory for LGBT persons and families as pertain to spousal benefits, protections, and privileges.

Implications for Inheritance, Estate Planning, and Power of Attorney

Potentially, the repeal of DOMA has paved the way for less complicated processes for LGBT persons in inheritance and estate planning; however, caution in these matters is urged. Issues of life and estate planning are typically the purview of state rather than federal law. Although marriage equality and relationship recognition for LGBT elders are making rapid changes, many states still do not provide protections for LGBT people and relationships. Life and estate planning is particularly important for the LGBT community. State laws dictate an order of succession regarding what happens to a person's assets if he or she dies without a will. Usually, if the person is married, his or her assets will be disbursed to the surviving spouse and children. If the person has no surviving spouse or children, his or her assets will go to other relatives. In a marriage equality state, this scenario holds regardless of the gender of the spouses. This chain of succession may provide a modicum of protection, although not to the same extent as a comprehensive estate plan. Difficulties could arise if a same-sex couple marries in a marriage equality state and then moves to a non-recognition state. There, should one spouse die without a will, the surviving spouse will likely *not* receive the deceased spouse's assets, and surviving children might not either. The deceased spouse's assets could then be distributed to his or her relatives, often contrary to his or her intent (Human Rights Campaign 2013).

Consequently, contents on the Web site of the Human Rights Campaign (2013) urge the LGBT community to treat such matters formally, without relying on default rules of state law. The Web site emphasizes that eliminating DOMA addressed only some life and estate planning concerns of married same-sex couples while creating complexities for others. For instance, federal benefits and protections available to same-sex couples may depend on where the couple was married or on where they currently live. Moreover, the Web site emphasizes that although overturning DOMA was a major victory for the LGBT community, it does not reduce or eliminate the need for comprehensive life and estate planning. In light of the DOMA ruling, it is critically important that all same-sex couples work with their financial and legal advisers to review their life and estate plans (Human Rights Campaign 2013). In addition, the National Center for Lesbian Rights (NCLR 2011) recommends the person selected as the surrogate decision-maker should be the person most likely to be knowledgeable about the individual's wishes. In comments submitted to the Centers for Medicare and Medicaid Services for a model for determining medical decision-making and advance directives for LGBT patients, NCLR stated the policy should not rely on an arbitrary ranking of family members. Instead, "determination should be based on proof of a close, personal relationship such as proof of shared residence, a shared social or personal life, and a relationship that exhibits a particularly high level of closeness and care" (p. 7). In other words, consideration for surrogacy should not be based simply on biological relationship as opposed to family of choice.

Families of Choice in Hospital Visitation and Medical Decision-Making

The right to make medical decisions is a protected individual right held solely by a patient who is competent and able to make such decisions. The expanded scope of exclusivity of this right to privacy of patient information and records has limited a patient's spouse, domestic partner, and other family members' access (Vergari 2007). In 2010, President Obama issued a presidential memorandum on hospital visitation that called for "appropriate rulemaking … to ensure that hospitals that participate in Medicare or Medicaid respect the rights of patients to visitors." The recommendation was for the US Department of Health and Human Services (HHS) to develop guidelines for hospital visitation that prohibit discrimination based on race, color, national origin, religion, sex, sexual orientation, gender identity, or disability. Later that year, HHS issued regulations that prohibit these types of discrimination in hospital visitation and make it clear that designated visitors should be permitted access to patients regardless of whether or not they have a legally recognized relationship. In addition, these regulations require hospitals to have written guidelines and inform patients of their visitation rights. A year later, HHS released a guidance letter to implement and enforce visitation, healthcare proxy, and advance directive requirements. In tandem with the presidential memorandum and HHS guidelines, additional non-discrimination protections are in the ACA's non-discrimination provision, Section 1557 (Riou 2014). For hospitals participating in Medicaid and Medicare, see Table 36.2 for requirement of written policies and procedures regarding patients' visitation rights.

The law explicitly grants same-sex couples equal or substantially equivalent standing to other family members in 36 states, and D.C. Law offers limited recognition of same-sex partners through broad language in five states. Same-sex couples are treated as legal strangers in nine states. Of LGBT persons covered by laws, 75 % live in states with inclusive medical decision-making laws, 4 % live in states with limited recognition of same-sex couples, and 23 % live in states where same-sex couples are treated as legal strangers (Movement Advancement Project 2015).

It is especially important for LGBT persons to take steps to ensure that the people whom they choose may visit them and make medical decisions on their behalf in an emergency situation and to protect visitation and decision-making rights: (a) complete advance healthcare directives and visitation authorization forms, (b) talk with a primary care physician about preferred visitors and advance healthcare directives, (c) work with local hospitals to file completed forms, and (d) carry information related to advance healthcare directives and visitation authorization forms in a wallet or other readily accessible area for emergencies (Human Rights Campaign 2011). Additional information on living will, healthcare proxy, and other medical decision-making tools is available at http://www.hrc.org under the tag, working for LGBT equal rights.

Despite pro-LGBT healthcare decision-making rights recommendations and policy released by the Obama administration, the Institute of Medicine, and HHS, Wahlert and Fiester (2013) warn of a false sense of security concerning surrogate decision-making rights for LGBT patients and families in the American healthcare system. The authors proposed that, "new regulations on surrogate decision-making merely invoke a sense of universal patient rights rather than actually generating them" (p. 802). LGBT patients are vulnerable to being mislead into believing that their rights extend further than they do in specific areas of medical practices, particularly misinterpretation of surrogate decision-making. For example, "many LGBT patients mistakenly believe that they have been granted additional federal rights to make end-of-life decisions for their loved ones when, in fact, they have not" (p. 802). Wahlert and Fiester urged that, as policies are being developed and implemented, policymakers must be careful not to overstate the ground being gained.

Summary

Certainly, the impending US Supreme Court decision concerning DOMA will be a landmark civil rights decision concerning the rights of all LGBT persons, especially those who are elderly. Historically, marriage and its attendant benefits have been the purview of states, and as such, the federal government has been loathe to interfere. However, in the *USA v. Windsor*, the US Supreme Court held that "the federal government could not refuse to recognize or provide benefits to people in same-sex marriages that were conducted in states where they were legal" and that withholding federal recognition of same-sex married couples "places them in an unstable position of being in second-tier marriages" and "demeans the couple." Also, the military has liberalized its policy to allow same-sex couples to have rights commensurate to those of different-sex couples. And with the Supreme Court ruling on same-sex marriages, other rights and benefits should follow. Still, in every domain —Medicare, Medicaid, Social Security, estate planning, surrogate decision-making, and immigration—the law is "not quite there" yet, and so caution is urged. At the time of this writing, the best defense appears to be a formal and legal one rather than relying on any other mechanism. Of course, the US Supreme Court ruling that DOMA is unconstitutional, such cautionary advice may not be needed.

Resources

American Civil Liberties Union: www.aclu.org/
   lgbt
Coalition Comments to the Centers for Medicare
   and Medicaid Services Concerning Medical
   Decision-Making for LGBT Patients (2011,
   June 8): www.aclu.org/files/assets/coalition_
   comments_to_cms_on_advance_dietives_
   and_medical_decision_making.pdf
Gay & Lesbian Advocates & Defenders: www.
   glad.org
Lambda Legal: www.lambdalegal.org
National Center for Lesbian Rights: www.
   nclrights.org
National Resource Center on LGBT Aging: The
   Legal Documents Every LGBT Older Adult
   Needs: www.lgbtagingcenter.org/resources/
   print.cfm?r=3

Learning Exercises

Self-Check Questions

1. Why is a comparison made between Loving
   v. Virginia (1967) and the US Supreme Court
   ruling that Section 3 of DOMA as
   unconstitutional?
2. What was decided in US v. Windsor? What is
   its significance?
3. In issues concerning same-sex marriages,
   what level of government has precedence,
   federal or state laws? Why?
4. What is the position of the Department of
   Defense on same-sex marriages?

Experiential Exercises

1. What is your state's position on same-sex
   marriages? Who are proponents of this position and who are opponents?
2. Examine what policies of some of your state's
   local churches are regarding same-sex
   marriages.

3. Search the Web for recent decisions that may
   be a bellwether concerning the impending
   Supreme Court decision.

Multiple-Choice Questions

1. What Supreme Court decision may be
   instructive concerning its decision related to
   DOMA?
   (a) Roe v. Wade
   (b) USA v. Winsor
   (c) Gideon v. Wainwright
   (d) Brown v. Board of Education
2. The US Supreme Court declared which section of DOMA unconstitutional?
   (a) Section 1
   (b) Section 2
   (c) Section 3
   (d) Section 4
3. The Defense of Marriage Act was passed in
   1996 under which president?
   (a) Reagan
   (b) Bush the Elder
   (c) Bush the Younger
   (d) Clinton
4. The chain of succession for inheritance when
   no will has been made gives primacy to the
   (a) Spouse
   (b) First-born son
   (c) First-born daughter
   (d) Sister or brother of the deceased
5. The US Supreme Court will pass down its
   decision on DOMA in what month?
   (a) April
   (b) July
   (c) May
   (d) June
6. The decision that the court is making
   concerns
   (a) Recognition of same-sex marriages as
       legal in all states
   (b) Recognition of same-sex marriages as
       legal in previously legalized states
   (c) Recognition of same-sex marriages in
       federal law only
   (d) Recognition of same-sex marriages in
       localities

7. What country outside of Europe has legalized same-sex marriage nationally?

   (a) Iran

   (b) Australia

   (c) Germany

   (d) Canada

8. What department of government does effectively recognize same-sex marriages for the purposes of receiving spousal benefits?

   (a) Health and Human Services

   (b) Department of Agriculture

   (c) Postal Service

   (d) Department of Defense

9. What government program provides insurance to poor people?

   (a) Social Security

   (b) Medicare

   (c) Medicaid

   (d) SSI

10. What government program provides long-term care payments for poor people?

   (a) Social security

   (b) Medicare

   (c) Medicaid

   (d) SSI

Key

1-B
2-C
3-D
4-A
5-D
6-A
7-D
8-D
9-C
10-C

References

Barnes, R. (2015, January 16). *Supreme Court agrees to hear gay marriage issue*. Retrieved March 10, 2015 from http://www.washingtonpost.com/politics/courts_law/supreme-court-agrees-to-hear-gay-marriage-issue/2015/01/16/865149ec-9d96-11e4-a7ee-526210d6.

GLAAD. (2015). *Frequently asked questions: Defense of Marriage Act (DOMA)*. Retrieved March 10, 2015 from http://www.glaad.org/marriage/doma.

Human Rights Campaign. (n.d.). *Overview of federal benefits granted to married couples*. Retrieved March 11, 2015 from www.hrc.org/resources/entry/an-overview-of-federal-rights-and-rpotections-granted-to-married-couples.

Human Rights Campaign. (2011). *Protecting your visitation and decision-making rights*. Retrieved March 12, 2015 from http://www.hrc.org/resources/entry/protecting-your-visitation-decision-making-rights.

Human Rights Campaign. (2013). *Protect yourself and those you love: A step-by-step guide to life and estate planning for LGBT Americans and their families*. Retrieved March 16, 2015 from https://dl.dropboxusercontent.com/u/39471968/clients/HRC/1213/HRC_Life_and_EstatePlanning_Guide.pdf.

Movement Advancement Project. (2015). *Medical decision-making policies*. Retrieved March 12, 2015 from http://www.lgbtmap.org/equality-maps/medical_decision_making.

National Center for Lesbian Rights. (2011, June 8). *Coalition comments to the centers for medicare and medicaid services concerning medical decision-making for LGBT patients*. Washington, DC. Retrieved March 12, 2015 from http://www.aclu.org/files/assest/coalition_comments_to_cms_on_advance_directives_and_medical_decision_making.pdf.

Pew Research Center. (2015). *Same-sex marriage state-by-state*. Retrieved March from www.pewforum.org/2015/02/09/same-sex-marriage-state-by-state/.

Riou, G. (2014, April 14). *Hospital visitation and medical decision making for same-sex couples*. Retrieved March 12, 2015 from http://ww.americanprogress.org/issues/lgbt/news/2014/04/15/88015/hospital-visitation-and-medical-decision-making-for-same-sex-couples/.

Sherman, M. (2015, January 16). *Gay marriage: High court sets stage for historic ruling*. Retrieved March 10, 2015 from www.lenconnect.com/article/20150116/News/150119223.

Vergari, C. (2007). Providing spouses with the power to make healthcare decisions. *Los Angeles Lawyer, 30*(8), 18–21.

Wahlert, L., & Fiester, A. (2013). A false sense of security: Lesbian, gay, bisexual, and transgender (LGBT) surrogate health care decision-making rights. *Journal of American Board of Family medicine, 26*, 802–804.

Glossary

These definitions are compiled from theoretical, practical, and cultural perspectives as commonly used. This list is not intended to be all-inclusive or representative of LGBT terminology. As with any terminology, definitions are influenced by the user, geographical location, and context. The intent of this glossary is to provide the reader with an understanding of terminology found in this book. In addition, each chapter defines specific terminology within the context in which it is used.

Biphobia	Aversion to, fear of, hatred of, or discrimination against people who are bisexual, which is typically based on the binary standard of male and female.
Bisexual	A person who is attracted to both people of their own gender and another gender. Bisexuality can occur simultaneously or concurrently.
Cisgender	Someone who is comfortable with the gender identity and gender expression expectations assigned to him or her based on his or her physical sex.
Coming out	The process of acknowledging one's sexual orientation and/or gender identity and/or revealing one's sexuality, gender

identity, or intersexed status with others.

FMT/F2M	Abbreviation for female-to-male transgender or transsexual person.
Gay	(1) A person who is primarily attracted to persons of the same gender; (2) typically refers to males who are attracted to males in a romantic, erotic, and/or emotional way; or (3) refers to the LGBTQI community as a whole.
Gender binary	The concept that there are only two genders—male and female and that a person must be strictly gendered as either/or.
Gender confirming surgery	Medical surgeries used to modify one's body to be more congruent with one's gender identity. Also referred to as gender reassignment surgery.
Gender expression	Refers to ways in which each individual manifests masculinity or femininity and expresses it through clothing, hair style, body movement, behavior, appearance, etc.
Gender identity	A person's sense of being masculine, feminine, or gendered.

© Springer International Publishing Switzerland 2016
D.A. Harley and P.B. Teaster (eds.), *Handbook of LGBT Elders*,
DOI 10.1007/978-3-319-03623-6

Gender variant	A person who, by nature or by choice, does not conform to gender-based expectations of society.	**MFT/M2F**	Abbreviation for male-to-female transgender or transsexual person.
Heteronormativity	The assumption is, in individuals and in institutions, that everyone is heterosexual and that heterosexuality is superior to being lesbian, gay, or bisexual.	**Outing**	Involuntary disclosure of one's sexual orientation, gender identity, or intersex status. Outing is usually done by someone else.
Heterosexism	Prejudice against those who exhibit non-heterosexual behaviors or identities commonly combined with the majority to impose such prejudice.	**Queer**	An umbrella term often used interchangeably with LGBT, which embraces a matrix of sexual preferences, orientations, and behaviors of the not-exclusively-heterosexual-and-monogamous majority. The term may have negative connotations for some, but is accepted by many younger people.
Homophobia	A range of negative attitudes, feelings, fear, hatred, or discomfort with people who identify as LGBT.	**Questioning**	The process of exploring and discovering one's own sexual orientation, gender identity, or gender expression.
In the closet (closeted)	Refers to LGBT or intersexed persons who have not disclosed their sex, sexuality, sexual orientation, or gender identity to others.	**Same gender loving**	A term used by the African-American/Black community to refer to an alternative sexual orientation without using terms and symbols associated with Europeans.
Intergender	A person whose gender identity is between genders or a combination of genders.		
Intersexed person (formally called hermaphrodites)	Someone born with both chromosomal and/or physiological abnormalities, and/or ambiguous genitalia.	**Sexual orientation**	The type of sexual, romantic, and/or physical attraction someone feels toward others.
Lesbian (gay woman)	A woman who has an emotional, social, psychological, and physical commitment and response to other women.	**Stealth**	A person chooses not to disclose in the public sphere about his or her gender history, either after transitioning or while successfully passing.
LGBTQI	Abbreviation for lesbian, gay, bisexual, transgender, queer, and intersexed community.	**Transgender (trans)**	An umbrella term to refer to those who do not identify with their assigned

	gender or anatomical sex at birth or binary gender system.
Transphobia	The irrational fear of those who are gender variant and/or the inability to deal with gender ambiguity.
Transsexual	Persons who have had their bodies surgically and hormonally reconstructed to match their gender identity.
Two-spirit	A Native/American/ Indian-First Nation term for people who blend the masculine and the feminine. Two-spirit persons are accepted or revered by Native/First Nation cultures.
Ze/Hir/Hirs	Alternate pronouns that are gender neutral and preferred by some gender variant persons. Pronounced /zee/ and /here/ and they replace "he"/ "she" and "his"/"hers" respectfully.

Human Rights Campaign: http://www.hrc.org/resources/entry/glossary-of-terms

International Spectrum: http://www.internationalspectrum.umich.edu/life/definitions

PFLAG Atlanta: http://www.pflag.org/lgbt-glossary/

UCLA LGBT Resource Center: www.lgbt.ucla.edu/documents/LGBTTerminology.pdf

Resources

These definitions have been compiled from the following Web sites, which are recommended for additional definitions:

Gender Equity Resource Center: http://geneq.berkeley.edu/lgbt_resources_definition_of_terms

Index

CPSIA information can be obtained
at www.ICGtesting.com
Printed in the USA
LVOW09*1918301117
558163LV00006B/24/P